CW01272585

Oxford Textbook of
The Newborn

Oxford Textbook of
The Newborn
A Cultural and Medical History

Michael Obladen

Professor of Pediatrics, Former Director, Department of Neonatology, Charité University Medicine, Berlin, Germany

OXFORD
UNIVERSITY PRESS

OXFORD
UNIVERSITY PRESS

Great Clarendon Street, Oxford, OX2 6DP,
United Kingdom

Oxford University Press is a department of the University of Oxford.
It furthers the University's objective of excellence in research, scholarship,
and education by publishing worldwide. Oxford is a registered trade mark of
Oxford University Press in the UK and in certain other countries

© Oxford University Press 2021

The moral rights of the author have been asserted

First Edition published in 2021

Impression: 1

All rights reserved. No part of this publication may be reproduced, stored in
a retrieval system, or transmitted, in any form or by any means, without the
prior permission in writing of Oxford University Press, or as expressly permitted
by law, by licence or under terms agreed with the appropriate reprographics
rights organization. Enquiries concerning reproduction outside the scope of the
above should be sent to the Rights Department, Oxford University Press, at the
address above

You must not circulate this work in any other form
and you must impose this same condition on any acquirer

Published in the United States of America by Oxford University Press
198 Madison Avenue, New York, NY 10016, United States of America

British Library Cataloguing in Publication Data
Data available

Library of Congress Control Number: 2020950918

ISBN 978–0–19–885480–7

DOI: 10.1093/med/9780198854807.001.0001

Printed in Great Britain by
Bell & Bain Ltd., Glasgow

Oxford University Press makes no representation, express or implied, that the
drug dosages in this book are correct. Readers must therefore always check
the product information and clinical procedures with the most up-to-date
published product information and data sheets provided by the manufacturers
and the most recent codes of conduct and safety regulations. The authors and
the publishers do not accept responsibility or legal liability for any errors in the
text or for the misuse or misapplication of material in this work. Except where
otherwise stated, drug dosages and recommendations are for the non-pregnant
adult who is not breast-feeding.

Links to third party websites are provided by Oxford in good faith and
for information only. Oxford disclaims any responsibility for the materials
contained in any third party website referenced in this work.

Cover illustration: Picture from 'Le Petit Parisien' of 19 October 1902, Vol. 14, issue 715, p. 333.
Accompanying text: 'At the [Hospital of] Assisted Infants. For some time, several incubators have been
installed in the nursery pavilion of the [Hospital of] Assisted infants, rue Denfert-Rocherau [formerly:
Foundling Hospice], designed to rear infants born before term or weak, during the first days following birth.
The apparatus consists of an iron box containing a sort of earthenware cradle lined with cotton wool,
in which the infant is wrapped. The box is closed with a lid in which a window allows to observe the infant.'

Foreword

As a German medical student with a keen interest in paediatrics and neonatology, one book was our point of reference. Everybody called it 'The Obladen'. First published in 1978 with the title *Neonatal Intensive Care Medicine*, the book essentially laid out clinical practice guidelines for neonatal intensive care units in the German-speaking world. It experienced phenomenal success. With a wide target audience of clinicians, midwives, nurses, and other professionals involved in the care of sick infants and their families, it fostered a much-needed holistic approach to neonatal intensive care. And in a field that was still maturing, its commitment to being evidence based assured readers that they could rely on the guidance provided. The current, ninth edition—now co-edited with Rolf F. Maier—retains these attractive features. It remains the go-to handbook for busy clinicians and other team members on neonatal intensive care units across Germany.

Michael Obladen, the book's author, had an outsize reputation as one of the founders of neonatology in Germany. By 1995, he led the country's largest neonatal intensive care unit at the pioneering Charité University Hospital in Berlin. When I met the great Obladen for the first time in 2004, my knees were wobbly and my throat dry. I had just completed medical school and was interviewing for a junior clinical position in his unit at the Charité. The conversation duly tested my limited medical credentials; however, Michael Obladen was equally interested in how my additional training in philosophy and history might bear on the ethical dilemmas of making treatment decisions for critically ill newborns. His questions betrayed a deeply humane approach to providing clinical care for some of the most vulnerable patients in modern medicine. Indeed, the short year that I ended up spending on Michael Obladen's clinical team taught me not only how difficult it is to be a responsible clinician in a rapidly evolving and complex discipline like neonatal intensive care; it also taught me to be kind, compassionate, and respectful in the face of relentless clinical and moral uncertainty.

The present book, the *Oxford Textbook of the Newborn: A Cultural and Medical History*, is bound to become a different kind of 'The Obladen'. Informed by the author's unique approach to neonatal intensive care, his almost 40 years of bedside experience, as well as his studies in history and philosophy, the book takes a deep dive into how Western societies have conceived of and treated the newborn over time. It covers a dazzling array of topics: among them, the history of ideas about life before birth, rites of passage for the newborn, infanticide and other forms of premature death in infancy, and of course, the history of various conditions and illnesses affecting newborns. Each chapter rests on a careful analysis of fiendishly hard-to-find sources, some in obscure languages, many tapped for the first time. Each chapter is also illustrated with poignant, often startling images.

The topics of this book are too varied to summarize in a foreword, but some overarching themes readily emerge. One theme is that neonatology—taken literally as the branch of knowledge ('ology') of the newborn ('neonate')—is a much older field than is commonly thought. It did not emerge in the 1960s, when the term 'neonatology' was first coined to summarize the knowledge that paediatricians had recently been accumulating about newborn care, previously provided by obstetricians and midwives. Rather, as this textbook amply demonstrates, neonatology has much deeper roots in religious, philosophical, medical, ethical, and legal thought, as well as in art and literature, which go back for millennia. It is perhaps not entirely surprising that humans throughout the ages have sought to accumulate knowledge of newborn life. How to think about and attend to newborns—especially those arriving too early or in unusual shapes, or those delivered after difficult births—are questions of enduring personal, social, and clinical importance. They are also questions that touch on what it fundamentally means to be human. However, what *is* surprising is the level of depth with which these questions have been pondered in the West, and just how much of that thinking the *Oxford Textbook of the Newborn* has unearthed from libraries and archives around the world.

Another overarching theme is that progress in neonatology has not been linear. While the prospects of newborns have improved dramatically over time, there have also been setbacks. Sometimes important clinical lessons, such as the need to avoid prone sleeping in infants, took years or decades to implement. Other times, clinicians and midwives relied for centuries on interventions that eventually proved harmful, such as the loosening of the tongue to promote better nursing.

Readers will discover many other themes that run through these fascinating pages. As the evolution of Western thinking about the newborn is laid bare before them, readers will also question their own assumptions about clinical norms, social practices, and cultural meanings related to human life around birth. I have no doubt that the *Oxford Textbook of the Newborn* will find the wide readership it deserves, and that it will become an even more iconic 'The Obladen'—not just for historians and philosophers of science and medicine as well as bioethicists, but again for clinicians, nurses, midwives, and others who are dedicated to making this world a better place for those who have just entered it.

Annette Rid, MD, PhD
Department of Bioethics
National Institutes of Health
Bethesda, MD, USA

Preface

'The babe, like to the castaway of raging surf,
Lies naked on the ground, speechless, in want
Of every help for life, when nature first
Hath poured him forth upon the shores of light
With birth-pains from within the mother's womb
And with a plaintiff wail he fills the place.
As well befitting one for whom remains
In life a journey through so many ills.'

Lucretius, 55 B.C.E.

'Miserable indeed is the lot of man in the state of infancy. He comes into the world more helpless than any other animal, and stands much longer in need of the protection and care of his parents; but, alas! this care is not always bestowed upon him; and when it is, he often suffers as much from improper management as he would have done from neglect.'

William Buchan, 1774

Since 1970, I have been collecting books and evaluating sources on neonates, and since 2008, I have been writing this book, an effort which soon proved presumptuous, even though I had studied medicine, philosophy, and history and had spent 39 years of my professional life with newborn infants. It was my aim to identify the technical, medical, social, and political conditions that improved—or worsened—the baby's quality of life. The breakthroughs. Also painful delays, and the catastrophe that an important scientific finding was lost and had to wait to be rediscovered deserved special attention. The book's main target groups are physicians, midwives, and nurses. However, medical terminology has been used cautiously, and a glossary has been added to the end matter to make the text accessible outside the health professions. The book's structure is neither chronological nor does it aim for completeness. Instead, it is arranged according to specific problems of the baby. It was not a major goal to list who detected what first or to compile another hagiography of pioneer physicians. Biographical notes have been kept to a minimum and assembled in the end matter. To avoid redundancies, important cultural implications have been summarized in a synchronoptic timetable in Appendix 3.

Rather than being merely young children, newborns have very specific problems and their history has multiple cultural implications. Procreation, fetal life, childbirth, and postnatal adaptation go beyond biological comprehension. Childbirth is a highly emotional topic, revealed by religious rituals of transition and benediction at birth. Parental bonding is not yet complete; in some cultures biological and social birth are not identical. Newborns depend on maternal care, breastfeeding, and cleanliness. Their mortality was higher than that in all other age groups, causing despair and indifference. Legislation provided specific protection as lawmakers tried to prevent infanticide and define the viability of preterm or malformed infants. Understanding the newborn requires insight into family structure; the psychology of infancy; the changing role of the woman and mother, but also of the infant, in society. Christianization promoted foundling hospitals, where good intentions and bad hygiene merged into a dubious partnership. Royal deliveries were confided to *accoucheurs*, men-midwives, who took the opportunity to graduate from barber-surgeons to obstetricians. The newborns' fate was influenced by religious history, as the Council of Trent or emancipation from the church following the French Revolution attest. Sometimes the newborn was assigned a legal position between fetus and adult. The infant was affected by the long-standing professional competition between midwives and surgeons, by the development of modern obstetrics, and by the medicalization of childbirth. Survival included nutritional aspects, especially the question as how to nurture the infant when the mother could not or would not breastfeed. Artificial nutrition improved with technical innovations such as pasteurization, evaporation, and cooling. Finally, the history of the neonate also embraced infanticide and abandonment, painful passage rites and mutilations of the body, and iatrogenic nonsense like tight swaddling, loosening the tongue, or shaping the head. Modern research on neonates originated from Napoleon's edict of 1811 establishing medical services at the foundling hospitals. Considering these manifold frameworks is essential for the historian of infant culture, but implies risks for the historian of infant medicine: where progress occurred (examples are infection control and care for preterm infants), the celebration of researchers may hinder the view of the suffering infant. Where religious or cultural habits differ from the present system of values (examples are abandoning, breastfeeding, and circumcision), emotional or polemic approaches may prejudice the view onto the social framework.

Studying history helps us understand the origins of current practice and to set signposts for future endeavours. I hope that much of the pleasure that I experienced exploring the newborn's path through history will be transmitted to my readers, especially to young researchers, whose task it will be to ensure that future neonatology remains part of the human culture.

Michael Obladen, MD, PhD
Berlin, March 2021

PART 1
Early life

1.1 **Animatio: ideas about the beginning of personhood** 3

1.2 **Hepar uterinum: ideas about fetal nutrition** 11

1.3 **Pulmo uterinus: ideas about fetal respiration** 17

INTRODUCTION

Identity of the human fetus, his life's conditions, and development have always fascinated researchers. Usually, the fetus was not considered a complete person. Aristotle attributed three different souls to subsequent developmental stages of the unborn. The rational soul was associated with the formed fetus, and dated to fetal movements. His concept of delayed ensoulment remained mainstream opinion throughout the Middle Ages. Contemporary philosophers replaced the soul by personhood, which was not assumed for the early stages of totipotent cells. Up to the 16th century, maternal and fetal vessels were believed to be connected in the placenta, and up to the 19th century a key nutritive function was attributed to amniotic fluid. The concept of active transport across the placental membrane originated in cell theory in the early 20th century. Research on fetal gas exchange began a century before oxygen was discovered. With the invention of the spectroscope, fetal oxygenation could be measured and fetal blood's increased affinity for oxygen was detected.

Abbreviations

B.C.E.	before the common era
C.E.	common era
ca.	circa
CRVI	Cardiovascular Research Institute
DPPC	dipalmitoylphosphatidylcholine
EEG	electroencephalogram
FDA	Food and Drug Administration
IMR	infant mortality rate
NEC	necrotizing enterocolitis
NICHD	National Institute of Child Health and Development
PDA	patent ductus arteriosus
RDS	respiratory distress syndrome
TRAP	twin reversed arterial perfusion
TTTS	twin–twin transfusion syndrome
UK	United Kingdom
US	United States
WHO	World Health Organization

PART 6
Breast is best

- 6.1 Bad milk: medical doctrines that impeded breastfeeding 213
- 6.2 Regulated wet nursing: managed care or organized crime? 221
- 6.3 Guttus, tiralatte, and téterelle: breast pumps 227
- 6.4 Pap, gruel, and panada: early approaches to artificial feeding 233
- 6.5 Milk demystified by chemistry 241
- 6.6 From swill milk to certified milk: progress in cow's milk quality 247
- 6.7 Technical inventions that enabled artificial infant feeding 253
- 6.8 Selling safety: commercial production of infant formula 259
- 6.9 Feeding the feeble: steps towards nourishing preterm infants 265
- 6.10 Much ado about nothing: controversies on tongue-tie 273
- 6.11 Lethal lullabies: opium use in infants 279

PART 7
Disease

- 7.1 Innocent blood: haemorrhagic disease of the newborn 291
- 7.2 Yellow brains and blue light: neonatal jaundice 297
- 7.3 Weak giants: infants of diabetic mothers 305
- 7.4 Filth, impurity, and threat: meconium 311
- 7.5 Necrotizing enterocolitis: 150 years of fruitless search for the cause 317
- 7.6 Better baby bones: attacking rickets and scurvy 325
- 7.7 Curse on two generations: congenital syphilis 333
- 7.8 Thrush: nightmare of the foundling hospitals 339
- 7.9 Systemic infection: sepsis 345

PART 8
Early death

- 8.1 From right to sin: laws on infanticide in antiquity 353
- 8.2 From sin to crime: laws on infanticide in the Middle Ages 359
- 8.3 From crime to disease: laws on infanticide in the modern era 365
- 8.4 Despising the weak: long shadows of infant murder in Nazi Germany 371
- 8.5 Cot death: history of an iatrogenic disaster 377
- 8.6 Theirs is the kingdom of heaven: infant mortality statistics 383
- 8.7 For whom no bell tolled: infant burials 391
- 8.8 Revived for paradise: respite sanctuaries 397

APPENDICES

1. Methodical limitations 403
2. Early special care baby units and their scientific achievements 405
3. Synchronoptic timetable 413

Glossary of abbreviations and medical and foreign language terms 417
Biographical notes on frequently cited authors 423
Index of Personal Names 439
Index of Locations 445
Index of Subjects 447

Contents

Abbreviations xiii

PART 1
Early life

1.1 Animatio: ideas about the beginning of personhood 3

1.2 Hepar uterinum: ideas about fetal nutrition 11

1.3 Pulmo uterinus: ideas about fetal respiration 17

PART 2
Birth

2.1 From apparent death to birth asphyxia 25

2.2 Resuscitation 1: artificial ventilation 33

2.3 Resuscitation 2: oxygen and other drugs 39

2.4 Resuscitation 3: endotracheal intubation 45

2.5 Umbilical cord and umbilical care 51

2.6 Postverta, Agrippa, Caesarea: born feet-first 57

2.7 Social birth: rites of passage for the newborn 63

PART 3
Prematurity

3.1 Measures of viability 71

3.2 Surviving against the odds 79

3.3 Respiratory distress: understanding surfactant deficiency 85

3.4 Holding breath: the development of surfactant substitution 91

3.5 Anatomy and spontaneous closure of the ductus arteriosus 95

3.6 Persisting patency of the ductus arteriosus in the preterm infant 101

3.7 Intraventricular haemorrhage 107

PART 4
Multiple birth

4.1 Unwelcome: the abominable twins 115

4.2 Fertility and fatality: higher-order multiples 123

4.3 Unequal but monozygotic: twin–twin transfusion syndrome 129

4.4 From monster to reversed perfusion: acardiac twins 137

PART 5
Odd shape

5.1 Cats, frogs, and snakes: concepts of neural tube defects 145

5.2 In God's image? The tradition of infant head shaping 155

5.3 Lame from birth: concepts of cerebral palsy 165

5.4 Possessed by evil spirits: seizures in infancy 173

5.5 Birthmark and blemish: the doctrine of maternal imagination 183

5.6 Cast aside: infants with Down's syndrome 191

5.7 Crooked limbs: the thalidomide catastrophe 197

5.8 A wretched condition: cleft urinary bladder 205

Acknowledgements

Termed by Alexander Schaffer in 1960, *neonatology* is a young field that evolved within the last 50 years, mostly in the US. Research is progressing rapidly, shaping and changing this field at an unthinkable speed. A free-rider of obstetrics, *neonatal care* had a 3000-year-old and not always glorious history, whereas paediatrics branched off from internal medicine in the latter half of the 19th century. Well into the 20th century, newborns remained within the realm of midwives, *accoucheurs*, and obstetricians. However, neither the excellent historians of obstetrics nor those of paediatrics paid them specific attention. A comprehensive history of the newborn has not yet been written. From ethnological, cultural, and psychological perspectives, Payne, Ploss, and deMause described children of all ages. The monographs of Cone, Silverman, and Baker focused on specific aspects of infant care and their development in the US. Wickes, Fildes, and Apple focused on the history of infant nutrition. The series of articles by Dunn in the *Archives of Diseases of Children* provided biographical notes on the pioneers of perinatal medicine. Many ideas from these authors were gratefully incorporated in the chapters of this book.

It is a genuine pleasure to thank those who helped me in writing this book. But it is impossible to list all those who contributed sources, stimulated my thinking, and deepened my knowledge during the decades of assembling this material. Some of the chapters have already been published in scientific journals. That guaranteed conciseness and gave me the benefits of peer review, and I am deeply grateful to the editors Henry Halliday and Christian Speer (*Neonatology*), Joachim W. Dudenhausen (*Journal of Perinatal Medicine*), Roger Brumback (*Journal of Child Neurology*), and Anne Merewood (*Journal of Human Lactation*) who encouraged me to continue and generously gave permission for republishing. I am also grateful to dozens of reviewers who donated their time to shorten the texts, correct the mistakes, and improve the style.

Many literature sources are in my personal library, but still more had to be sought in specialized libraries and museums, which often required help. *Au lieu* of a great number of librarians, I want to specifically thank Bernadette Molitor, fonds ancien, Bibliothèque Interuniversitaire de Medicine, Descartes University Paris; Dr Angela Karasch, Director of the Historic Collection, and Rita Matysiak, Director of the Division of Remote Retrieval, University Library of Freiburg; and Heike Breuer, Institute of Ethics and History of Medicine, Freiburg University. Other institutions I frequently visited include the University Library, Basel; Staatsbibliothek Berlin; Steiermärkisches Landesarchiv Graz; Wellcome Library London; Germanic National Museum, Nürnberg; Archives of the Assistance Publique, Paris; and Anna Amalia Library, Weimar.

While writing these chapters, I have become deeply indebted to many people for their help and guidance during a difficult journey. The following persons who have contributed greatly are mentioned as *pars pro toto*: Carole Gustely Cürten, Freiburg, transformed my thoughts into readable English, and in many instances helped to find the appropriate wording when nuances were important. Sieghard Irrgang, Kassel, generously shared his proficiency in Latin with me when grappling with the ancient texts. Gabi Völker and Boris Metze, Department of Neonatology, Charité University Medicine, Berlin, taught me how to construct graphics, and helped when the computers failed. Editorial assistance by Oxford University Press was a pleasure. Editor-in-chief Nicola Wilson believed in the project from the beginning and paved the way towards its realization. Rachel Goldsworthy helped me amiably when difficulties arose and ensured a perfect form of the edition. For decades, 'the book' was part of my family life. My wife, Dr Brigitte Stiller, a paediatrician and scientist herself, has read and reread all chapters and contributed a large number of suggestions, discussions, and clarifications. Whatever errors and unjustified conclusions are left are mine and mine alone.

Michael Obladen, MD, PhD

1.1

Animatio

Ideas about the beginning of personhood

Introduction

Most cultures attributed a spiritual identity to the human, reborn in another individual, or living eternally in paradise or nirvana. The ontological status of the human unborn has been subject to intense debate in many cultures and for millennia. Theologists grappled with the question of whether and how to baptize fetuses or malformed infants. Obstetricians needed to justify dismembering or perforating operations in cases of oblique pelvis or hydrocephalus, a frequent dilemma before Caesarean delivery became possible. Other issues included assisted reproduction, preimplantation diagnostics, abortion, the use of fetal tissues, and postnatal support for immature infants. The availability of genome editing will soon reignite moral indignation sentiments and unsolved legal arguments. Most of these topics are developing dynamically, and it is worth studying the history of this controversy. The field of reproduction is a minefield of linguistic and semantic uncertainties: seemingly specific terms (embryo, life, person, human, individuum, soul, etc.) may have different meanings in philosophical, theological, jurisprudential, medical, and biological contexts. Historical perspectives have been addressed in many publications on the topic. The excellent monographs of the theologians John Noonan [1] and Norman Ford [2] combined the resources of theology, philosophy, clinical medicine, and basic science. The present chapter aims to broaden the historical perspective in order to shed light on the development of this controversy. It was not aimed to promulgate my own views and values, but to fulfil the historian's duty of reporting the thoughts of others as objectively and as honestly as possible. I will not review the debates or legislation concerning abortion and reproductive technologies, and will avoid the poorly defined term *conception*. Much of early embryogenesis was clarified recently: as late as 1672 de Graaf confused follicle and oocyte. I have assiduously tried to avoid projecting current knowledge into the thoughts of the past: ancient authors cannot answer modern questions.

Antique concepts of soul and ensoulment

In *Egypt*, as in many other cultures, the placenta was attributed a soul of its own, or a part of the infant's soul, a second self. Narmer, the Pharaoh who united Upper and Lower Egypt, was depicted in the 31st century B.C.E. (**Fig. 1.1.1**). Identified by his seal and the red crown of Lower Egypt, the king is shown in a state procession, preceded by the official Tshet and four standard bearers. The first two of them carry Horus falcons, the next a canine-shaped Anubis, the god of mummification. The last carries a standard representing the pharaoh's placenta [3], a secret helper granting the kingdom's prosperity. This remained a ritual accessory until the Ptolemies [4]. As pronounced in the hymn to the sun-god Aton, Akhenaton's monotheistic religion attributed sensation to the fetus in 1340 B.C.E. [5]: 'Giving life to the son in the body of his mother, soothing him that he may not weep, nursing him in the womb, giver of breath to animate every one that he maketh, when he cometh forth from the womb on the day of his birth.'

To the *Jews*, life and soul were synonymous [Genesis 2:7]: 'The Lord God formed man of the dust of the ground and breathed into his nostrils the breath of life, and man became a living soul.' A distinction arose when a moral faculty was attributed to the soul, as in Deuteronomy 4:9: 'Keep thy soul diligently, lest thou forget the things which thine eyes have seen.' The Talmud prescribed [Yebamoth 69b]: 'If she is found pregnant, the semen, until the fortieth day, is only a mere fluid.' The *Hindus* believed in reincarnation, with the spirit (*atman*) present in the embryo from fertilization. In the Rg Samhita (before 1200 B.C.E.), the deity Vishnu was regarded the 'protector of the child-to-be' [VII.36.9]. The Caraka Samhita (200–500 C.E.) specified the origin of human personhood [6]: 'Conception occurs when intercourse takes place in due season between a man of unimpaired semen and a woman whose generative organs are unvitiated, when the individual soul (*jiva*) descends into the union of semen and [menstrual] blood in the womb.'

Buddhists also believed in a cyclic course of human existence, either eternally or leading into nirvana. They did not postulate an

Reproduced with permission from Obladen M. Animatio: A history of ideas on the beginning of personhood. *Journal of Perinatal Medicine*, 46(4):355–364. Copyright © 2017 Walter de Gruyter GmbH, Berlin/Boston.

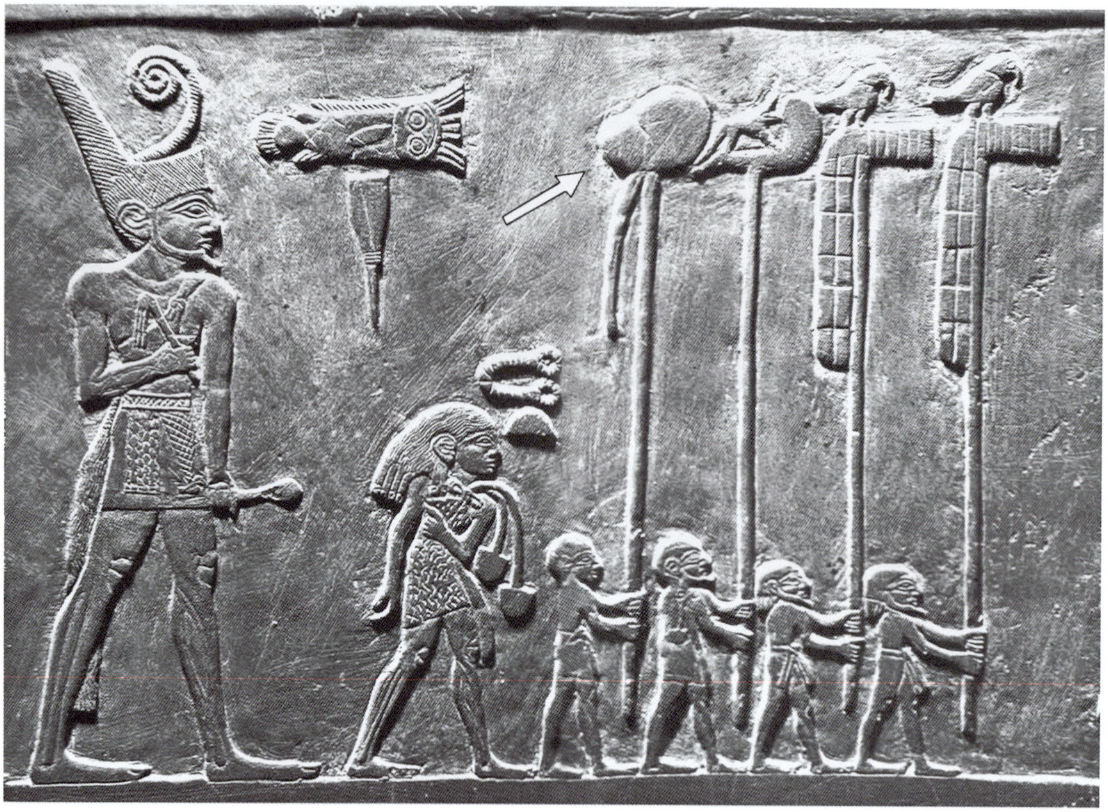

Fig. 1.1.1 Standard representing Pharaoh Narmer's placenta (arrowed), from a palette of the 31st century b.c.e. found in the Horus temple, Hierakonpolis. See text for details.
Modified from inv. JE 14716/CG 32169. Egyptian museum, Cairo.

initial starting point to an individual's series of lives and held the view that occurs instantaneously upon death [7]. In 188 B.C.E., the Chinese prescribed specific diets for each gestational month on a silk manuscript [8]: 'In the first month [the embryo] is called 'flowing into the form.' Food and drink must be the finest ... In the fifth month, vapor [*qi*] forms from fire.' Confucianism assumed a liberal position towards abortion. The Qur'an does not mention ensoulment of the unborn and the embryo's ontologic standing is controversial among Muslims.

Greek and Roman philosophy

The *Greeks* did not regard the fetus as a human person, and believed animation occurred either at birth or at a specific date during gestation. The unborn soul's immediate function was to form and activate the body. The Hippocratic corpus (ca. 400 B.C.E.) ruled in *On the Nature of the Child* [9] 'the fetus is *formed*. This stage is reached, for the female fetus, in 42 days at maximum, and for the male, in 30 days at maximum.' This sex difference may be due to confusing the penis with the embryonal tail, which is prominent at 35 days but has disappeared by 56 days after fertilization [10]. Athen's philosopher Plato (ca. 360 B.C.E.) timed ensoulment at birth and discerned three souls ruling and serving the body [11]: 'two kinds in the soul, the rational and the appetitive. ... there exists a third kind, this principle of high spirit, which is the helper of reason by nature unless it is corrupted by evil nurture.' In *Generation of Animals* [12], Aristotle (ca. 340 B.C.E.) attributed to the earliest embryo a vegetative existence animated by a *nutritive* soul; to the more mature embryo a *sentient* soul ... 'in virtue of which an animal is an animal' and to the 'formed fetus, a *rational* soul'. He justified delayed *rational* ensoulment 'because the end or completion is formed last of all, and that which is peculiar to each thing is the end of its process of formation'. Aristotle dated rational ensoulment to the time of fetal movements [13]: 'If the child is male, movement is usually felt on the right side of the groin, in about forty days; if female, the movement occurs on the left side, in about ninety days ... All these things vary in a greater or less degree.' Aristotle's teachings including the attribute *formed* dominated the opinion for 2000 years. The equation of *formedness* and animation was not debated until the 19th century.

Romans believed the fetus to be without soul, a part of the mother's body (*portio mulieris*), whereas ensoulment occurred with the inspiration of (cold) air at birth. An exception was T. Lucretius Carus, who around 60 B.C.E. wrote [14]: 'This the joint contact of the body and soul/Learn from their earliest age the vital motions/ Even when still buried in the mother's womb;/So no dissevering can hap to them.' Galen, teaching in Rome (200 C.E.), also incorporated three souls in his system of physiology (Fig. 1.1.2), locating the *natural spirit* in the liver, the *vital spirit* in the left heart, and the *animal spirit* in the brain. He believed that inhaled air cooled down the vital spirit before its journey to the brain [15]. Concerning the soul, he confessed in *De Foetuum Formatione* [16]: 'Not finding a scientifically proven view, I confess being in a hopeless situation regarding the essence of the soul, not even reaching the step of conviction.'

CHAPTER 1.1 Animatio: ideas about the beginning of personhood

From delayed to immediate ensoulment: Christian positions

The Church Fathers held heterogeneous opinions, mainly relating to original sin and based on conflicting views as to whether the soul is newly created or transmitted from Adam. In *A Treatise on the Soul*, Tertullian (ca. 200 C.E.) expressed two opposing positions [17]: In chapter 27: 'Life begins with conception, because we contend that the soul also begins from conception' and in chapter 37: 'The embryo becomes a human being in the womb from the moment that its form is completed.' Around 300 C.E., Lactantius likewise was ambivalent [18]: '[the soul] is not introduced into the body at birth, but immediately [*protinus*] after conception, when the divine necessity has formed the fetus', specifying: 'the whole work is completed at 40 days'.

Also, Augustine (of Hippo, North Africa, ca. 400 C.E.) distinguished between unformed (*inanimati*) and formed (*animati*) fetuses, stating that unformed fruits cannot be animated [19]: 'To kill an unformed [embryo] is not homicide … because it cannot be imagined that a soul lives in a body which lacks sensation, form, and mind.' But Augustine retained doubts [20]: 'I do not know whether it is in the power of researchers to resolve [the question] as to when the human begins to live in the womb, and whether there may be occult life not yet discernable by movements.' In his (1100 C.E.) chapter on the transmission of original sin, Anselm of Canterbury stated [21]: 'No human mind can accept that [the embryo] has a rational soul soon after conception.' In 1147, Hildegard von Bingen, in her vision 'The soul and its tent' [22] described delayed ensoulment in a formed fetus (Fig. 1.1.3): 'And I saw, as it were, a woman having a complete human form within her womb. And then, by a secret disposition of the Highest Creator, a fiery sphere having none of the lineaments of a human body possessed the heart of the form, and reached the brain and transfused itself through all the members.' In 1265, Thomas Aquinas adopted Aristotle's biology, assuming three subsequent souls [23] and delayed, stepwise ensoulment [24]: 'It cannot be said that the soul in its complete essence is present in the semen from the very beginning, though its operations are not manifested because of the lack of organs.'

In 1312, the Council of Vienne 'declared that the substance of the rational or intellectual soul is of itself and essentially the form of the human body' maintaining the theory of delayed hominization [25]. Immediate ensoulment, as illustrated by Jean Mansel in 1493 (Fig. 1.1.4) was associated with the dogma of original sin. In 1439, the Council of Florence rigidified this dogma and declared invalid Thomas Aquinas' proposal of 'an edge of hell' (*limbus puerorum*) for infants who died without baptism [25]: 'the souls of those who depart this life in original sin alone, go down straightway to hell to be punished.' This harsh verdict was confirmed by the Council of Trent in 1546 (see Chapter 8.2), although the catechism of this Council tried to solve the dilemma in 1567 [26]: 'In the natural order, no body can be provided with a human soul except after the prescribed space of time.' Paolo Zacchia, Roman physician and legal advisor to Pope Innocent X, proposed a pragmatic compromise around 1630 [27]: 'From the 60th day the fetus, no matter if male or female, must always be regarded as animated … To avoid controversies, each abortus has to be inspected by a physician to decide if it could have been animated, or not.' But with the Inquisitor

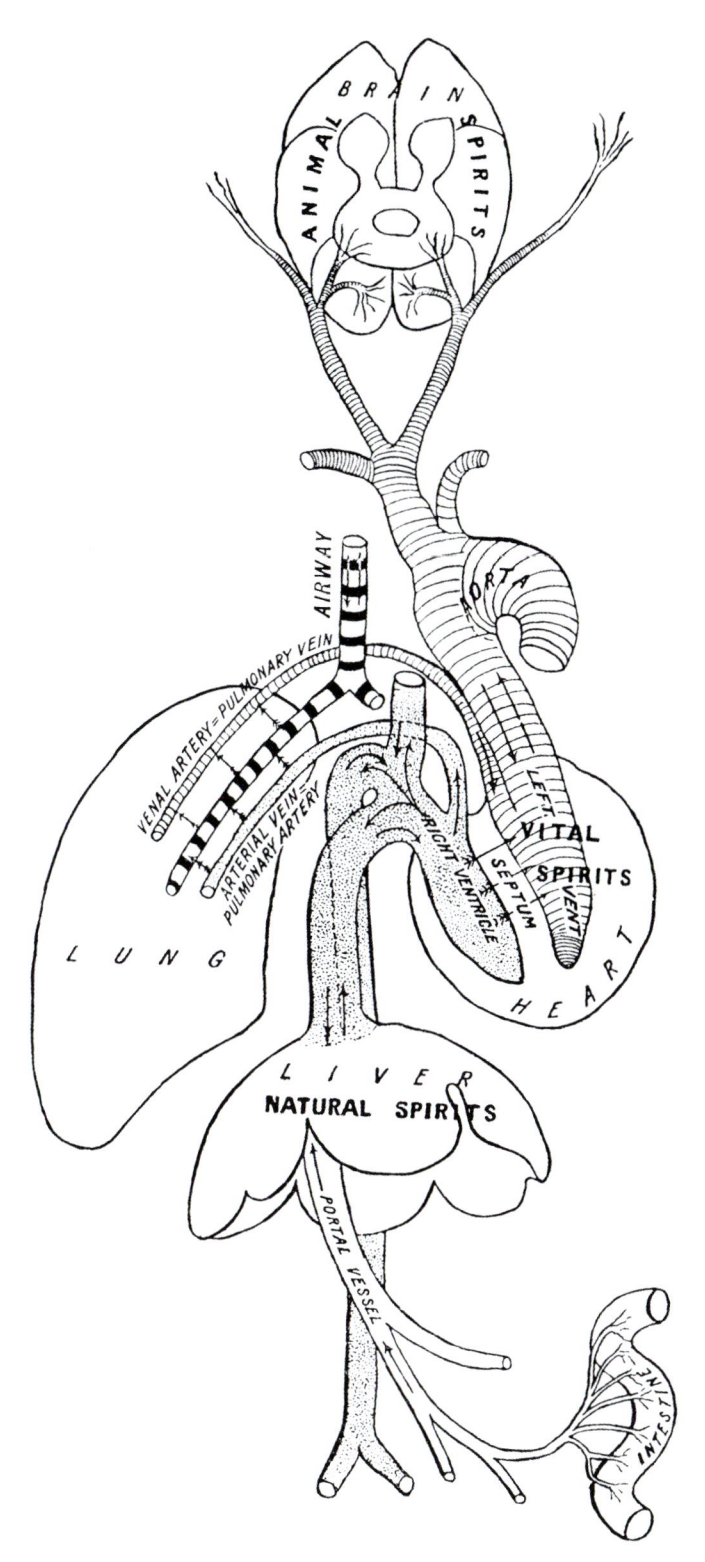

Fig. 1.1.2 Galen's physiological system (2nd century c.e.) as depicted by Charles Singer 1922 [59]. Note three different types of soul ('spirits') and their location. See text for details.

Christianization was associated with a division of *ensoulment*: biologically, it became a developmental process, and theologically a transcendental act. Attempts to reconcile the two perspectives failed.

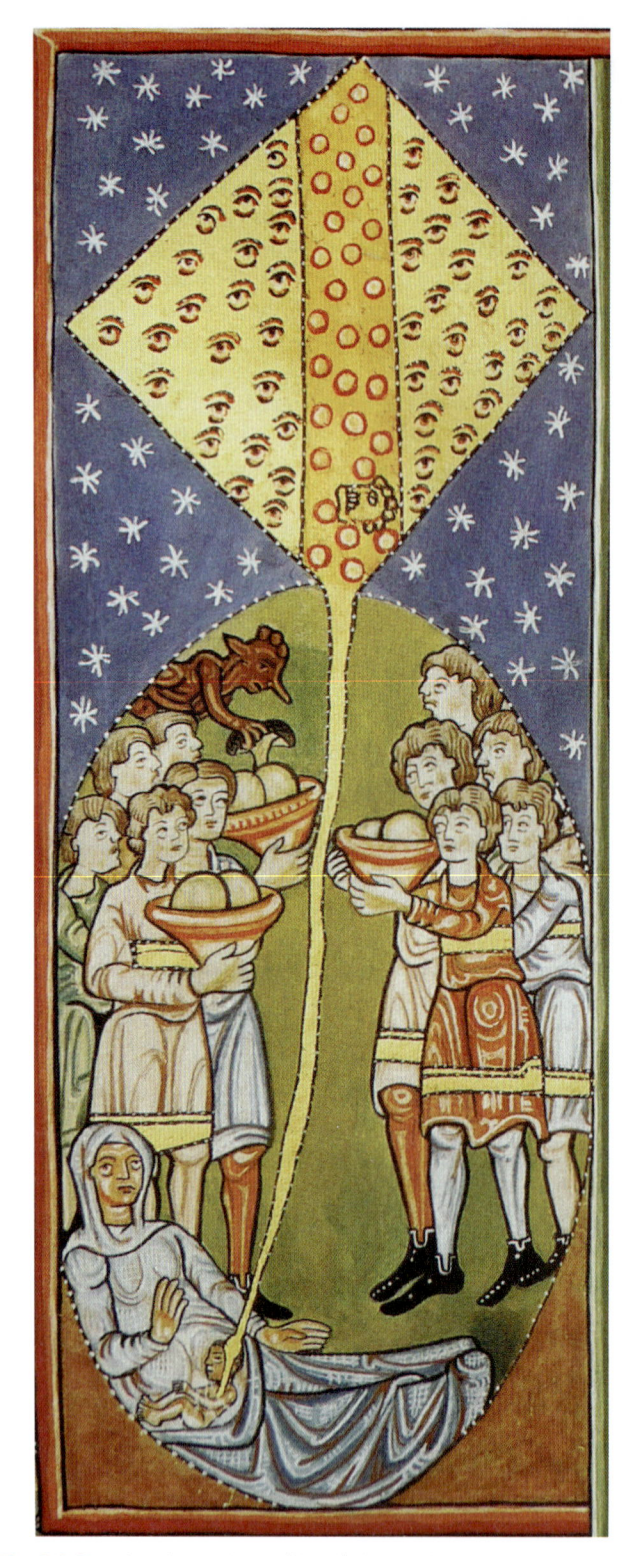

Fig. 1.1.3 Delayed ensoulment (detail), depicted around 1147 c.e. in Hildegard von Bingen's *Liber Scivias*. The soul, coming from the square-shaped wisdom of God, enters a well-formed fetus while *in utero*. Ten persons carry vessels with cheese, representing their souls; above and left: the devil puts a poisonous mushroom into a soul. See text for details. Rupertsberg Codex, Rüdesheim, Abtei St. Hildegard, Fol. 22r, with permission.

In 1766, Albrecht von Haller summarized 'there is no time at which the fetus does not live' [29]. This view was corroborated in 1857 by the French Jesuit John Gury [30]: 'Providing abortion is homicide irrespective of the circumstances: Even if the foetus were not ensouled, it is anticipated homicide … because the foetus is directed to the formation of man.' This position was adopted by Pope Pius IX, who in 1869 with the *Constitutio Apostolicae Sedis* dropped the reference to the 'ensouled fetus,' ordering automatic excommunication for any abortion [31]. This has remained the Catholic stance. The Protestant position was not substantially different. Luther decreed in 1536 [32]: 'The child in the womb has a soul from the beginning.' Calvin wrote in 1545 [33]: 'For the fetus, though enclosed in its mother's womb, is already a human being, and it is almost a monstrous crime to rob it of the life which it has not yet begun to enjoy.'

Enlightenment: rational soul versus personhood

When the Aristotelian transmutation from vegetative to rational soul became obsolete, philosophers began to equate the rational soul with personhood. Concepts of personhood were by no means monolithic, and neither life nor soul was defined unanimously. In his *Discours de la Methode*, René Descartes expressed a dualistic view in 1637 [34]: 'This self, that is to say the soul, by which I am what I am, is entirely distinct from the body.' In 1677, Spinoza opposed Descartes' dualism but rejected the soul's immortality [35]. Immanuel Kant wrote in 1788 [36] 'The soul exists as substance … What is conscious of the numerical identity of its Self in different times, is to that extent a person.' He viewed the embryo as 'developing into a human being' [37].

Contemporary philosophers' views

Defining humanity or even personality of an individuum remained difficult when ethics of principles were replaced by utilitarianism, which aimed to minimize harm and maximize utility. Contemporary ontologists began to base personhood on self-consciousness, with different reasoning: in 1974, Houston philosopher Tristram Engelhardt denied personhood to fetuses, premature infants, and patients in a persistent vegetative state [38]: 'As more can be done for the survival of premature infants, social action can obscure the moment when the fetus becomes socialized and appreciated as a child.' American ethicist Michael Tooley stated in 1983 that fetuses and newborns are no human persons, because they show no evidence for a capacity for thought, self-consciousness, or rational deliberation [39]: 'What makes an individual a person … is the property of being an enduring subject of non-momentary interests.' Melbourne theologian Norman Ford discerned in 1988 [2] 'genetic individuality begins at fertilization; unique ontological individuality means to find out how far we can trace back our personal identity as the same continuing individual living body or entity.' Ford justified his concept, that the human individual begins with the appearance of the primitive streak, with the embryo's potential [2]: 'A human person begins as a living individual with the inherent active potential to develop towards human adulthood without ceasing to be the same ontological individual.' For pre-embryonic stages the potentiality argument is less convincing and depends on probability.

Cangiamila's 1000-page 'Holy Embryology' (*Embryologia Sacra*) (1745) the Aristotelian doctrine faded [28]: He admitted that 'one cannot be sure that the embryo is ensouled', but nevertheless demanded draconic punishment for everyone assisting an abortion.

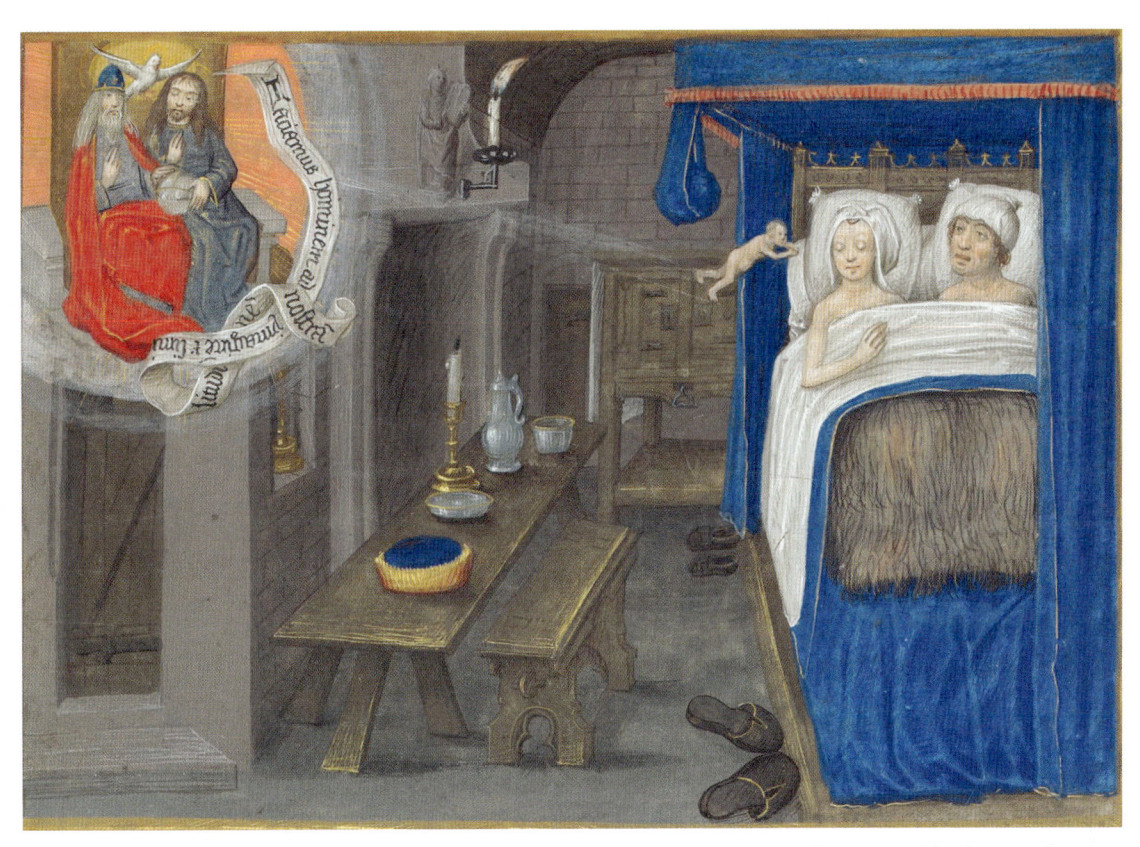

Fig. 1.1.4 Immediate ensoulment depicted around 1493 in a miniature by Jean Mansel. At the alleged moment of fertilization, the trinity appears through the opened wall, sending the infant's soul on a beam of light, and holding a scroll with the words from Genesis 1:26: 'Let us make man in our image, after our likeness.'
Bibliothèque Nationale de l'Arsenal, Paris, inv. 5206, fol. 174, with permission.

Also in Melbourne, the philosopher Peter Singer [40] denied personhood not only to fetuses, but also to infants 'who lack rationality, autonomy, and self-consciousness … No infants—disabled or not—have as strong a claim to life as beings capable of seeing themselves as distinct entities, existing over time.' In 1989, Hans-Martin Sass, a philosopher in Bochum, claimed that personal life begins with 'neuromaturation', meaning sometime between days 16 and 70 [41]. The American College of Obstetrics and Gynecology recommended in 1994 [42]: 'the human preembryo does not possess the biologic individuality necessary for concrete potential to become a human person.' Many modern ontologists maintained the principle of human dignity, as did Frankfurt philosopher Jürgen Habermas [43]: 'Human rights derive their moral content, which they spell out in the language of positive laws, from a universalistic and individualistic concept of human dignity.'

None of these positions has found general acceptance, but most ethicists and scientists assume a clear change in ontological status at birth. The argumentation chain—no (functional) brain > no mind > no personhood > no right to life—assigns different values to different individuals, which inevitably leads down the slippery slope of intellectual abilities. Excluding minorities is a dilemma for all societies, not only in medicine. The mass murder of handicapped infants in Nazi Germany (see Chapter 8.4) reminds us that the threat is not just theoretical. As reported by Annie Janvier in Montreal [44], modern health professionals place less value on the life of premature infants than on that of older children and adults—even when they have a better prognosis.

A soul in one cell? Biological facts

Modern research has not alleviated the dilemma, but it has somewhat de-emotionalized the debate. Inquisitor Cangiamila saw but four possibilities for animation in 1765 [28]: 'Undoubtedly our body receives a soul while *in utero*. We must discuss at which time this occurs. Four stages have to be considered: (1) when after conception it begins to form; (2) when its vital organs heart and brain have been formed; (3) when all parts of the body are distinguishable; (4) when the fetus is not only formed, but is so much grown and corroborated, that respiration and birth are possible.' This dispute has not been settled, but the number of possibilities for the onset of individual life has risen to at least 16, as summarized in Table 1.1.1.

These biological steps show that there is no single moment when individual human life begins; rather, development is a gradual process. Presently, there are three biological arguments to assume personhood on day 15:

1. The *substrate* argument: the greatest part of the pre-embryo is trophoblast, indistinct from the embryoblast. Can a trophoblast—the future placenta—possess dignity? A similar question was posed by John Burn in 2008 [45]: 'Can a cell have a soul?' In Western societies there is a tendency to equate personhood with the genome as the secular equivalent of the soul, as defined by Alex Mauron [46]: 'Our genome is synonymous with our humaneness.' But the seemingly simple definition is problematic: genetic identity is not the same as ontological identity.

Table 1.1.1 Proposed definitions of the onset of individual human life arranged according to the age of the conceptus

Age, Carnegie stage	Definition	Rationale	Objections	Proponents
0	Sperm penetrates the oocyte	Beginning of fertilization	No individual life	Rager 2009 [47]
1 d, CS01	Fertilization. Chromosome sets fuse. Syngamy. Zygote	Haploid gametes have fused. End of fertilization	Divisibility, no identity, no implantation, waste	Catholic position since 1869 [31]
2 d, CS02	Pre-embryo; zygote divides	Blastomere has the potential to become an embryo	Translation of DNA not before 24–48 h	Beller 1994 [48] Moraczewski 1983 [49]
4 d, CS03	Morula: 8–16 cells	Paternal genome expressed	No ongoing identity	
5 d, CS04	Early blastocyst. Implantation begins	Most zygotes perish before implantation	Perspective overturns probability	Mendiola 1999 [50]
8–9 d, CS05	Implantation in uterine mucosa completed	Until this time zygote may become several persons	Divisibility precludes ensoulment	Shannon and Wolter 1990 [51]
14 d, CS06a	Embryoblast/trophoblast separate. Placenta stalk	Before: undifferentiated cell cluster. Now distinct	Divisibility precludes ensoulment	Ford 1988 [2], Koch-Hershenov 2006 [52]
15–16 d, CS06b	Embryo. Primitive streak appears	No more totipotent cells	Half of all zygotes are lost by now	Eberl 2000 [54] Noonan 1970 [1]
24 d, CS11	Neural tube closed	No brain, no soul	Brain function more important	Kuljis 1994 [55]
30 d male, 42 d female, CS18	'Formed' fetus	Feeling the life: movements	Movements usually not before 12 weeks	Hippocrates 429 b.c.e. [9]
56 d, CS23	Organogenesis complete. End of embryonic period	Approaching human shape	No sharp boundary	Zacchia 1621 [27]
40 d male 80 d female	Ensoulment; 'formed' fetus	'Quickening', feeling life	Requires a sequence of 3 souls	Aristotle 340 b.c.e. [13]; Thomas Aquinas 1265 [24]
70 d	Synaptogenesis begins	No identity without nervous conduction	Problematic analogy to brain death	Sass 1994 [41]
16 wks	Cortical plate 6 layers	Essential species difference; merely a potential person	Sufficiently organized to embrace rationality	Donceel 1970 [56]
23/24 wks	Extrauterine viability	Viable fetus is a patient	Different among countries	Kurjak 2007 [57], Chervenak 2007 [58]
At birth	Autonomous life. Change in legal status	Onset of breathing. Change in legal status	Extensive dependency	Plato 360 b.c.e. [11]
12 mo	Self-awareness = personhood	No personhood without language	Excludes mentally impaired. Slippery slope	Engelhardt [38]; Singer 1993 [40]

CS, Carnegie stage; d, days from fertilization; mo, months from birth; wks, weeks from last menstruation. Definitions: [42, 53].

If personhood is assumed for the zygote, why not for a hydatidiform mola or a teratoma?

2. The *totipotency* argument: a serious dilemma is that a totipotent cell may split into several individuals and therefore must have several souls. It is difficult to imagine an organism—let alone a person—of which each cell has the capacity to develop into an individuum. As pointed out by Rose Koch-Hershenov [52]: 'Monozygotic twinning renders implausible the existence of the human being during the earliest stages of embryonic development.'

3. The *wasting* argument: most pre-embryos do not implant into the uterine mucosa and never develop into a newborn. This converts the potential of human development into a matter of probability. It is difficult to claim personhood for pre-embryos knowing that most of them will die before ever becoming conscious.

Ethical perspectives on individual human life have always been influenced by medical progress. This became obvious in the debates on perforating operations in the 19th century; contraceptives since the 1960s; neonatal intensive care for immature infants since the 1980s; and preimplantation diagnostics nowadays. Sound philosophy cannot be based on dubious or false biological premises. However, procreation, fetal life, and childbirth extend beyond scientific comprehension, and the beginning of individual life is not only matter of biological definitions.

Conclusion

The question as to when the soul is infused during development remained unsettled for more than 2000 years. It was a metaphysical claim unsupported by biological knowledge. The Christian position was inconsistent, mostly supporting the Aristotelian concept of delayed ensoulment. After the Reformation, theology and biology took different paths, and centuries of discussion precluded consensus on definitions. Also, modern philosophy, by replacing the soul with personhood, had to adapt to modern—and rapidly changing—biological knowledge. Presently it seems that embryogenesis is a continuous process without sharp boundaries. There is no doubt: the zygote has life, and it is human. But our historical perspective does not answer the key question: is it a person? Biological facts suggest that personhood is acquired at implantation, and not at fertilization. But biological facts alone cannot determine the embryo's moral status, and science alone cannot determine human values. Seemingly a philosophical, a priori defined matter, the definitions of life—even more of fetal life—were always pragmatic, purpose driven, revealed intercultural variation, and underwent multiple modifications due to social, political, and medical needs. It is up to societies to decide when and how fetuses achieve the status of persons. Arguments will promote agreement more than convictions, and not all societies will reach the same consensus. The obligation to protect the conceptus is negotiated and determined by legislators, keeping societal acceptability and moral consistency in mind. It would be naive to discuss the problem without considering the earth's overpopulation and the poor control that many women are allowed regarding reproduction. In most countries the fetus is not considered a person, but is granted certain rights. The never-ending abortion debate has revealed deep moral ambiguity and uncertainty within American and European societies. This chapter does not argue for or against any side; rather, it shines a historical flashlight on the origins of the ongoing debate. There are no simple answers to difficult questions.

REFERENCES

1. Noonan JT: The morality of abortion. Legal and historical perspectives. Cambridge, MA: Harvard University Press, 1970: p. 1–59.
2. Ford NM: When did I begin? Conception of the human individual in history, philosophy and science. Cambridge: Cambridge University Press, 1988, p. 85.
3. Blackman AM: The pharaoh's placenta and the moon-god Khons. J Egypt Archaeol 1916;**3**:235–49.
4. Seligmann CG, Murray MA: Note upon an early Egyptian standard. Man 1911;**11**:165–71.
5. Breasted JH: Akhenaton's hymn to Aton. In: Gressmann H: Cambridge ancient history. Cambridge: Cambridge University Press, 1925: Vol **2**, p. 118.
6. Lipner JJ: The classical Hindu view on abortion and the moral status of the unborn. In: Coward HG: Hindu ethics. Albany, NY: State University of New York Press, 1989: p. 41–69.
7. Keown D: Buddhism and bioethics. Basingstoke: Macmillan, 1995: p. 72–93.
8. Harper DJ: MSV Taichan shu: book of the generation of the fetus. In: Early Chinese medical literature. London: Routledge, 2009: p. 372–84.
9. Lonie IM: The Hippocratic treatises 'On generation', 'On the nature of the child', 'Diseases IV': Ars medica 2:7. Berlin: de Gruyter, 1981: p. 7–9, 13–9.
10. Hashimoto R: Development of the human tail bud and splanchnic mesenchyme. Congenit Anom (Kyoto) 2013;**53**:27–33.
11. Plato: The republic, Book IV. Loeb Classical Library 237. London: Heinemann, 1988: p. 403.
12. Aristotle: Generation of animals: Loeb Classical Library 366. Cambridge, MA: Harvard University Press, 1942: 736a35-b5.
13. Aristotle: Historia animalium, Book VII. Loeb Classical Library 439. Cambridge, MA: Harvard University Press, 1991: Vol. **VII**, 583b2–5.
14. Lucretius Carus T: Of the nature of things. A metrical translation by WE Leonard. London: Dent, 1916: p. 104.
15. Singer C: Galen as a modern. Proc R Soc Med 1949;**42**:563–70.
16. Galen: Über die Ausformung der Keimlinge (de foetuum formatione liber). Übersetzt und erläutert von D. Nickel: Corpus medicorum Graecorum 5.3.3. Berlin: Akademie-Verlag, 2001: p. 97–8.
17. Tertullianus QSF: A treatise on the Soul. In: Alexander Roberts: The ante-Nicene fathers, Vol. III: Latin Christianity. Peabody, MA: Hendrickson, 1995: p. 374, 394.
18. Lactantius LCF: De opificio Dei (304 C.E.). In: Migne JP: Patrologia latina. Paris: Vrayet, 1844: Vol. **7**, cap. 12, col. 69, 55.
19. Sancti Aurelii Augustini: Quaestionum in Heptateuchum libri 7 (ca. 400 C.E.). In: Migne JP: Patrologia latina. Paris: Apud Editorem, 1845: Vol. **34**, col. 626.
20. Sancti Aurelii Augustini: Enchiridion ad Laurentium, sive de fide, spe et charitate (ca. 400 C.E.). In: Migne JP: Patrologia latina. Paris: Apud Editorem, 1841: Vol. **6**, col. 272.
21. Anselmi Cantuariensis: De conceptu virginali et originali peccato. In: Gerberon: Sancti Anselmi Opera Omnia. Venetiis: Joseph Corona, 1744: Vol. **1**, p. 147.
22. Sanctae Hildegardis: Scivias, sive visionum ac revelationum libri tres. In: Patrologia latina. Paris: Migne JP: 1855: Vol. **197**, col. 413–7.
23. Thomas Aquinas: Summa Theologiae, pars I, qu. 118: Human reproduction with respect to the soul. Cambridge: Blackfriars, 1970: Vol. **15**, p. 146–54.
24. Thomas Aquinas: Summa contra gentiles. Book 2: Creation. Notre Dame, London: University of Notre Dame Press, 1975: p. 300–1.
25. Tanner NP: Decrees of the Ecumenical Councils. Washington, DC: Georgetown University Press, 1990: p. 360, 528, 666.
26. Pius V. Pont. Max.: Catechismus Romanus, ex decreto Concilii Tridentini. Lugduni: Apud Guliel. Rovilium, 1567: **Pars I**, p. 36.
27. Zacchia P: Quaestionum medico-legalium (1st ed. 1621). 4. ed. Avenione: Joannis Piot, 1655: Vol. Tit. 2, quaest. 9, p. 56–8.
28. Cangiamila FE: Embryologia sacra sive de officio sacerdotum, medicorum, et aliorum circa aeternam parvulorum in utero existentium salutem (1st ed. Milan 1745). 3. ed. Augustae Vindelicorum: Mauracher, 1765: p. 70, 136.
29. Haller A: Elementa physiologiae corporis humani. Lugduni Batavorum: Haak, 1766: Vol. **8**: Fetus hominisque vita, p. 334.
30. Gury JP: Compendium theologiae moralis. 2. ed. Ratisbonae: Manz, 1857: p. 114.
31. Pius XI Papa: Constitutio Apostolicae Sedis moderationi. In: Acta Sanctae Sedis/Acta Pii IX 1869–70. Rome: Libreria Editrice Vaticana, 1911: Vol. **5**, p. 305–17.
32. Luther M: Disputatio de homine (1536). Weimar: Böhlau, 1926: Vol. **39-1**, p. 174–80.
33. Calvin J: Commentaries on the last four books of Moses (1545). Vol **3**. Grand Rapids, MI: Eerdmans, 1950: p. 51–2.
34. Anscombe GE, Geach PT: Descartes: philosophical writings. London: Nelsons University Paperbacks, 1975: p. 32.
35. Spinoza B: Ethica, ordine geometrico demonstrata, et in quinque partes distributa. In: Opera posthuma, tract. 1. Amsterdam: [N.N.], 1677.
36. Kant I: Critique of pure reason (1st ed. 1788). Translated and edited by: Paul Guyer and Allen W. Wood. Cambridge: Cambridge University Press, 1998: p. 422.
37. Kant I: Religion innerhalb der Grenzen der bloßen Vernunft (1793). Wiesbaden: Insel, 1960: Vol. **4**, p. 785 = A170.
38. Engelhardt HT: The ontology of abortion. Ethics 1974;**84**:217–34.

39. Tooley M: Abortion and infanticide. Oxford: Clarendon Press, 1983: p. 303.
40. Singer P: Practical ethics. Cambridge: Cambridge University Press, 1993: p. 182.
41. Sass H-M: The moral significance of brain-life criteria. In: Beller FK, Weir RF: The beginning of human life. Dordrecht: Kluwer, 1994: p. 57–70.
42. American College of Obstetrics and Gynecology: Preembryo research: history, scientific background, and ethical considerations. Committee on Ethics. Int J Gynecol Obstet 1994;**45**:291–301.
43. Habermas J: The concept of human dignity and the realistic utopia of human rights. Metaphilosophy 2010;**41**:464–80.
44. Janvier A, Leblanc I, Barrington KJ: Nobody likes premies: the relative value of patients' lives. J Perinatol 2008;**28**:821–6.
45. Burn, J: Can a cell have a soul? BMJ 2008;**336**:1132.
46. Mauron A: Essays on science and society. Is the genome the secular equivalent of the soul? Science 2001;**291**:831–2.
47. Rager G: Beginn, Personalität und Würde des Menschen. 3. ed. Freiburg: Alber, 2009: p. 82.
48. Beller FK, Zlatnik GP: Medical aspects of the beginning of individual lives. In: Beller FK, Weir RF: The beginning of human life. Dordrecht: Kluwer, 1994: p. 3–16.
49. Moraczewski AS: Human personhood: a study in personalized biology. In: Bondeson WB et al.: Abortion and the status of the fetus. Dordrecht: Reidel, 1983: p. 301–11.
50. Mendiola MM, Peters T, Young EWD, Zoloth-Dorfman L: Research with human embryonic stem cells: ethical considerations. Hastings Center Report 1999;March:31–6.
51. Shannon TA, Wolter AB: Reflections on the moral status of the pre-embryo. Theol Stud 1990;**51**:603–26.
52. Koch-Hershenov R: Totipotency, twinning, and ensoulment at fertilization. J Med Philos 2006;**31**:139–64.
53. O'Rahilly R, Muller F: Developmental stages in human embryos: revised and new measurements. Cells Tissues Organs 2010;**192**:73–84.
54. Eberl J: The beginning of personhood. A Thomistic biological analysis. Bioethics 2000;**14**:134–57.
55. Kuljis RO: Development of the human brain: the emergence of the neural substrate for pain perception and conscious experience. In: Beller FK, Weir RF: The beginning of human life. Dordrecht: Kluwer, 1994: p. 49–56.
56. Donceel JF: Immediate animation and delayed hominization. Theol Stud 1970;**31**:76–105.
57. Kurjak A, Carrera JM, McCullough LB, Chervenak FA: Scientific and religious controversies about the beginning of human life. J Perinat Med 2007;**35**:376–83.
58. Chervenak FA, McCullough LB, Levene MI: An ethically justified, clinically comprehensive approach to peri-viability. J Obstet Gynaecol 2007;**27**:3–7.
59. Singer C: The discovery of the circulation of the blood. London: Bell, 1922: p. 9.

1.2

Hepar uterinum
Ideas about fetal nutrition

Introduction: oral versus parenteral

Although the placenta is the only readily accessible internal organ, it took millennia to even begin understanding its basic functions. Psalm 139:15 stated: 'My substance was not hid from thee, when I was made in secret, and curiously wrought in the lowest parts of the earth.' Superstition flourished where knowledge was wanting and metaphysical claims conflicted with biological discoveries. Romans imagined that the goddess Alemona nourished the unborn in the womb. As it obviously kept the fetus alive, many cultures revered the placenta, their rites aiming to perpetuate its poorly comprehended function of protecting the infant. In some cultures, placentas were buried, burned, eaten, used as a medicine, or ritually disposed of. Other rites required that a source of infection be removed, such as the Babylonian Talmud [Niddah 26a]: 'If a placenta is within the house, the house is unclean.' An enduring controversy arose already in the Hippocratic Corpus (4th century B.C.E.): in *De Carnis*, one author claimed [1] 'While the child is in utero, it sucks with compressed lips from the maternal uterus both nutriment [into the stomach] and attracts hot spirit [*pneuma*] into its heart.' In *De Octimestri Partu*, another Hippocratic author stated [2]: 'The umbilical cord is the only access to the infant's body, attached to the uterus, and through it the nutriment is taken. All other pathways are closed, and do not open until the child exits the womb.'

The historiography of embryology is extensive and the excellent works of Adams [3], Needham [4], De Witt [5], and Longo [6] drew attention to the placenta, albeit not specifically to its nutritive function. This chapter provides historical insights into fetal alimentation and identifies major steps in the perception of placental nutrient transfer. Its focus is on macronutrients, omitting embryology, placental anatomy, endocrine regulation, metabolism, and the pathology of intrauterine growth restriction. It also omits an abundance of lore and legend around the placenta, as has been assembled by Long [7]. The chapter is not organized chronologically, but according to the supposed routes of nutrient supply.

Menstrual blood

Since prehistory, the cessation of menstruation was associated with the formation of the *conceptus*. The Hippocratic book *De Natura Pueri* [1] suggested: 'The [menstrual] blood descends from the woman's whole body, and surrounds the [fetal] membrane. This blood is drawn into the membrane ... and by coagulating, it causes the growth of what is to become a living thing.' At a later stage, 'flesh begins to be formed, with the umbilicus, through which the embryo breathes and grows, projecting from the center.' Aristotle's *De Generatione Animalium* greatly influenced embryologic concepts up to the 17th century [8]. In 746a20, he opposed the Hippocratic view [9]: 'Those people who say that children are nourished in the uterus by means of sucking a bit of flesh are mistaken' and postulated a vascular connection between mother and fetus in 740a25: 'Now since the unborn is already an animal potentially, though an imperfect one, it must get its nourishment from elsewhere; and that is why it makes use of the uterus, i.e. of the mother, just like a plant makes use of the earth ... The blood-vessels join on to the uterus as though they were roots, and through them the fetation gets its nourishment.'

Galen (2nd century C.E.) believed the umbilical veins conveyed *alimentary blood* and the umbilical arteries supplied *vital spirit*. His opinion that 'the umbilical vessels are extensions of the uterine arteries' [10] was reiterated for 14 centuries. In 1194, Pope Innocent III, inspired by the elder Pliny [11], despised the fetus because of its unclean nutrition [12]: 'The menstrual blood ceases to flow after conception in order to feed the *conceptus*. This blood is so detestable and unclean that upon contact, grains don't germinate, trees wither ... and dogs turn rabid from eating it.' Realdo Colombo, professor of anatomy in Rome, used the term *placenta* [cake] for the 'thick round material at the umbilical vessels' origin' and stated in 1559 [13]: 'The fetus accepts nutriment through the navel, via the umbilical vein. It is a fairytale told by the great Hippocrates when he claimed that [the fetus] in the womb sucks with its mouth.' Vopiscus Plempius was professor of medicine in Louvain; his second name Fortunatus alluded to his birth by Caesarean section from a mother who died in childbirth. In 1644, he maintained that the fetus was

---

Reproduced with permission from Obladen, M. Hepar uterinum: a history of ideas on fetal nutrition. *Journal of Perinatal Medicine*, 45(7):779–786. Copyright © 2017 Walter de Gruyter GmbH, Berlin/Boston.

nourished directly by menstrual blood, but also accepted nourishment via umbilical vessels [14]: 'The placenta conveys nutriment to the foetus through the umbilical cord.' Leiden anatomist Franciscus Sylvius wrote in 1679 [15]: 'The monthly flow contributes more than the maternal [arterial] blood to the fetal nutrition.'

'Purified' maternal blood via umbilical cord

Assuming connected vessels, some authors believed the fetus was nourished by secretions from maternal blood, and not by the blood itself. Referring to ancient superstitions, Paris Royal Physician Jean Fernel assumed in 1555 [16]: 'Given the toxicity of menstrual blood it seems incredible that the fetus is nourished by this pestilential effluent.' In 1626, Adriaan van den Spieghel correctly described the flow direction in the umbilical vessels [17] and in 1672, Isbrand van Diemerbroeck, professor of anatomy in Utrecht, specified [18]: 'The uterus is directly connected to the placenta by open pores and small arterioles … and transfuses blood and milky juice into the placenta … However, most [umbilical] vessels have no anastomoses. Both arteries lead the fetal cardiac blood to the placental tissue, whereas the single [umbilical vein] transfuses the good part of the blood, refined and fermented, from the uterine vessels to the fetus … We hold it most likely that the placenta dissolves coarse and incompatible particles, mixes them with sulphur, and cooks them so that the blood the fetus requires is predigested.'

Fetal blood via umbilical cord

This route of nutrition was proposed by authors who maintained that circulations were distinct, being unaware of the intervillous space, but aware of absorbing vessels. Giulio Cesare Aranzio, professor of anatomy in Bologna, coined the term 'hepar uterinum' for the placenta, and denied any connections between maternal and fetal blood vessels in 1587 [19], even though he admitted: 'It is repugnant to sense that these [umbilical] vessels fail to reach the inner surface of the uterus, because the placenta's substance is located between their ramifications and the uterine wall.' Forty-one years before Harvey's discovery [20], Aranzio did not address circulation: it would take two more centuries, Bartholin's injection technique, and the Hunter brothers' experiments (Fig. 1.2.1) to prove that Aranzio was right. Nicolaas Hoboken in Utrecht stated in 1675 [21]: '[In early gestation] the embryo is entirely nourished by means of a gelatinous juice, which is secreted by the womb and imbibed by the pores of the chorion' (Fig. 1.2.2). In 1674, John Mayow believed [22]: 'Just as [in] the lacteal vessels which originate in the intestinal membranes … a nutritious juice, properly concocted, enters the openings of the umbilical vessels only by percolation through the membrane.'

By mouth in addition to the umbilical blood

In 1651, William Harvey agreed with Aranzio [23]: 'The extremities of the umbilical vessels are in no way conjoined to the uterine vessels by an Anastomosis; nor do extract blood from them, but are terminated in that white mucilaginous matter, attracting nourishment from it, as they did formerly draw Aliment from the white moisture concluded within the membranes.' Like most 17th-century researchers, Harvey did not use the microscope. He proposed that the mode of nutrition changes with development of the unborn: 'I believe that this *Colliquamentum*, or water wherein the foetus swims, doth serve for his sustenance; and that the thinner & purer part of it, being imbibed by the *Umbilical Vessels*, do constitute and supply the

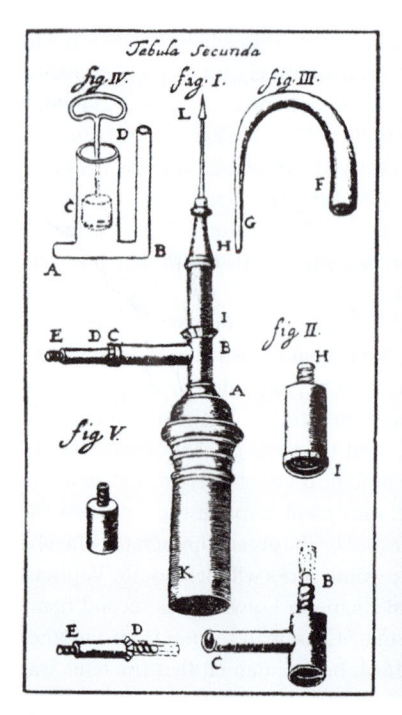

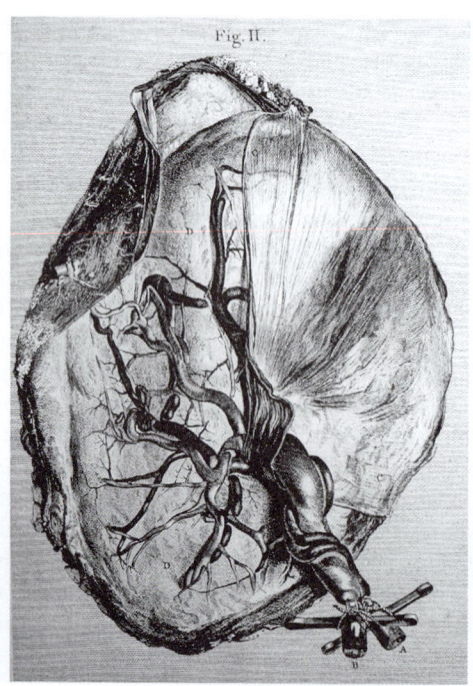

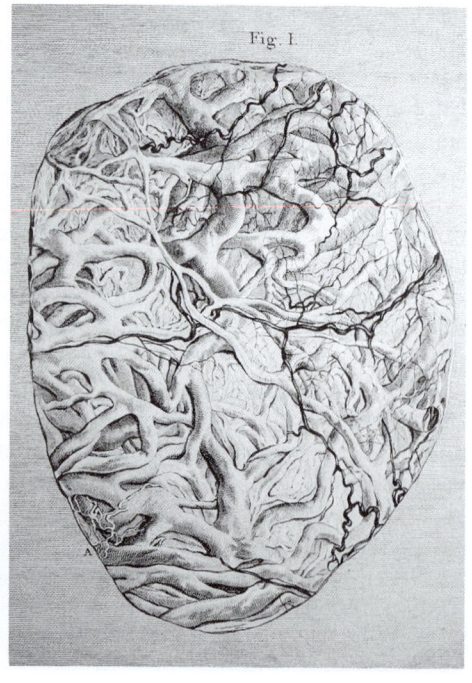

Fig. 1.2.1 Left: anatomical injection apparatus that could be recharged without disconnecting the syringe, from Caspar Bartholin 1679 [54]. Centre and right: William Hunter's injection experiments of 1774 [25]. Centre: inner side of the placenta. Umbilical arteries are injected with green, umbilical vein filled with blue wax. Right: uterine wall and outer side of the placenta showing the uterine vessels injected with yellow wax.

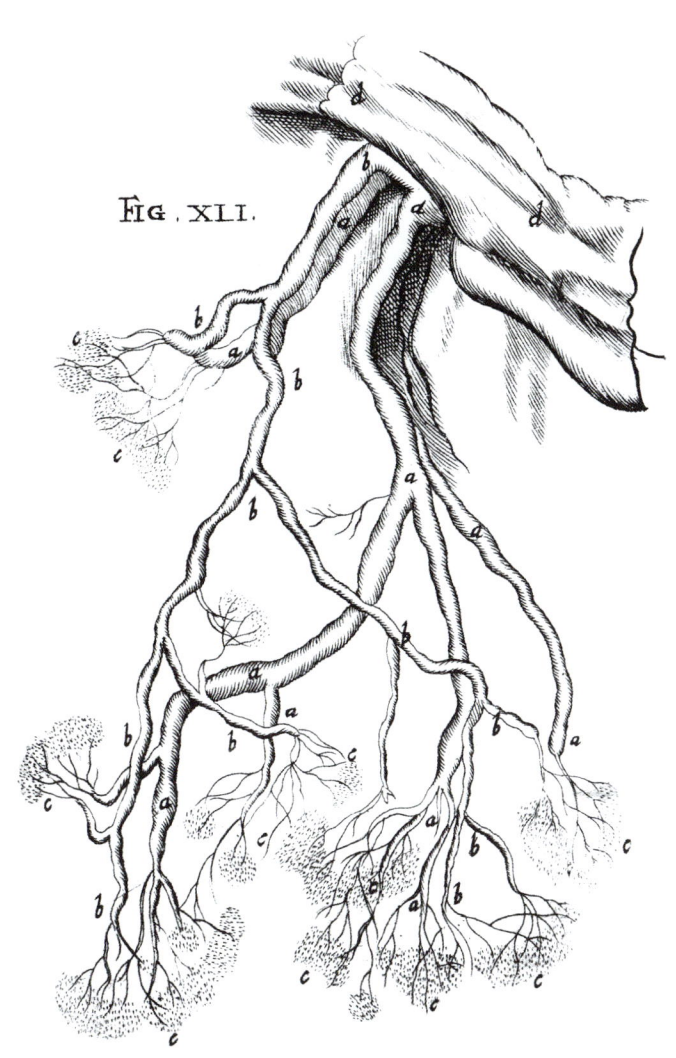

Fig. 1.2.2 Vascular ramifications in the placenta depicted by Nicolaas Hoboken 1669 [21]: aa, umbilical veins and cc, their ramifications with bb, the umbilical arteries; d, umbilical cord; 'The small dots represent liquid nutritional particles.'

primogenit parts: and the rest, like *Milk*, being by suction conveyed into the *Stomack*.'

In London, Walter Needham specified in 1667 [24]: 'It remains difficult to understand the secretion of the nutritious juice from the arteries. A fresh amount of the liquid is brought in as blood, from which some splits into the amnion, the rest returns into the veins.' Using injections of coloured melted wax, William Hunter [25] proved in 1774 finally and incontrovertibly that maternal and fetal circulations are distinct: 'Though the placenta be completely filled, none of the wax finds its way into any of the umbilical vessels.' Blood from the 'curling arteries' accumulated in the placenta in a space which he called 'sinus system'. An unbrotherly rivalry resulted from John Hunter's claim to have discovered the sinuses already in 1754 [26, 27]. The intervillous space was finally defined by William Carpenter in 1854 [28]: '[The vascular tufts] dip-down, as it were, into a cavity, whose inner wall is formed by … the large veins or sinuses of the uterus.' Albrecht von Haller was ambivalent in 1779 [29]: '§895: The nourishment of the fetus from the beginning to the end of the conception [pregnancy], is without doubt conveyed through the umbilical vein, gathering its roots from the exhaling vessels of the uterus … §897: But is the fetus also nourished by the mouth? Does it drink from the cavity of the amnios, the lymphatic lubricating liquor? … On every point, numberless difficulties occur; but it seems more probable, that this liquor is nutritious, especially in the early stages of the fetus, and is derived from the uterus.'

By mouth only with amniotic fluid or uterine milk

Greek authors believed the growing uterus pressed against the breasts, to pump milk into the uterine arteries, and thence to the 'uterine paps' [5]. Galen claimed a vessel led from the uterus to the breast, whereas Albertus Magnus (1193–1280) maintained there was flow in the other direction [30] 'The breasts are connected to the *secundines* in which the infant lies, by a vessel leading from the breasts to the infant's navel, through which the mother's milk nourishes the infant in utero.' Peter Stalpart van der Wiel opposed the idea of nutrition via the umbilical cord in 1686 [31]: 'The embryo takes in enough nutritional juice only by its mouth.' Anthony Everaerts of Middelburg also believed in uterine paps and propounded the theory that uterine milk was identical to the contents of the thoracic duct. Reasoning with tongue movements and presence of chylus in the stomach and meconium in the gut, Everard maintained in 1686 [32]: 'I do not doubt that fetuses in utero suck up the water in which they swim for their nutrition and growth.' In 1682, London physician Thomas Gibson distinguished nutrition in early and late pregnancy [33]: 'The Chorion imbibe[s] that albugineous liquor that from the first Conception encreases daily in it (and transudes through the Amnios wherein the Embryo swims) till the Umbilical vessels and the Placenta are formed, from and through which the fetus may receive nourishment. This liquor that it imbibes I take to be nutritious juice that ouzes into the Cavity of the Uterus out of the Capillary orifices of the Hypogastrick and Spermatick Arteries.' For Gibson, a case of oesophageal atresia with fistula seemed to prove the theory of oral nutrition [34]: 'About November 1696 I was sent to an infant that could not swallow … [died on day 3, postmortem] … we blew by a pipe down the gullet, but found no passage into the stomach. Then we made a slit in the stomach, and put a pipe in its upper orifice, and blowing, we found the wind had a vent … found an oval hole, half an inch long, opening into the [trachea] … Now, I say, this is a plain confirmation of the fetus's being nourished by the mouth; for the *Gula* being impervious, Nature had formed this hole in the wind-pipe and gullet, for the liquor contained in the *amnios* to pass into the Stomach.'

A new era of understanding began with the use of the microscope by Marcello Malpighi in 1685 [35]: 'I am disposed, I say, to believe that the fluid surrounding the fetus may serve it for nourishment; that the thinner and purer portions of it, taken up by the umbilical veins, may serve for the constitution and increase of the first formed parts of the embryo; and that the remainder or the milk, taken into the mouth by suction, passed on to the stomach by the act of deglutition, and there digested or chylified, the new being continues to grow and be nourished.' In 1802, Frédéric Lobstein, anatomist in Strasbourg, still supported the view that the main source of fetal nutrition was by amniotic fluid per os—despite the fact that he used the microscope and found arterioles and venules in the chorionic villi (Fig. 1.2.3) [36].

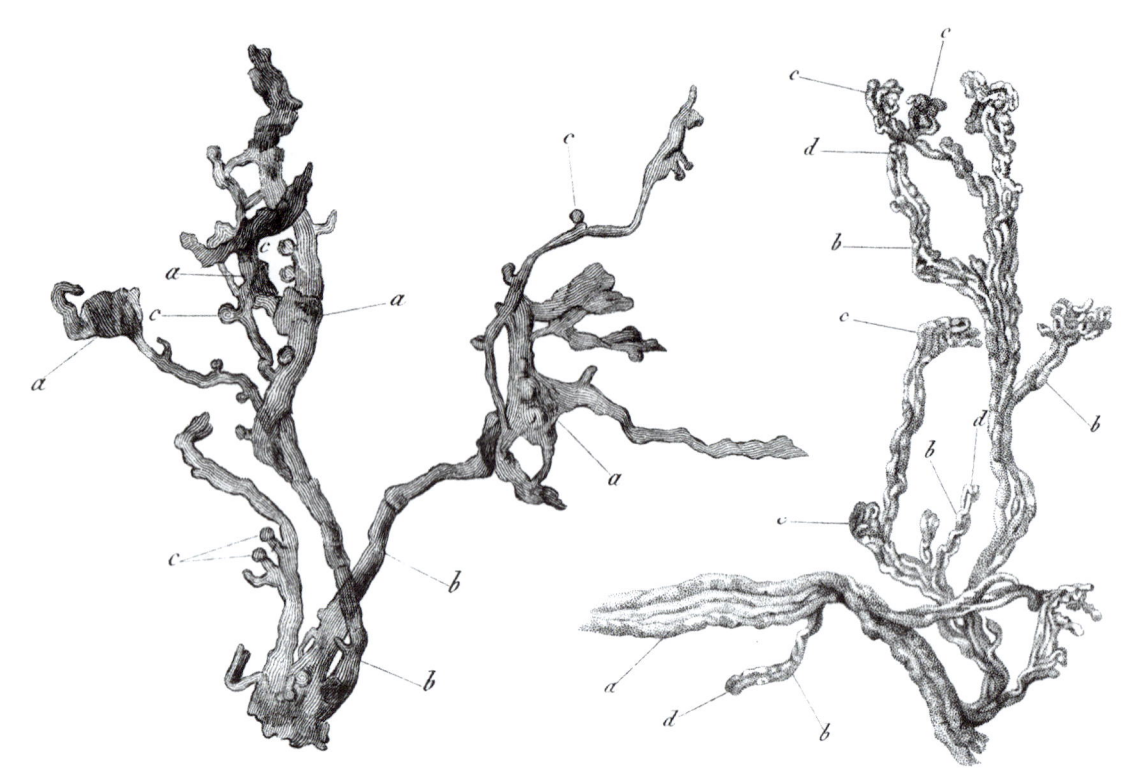

Fig. 1.2.3 Microscopic views of chorionic flakes, by Frédéric Lobstein 1802 [36]. Left: early gestation. Ramifications (aa) are thicker than their trunks (bb). Right: at term. Vessels have been injected with coloured resin, arteries and veins run parallel in pairs, their ends are twisted and dilated.

Molecular diffusion

In 1828, Henri Dutrochet described the passage of liquids through semipermeable membranes, naming it *endosmose* (inwards) and *exosmose* (outwards) of organs [37]. Matthias Schleiden formulated the cell theory in 1837, postulating a solid membrane and liquid contents [38]. In 1842, the London ophthalmologist John Dalrymple wrote [39]: 'Hence, while the blood, or nutrient material in the blood, brought by the uterine arteries, and previously aerated by the mother, enters by *endosmose* the absorbent capillaries of the foetal villi; that portion of the foetal blood that requires the action of oxygen escapes by *exosmose*, and returns via the uterine sinuses and veins to the maternal heart.' Another revolution came with the arrival of chemistry. In 1851 Joseph Hyrtl stated [40]: 'Its low protein content makes improbable that the amniotic fluid can serve as nourishment.' By iodine staining in sheep and calf fetuses, Claude Bernard ascertained the importance of carbohydrates for fetal development in 1859 [41]: 'During early fetal development the placenta seems destined to accomplish the glycogenic function of the liver, until the latter has assumed its function.' William Carpenter in 1854 described two cell layers covering the villi [28], 'first a fetal, than a maternal layer of cells'. The syncytial character of the outer was characterized by the pathologist Theodor Langhans in Bern [42], who showed that both layers were of fetal origin, the lower disappearing during gestation, the upper becoming a conglomerate. The combined barrier thickness of cyto- and syncytiotrophoblast, 35 μm in early, and still about 10 μm in mid-gestation [43], made a direct passage of molecules unlikely. But as late as 1922, Shimidzu, from the permeability of dyes, held the feto-maternal border to be a semipermeable membrane: 'The placenta seems to have no mysterious function as a special selector of materials in favor of the fetus, but merely the function of an ultra-filter [44].' Deeper understanding resulted from the structure of the cell membranes: using a Langmuir trough, Gorter and Grendel demonstrated in 1925 that cell membranes 'are covered by a layer of fatty substances that are two molecules thick' [45]. In 1958, Wilkin and Bursteijn found the total villus surface measured 14 m^2 and the capillary length in the villi 50 km at term [46]. The presently accepted 'fluid mosaic model' of the cell membrane was proposed in 1972 by Jonathan Singer and Garth Nicolson [47], with structural proteins integrated into the phospholipid bilayer that function as receptors and transport channels.

Active transport

Already in 1917, A. Morse observed that the *amino acid* nitrogen was higher in human cord blood than in maternal plasma [48]. Active transport against a gradient required a carrier-mediated process, and various transport systems were identified by Christensen and Streicher 1948 [49]. Using radioactive labelling, du Pan and colleagues demonstrated in 1959 the active transport of gammaglobulins to the fetus [50].

Glucose is not predominantly transported by diffusion either: in 1951 in London, Arthur Huggett and co-workers injected glucose into pregnant ewes and found: 'While possibly some glucose may pass across the placenta by a process of physical diffusion, there is, in addition, a chemical system within the placenta into which the glucose enters with induced formation of fructose' [51]. One year later

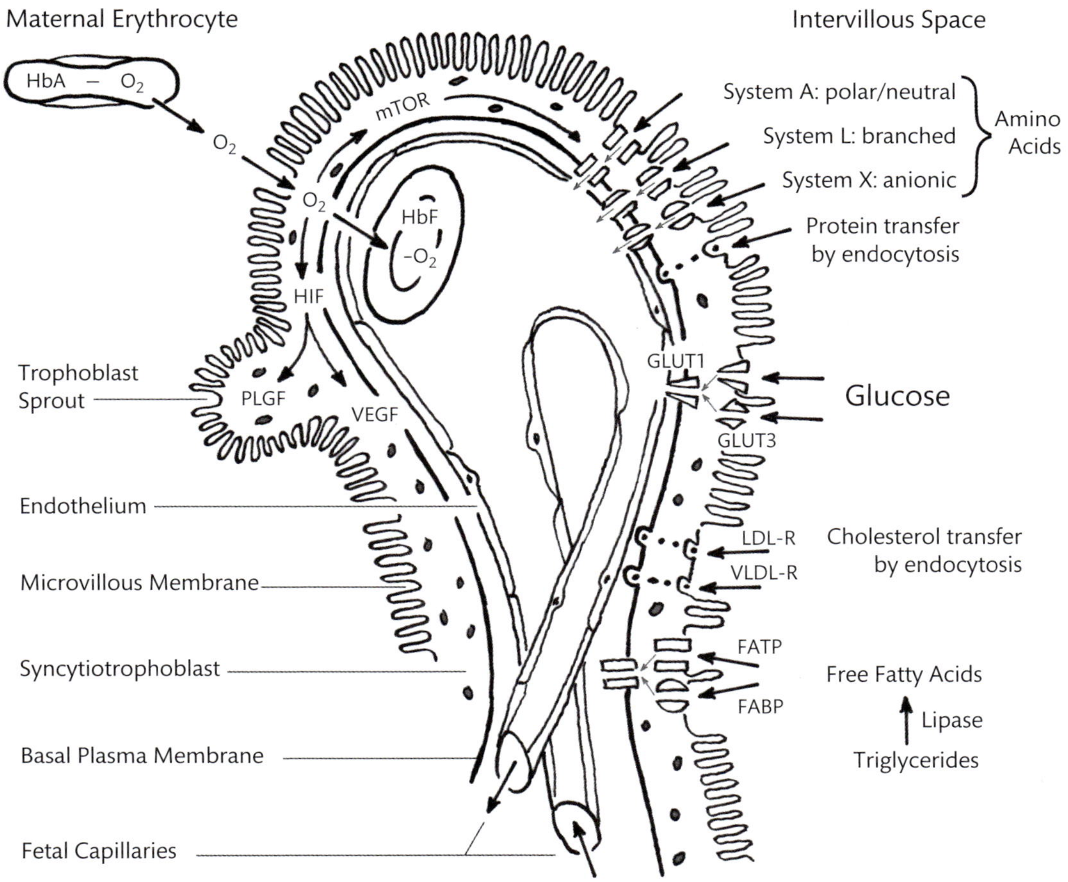

Fig. 1.2.4 Simplified sketch showing mechanisms of materno-fetal transport of macronutrients and oxygen across the syncytiotrophoblast in late gestation. Active amino acid transport is achieved by system A for small neutral, system L for branched-chain, and system X for anionic amino acids. Proteins (immunoglobulins) are transferred by endocytosis. Glucose is transported mainly by GLUT-1 and GLUT-3. Cholesterol transfer to the trophoblast is mediated by lipoprotein receptors LDL-R and VLDL-R. Maternal triglycerides are hydrolysed to free fatty acids by lipoprotein lipase before being transported by FATP (fatty acid transport protein) and FABP (fatty acid binding protein). Fetal haemoglobin (HbF) has greater oxygen affinity than maternal haemoglobin (HbA); HIF, hypoxia inducible factor, key activator of oxygen dependent gene expression; mTOR, mechanistic target of rapamycin, a nutrient sensor that upregulates amino acid transporters in hypoxia; PLGF, placenta growth factor; VEGF, vascular endothelial factor.
Source: Data from [53, 55–57].

and in the same institution, Wilfried Widdas identified the kinetics of the glucose carrier mechanism [52].

Many fatty acids are transported selectively by fatty acid binding proteins and fatty acid transport proteins [53]. Multiple and complex active transport systems are present on the trophoblast microvillous and basal membranes and on the endothelial membranes of fetal capillaries (**Fig. 1.2.4**). Among the reasons for net materno-fetal transfer are: (1) the fetal blood flow in the villous capillaries exceeds the maternal blood flow in the intervillous space; (2) the microvillous membrane is larger than the basal membrane; and (3) different transport systems exist on microvillous membrane and basal membrane.

Conclusion

It is hard to understand why the injection of easily accessible placental blood vessels, as well as microscopy, both powerful tools already available, remained largely unused up to the end of the 18th century, whereas formal, historic, or religious arguments dominated the discussion. Bitter controversies were fought out during the 17th century, based more on traditionalism and dogma than on critical observation. When with the discovery of oxygen the placenta's respiratory function became understood at the end of the 18th century, its nutritional function fell from grace. Scientists understood, albeit reluctantly, that the complex organ exerted multiple functions, of which nutrition is but one part. Deeper comprehension of this function began with cell theory. **Fig. 1.2.4** suggests that today we are nearer to recognizing the mechanisms, but not by much.

REFERENCES

1. Lonie IM: The Hippocratic treatises 'On generation', 'On the nature of the child', 'Diseases IV'. Berlin: de Gruyter, 1981: p. 7–9, 13–9.
2. Hippocrates: Über Achtmonatskinder. Edited by: Hermann Grensemann. Berlin: Akademie-Verlag, 1968: p. 87.
3. Adams F: On the construction of the human placenta. An historical sketch. Aberdeen: Brown and Company, 1858.

4. Needham JA: A history of embryology. Revised with the assistance of Arthur Hughes: 2. ed. Cambridge: Cambridge University Press, 1959.
5. De Witt F: An historical study on theories of the placenta to 1900. J Hist Med 1959;14:360–74.
6. Longo LD, Reynolds LP: Some historical aspects of understanding placental development, structure and function. Int J Dev Biol 2010;54:237–55.
7. Long EC: The placenta in lore and legend. Bull Med Libr Assoc 1963;51:233–41.
8. Aristotle: Generation of animals. Loeb Classical Library 366. Cambridge, MA: Harvard University Press, 1942: Vol. Book 2, 4.
9. Hippocrates: De carnibus. Edited by Anutius Foesius: Magni Hippocratis opera omnia. Frankfurt: Wechel, 1596: p. 209.
10. Galen: Über die Ausformung der Keimlinge (de foetuum formatione liber). In: Corpus medicorum Graecorum 5.3.3. Berlin: Akademie-Verlag, 2001: p. 97–8.
11. Robinson GW: Birth characteristics of children with congenital dislocation of the hip. Am J Epidemiol 1968;87:275–84.
12. Innocentii Papae Tertii: De contemptu mundi, sive de miseria humanae conditionis, libri tres. Lovanii: Wellenus, 1563: p. 4r.
13. Colombo R: De re anatomica libri XV. Venice: Bevilaqua, 1559: p. 247–9.
14. Plempius VF: Fundamenta medicinae. 1. ed. Lovanii: Zegers, 1644: p. 209.
15. Sylvius de le Boe F: Praxeos medicae liber tertius. In: Opera Medica. Amsterdam: Elsevier & Wolfgang, 1679: p. 481.
16. Fernel J: Universa Medicina (1st. ed. Paris 1554). Physiologiae libri VII; Liber 7, pars 3: De hominis procreatione.... Venice: Constantin, 1577: p. 178 v.
17. Spieghel A: De formato foetu liber singularis. Patavii: de Martinis, 1626: p. 18–22, Plate 7.
18. Diemerbroeck I: Anatome corporis humani (1st ed. Ultrajecti 1672). Lugduni: Huguetan, 1679: p. 196–200.
19. Arantius JCB: De humano foetu liber (1st ed. 1564). Venice: Brechtanus, 1587: p. 18.
20. Harvey W: An anatomical dissertation upon the movement of the heart and blood in animals. Frankfurt: Fitzer, 1628: p. 39.
21. Hoboken N: Anatomia secundinae humanae (1st ed. Utrecht 1669). Ultrajecti: Ribbius, 1675: p. 172, 441, Plate XLI.
22. Mayow J: On the respiration of the foetus in the uterus (1st ed. 1674). Edinburgh and London: Alembic club, 1907: p. 211–7.
23. Harvey W: Anatomical exercitations, concerning the generation of living creatures (1st Latin ed. 1651). London: Pulley, 1653: p. 358, 439, 483.
24. Needham W: Disquisitio anatomica de formato foetu (1st ed. London 1667). 2. ed. Amstelodami: le Grand, 1668: p. 20–5, 149–57.
25. Hunter W: Anatomia uteri humani gravidi tabulis illustrata. Birmingham: Baskerville, 1774: p. 48, plate X.
26. Hunter J: On the structure of the placenta. In: Observations on certain parts of the animal oeconomy. London: Leicester Square, 1786.
27. Corner GW: Exploring the placental maze. Am J Obstet Gynecol 1963;86:408–18.
28. Carpenter WB: Principles of comparative physiology. 4. ed. London: Churchill, 1854: p. 626–7.
29. Haller A: First lines of physiology. Edinburgh: Elliot, 1779: p. 129, 461–6.
30. Albertus Magnus: Ein Newer Albertus Magnus von Weibern und geburten der Kinder. Frankfurt/Main: Gülfferich, [1556]: Fol. 4r.
31. Stalpart van der Wiel P: Dissertatio medica inauguralis de nutritione foetus. Lugduni Batavorum: Elzevier, 1686: p. F4.
32. Cosmopolita (Anthony Everaerts): Historia naturalis, comprehendens humani corporis anatomiam. Lugduni Batavorum: Kellenaar, 1686: p. 133–44, 187–96.
33. Gibson T: The anatomy of humane bodies epitomized. 1. ed. London: Flesher, 1682: p. 181.
34. Gibson T: The anatomy of humane bodies epitomized (1st ed. London 1682). 6. ed. London: Awnsham & Churchill, 1703: p. 220.
35. Adelmann HB: Marcello Malpighi and the evolution of embryology. Ithaca, NY: Cornell University Press, 1966: Vol. 5, p. 2252.
36. Lobstein JF: Essai sur la nutrition du foetus. Strasbourg: Levrault, 1802: p. 91–4.
37. Dutrochet H: Nouvelles recherches sur l'endosmose et l'exosmose. Paris: Baillière, 1828:
38. Schleiden MJ: Beiträge zur Phytogenesis. Arch Anat Physiol Wiss Med 1838;5:137–76.
39. Dalrymple J: On the structure and functions of the human placenta. Med Chir Trans 1842;25:21–9.
40. Licetus F: De monstris (1.ed. Patavii 1616). Amstelodami: Frisius, 1665: p. 135, 185.
41. Bernard C: Sur une nouvelle fonction du placenta. J Physiol Homme Animaux 1859;2:31–40.
42. Langhans T: Über die Zellschicht des menschlichen Chorions. Beitr Anat Physiol 1882;Festschrift für Henle:69–79.
43. Jauniaux E, Burton GJ, Moscoso GJ, Hustin J: Development of the early human placenta: a morphometric study. Placenta 1991;12:269–76.
44. Shimidzu Y: On the permeability to dyestuffs of the placenta of the albino rat and the white mouse. Am J Physiol 1922;62:202–24.
45. Gorter E, Grendel F: On bimolecular layers of lipoids on the chromocytes of the blood. J Exp Med 1925;41:439–43.
46. Wilkin P, Burszteijn M: Étude quantitative de l'evolution de la superficie de la membrane d'échange du placenta humain. In: Snoeck J: Le placenta humain. Paris: Masson, 1958: p. 211–48.
47. Singer SJ, Nicolson GL: The fluid mosaic model of the structure of cell membranes. Science 1972;175:720–31.
48. Morse A: The amino acid nitrogen of the blood in cases of normal and complicated pregnancy and also in the newborn infant. Bull Johns Hopkins Hosp 1917;28:199–204.
49. Christensen HN, Streicher JA: Association between rapid growth and elevated cell concentration of amino acids. J Biol Chem 1948;175:95–100.
50. Du Pan RM, Wenger P, Koechli S, et al.: Étude du passage de la gamma-globuline marquée à travers le placenta humain. Clin Chim Acta 1959;4:110–5.
51. Huggett AStG: The origin of the blood fructose of the foetal sheep. J Physiol 1951;113:258–75.
52. Widdas WF: Inability of diffusion to account for placental glucose transfer in the sheep. J Physiol 1952;118:23–39.
53. Haggarty P: Placental regulation of fatty acid delivery and its effect on fetal growth—a review. Placenta 2002;23:S28–38.
54. Bartholin C: Administrationum anatomicarum specimen. Frankfurt: Haubold, 1679: p. 73, Tabula II.
55. Carter AM: Evolution of placental function in mammals: the molecular basis of gas and nutrient transfer, hormone secretion, and immune responses. Physiol Rev 2012;92:1543–76.
56. Cetin I, Alvino G, Radaelli T, Pardi G: Fetal nutrition: a review. Acta Paediatr Suppl 2005;94:7–13.
57. Larqué E, Ruiz-Palacios M, Koletzko B: Placental regulation of fetal nutrient supply. Curr Opin Clin Nutr Metab Care 2013;16:292–7.

1.3

Pulmo uterinus
Ideas about fetal respiration

Introduction

Three billion years ago, cyanobacteria began to photosynthesize, enriching the earth atmosphere with oxygen and enabling the evolution of complex multicellular organisms. In the Middle Ages, alchemists explained respiration, as did Michael Sendivogius in Prague in 1604, who pondered about a property of air, 'a nitrous substance' that supported respiration [1]: 'In it [aire] also is the vitall spirit of every Creature, living in all things … It nourisheth them, makes them conceive, and preserveth them … Man dies if you take Aire from him, &c. Nothing would grow in the world, if there were not a power of the aire, penetrating, and altering, bringing with it selfe nutriment that multiplies.' Researchers theorized on respiration of the unborn, as did John Mayow in 1674 [2]: 'It will not be out of place to inquire how it happens that the foetus can live though imprisoned in the straits of the womb and completely deprived of the access of air.'

Even more than its nutritive function, the placenta's role in gas exchange remained a mystery nearly into our times. This chapter aims to identify important steps in understanding fetal oxygenation; it omits embryology, placenta anatomy, fetal hypoxia, neonatal resuscitation, and the history of blood gas analysis. The history of placental functions was reviewed by Metcalfe and colleagues [3] and Longo [4]; the following chapter focuses on ancient and medieval sources on fetal respiration. I have attempted to avoid projecting modern ideas into the thoughts of past scientists as much as possible. Caution is needed with the prefix *nitro-*, which has changed its meaning: before 1779 it referred to what is now known to be oxygen.

The pneuma doctrine

The Hippocratic Corpus was not unanimous in the fourth century B.C.E. concerning fetal respiration. The author of *De Natura Pueri* stated [5]: '[The seed] acquires breath, since it is in warm environment and the mother breathes. When it is filled with breath, the breath makes a passage for itself in the middle of the seed and escapes… The seed, then, is contained in a membrane, and it breathes in and out.' The author of *De Octimestri Partu* stated [6]: 'All things are conferred to the embryo via [the umbilicus] only.' Concerning *pneuma*, Aristotle had different viewpoints in *De Generatione Animalium*, which for him were not contradictory [7]: in 736a1 he characterized *pneuma* as warm air, in 736b5 as a carrier of vital function and instrument of the soul. In Galen's system of physiology, the *vital spirit* was carried from the air to the heart via pulmonary arteries (see Fig. 1.1.2 in Chapter 1.1). The left ventricle was imagined as the warmest part of the body, whence the *vital spirit* was distributed by the aorta. Inspired air was believed to both feed and cool the flame in this furnace. Galen considered the fetus to be an animal, and the uterine and fetal vessels connected 'to bring it nutriment and *pneuma* from the mother' [8]. He assumed that the umbilical arteries convey vital spirit, and the umbilical vein the nutrients. The fetal circulation and its transition at birth were correctly described in William Harvey's masterpiece in 1628 [9]. In Christian theology, the difference between pneuma and soul vanished, and pneuma became an equivalent of the Holy Spirit [10].

Separate circulations and shades of red

Despite Aranzio's 1564 theory of distinct circulations [11], Adriaan van den Spieghel, professor of anatomy in Padua, believed that maternal and fetal vessels are connected in the placenta. He identified the flow direction in the umbilical vessels and in 1626 contradicted Galen [12]: 'In my opinion the [umbilical] arteries do not transport vital spirit from the mother to the fetus. Rather, the blood flow is directed from the fetal heart towards its external parts [the placenta] … to transmit vitality and heat to them.' Fig. 1.3.1 is Spieghel's publication of a drawing from his Padovan predecessor Giulio Casserio [13]. Described remarkably late and stubbornly debated was the fact that the umbilical vessels convey blood of a different colour. The Amsterdam anatomist Nicolaas Hoboken observed in 1669 [14]: '[On the placental surface] the ramifications of the veins appear in a lighter red than those of the arteries, which appear

---

Reproduced with permission from Obladen, M. Pulmo uterinus: a history of ideas on fetal respiration. *Journal of Perinatal Medicine*; 46(5):457–464. Copyright © 2017 Walter de Gruyter GmbH, Berlin/Boston.

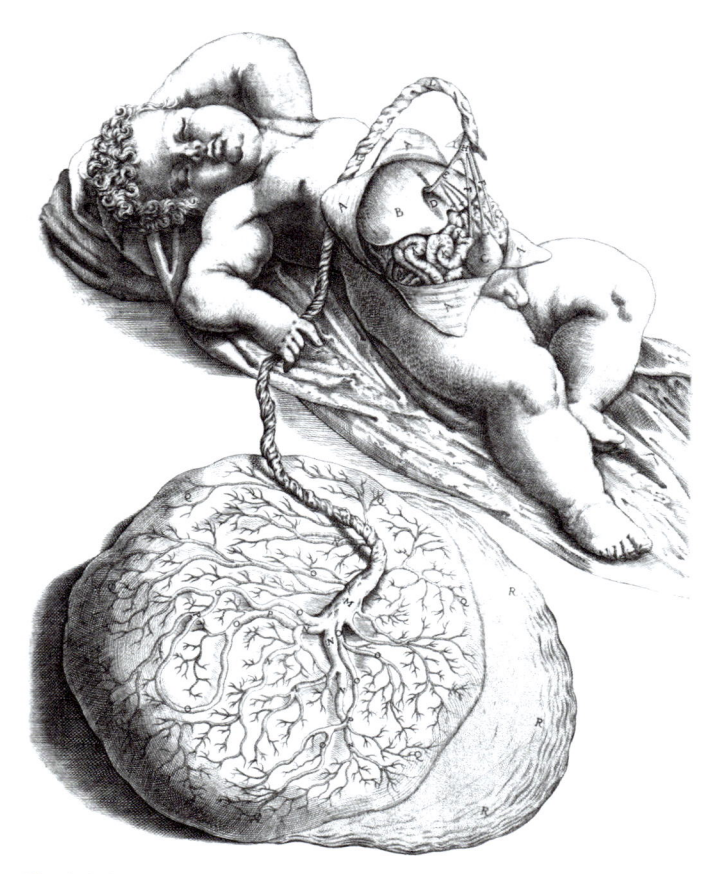

Fig. 1.3.1 Placental and umbilical vessels, published by Adriaan van den Spieghel 1626 [12] (originally drawn by his predecessor Giulio Casserio in 1616) [13]. E, umbilical vein passing the fetal liver. F, umbilical arteries deviating down to the iliac arteries; H, (assumed) extracorporeal fusion of umbilical vessels. M, trunk where the umbilical vein vessels (from the placenta) fuse. Placental ramifications of umbilical artery (O) and vein (N), and anastomoses between them (P).

violet.' In the same year, Oxford physiologist Richard Lower wrote [15]: 'The [bright] red color is due to small air particles accumulated in the blood when it returns from the lung where it has been thoroughly mixed with air … I ask myself how the nitrous vital spirit transits and accumulates in the blood during its passage through the lung.' In 1779, Albrecht von Haller observed [16]: 'Let us compare the blood of an adult person to that of a fetus … It appears then in a fetus, that the blood is destitute of its florid redness and solid density … therefore, all these properties, the blood acquires in the lung.' In 1799, Schütz and Autenrieth reported having disproved the observation of different blood colours in umbilical artery and vein by examining rabbit and cat fetuses [17].

Phlogiston and fire-air: Harvey's question

In his *De Generatione* of 1651, William Harvey queried [18]: 'In the mean time I shall propose this problem to the Learned, namely, how the embryo doth subsist after the seventh month in his mother's womb? when yet in case he were born, he would instantly breath[e]: nay he could not continue one small hour without it? and yet remaining in the womb … he lives, and is safe without the help of Respiration.' Already in the 17th century, several *Learned* tried to answer Harvey's question, but without the knowledge of oxygen their answers had to remain incomplete. The sixth chapter of Walter Needham's book of 1668 addresses respiration or *biolychnium* (a forerunner of *phlogiston*), and in it he opposed Galen's concept of a vital flame [19], 'which no mortal has ever seen … It may be imagined hidden in the heart's chamber … but blood, when thrown into the fire, does not ignite easily … The embryo does not go up in flames before it breathes, and when it draws air into its lungs.' The main work of Giovanni Borelli, a Roman physicist, was published in 1681 [20]: 'Without respiration, the fetal life can be preserved because this deficiency is compensated by the mother's respiration. Indeed, copious air particles are intermixed with the maternal blood from which it acquires vital mobility. This vitalized blood flows through the umbilical vessels to the fetal heart, acting as if the fetus were breathing himself.' In Leiden, Pieter Stalpart van der Wiel was still convinced by Galen's physiology in 1686 [21]: 'The air, which must cool the foetal blood, does not cross the placenta easily: in its tissue, which functions as do the lung cells, [the spirit of] each maternal breath is propelled through the membranes' pores.' John Ray, naturalist in Essex, wrote in 1691 [22]: '[The fetus] doth receive air, so much as is sufficient for it in its present state, from the maternal Blood by the placenta uterina, or the *Cotyledons*.'

Although logical, these explanations did not bear fruit, because Europe was enthralled with the vitalists' theories: based on ideas of Joachim Becher [23], Georg Ernst Stahl developed the phlogiston theory from 1697 [24]. He postulated a hypothetical substance, released from combustibles, which passed from air to plants and animals. Respiration consisted not in absorbing an air compound, but in giving off phlogiston. The consistent theory explained combustion, chemical reactions, and respiration, was adopted by most European chemists, and persisted for a century.

Sal-nitro, or whatever the blood receives

Richard Lower's colleague in Oxford, John Mayow, went one step further in 1674 by describing *sal-nitro*, the compound of air essential to burn a candle and for animal respiration. He modified Aranzio's statement: 'I think that the placenta should no longer be called a uterine liver but rather a uterine lung' [2] and answered Harvey's question: 'The blood of the embryo, conveyed by the umbilical arteries to the placenta or uterine carunculae, brings not only nutritious juice, but along with this a portion of nitro-aerial particles to the foetus for its support; so that it seems that the blood of the infant is impregnated with nitro-aerial particles by its circulation in the umbilical vessels, quite in the same way as in the pulmonary vessels.' Lower, Mayow, and Borelli revealed remarkable insight more than a century before the discovery of oxygen and in the dawning phlogiston era. At the same time, Isbrand van Diemerbroeck, professor in Utrecht, envisioned the placenta's metabolic needs in 1672 [25]: 'The [maternal] arterial blood supplies vital spirit to all parts of the fetus, also to his membranes, and the maternal spirited blood induces growth, nutrition, vitality, and activity of the placenta.' Philipp Verheyen, anatomist in Louvain who described fetal circulation in 1693, was impressed by the blood flow in the umbilical vessels [26]: 'It is worth inquiry for what purpose the blood of the fetus is sent in such great quantity out of its body into the

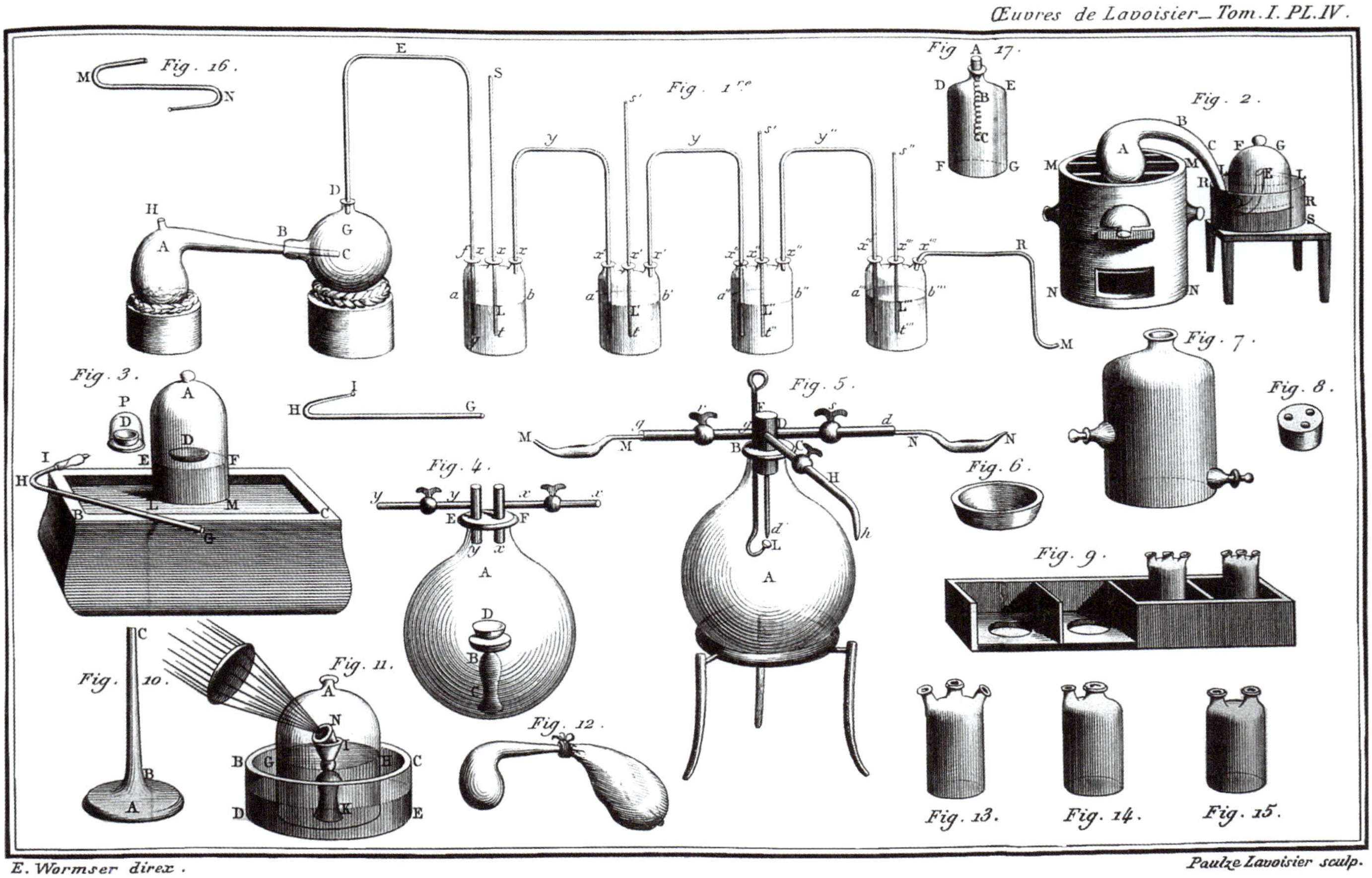

Fig. 1.3.2 Antoine Lavoisier's equipment to analyse oxygen in the atmosphere, 1789 [30].

placenta: As certainly a far less quantity of blood would suffice for its nourishment.'

From the same observation, the London surgeon William Cheselden suspected fetal respiration in 1713 [27]: 'But for what end such a quantity flows continually and back again, I cannot conceive, unless it is that the Foetus not breathing for itself, it is necessary that as much blood of the mother should flow continually to the Foetus, as can leave enough air, or whatever our blood receives in the lungs [,] for the Foetus.' In 1737, Giovanni Battista Mazzini, professor in Brescia, published a monograph on fetal respiration [28]: 'Everyone knows that air dissolved in liquids consists of liquid and elastic particles which are able to move, to react, and to expand.'

Oxygen and gas exchange: the chemistry of air

Scheele, who distinguished *fire-air* and *foul air*, Priestley, who called oxygen *dephlogistated air*, and Cavendish, who named hydrogen *inflammable air*, were prisoners of the phlogiston theory [29]. However, in 1779 Antoine Lavoisier, who understood their discoveries, named the new gas *oxygène*. He published his monumental *Traité Elémentaire* in 1789 [30] (**Fig. 1.3.2**), founding modern chemistry and basing respiration physiology on gas exchange. The following steps came fast: Christoph Girtanner wrote in 1792 [31]: 'Fetal blood receives some of the oxygen contained in the maternal arterial blood' and Erasmus Darwin proposed in 1794 [32]: 'By the late discoveries of Dr. Priestley, M. Lavoisier, and other philosophers, it appears, that the basis of atmospherical air, called oxygene, is received by the blood through the membranes of the lungs … The placenta consists of arteries carrying the blood to its extremities, and a vein bringing it back, resembling exactly in structure the lungs and gills above mentioned; and that the blood changes its color from a dark to a light red in passing through these vessels.' In Copenhagen, Poul Scheel noted in his dissertation in 1798 [33]: 'The fetal blood exposed to placental action and returning by the umbilical vein is of a (slightly) brighter red that the venous blood in the umbilical arteries … In utero, the fetal blood either absorbs less oxygen, or is in less contact with it than in the lungs.'

Oxygenation of maternal and fetal haemoglobin

In 1860, Gustav Kirchhoff and Robert Bunsen invented the spectroscope, using it to analyse gases [34] (**Fig. 1.3.3**). In 1862, Felix Hoppe-Seyler used the instrument to study oxygenated and deoxygenated haemoglobin [35]. In 1866, Ernst Körber demonstrated that compared to adult human blood, fetal hematin was alkali resistant and lost its oxygenation band slower [36]. Using a Browning spectroscope in Hoppe-Seyler's Institute of Physiological Chemistry in Strasbourg in 1876, the Swiss gynaecologist Paul Zweifel measured

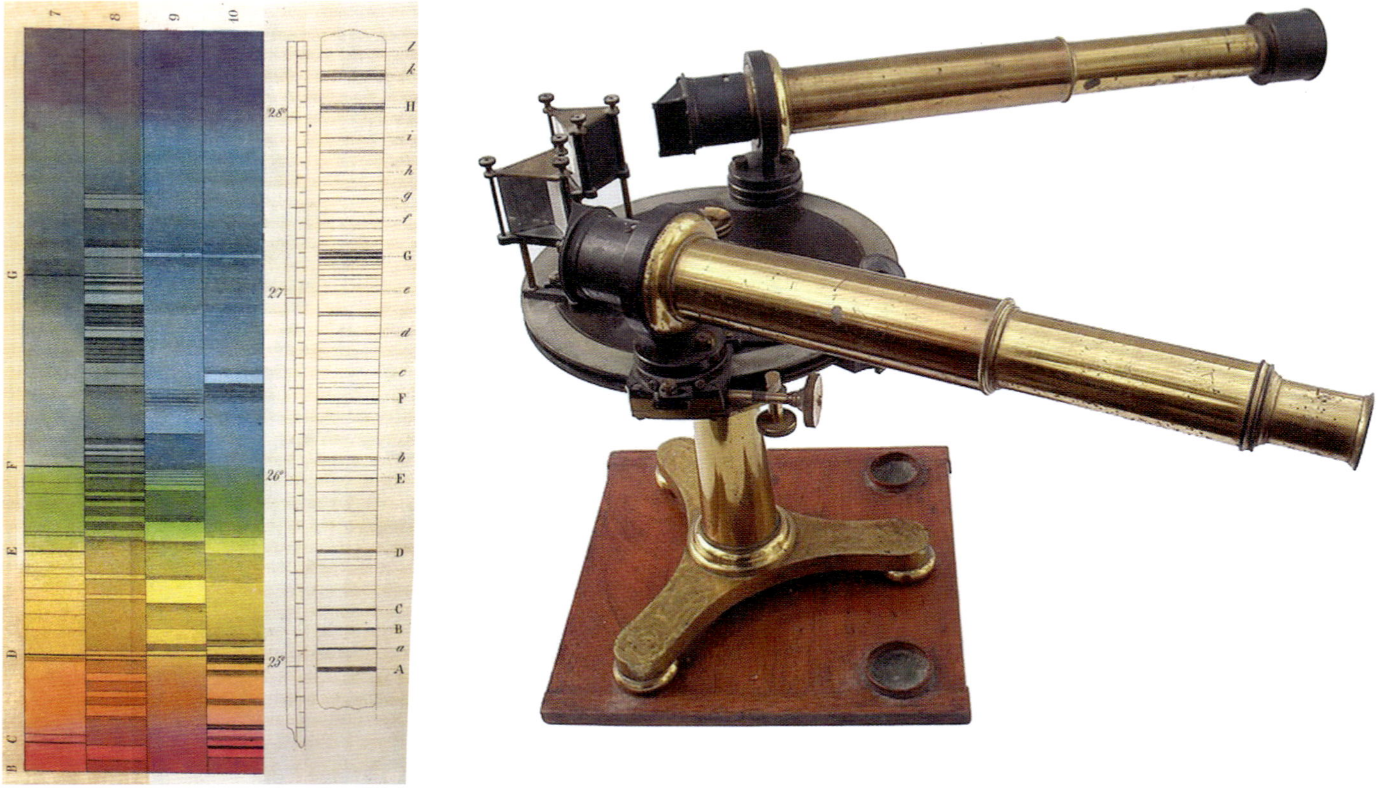

Fig. 1.3.3 Spectroscopy for oxygen analysis. Left: light spectra published by Gustav Kirchhoff and Robert Bunsen in 1860 [34], oxygen absorption lines are A, a, and B. Right: Browning spectroscope used by Paul Zweifel to measure oxyhaemoglobin in fetal blood in 1876 [37].

oxyhaemoglobin in rabbit fetuses, proving their oxygen consumption [37]: 'Fetal breathing in the placenta is subjected to the same conditions as in the animal that is born.' In 1884, Cohnstein and Zuntz confirmed chemically that fetal umbilical venous blood contains more oxygen and less carbon dioxide than that returning to the placenta [38]. Using van Slyke's constant pressure blood gas pump, Arthur Huggett measured absolute partial pressures of oxygen and carbon dioxide in goat fetuses in 1927. He constructed dissociation curves for these gases, demonstrated a maternal–fetal oxygen gradient, concluding [39]: 'The gases diffuse across the placenta and are not secreted by placenta activity.' Gideon Dodds determined perimetrically that the total villi surface measured 6.5 m² in 1922 [40].

In 1927, Joseph Barcroft measured impaired oxygenation using a mobile laboratory in adults during excursions on high mountains [41]. In 1933, he described a similar change in goat fetuses of different maturity from the Cambridge Physiological Institute. The fetal oxygen dissociation curve was left of the maternal curve, the gap increasing during pregnancy (**Fig. 1.3.4**) [42]: 'The foetus then grows in an environment the oxygen concentration of which is falling all the time – an uphill business you may say. True indeed, for is it not the problem of Everest, the maintenance of the organism in an atmosphere becoming progressively rarer?' Barcroft continued 'researches on pre-natal life' and published this *magnum opus* [43] in 1946, the greatest contribution to fetal physiology in the 20th century.

In 1946, Donald Barron discovered in sheep that the maternal–fetal oxygen gradient increased during gestation [44]. In 1948, Rodney Porter and Frederick Sanger at Cambridge identified the terminal amino acids of haemoglobins, finding 2.6 valine residues in the fetal and five in the adult human haemoglobin [45]. In 1955, Seymour Romney and colleagues determined human diaplacental oxygen transfer as 5 mL/kg/min during Caesarean section at term [46].

In 1964, Heinz Bartels and Waldemar Moll in Tübingen demonstrated that human placental flow resembled a multivillous stream system which was less effective than the countercurrent system of sheep and rabbits [47]. They identified an absolute oxygen diffusion capacity of the human placental membrane of 0.5 mL/min/mmHg. Geoffrey Dawes and colleagues observed in 1969 that in hypoxic fetal lambs the blood pressure (and hence the umbilical flow) increased and concluded [48]: 'The fetal circulation is under reflex control by the aortic chemoreceptors.'

Oxygen and gene expression

There are several advantages to the embryo's development in low oxygen. It minimizes the production of reactive oxygen species, which would trigger widespread apoptosis incompatible with fetal development. When the maternal circulation within the placenta is established at 3 months of pregnancy, a major rise in oxygenation occurs which initiates active transport and protein synthesis [49]. Oxygen-dependent transcription factors regulate the expression of multiple genes required to regulate embryonal (e.g. vascular endothelial growth factor (VEGF)) and placental (e.g. placental growth factor (PLGF)) development; and they suppress the genes

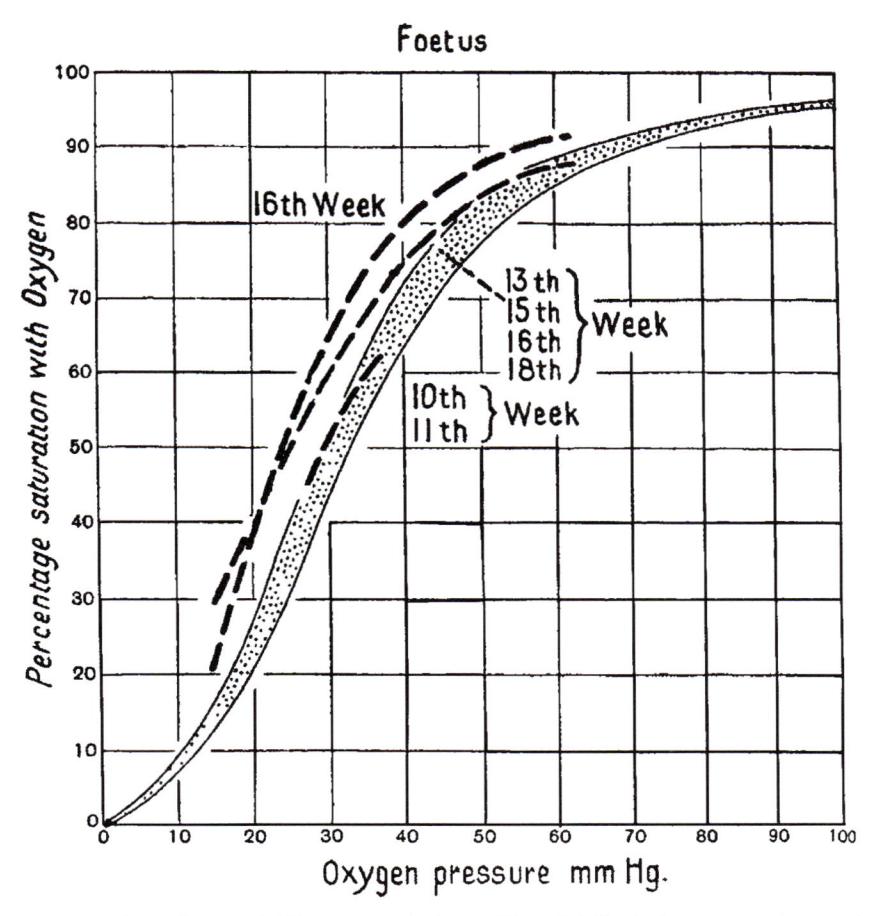

Fig. 1.3.4 Oxygen dissociation curves of goat fetuses of different maturity (term: 21 weeks). Shaded area: normal, anaesthetized pregnant goats; dashed: fetal blood at various gestational ages. Partial pressure of carbon dioxide adjusted to 50 mmHg.
Reproduced from Barcroft, J. The conditions of foetal respiration. *The Lancet*, 222:1021–4. Copyright © 1933 Elsevier, with permission.

that regulate pathways required immediately after birth, when in an oxygen-rich environment the fetal gene programme is replaced by the adult system within minutes. Hypoxia-inducible factor 1 (HIF-1) is a transcription factor that functions as a master regulator of oxygen homeostasis. Its oxygen-dependent action on over 40 target genes was reviewed by Semenza [50]. The postnatal metabolic shift from glucose to fatty acid oxidation, the closure of the ductus arteriosus, and the switch from fetal to adult haemoglobin production are just a few familiar examples of this dramatic change.

Conclusion

The placenta's respiratory function is far from being well understood. The dilemma was that although easily accessible for anatomical study, the organ is essentially inaccessible for functional studies. Another problem was that placenta anatomy, vascularization, and function as well as fetal partial pressure of oxygen vary greatly between different species, and that data from animal experiments were applicable to humans only with utmost caution. Amazingly, serious research on fetal respiration began more than a century before the discovery of oxygen. All five comprehension steps had to be taken before even basic understanding was achieved, namely: (1) that maternal and fetal vasculatures are distinct (Aranzio, 1564); (2) that blood flows sequentially through systemic and pulmonary circulation (Harvey, 1628); (3) that oxygen is absorbed from air and enables metabolism (Lavoisier, 1779); (4) that gases diffuse through the placental membrane (Zweifel, 1876); and (5) that oxygen affinity is higher in fetal than in maternal blood (Barcroft, 1933). The acquisition of knowledge of fetal respiration is an example of arduous translational research with direct benefit for the pregnant mother and her newborn infant.

REFERENCES

1. Sendivogius M: A new light of Alchymie (1st lat. ed. 1604). London: Cotes, 1650: p. 96.
2. Mayow J: On the respiration of the foetus in the uterus (1st ed. 1674). Edinburgh: Alembic Club, 1907: p. 211–7.
3. Metcalfe J, Bartels H, Moll W: Gas exchange in the pregnant uterus. Physiol Rev 1967;**47**:782–838.
4. Longo LD, Reynolds LP: Some historical aspects of understanding placental development, structure and function. Int J Dev Biol 2010;**54**:237–55.
5. Lonie IM: The Hippocratic treatises 'On generation', 'On the nature of the child', 'Diaseases IV'. Berlin: de Gruyter, 1981: p. 7–9, 13–9.
6. Hippocrates: Über Achtmonatskinder. Edited by Hermann Grensemann. Berlin: Akademie-Verlag, 1968: p. 87.

7. Aristotle: Generation of animals. Loeb Classical Library 366. Cambridge, MA: Harvard University Press, 1942: Book 2, 4.
8. Galen: On the usefulness of the parts of the body. Ithaca, NY: Cornell University Press, 1968: Vol. **2**, p. 637, 661, 712.
9. Harvey W: An anatomical dissertation upon the movement of the heart and blood in animals. Frankfurt: Fitzer, 1628: p. 39.
10. Ratzinger J: The Holy Spirit as communio: concerning the relationship of pneumatology and spirituality in Augustine. Communio 1998;**25**:324–37.
11. Arantius JCB: De humano foetu liber (1st ed. 1564). Venetiis: Brechtanus, 1587: p. 18.
12. Spieghel A: De formato foetu liber singularis. Patavii: de Martinis, 1626: p. 18–22, Plate 7.
13. Casserio G: Tabulae anatomicae; de formatio foetu tabulae (1st ed. 1627). Francofurti: Merian, 1632: Tab. VII.
14. Hoboken N: Anatomia secundinae humanae (1st ed. Utrecht 1669). Ultrajecti: Ribbius, 1675: p. 172, 441, Plate XLI.
15. Lower R: Tractatus de corde. Item de motu, colore, & transfusione sanguinis. Lugduni Batavorum: Willeke & de Beunje, 1669: p. 178.
16. Haller A: First lines of physiology. Edinburgh: Elliot, 1779: p. 129, 461–6.
17. Schütz GF, Autenrieth J: Dissertatio inauguralis medica sistens in experimenta circa colorem foetus et sanguinem ipsius. Inaug. Diss: Tübingen, 1799.
18. Harvey W: Anatomical exercitations, concerning the generation of living creatures (1st Latin ed. 1651). London: Pulley, 1653: p. 358, 439, 483.
19. Needham W: Disquisitio anatomica de formato foetu (1st ed. London 1667). 2. ed. Amstelodami: le Grand, 1668: p. 20–5, 149–57.
20. Borelli GA: De motu animalium. Pars secunda (1st ed. 1681). 2. ed. Lugduni Batavorum: van der Aa, 1685: p. 167.
21. Stalpart van der Wiel P: Dissertatio medica inauguralis de nutritione foetus. Lugduni Batavorum: Elzevier, 1686: p. F4.
22. Ray J: The wisdom of God manifested in the works of the creation. 1. ed. London: Smith, 1691: p. 56–7.
23. Becher JJ: Actorum laboratorii chymici Monacensis. Francofurti: Zunner, 1669.
24. Stahl GE: Zymotechnica fundamentalis. Halle, Saale: Salfeldius, 1697.
25. Diemerbroeck I: Anatome corporis humani (1st ed. Ultrajecti 1672). Lugduni: Huguetan, 1679: p. 196–200.
26. Verheyen P: Corporis humani anatomia. Lovanii: Aegidius Denique, 1693: p. 116.
27. Cheselden W: The anatomy of the human body (1st ed. 1713). 4. ed. London: Bowyer, 1730: p. 272.
28. Mazzini GB: Conjecturae physico-medico-hydrostaticae de respiratione foetus. Brixiae: Rizzardi, 1737: p. 3, 15.
29. Astrup P, Severinghaus JW: The history of blood gases, acids and bases. Copenhagen: Munksgaard, 1986: p. 28–49.
30. Lavoisier A: Traité élémentaire de Chimie (1st ed. 1789). Oeuvres de Lavoisier, Tome I. Paris: Imprimerie Impériale, 1864: p. Fig. 2.
31. Girtanner C: Anfangsgründe der antiphlogistischen Chemie. Berlin: Unger, 1792: p. 255.
32. Darwin E: Zoonomia; or the laws of organic life. London: Johnson, 1794: Vol. **1**, p. 470–5.
33. Scheel P: Dissertation inauguralis de liquore amnii asperae arteriae foetuum humanorum. Hafniae: Christensen, 1798: p. 18–24, 48.
34. Kirchhoff GR, Bunsen RWE: Chemische Analyse durch Spektralbeobachtungen. Leipzig: Engelmann, 1860: plate II.
35. Hoppe-[Seyler] F: Über das Verhalten des Blutfarbstoffes im Spectrum des Sonnenlichtes. Virchows Arch Path Anat 1862;**23**:446–9.
36. Körber E: Ueber Differenzen des Blutfarbstoffes. Dorpat: Mattiesen, 1866: p. 37–9.
37. Zweifel P: Die Respiration des Foetus. Arch Gynecol 1876;**9**:291–305.
38. Cohnstein J, Zuntz N: Untersuchungen über das Blut, den Kreislauf und die Athmung beim Säugethier-Fötus. Pflügers Arch Physiol 1884;**34**:173–233.
39. Huggett AStG: Foetal blood-gas tensions and gas transfusion through the placenta of the goat. J Physiol 1927;**62**:373–84.
40. Dodds GS: The area of the chorionic villi in the full term placenta. Anat Rec 1922;**24**:287–94.
41. Barcroft J: Die Atmungsfunktion des Blutes. 1. Erfahrungen in großen Höhen. Berlin: Springer, 1927: p. 1–182.
42. Barcroft J: The conditions of foetal respiration. Lancet 1933;**222**:1021–4.
43. Barcroft J: Researches on pre-natal life. 2. ed. Springfield, IL: Thomas, 1947: Vol. **1**.
44. Barron DH: The oxygen pressure gradient between the maternal and fetal blood in pregnant sheep. Yale J Biol Med 1946;**19**:23–7.
45. Porter RR, Sanger F: The free amino groups of haemoglobins. Biochem J 1948;**42**:287–94.
46. Romney SD, Reid D, Metcalfe J, Burwell S: Oxygen utilization by the human fetus in utero. Am J Obstet Gynecol 1955;**70**:791–9.
47. Bartels H, Moll W: Passage of inert substances and oxygen in the human placenta. Pflügers Arch Physiol 1964;**280**:165–77.
48. Dawes GS, Duncan SL, Lewis BV, et al.: Hypoxaemia and aortic chemoreceptor function in foetal lambs. J Physiol 1969;**201**:105–16.
49. Carter AM: Evolution of placental function in mammals: the molecular basis of gas and nutrient transfer, hormone secretion, and immune responses. Physiol Rev 2012;**92**:1543–76.
50. Semenza G: Signal transduction to hypoxia-inducible factor 1. Biochem Pharmacol 2002;**64**:993–8.

PART 2
Birth

2.1 **From apparent death to birth asphyxia** 25

2.2 **Resuscitation 1: artificial ventilation** 33

2.3 **Resuscitation 2: oxygen and other drugs** 39

2.4 **Resuscitation 3: endotracheal intubation** 45

2.5 **Umbilical cord and umbilical care** 51

2.6 **Postverta, Agrippa, Caesarea: born feet-first** 57

2.7 **Social birth: rites of passage for the newborn** 63

INTRODUCTION

Assisting at birth was an entirely female activity for millennia, without written instructions. Male surgeons entered obstetrics in the 17th century following the invention of the forceps: midwives were forbidden to use instruments. Effective resuscitation techniques developed when books on midwifery became available in the 18th century, such as mouth-to-mouth ventilation. Apparent death was attributed to a lack of vitality until oxygen became known at the end of the 18th century. Within 7 years of its discovery, oxygen was being used in neonatal resuscitation. Continuous distending airway pressure was available at the beginning of the 20th century, falling into oblivion during World War I and waiting to be rediscovered 60 years later. Newborns were regarded as unfinished. In many cultures, rites of passage accompanied the postnatal transition. They usually included cleansing, exorcism of evil spirits, and a name-giving ceremony that assigned the infant a right to live.

2.1 From apparent death to birth asphyxia

Introduction

Birth asphyxia is neither the most dangerous nor most frequent life-threatening condition patients and doctors encounter, yet it is the most frequent cause of litigation [1, 2]. Although not compatible with scientific evidence, birth asphyxia was and is frequently believed to be associated with cerebral palsy. It was hypothesized that lack of definition and interprofessional blaming contributed to the belief that birth asphyxia is preventable. By delineating the path from a non-entity to a condition suspected of resulting from malpractice, the following chapter seeks to explain this phenomenon from a historical perspective. Its focus is the definition of birth asphyxia and the interprofessional controversy. It omits the history of neonatal resuscitation (see Chapters 2.2–2.4) and is short on historic aspects described elsewhere, such as obstetric forceps [3] and electronic fetal monitoring [4, 5]. The use of the term 'birth asphyxia' in the German literature was addressed by Stiller [6].

Obstetrics before the printing era

Hellas and Rome showed little sympathy for weaklings: malformed or premature infants were abandoned at the Taygettos canyon or the columna lactaria, respectively. The Greek goddesses Hera and Artemis and the Roman goddess Juno Lucina were believed to protect childbirth, and midwives enjoyed high esteem. A tombstone from Menidi, 4th century B.C.E., reads [7]: 'Phanostrate, a midwife and physician, lies here. She caused pain to none, and all lamented her death.'

Postnatal difficulties were believed to result from intrauterine conditions, and maintaining placental circulation was the main therapy. For poorly adapted neonates, the Corpus Hippocraticum recommended in the 5th century B.C.E. [8]: 'You should not remove their umbilical cord before they pass urine or sneeze or give voice, instead leaving it connected … If the umbilical cord puffs up with air like a pouch, the child will move or sneeze and give voice; then you should remove the cord while the child is taking a breath. If, after a certain time, the umbilical cord does not puff up with air nor the child move, it will not survive.' In the 4th century B.C.E., Aristotle reported [9]: 'Often the baby seemed to be born dead when … the blood happens to run out into the umbilicus and the surrounding part; but certain midwives who have acquired this skill, squeezed the blood back inside, out of the umbilical [cord], and immediately the baby … has revived again.'

Roman midwives often began their career as slaves and were freed after a happy delivery. Soranus did not favour resuscitation in disturbed respiration in the 2nd century C.E. [10]: '[the newborn is worth raising] who immediately cries with proper vigor; for one that lives for some length of time without crying, or cries but weakly, is suspected of behaving so on account of some unfavourable condition.' With the advent of Christianity, Greek and Roman ideas about human life changed. In 319 C.E., Roman Emperor Constantine decreed that the state provide maintenance and education for poor children and prevent the exposure, sale, and murder of infants [11]. From Soranus [10] until Scipio Mercurio [12], the Middle Ages brought 1400 years of stagnation in midwifery, the main reason being the 'dead hand of Galen', as Radcliffe characterized the medieval hostility towards research [13]. Another reason was the century-long divorce of surgery from medicine that excluded barber-surgeons and midwives from academic training. Not until the printing press became available around 1500 did obstetric knowledge dissipate and improve, despite the fact that most midwives and barber-surgeons were illiterate.

Interprofessional competition and blame

Interprofessional conflicts were common even before book printing weakened the privileges of learning. Rights and duties of midwives were regulated since the 14th century; a typical example is the Freiburg order of 1557 [14]: 'They shall not use any gruesome or clumsy instrument to break or extract the infant.' As late as 1786, Jean-François Icart listed four instruments that midwives were allowed to use and had been loaned by the diocese of Castres [15]: (1) a clyster-syringe for enemas; (2) a catheter to empty the bladder; (3) a small syringe for intrauterine baptism; and (4) a tube to ventilate the baby.

Barber-surgeons, all male, became active in obstetrics in the 13th century, their activities regulated by the guild. In London, the company of barber-surgeons was founded in 1540 [16], whereas midwives were legally regulated as late as 1902 [17]. The surgeons' arrival on the birth scene, however, heralded the death of mother or child, if not both: it was their privilege to use hooks (crochets), their duty to remove the dead fetus following prolonged or obstructed labour, oblique pelvis, or hydrocephalus, in an attempt to save the mother's life (Fig. 2.1.1). Not until the Chamberlen family's secret—the obstetric forceps—leaked out around 1720, did that instrument become the key that opened the lying-in room for men [3]. Benjamin Pugh, surgeon in Chelmsford, Essex, justified his treatise of midwifery 'with regard to the operation' in 1754 [18] 'as every young Surgeon now intends practicing Midwifery, and it is become almost as universal in this Kingdom, as ever it was in France'. Male assistance first became fashionable in delivery rooms of the nobility: in 1670, Julien Clément delivered Madame Montespan, future mistress of Louis XIV; in 1688, Hugh Chamberlen the future wife of James II; in 1738, William Hunter attended the birth of George III, and so on. Midwives and surgeons who published texts on obstetrics remained rare, as publishing was a strictly regulated privilege. Usually they were appointed to the royal courts, who gave them permission to publish without the need for consent by the medical faculties.

The respect for midwives waned immediately and bitter competition arose when men entered 'real' obstetrics in which both mother and child were expected to survive. Named *accoucheurs* or *man-midwife*, they used their publications to blame the midwives for everything that could go wrong during a delivery. Eucharius Rösslin's book first appeared in 1513, was frequently reprinted, and translated into English by Thomas Raynald in 1540 [19]: The bellicose introductory poem stated:

> 'I mean the midwives each and all,
> who know so little of their call,
> that through neglect and oversight,
> they destroy children far and wide.'

In Paris, a statute of 1560 regulated supervision of the five *matrones jurées* (sworn matrons) by the Royal Barber Surgeon [20]. In 1620, Royal accoucheur Jacques Guillemeau in Paris criticized impatient midwives [21], 'who with their fingernails break the membranes, have caused the death of many women and numberless infants' and in 1627 branded Royal midwife Louise Bourgeois as 'presumptuous, ignorant, and brutal' [22]. Ambroise Paré, surgeon at the Hôtel-Dieu—which served as school of midwifery—stated condescendingly in 1573 [23]: 'Midwives are to be admonished that as often as they perceive the childe to be comming forth either with its bellie or his back forwards ... that they should turn it, and draw it out by the feet; for the doing whereof, if they be not sufficient, let them crave the assistance and help of some expert Chirurgian.' In 1672, Percival Willughby of Derby [24] moaned

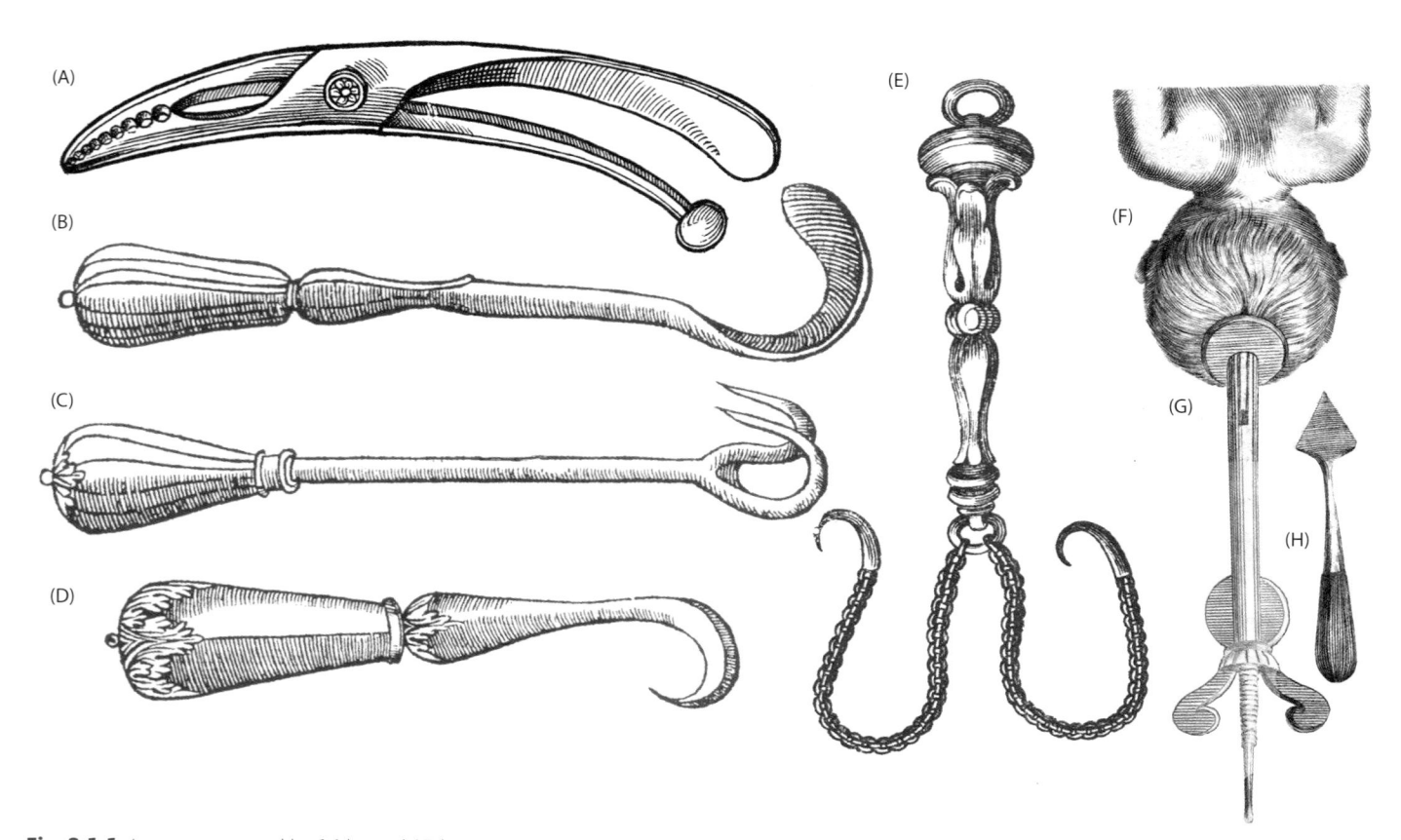

Fig. 2.1.1 Instruments used by 16th- and 17th-century surgeons to dismember and extract dead fetuses. A, duck's beak, depicted by Jacob Rueff, 1587 [83]; B–D, blunt and sharp hooks (crotchets) depicted by Jacques Dalechamps, 1573 [84] and Ambroise Paré, 1573 [23]; E, double hook with chains, depicted by Johannes Scultetus, 1666 [85]; F, infant head, with extractor (*tire-tête*) applied to the sagittal suture; G, extractor (*tire-tête*); and H, fontanelle-lancet depicted by François Mauriceau, 1668 [33].

'midwives will follow their own wayes, and will have their own wills'. Constantly attacked by surgeons, the midwives retaliated, usually by claiming overuse of and complications using the forceps, and avarice of the *accoucheur*, who received higher wages than the midwife. In Prussia, the book of Royal Midwife Justine Siegmundin, first published in 1690, set the German standard for a century [25]. She defined *weakness* as a form of suffocation, due to delayed onset of breathing. Andreas Petermann, professor of surgery at Leipzig University, attacked the book as 'speculation-based, illogical, and dangerous for midwives and parturients' and tried to have the censor forbid it, without success. The 5-year controversy is reproduced in later editions of Siegemundin's book. In England, Elizabeth Nihell attacked William Smellie in 1760 [26]: 'Pernicious quackery of those instruments [Smellie's forceps, **Fig. 2.1.3c**] has been artfully made the pretext of an innovation set on foot by Interest, adopted by Credulity, and fostered by Fashion.' The frontispiece of Samuel Fores' book of 1793 (**Fig. 2.1.2**) gives us an idea of the pamphlet wars between the two health professions [27]. There are many other examples. The persistent controversy was described by Hagen in 1791 [28] and Donnison in 1977 [17]. After two centuries of blaming, the stage was set for the courts. Midwives' textbooks meticulously regulated every detail, as Hauck explained in 1815 [29], 'to prove punishable offences'. A century later, Ahlfeld stated similar purposes in 1905 [30]: 'The official textbook of midwifery also serves as a guide for disciplinary avengement and decisions *in foro* [court trial].' The German textbook on forensic medicine resumed in 1872 [31]: 'Most frequently sued for alleged malpractice are obstetricians and midwives.' The surgeons had won a pyrrhic victory that maintained the hierarchy, but undermined the respect for both professions.

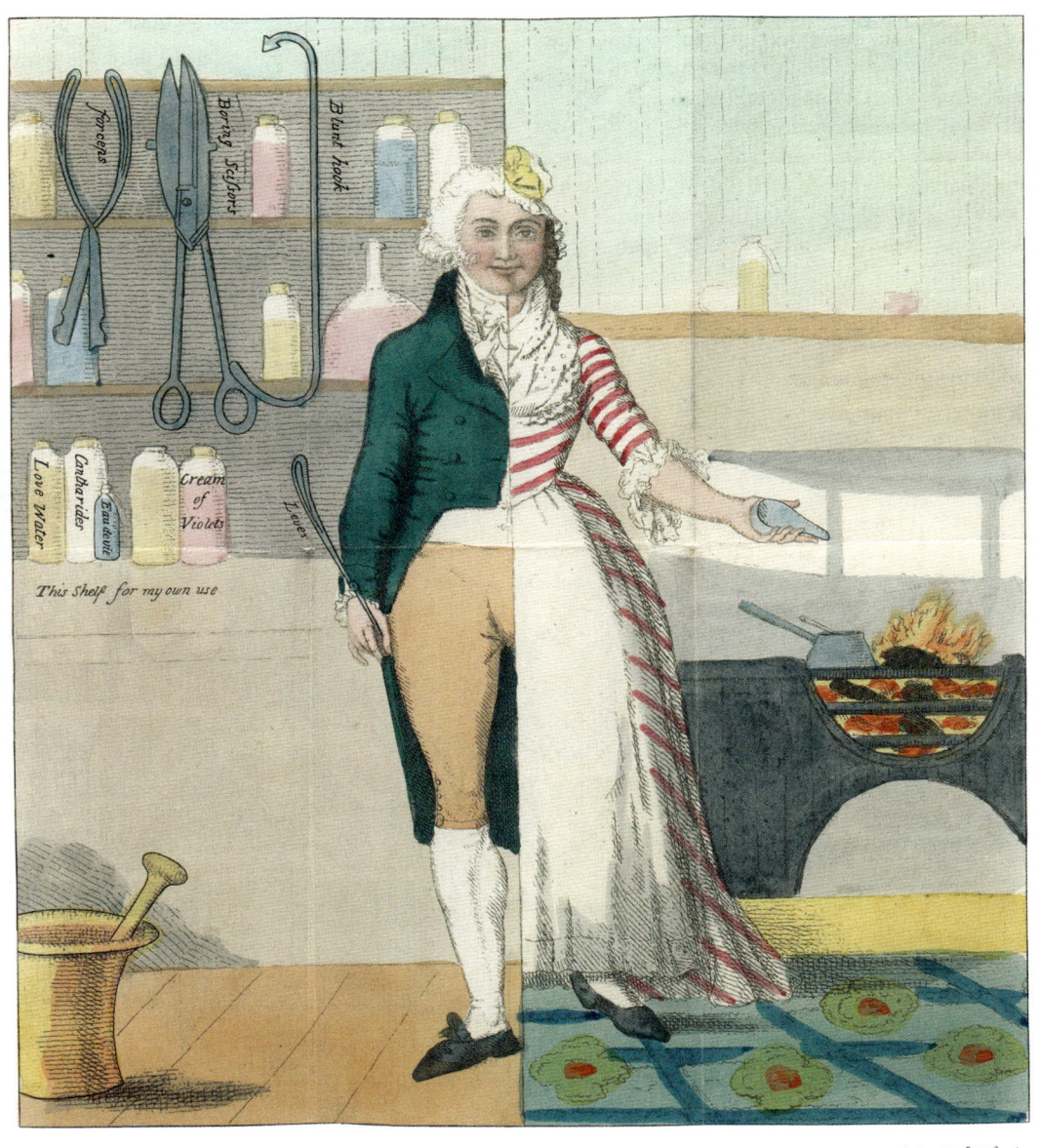

Fig. 2.1.2 Example of a pamphlet deriding male obstetricians. Frontispiece of Samuel Fores: *Man-Midwifery Dissected*, 1793 [27]: the instruments (lever, forceps, boring scissors, blunt hook) allude to the man-midwife's cruelty, the aphrodisiacs on the shelf to his lechery.

'Apparent death' classified by alleged causes

Apparent death (*mors apparens*) of the neonate was addressed in early printed books on obstetrics. In 1472, Padovan professor Paolo Bagellardo described birth asphyxia quite precisely [32]: '[The midwife should examine] whether the infant is alive or not, or spotted, that is: whether black or white or of livid color, and whether it is breathing or not. If she finds it warm, not black, she should blow into its mouth, if it has no respiration, or into its anus.' Had he omitted the last words, we would praise Bagellardo as pioneer of neonatology. Whereas birth asphyxia was not differentiated from immaturity or weakness in the preterm infant, inability to breathe was regarded a treatable condition in the term infant. A century before the discovery of oxygen, several researchers were aware of normal and disturbed fetal gas exchange: Parisian accoucheur François Mauriceau described a prolapsed umbilical cord in 1668 [33]: 'Lacking placental respiration, the fetus now should inspire by the mouth, to refresh its heart ... secluded in the womb, however, this path is not available, and the infant must soon die from suffocation, because both ways [placenta and lungs] are unavailable.' Mauriceau reported that more than half of young infants died, and discerned several *accidents* leading to apparent death: (1) weakness in prematures; (2) violence due to difficult labour; and (3) sudden suffocation.

Physiologist John Mayow of Oxford wrote in 1674 [34]: 'The foetus in the uterus, whose blood does not pass through the lungs but through special ducts, does not need to breathe at all ... With respect, then, to the use of respiration, it may be affirmed that an aerial something [sal-nitro] essential to life, whatever it may be, passes [from the placenta] into the mass of the blood.' Philipp Verheyen, anatomist in Louvain, was aware of the placenta's respiratory function in 1693 [35]: 'In the fetus, whose lungs repose, this substance, which feeds the flame of life, is extracted by the placenta from the maternal blood, and admixed with the fetal blood (Fig. 2.1.3).' Seven years after Lavoisier named oxygen, Swiss scientist Christoph Girtanner associated its deficiency with fetal asphyxia in 1792 [36]: 'The fetal lung is outside the body: It is the placenta ... The infant dies suddenly, when during birth the cord is compressed, and the circulation to and from the placenta is interrupted.' In 1819, Alexandre Lebreton published a book on neonatal diseases in which he classified apparent death according to six causes [37]: (1) brain compression; (2) venous brain congestion; (3) spinal cord trauma; (4) anaemia or emptiness of blood vessels; (5) weakness; and (6) syncope, which meant overload with blood. From 1840 to 1874, several French obstetricians proposed returning to the term 'apparent death' rather than the ill-defined terms *syncope, apoplexy, weakness, suffocation*, and so on [38].

In Prussia, Christoph Hufeland used the term asphyxia in 1836 [39] for 'a perfect image of death ... cessation of circulation and respiration, and motion. It is often a continuance of the fetal state (water-life), a failure to commence atmospherical, independent existence.' He assumed three specific causes according to the infant's appearance: (1) true weakness due to immaturity; (2) overload of blood in brain and heart due to prolonged labor or cord entanglement; and (3) suffocation due to mucus obstruction.

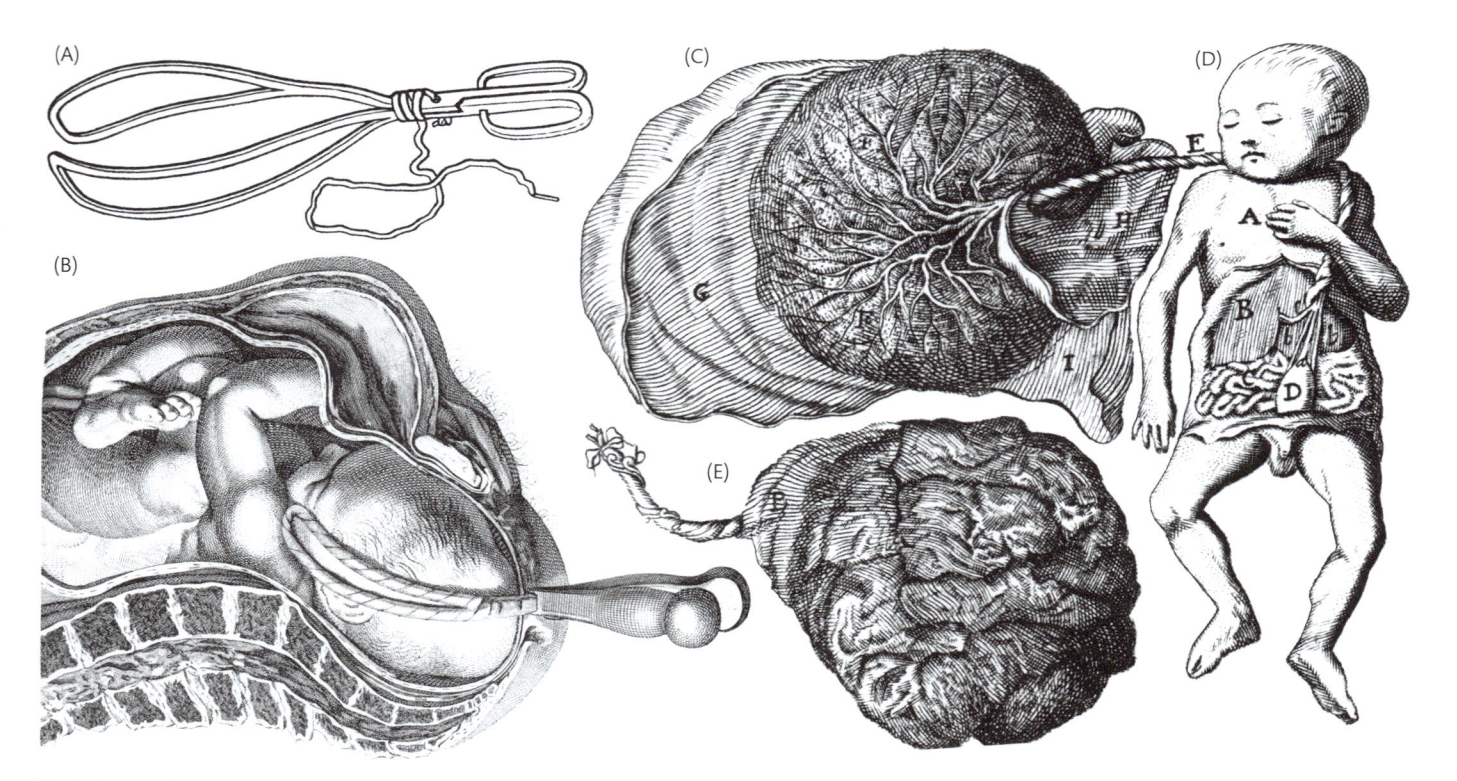

Fig. 2.1.3 Asphyxia was related to respiratory placental insufficiency at the end of the 17th century. A, Chamberlen forceps type 2, around 1650 [3]; B, Prolonged birth (longish head and vertex tumor) with William Smellie's curved forceps, depicted in 1754 [86]; D, asphyctic infant at autopsy; C, fetal side, E, maternal side of placenta, depicted by Philipp Verheyen, 1693 [35].

Vitalism, burying alive, and the diagnosis 'asphyxia'

During the 18th century, philosophical theories still exerted great influence in medicine. 'Apparent death' was related to 'viability' or 'life force'—philosophical terms that originated with vitalism. To discern living and dead matter, Georg Ernst Stahl postulated an *energia operandi* (energy of action) in 1733. Albrecht von Haller defined life as the *irritability* of tissues, especially nerves and muscles in 1752. Johann Wolfgang Goethe, a vitalist himself, combined this concept by again blaming the midwife, when describing his own birth on 28 August 1749 [40]: 'The midwife was so unskilled that I was brought into the world as good as dead, and only with great difficulty could I be made to open my eyes and see the light … my grandfather, Johann Textor, who was chief magistrate, was moved by this to appoint an official birth-assistant and to reintroduce the instruction of midwives.'

The mass phobia of apparent death began with the books of Lancisi 1707 [41] and Winslow and Bruhier 1742 [42]; these books went through many editions and translations, and accompanied the Europe-wide obsession of 'being buried alive'. Humane Societies were founded to teach resuscitation [43] and pamphlets were distributed by Royal order to the public at governmental expense, as that of de Gardane 1774 in France [44] and Prussia; and it was those very pamphlets that introduced incorrectly the term *asphyxia* (pulselessness) into medical texts as in John Aitken's book on midwifery that appeared in 1784 in Edinburgh [45] and 1789 in Nürnberg [46]. The term 'asphyxia' was criticized from the beginning, but 'apparent death' had fallen from grace and could no longer be used for a baby having difficulty breathing at birth. This change did not put forward a definition, but was understood as a shift from unavoidable fate to preventable condition.

Asphyxia classified by alleged grades

The textbook on obstetrics by Heidelberg obstetrician Hermann Naegele exemplifies how the interpretation of birth asphyxia changed in the second half of the 19th century. In the fifth edition of 1863 [47], he proposed the traditional classification: '1, *asphyxia livida suffocatoria*, due to compressed placenta or cord; 2, *asphyxia livida apoplectica* due to compressed brain; 3, *asphyxia pallida* due to exhausted nervous activity, blood loss, and placental insufficiency.' In the eighth edition of 1872 [48], Naegele equated asphyxia and apparent death, defined as minimal signs of life with some vitality preserved, and specified three grades: (1) mild: skin blue, but some respiratory efforts; (2) medium: skin pale, gasping, and poor reflex activity; and (3) severe: slow heart action, no respiratory effort, and no reflex activity. In 1931, New York anaesthesiologist Paluel Flagg classified neonatal asphyxia in three grades according to reflex excitability [49]—mild: depression; moderate: spasticity; and severe: flaccidity.

Retrospective brain damage

In 1784, London surgeon and male midwife Micheal Underwood described *palsy of the lower extremities*: 'It seems to arise from debility … and usually attacks children one year old … The first thing observed is debility of the lower extremities, which gradually become more infirm' [50]. In 1826, Johann Christian Jörg noted [51]: 'In too early and unripe born children a state of weakness may persist … in the muscles until puberty or even longer. It hinders the child in the use of its limbs and in holding head and trunk.' In 1862, London orthopaedist William John Little published his influential paper relating *deformities* to 'abnormal parturition, difficult labours, premature birth, and asphyxia neonatorum' [52]: 'A larger proportion of infants, either dead, stillborn, apoplectic, or asphyxiated at birth, have been rendered so by interruption of the proper placental relation of the fetus to the mother, and non-substitution of pulmonary respiration, than from direct mechanical injury to the brain and spinal cord.' A closer look into this paper reveals that half of Little's 49 infants were preterm, and that only five had been both term and asphyctic; no postmortem findings were reported. From one case involving a traumatic breech delivery and a literature search on 34 cases with cerebral palsy, Sarah McNutt concluded in 1885 [53] that 'meningeal hemorrhage at parturition [is] one of the commonest agencies in the production of spastic hemiplegia'. William Osler used the term *cerebral palsy* in 1889 for hemiplegia and diplegia in 140 children [54], ascribing its aetiology to trauma and infection, but not to birth asphyxia. In 1897, Sigmund Freud contradicted Little [55]: 'Premature, precipitate and difficult birth and asphyxia neonatorum are not causal factors in the production of diplegia; they are only associated symptoms of deeper lying influences which have dominated the development of the foetus or the organism of the mother.' But his criticism went unheeded: Little's hypothesis fulfilled an obvious need for causality all too well.

Eastman and DeLeon compared 96 children with cerebral palsy and a control group in 1955 [56]: 41% of the patients with cerebral palsy had 'poor' adaptation (controls: 2%); 34% were born preterm (controls: 9%); 50% had fever at birth (controls: 6%); and 15% had malformations (controls: 2%). The population-based prospective study from Australia [57] showed that less than 10% of cerebral palsies were associated with birth asphyxia. Considerable evidence has accumulated in recent decades that rather than birth asphyxia, prenatal events such as growth retardation, infections, or genetic abnormalities are what cause cerebral palsy [58].

Measurements and definitions

The era of measurement dawned in the 20th century, and blood gas analysis helped to better understand birth asphyxia: in 1928, Blair Bell and his associates in Liverpool reported a mean oxygen content of 9.02 vol.% in blood of the umbilical vein and of 5.85 vol.% in that of the umbilical artery at birth [59]. In Baltimore in 1932, Nicholson Eastman published cord blood gas analyses of infants with and without asphyxia [60]: 'The primary blood chemical change in asphyxia neonatorum is a reduction in the oxygen content of the fetal blood to extremely low levels, the blood of the umbilical vein falling in fatal cases below one volume per cent … The serum pH of asphyxiated infants is reduced to the lower limits compatible with life.'

The New York anaesthesiologist Virginia Apgar, disturbed by the lack of specificity in resuscitation and by the poor quality of asphyxia studies, devised a clinical score in 1953 to quantify the degree of asphyxia and improve resuscitation efforts in the neonate [61]. In a

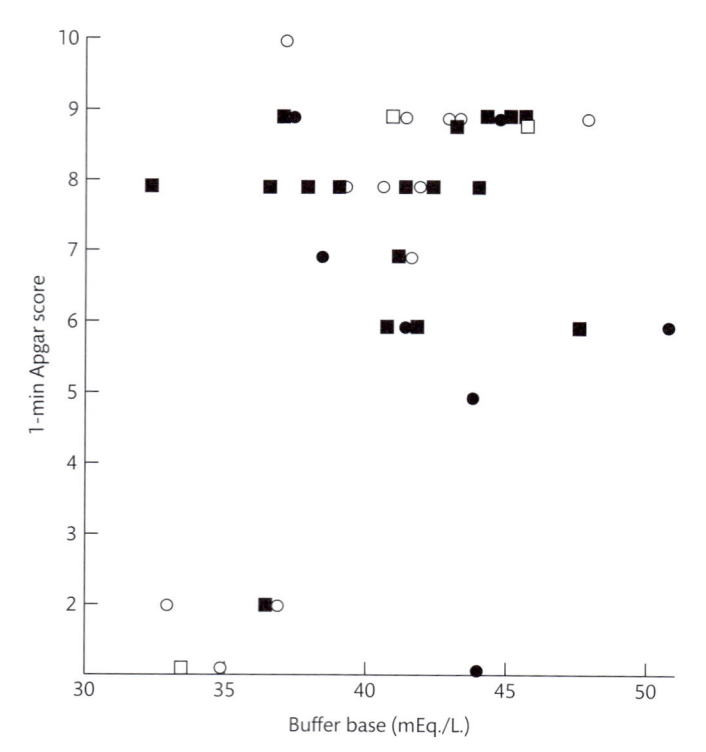

Fig. 2.1.4 Correlation between Apgar score at 1 min and buffer base in umbilical artery blood in 43 infants with a low oxygen saturation and high carbon dioxide tension, signalling 'some degree of asphyxia' [63]. Open/closed circles, regional/inhalation anaesthesia at vaginal delivery; open/closed squares, regional/inhalation anaesthesia at Caesarean section.

Reproduced with permission from James, L.S., Weisbrot, I.M., Prince, C.E., et al. The acid-base status of human infants in relation to birth asphyxia and the onset of respiration. J Pediatr, 52:379–394. Copyright © 1958 Published by Mosby, Elsevier.

neurodevelopmental follow-up in 215 infants she found 'no significant correlation between intelligence quotient and oxygen content or saturation at any time during the first three hours of life' [62]. Apgar's associate L. Stanley James published blood gas measurements of umbilical venous and arterial blood in infants with and without asphyxia in 1958 [63]: 'Some degree of asphyxia, usually of brief duration, is a normal finding in all births ... asphyxia produces a respiratory acidosis followed by a superimposed metabolic acidosis.' However, the Apgar score and base deficit correlated poorly (Fig. 2.1.4). In 1959, Geoffrey Dawes and his co-workers in Oxford found that severely hypoxic lamb fetuses survived up to 1 h by raising their blood pressure and heart rate [64]. Apgar's and James' work paved the way towards a definition of asphyxia, but it remains difficult to understand how and why the Apgar score and cord blood gases were mistakenly employed for neurodevelopmental prognostication [65] and to justify bicarbonate buffering [66]. Whereas the International Classification of Diseases continued to derive the birth asphyxia diagnosis from the Apgar score, the American Academy of Pediatrics stated in 1986 that the Apgar score alone suffices for neither diagnosis nor prognosis [65]. The first clear definition of birth asphyxia was provided by the American College of Obstetrics and Gynecology in 1992 [67], demanding each of four criteria: pH less than 7.00; Apgar score less than 4 for more than 5 min; neonatal neurologic sequelae; and multiorgan dysfunction. Endorsed by 16 scientific societies, this template was further specified in 1999 by MacLennan [68]: 'Essential criteria defining an acute intrapartum hypoxic event: pH <7.0, base excess >12 mmol/l, early symptoms of neonatal encephalopathy, later cerebral palsy. Additional non-specific criteria that help to time the lesion are: a sentinel hypoxic event, sudden sustained decrease of fetal heart rate, Apgar 0–6 for longer than 5 min, early multiorgan failure, early cerebral imaging with evidence of brain damage.' In 2005, the American College of Obstetrics and Gynecology decreed [69]: 'The term birth asphyxia is nonspecific and should not be used.'

Electronic fetal monitoring and litigation

Information on the fetal state was scarce up to the 19th century. In 1766 Wrisberg [70] and in 1818 Mayor [71] used direct auscultation, but fetal heart rate monitoring became generally accepted with Lejumeau de Kergaradec's use of the stethoscope in 1822 [72]. Electric augmentation and graphic registration were used by Sampson and co-workers in 1926 [73]. Continuous electronic fetal heart rate monitoring was developed in the late 1950s by Edward Hon (New Haven), Roberto Caldeyro-Barcia (Montevideo), and Konrad Hammacher (Düsseldorf). Its history has been detailed by Goodlin [4] and Banta [5]. Electronic monitoring during birth was generally introduced in the 1970s without scientific validation, but with strong support by the monitoring industry. In 1985, Devoe and Castillo collected 21 different analysis criteria used in 45 studies [74], many without calculating sensitivity, specificity, and predictive values. Controlled studies shed doubts on this technique, as was reported by Banta and Thacker in 1978 [75]: 'No decrease in perinatal deaths, no fewer admissions to NICU [neonatal intensive care unit], no less cerebral palsy ... We found no benefit but substantial risk due to increased incidence of Caesarian delivery.' A fierce controversy began [5]: 'Obstetricians were outraged at the conclusions of this report.' An editorial stated: 'The findings were sweeping, poorly thought out, and extremely negative.' This did not change the facts, and 40 years later the 2017 Cochrane review, which included 13 randomized trials involving over 37,000 women, gave no better news [76]: 'Compared with intermittent auscultation, continuous cardiotocography reduced the neonatal seizure rate, but showed no improvement in perinatal deaths and cerebral palsy rates ... There was an increase in Caesarean sections [by 63%] and instrumental vaginal deliveries.' Meanwhile from 5% in 1970, the rate of Caesarean deliveries skyrocketed to 20% in Asia, 26% in Europe, 33% in North America, and 42% in Latin America [77]. Also, the number of malpractice tort trials rose. However, electronic fetal monitoring persisted, as did cerebral palsy, which remained constant at 2 per 1000 [78]. Rapidly, they both made their way into litigation. Obstetricians became the most frequently sued physicians in the US [2]. In 2006, their insurance premiums had risen up to US$299,420 per year [1], and 60% of the malpractice insurance premiums covered lawsuits for allegedly birth-related cerebral palsy [79]. In Australia, obstetricians (2% of the physician group) account for 18% of all payments [80], while they are becoming an endangered species in the US [81]. In Germany, midwives could no longer afford the insurance premiums [82] and have disappeared from some regions.

Conclusion

Birth and birth asphyxia have been accompanied by 500 years of bitter competition between midwives and surgeons. The diagnosis 'asphyxia' originated around 1774, not on scientific grounds but linked to the obsession of being buried alive, to avoid the emotionally charged 'apparent death'. It is philosophically interesting that the term 'asphyxia' was criticized from the very beginning because of its semantical incorrectness (pulselessness), but never for the more important lack of a definition. William Little's unproven hypothesis of 1862 fulfilled perfectly the need for causality in families burdened with a child suffering from cerebral palsy. This tragic disease, sometimes accompanied by mental impairment, became less tolerated when infant deaths waned. As decried by Virginia Apgar, the poor definition of birth asphyxia precluded scientific studies for a long time. The unjustified linking of asphyxia to cerebral palsy, ascribing unproven diagnostic power to electronic monitoring, and the belief in prevention via Caesarean section transformed common delivery techniques into malpractice. This may have been promoted by age-old competition between midwives and surgeons, which created a culture of blame and undermined the respect for both professions.

REFERENCES

1. Hankins GD, MacLennan AH, Speer ME, et al.: Obstetric litigation is asphyxiating our maternity services. Obstet Gynecol 2006;**107**:1382–5.
2. Studdert DM, Mello MM, Gawande AA, et al.: Claims, errors, and compensation payments in medical malpractice litigation. N Engl J Med 2006;**354**:2024–33.
3. Aveling JH: The Chamberlens and the midwifery forceps. London: Churchill, 1882: p. 222–3.
4. Goodlin RC: History of fetal monitoring. Am J Obstet Gynecol 1979;**133**:323–52.
5. Banta HD, Thacker SB: Historical controversy in health technology assessment. Obstet Gynecol Surv 2001;**56**:707–19.
6. Stiller S: Entstehung und Wandel der Diagnose 'Geburtsasphyxie'. Freiburg: Med. Diss., 2015.
7. Kaibel G: Epigrammata Graeca: ex lapidibus conjecta. Berlin: Reimer, 1878: p. 17.
8. Hippocrates: Superfetation. Loeb Classical Library 509. Cambridge MA: Harvard University Press, 2010: p. 329.
9. Aristotle: Histora of animals. Loeb Classical Library 439. Cambridge MA: Harvard University Press, 1991: Vol. **9**, p. 588a5; 587a20–24.
10. Temkin O: Soranus' Gynecology. Baltimore, MD: The Johns Hopkins Press, 1956: p. 80.
11. Theodosiani: Libri XVI cum constitutionibus Sirmondianis. Edited by: Thomas Mommsen: Dublin: Weidmann, 1971: Vol. **XI**, Title 27, p. 616.
12. Mercurio S: Kinder-Mutter oder Hebammen-Buch (1st Ital. ed. 1595). Wittenberg: Tobias Mevii, 1671.
13. Radcliffe W: Milestones in midwifery. Bristol: Wright, 1967: p. 11.
14. Burckhard G: Studien zur Geschichte des Hebammenwesens. Leipzig: Engelmann, 1912: p. 162.
15. Icart J-F: Mémoire sur le besoin indispensable de quelques instruments simples et faciles à employer, dont les Sages-Femmes de la Campagne devraient etre pourvues. Castres: Robert, 1786.
16. Robinson JO: The barber-surgeons of London. Arch Surg 1984;**119**:1171–5.
17. Donnison J: Midwives and medical men. New York: Schocken, 1977.
18. Pugh B: A treatise of midwifery, chiefly with regard to the operation. London: Buckland, 1754: p. 48–51, 133.
19. Rösslin E: Der Swangern Frauwen und hebammen Rosegarten (Engl. transl. Thomas Reynald 1540). Straßburg: Flach, 1513: p. A I, 94.
20. Petrelli RL: The regulation of French midwifery during the Ancien Régime. J Hist Med Allied Sci 1971;**26**:276–92.
21. Guillemeau J: De la grossesse et accouchement des femmes. Paris: Pacard, 1620: p. 174.
22. Perkins W: Midwives versus doctors: the case of Louise Bourgeois. Seventeenth Century 1988;**3**:135–57.
23. Paré A: The generation of man (1st ed. Paris 1573). In: Thomas Johnson: The workes of that famous chirurgion Ambrose Parey. London: Cotes & Du-gard, 1649: Vol. **67**, p. 603, 614, 647.
24. Willughby P: Observations on midwifery (1672). Wakefield, Yorkshire: S.R. Publishers, 1972: p. 126.
25. Siegemundin J: Königl.-Preußische und Chur-Brandenburgische Hof-Wehe-Mutter (1st ed. 1690). Berlin: Voß, 1752: p. 246.
26. Nihell E: A treatise on the art of midwifery. London: Morley, 1760: p. 245.
27. Fores SW: Man-midwifery dissected; or, the obstetric family-instructor. Pseudonym: John Blunt. London: Fores, 1793.
28. Hagen JP: Versuch eines allgemeinen Hebammen-Catechismus. 4. ed. Berlin: Maurer, 1791: p. XII–XVIII.
29. Hauck GP: Lehrbuch der Geburtshülfe zum Unterricht für die Hebammen. Berlin: Enslin, 1815.
30. Ahlfeld F: Buchanzeige: Hebammen-Lehrbuch. Monatsschr. für Geburtshülfe und Gynäkologie 1905;**21**:123–31.
31. Buchner E: Lehrbuch der gerichtlichen Medizin für Ärzte und Juristen. 2. ed. München: Finsterlin, 1872: p. 449.
32. Bagellardo P: Opusculum recens natum de morbis puerorum (1st ed. 1472). Lyon: Barbou, 1538: p. 4, 31, 43.
33. Mauriceau F: Traité des maladies des femmes grosses, et de celles qui sont accouchées (1st ed. 1668). 7. ed. Paris: Compagnie des Libraires, 1740: Vol. **1**, p. 329, 367, 481.
34. Mayow J: On the respiration of the foetus in the uterus (1st Latin ed. 1674). Edinburgh: Alembic Club, 1907: p. 203–4.
35. Verheyen P: Corporis humani anatomia. Lovanii: Denique, 1693: p. 116, Tabula 11.
36. Girtanner C: Anfangsgründe der antiphlogistischen Chemie. Berlin: Unger, 1792: p. 248–53.
37. Lebreton A: Untersuchungen über die Ursachen und die Behandlung mehrerer Krankheiten der Neugeborenen (1st French ed. 1819). Leipzig: Industrie-Comptoir, 1820: p. 1.
38. Martel J: De la mort apparente chez le nouveau-né. Paris: Baillière, 1874.
39. Hufeland CW: Enchiridion medicum or the practice of medicine (1st German ed. Berlin 1836). New York: Radde, 1855: p. 261, 537.
40. Goethe JW: From my life. Poetry and truth. (1st German ed. Stuttgart 1811). New York: Suhrkamp, 1987: p. 21.
41. Lancisi GM: Abhandlung von plötzlichen und seltsamen Todesfällen und ihren Ursachen (Lat. ed. Rome 1707). Leipzig: Weygand, 1785.
42. Winslow J: Dissertation sur l'incertitude des signes de la mort, et l'abus des enterrements. Paris: Morel, 1742.
43. Ackerknecht EH: Death in the history of medicine. Bull Hist Med 1968;**42**:19–23.

44. De Gardanne JJ: Catechisme sur les morts apparentes dites asphyxiés (1st ed. 1781). Imprimé et publie par ordre du gouvernement. Dijon: Defay, 1783.
45. Aitken J: Principles of midwifery, or puerperal medicine (1st ed. Edinburgh 1784). Edinburgh: Edinburgh Lying-in Hospital, 1785.
46. Aitken J: Grundsätze der Entbindungskunst. Nürnberg: Raspische Buchhandlung, 1789.
47. Naegele HF: Lehrbuch der Geburtshülfe. 5. ed. Mainz: Von Zabern, 1863: p. 784–7.
48. Naegele HF: Lehrbuch der Geburtshülfe. 8. ed. Mainz: Von Zabern, 1872: p. 811–21.
49. Flagg PJ: The treatment of postnatal asphyxia. Am J Obstet Gynecol 1931;**21**:537–41.
50. Underwood M: A treatise on the disorders of childhood, and management of infants from the birth (1st ed. 1784). 2. ed. London: Matthews, 1801: Vol. **1**, p. 13, 91.
51. Jörg JCG: Handbuch zum Erkennen und Heilen der Kinderkrankheiten. Leipzig: Cnobloch, 1826: Vol. **1**, p. 369.
52. Little WJ: On the influence of abnormal parturition, difficult labours, premature birth and asphyxia neonatorum on the mental and physical condition of the child, especially in relation to deformities. Trans Obstet Soc London 1861–1862;**3**:293–344.
53. McNutt SJ: Double infantile spastic hemiplegia, with the report of a case. Am J Med Sci 1885;**89**:58–79.
54. Osler W: The cerebral palsies of children. London: Lewis, 1889: p. 91, 96.
55. Freud S: Die infantile Cerebrallähmung. In: Nothnagel H: Specielle Pathologie und Therapie. Wien: Hölder, 1897: Vol. **9**, p. 11.
56. Eastman NJ, DeLeon M: The etiology of cerebral palsy. Am J Obstet Gynecol 1955;**69**:950–61.
57. McIntyre S, Blair E, Badawi N, Keogh J, Nelson KB: Antecedents of cerebral palsy and perinatal death in term and late preterm singletons. Obstet Gynecol 2013;**122**:869–76.
58. Nelson KB, Blair E: Prenatal factors in singletons with cerebral palsy born at or near term. N Engl J Med 2015;**373**:946–53.
59. Blair Bell W, Cunningham L, Jowett M, et al.: The metabolism and acidity of the foetal tissues and fluids. BMJ 1928;**1**:126–31.
60. Eastman NJ: Foetal blood studies III. The chemical nature of asphyxia neonatorum and its bearing on certain practical problems. Bull J Hopkins Hosp 1932;**50**:39–50.
61. Apgar V: A proposal for a new method of evaluation of the newborn infant. Curr Res Anesth Analg 1953;**32**:260–7.
62. Apgar V, Girdany BR, McIntosh R, Taylor HC Jr: Neonatal anoxia. I. A study of the relation of oxygenation at birth to intellectual development. Pediatrics 1955;**15**:653–62.
63. James LS, Weisbrot IM, Prince CE, Holaday DA, Apgar V: The acid-base status of human infants in relation to birth asphyxia and the onset of respiration. J Pediatr 1958;**52**:379–94.
64. Dawes GS, Mott JC, Shelley HJ: The importance of cardiac glycogen for the maintenance of life in foetal lambs and new-born animals during anoxia. J Physiol 1959;**146**:516–38.
65. American Academy of Pediatrics Committee on Fetus and Newborn: Use and abuse of the Apgar score. Pediatrics 1986;**78**:1148–9.
66. Usher R: Reduction of mortality from respiratory distress syndrome of prematurity with early administration of intravenous glucose and sodium bicarbonate. Pediatrics 1963;**32**:966–75.
67. American College of Obstetrics and Gynecology: Fetal and neonatal neurologic injury. Int J Gynecol Obstet 1993;**41**:97–101.
68. MacLennan A, International Cerebral Palsy Task Force: A template for defining a causal relationship between acute intrapartum events and cerebral palsy. BMJ 1999;**319**:1054–9.
69. American College of Obstetrics and Gynecology: Committee Opinion Nr. **326**: Inappropriate use of the terms fetal distress and birth asphyxia. Obstet Gynecol 2005;**106**:1469–70.
70. Roederer JG: Elementa artis obstetriciae in usum auditorium (1st ed. Goettingiae 1753). Edited by Heinrich August Wrisberg: 2. ed. Goettingiae: Vandenhoeck, 1766: p. 69, note 63.
71. Laennec RTH: Traité de l'auscultation médiate et des maladies des poumons et du coeur (1st ed. Paris 1819). 4. ed. Paris: Chaudé, 1837: Vol. **3**, p. 520–1.
72. Lejumeau de Kergaradec J-A: Mémoire sur l'auscultation appliquée a l'étude de la grossesse. Paris: Méquignon-Marvis, 1822.
73. Sampson JJ, McCalla RL, Kerr WJ: Phonocardiography of the human fetus. Am Heart J 1926;**1**:717–34.
74. Devoe LD, Castillo RA, Sherline DM: The nonstress test as a diagnostic test. Am J Obstet Gynecol 1985;**152**:1047–53.
75. Banta HD, Thacker SB: Costs and benefits of electronic fetal monitoring. Hyattsville, MD: National Center for Health Services Research, 1978.
76. Alfirevic Z, Devane D, Gyte GML, Cuthbert A: Continuous cardiotocography (CTG) as a form of electronic fetal monitoring (EFM) for fetal assessment during labour. Cochrane Database Sys Rev 2017;**2**:CD006066.
77. Betran AP, Ye J, Moller A-B, Zhang J, Gülmezoglu AM, Torloni MR: The increasing trend in Caesarean section rates: global, regional and national estimates: 1990–2014. PLoS One 2016;**11**:1–12.
78. Emond A, Golding J, Peckham C: Cerebral palsy in two national cohort studies. Arch Dis Child 1989;**64**:848–52.
79. Freeman JM, Freeman AD: No-fault neurological compensation: perhaps its time has come, again. Harvard Med Inst Forum 2003;5–6.
80. Johnson SL, Blair E, Stanley FJ: Obstetric malpractice litigation and cerebral palsy in term infants. J Forensic Leg Med 2011;**18**:97–100.
81. Sartwelle TP, Johnston JC: Cerebral palsy litigation: change course or abandon ship. J Child Neurol 2015;**30**:824–41.
82. Peters M, Dintsios CM: Marktversagen im Haftungsbereich: Die aktuelle Haftpflichtversicherungssituation der Hebammen in Deutschland. Gesundh Ökon Qual Manag 2015;**20**:157–62.
83. Rueff J: De conceptu, et generatione hominis: de matrice et eius partibus, nec non de conditione infantis in utero... Frankfurt: Feyerabend, 1587: p. 25.
84. Dalechamps J: Chirurgie Francaise (1st ed. 1573). Paris: Olivier de Varennes, 1610: p. 323–36.
85. Scultetus J: Wund-Artzneyisches Zeug-Hauß. Franckfurt: Gerlin, 1666: p. 42.
86. Smellie W: A set of anatomical tables, with explanations, and an abridgement, of the practice of midwifery, with a view to illustrate a treatise on that subject, and collection of cases. London: Freeman, 1754: p. Table 21.

2.2

Resuscitation 1
Artificial ventilation

Introduction

Neonatal asphyxia has been mentioned in the literature since the dawn of writing. In the 16th century B.C.E., the Papyrus Ebers [1] gave the prognosis for a neonate on the day of its birth, perhaps alluding to expiratory grunting in respiratory distress: 'If it cries nee, it will live. If it moans bá, it will die.' Whereas birth asphyxia was not discriminated from immaturity or weakness in the preterm infant, inability to breathe was considered a treatable condition in the term infant. As Hellas and Rome felt little sympathy for weaklings, treatment of birth asphyxia (apparent death) was seldom mentioned in the ancient literature and before Emperor Constantine's Christian edicts, infanticide was frequent. Obstetrics and the care for neonates remained in the hands of more or less illiterate midwives and barber-surgeons until the Middle Ages.

Stimulation

Literate midwives (some male) were the first to set standards for treating the neonate when printed books became available. Eucharius Rösslin's book appeared in 1513 and was frequently reprinted and translated. Midwife authors remained rare as publishing was a strictly regulated privilege. They were usually appointed to the courts, who gave them permission to publish without requiring approval by the medical authorities. Famous midwifery authors included the Chamberlen family in England, Louise Bourgeois, Marie Boivin, Marie-Louise Lachappelle, François Mauriceau in France, and Justine Siegemundin in Germany.

Louise Bourgeois described resuscitation in 1609 [2]: 'I saw the most experienced physicians put a small spoonful of pure wine into the neonate's mouth, explaining that that would help the infant to regain its spirits after being agitated by the labours, which sometimes make it so weak that it seems more dead than alive. The wine's other advantage is that it loosens the phlegm they usually have in the throat.' Half a century later, François Mauriceau was still using wine, but changed its application [3]: 'To render the infant the help needed, it should be rested on a warmed bed and brought near the fire, where the midwife having taken some wine into her mouth shall blow it into the infant's mouth, which can be repeated several times if necessary... She should warm all the parts of the body to recall the blood and spirits which retired during the weakness and endangered suffocation. The infant regains its strength and begins to move one limb after the other; after which it will expel some small weary cries, which will augment and become lauder when it breathes easier.'

Mouth-to-mouth ventilation

For centuries, mouth-to-mouth ventilation was a widespread and successful method of resuscitation. Paolo Bagellardo specified in 1472 [4]: 'If she finds [the newborn] warm, not black, she should blow into its mouth if it is not breathing.' Mouth-to-mouth breathing was refined during the following centuries and was praised by the Royal Accoucheur Levret in 1766 [5] as follows: 'It should not be forgotten, in such cases, to use the most vivid *errhines* [mucus increasing drugs] or sneezing powders, to apply a bit of salt into the infant's mouth, to tickle his throat with a new feather's tail, and to keep him moving continuously until he breathes freely. There is one more means which sometimes works as by magic, that is to place one's mouth on that of the infant and to blow into it, taking care to pinch the tip of the nose simultaneously. This method is so effective, that it is really seldom that others will help if it fails.'

Until the French Revolution, the Church dominated medical teaching. When Benedict XIV ascended the Holy Chair in 1740, he noted the need to set rules for baptism throughout Europe and appointed the theologian, lawyer, and physician Francesco Cangiamila as inquisitor. He wrote a comprehensive textbook that was translated into seven languages and remained a compulsory requisite to the clergy and most physicians through numerous editions for nearly 100 years. Successful efforts to resuscitate the neonate were mandatory before baptism was allowed, and the sequence of efforts described by the inquisitor was [6]: 'Most importantly and before all other procedures warm human breath should be insufflated through a tube into the infant's mouth. Its nostrils should be closed so that the air cannot escape; the air should be warm and come from a healthy and virtuous person.' The following six steps the inquisitor recommended were: to suck the infant's nipples, tickle its soles, give a warm bath, burn the umbilical cord, insufflate the rectum with tobacco smoke, and place the infant inside a chicken carcass.

The proper sequence of resuscitating measures was considered to be important, as emphasized in Rau's 1807 teaching book for midwives in 1807 [7]: 'Do not cut the umbilical cord immediately unless it has ruptured from the placenta, but start to resuscitate the infant before … You may have the pleasure to see life returning even after hours. Therefore, you should not give up too early in your efforts … The proper measures are as follows: 1. Remove any mucus from the infant's mouth; 2. Wrap the infant's extremities in warm towels and rub his chest with a cloth soaked in warm wine; 3. When no effect appears within five minutes, put the infant into a lukewarm bath. The water should reach the arms, the head is to be held upright … 5. Blow air into the mouth, using a specifically designed tube or a quill, while closing its nostrils. This must be done by a healthy person, and a small quantity of air should be blown only, but repeatedly; 6. Apply an enema of water and wine, or of pure wine; 7. Take the infant out of the bath, place it on a dry towel, and drip cold water onto its chest; 8. Hold strong smelling things close to its nose, e.g. ammonia, spirit, a fresh-cut onion, or horseradish; 9. Drip some warm wine or brandy into its mouth; 10. If all that fails to help, burn its foot soles with a hot iron or with glowing coal; if you reach your goal earlier on and life returns, omit the stronger procedures, but return the infant to the lukewarm bath and gently rub its chest until the breathing becomes regular.'

Vitalism and *balneum animale*

Concurring with the vitalist doctrine of weakness (see Chapter 2.1) and from the early Middle Ages, animals were slaughtered in order to transmit their life force, equated with warmth, to the asphyctic baby. At the birth of Purchart I, later abbot of Saint Gall, around 925 C.E., 'the mother passed away. The child, cut from the mother's womb, was wrapped in the fat freshly removed from a pig' [8]. In 1565, Simon Vallambert mentioned the midwives' custom [9] 'to wrap the infant immediately in the skin of a sheep or a lamb, freshly skinned and still warm, with the intention to alleviate the trauma suffered during birth'. The Swiss physician Johannes Fatio derided the habit in 1752 [10], insisting that mouth-to-mouth ventilation is more efficient than 'placing boiling-hot meat on the infant's head and chest'. Gustav Jägerschmidt proposed to stabilize preterm infants in 1776 [11] 'wrapping in warmed towels or in freshly slaughtered animals as long as these maintain their natural warmth'. As late as 1837, Christian Hufeland proposed [12] 'to place such asphyctic newborn inside the carcass of a freshy slaughtered animal, thus providing a true *balneum animale* [animalic bath]'.

Early ventilators

In 1755, John Hunter built a double-chambered bellows-type ventilator with pressure-limiting valves [13]. Shortly thereafter followed the ventilators of Chaussier [14] and Gorcy [15] which replaced mouth-to-mouth by bag or bellows ventilation to mask or tube, and at the end of the 18th century the stage seemed set for artificial ventilation of the neonate. Hufeland referred to Gorcy's ventilator in 1791 [16] as a 'new instrument to restore respiration in apparent death … The inventor is Mr Gorcy, physician at the military hospital at Neu-Breisach, and Mr Rouland in Paris has made it more comfortable and affordable … Both bellows end below the valve in a common curved tube. During use one brings the ivory tube into one of the nostrils or into the mouth and closes in the first case the other, in the latter both of the nostrils. During opening, one of the bellows receives fresh atmospheric air, the other expires air from the curved tube. During compression one of the bellows expels the expiratory gas into the atmosphere, the other moves the atmospheric air into the infant's lung.'

Scientific progress accelerated in Paris following the revolution. Legallois investigated survival time of animals kept from breathing. He detected the breathing centre by cutting the medulla and found that fetuses separated from their mothers survived longer than adult animals. As early as 1820, Capuron added electrodefibrillation or electric stimulation of the phrenic nerve to traditional resuscitation methods [17]: 'Finally you should seek the aid of electricity, which has been so much recommended … and apply it to the stomach region. You can also try galvanism applying the current to one of the ears and place one of the infant's hands into a saturated salt solution … To tell the truth, it is not always easy to obtain an electric apparatus or a galvanic battery.' Electric stimulation was never given up entirely as seen from Cross' recommendation in 1951 [18].

Academy verdict and indirect methods

In 1828, the Paris surgeon Jean-Jacques Leroy d'Etiolles wrote an influential article which virtually put an end to resuscitation by the insufflation of air [19]. He ventilated the lungs of different living animals, of adults drowned in the Seine River, and of stillborn or deceased neonates, and measured the inflation pressure required to cause pneumothorax. Without using a pressure-reducing valve, he found that the lungs of stillborn infants always tolerated a given pressure, whereas pneumothorax occurred in adults or animal lungs. He concluded 'the reason may be that the neonate's lung is more compact … the diaphragm is displaced downwards and forms an elastic tumor …: In artificial respiration, the air which enters the lung distends the chest, whereas in natural respiration it is the chest and perhaps the lung which dilate to admit the air.'

The powerful Académie des Sciences appointed a commission headed by Magendie and Dumeril to verify Leroy's findings and when they confirmed them in 1829, artificial ventilation was discredited [20]: 'If blown brusquely into the trachea, the air can cause sudden death, even if this insufflation is done by mouth … Only if applied gently with the mouth or bellows, in experienced hands it is an important help for asphyctic persons.' Except in Britain, where John Snow constructed 'a little instrument adapted to the size of newborn children' in 1841 [21], artificial ventilation was abandoned for neonates as well, and when Schwartz wrote a book on the apparent death of the neonate in 1858, he mentioned it as an outdated technique [22]: 'I found efficacious only those procedures which stimulate peripheral nerves: Warm bathing, dripping cold water, stimulating the skin, and so forth. I have not seen any benefit from artificial ventilation which has been so strongly advocated.' Among the various methods of indirect ventilation, the resuscitation method published by Silvester in 1858 became most popular and was still taught after World War II [23]: 'Raise the patient's arms upwards by the sides of his head, and then extend them gently and steadily upwards and forwards for a few moments. (This movement enlarges the chest's capacity by elevating the ribs, and induces inspiration.) Next, move down the patient's arms and press them gently and firmly for a few moments against the sides of the chest. (This action diminishes the cavity of the thorax, and produces a forcible expiration).'

In this anti-ventilation era, the obstetrician Schultze in Jena proposed a swinging manoeuvre for resuscitation in 1871 [24]: 'After cord clamping the obstetrician holds the infant's shoulders, his thumbs hold the thorax frontally, his index fingers the axillae from behind, and the other three fingers the back of the thorax … He swings the infant from this hanging position upwards. When the obstetrician's arms are elevated horizontally, he stops gently, so that the infant's body slowly sinks forwards, and the abdomen is compressed by the weight of the breech … The infant's body is now straightened out in one swing; its thorax, free of any pressure, will enlarge due to its elasticity, the diaphragm descends due to the swing's action on the bowels triggering a deep inspiration' (Fig. 2.2.1).

With today's knowledge, this manoeuvre, done in an infant in severe birth asphyxia, cannot have led to anything but hypothermia and intraventricular haemorrhage. However, being so much easier than endotracheal intubation, the swingings, sadly, continued to be en vogue until after World War II, despite the side effects described by Ylppö in 1919 [25]: 'I strongly advise against the use of Schultze swingings in preterm infants, especially in small ones. I showed what a large trauma the preterm delivery means for the child and what disastrous consequences it carries in form of brain and spinal cord hemorrhage … Except in preterm infants born in breech position, it is mostly in preterm infants resuscitated by Schultze swingings that I have seen the most extensive cerebral hemorrhages.'

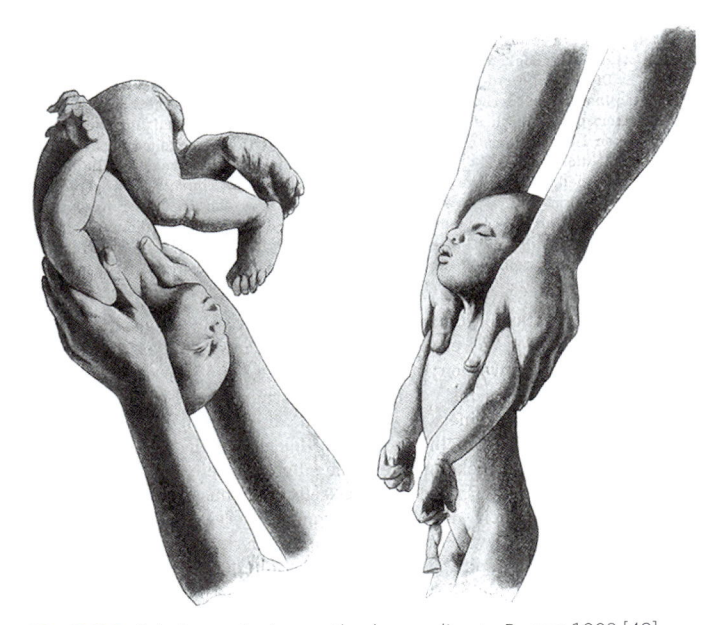

Fig. 2.2.1 Schultze swinging method according to Bumm 1903 [42].

In addition to the risk of pneumothorax, infectious diseases passing both to and from the newborn infant prevented further development of mouth-to-mouth breathing. Indeed, it was this method, which revealed the infectivity of tuberculosis in South Germany 7 years before Koch isolated the bacillus [26]: 'In Neuenburg, ten infants fell ill and died (most at three months of age) from meningitis tuberculosa, all born between April 1875 and May 1876. None of them had a genetic disposition for tuberculosis. They all had been delivered by the midwife S. In midwife R's practice, not a single infant died from meningitis tuberculosa or other tuberculous disease. Midwife S. suffered from lung phthisis; in July 1875 the presence of caverns and of putrid sputum was diagnosed, in July 1876 she succumbed to the disease. Midwife S. had the habit of aspiring mucus from the neonates' airways with her mouth, to inflate air even at low degrees of asphyxia, and to treat the infants in a manner that probably contaminated the infants' lungs with her expired air … Meningitis tuberculosa had not been an endemic disease in Neuenburg. Within nine years from 1866 to 1874, only 2 infants died from meningitis tuberculosa.'

Using plethysmography, Champneys compared the efficacy of nine different indirect ventilation methods (Marshall Hall, Howard, Silvester, Pacini, Bain, Schücking, Schüller, Schroeder, Schultze), and concluded in 1887 [27]: 'The ventilation of the lungs is secured by various methods of manipulation, of which, for stillborn children, only two are trustworthy, namely, the method of Schultze, and that of Silvester, with its modifications by Pacini and Bain.' As late as 1960, after a century without evidence, it became obvious that Silvester's method neither aerated the lungs nor improved oxygen saturation in neonates [28].

Tank ventilators

Following the banning of intermittent positive pressure ventilation, body-enclosing, tank-type ventilators were constructed which avoided intubation and overinflation. Knapp [29] described Woillez' 1876 model [30] (Fig. 2.2.2): 'Woillez' apparatus is a metal sheet cylinder. One end is hermetically closed; the apparent dead patient is pushed up to his neck into the other, open end. Rubber tissue is fastened to the neck at this end, so that the cylinder closes as air tightly as possible. A rubber tube connects the inside of the cylinder to a bellows. By forced movement of the latter, the air in the cylinder is alternatively rarefied or put under augmented pressure. In the first case, a strong inspiration results; in the latter, a vigorous expiration takes place which forces any bronchial liquid out of mouth and nose.'

Alexander Graham Bell, who after his emigration from Britain became famous for inventing the telephone, invented a negative pressure jacket to ventilate neonates in 1869 [31]. Tank ventilators proliferated in the poliomyelitis epidemics in the 20th century [32], allowed long-term ventilation, but were somewhat clumsy in the delivery room [33]. A clear disadvantage of tank- and cuirass-type respirators was their immobility, which led Trueheard [34] to construct a portable ventilator providing intermittent positive pressure. It consisted of an air reservoir with several valves and regulators, connected to a glottis catheter, which serves both for aspiration and inflation, while pressure and quantity of the air can be adjusted as required. The air reservoir was carried with a forehead ribbon (Fig. 2.2.3).

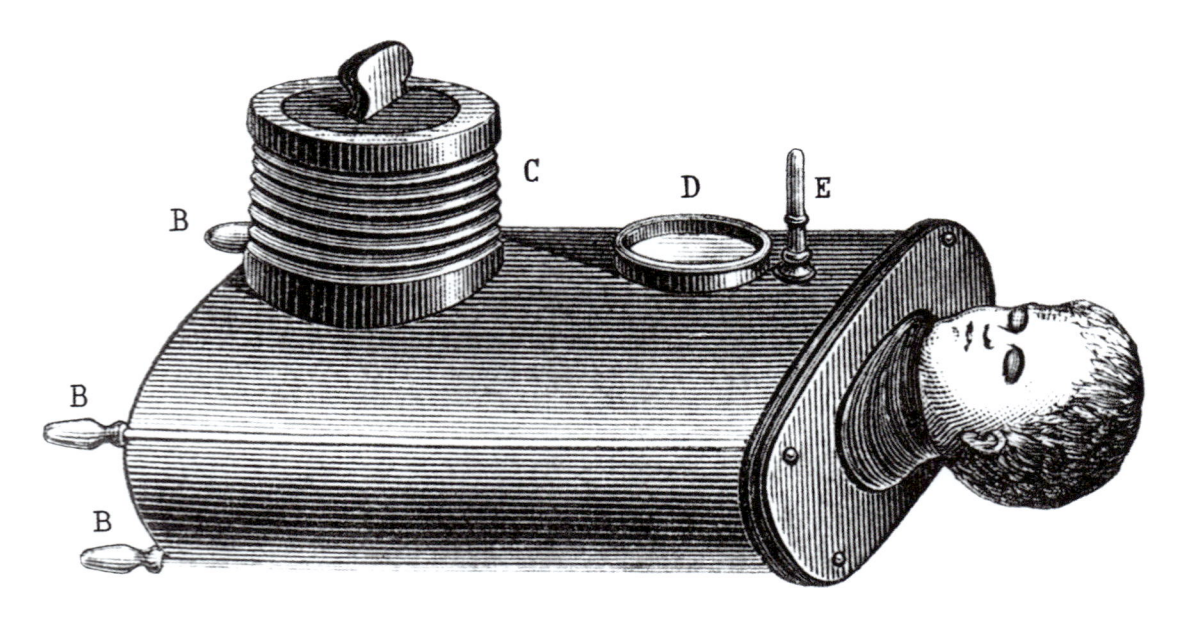

Fig. 2.2.2 Body-enclosing tank respirator of Woillez 1876 [30].

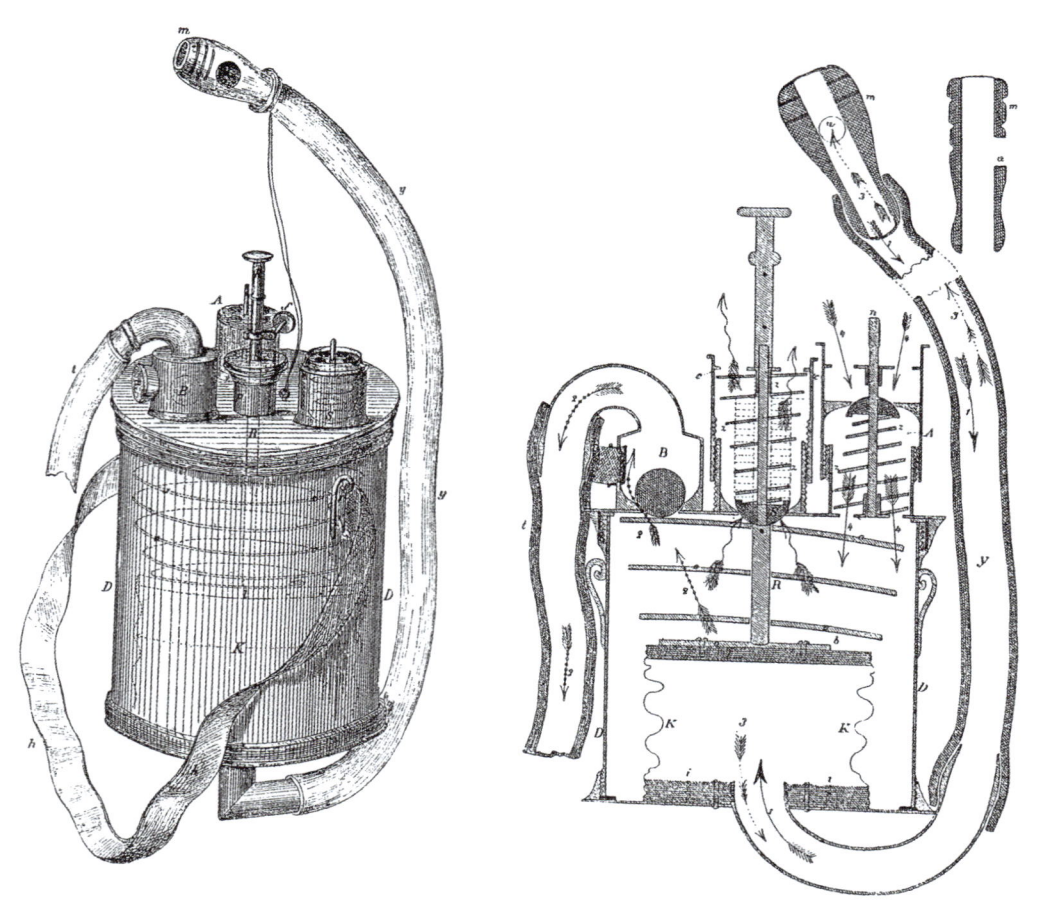

Fig. 2.2.3 Trueheard's mobile respirator for neonates 1872 [34].

Modern ventilators

In 1907, Draeger developed the Pulmotor, a mobile, short-term respirator that applied alternating positive–negative pressure [35]. Despite being commended and condemned [36], the neonatal version remained in use in most European delivery rooms for half a century, as Keuth reported in 1958 [37]: 'For automated ventilation with changing pressure we use the Baby Pulmotor with double tubing (to minimize dead space). It works either with pure oxygen or with air and is regulated by pressure (turning points +20 and −15 cm of water). The tidal minute volume applied depends on the infant's size, degree of lung expansion, and the rate.' Intermittent mandatory ventilation began with Flagg's devices [38] and Kreiselmans apparatus [39], volume control with the huge Engström device [40]. In 1960, Abramsons book listed 21 ventilators for neonates produced in North America [41].

Conclusion

The early rise, deep fall, and slow resurrection of mechanical ventilation for neonatal asphyxia demonstrates how a strong recommendation from scientific authorities based on weak scientific evidence can delay medical progress for many decades.

REFERENCES

1. Bryan CP: The Papyrus Ebers. New York: Appleton, 1931: p. 341.
2. Bourgeois L: Observations diverses sur la sterilite, perte de fruits, fécondité, accouchments, et maladies de femmes, et enfants nouveaux-naiz. Paris: Dehoury, 1609: p. 95.
3. Mauriceau F: Traité des maladies des femmes grosses, et de celles qui sont accouchées (1st ed. 1668). 7. ed. Paris: Compagnie des Libraires, 1740: Vol. **1**, p. 329, 367, 481.
4. Bagellardo P: Opusculum recens natum de morbis puerorum (1st ed. 1472). Lyon: Barbou, 1538: p. 4, 31, 43.
5. Levret A: L'art des accouchemens. 3. ed. Paris: Didot Jeune, 1766.
6. Cangiamila FE: Embryologia sacra sive de officio sacerdotum, medicorum, et aliorum circa aeternam parvulorum in utero existentium salutem. 3. ed. Augustae Vindelicorum: Mauracher, 1765: p. 562.
7. Rau GMWL: Handbuch für Hebammen. Gießen und Darmstadt: Heyer, 1807: p. 183–6.
8. Duft J: Notker der Arzt. Klostermedizin und Mönchsarzt im frühmittelalterlichen St. Gallen. St. Gallen: Buchdruckerei Ostschweiz, 1972: p. 21–2.
9. Vallambert Sd: Cinq livres de la manière de nourrir et gouverner les enfants dès leur naissance. Poitiers: Manefz et Bouchetz, 1565: p. 127.
10. Fatio J: Helvetisch-vernünftige Wehe-Mutter. Basel: Imhof, 1752: p. 334.
11. Jägerschmid GF: Unterricht für die Hebammen in den Badischen Landen. 2. Theil, welcher die Verpflegung der Schwangeren, Kindbetterinnen und Kinder enthält. Carlsruhe: Macklot, 1776: Vol. **2**, p. 82.
12. Hufeland CW: Tödtliche Zufälle der Neugeborenen in den ersten vierzehn Tagen des Lebens. In: Sammlung auserlesener Abhandlungen über Kinder-Krankheiten. Prag: Haase, 1837: Vol. **6**, p. 3–17.
13. Hunter J: Double chambered bellows for artificial respiration. J Phil Trans 1776;**66**:412.
14. Chaussier F: Reflexions sur les moyens propres a déterminer la respiration dans les enfants qui naissent sans donner aucune signe de vie. Paris: Histoire de la Société Royale de Médecine, 1780–1781: Vol. **4**, p. 346–54.
15. Gorcy PC: Nouveau instrument pour rétablir la réspiration dans le mort apparent. Gren Journal De Physique 1790.
16. Hufeland CW: Neues Instrument zu Wiederherstellung der Respiration im Scheintod. Neueste Annalen der Französischen Arzneikunde 1791–1799;**1**:359–62.
17. Capuron J: Traité des maladies des enfans. 2. ed. Paris: Croullebois, 1820: p. 21.
18. Cross K, Roberts P: Asphyxia neonatorum treated by electrical stimulation of the phrenic nerve. BMJ 1951;**1**:1043.
19. Leroy d'Etiolles JJJ: Second mémoire sur l'asphyxie. J Physiol Exp Path 1828;**8**:97–135.
20. Magendie F, Duméril AMC: Rapport sur un mémoire de M. Leroy d'Etioles, relatif a l'insufflation du poumon. J Chim Med Pharm Tox, Paris 1829;**5**:335–44.
21. Snow J: On asphyxia, and on the resuscitation of stillborn children. Lond Med Gaz 1841;**29**:222–7.
22. Schwartz H: Die vorzeitigen Athembewegungen. Leipzig: Breitkopf und Härtel, 1858: p. 283.
23. Silvester HR: A new method of resuscitating still-born children, and of restoring persons apparently drowned or dead. BMJ 1858;**I**:576–9.
24. Schultze BS: Der Scheintod Neugeborener. Jena: Mauke, 1871: p. 162.
25. Ylppö A: Pathologisch-anatomische Studien bei Frühgeborenen. Zeitschr Kinderheilk 1919;**20**:212–431.
26. Reich H: Die Tuberculose, eine Infectionskrankheit. Berl Klin Wochenschr 1878;551–3.
27. Champneys FH: Experimental researches in artificial respiration in stillborn children. London: Lewis, 1887: p. 140.
28. Saling E: Über die Wirksamkeit von älteren und neuen Asphyxiebehandlungsmethoden. Geburtsh Frauenheilk 1960;20: 325–39.
29. Knapp L: Der Scheintod des Neugeborenen. **2**. klinischer Teil. Wien: Braumüller, 1904: p. 169.
30. Woillez EJ: Du spirophore, appareil de sauvetage pour le traitement de l'asphyxie. Bull Acad Méd 1876;**5**:611–27.
31. Baskett T: Alexander Graham Bell and the vacuum jacket for assisted respiration. Resuscitation 2004;**63**:115–17.
32. Drinker P, Shaw LA: An apparatus for the prolonged administration of artificial respiration: I. a design for adults and children. J Clin Invest 1929;**7**:229–47.
33. Murphy D, Wilson R, Bowman J: The Drinker respirator treatment of the immediate asphyxia of the newborn. Am J Obstet Gynecol 1931;**21**:528–36.
34. Trueheard: Ein Apparat zur künstlichen Respiration bei Asphyxie. Beiträge zur Gebh u Gyn (Berlin) 1872;**I**:154–6.
35. Draeger L, Blume G: Zur Geschichte des Drägerwerkes von 1889 bis 1936. Lübeck: Verlag Graphischen Werkstätten, 1994: p. 24.

36. Wiggin SC, Saunders P, Small GA: Resuscitation (concluded): Asphyxia neonatorum. N Engl J Med 1949;**241**:413–20.
37. Keuth U: Trachealintubation und Wechseldruckbeatmung bei atemgestörten Frühgeborenen. Zeitschr Kinderheilk 1958;**81**:660–74.
38. Flagg PJ: Treatment of asphyxia in the newborn. JAMA 1928;**91**:788–91.
39. Kreiselman J, Kane H, Swope R: A new apparatus for resuscitation of asphyxiated newborn babies. Am J Obstet Gynecol 1928;**15**:552.
40. Engström CG: Treatment of severe cases of respiratory paralysis by the Engström Universal Respirator. BMJ 1954;**II**: 666–9.
41. Abramson H: Resuscitation of the newborn infant. St. Louis, MO: Mosby, 1960: p. 274.
42. Bumm E: Grundriß zum Studium der Geburtshilfe. 2. ed. Wiesbaden: Bergmann, 1903.

2.3

Resuscitation 2
Oxygen and other drugs

Introduction: tobacco smoke

This chapter is devoted to drugs used to resuscitate newborn babies at birth. Tobacco had barely found its way from America to Europe, when it began to be used in medicine. In 1661, Thomas Bartholin described and depicted [1] a device for resuscitating drowned persons via rectal insufflation of tobacco smoke. In 1766, the Abbé Dinouart translated Cangiamila's *Embryologia Sacra* [2], inserting a paragraph on apparent death recommending the tobacco clyster to resuscitate newborns (Fig. 2.3.1, left). The Berlin obstetrician Christian Mursinna wrote in 1786 [3]: 'Insufflating air into the lungs is the first and best measure… Then tobacco smoke is blown into the baby's anus… sometimes it helps to blow some of the smoke into the baby's mouth.' In his 1787 textbook [4], the Tübingen obstetrician Friedrich Osiander devoted 12 pages to a tobacco clyster for resuscitating newborns, with the amount of smoke varying according to the baby's size (Fig. 2.3.1, right). Picasso's biographer Norman Mailer reported [5]: 'On October 25, 1881, the baby came out stillborn; he did not breathe; neither did he cry. If it had not been for the presence of his uncle, Dr. Salvador Ruiz, the infant might never have come to life. Don Salvador, however, leaned over the stillbirth and exhaled cigar smoke into its nostrils. Picasso stirred. Picasso screamed. A genius came to life.'

Phlogiston and oxygen

Sendivogius and Scheele had isolated oxygen before, but when the ingenious Birmingham reverend Joseph Priestley published his experiments 'on different kinds of air' performed with mercuric oxide in his bathroom in 1772 [6], two French gentlemen understood their meaning immediately: The young Dijon physiologist François Chaussier was developing a device to resuscitate neonates. He published a paper on oxygen in 1777 [7] and proceeded to construct a pressure-limited ventilator for the use of oxygen in neonatal resuscitation in 1781 [8]. Chaussier made oxygen, called 'dephlogistated air' according to Stahl's theory, the first drug used specifically in neonates.

The other person who understood Priestley's discovery, was the Parisian chemist Antoine Lavoisier. He possessed a letter of the Swedish pharmacist Carl Wilhelm Scheele, in which the naive apothecary had reported his unpublished observation of 'fire-air'. Lavoisier now appreciated the significance of Scheele's discovery, discarded the phlogiston theory [9], and named the new gas 'oxygine' [10]. In his *Traité Élémentaire de Chimie* he showed that it maintained metabolism in living organisms, without mentioning Scheele's contribution [11]. In 1992, Scheele's letter was found in Madame Lavoisier's estate [12]. The fate of the two French oxygen specialists turned out to differ remarkably: Lavoisier was guillotined in 1794, not for scientific fraud, but for blackmail when he had been a tax tenant during the Ancien Régime. Chaussier was awarded the Paris chair of anatomy in 1794 and was appointed director of the Maternité, the largest obstetric hospital in the world, by Napoleon in 1804. Still in Dijon, he wrote in 1781 an article for the Paris faculty [8]: 'Some apply their lips onto those of the infant and blow into its chest exhaled air, which is well known to have acquired a poor quality having passed the lung. The nicely done experiments of Mr Priestley and Mr Fontana have shown that exhaled air contains large amounts of phlogistated air and fixed air, neither of which aides respiration … To overcome all these problems, I have constructed a simple machine with which one can easily and safely apply fresh and salutary air into the infant's lung [see Chapter 3.3, Fig. 3.3.3] … During a difficult delivery it is easy to predict when the infant will be born in a state of weakness sufficient to arrest the organs of respiration: Therefore the prudent obstetrician can prepare in advance all the equipment required to restore its life. It is, I confess, more comfortable to have a flacon of volatile alkali in the pocket; but I do not demand that an obstetrician carries with him the large canister of dephlogistated air which I just described: it can be manufactured in a much smaller, portable, and less annoying way. Moreover, one can acquire dephlogistated air from the depots, or chemistry laboratories. Finally, as we are dealing with a matter of life, can one ignore any effort to preserve it?'

Reproduced with permission from Obladen, M. History of neonatal resuscitation. Part 2: Oxygen and other drugs. *Neonatology*, 95:91–96. Copyright © 2009 S. Karger AG, Basel.

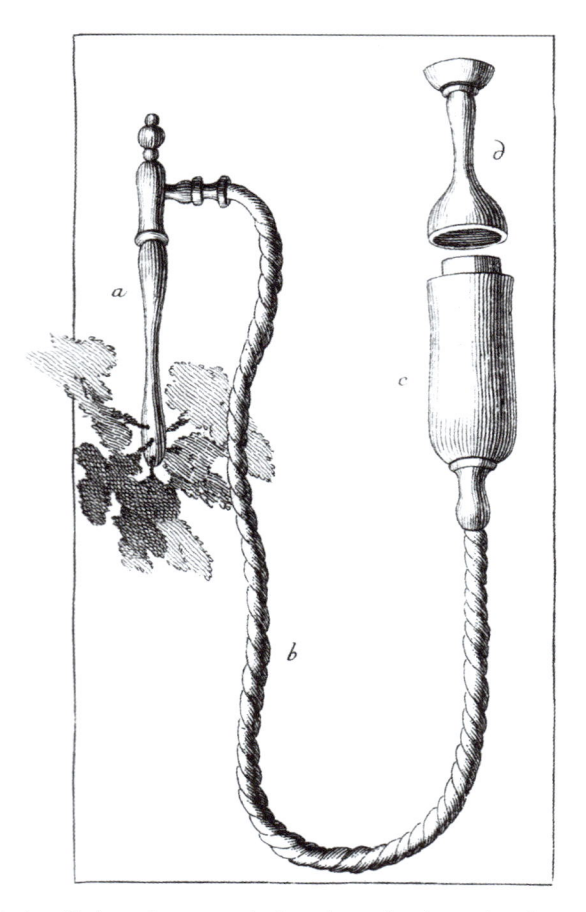

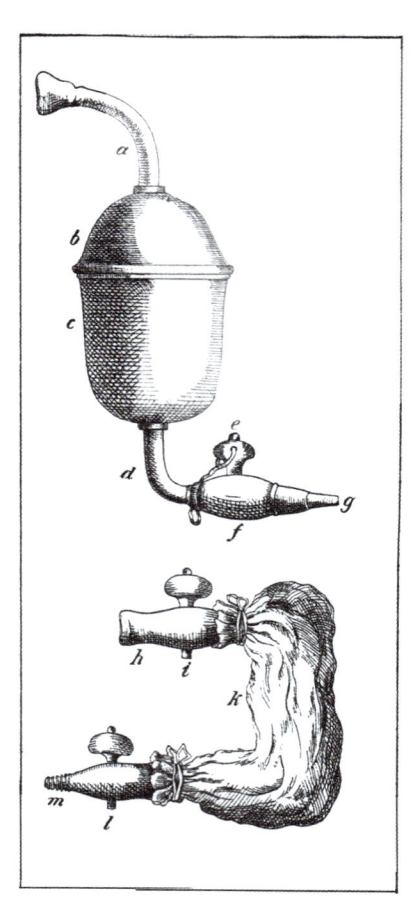

Fig. 2.3.1 Clysters for insufflating tobacco smoke into the asphyctic newborn's anus. Left: device published by Dinouart 1766 [2]. Right: device published by Osiander in 1787 [4].

Within a few years, the use of oxygen in neonatal resuscitation became popular throughout Europe, as described by Joseph Jakob von Plenk in Vienna in 1807 [13]: '3. Most helpful is the galvanic bath in which one pole of the column is placed in the water, and the other on the infant's chest. 4. Ventilation of the lung: A highly effective and specific treatment is the inflation of oxygen gas, which can be performed with a curved cannula through the nostrils. (It is advisable that every pharmacy has at all times a galvanic column and an oxygen balloon available to the obstetrician foreseeing a difficult delivery).'

When Little in 1861 and Mitchell in 1862 reported brain damage in infants who had survived birth asphyxia, oxygen use in the delivery room proliferated further. A century later, an unfounded belief in perinatal brain damage resulting from birth asphyxia was deeply rooted in the mind of paediatricians and obstetricians [14], Russ and Strong [15] even specified that 'prolongation of anoxia for more than two minutes after delivery of an infant will cause serious cerebral damage'.

In the early 20th century, intravenous injection of oxygen was performed in cyanotic adults [16], and it was also infused into the umbilical vein of asphyctic neonates [17], as cited by Reuss [18]: 'A metal syringe with a stopcock is filled with oxygen by connection with a rubber tube to an oxygen tank whereby the inflowing gas pushes back the piston. The cock is closed and the sterilized blunt adaptor of the syringe is ligated into the umbilical vein; then 10–20 cc of oxygen are injected within several minutes. This method is regarded as promising, but it also carries risks (heart dilatation).'

Gastric administration of oxygen was described by Arvo Ylppö in Berlin [18]: 'In experiments on myself I observed that the human gastric mucosa absorbs oxygen remarkably well.' Pharyngeal oxygen administration became Ylppö's method of choice in 1919 [19]: 'A small Nélaton-catheter is inserted through the nose into the pharynx and a small, weak oxygen stream is directed into the pharynx for shorter or longer periods of time as needed. Because of the rapid diffusion of oxygen it makes no sense to put a funnel in front of the infant's mouth. With this technique the air contains barely more oxygen than it otherwise would.' **Fig. 2.3.2** shows the huge cooking pan serving as an incubator for preterm infants at the Kaiserin Auguste Victoria Haus in Berlin—side by side with a large oxygen tank [20]. Gastric oxygen did not gain widespread acceptance, but still was in use after the Second World War [21–23].

Continuous distending airway pressure

Positive end expiratory pressure via an endotracheal tube to apply oxygen is cited by Reuss [24] as having been published by Hoerder in 1909 [25], but Hoerder's original publication is not compatible with the citation: 'Hoerder recommends a modified so-called "overpressure apparatus" of Brat and Schneider. With the right pressure,

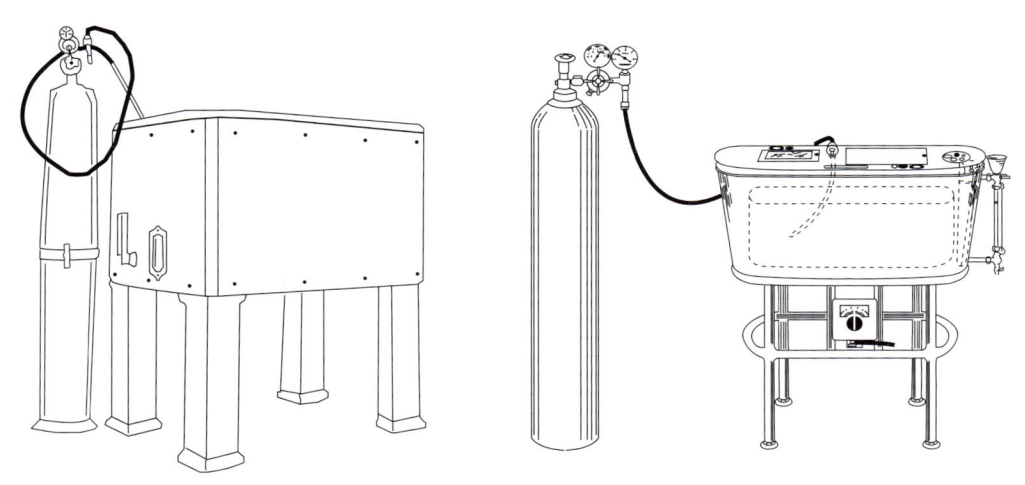

Fig. 2.3.2 Continuous oxygen administration to preterm infants. Left: heated open bed used in Berlin by Ylppö, 1919 [20, 40]. Right: Hess bed used in Chicago from 1921 [55, 56].

the method enables the lung to be expanded during the expiration phase without hindering the retraction required for ventilation. The excess pressure is produced by cautiously obtruding the expiratory valve, which impedes breathing. A marked tracheal tube is inserted shortly above the bifurcation. The mucus is aspirated into a small glass bowl and oxygen is insufflated. The pressure is regulated by a water trap. The insufflation of oxygen (at a rate of 30 to 40 per minute) should only be stopped once the child has obtained a healthy colour, and the catheter should only be removed when the child is able to breathe spontaneously and rhythmically.'

'Oxygen pressure breathing' meant the use of continuous positive airway pressure via mask and bag and was published by Engelmann in 1911 [26]: 'The apparatus I constructed with the help of Dr. Tiegel consists of a normal oxygen tank, a simple water valve, and a modified Wantscher-Tiegel [face] mask. [The latter] … is sealed to the face with a hermetically closing rubber ring. A large rubber bag is screwed to the mask roof and communicates with it through a wide opening and is an essential part of the apparatus. Without the bag, breathing—especially inspiration—would be impeded, because the flow from the tube could not quickly enough provide the gas volume required for inspiration … Inside the mask an ascending tube delivers the stream of gas from the tank to the bag. From here it is partly inspired, and partly mixed with the expiratory air, which is guided through the lower part of the mask and a metal tube inserted into a calibrated water valve. Pressure in the whole system is regulated by shifting the metal tube' (**Fig. 2.3.3**). Continuous distending airway pressure was rediscovered by Gregory in 1971 [27] and became the standard treatment of respiratory distress syndrome. It was only recently established that early continuous positive airway pressure in the delivery room can actually prevent the need for mechanical ventilation [28].

When oxygen became uncovered as a key accomplice to the retinopathy tragedy in preterm infants [29, 30], its use became somewhat curtailed in the nurseries, but it continued to prevail in the delivery rooms.

In 1953, New York anaesthesiologist Virginia Apgar described a score quantifying the degree of asphyxia in the neonate [31]. The score was intended to specify the resuscitation efforts and to prognosticate the infant's chance of survival: 'Resuscitation of infants at birth has been the subject of many articles. Seldom have there been such imaginative ideas, such enthusiasm, and dislikes, and such unscientific observations and study about one clinical picture. There are outstanding exceptions to these statements, but the poor quality and lack of precise data of the majority of papers concerned with infant resuscitation are interesting … The time for judging the five objective signs was varied until the most practicable and useful time was found. This is sixty seconds after the complete birth of the baby … Oxygen was used freely if the infant's condition was not good. In 217 of 336 infants who received oxygen, ratings were obtained and the method of administration was recorded: Face oxygen (n = 117), score 6.7; positive pressure mask (n = 90), score 3.9; endotracheal oxygen (n = 10), score 2.1.'

With her associate L. Stanley James, Apgar compared her score with acid–base biochemical correlates [32]: 'If, on the other hand, the asphyxia is prolonged, a marked reduction in the buffer base occurs (depressed infants Apgar score 0–4, Table I), indicating a metabolic acidosis which has become superimposed on the respiratory acidosis.' Both authors may have unintentionally augmented the use of oxygen and of bicarbonate, when high scores and pink babies became fashionable worldwide. A typical recommendation in 1966 [33] was given by Klaus: 'There is no contraindication to the use of warm 100 per cent oxygen during resuscitation. The birth process is an asphyxial episode, and high concentrations of oxygen during the first minutes of life can only be helpful.'

Ever since the Oslo neonatologist Ola Saugstad proposed that hypoxanthine and oxygen may cause lung injury [34], a growing body of evidence suggested that oxygen indeed may be harmful. After two centuries without evidence, the Resair 2 study in 1998 put an end to the belief that neonates are best resuscitated with oxygen [35]: 'This study with patients enrolled primarily from developing countries indicates that asphyxiated newborn infants can be resuscitated with room air as efficiently as with pure oxygen. In fact, time to first breath and first cry was significantly shorter in room air- versus oxygen-resuscitated infants. Resuscitation with 100% oxygen may depress ventilation and therefore delay the first breath.'

When François Chaussier initiated oxygen treatment for neonatal asphyxia in 1780, it merely seemed logical to him [8]. When, in 2005, the International Liaison Committee on Resuscitation guidelines

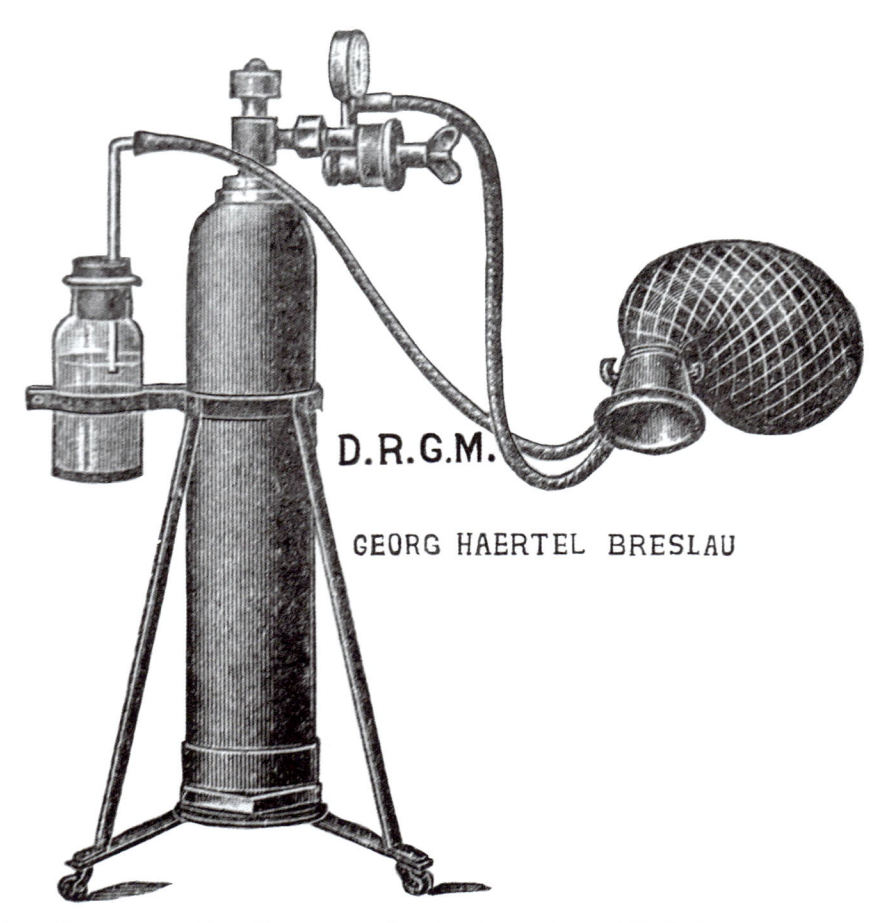

Fig. 2.3.3 Oxygen application with continuous distending pressure, described by Engelmann 1911 [57].

[36], European guidelines [37], and Cochrane database [38] gave three different recommendations for the use of oxygen in neonatal resuscitation, the weakness of modern, purportedly evidence-based medicine was revealed.

Alkali

Following experiments in 1902, Schücking concluded that it was not the lack of oxygen but accumulated carbon dioxide that was the lethal mechanism in asphyxia. He injected carbon dioxide-binding sodium saccharate into the umbilical vein [39]. Severe neonatal acidosis was observed by Ylppö in 1919 [40]: 'Even when the infant is still alive, the blood of preterm infants may possess such high acidity as has never been observed in adult blood.'

Sodium bicarbonate administration was proposed by Robert Usher [41] to reduce mortality in preterm infants, and was shown to reduce brain damage in asphyxiated animals by Dawes [42]: 'The brains of mature fetal rhesus monkeys which had been asphyxiated at birth under standard conditions, with subsequent resuscitation and recovery, were examined microscopically and the degree of permanent damage was assessed. Of the brain stem nuclei, that of the inferior colliculus proved the best guide. Administration of alkali [sodium bicarbonate and Tris] and glucose reduced the incidence and the extent of brain damage.' Clinical non-randomized studies seemed to confirm the benefit of buffers, and when several prominent obstetricians recommended bicarbonate and THAM (tromethamine) for birth asphyxia [43, 44], the widespread use of alkali took over textbooks and delivery rooms [45]. Even though Corbet's randomized trial [46] showed that giving bicarbonate to asphyctic infants neither accelerated correction of acidaemia nor reduced mortality, it took many more years to stop 'blind buffering' in delivery rooms.

Analeptics

Attempts to stimulate the breathing centre in the medulla are even older than its detection by Legallois [47]. Underwood [48] recommended in 1784: 'Many new-born infants, it is well known, from some difficulty in the birth, lie for a time in a very feeble and uncertain state, with no other sign of animation than a weak pulsation of the heart, and the arteries of the navel-string … The proper remedies are gentle stimulants and cordials; such as rubbing the nostrils, temples, and the feet and hands, with sal volatile; and as soon as the infant becomes capable of swallowing, a few drops of the volatile tincture of valerian should be administered in some generous white wine, and repeated every two to three hours, until the child shall appear perfectly recovered.' Knapp recommended in 1906 [49]: 'Among the analeptics, subcutaneous injections of camphor oil or camphorated ether occasionally render good services according to my own experience.'

In the years 1958–1960, at the Leipzig Obstetrical Hospital, 461 neonates with assumed asphyxia received intramuscular injections of 20 mg/kg of micoren without a control group. When 94% of them began breathing spontaneously within 3 min, the author concluded [50]: 'Respiratory and circulatory stimulants, such as micoren which we use, are a great advancement in the therapy of intra-uterine and postpartum asphyxia. They are distinguished by inducing a rapid effect and almost negligible toxicity.'

In the UK, analeptics were propagated by Barrie [51, 52]: 'Recent studies here have shown that nikethamide ("Coramine") and vanillic acid diethylamide ("Vandid") are of potential value in the resuscitation of the asphyxiated baby … Neonatal resuscitation should follow an agreed and well-rehearsed sequence, like the drill for fire or accident. Place baby in warmed cot. Apnoea 1 minute: Oxygen by funnel, 4 litres per minute. Nalorphine (0.25 mg) and vitamin K (1 mg) intramuscularly when indicated. Apnoea 2 minutes: nasal oxygen, 1 liter per minute. Apnoea 3 minutes: "Vandid" 25 mg (0.5 ml of 5% solution) on to tongue; premature babies half dose. Apnoea 4 minutes: Intubate and inflate lungs, half-second puffs of oxygen at 40 cm water-pressure; reduce to 10 cm when lungs fully inflated.' Following the study by Barr and Barr [53] it became popular to "antagonize" neonatal effects of maternal analgesics and sedatives as described by Bretscher [54]: 'Undisputed is the great value of the opiate antagonist N-allyl-normorphine (Lethidrone, Lorfane). The antagonism acts primarily on the breathing depressing effect of opiates.'

Conclusion

An armada of drugs has been used to prevent or treat neonatal asphyxia, including alpha lobelin, micoren, methamphetamine, theophylline, doxapram, almitrine, and dimenhydrinate. There is little evidence that we have made substantial progress during the half century since Virginia Apgar complained about the poor quality of studies and lack of solid data in most papers on infant resuscitation.

REFERENCES

1. Bartholin T: Historiarum anatomicarum rariorum Centuria V–VI. Hafniae: Henrici Gödiani, 1661: p. 310, 357.
2. Dinouart JA: Abregé de l'embryologie sacrée, ou traité des devoirs des prêtres, de médecins, des chirurgiens et des sages-femmes envers les enfants qui sont dans le sein de leurs mères. 2. ed. Paris: Nyon, 1766: p. 245–9.
3. Mursinna CL: Abhandlung von den Krankheiten der Schwangern, Gebärenden und Wöchnerinnen. Berlin: Himburg, 1786: Vol. **2**, p. 289–92.
4. Osiander FB: Beobachtungen, Abhandlungen und Nachrichten, welche vorzüglich Krankheiten der Frauenzimmer und Kinder und die Entbindungswissenschaften betreffen. Tübingen: Cotta, 1787: p. 273–84.
5. Mailer N: Portrait of Picasso as a young man. New York: Atlantic Monthly Press, 1995: p. 3.
6. Priestley J: Observations on different kinds of air. Phil Trans Royal Soc Lond 1772;**62**:147.
7. Chaussier F: Mémoire de physique expérimentale sur quelques propriétés de l'air inflammable. J Physique 1777;**10**:309–21.
8. Chaussier F: Reflexions sur les moyens propres a déterminer la respiration dans les enfants qui naissent sans donner aucune signe de vie. Paris: Histoire Société Royale de Médecine, 1780–1781: Vol. **4**, p. 346–54.
9. Lavoisier AL: Mémoire sur la nature du principe qui se combine avec les métaux pendant leur calcination, et qui en augmente le poix. Hist Acad Roy Sci 1778;520–6.
10. Lavoisier AL: Mémoire sur l'affinité du principe oxigine avec les differentes substances auxquelles il est susceptible de s'unir. Hist Acad Roy Sci 1785;530–40.
11. Lavoisier AL: Traité élémentaire de chimie. Paris: Couchet, 1789.
12. Severinghaus JW: Fire-air and dephlogistation. Adv Exp Med Biol 2003;**543**:7–19.
13. Plenk J: Lehre von der Erkenntniß und Heilung der Kinderkrankheiten. Wien: Binz, 1807: p. 13.
14. Roberts MH: Emergencies encountered in neonatal period. JAMA 1949;**139**:439–44.
15. Russ JD, Strong RA: Asphyxia of newborn infant. Am J Obstet Gynecol 1946;**51**:643–51.
16. Tunnicliffe FW, Stebbing MB: The intravenous injection of oxygen gas as a therapeutic measure. Lancet 1916;**II**:321–3.
17. Offergeld: Zur Behandlung asphyktischer Neugeborener mit Sauerstoffinfusionen. Zentrabl Gynäk 1906;**30**:1417.
18. Ylppö A: Über Magenatmung beim Menschen. Biochem Zeitschr 1917;**78**:273.
19. Little WJ: Course of [18] lectures on deformities of the human frame. Lancet 1843–1944;41:Lecture 8: pp 318–22; Lecture 9: pp 350–3.
20. Ylppö A: Pathologie der Frühgeborenen einschliesslich der 'debilen' und 'lebensschwachen' Kinder. In: Pfaundler M, Schlossmann A: Handbuch der Kinderheilkunde. 3. ed. Leipzig: Vogel, 1923: Vol. **1**, p. 580.
21. Akerrén Y, Fürstenberg N: Gastro-intestinal administration of oxygen in treatment of asphyxia in the newborn. I. J Obstet Gynaecol Br Emp 1950;**57**:705–13.
22. Saling E: Über die Wirksamkeit von älteren und neuen Asphyxiebehandlungsmethoden. Geburtsh Frauenheilk 1960; 325–39.
23. James LS, Apgar V, Burnand ED, et al.: Intragastric oxygen and resuscitation of the newborn. Acta Paediatr Scand 1963;**52**:245–51.
24. Reuss A: Die Krankheiten des Neugeborenen. Berlin: Springer, 1914: p. 253–4.
25. Hoerder C: Wesen und Bekämpfungsmethoden der asphyxia neonatorum. Med Klin 1909;**44**:1657–61.
26. Engelmann F: Die Sauerstoffdruckatmung zur Bekämpfung des Scheintodes Neugeborener. Zentralbl Gynäk 1911;**35**:7–13.
27. Gregory GA, Kitterman JA, Phibbs RH, Tooley WH, Hamilton WK: Treatment of idiopathic respiratory distress syndrome with continuous positive airway pressure. N Engl J Med 1971;**284**:1333–40.
28. Ho JJ, Henderson-Smart DJ, Davis PG: Early versus delayed initiation of continuous distending pressure for respiratory distress syndrome in preterm infants. Cochrane Database Syst Rev 2002;**2**:CD002975.
29. Campbell K: Intensive oxygen therapy as a possible cause of retrolental fibroplasia: a clinical approach. Med J Aust 1951;**2**:48–50.
30. Patz A, Hoeck LE, De La Cruz E: Studies on the effect of high oxygen administration in retrolental fibroplasia. Am J Ophthalmol 1952;**35**:1248–53.

31. Apgar V: A proposal for a new method of evaluation of the newborn infant. Curr Res Anesth Analg 1953;**32**:260–7.
32. James LS, Weisbrot IM, Prince CE, Holaday DA, Apgar V: The acid-base status of human infants in relation to birth asphyxia and the onset of respiration. J Pediatr 1958;**52**:379–94.
33. Klaus M, Meyer BP: Oxygen therapy for the newborn. Pediat Clin N Am 1966;**13**:731–52.
34. Saugstad OD, Hallman M, Abraham JL, et al.: Hypoxanthine and oxygen induced lung injury. Pediatr Res 1984;**18**:501.
35. Saugstad OD, Rootwelt T, Aalen O: Resuscitation of asphyxiated newborn infants with room air or oxygen. Pediatrics 1998;**102**:e1–7.
36. International Liaison Committee on Resuscitation (ILCOR): Part 7: Neonatal resuscitation. Resuscitation 2005;**6**:293–303.
37. Biarent D, Bingham R, Richmond S, et al.: European Resuscitation Council guidelines for resuscitation. Section 6. Paediatric life support. Resuscitation 2005;**67S1**:S97–133.
38. Tan A, Schulze A, O'Donnell CPF, Davis PG: Air versus oxygen for resuscitation of infants at birth. Cochrane Database Syst Rev 2005;**2**:CD002273.
39. Schücking A: Infusion durch die Nabelvene. Zentralbl Gynäk 1902;**26**:601–3.
40. Ylppö A: Zur Physiologie, Klinik und zum Schicksal der Frühgeborenen. Zeitschr Kinderheilk 1919;**24**:56.
41. Usher R: Reduction of mortality from respiratory distress syndrome of prematurity with early administration of intravenous glucose and sodium bicarbonate. Pediatrics 1963;**32**:966–75.
42. Dawes GS, Hibbard E, Windle WF: The effect of alkali and glucose infusion on permanent brain damage in rhesus monkeys asphyxiated at birth. J Pediatr 1964;**65**:801–23.
43. Cosmi EV, Carenza L, Gozzi G: Management of acidosis in the newborn using an organic 'buffer-substance'. Acta Anaesthesiol 1967;193–205.
44. Berg D, Mulling M, Saling E: Use of THAM and sodium bicarbonate in correcting acidosis in asphyxiated newborns. Arch Dis Child 1969;**44**:318–22.
45. Roberton C: Use of THAM in the newborn. Arch Dis Child 1969;**44**:544.
46. Corbet AJ, Adams JM, Kenny JD, Kennedy J, Rudolph AJ: Controlled trial of bicarbonate therapy in high-risk premature newborn infants. J Pediatr 1977;**91**:771–6.
47. Legallois JJC: Expériences sur le principe de la vie, notamment sur celui des mouvements du coeur. Paris: D'Hautel, 1812.
48. Underwood M: A treatise on the disorders of childhood, and management of infants from the birth (1st ed. London 1784). 2. ed. London: Matthews, 1801: Vol. **1**, p. 13, 91.
49. Knapp L: Der Scheintod des Neugeborenen. 2. klinischer Teil. Wien und Leipzig: Braumüller, 1904: p. 169.
50. Tosetti K: Behandlung der kindlichen Asphyxie mit einem Atmungs- und Kreislaufstimulans. Schweiz Med Wochenschr 1961;**91**:1373–6.
51. Barrie H, Cottom D, Wilson BDR: Respiratory stimulants in the newborn. Lancet 1962;**II**:742–6.
52. Barrie H: Resuscitation of the newborn. Lancet 1963;**I**: 650–5.
53. Barr W, Barr GTD: N-Allylnormorphine in the treatment of neonatal asphyxia. J Obstet Gynaecol Br Emp 1956;**63**:216.
54. Bretscher J: Über die Reanimation asphyktischer Neugeborener. Gynaecologia 1964;**157**:215–31.
55. Hess JH: An electric-heated water-jacketed infant incubator and bed. JAMA 1915;**64**:1068–9.
56. Hess JH: Premature and congenitally disabled infants. London: Churchill, 1923.
57. Engelmann F: Die Sauerstoffdruckatmung zur Bekämpfung des Scheintodes Neugeborener. Zentralbl Gynäk 1911;**35**: 7–13.

2.4

Resuscitation 3
Endotracheal intubation

Introduction

Direct intratracheal ventilation was used in Padua by the anatomist Andreas Vesalius in 1543 to avoid death due to pneumothorax in an animal, whose chest he had opened to study the heart [1]: 'But that so to speak life is maintained in the animal, an opening must be made in the trunk of the trachea, into which a tube of reed or cane should be inserted; you must then blow into this, so that the lung can rise again and the animal takes in air. Already with a slight breath, the living animal's lung will swell to the full extent of the thoracic cavity, and the heart becomes strong and shows a marvellous variety of motions. With the lung inflated once and a second time, you can examine the motion of the heart by sight and touch as much as you wish.'

Tracheal intubation in adults

In the 10th century C.E., Avicenna recommended to resuscitate drowned persons by 'inserting into the throat a cannula made of gold or silver and to blow into it' [2]. Given his canon's wide distribution, it can be assumed that tracheal intubation persisted for this indication for the following 600 years. In 1787, the Gravesend surgeon Charles Kite was awarded a silver medal from the Humane Society for his essay describing intubation in adults [3]: 'Should any further impediment occur, the crooked tube, bent like a male catheter, recommended by Dr Monro and mentioned by Mr Portal, Mr LeCat, and others, should be introduced into the glottis, through the mouth or the nostril; the end should be connected to a blow-pipe according to the plan mentioned in the description of a pocket-case of instruments for the recovery of the apparently dead by Mr Savigny.'

Monro and Portal were cited by Pagenstecher [4] to have invented endotracheal tubes for infants, but that information has been difficult to verify. William Smellie was given credit for describing endotracheal intubation in the neonate. However, the Sydenham reprint of his 1788 edition [5] suggests that he merely used a tube to ventilate the mouth, a technique not different from that applied by Mauriceau or Cangiamila: 'Sometimes a great many minutes are elapsed before it begins to breathe. Whatever augments the circulating force, promotes respiration; and as this increases, the circulation grows stronger, so that they mutually assist each other. In order to promote the one and the other, the child is kept warm, moved, shaken; whipt; the head, temples, and breast rubbed with spirits, garlic, onion, or mustard, applied to the mouth and nose; and the child has been sometimes recovered by blowing into the mouth with a silver cannula, so as to expand the lungs.'

Benjamin Pugh's 'air-pipe' was probably not inserted into the trachea [6]: He used the flexible tube (Fig. 2.4.1A) in prolonged breech delivery, 'introduced into the child's mouth, as near to the larynx as I could'. His report of 1754 sheds light on the lack of elastic materials: '[The air-pipe] is made of a small common wire, turned very close (in the manner of wire-springs), and covered with thin soft leather, one end is introduced up the palm of the hand, and between the fingers that are in the child's mouth, as far as the larynx, the other end external.' The London surgeon Michael Underwood, in 1784 [7], was aware of a blow-pipe without precisely stating that it should be introduced into the larynx: 'To these ends, I have depended above all upon blowing into the windpipe, through the mouth; which I am satisfied, may be more effectually done by the mouth of the assistant being placed immediately upon the child's, than by means of a blow-pipe; (although the air is, indeed, certainly less pure;) at the same time, preventing a premature return of the air, by the fingers of one hand placed at the angles of the mouth, and those of the other on each side of the nose. But I have sometimes imagined, that I might attribute much of my success not only to the *continuance* of this, but to the *manner* of doing it, by attempting to imitate *natural* respiration, by forcing out the air I have thrown in, by a strong pressure against the pit of the stomach.'

Intubation in newborns

Endotracheal intubation in the newborn was definitely used in neonates by the Copenhagen obstetrician Paul Scheel in 1798 [8]: 'Having

---

Reproduced with permission from Obladen, M. History of neonatal resuscitation. Part 3: Endotracheal intubation. *Neonatology*, 95:198–202. Copyright © 2009 S. Karger AG, Basel.

cleaned the throat (of mucus, with a feather or the little finger) we come to the trachea itself. I believe it is best evacuated with a syringe attached to a long flexible tube (e.g. Pickeli's catheter made of elastic resin), the diameter of which fits in the trachea. Once inserted and connected, it is with its help that the intratracheal liquid is evacuated by suctioning. Once that is finished, atmospheric air can be pushed into the lungs in the same manner without the danger of expanding the gastrointestinal tract with gas through the esophagus.'

Endotracheal intubation was introduced in the Paris Maternité by Francois Chaussier in 1806 [9]: 'The presented instrument [Fig. 2.4.1B] which we call sonde of the larynx or laryngeal tube, seems to meet all conditions required. Its construction is simple, its use not very difficult. It is a small conic metal tube (of silver or copper), 18 to 20 cm long, which by volume and form differs little from a urinary bladder sonde. Only it is somewhat flattened at the sides to avoid vacillating between the fingers, and to accommodate the elongated glottis opening. The thicker end is round and dilated to adapt to the lips or a bellow's pipe. The other end is smaller, flattened, and perforated on both sides by two eyes or oblong openings... At the curvature height a small transversal disc is welded which is perforated by several holes serving to fix a delicate soft sponge or, what we prefer, a more or less compressed slice of agaric or a small piece of buffalo skin. Because of its construction, the instrument adapts to the oblique cup of the larynx. It closes its opening precisely making sure that the inflated air cannot flow back but necessarily dilates the lungs.'

As reported by Madame Boivin [10], Chaussier propagated and taught all midwives in training how to use endotracheal tubes: 'Insufflating air into the lungs using a laryngeal tube, either by mouth, or by a little ventilator which can rapidly be adapted to it. During this operation, the infant's head and chest should be positioned somewhat elevated and breathing action should be imitated by gentle compression of the chest, letting the air escape which one has insufflated ... It resembles a urinary catheter; the tip, more curved, is introduced into the larynx entry, as the name indicates. This instrument, invented by Professor Chaussier, brought back to life many infants. It is in the hands of all midwives trained at the Maternité, and is sold in Paris by the cutler *Grangeret*, rue des St. Pères, suburb Saint-Germain.'

At Guy's Hospital, the obstetrician James Blundell disregarded the Paris Academy's ban and continued to use an endotracheal catheter, which he described in 1834 [11]: 'The only mode of performing this operation effectually is by means of a small instrument, the tracheal pipe, which I think every accoucheur should carry along with him to a labour. The tracheal pipe is a little tube of silver, designed to pass into the trachea, its end closed like a catheter, with a long, broad fissure on either side to give free vent to air and mucus. The closed extremity and lateral openings I prefer, as there is less risk of injuring the delicate membrane of the trachea, if a terminal aperture does not exist. In introducing this instrument there is some difficulty at first, if you do not manoeuvre rightly; yet every moment is of the greatest importance, for while you are blundering the child is dying. Now not to detain you needlessly, I may be allowed to observe, that my own method of operating is the following: I pass the fore-finger of my left hand down upon the roof of the tongue and into the rima glottidis, and then using the tube with the right hand, I slide it along the surface of the finger, used as a director, till reaching the rima. I insert the tube at the moment when the finger is with-drawn from it, afterwards feeling on the front of the neck whether the instrument is lying in the trachea or the oesophagus.'

Twelve years later and obviously under the influence of Leroy's anti-ventilation campaign [12, 13], the Paris paediatrician Bouchut

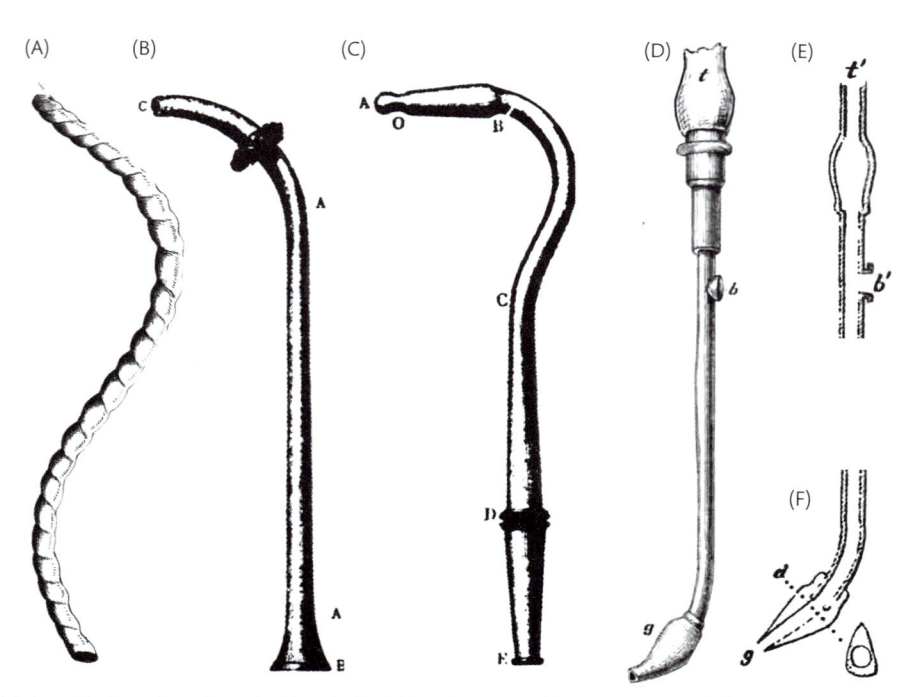

Fig. 2.4.1 Tubes for artificial ventilation of newborn babies. A, Pugh's leather-coated 'airpipe' of 1754 [6]; B, Chaussier's curved silver endotracheal tube of 1806, with stop-ring at larynx entry. [9]; C, Ribémont's modified silver tube of 1878; D, Trueheard's tube with conical tip for position at larynx entry or nostril, 1870 [28]; E, detail of D, the opening b is closed and opened intermittently to allow expiration; F, detail of D showing triangular diameter.

found endotracheal intubation more difficult [14]: 'Some authors recommend putting the mouth on that of the infant, and blowing into the deep pharynx. It is better to practise insufflation with a curved tube placed into the larynx. This operation must be performed with great caution, on the one hand to avoid a false position and to inflate the esophagus, on the other hand to avoid excessive dilation of the lungs and prevent pulmonary emphysema.'

Various endotracheal tubes were invented in Germany [15, 16]. The Krefeld obstetrician Hecking proposed intrauterine intubation and ventilation of the asphyctic yet unborn infant [15], truthfully admitting the absence of a control group in his 1827 study: 'After version (from breech position) I pushed this tube into the child's mouth and fixed it in this position; if a flame located in front of the tube's opening indicated no respiration within 2 or 3 minutes, I blew into it atmospheric air collected in my mouth. Several times I realized continuing in- and expiration up to the complete delivery of the infant … I must honestly confess that it is possible several infants would have been delivered alive without use of the instrument. I am convinced that with its use I saved 6 infants within 6 years and maintained their life.'

At Heidelberg in 1856, Pagenstecher still advocated artificial ventilation and used an insertion technique similar to Blundell's, despite acknowledging its drawbacks [4]: 'The consequences are profound: Even when the air does not enter the pleural cavity, where only unnatural communication with the lung exists, and the air so to speak crawls along the bronchi and the edges, severe symptoms appear. The respiring space shrinks, the healthy parts are squeezed, and the consequences of injury and inflammation are added on … Compared with mouth-to-mouth breathing, well-constructed tubes have the advantage of guiding the air more safely. They always cause considerable local irritation. They are best guided with an accompanying finger under the epiglottis, and then palpated externally at the larynx to assure their proper position. We admit that in some cases the resistance of epiglottis and glottis can only be overcome with the cannula … Deciding on the right measure to take here is not easy. One should not disturb the infant's own movements, not extinguish the faint spark, but also not interrupt for too long. When respiration is weak or slow but otherwise normal, ventilation cannot be recommended at all.'

Throughout the 19th century, neonates were intubated with the fingers. Following anatomic studies with frozen sections (Fig. 2.4.2), a sophisticated and more steeply curved laryngeal tube was proposed by Ribémont in 1878, which was easier to introduce and was attached to an India rubber balloon for ventilation [17].

In the US, artificial ventilation continued to be practised in addition to Schultze's swinging method. In 1870 and together with his mobile ventilator, Dr Trueheard of Galveston published a tube with a conical tip (lit) that could be inserted into the larynx entry or into a nostril (Fig. 2.4.1D–F). Joseph de Lee recommended in 1897 [18]: 'In the more severe cases (asphyxia livida) the deeper passages must be cleared, and this is best done by means of a soft woven catheter open at the end, No. 14 French. This little instrument ought to be found in the satchel of every obstetrical attendant. With a little practise its use becomes easy. The index finger of the left hand pulls the epiglottis forward and comes to touch the arytenoid cartilages. The catheter is then passed along the finger, the end is pulled against the posterior surface of the epiglottis with the finger, and is then pushed into the trachea with a gentle twisting motion of the right hand … Slapping on the back, cold water on the chest, the cold plunge-bath, are almost never necessary, and the latter two are distinctly harmful. In the severest cases (asphyxia pallida) the diagnostic criterion of which is the absence of reaction in the throat, this simple treatment does not suffice. One must waste no time with trying the skin reflexes, but immediately after the air passages are cleared artificial respiration must be begun. Of all the methods of artificial respiration only three have proven of service in my hands: Rhythmical compression of the chest, the Schultze swingings, and mouth-to-mouth insufflation with the tracheal catheter.'

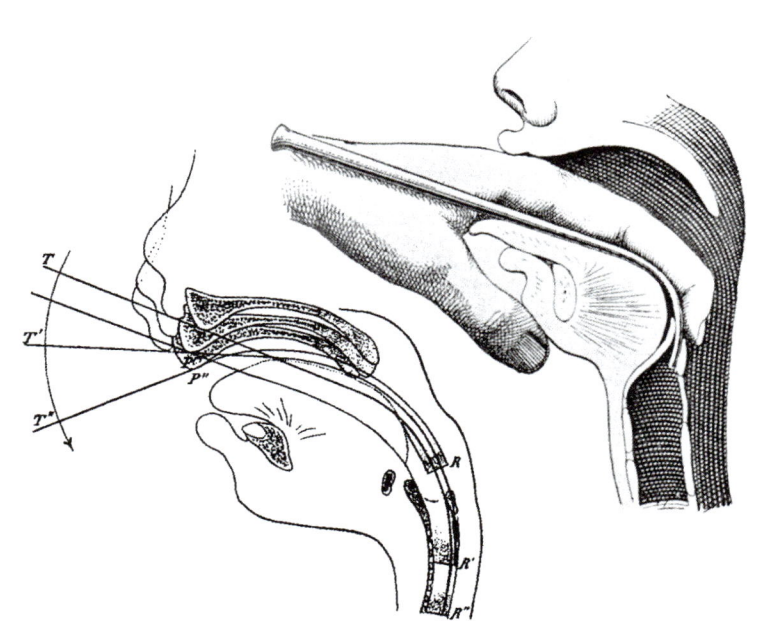

Fig. 2.4.2 Studies in frozen sections of the upper airway by Ribémont aiming to optimize the tube curvature and the insertion technique during finger intubation [17].

Modern developments: the laryngoscope

A wide variety of endotracheal tubes were developed in conjunction with the triumphal march of endotracheal anaesthesia in the 20th century. O'Dwyer recognized the need to build a device for the insertion of small metal tubes in children with croup [19], but a laryngoscope was not used. Nasotracheal intubation was reported by Kuhn in 1902 [20] (who also invented the self-inflating ventilation bag), and was popularized by Magill, who developed the intubation forceps in 1920 [21], still using the blind insertion technique.

In 1928, New York anaesthetist Paluel Flagg described a battery-powered infant laryngoscope with a straight blade [22]: 'The problem of scientific artificial respiration, both in infants and in adults, revolves on the ease with which the larynx may be exposed and intubated … The chief resistance to the popularization of laryngoscopy appears to be the uncertain function of the usual delicate electrical equipment commonly used for laryngeal and bronchial works. Laryngoscopy at the bedside, in the office, and in the ordinary emergency is well covered by ordinary pocket flashlight facilities, and, furthermore, permits of the use of the large lamp which seldom burns out. The author's baby speculum was constructed on data furnished by the new-born still-born infant and in babies in whom postpartum deaths had occurred within a few hours. The weight of the babies observed varied between 6 and 10 pounds (2.7 and 4.5 Kg.). The distance from the upper gums to the glottis averaged 2 1/2 inches (6.3 cm).'

Shortly thereafter, Richard Foregger developed and manufactured different types of infant laryngoscopes and endotracheal tubes [23], which initially were made of rubber.

Due to inherently high airway resistance in neonates, thin-walled tubes were needed, and some had to be reinforced with metal spirals to avoid kinking (Woodbridge) or were fitted with shoulders (Cole) or bulges (Loennecken) to prevent them from slipping down too deep. Endotracheal tubes were better tolerated by the tissue when rubber was replaced by polyvinyl chloride and later polyethylene or polyurethane. The history of anaesthesia equipment was compiled by Jackson [24], and the further specific development of endotracheal tubes was described in detail by White [25]. Barrie summarized the requirement for a endotracheal tube for neonates in 1963 [26]: 'The ideal endotracheal tube for infants is soft enough to do no injury, yet rigid enough to be unkinkable; it must maintain its curve so that it can be inserted with ease and without need for an introducer; its internal diameter must be large enough to allow perfect air-flow, yet its dead-space must be minimal; it must be suitable for babies weighing from as little as 2 lb. to as much as 10 lb.; it must be non-irritant, sterile, easily connected to standard equipment and preferably also cheap and disposable.' More recently, fibreoptic instruments have been developed but have not yet proven to be superior to rigid laryngoscopes [27].

Conclusion

The development of tissue-friendly endotracheal tubes suitable for neonates did not dramatically change the treatment of birth asphyxia, but they proved indispensable to progress in neonatal intensive care and long-term ventilation. Regarding neonatal asphyxia, it remains unclear whether initial resuscitation is better performed with mask and bag or with an endotracheal tube, and if tubes are better applied orally or nasally. As elegantly mentioned by Underwood in 1801 [5], all these techniques require great dexterity, skill, and exercise, all of which are variable and unequally distributed among staff in the delivery room. The difficulty in adjusting for these variables offers a key explanation as to why valid scientific studies on endotracheal intubation have been lacking in the more than 200 years since it was first taught to Parisian midwifes.

REFERENCES

1. Vesalius A: De humani corporis fabrica. Lib. VII Cap. XIX: De vivorum sectione nonnulla. Basel: Oporinus, 1543: p. 658 (recte 662).
2. Avicenna: Liber canonis Avicennae revisus et ab omni errore purgatus. Venetiis: Heredum Octaviani Scoti, 1505: Vol. **3**, p. Fol. 237r.
3. Kite C: An essay on the recovery of the apparently dead. London: Dilly, 1788: p. 146.
4. Pagenstecher HA: Über das Lufteinblasen zur Rettung scheintodter Neugeborner. Heidelberg: Mohr, 1856: p. 47–50.
5. Smellie W: A treatise on the theory and practise of midwifery. London: Sydenham Society, 1878: Vol. **1**, p. 226.
6. Pugh B: A treatise of midwifery, chiefly with regard to the operation. London: Buckland, 1754: p. 48–51, 133.
7. Underwood M: A treatise on the disorders of childhood, and management of infants from the birth (1st ed. London 1784). 2. ed. London: Matthews, 1801: Vol. **1**, p. 13, 91.
8. Scheel P: Dissertation inauguralis de liquore amnii asperae arteriae foetuum humanorum. Hafniae: Brummer, 1798: p. 60.
9. Chaussier F: Proces-verbaux des distributions des prix, faites aux elèves sages-femmes de la Maternité, 1805–1824. Paris: Archives de l'Assistance publique de Paris, 1806: Vol. Cote 678, FOSS 1, Liasse 678, p. 54–113.
10. Boivin MAV: Mémorial de l'art des accouchements. 3. ed. Paris: Méquignon, 1824: p. 397.
11. Castle T: The principles and practise of obstetricy as at present taught by James Blundell. London: Cox, 1834: p. 246–50.
12. Leroy d'Etiolles JJ: Second mémoire sur l'asphyxie. J Physiol Exp Path 1828;**8**:97–135.
13. Magendie F, Duméril AMC: Rapport sur un mémoire de M. Leroy d'Etioles, relatif a l'insufflation du poumon. J Chim Med Pharm Tox, Paris 1829;**5**:335–44.
14. Bouchut E: Manuel pratique des maladies des nouveau-nés et des enfants à la mamelle. Paris: Baillière, 1845: p. 384.
15. Hecking P: Abbildung und Gebrauch eines von mir erfundenen Luftleiters. Crefeld: Schüller, 1827: p. 79.
16. Hüter V: Die Katheterisation der Luftröhre bei asphyctisch geborenen Kindern. Mschr Geburtsh Gynäk 1863;**21**:123–51.
17. Ribémont A: Recherches sur l'insufflation des nouveau-nés et description d'un nouveau tube laryngien. Progrès Médical 1878;**16**:293–5; 17:316–7; 19:355–7; 20:376–8: 21:395–6.
18. De Lee J: Asphyxia neonatorum: causation and treatment. Medicine (Detroit) 1897;**3**:643–60.
19. O'Dwyer JP: Intubation of the larynx. New York Med J 1885;**42**:145–7.
20. Kuhn F: Die pernasale Tubage. München Med Wochenschr 1902;**49**:1456.

21. Magill IW: Forceps for intratracheal anaesthesia. BMJ 1920;**II**:670.
22. Flagg PJ: Treatment of asphyxia in the newborn. JAMA 1928;**91**:788–91.
23. Foregger R: Richard von Foregger, 1872–1960. Manufacturer of anesthesia equipment. Anesthesiology 1996;**84**:190–200.
24. Jackson DE: Anesthesia equipment from 1914 to 1954 and experiments leading to its development. Anesthesiology 1955;**16**:953–61.
25. White GMJ: Evolution of endotracheal and endobronchial intubation. Br J Anaesth 1960;**32**:235–46.
26. Barrie H: Resuscitation of the newborn. Lancet 1963;**I**:650–5.
27. Roth AG, Wheeler M, Stevenson GW, Hall SC: Comparison of a rigid laryngoscope with the ultrathin fiberoptic laryngoscope for tracheal intubation in infants. Can J Anaesth 1994;**41**:1069–73.
28. Trueheard: Ein Apparat zur künstlichen Respiration bei Asphyxie. Beitr Geburtsh Gynäk (Berlin) 1872;**I**:154–6.

2.5
Umbilical cord and umbilical care

Introduction

The navel is the human body's centrepiece. Its life-sustaining function before birth was well known, as was its life-robbing dysfunction in cord coiling, entangling, prolapse, or rupture [1]. Adriaan Spieghel detected the two-directional blood flow within the umbilical cord in 1626 [2]. It is no wonder the umbilicus and navel-string were considered living parts of the infant's body, or a living being, the child's brother or sister, or that they were mystified in multiple ways and in many societies. Bewailing the fate of Jerusalem, the prophet Ezekiel reported around 486 B.C.E. [Ezekiel 16:4–6]: 'As for thy nativity, in the day thou wast born thy navel was not cut, neither wast thou washed in water to supple thee … None eye pitied thee, to do any of these unto thee, to have compassion upon thee; but thou wast cast out in the open field, to the loathing of thy person … polluted in thine own blood.'

Cutting the navel-string symbolized the transit from intra- to extrauterine life, was associated with wound and pain, and elicited multiple rites and superstitions. Focusing on umbilical infection, this chapter describes techniques of cutting and ligating the navel-string and caring for the stump. It omits anatomy, embryology, and malformations of the navel which have been described [3]; and umbilical haemorrhage which is addressed in Chapter 7.1.

Omphalos, centre of the world

In various societies and epochs, sacred stones were venerated as designating the centre of the world, as the earth was believed to be a round disc. Many peoples kept, in their own territory, an *omphalos* or *regio media* (navel or centre of the earth), consecrated and believed to confer protection. The Gauls had the *Carnutes*' land, the Irish Celts the *Ushriagh* hill [4]. Jews believed the sacred space in the Jerusalem temple to be Jahweh's resting place, located on a site representing the navel of the earth [5]. The most venerated *omphalos* in the Greek world was a conoidal marble decorated with bands, associated with Apollo's temple in Delphi, and located close to Pythia's tripod where the oracles were announced [6]. Etruscan omphalos bowls with large hemispherical navels were in fashion from the 8th to 5th century B.C.E., possibly used as incense burners in a ritual context [7].

Cutting and ligating the cord

Tying and cutting the navel-string is an almost universal human behaviour, separating mother and child both physically and symbolically. This is remarkable, as animals don't bother much about the navel-string: the mother animals tear or gnaw it off, even in species that are strict vegetarians. Human neonates are functionally less mature than most other mammal infants and cannot walk at birth, making it difficult to get rid of the cord with the placenta attached. A major goal of ligating was therefore to prevent fatal haemorrhage. However, haemorrhage occurs seldom even when the cord is not ligated [8], and crushing the cord stops bleeding more effectively than cutting the vessels. In the Hippocratic world, the cord was not severed before the placenta was born [9]; the need for ligating the cord was mentioned by Aristotle [10].

The customs of ligating and cutting the cord most probably evolved among humans for cultural and ritual purposes rather than health aspects. It was meant to honour, support, or maintain the mother's compassionate connection with her child after birth. Soranus of Ephesus, whose words remained highly influential up to the 18th century, wrote in the 2nd century in Rome [11]: 'One must cut off the navel cord at a distance of four fingerbreadths from the abdomen, by means of something sharp-edged, that no bruising may arise. And of all material, iron cuts best; but the majority of the midwives approve of the section by means of glass, a reed, a potsherd, or the thin crust of bread; or by forcefully squeezing it apart with a cord, since during the earliest period, cutting with iron is deemed of ill omen.'

Since antiquity, highly varied techniques of cutting the umbilical cord evolved, and instead of knives or scissors, living materials such as biological products, plant leaves, breadcrust, mussel shells, or wooden saws were used to severe the cord, as were natural products such as plant fibres or sinews to tie it, some before, some after expulsion of the placenta (Table 2.5.1). These materials often were contaminated with bacteria or spores, which explains the high incidence of omphalitis and neonatal tetanus in olden times.

In 1709, Veit Riedlin, city physician of Ulm, was expert witness in a malpractice trial against a midwife accused 'of having ligated the umbilical cord too close to the belly, constricting part of the abdominal skin … she defended the mistake as having resulted not from ignorance or neglect, but from poor vision' [1]. Today, we can scarcely imagine how dark it was in 18th century cottages with their tiny

Table 2.5.1 Examples of cutting instruments and umbilical cord care during the 18th and 19th century, by regions

Region/country	Cord care	Stump care
Europe		
England	Hollister clamp	Covering with zinc powder or starch
France	Ligation not before infant cries. Longer cord for boys to promote penis growth	Cord preserved for long time
Germany	Ligation with linen band. Midwives ordered to carry rounded scissors	Abdomen binding. Franconia: stump kept for several years, then fed to child
Africa		
North Africa	Crushing with stones, broken glass, used razor blade	Morocco: stump sewed into cushion to protect against the devil
Central Africa	Cutting with palm leave-stalk or blade of grass	Petroleum jelly, human milk, ash (black powder)
South Africa	Ligation with a sinew	Cow dung poultices
America		
North America	Cutting with obsidian fragment	Belly bands
Mexico	Thread tying, cutting with candle-heated scissors	Carbonized with candle. Grease application
South America	Crushing with a stone, cutting with mussel shell	Ash or fishbone powder
Asia and Australia		
India	Wooden knife or saw. Ligated with woollen thread	Stump rubbed with musk
Bangladesh/Pakistan	Cutting with bamboo slip, tying with a thread	Repeated application of *ghee* (clarified butter)
Nepal	Blades of grass, bark, fibres, reeds	
China/Vietnam	Cutting with a piece of porcelain	Stump buried in a special jar, retaining the child at this location
Japan	Broken piece of pottery	Oak-gall powder
New Zealand/Central Australia	Knot in navel-string; cut with a shell; ligation with flax	Stump swathed in fur-string, worn as amulet around child's neck
Papua New Guinea	Sharp-edged shell	Mother ties string at net in which baby is carried

Data compiled from Kolb 1731 [16], Engelmann 1884 [18], Frazer 1890 [19], Ploss 1902 [8], Roscher 1913 [20], Buschan 1941 [21], Romney 1963 [22], Traverso 1989 [17], and Dhingra 2014 [23].

windows and candlelight. Joseph Raulin, obstetrician in Paris, described the procedure in 1770: [12]: 'Take three or four wax-coated threads, make a knot on each end, wind them around the navel-cord and make a double knot. The threads must be pulled together to stop the bleeding, but not too tightly to avoid inflammation … Very thin umbilical cords are better ligated with a broad linen bandage, which does not cut into the cord tissue.'

The Regensburg midwives' order detailed the same practice in 1779 [13]: 'She must bring a round, sharp scissors and several wax-coated strings, or small linen bands.' All practices were influenced by superstition. Most recent is the Lotus birth [14], in which the umbilical cord is not cut and the placenta remains attached to the baby, covered with herbs to suppress the smell.

Care of the umbilical stump

Historically, many methods of caring for the umbilical stump were propagated, varying widely according to culture, ritual, and location. They were certainly associated with postpartum infection, at all times leading cause of infant mortality worldwide. Soranus recounted the Roman habit in the 2nd century C.E. [11]: 'Most women burn and grind the ankle-bone of a pig … and sprinkle this over while others use lead which has been heated and washed … Since the material is cooling, the wound will cicatrize and since it is heavy, the umbilicus will be properly moulded into a cavity.' Avicenna, teaching in Persia during the 11th century C.E. [15], proposed: 'The umbilical cord should be severed four fingers' breadth from the umbilicus after it has been well but gently tied with a clean woollen ligature, so as to inflict no pain, and that an oiled cloth should be placed upon it. To help the separation of the cord, apply equal parts of the following: turmeric, dragon's blood, Persian gum, caraway, sweet scented moss, myrrh. These are ground together and applied.'

In 1731, Peter Kolb reported from the South African Khoi-San [16]: 'If a Child is born alive, the First Thing they do is to rub it gently all over with fresh Cow-Dung. They say, 'tis dangerous to wash it with warm water … The Child's Navel String is tied with a Sheep's sinew, so long that it hangs down a considerable Length below the Knot: And there it is to remain till it rots off. The Belly-Band for the Keeping down of the Navel is a narrow Piece of Sheep-Skin.'

In case the navel-string was torn off, the Regensburg midwives' order of 1779 mandated 'she should moisten a strong swab with vinegar, insert a coin, place it on the navel and fix it with a bandage until the surgeon arrives'. A similar procedure was used in India to prevent umbilical hernia. Table 2.5.1 shows how difficult it was for midwives and mothers to refrain from manipulating the umbilical stump. They applied substances like ash, zinc powder, ground pig- or fishbones, oak-gall powder, grease, musk, and others. Oily materials such as petroleum jelly, or *ghee* [clarified butter] were especially dangerous as they blocked the access of oxygen to the wound [17].

Even in today's rational times and in developed countries there is little consensus on how to handle the umbilical cord after birth. In

Britain, dry care exists besides time-honoured binding with Steret or Ster-Zac [24]. In the US, cord care includes alcohol application, triple dye, and a belly band taped over the navel [25]. Randomized trials on topical cord care were conducted. In developed countries, no difference in systemic infections appeared between cords treated with antiseptics compared with dry cord care [26]. The American Academy of Pediatrics recommended in 2016 that 'in resource-limited populations, the application of prophylactic antimicrobials to the umbilical cord remains appropriate' [27].

Spontaneous cord separation

Under normal circumstances, the cord dries by mummification and is sloughed off like a foreign body. In this process, immigrating white blood cells and reactive inflammation of the lymph vessels play a major role, as demonstrated by Herzog in 1891 [28] (Fig. 2.5.1). With 'Western' cord care (alcohol cleansing and daily triple-dye), the cord stump separated at a mean age of 13 days after vaginal, and 16 days after Caesarean delivery [29].

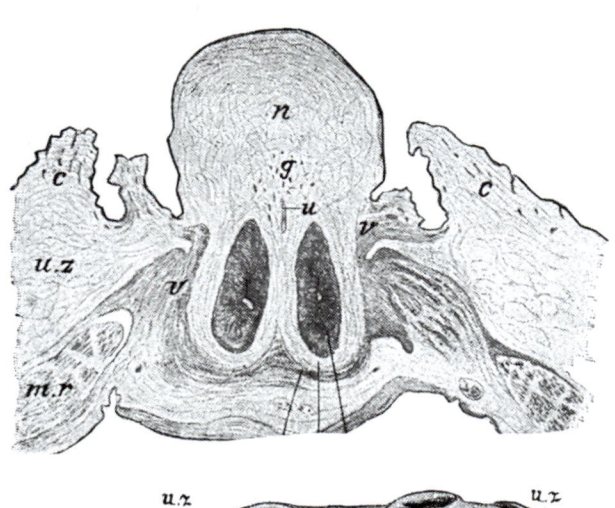

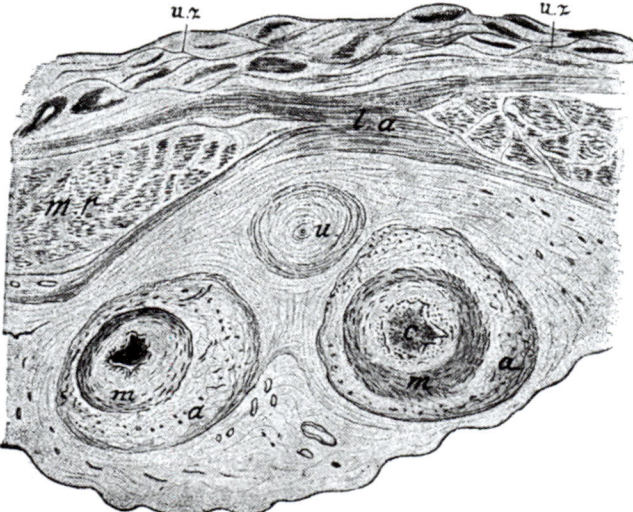

Fig. 2.5.1 Histology of severing, cuts through abdominal wall, depicted by Herzog in 1891 [28]. Top: at birth, entry of arteries into the umbilical cord. Bottom: 4 weeks of age, cut 2 cm below the navel.

Neonatal omphalitis

Before bacteria became known to cause infection [30], the hygienic conditions of cord care were usually poor, and omphalitis was frequent. In the Vienna Foundling Hospital, Alois Bednar characterized its symptoms in 1853 [31] and, also in Vienna, Hermann Widerhofer distinguished in 1862 superficial inflammation (excoriation), mucus effusion (blenorrhoe), granulating inflammation (fungus), deep inflammation (omphalitis, Fig. 2.5.2), and lethal omphalitis once the peritoneum is affected. Heinrich Finkelstein, Berlin, described two progressing vascular forms of deep navel infection [32]: local purulent thrombosis of the umbilical arteries (Fig. 2.5.3, left) and infection advancing via the lymphatic vessels, which he termed periarteriitis umbilicalis (Fig. 2.5.3, right). All deep infections could invade the bloodstream leading to sepsis (see Chapter 7.9).

Neonatal tetanus

An unusual type of infection was transmitted by anaerobic bacteria that produced a neurotoxin acting on the spinal cord and suppressing relaxation which led to terrible spasms and painful contractions. Its mortality approached 100%. *Clostridium tetani* and its spores are found ubiquitously in soil and manure, and are unlikely to be eradicated. Devastating epidemics of neonatal tetanus occurred on remote tropical islands, where age-old customs persisted well into the 19th century. Tetanus was a nightmare among Caribbean infants born into slavery. Jean-Louis Fourcroy, artillery officer in St. Domingue (now Haiti, then a profitable French colony producing sugar and indigo),

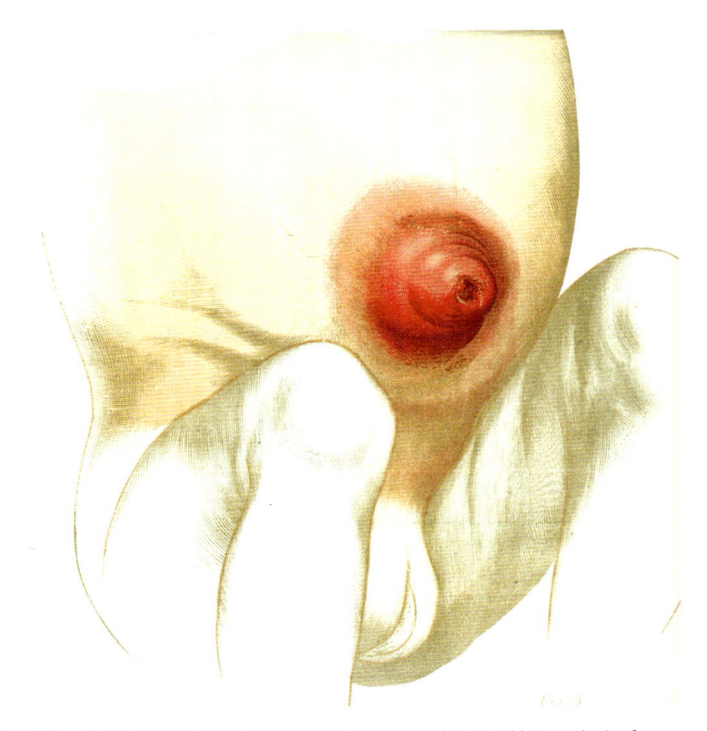

Fig. 2.5.2 Omphalitis with deep phlegmone depicted by Widerhofer in 1862 [47]. Note infant's flexed knees to relieve tension in the abdominal wall.

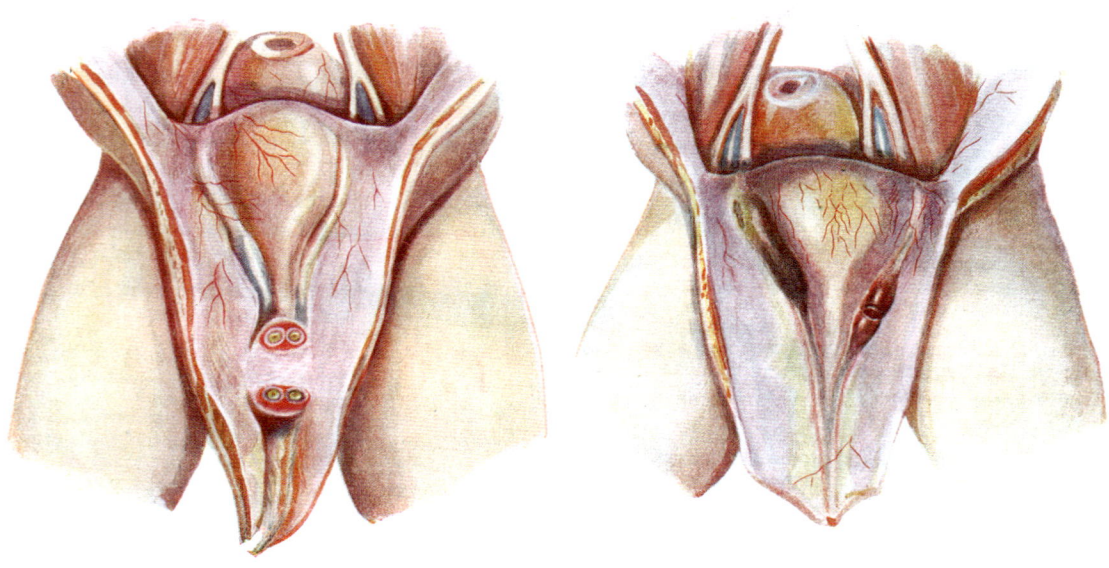

Fig. 2.5.3 Deep navel infections, depicted by Finkelstein in 1921 [32]. Left: purulent thrombosis of umbilical arteries. Right: inflammation of arteries and lymphatic vessels.

reported [33]: 'When I arrived in 1744, infants could not be raised in the Cap François Plane: nearly all of them, precisely 80%, died of a disease called *mal de mâchoire* [lockjaw] or *tetanos*, which carried them away within nine days after birth, even though all Negro mothers breastfed their infants.' Epidemics of neonatal tetanus were described in Menorca 1751 [34], and in Guinea and other parts of Africa in 1778 [35]. In 1784, Jean-Jacques Gardanne ascribed lockjaw in the newborn 'to the mothers imagination and lifestyle during pregnancy ... without excluding excessive ligation of the cord or other irritant cause' [36]. Joseph Clarke, master of the Dublin Lying-in Hospital, reported in 1789 [37]: 'At the conclusion of the year 1782, of 17,650 infants born alive, 2,944 died within the first fortnight ... The disease which carried off most of these children, perhaps nineteen of twenty, was general convulsions, or what our nurse-tenders have been long in the habit of calling the nine-day fits ... twisting of the upper extremities while awake ... screwing and gathering of the mouth into a purse ... irregular contractions and relaxations of their muscular frame ... the jaws locked from the commencement, so as to prevent the actions of sucking and swallowing.'

In 1812, the British physician Henry Holland after a voyage to Iceland [38] described 'a singular disease, eminently disastrous, called *Ginklofe* by the Icelanders: the Tetanus or Trismus Neonatorum of medical writers ... The population of the [small island of Heimaey] does not amount at present to 200 souls, and is almost entirely supported by migration from the mainland; scarcely a single instance having been known, during the last twenty years, of a child surviving the period of infancy ... Very soon after birth, strabismus and rolling of the eyes are observed; the sinews contract, and the muscles of the back are drawn together and stiffened ... *trismus* [lockjaw] generally comes on sometimes attended by *Opisthotonus* ... the infant is speedily carried off ... [During] a period of twenty-five years, 184 infants died [on Heimaey island] upon this disease, most frequently on the 7th day of life.'

In 1817, Abraham Colles of Dublin, after many 'careful dissections of children which had died of locked jaw' established the identity of *trismus nascentium* (neonatal tetanus) and *trismus traumaticus* of adults, and demonstrated umbilical infection as the former's cause [39]. At the St. Petersburg Foundling Hospital [40], Philipp Doepp observed from 1830 to 1833 'around 20 infants affected by trismus per year, and I must confess that I could not save a single one ... sucking becomes impossible early, because the mouth remains immobile and half-open due to the upper lip contracted in folds. The resulting facial expression is unmistakable for those who ever witnessed it.'

The anaerobic pathogen *Clostridium tetani* was detected in 1884 [41], the protective effect of passively transferred antitoxin was demonstrated in 1897 [42], and in 1924, Pierre Descombey detoxified tetanus bacteria with formaldehyde and developed a highly effective vaccine [43]. In 1961, Newell and co-workers started a randomized, double-blind field trial in a rural area of Colombia suffering a high tetanus rate: in 341 fully immunized mothers, the infants' tetanus death rate was zero, whereas in the unimmunized control group it was 8% [44]. Also, a meta-analysis in 2015 confirmed if the mother was immunized before or during pregnancy, her antibodies protected the infant [45]. Thanks to preventive immunization and improved obstetric care, the gruesome disease virtually disappeared from developed countries, but the case fatality rate remained around 85% and tremendous differences persisted between developed and developing regions in the world. Neonatal tetanus is vastly underreported and 24 countries have not yet eliminated the disease. Following repeated World Health Organization campaigns, the number of newborns dying from tetanus dropped from 800,000 in the year 1987 to 58,000 in 2010 [46].

Conclusion

The navel-string was considered a living part of the infant's body and treated with great scrutiny and poor hygiene. Since antiquity, the superstition that the cord not be cut with an iron knife caused a myriad of unclean and dangerous practices. As in all retrospective diagnoses, and as remarked in the confusion of difficult teething and infantile scurvy (see Chapter 7.6), caution is needed: in some cases, especially in survivors, tetanus may have been confused with tetany, a frequent and usually non-lethal metabolic condition caused by low calcium concentration in blood, which leads to jitteriness and increased muscle tone. Navel tetanus was conquered by improved hygiene and public health policies including immunization and educational programmes. In developing countries, umbilical infections remained a significant problem.

REFERENCES

1. Riedlin V: Curarum medicarum millenarius. Ulm: Kuhn, 1709: p. 467.
2. Spieghel A: De formato foetu liber singularis. Patavii: de Martinis, 1626: p. 18–22, plate 7.
3. Fahmy M: Umbilicus and umbilical cord. New York: Springer, 2018.
4. Loth J: La croyance a l'omphalos chez les Celtes. Compt Rend Acad des Inscriptions et Belles-Lettres 1914;**58**:481–2.
5. Terrien S: The omphalos myth and Hebrew religion. Vetus Testamentum 1970;**20**:315–38.
6. Scott M: Delphi: a history of the center of the ancient world. Princeton, NJ: Princeton University Press, 2014: p. 10–39.
7. Cook BF: A class of Etruscan bronze omphalos-bowls. Am J Archaeol 1968;**72**:337–44.
8. Ploss H: Das Weib in der Natur- und Völkerkunde. 7. ed. Leipzig: Grieben, 1902: Vol. **2**, p. 206–24.
9. Hippocrates: De morbis mulierum. Foesius A: Francofurti: Andreas Wecheli, 1596: p. 659, 685.
10. Aristotle: History of animals. Loeb Classical Library 439. Cambridge, MA: Harvard University Press, 1991: Vol. **7**, p. 587a9.
11. Temkin O: Soranus' Gynecology. Baltimore, MD: The Johns Hopkins Press, 1956: p. 79–117.
12. Raulin J: Von Erhaltung der Kinder (1st French ed. 1768). Leipzig: Crusius, 1769: Vol. **2**, p. 10–7.
13. Regensburgische: Erneuerte und vermehrte Hebammenordnung. Regensburg: Montag, 1779: p. 20–4.
14. Monroe KK, Rubin A, Mychaliska KP, et al.: Lotus birth: a case series report on umbilical nonseverance. Clin Pediatr 2019;**58**:88–94.
15. Gruner OC: A treatise on the canon of medicine of Avicenna, incorporating a translation of the first book. London: Luzac & Co., 1930: p. 363.
16. Kolb P: The present state of the Cape of Good-Hope (1st German ed. 1719). London: Innys, 1731: p. 139–46.
17. Traverso HP, Kahn AJ, Rahim H, et al.: Ghee application to the umbilical cord: a risk factor for neonatal tetanus. Lancet 1989;**333**:486–8.
18. Engelmann GJ: Die Geburt bei den Urvölkern. Wien: Braumüller, 1884: p. 171–5.
19. Frazer JG: The magic art and the evolution of kings. In: The golden bough (1st ed. 1890). London: Macmillan, 1963: Vol. **1**, p. 182–201.
20. Roscher WH: Omphalos. Leipzig: Teubner, 1913: p. 6–30.
21. Buschan G: Über Medizinzauber und Heilkunst im Leben der Völker. Berlin: Arnold, 1941: p. 538–47.
22. Romney K, Romney R: The Mixtecans of Juxtlahuaca, Mexico. New York: Wiley, 1966: p. 89–95.
23. Dhingra U, Gittelsohn J, Suleiman AM, et al.: Delivery, immediate newborn and cord care practices in Pemba, Tanzania. BMC Pregnancy Childbirth 2014;**14**:173.
24. Salariya EM, Kowbus NM: Variable umbilical cord care. Midwifery 1988;**4**:70–6.
25. Perry DS: The umbilical cord: transcultural care and customs. J Nurse Midwifery 1982;**27**:25–30.
26. Zupan J, Garner P, Oman AA: Topical umbilical cord care at birth. Cochrane Database Syst Rev 2004;**3**:CD001057.
27. Stewart D, Benitz W: Umbilical cord care in the newborn infant. Pediatrics 2016;**138**:e20162149.
28. Herzog W: Die Rückbildung des Nabels und der Nabelgefässe. München: Lehmann, 1891: p. 21–32, figs. 10 and 18.
29. Novack AH, Mueller B, Ochs H: Umbilical cord separation in the normal newborn. Am J Dis Child 1988;**142**:220–3.
30. Pasteur L: La théorie des germes et ses applications a la médicine et a la chirurgie. Bull Acad Nat Med, 2e série 1878;**7**:166–7.
31. Bednar A: Die Krankheiten der Neugeborenen und Säuglinge. Wien: Gerold, 1853: Vol. **3**, p. 173.
32. Finkelstein H: Lehrbuch der Säuglingskrankheiten. 2. ed. Berlin: Springer, 1921: p. 161–3.
33. Fourcroy JL: Les enfans élevés dans l'ordre de la nature. Paris: Frères Estienne, 1774: p. 61–2, 302–5.
34. Cleghorn G: Observations on the epidemical diseases in Minorca. London: Wilson, 1751.
35. Ackermann JC: Abhandlung über die Kenntnis und Heilung des Trismus oder des Kinnbackenzwanges. Nürnberg: Bauer, 1778: p. 29–42.
36. Gardanne JJ: Des maladies des créoles en Europe. Paris: Valade, 1784: p. 176–7.
37. Clarke J: An account of a disease which, until lately, proved fatal to a great number of infants in the Lying-In Hospital of Dublin. Trans Roy Irish Acad 1789;**3**:89–109.
38. Holland H: On the diseases of the Icelanders. Appendix to: Mackenzie GS: Travels in the Island of Iceland. 2. ed. Edinburgh: Constable, 1812: p. 404–6.
39. Colles A: On the cause of the disease termed trismus nascentium. Dublin Hosp Rep 1817;**1**:285–91.
40. Doepp P: Bemerkungen über einige Krankheiten der Säuglinge. Analekt Kinderkrankh 1835;**1**:150–68.
41. Nicolaier A: Über infectiösen Tetanus. Dtsch Med Wochenschr 1884;**1**:842–4.
42. Nocard E: Serum therapy of tetanus, experimental and clinical researches. Recueil de Medicine Veterinaire 1897;**21**:453–62.
43. Descombey P: L'anatoxine tétanique. Compt Rend Soc Biol 1924;**91**:239–41.
44. Newell KW, Duenas Lehmann A, Leblanc DR, Garces Osorio N: The use of toxoid for the prevention of tetanus neonatorum. Bull World Health Org 1966;**35**:863–71.
45. Demicheli V, Barale A, Rivetti A: Vaccines for women to prevent neonatal tetanus. Cochrane Database Syst Rev 2015;**2**:CD002959.
46. Thwaites CL, Beeching NJ, Newton CR: Maternal and neonatal tetanus. Lancet 2015;**385**:362–70.
47. Widerhofer H: Die Krankheiten am Nabel des Neugeborenen. Jahrb Kinderheilk 1862;**5**:181–212.

2.6

Postverta, Agrippa, Caesarea
Born feet-first

Introduction

The frequency of breech delivery is 3% among singletons at full term. In babies born prematurely it is up to 25% [1, 2]. Breech is a normal presentation during the early phases of pregnancy. Why spontaneous intrauterine version occurs is not well understood: the process involves fetal movements, amniotic fluid volume, and the maternal pelvis diameter. The following chapter deals with this presentation's dangers for the child and with protective strategies developed by midwives and obstetricians through history.

Hindu medicine

In the Hindu textbook *Susruta Samhita* (600 B.C.E.), chapter 15 explained how to extract a fetus from the breech position [3]. When the fetus could not be extracted, the following mantra had to be uttered: 'O thou beautiful damsel, may the divine ambrosia and the Moon god with Chitrabhánu and the celestial horsemen Uchchaih-Sravas take their residence in thy room; may this water-begotten nectar, help thee, O lady, in swiftly casting off thy womb.' The text specifies: 'In the case of leg presentation the [dead] fetus should be drawn downward by pulling its legs … in full breech presentation the buttocks should be first pressed and lifted up and then the fetus should be drawn downwards by the legs.' After the warning 'surgical operations should not be made if the fetus could be detected alive in the womb', the text explains how to sever the fetal skull, and dismember and extract the fetus with the hook.

Greece: somersault theory

Hippocratic authors (5th century B.C.E.) regarded the fetal version from the breech into the vertex position a traumatic process [4]: in the eighth month, the fetus suffers the 'intrauterine disease … The fetal precipitation from breech into vertex presentation is most dangerous' (Fig. 2.6.1). Assumed fetal trauma initiated the enduring theory that preterm infants of 7 months' gestation have better chances than those of 8 months' gestation. Even though never proven, the doctrine of the traumatic fetal version persisted, and as late as 1766, Royal accoucheur André Levret wrote [5]: 'One must admit that in certain circumstances the *culbute* [somersault] is dangerous.' Albrecht von Haller's *Génération* of 1774 [6] stated: 'Towards the seventh or eighth month, the fetus hurls himself into the pelvis and presents his head to the uterine mouth … It is this fall of the head into the pelvis that causes the woman's belly to drop at the end of pregnancy.' For delivery from double footling presentation, the author of the Hippocratian work 'de superfetatione' offered little practical help [7]: 'When both legs come into view and remain there, but there is no progress on either side, employ a vapour-bath by which the uterus will be moistened.' The book 'Of women's diseases' provided more specific instructions how to turn and deliver the fetus from various breech and footling positions [8] and the book 'Excision of the fetus' described embryotomy in detail [9].

Rome: Postverta and Agrippa

Pliny the elder (23–79 C.E.) cautioned [10]: 'It is contrary to nature for children to come into the world with their feet first, for which reason such children are called *Agrippae*, meaning that they are born with difficulty.' The Romans used to perpetuate the birth history in the *cognomen* (middle name) as in: *Felix*, *Fortunatus* (survived a difficult birth); *Lucius* (born at sunrise); *Caesar* (cut out from the dead mother's womb); *Opiter* (born after the father's death); *Geminus /Gemellus* (born as a twin); *Vopiscus* (surviving twin, the other deceased before birth), and so on [11]. In addition to *Juno Lucina*, the protectress of childbirth, Romans relied on the goddesses *Carmentes*, who presided over births depending on the infant's presentation: *Anteverta* (Proverta, Prorsa) for cephalic, *Postverta* (Porrima) for breech delivery, as described by Aulus Gellius (130–170 C.E.) [12]: 'They at whose birth the feet appeared before the head, which is the most difficult and dangerous mode of delivery, are called *Agrippa*, from *aegritudo* [difficulty] … When, contrary to nature they are turned upon their feet, and retained in the womb, with their arms extended, women are delivered with great difficulty … For the purpose of deprecating this calamity, altars were erected at Rome, near the two temples of *Carmentes*, one of which was called *Postverta*, the other *Pro[r]sa*, from the different power and names of the different births, natural and the contrary.'

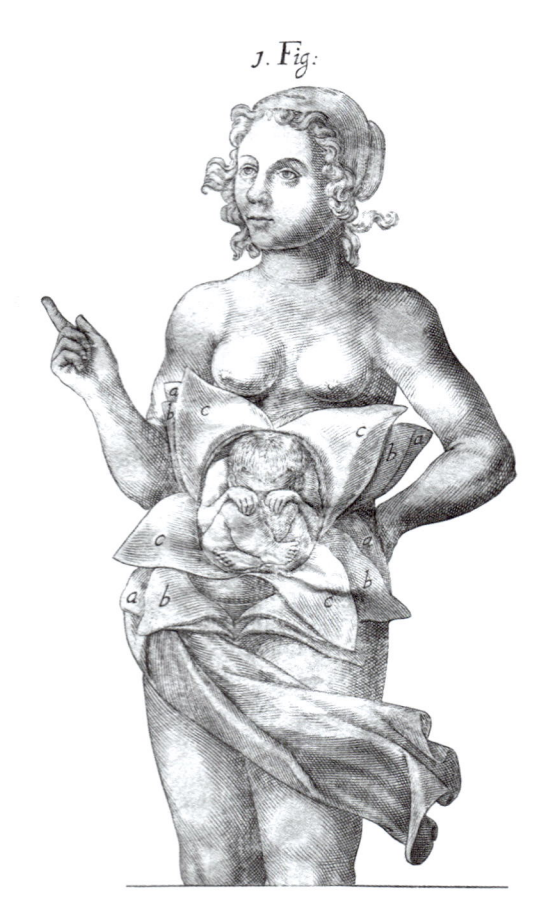

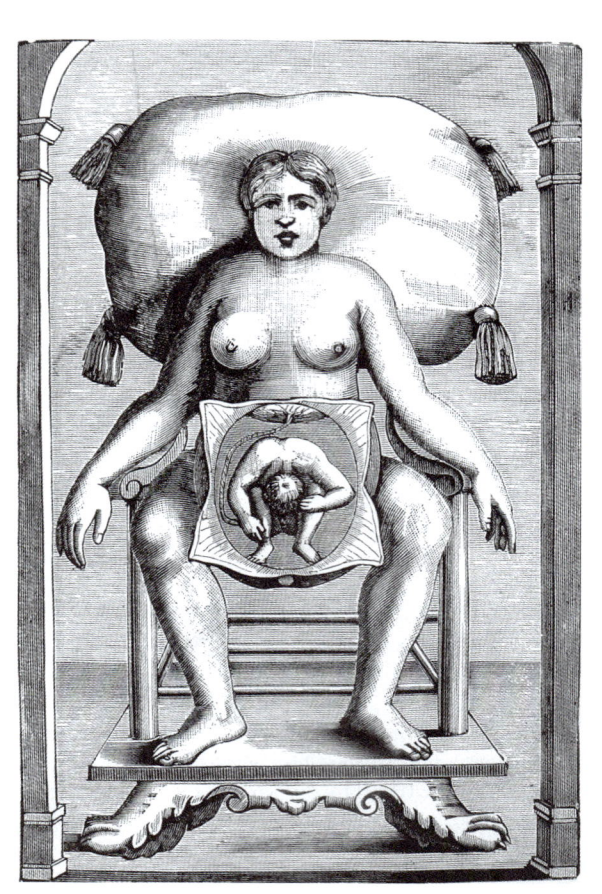

Fig. 2.6.1 Left: typical fetal breech position in early pregnancy, depicted in a crosswise dissected pregnant woman by Scipio Mercurio in 1671 [55]; a, abdominal wall; b, uterine wall; c, fetal membranes. Right: the 'somersault' (*culbute*) of the fetus believed to occur during the eighth month of gestation, depicted by an unknown author around 1766 [56].

Soranus (2nd century C.E.) classified various forms of breech presentation [13]: 'Women have difficult labor in whom the fetus does not present by the head but by the feet, or is doubled up upon the hips or side.' After describing podalic version in the various types of breech presentation, he continued: 'If the fetus does not respond to manual traction, because of its size, or death, or impaction in any manner, one must proceed to the more forceful methods, those of extraction by hooks and embryotomy.'

Middle Ages and podalic version

In the 6th century C.E., Muscio brought Soran's knowledge into the Middle Ages. The Salternitan *Trotula* trilogy stated in the 12th century C.E. [14]: 'If the child does not come out in the manner in which it ought, as when the legs or arms exit first, let a midwife assist with a small and smooth hand moistened in a decoction of linseed and fenugreek, and let her replace the child in its place and let her put it in its correct position.'

Cephalic and podalic version and breech extraction were widely used in the Middle Ages and have been discussed by Thomas of Cantimpré in 1263 [15], who advocated internal version onto the head, and by Jacques Guillemeau [16], who confessed in 1643: 'Personally, I feel that it is easier and safer to extract the infant by the feet than to turn it and bring the feet up and the head down.' Ulysses Aldrovando was professor of medicine in Bologna from 1571 to 1600. He discerned and illustrated 15 forms of 'non-natural' birth presentations and was most impressed by the third, incomplete footling [17] (**Fig. 2.6.2**): 'In this case, the wise midwife should reposition the mother in her bed and try to make the fetus retract the prolapsed foot. This can be achieved by rolling and turning the mother in her bed, so that the fetus assumes another position.' François Mauriceau, accoucheur in Paris, gave a realistic report [18]: 'On August 18, 1669, I delivered a woman who had lost much blood by placenta detachment, which appeared first in the passage, with the infant's foot and knee … But the feet were firmly held back by the membranes, and I could pull the legs forward only after pushing back the prolapsed part of the placenta … The infant was born alive, but so feeble that it died one hour later … the mother could be saved.' At the same time, Percival Willughby had observed dreadful deliveries in Derby and concluded in 1672 [19]: 'All births, comming by the back, belly, buttock, sides, or knees, or with head, and neck distorted; and all unnaturall births whatsoever, with all difficult births, bee ever the best, easiest, and safest laid by the feet of the infant. It is impossible to lay any unnatural birth by the infant's head' (**Fig. 2.6.3**).

CHAPTER 2.6 Postverta, Agrippa, Caesarea: born feet-first

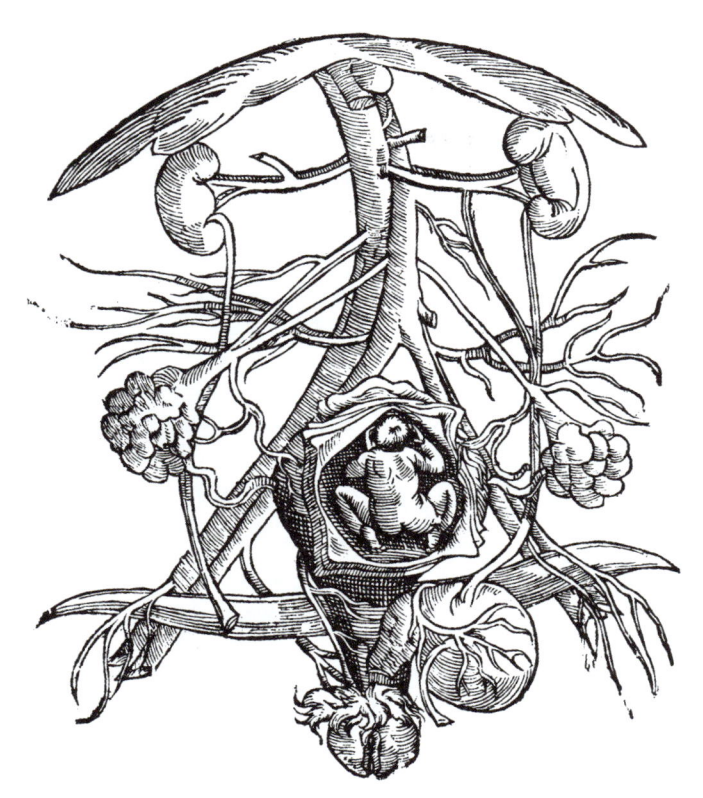

Fig. 2.6.2 Fetal breech position in early pregnancy, depicted by Ulysse Aldrovando in 1642 [17].

Infant trauma and mortality

During the 18th and 19th centuries, the situation did not change much, especially for large babies and a narrow pelvis, a frequent condition before rickets prevention was introduced in early 20th century. Adalbert Vysin reported in 1882 [20]: 'The fetus was in second breech presentation and female. The greater part of the breech passed the pelvic cavity, but then got stuck, despite forceful contractions and good cooperation of the mother. Nor did the delivery make any progress … the blunt hook and an elastic band did not help … the blood circulation between mother and fetus ceased due to cord compression, and the fetus died. Resuscitation was without success … The infant weighed 9.8 kg [17.5 Vienna pounds].' Breech delivery was associated with high infant mortality, trauma to the hyperextended neck and to the unmoulded aftercoming head, and with asphyxia from cord compression and prematurity. In breech presentation, the cord prolapses easily, and once the navel is born, the infant no longer receives fresh blood from the placenta. Prosper-Sylvain Denis, after more than 300 autopsies of neonates at the Paris Foundling Hospital, described cerebral haemorrhages in 1826 [21]: 'It is strange to see parts of the meninges partially destroyed, reduced to disintegrated white shreds. The site of these alterations is generally the cerebellar tentorium. They are due to the violent distension and final rupture of the fold, consequent to the head's straining during delivery.' A century later, J. R. Cameron evaluated breech deliveries at Edinburgh Simpson Memorial Hospital and found [22]: 'A high incidence of tentorial tears, tears of the falx, and intracranial hemorrhages.' Injury to the pituitary stalk resulting in diminished growth, as described by Van der Werf ten Bosch in 1962 [23]. Recent work has confirmed that most cases of 'idiopathic' hypopituitarism (non-genetic, no tumour) result from perinatal trauma to the hypothalamus or pituitary stalk, usually from breech delivery [24]. Both podalic version and extraction from breech presentation remained dangerous in the 20th century: The collaborative study of the National Institute of Health revealed that in 1959–1962, 'only 77% of the infants delivered by breech survived the neonatal period' [25] and in the 1960s, the mortality of infants delivered from breech presentation was five times higher than that from cephalic (vertex) presentation [26]. In addition to greater mortality, breech infants frequently suffered 'birth injuries', some of which are listed in Table 2.6.1. As in 'postasphyctic' brain damage (see Chapter 2.1), midwives and obstetricians were unjustifiably blamed, even if the lesion was not the result of, but an underlying precondition for breech presentation, as was typical for wry-neck with sternocleidomastoid tumour [27]. In 1944, Chandler and Altenberg studied 101 infants operated for wry-neck in Chicago, half of whom were in the breech position [28]: 'Intrauterine malposition, pressure, and ischemia contribute to causing muscular torticollis by rendering the muscle atrophic, maldeveloped, shortened, and ischemic.' The grim prognosis of the breech infant did not just result from the rough delivery: often breech presentation was the result of an underlying pathology persisting beyond the neonatal period—failed cephalic version may result from neuromuscular or musculoskeletal dysfunction.

Breech delivery and infanticide

Historically, infanticide was a worldwide phenomenon, and sometimes the rule rather than the exception. Hrdy and Hausfater demonstrated [38] that 'virtually all infanticides ultimately relate to competition for resources' and are, by curtailing parental investment, an adaptive behaviour. In many societies, infants with elevated perinatal risk were considered dangerous, as were twins, infants with connatal teeth, premature and malformed infants, and those born feet-first. The infant whose mother had died in childbirth was considered a witch who killed his or her mother [39]. In 1649, Archbishop Pedro de Villa Gomez complained that Peruvian Incas offer the child that is born feet first which they call *Chacpa* [40]. The Plateau Tonga of Zambia considered breech deliveries as *malweza* (cursed) [41] and the Kaguru of east-central Tanzania considered all breech deliveries as *chigego* (unnatural) [42]: the mother was obliged to consult a diviner to find out why the infant failed to assume the vertex position, and if the child was allowed to live, to perform the necessary cleansing ritual [42]. The Bantu tribes of Central Kenya suffocated infants born feet-first [43]. The Bariba of Benin classified infants born from the breech position as witch children and used to kill them; they later handed them over to the Fulbe as slaves [44]. Still today, the Kasena of East Ghana regard breech-born infants as *chuchuru* (spirit child), dangerous and bringing misfortune to the family [45]. *Chuchuru* infants were often killed, neglected, or poisoned by the concoction man [46]. Malformed and handicapped infants remained a sociocultural burden for poor African societies, even though infanticide has recently been largely replaced by entrusting 'extraordinary' children to foster homes or shelters [47].

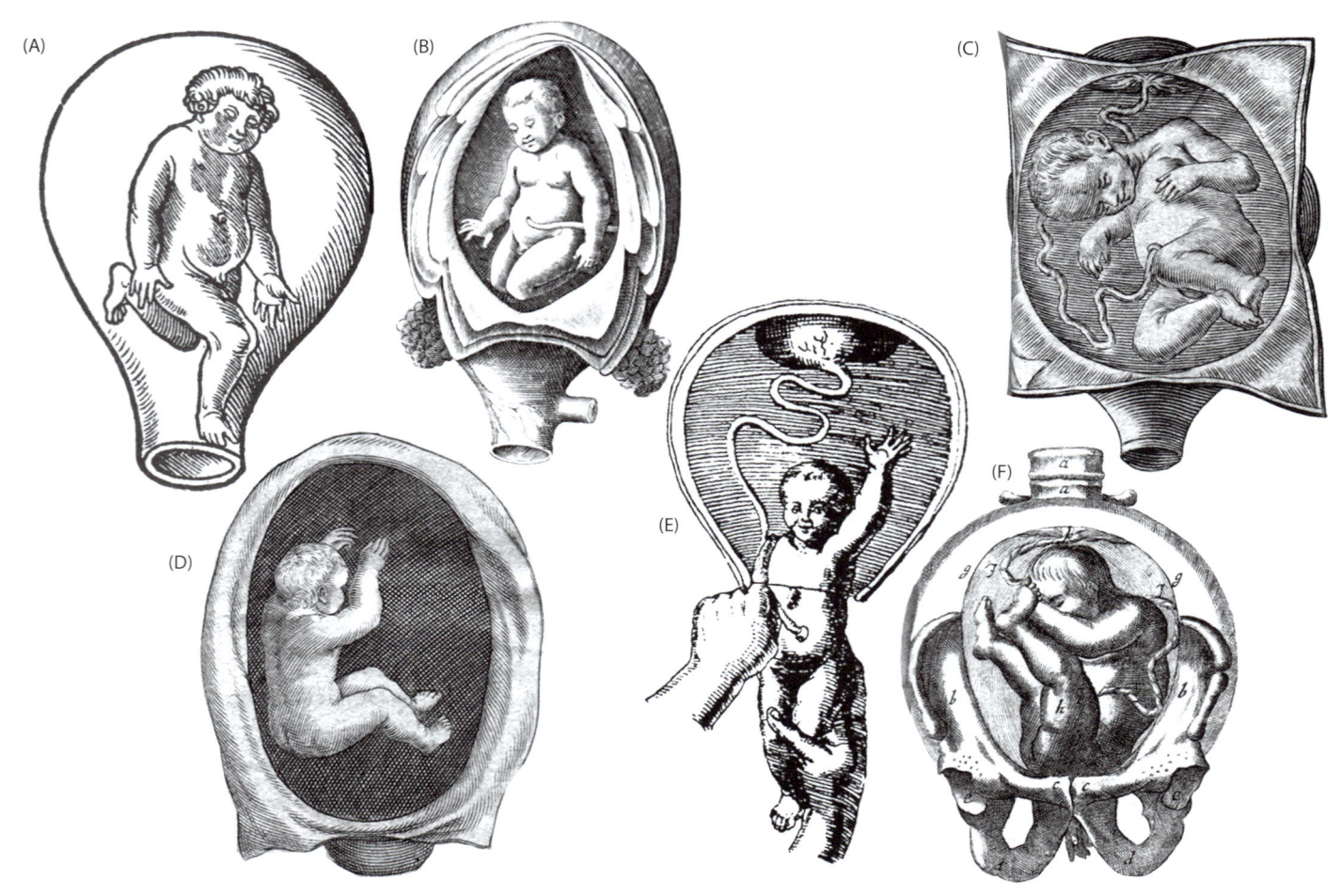

Fig. 2.6.3 Types of breech presentation as depicted in 16th- and 17th-century midwifery books. A, single footling, Eucharius Roesslin 1513 [57]; B, kneeling breech, Jacques Guillemeau 1643 [16]; C, incomplete kneeling breech, François Mauriceau 1680 [58]; D, complete breech, Scipio Mercurio 1671 [55]; E, extraction from double footling presentation, Johannes Muralt 1697 [59]; F, frank breech, Hendrik van Deventer 1761 [60].

Table 2.6.1 Neonatal disorders associated with breech presentation and delivery

Conditions before birth	Reference	Conditions at birth	Reference
1. Neuromuscular dysfunction Prematurity Anencephaly Spina bifida Hydrocephalus Spinal muscular atrophy Fetal alcohol syndrome Prader–Willi syndrome Trisomy 18	[29] [32] [25]	**1. Hypoxia, ischaemia** Umbilical cord prolapse Cord compression once the umbilicus is born Entrapment of the aftercoming head	[33] [34]
2. Uterine anomalies Uterus bicornis Polyhydramnios, e.g. Oesophageal atresia	[29]	**2. Rapid passage, traction** Fractures of arm, leg, or clavicle Brain haemorrhage	[22] [34]
3. Narrowness/oversized fetus Twins Oligohydramnios Torticollis Potter sequence Hip dysplasia	[28] [30] [1]	**3. Hyperextension** Sternocleidomastoid fibrosis Arm plexus palsy Tentorium or cerebellum injury Pituitary stalk injury, dwarfism	[21] [35] [36] [23] [37]

'The lost art of obstetrics'

Abdominal delivery of the living woman became an option when, in 1899, a Caesarean section was done in a breech presentation in Boston [48]: 'Because of rupture of the uterus in a previous labor of a woman [with oblique pelvis] who had had two stillbirths and one neonatal death. The cesarean section yielded a living infant that weighed 3900 g.' However, up to the middle of the 20th century, the operation was associated with considerable risk for the mother. In 1959, Ralph Wright of New Britain postulated [49]: 'Any patient over 35 weeks' gestation who enters labor with a living baby in breech presentation should be delivered by cesarean section, providing there is no maternal disease that contraindicates abdominal delivery.' Within a nationwide study, the American Medical Association investigated 16,327 breech births in 1962. When corrected for prematurity and limited to babies weighing greater than 2500 g, perinatal mortality was 3.5 times the expected value, and the perinatal mortality rate after vaginal delivery twice that of elective Caesarean section [26]. Despite several small randomized trials in the 1970s [50, 51], the debate on infant benefit versus maternal risks went on for another 25 years among obstetric authorities: 'Vaginal delivery of an infant in breech position is the main technique left in the art of obstetrics.' With routine Caesarean section for breech, 'we would be relegating ourselves to the role of either midwife or surgeon' [52]. Gimovski insisted that the vaginal management of breech labour and delivery was 'the measure of an obstetrician' [51], and as late as 1985, Confino and colleagues warned [53] 'the more we operate on breeches, the less experienced obstetricians will deliver them vaginally'. Finally, in 1997–2000, Mary Hannah in Toronto coordinated a group of 121 centres in 26 countries to perform a sufficiently powered randomized multicentre trial in 2088 breech deliveries at term [31], which yielded evidence: after elective Caesarean delivery, perinatal/neonatal mortality (0.3 versus 1.3%) or serious neonatal morbidity (1.4 versus 3.8%) were significantly lower than after planned vaginal birth. And, importantly: no maternal disadvantage whatsoever was observed with elective Caesarean delivery in term presentation. Those results were confirmed by a population-based study of all deliveries in Sweden published by Ekéus in 2017 [54]: compared to elective Caesarean section, the risk of vaginally delivered breech infants was eight times higher for perinatal mortality, seven times higher for intracranial haemorrhage or seizures, and 24 times higher for brachial plexus injury. Today, vaginal delivery from the breech position has largely disappeared.

Conclusion

Throughout history, breech presentation was the main cause of 'difficult' delivery, maternal mortality, and perinatal death. Embryotomy to save the mother was a dreaded intervention—and a major reason for men entering the previously female profession of midwifery. Long-term sequelae after breech delivery cannot be understood apart from considering the underlying causes of breech presentation and their interaction. They are not just obstetric accidents, let alone poor obstetric management. Only recently was the threat of malpresentations overcome by Caesarean delivery. That this mode of birth was accepted so reluctantly illustrates how the interests of professional organizations can perpetuate suboptimal treatment contrary to scientific evidence.

REFERENCES

1. Smith WB: Breech presentation sequence. In: Recognizable patterns of human deformation. Philadelphia, PA: Saunders, 1981: p. 66–75.
2. Mostello D, Chang JJ, Bai F, et al.: Breech presentation at delivery: a marker for congenital anomaly? J Perinatol 2014;**34**:11–15.
3. Sushruta Samhita: An English Translation. Edited by: Kavirai Bhishagratna. Calcutta: Bhishagratna, 1911: Vol. **2**, p. 404–7.
4. Hippokrates: Über Achtmonatskinder. Edited by: Hermann Grensemann. Berlin: Akademie-Verlag, 1968: p. 83.
5. Levret A: L'art des accouchemens (1st ed. 1753). 3. ed. Paris: Didot Jeune, 1766: p. 76, 261, 445.
6. Haller A: La génération; ou exposition des phénomènes relatifs a cette fonction naturelle. Paris: Doué, 1774: Vol. **2**, p. 424–7.
7. Hippocrates: De superfetatione. Loeb Classical Library 509. Cambridge, MA: Harvard University Press, 1923: Vol. **9**, p. L8, 476–508, 313–54.
8. Fasbender H: Entwickelungslehre, Geburtshülfe und Gynäkologie in den Hippokratischen Schriften. Stuttgart: Enke, 1897: p. 148–65.
9. Hippocrates: Excision of the fetus. Hippocrates Works Loeb Classical Library. Cambridge, MA: Harvard University Press, 2010: Vol. **9**, p. 368–73.
10. Plinius the Elder: Natural history. Translated by: Philemon Holland. London: Wernerian Club, 1847: Vol. **1**, Book 7, cap. 3, p. 187, 192–9.
11. Heiß JB: Ueber die römischen Personen-Namen. Straubing: Mauter, 1873: p. 6–10.
12. Aulus Gellius: The attic nights. London: Johnson, 1795: Vol. **2**, p. 245.
13. Temkin O: Soranus' Gynecology. Baltimore, MD: The Johns Hopkins Press, 1956: p. 37, 176, 189.
14. The Trotula: An English translation of the Medieval compendium of women's medicine. Philadelphia, PA: University of Pennsylvania Press, 2002: p. 80.
15. Cantimpratensis T: Liber de natura rerum. Edited by: Helmut Boese. Berlin: de Gruyter, 1973: p. 99.
16. Guillemeau J: De la grossesse et accouchement des femmes. Paris: Jost, 1643: p. 190–8.
17. Aldrovando U: Monstrorum historia. Bononiae: Tebaldini, 1642: p. 56, 85.
18. Mauriceau F: Observations sur la grossesse et l'accouchement des femmes. Paris: Compagnie des Libraires Associés, 1738: Vol. **2**, p. 8, 42, 249.
19. Willughby P: Observations on midwifery [1672]. Edited from the original manuscript by: Henry Blenkinsop. Wakefield, Yorkshire: S.R. Publishers, 1972: p. 102, 120.
20. Vysin A: Die Geburt einer ungewöhnlich stark entwickelten Frucht. Wiener Medizinische Presse 1880;**23**:1297–8.
21. Denis P-S: Recherches d'anatomie et de physiologie pathologique sur plusieurs maladies des enfants nouveau-nés. Commercy: Denis, 1826: p. 392.
22. Cameron JR: A discussion on intracranial injury in the newly born and its relationship to breech delivery. Trans Edinb Obstet Soc 1931;**51**:137–52.
23. Van der Werf ten Bosch JJ: Hypofysaire dwerggroei. Ned Tijdschr Geneeskd 1962;**106**:1282–94.

24. Craft WH, Underwood LE, Van Wyk JJ: High incidence of perinatal insult in children with idiopathic hypopituitarism. J Pediatr 1980;**96**:397–402.
25. Berendes HW, Weiss W, Deutschberger J, Jackson E: Factors associated with breech delivery. Am J Public Health 1965;**55**:708–19.
26. Morgan HS, Kane SH: An analysis of 16,327 breech births. JAMA 1964;**187**:262–4.
27. Illingworth RS: Why blame the obstetrician? A review. BMJ 1979;**1**:797–801.
28. Chandler FA, Altenberg A: 'Congenital' muscular torticollis. JAMA 1944;**125**:476–83.
29. Braun FHT, Jones KL, Smith DW: Breech presentation as an indicator of fetal abnormality. J Pediatr 1975;**86**:419–21.
30. Vartan CK: The behaviour of the foetus in utero with special reference to the incidence of breech presentation at term. J Obstet Gynecol Br Emp 1945;**52**:417–34.
31. Hannah ME: Planned caesarean section versus planned vaginal birth for breech presentation at term: a randomised multicentre trial. Lancet 2000;**356**:1375–83.
32. Brenner WE, Bruce RD, Hendricks CH: The characteristics and perils of breech presentation. Am J Obstet Gynecol 1974;**118**:700–12.
33. Hall JE, Kohl S: Breech presentation, a study of 1,456 cases. Am J Obstet Gynecol 1956;**72**:977–90.
34. Robinson GW: Birth characteristics of children with congenital dislocation of the hip. Am J Epidemiol 1968;**87**:275–84.
35. Capon NB: Intracranial traumata in the newborn. Br J Obstet Gynaecol 1922;**29**:572–90.
36. Wigglesworth JS, Husemeyer RP: Intracranial birth trauma in vaginal breech delivery. Br J Obstet Gynaecol 1977;**84**:684–91.
37. Tan KL: Brachial palsy. J Obstet Gynaecol Br Commonw 1973;**80**:60–2.
38. Hausfater G, Hrdy SB: Infanticide: comparative and evolutionary perspectives. New York: Aldine, 1984: p. VII.
39. Scrimshaw SCM: Infanticide in human populations: societal and individual concerns. In: G. Hausfater: Infanticide: comparative and evolutionary perspectives. New York: Aldine, 1984: p. 170–93.
40. Rivero ME, Tschudi JJ: Peruvian antiquities. New York: Putnam, 1853: p. 173–7.
41. Colson E: Marriage and the family among the Plateau Tonga of Northern Rhodesia. Manchester: Manchester University Press, 1958: p. 161.
42. Beidelman TO: Kaguru omens. An East African people's concepts of the unusual, unnatural and supernormal. Anthropol Q 1963;**36**:43–59.
43. Middleton J, Kershaw G: The central tribes of the North-Eastern Bantu. In: East Central Africa, Part V. London: International African Institute, 1965: p. 55.
44. Sargent CF: Born to die: witchcraft and infanticide in Bariba culture. Ethnology 1988;**27**:79–95.
45. Awedoba AK, Denham AR: The perception of abnormality in Kasena and Nankani infants: clarifying infanticide in Northern Ghana. Ghana Stud 2012;**15**:41–67.
46. Denham AR, Adongo PB, Freydberg N, Hodgson A: Chasing spirits: clarifying the spirit child phenomenon and infanticide in Northern Ghana. Soc Sci Med 2010;**71**:608–15.
47. Delaunay V: Improving knowledge on child abandonment and care in Africa. Afr Popul Stud 2011;**25**:73–94.
48. Goethals TR: Cesarean section as method of choice in management of breech delivery. Am J Obstet Gynecol 1956;**72**:536–52.
49. Wright RC: Reduction of perinatal mortality and morbidity in breech delivery through routine use of cesarean section. Obstet Gynecol 1959;**14**:758–63.
50. Collea JV, Chein C, Quilligan EJ: The randomized management of term frank breech presentation. Am J Obstet Gynecol 1980;**137**:235–42.
51. Gimovsky ML, Wallace RL, Schifrin BS, Paul RH: Randomized management of the non-frank breech presentation at term: a preliminary report. Am J Obstet Gynecol 1983;**146**:34–40.
52. Patterson SP, Mulliniks RC, Schreier PC: Breech presentation in the primigravida. Am J Obstet Gynecol 1967;**98**:404–10.
53. Confino E, Gleicher N, Elrad H, et al.: The breech dilemma. Obstet Gynecol Surv 1985;**40**:330–7.
54. Ekéus C, Norman M, Aberg K, et al.: Vaginal breech delivery at term and neonatal morbidity and mortality. J Matern Fetal Neonatal Med 2019;**32**:265–70.
55. Mercurio S: Kinder-Mutter oder Hebammen-Buch (Ital. ed. 1601). Wittenberg: Mevius, 1671: p. **54**, plate 3.
56. Ploss H: Das Weib in der Natur- und Völkerkunde. 7. ed. Leipzig: Grieben, 1902: Vol. **1**, p. 756.
57. Rößlin E: Der Swangern Frauwen und hebammen Rosegarten. Straßburg: Flach, 1513: p. 30.
58. Mauriceau F: Tractat von Kranckheiten schwangerer und gebärender Weibspersonen (1st French ed. 1668). Basel: Bertsche, 1680: p. 194, 226.
59. Muralt J: Kinder- und Hebammenbüchlein. Basel: König, 1697: p. 39.
60. Deventer Hv: Neues Hebammen-Licht (1st Latin ed. 1701). 5. ed. Jena: Cröker, 1761: p. 261, 325, fig. 27.

2.7

Social birth

Rites of passage for the newborn

Introduction

To accept and welcome the infant, most cultures developed postnatal rites that were often ceremonially complex, painful, or risky, and faithfully performed for centuries. These rites typically adopted the three-phase pattern identified by ethnographer Arnold van Gennep in 1909 [1]: (1) separation from the previous world (neonate: from the mother); (2) liminality and transition (neonate: purgation); and (3) incorporation into the new world (neonate: name giving). Blood and meconium were greatly feared, and the primary goal of neonatal rites was that of cleaning, understood in more than a corporal sense. Consequently, they embraced exorcism to remove or incantations to protect from evil spirits. The rite, especially the name giving, regulated the infant's relation to other individuals and to the society, and usually granted the right to live. The time interval from biological to social birth was 3–8 days, which excluded most of those born, who died in the very first days of life.

Familiarity with more than one culture may help to understand why aborting a malformed fetus or foregoing life support for an immature infant may be or may not be an option for a family. By cursorily comparing the age-old rites of different cultures, the following chapter aims to shed light on the difficulties infants encounter to be accepted in society, especially when born prematurely or malformed. Cultures were selected that persisted for several centuries and for which written or pictorial sources were available. This chapter does not address infanticide (see Chapters 8.1–8.3) nor postnatal adaptation.

Mesopotamian, Egyptian, and Jewish rites

In Sumerian times (third millennium B.C.E.) *Ninhursag*, the goddess of childbirth, was believed to protect the newborn, whereas a demon named *Dimme* lurked nearby after delivery seeking an opportunity to destroy the infant [2]. The Mesopotamian societies developed highly constant exorcisms and protective rituals for the newborn. Phoenicians tried to guard their infants from the 'pack of the night' by specific incantations against the 'she-who-flies' and 'she-who-strangles-the-lamb' demons (Fig. 2.7.1A). Babylonians and Assyrians feared the lion-headed *Lamashtu*, whose principal victims were fetuses and neonates (Fig. 2.7.1C). She was depicted with blood-stained hands, prehensile feet, holding snakes, and with a piglet suckling her right and a whelp her left breast. Part of the canonical incantation is shown in Fig. 2.7.1B [2, 3]: 'She is fierce, violent, divine, the daughter of Anu! Terrifying, she emerged from the marshes. I conjure her, that she will not take to her breast the infant which I take to my breast.' The rite included anointing with various fats and: 'You make a clay figurine of Lamashtu ... take seven strands of dyed wool, a bristle of a donkey's hair ... twist all these into three coils, place it around the infant's neck ... speak the incantation over its head, hands, chest, hips, and feet.'

The Ancient Egyptians believed the child was protected by the goddesses *Isis* and *Hathor*, to whom offerings were given. After birth, the infant was washed; cutting the umbilical cord was associated with religious purification, as specified in spell 17 of the *Book of the Dead* (1550 B.C.E.) [4]: 'I destroy what was done wrongly against me, I dispel what was done evilly against me. What does it mean? It means that the navel-string of N ... will be cut. All the ill which was on me has been removed. It means that I was cleansed on the day of my birth.'

The Jewish religion had several rites to remove maternal uncleanness after birth [Leviticus 12:1–8]. The rite for the newborn included the *brit milah* (Jehova's covenant of circumcision) for male infants on the eighth day of life. It replaced the firstborn sacrifice performed in Phoenician cultures and represented not only a rite of passage, but a physical sign of belonging to the Chosen People. Rules on how to circumcise were specified in the Mishnah Shabbat 19. Initially, only a small portion, from the 2nd century C.E. a larger portion (*peri'ah*) of the preputium (foreskin) was removed by the *mohel* (ritual circumciser). The infant was held by the godfather and placed on the lap of the *sandaq* (holder); specific prayers were spoken, and the rite usually included the naming ceremony [5] (Fig. 2.7.2, left). The ancient *metzitzah* (sucking the blood by the mohel's mouth) is no longer practised by many Jews.

Reproduced with permission from Obladen M: Social birth: rites of passage for the newborn. *Neonatology*, 112:317–323. Copyright © 2017 S. Karger AG, Basel.

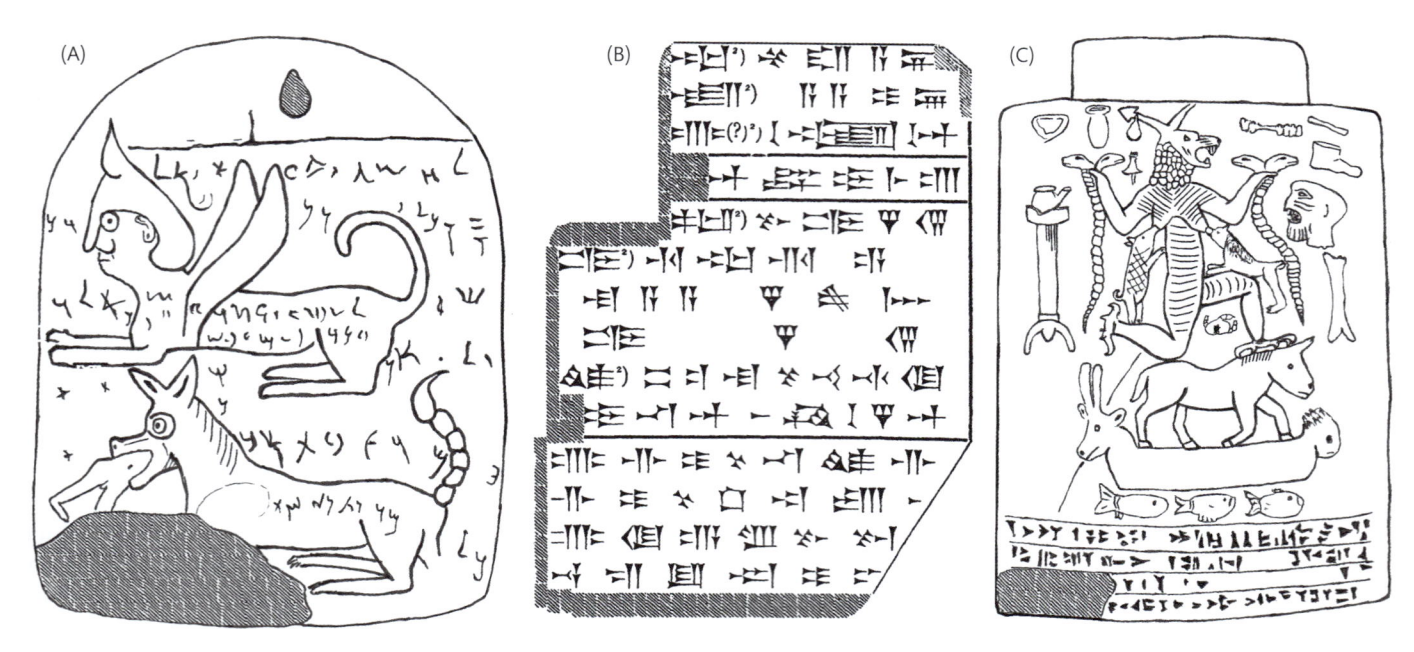

Fig. 2.7.1 Mesopotamian incantations to protect the newborn. A, clay tablet from the 7th century b.c.e. found in Arslan Tash, Syria. The upper figure is the sphinx-shaped 'she-who-flies', the lower figure devouring an infant is the wolf-shaped 'she-who-strangles-the-lamb'. The Phoenician inscription reads: 'The house I visit you shall not visit and the court I enter you shall not enter. O flyers, goddesses: from the dark room pass away' [42]. B, clay tablet with Babylonian cuneiform scripture from the 13th century b.c.e., found in Assurbanipal's Niniveh library (modified and redrawn from Tablet K 2543, British Museum). See text for Lamashtu incantation [3]. C, Babylonian Lamashtu amulet from ca. 1000 b.c.e.; private collection, modified and redrawn from Farber [43]. It shows the lion-headed goddess holding snakes, kneeling on a donkey (who stands in a boat), and suckling animals regarded as unclean.

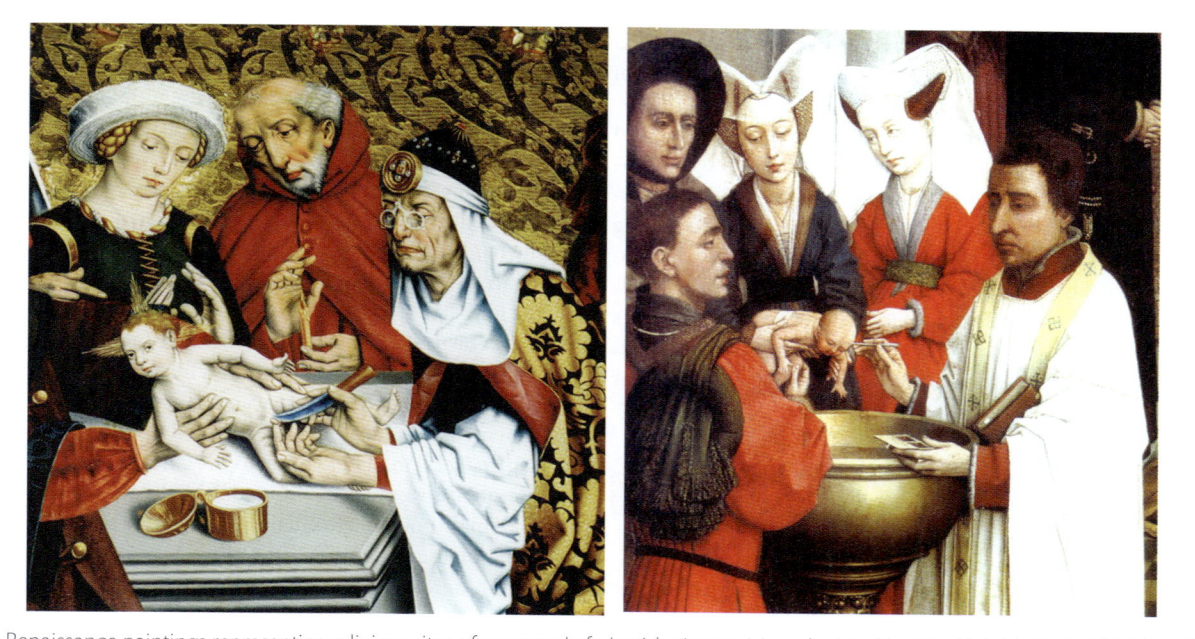

Fig. 2.7.2 Renaissance paintings representing religious rites of passage. Left: Jewish circumcision, depicted by Friedrich Herlin in 1466 (detail); note the mohel's riveted glasses, a novelty at that time. Altarpiece from St. Jacob Church, Rothenburg. Right: Christian baptism, depicted by Rogier van der Weyden ca. 1445 (detail); the Seven Sacraments altarpiece illustrates §12 of the Roman Ritual, when the priest inserts his own saliva into the infant's ear, speaking *ephphata* (be opened).
Left: © Dia archive St. Jacob, Rotenberg, with permission. Right: Rogier Van der Weyden, The Seven Sacraments: Baptism, Confirmation and Confession (detail), left panel, 119 × 63 cm. Royal Museum of Fine Arts Antwerp, photo Hugo Maertens, with permission.

Circumcision originated in many cultures, mostly as an initiation rite in adolescents. Female genital mutilation was and is practised in some cultures, but usually not in the neonatal period. Neonatal male circumcision for medical, non-ritual purposes has been described by Gollaher [6], and continues to be hotly debated [7]. In the US, where two-thirds of men are circumcised, the American Academy of Pediatrics stated in 2012 [8]: 'The health benefits of newborn male circumcision outweigh the risks', referring mostly to protection against sexually transmitted viral infections. Dutch and Swedish paediatric societies have opposed infant male circumcision [9, 10], whereas Canadian, British, and German physicians have taken an intermediate position [11–13]. Courts and legislators have been involved. Style and duration of the debate suggest that it has more to do with cultural than with medical issues.

Greek and Roman purification rites

Aristotle explained (ca. 340 B.C.E.) [14]: 'Most [newborns] are carried off before the seventh day, that is why they give the child its name then from the belief that it has now a better chance of survival.' The Greek *amphidromia* (running around) was described by Plato [15]: 'They carry the baby around the hearth while they run around in a circle, and give the child its name. Friends, acquaintances and relatives send presents to the child, most often octopuses.' A garland of olive leaves for boys or a tuft of wool for girls was suspended on the home's door [16].

Romans called the neonate *sanguinolentus* (the blood-stained). As Plutarch reported [17], the *dies lustricus* (day of purification) was held 'when the boys were 9 days old, Girls 8 … for the Female grows up and comes to full perfection before the Male. They take the Days after the seventh which is dangerous by reason of the navel-string, which falls off at seven Days old, and before an infant is more like a Plant than an Animal.' The ceremony included washing and cleansing rituals to protect against evil spirits, and giving the *praenomen*, to be completed by the family name. Part of the ceremony was the *defascinatio* (disenchantment) via the aunt's saliva, recounted by Persius in 61 C.E. [18]:

> 'Lo! from his little crib, the grandam hoar,
> Or aunt, well vers'd in superstitious lore,
> Snatches the babe; in lustral spittle dips
> Her middle finger, and anoints his lips,
> And forehead: – Charms of potency, she cries,
> to break the influence of evil eyes!'

Ritual swaddling, meticulously described by Soranus [26], was believed to promote health and beauty and was adopted by several cultures. Protectress of the newborn was *Juno Lucina*; the birth was announced by placing a laurel wreath on the front door [19].

Other non-Christian rites

The Vedic scriptures mentioned Hindu rites from the second millennium B.C.E. [20]: the *Namakarana* (naming ceremony) was performed on the tenth day after birth, the last on which the mother had to be secluded. A talisman of *putrudu* [a resinous wood] was attached to the infant and the hymn recited: 'Accept this amulet of immortality … I bring you breath and life, do not go to the dark shadows, stay in safety, go to the light of those living before you.' Two names were then given to the infant.

There is little information on the passage rites of Germanic and Nordic peoples. Roman physician Soranus claimed in the 2nd century C.E. [21] 'after omphalotomy, the barbarians, as Germans and Scythians, put the newborn into cold water in order to make it firm and to let die, as not worth rearing, one that cannot bear the chilling.' Sprinkling water on the newborn was a Druidical rite before the Norse incursions. For the Norse and Icelandic Celts it has been described in the Edda in 1220 C.E. [22]: 'Edda a child brought forth: they with water sprinkled its swarthy skin, and named it Thrael.'

Muslim rites varied according to the epoch and region. They usually included the *adhan* (speaking the testimony into the infant's ear); the *tahneek* (rubbing a softened date on the infant's palate); and the *taweez*, an amulet with a prayer or Q'uran sura, fixed at the wrist or neck [23]. *Subu*, the naming ceremony, was performed a week after birth; the baby was bathed, dressed in new clothes, and henna was applied to its face, hands, and feet. In Morocco, the naming ceremony was accompanied by the *aqiqah*, the ritual sacrifice of a sheep or goat, a feast of male relatives, and the infant's first haircut [5]. *Khitan*, the male circumcision, took place within a few weeks after birth, but could be delayed up to the age of 7 years.

The rites of the Mayas in Yucatan before the conquistadores' arrival were described by Bancroft [24]: 'The midwife washed the child, placed a bow and arrow in its hands, if a boy, a spindle, if a girl, and drew a mark upon its right foot, so that it might become a good mountaineer.' 'Feasts that took place on the day when the umbilical cord was to be cut … the cord was laid upon an ear of maize … one half of the yield for the first food of the child aside from the mother's milk.' 'The naming of the child … on the twelfth day … On conclusion of the ceremonies, infant and mother were taken to a fountain or river to be bathed, and during the bath incense, birds, or cacao were offered.' This ceremony must not be confused with the Mayan *caputizihil* (to be born anew) performed at 3–12 years, which involved exorcising the devil, blessing prayers, and anointing of the forehead, hands, and feet with water and cacao [25].

Christian baptism

During the first centuries of Christianity, newborns were not baptized and older children only in an emergency, as suggested by a Hybla tombstone from 314 C.E. [26]: 'for Julia Florentina, their sweet and most innocent infant … She lived 18 months and 22 days and was baptized in the 8th hour of the night, four hours before her last breath.' The desire for neonatal baptism arose with Augustine's dogma of original sin, and the Council of Carthago declared in 418 [27]: 'Whosoever denies that infants newly from their mother's wombs should be baptized, or says that baptism is for remission of sins, but that they derive from Adam no original sin, which needs to be removed by the laver of regeneration … is to be understood as false, let him be *anathema* [excommunicated].'

For the 'unclean' newborn, baptism had three purposes: (1) to eliminate original sin; (2) to ensure the soul's resurrection after death; and (3) accepting the infant into the church. The ancient fear of demons was integrated into the baptismal sacrament. Twenty-five steps of the rite were meticulously detailed by Pope Benedict XIV in the Roman Rituale of 1760 [28] and included specific prayers and benedictions; salting the lips; inserting the priest's saliva into the infant's ear (Fig. 2.7.2 right); exhaling onto its face; anointing chest and shoulders; and pouring the baptismal water over the infant's head or immersing the infant in the font. The rite embraced exorcism until 1786, when the Leipzig tailor Höhn rejected for his child the phrase 'come out, unclean spirit', which the church conceded after some debate [29].

Abode of deceased unbaptized infants

The Bible was clear in John 3:5: 'Except a man be reborn of water and of the Spirit, he cannot enter into the kingdom of God.' In 418, the Council of Carthago confirmed that there is no abode for the blessed other than in heaven [27]. But this harsh verdict was difficult to bear in the context of newborn infants who died without any sin of their own, and in 1265, Thomas Aquinas conceded they may enjoy perpetual bliss without punishment in the *limbus puerorum*, an atrium of hell [30]. In 1536, reformer Martin Luther taught [31]: 'What is not said in the Bible, must be left to God's grace and power … I do not contradict those who imagine the infants' place in the middle between redeemed and condemned.' John Calvin rejected the 'papistic' belief in limbo as the abode of innocent souls denied access to heaven [32]. Other reformed Christian Churches, and especially Baptists, held different views on baptism and limbo, which are beyond the limits of this chapter. The councils debated and redebated the matter for centuries. In the absence of theological guidance, people were obsessed by the superstition that the infant's soul would find no peace, but stray about. Region-specific beliefs included were-wolves, the wild hunt, will-o'-the-wisp, spook-lights, and many others. As late as 2007 the Catholic church in effect abandoned the limbo doctrine, declaring 'hope for salvation for infants who die without being baptized' [33].

Emergency and conditional baptism

In the 12th century, the Catholic church developed a shortened rite for hospitals or at birth in case of impending death (Fig. 2.7.3A). Catholics but not Protestants allowed lay persons—including females—to carry out emergency baptism to newborns believed endangered. To ensure emergency baptism, Louis XIV excluded in 1680 [34] 'from midwifery all those, male or female, who profess the religion that pretends to be reformed'. Two controversies remained: the baptism of severely malformed neonates, believed non-human in the Middle Age; and the Caesarean delivery in case of

Fig. 2.7.3 European equipment used for baptism. A, parchment ritual of ca. 1190 c.e. from Codex CmI LXXIII, Benedictine Abbey in Lambach, Austria. Top inscription: 'Accept the white cloth of innocence and preserve it until you stand before Christ's throne of judgement.' Bottom inscription requests the grace of baptism for a person who is dying. B, bronze baptismal font that could be heated to avoid hypothermia (Taufgrapen); 14th century, Bovenau, German state of Schleswig-Holstein. C, syringe for intrauterine baptism published by Parisian accoucheur François Mauriceau in 1680 [39]. D, syringe for intrauterine baptism published by Augsburg midwife Barbara Wiedenmann in 1735 [41].
Reproduced from Codex CmI LXXIII, Benedictine Abbey in Lambach, Austria with permission.

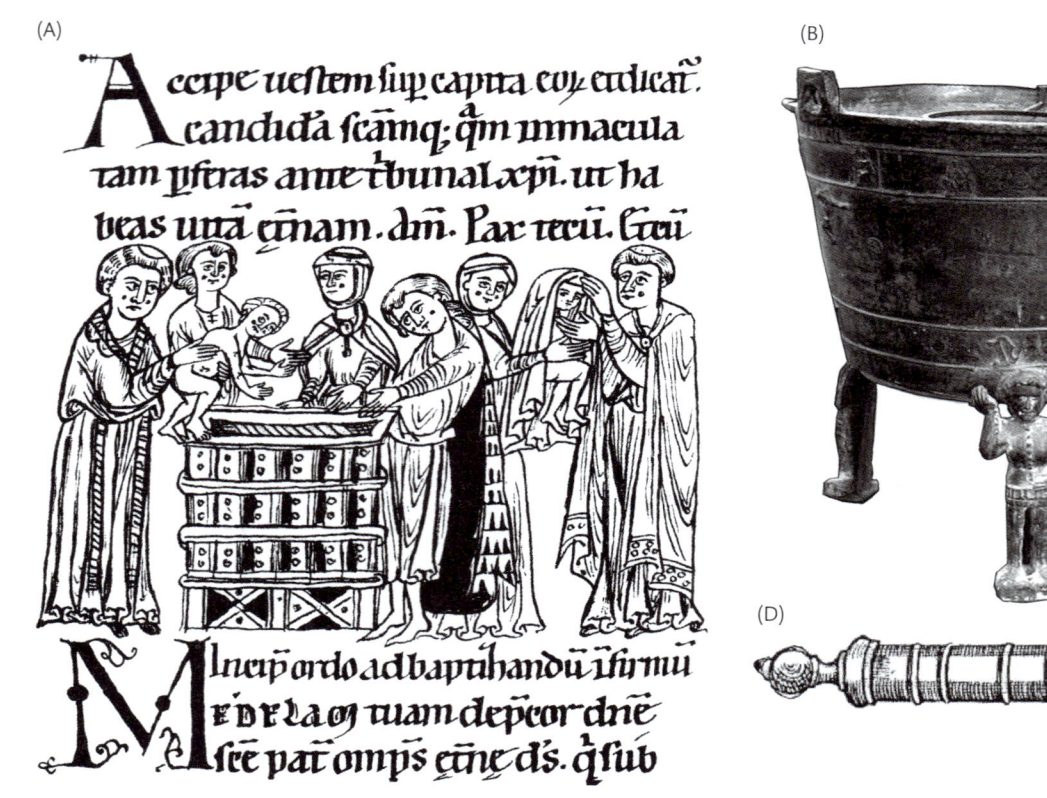

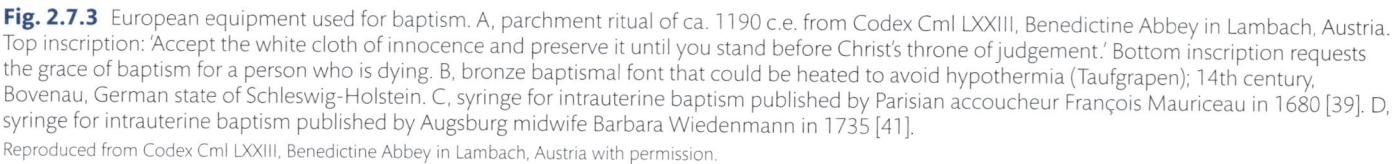

maternal death. As the rites varied within countries, Pope Benedict XIV appointed the inquisitor Francesco Cangiamila in 1744 to standardize baptism, which resulted in the voluminous *Embryologia Sacra* [35]. The inquisitor introduced conditional baptism for the malformed (if you are human …).

Caesarean delivery has been ascribed to the birth of Buddha and Asklepios, and has been reported by Pliny [36] for Scipio Africanus and Manilius. Since the Justinian Digests (533 C.E.) [37] the *lex regia* [royal law] was cited 'which forbids to bury a deceased pregnant woman, before the infant has been excised'. Such 'Caesarean' sections aimed to save the fetal life, but fell into oblivion in the Early Middle Ages. The procedure was rediscovered by the Catholic Church with the aim to save the infant's soul. The midwifes order of Regensburg decreed in 1452 [38]: 'If [in case the mother dies] the midwife did not call the surgeon in time, she must help the soul of the infant herself with the cut.' Cangiamila reinforced the midwives' (and the priests'!) duty to perform a Caesarean section in the dead mother for the child's sake, but overall the operation was seldom performed.

Baptism of the unborn

Whole-body immersion persisted well into the Middle Ages, when the risk of hypothermia due to the procedure was recognized, foremost in northern Europe. As the churches were usually unheated, baptismal fonts of bronze were constructed that could be heated from below (Fig. 2.7.3B). When François Mauriceau invented a syringe for intrauterine baptism in 1680 [39] (Fig. 2.7.3C), another theological dilemma arose: a committee set up by the Sorbonne to investigate the matter found that even though technically possible, the unborn could not be considered to be 'reborn by water', and referred the matter to the Pope [40]. Cangiamila defined another form of conditional baptism, *si es capax* [if you are capable …] [35], and declared intrauterine baptism to be valid, but to be repeated after birth if the newborn was still alive. Although theological doubts persisted, most midwives' textbooks accepted the baptismal syringe, as did Augsburg midwife Barbara Wiedenmann [41] (Fig. 2.7.3D).

Conclusion

In neonates, a liminal status persisted up to the rites of passage. These possibly originated as a culturally accepted disguise for infanticide during the first days of life. When performed, the rites granted the right to life as an ethical concept. Today, neonatologists are well acquainted with the time interval between biological and social birth: a postponed birth announcement of the preterm infant and reluctant paternal visits to the intensive care unit suggest the infant's ambivalent status. Rites of passage were remarkably similar across different cultures, as exorcism or the use of saliva from a venerated person prove. Allegedly nourished by menstrual blood, and polluted with blood and meconium, the newborn was regarded as impure, possessed by evil spirits, or at least in need of purification. The derision of other religion's rites was and is frequent, and knowledge of their history may help us better understand parental spiritual needs. Circumcision changed from being a religious commandment to an alleged health benefit. As observed in conjunction with tongue-tie and head shaping (see Chapters 5.2 and 6.10), the debate on male circumcision is another example of how yesterday's ritual evolved into today's medical recommendation. Due to secularization, less family cohesion, childbirth in hospital, and lowered infant mortality, the importance of rites of passage has diminished in modern societies.

REFERENCES

1. Gennep Av: Übergangsriten (Les rites de passage; 1st ed. 1909). Frankfurt: Campus, 1986.
2. Farber W: Lamashtu: An edition of the canonical series of Lamashtu incantations and rituals and related texts from the second and first millennia B.C. Winona Lake: Eisenbrauns, 2014: p. 1–6, 151–79.
3. Myhrman DW: Die Labartu-Texte. Zeitschrift für Assyrologie 1902;**16**:141–200.
4. Andrews C: The ancient Egyptian book of the dead. Austin, TX: University of Texas Press, 1990: p. 45.
5. Eliade M: Rites of passage. In: The encyclopedia of religion, Vol. **12**. New York: Macmillan, 1987: p. 388–400.
6. Gollaher DL: Circumcision: a history of the world's most controversial surgery. New York: Basic Books, 2000.
7. Svoboda JS, Van Howe RS: Out of step: fatal flaws in the latest AAP policy report on neonatal circumcision. J Med Ethics 2013;**39**:434–41.
8. American Academy of Pediatrics: Male circumcision. Technical report. Pediatrics 2012;**130**:e756–85.
9. Sheldon T: Dutch medical alliance moves to change thinking on male circumcision. BMJ 2010;**340**:c2987.
10. Hofvander Y: New law on male circumcision in Sweden. Lancet 2002;**359**:630.
11. Sorokan ST, Finlay JC, Jefferies AL, Canadian Pediatric Society: Newborn male circumcision. Paediatr Child Health 2015;**20**: 311–5.
12. British Medical Association: The law and ethics of male circumcision: guidance for doctors. J Med Ethics 2004;**30**:259–63.
13. Merkel R, Putzke H: After Cologne: male circumcision and the law. J Med Ethics 2013;**39**:444–9.
14. Aristotle: Historia animalium, Book VII–X. Loeb Classical Library 439. Cambridge, MA: Harvard University Press, 1991: Vol. **9**, p. 588a5.
15. Plato: Theaetetus. London: Routledge & Kegan Paul, 1979: p. 160 E.
16. Dasen V: Childbirth and infancy in Greek and Roman antiquity. In: Rawson B: A companion to families in the Greek and Roman world. Malden, MA: Wiley-Blackwell, 2011: p. 291–314.
17. Plutarch: The Roman Questions, Nr. 102. Morals. London: Bradyll, 1704: Vol. **2**, p. 388.
18. Aulus Persius Flaccus: The satires. London: Bulmer and Nicol, 1821: Vol. Sat. II, verse 55, p. 69–71.
19. Dasen V: Roman birth rites of passage revisited. J Rom Archaeol 2009;**22**:199–214.
20. Oldenberg SH: The religion of the Veda (1st ed. Berlin 1894). Delhi: Motilal Banarsidass, 1988: p. 247.
21. Temkin O: Soranus' Gynecology. Baltimore, MD: The Johns Hopkins Press, 1956: p. 79–117.
22. Saemund the Learned: The Edda. Edited and translated from the old Norse or Icelandic. London: Trübner, 1866: Vol. **1**, p. 86.
23. Gatrad AR, Sheikh A: Muslim birth customs. Arch Dis Child Fetal Neonatal Ed 2001;**84**:F6–8.

24. Bancroft HH: The native races of the pacific states. Vol. II: Civilized nations. 1875: Vol. **2**, p. 679–80.
25. Landa Dd: Account of the affairs of Yucatán (1st ed. 1566). Chicago IL: O'Hara, 1975.
26. Diehl E: Inscriptiones Latinae Christianae Veteres. Berlin: Weidmann, 1925: Vol. **1**, p. 296.
27. Council of Carthago: The canons of the 217 blessed fathers who assembled at Carthage, AD 419. Nicene and Post-Nicene Fathers: Second Series. New York: Cosimo, 2007: Vol. **14**, Canon 110, p. 496.
28. Benedicti Papae XIV: Ordo baptismi parvulorum. In: Rituale Romanum, Tomus I. Patavii: Typis Seminarii, apud Joannem Manfre, 1760: Vol. **1**, p. 85–114.
29. Buchner E: Religion und Kirche (16. bis 18. Jahrhundert). München: Langen, 1925: p. 133.
30. Thomas Aquinas: On evil. Question 5, article 3. Notre Dame, Indiana: University of Notre Dame Press, 1995: p. 220.
31. Luther M: Die Disputation de homine. Weimar: Böhlau, 1932: Vol. **39.1**, p. 174–80.
32. Calvin J: Institutes of the Christian Religion (ed. 1559). Louisville, KY: John Knox, 1960: Vol. Book 4, p. 1320–23.
33. Sullivan FA: The development of doctrine about infants who die unbaptized. Theol Stud 2011;**72**:3–14.
34. Louis XIV: Declaration du Roy, portent défenses a ceux de la Réligion Prétendue Reformée, de faire des fonctions de Sages-Femmes. Lyon: Jullieron, 1680: p. 1–4.
35. Cangiamila FE: Embryologia sacra sive de officio sacerdotum, medicorum, et aliorum circa aeternam parvulorum in utero existentium salutem. 3. ed. Augustae Vindelicorum: Mauracher, 1765: p. 420–9, 482–90.
36. Pliny: Natural history, Books 3–7. Cambridge, MA: Harvard University Press, 2006: Vol. 7, IX, p. 537.
37. Justinian: Digesta Justiniani Augusti; XI, 8.2. Edited by: Paul Krüger and Theodor Mommsen. Berolini: Weidmann, 1868: Vol. **1**, p. 213.
38. Niedermeier H: Die Regensburger Hebammenordnung von 1452. Verhandlungen Histor Verein Oberpfalz Regensburg 1975;**115**:253–66.
39. Mauriceau F: Tractat von Kranckheiten schwangerer und gebärender Weibspersonen. Basel: Bertsche, 1680: p. 268–70.
40. Astruc J: L'art d'accoucher réduit a ses principes. Paris: Cavelier, 1766: p. 336–41.
41. Wiedenmann B: Kurtze, jedoch hinlängliche und gründliche Anweisung Christlicher Hebammen. Augsburg: Lotter, 1735: p. 195–7.
42. Röllig W: Begegnungen mit Göttern und Dämonen der Levante. In: T. Hölscher: Gegenwelten zu den Kulturen Griechenlands und Roms in der Antike. München, Leipzig: Saur, 2000: p. 47–66.
43. Farber W: Istu api ilamma ezezu ezzet: Ein bedeutsames neues Lamashtu-Amulett. In: Festschrift für Wolfgang Röllig. Kevelaer: Butzon & Bercker, 1997: p. 115–28.

PART 3
Prematurity

3.1 **Measures of viability** *71*

3.2 **Surviving against the odds** *79*

3.3 **Respiratory distress: understanding surfactant deficiency** *85*

3.4 **Holding breath: the development of surfactant substitution** *91*

3.5 **Anatomy and spontaneous closure of the ductus arteriosus** *95*

3.6 **Persisting patency of the ductus arteriosus in the preterm infant** *101*

3.7 **Intraventricular haemorrhage** *107*

INTRODUCTION

The premature infant was considered even more unfinished than the term infant. Legally assuming a position between fetus and child, it was assigned a diminished right to live. Birthweight and length were not measured until the end of the 18th century. Immature infants who survived without handicaps have been described at all times. When surfactant deficiency in the immature lung was identified, a causal treatment for this most lethal disease of prematurity became available. Anatomically known since antiquity, the role of the ductus arteriosus remained unclear until Harvey's discovery of circulation. When it became understood that prostaglandins prevent its closure in the preterm infant, effective interventions became available. Retinopathy of prematurity was an example of an iatrogenic disease resulting from uncontrolled introduction of a new treatment (oxygen) to a vulnerable population without a control group or systematic follow-up. Devices maintaining the premature's body temperature were developed in France and Russia in the first half of the 19th century, and closed incubators made the development of neonatal intensive care in the second half of the 20th century possible.

3.1 Measures of viability

Introduction: an interest in viability

The neonatologist is asked no question more frequently, and none has exhausted the printing press as much as: 'What is the border of viability for preterm infants?' This question is not at all new. Before being called *premature*, the infants were described as 'weak' or 'lebensschwach', and Budin's special care unit in Paris was referred to as 'pavillon des débiles' in 1883. During the 20th century, *weak*, *feeble*, *untimely*, *previable*, and *premature* were not used synonymously, but remained poorly defined. However, human beings seem to need precise borders and for various reasons a clear definition of viability was sought:

1. *Legal* definitions were required to distinguish preterm infants from miscarriages, in making the accusation of infanticide, and to determine the legitimacy of offspring, especially after the father's death, and to secure the inheritance of estate and title [1].
2. Rejection of the *technical* and intimidating setting in which immature infants are reared [2]; the naive wish for a 'natural' childbirth despite awareness of high natural infant mortality (at the begin of the 20th century, one in four infants died during the first year) and despite the observation that most medical interventions are far from 'natural'.
3. Medical care for the poor was notoriously underfinanced, and the high *cost* of maintaining preterm infants elicited utilitaristic considerations and competition for resources. Adalbert Czerny, directing the children's hospital at the Berlin Charité from 1913, strongly opposed the preterm infants' special care unit at the Kaiserin Auguste Victoria Haus in the same city, 'which proved that much money can maintain a few infants. This achievement cannot be regarded as social … No medical progress came from that institution' [3]. Not long ago, even Los Angeles neonatologist Jeffrey Pomerance worried about the allegedly high cost of caring for preterm infants, stating 'Society, however, must be the ultimate judge' [4].
4. Pessimistic views about *handicaps* or lifelong impairment [5, 6] were extensively debated with authors with more optimistic expectations [7, 8]. This discussion gradually replaced survival by survival without handicap [9]. In modern neonatology, definitions of viability (sometimes reduced to simple figures indicating gestational age) were used to decide whether to resuscitate a preterm infant [10, 11].
5. The proximity to the *fetal state* with its limited rights rendered the neonate (and even more so the premature infant) a lower moral status than other patients [12] with the consequence of 'special' ethics for newborns.

Gestational age: from creed to science

Egyptians, Assyrians, Babylonians, Hebrews, and Greeks established lunar months of 29–30 days, with different ways of intercalating additional months adapting to the solar year. This explains Solomon's statement in the 10th century B.C.E. [Wisdom 7:2]: 'And in my mother's womb I was fashioned to be flesh in the time of ten months.' Shorter gestation, *out of due time*, was associated with ill fortune: 'A hidden, untimely birth, as infants who never saw light' [Job 3:16]. Based on mystic numbers, the Hippocratic writers (5th to 3rd century B.C.E.) divided the pregnancy into seven phases of 40 days (tessarakontads) adding to 280 days, besides the classification into 10 (lunar) months. A crisis was believed to occur at 8 months when the fetus 'precipitated' from the breech into the cephalic position. Hippocrates' *The Eight Month Infant* established the tenacious idea that 7-, but not 8-month-old infants could survive [13]: 'It is impossible that the infant overcomes two subsequent diseases, that is why the eight month infants don't come through. Because in them it occurs that they subsequently suffer an intrauterine disease and a disease occurring after birth … For all these reasons it is necessary for most women to conceive at full moon (around the middle of the month), so that the 280 days—which is seven tessarakontads—may reach into the eleventh [lunar] month.'

When the Julian reform of 46 B.C.E. fixed the solar month at 30–31 days, confusion arose as to the Hippocratic gestational definition, and Galen (131–201 C.E.) felt the need to comment on Hippocratic teachings [13, 14]: 'Hippocrates: Whether one was to count nine months from the woman's disease or from conception? Whether these are Greek months adding to 270 days, or if there is something to add? Galen: By woman's disease he means the monthly [menstruation]. He says, that one has to discriminate if the duration of pregnancy is calculated from the day when the monthly last appeared, or

---

Reproduced with permission from Obladen, M. Historical notes on immaturity. Part 1: Measures of viability. *Journal of Perinatal Medicine*, 39:563–569. Copyright © 2011 Walter de Gruyter GmbH, Berlin/Boston.

from the day of conception … In the book of the eight month infant it has been explained, that the months shall not be calculated with thirty days.'

But it was not that easy to correct the mistakes due to translation, calendar change, and use of the first day of menstruation. The Hippocratic dogma that the 8-month infant invariably dies relieved parents and caretakers from feelings of guilt in times of extremely high perinatal mortality, which may explain its persistence into the 18th century, when Albrecht von Haller [15] stated in 1774: 'To the errors of the Hippocratic author the claim must be added that infants born at eight [months] are not viable, and his explanation is strange … The less an infant approaches the time of seven months, the more I have difficulty to believe that it could be perfect and viable, and that it will live for some time.'

As pointed out by Baskett [16], Naegele's rule (counting back 3 months and adding 7 days), is only correct when applied to the last day of menstruation. Herman Boerhaave, who published the rule in 1744 [17], and Franz Carl Naegele, who referred to that work in 1812 [18], probably meant it like this and Edinburgh obstetrician Thomas Denman (first ed. 1782) remained unclear [19]: 'In order to avoid any great error it is customary to reckon forty-two weeks from the last act of menstruation.' Further inaccuracy arose from confusion ongoing with completed weeks and from combining months, weeks, and days as pointed out by the Chicago neonatologist Julius Hess in 1923 [20]: 'Great confusion exists in a study of various statistics because of the misapplication of the term "months"; the latter should apply to lunar months (28 days) and not calendar months or better the age should be stated in days or weeks.' Last but not least: in firstborn infants, gestational age was sometimes derived from the date of marriage and many famous personalities were reported to have been preterm, but had normal birthweight.

Little interest in measurement

In 1838, Adolphe Quetelet, director of the Brussels Observatory and a pioneer of statistics, rightly bemoaned [21], that neonates were usually neither measured nor weighed. As scales were available since antiquity and had been specifically adapted for neonates (Figs. 3.1.1 and 3.1.2), it is worthwhile to explain this remarkable disinterest:

1. The *evil eye* superstition: in many regions of Europe, especially in Ireland and Scotland [22, 23], measuring or weighing a baby was thought to bring bad luck.

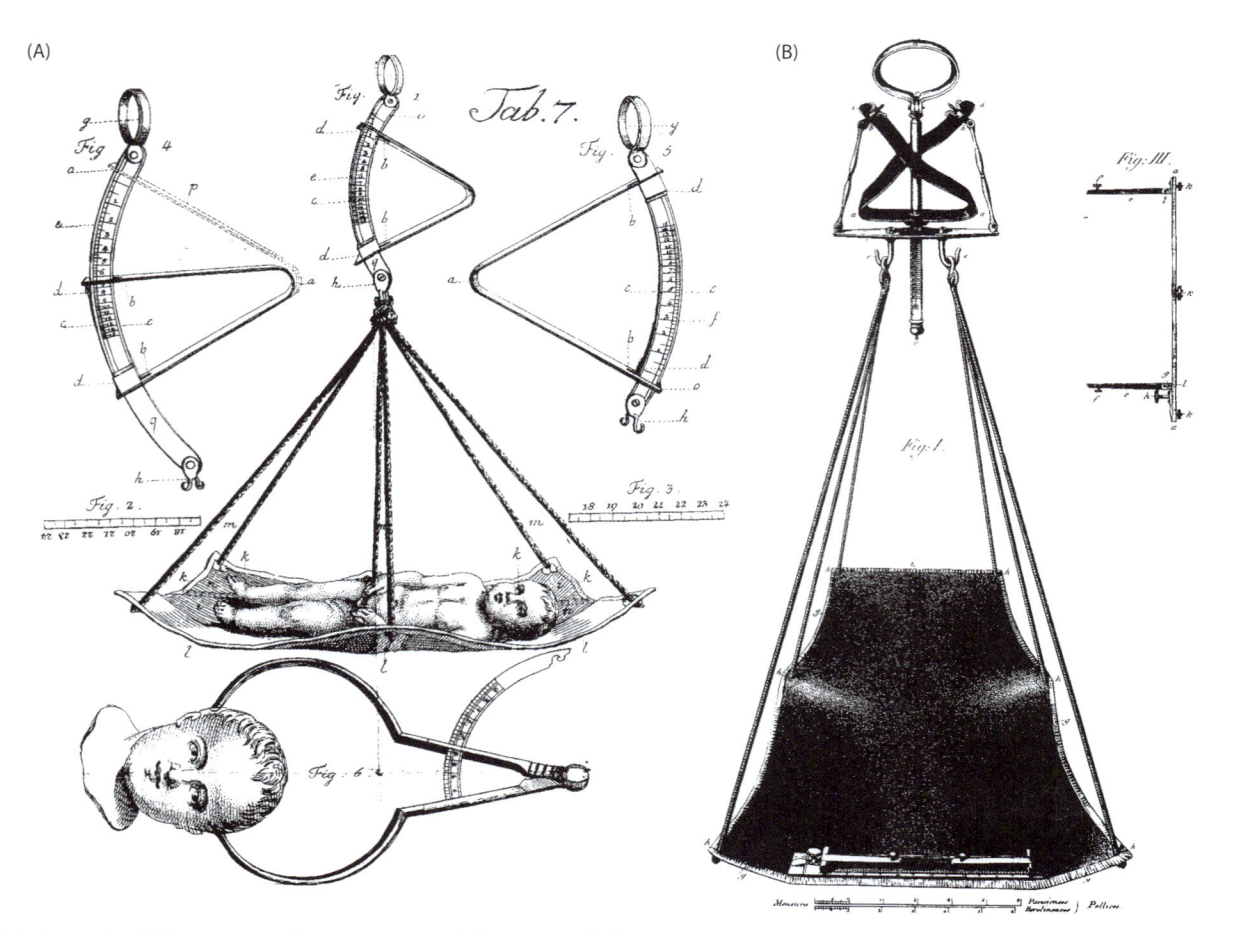

Fig. 3.1.1 Infant scales, 18th century: A, 'baromacrometer' of Stein 1775 [29], a portable scale operated with steel springs and three different rulers. Bottom: cephalometer, consisting of calliper circle and quadrant. B, 'pediometer' of Siebold 1815 [53]; portable spring scale with flexible pan. a, c, graduated rulers show the length in Berlin and Paris units (pollices).

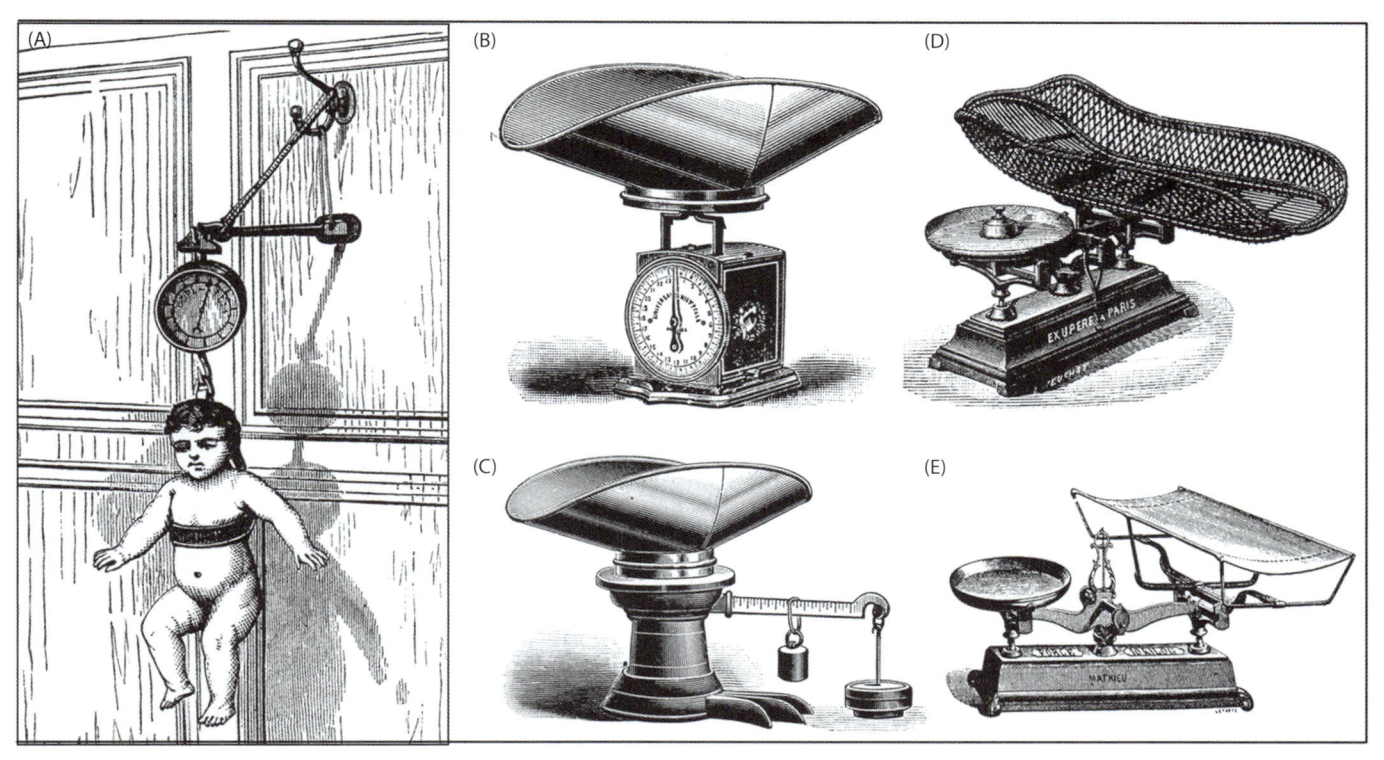

Fig. 3.1.2 Infant scales, 19th century: A, spring-loaded baby scale according to Bouchut 1867 [54]; B, universal family scale, and C, precision scale for use in hospitals according to Holt 1898 [55]; D, basket-type, and E, hammock-type scales according to Auvard 1905 [56].

2. Grossly inaccurate measurements by the authorities discouraged measuring altogether, as Cone pointed out [24]. François Mauriceau wrote in 1668 [25]: 'One will find that [the fetus] of nine months ordinarily weighs about 12 pounds [approximately 5874 g]. I have even seen some to weigh as much as 14 pounds [approximately 6853 g].' It is unclear if his scale did not work properly, or if he used measures deviating from the official Paris definitions. His textbook, frequently re-edited and translated, remained the authoritative reference for over a century, and everyone who reported birthweight found himself disagreeing with Mauriceau. The London physician Theophilus Lobb reported in 1747 [26]: 'I have weighed a Child, and Placenta soon after Delivery: the Child weighed sixteen Pounds, and seven Ounces, which is a large Child, but have seen some larger; and the Placenta weighed one Pound, four Ounces with the umbilical Chord.' The Scottish authority William Smellie noted in 1752 [27], 'at nine months the infant would weigh from ten to twelve, and sometime sixteen pounds', which casts doubt on the correct use of the avoirdupois units for infant weighing at birth. These authors' incorrect data partly explain the reluctance to weigh neonates at all. As late as 1753, the Göttingen obstetrician Johann Georg Roederer reported longitudinal weight measurements of neonates [28] and his pupil Georg Wilhelm Stein (the elder), director of the Kassel Foundling Hospital, designed an infant scale [29] (Fig. 3.1.1), with which he characterized different groups of infants at birth: mean birthweight/body length was 3274 g/53 cm in term liveborn infants, 2046 g/43 cm in preterm (viable) infants, 779 g/33 cm in 'untimely' (previable) infants, and 1450 g/39 cm in firstborn, 1333 g/38 cm in secondborn 'preterm' twins.

The metric dilemma

The ignorance of birthweight and body length leads us back into the conversion chaos of the pre-metric era. In Europe, hundreds of different measures were used, carved on a stone at the market place and changed from city to city, with time, and with political affiliation. Units were derived from human limbs like finger breadths = 1/4 palm, 1/12 span, 1/16 foot, digits, shoes, ells, and so on. The English avoirdupois definition of pounds and ounces was passed from the Saxons and remained constant in the UK and US since standardization under Elizabeth I. The metric system (g and cm), adopted in France during the Revolution, was gradually accepted in many European countries. George Washington and Thomas Jefferson proposed it to the US congress in 1790 in vain. The battle between the avoirdupois and metric systems continued throughout the 19th century and came to an end in most European countries with the Paris Meter Convention of 1875. Table 3.1.1, far from complete, gives an overview of mass and length units previously used in various regions and times. One can imagine that textbook authors refrained from reproducing body measurements which most of their readers could not understand.

Charts of fetal growth

In contrast to former times, the 20th century did not fall short in taking neonatal measurements, and many authors felt a need to standardize intrauterine growth. Given that surviving preterm infants were often small for gestational age, they changed remarkably

PART 3 Prematurity

Table 3.1.1 Conversion units. Historic mass and length units allowing the determination of weight and body length at birth, as well as the years from which the metric system was adopted in selected states [30–32]. Regional and local variations were considerable

States Metric adopted	Traditional mass units	Traditional length units
UK, US, Canada (1971)	1 pound = 16 ounces = 453.6 g (1 ounce = 28.35 g)	1 foot = 12 inches = 30.48 cm (1 inch = 2.54 cm)
France (1789) 1839	1 livre =16 ounces = 489.5 g (1 ounce = 30.59 g)	1 pied = 12 pouces = 32.5 cm (1 pouce = 2.7 cm = 12 lignes; 1 ligne = 2.26 mm)
Switzerland (Basel) (1835) 1868	1 Pfund/livre = 500g = 16 Unzen (since 1853, 493 g before 1853). 1 Unze = 31.25 g (since 1853, 30.8 g before 1853)	1 Fuß = 10 Zoll = 30.00 cm (1 Zoll = 3.00 cm)
Italy (Rome) (1803) 1861	1 libbra = 12 oncie = 327.5 g (1 oncia = 27.3 g)	1 piede = 12 pollici = 51.37 cm (1 pollice = 4.28 cm) 1 bracchio = 54 cm
Spain 1860	1 libra = 16 onza = 460.1 g (1 onza = 28.76 g)	1 pie = 12 pulgada = 27.86 cm (1 pulgada = 2.32 cm) 1 vara = 3 pie = 83.59 cm
Greece (1836) 1922	1 Oka = 5/2 pound = 1280 g	1 piki = 0.648 cm
Prussia (Berlin) 1872	1 Pfund = 32 Loth = 16 Unzen (1 Loth = 14.61 g; 1 Unze = 29.22 g)	1 Alter Fuß = 12 Zoll = 31.38 cm (1 Zoll = 2.615 cm) 1 Elle = 2 Spannen = 66.68 cm
Saxonia (Leipzig) 1872	1 Leipziger Pfund = 32 Loth = 467.6 g (1 Loth = 14.61 g)	1 Fuß = 12 Zoll = 28.77 cm (1 Zoll = 2.36 cm) 1 Elle = 2 Spannen = 56.64 cm
Hesse (Cassel) 1869	Before 1860: 1 Pfund = 32 Loth = 467.7 g (1 Loth = 14.16 g) From 1860: 1 Pfund = 30 Loth = 500 g (1 Loth = 16.66 g)	1 Fuß = 12 Zoll = 28.77 cm (1 Zoll = 2.397 cm)
Bavaria (Munich) 1872	1 Pfund = 32 Loth = 16 Unzen = 560.9 g (1 Loth = 17.53g; 1 Unze = 35.06 g)	1 Bayerischer Fuß = 12 Zoll = 29.19 cm (1 Zoll = 2.43 cm) 1 Elle = 2 Spannen = 83.3 cm
Austria (Vienna) 1871	1 Wiener Pfund = 16 Unzen = 561.3 g (until 1811: One Unze = 35.08 g; thereafter: 35.0 g)	1 Wiener Fuß (=Schuh) = 12 Zoll = 31.61 cm (1 Zoll = 2.63 cm)
Netherlands 1820	1 Pond = 16 Unzen = 494.1 g (1 Unze = 494.1 g)	1 Voeten = 12 Duime = 28.31 cm (1 Duime = 2.36 cm) 1 Elle = 5/2 Voeten
Denmark 1907	1 pund = 16 unze = 32 loth = 500 g (1 unze = 31.25 g)	1 fod = 12 tomme = 31.39 cm (1 tomme = 2.62 cm)
Sweden 1889	1 skålpund = 32 lod = 16 uns = 425.1 g (1 lod = 13.28 g, 1 uns = 26.56 g). Since 1855: 1 skålpund = 100 ort = 454 g (1 ort = 45.4 g)	1 fot = 10 tum = 29.69 cm (1 tum = 2.97 cm)
Poland 1919	1 funt = 16 uncja = 405.5g (1 uncja = 35.34 g)	1 stopa = 12 cali = 28.80 cm (1 cal =2.40 cm)
Russia 1917	1 Funt = 16 Once = 32 Loth = 409.5 g (1 Once = 25.59 g)	1 Foute = 12 Duime = 30.48 cm = 12/7 Tchevert (1 Duime = 2.54 cm, 1 Tchevert = 17.78 cm)

(Year), incomplete use.

little during the when measured correctly: **Fig. 3.1.3** compares the medians of fetal weight and length, based on data of André Levret from Paris 1747 [33], Hermann Franz Naegele from Heidelberg 1843 [34], and Lula Lubchenco from Denver 1966 [35, 36].

Empirical threshold definitions

A host of short-lived definitions has been coined for viability, several of which follow. Aristotle (384–322 B.C.E.) [37]: 'Now those that are born earlier than the seven [lunar] months can in no case live.' In 1668, Mauriceau bemoaned [25]: 'It is so rare to see an infant survive longer who is truly born at seven months, that of a thousand one will hardly find one to get away.' Alluding to the obstinate habit of counting ongoing instead of completed months or weeks, Levret (first ed. 1753) felt a need to clarify this statement [33]: 'Mauriceau undoubtedly speaks of those really lacking two entire months.' His Parisian colleague Joseph Raulin discerned preterms and prematures among the 7-month infants in 1768 [38]: 'The formation of their fingernails reveals if they can live or not.' Debility, immaturity, and asphyxia were neither defined nor distinguished and in vain Christian Stempel tried to discern 'natural' from 'morbid' forms of *weakness* in 1754 [39]: Joseph Capuron, professor of obstetrics in Paris, stated in 1820 [1]: 'Truly, there never can be any viability of the fetus born before the end of the fifth [solar] month of pregnancy … During the following two months, from the end of the fifth until the end of the seventh, the infants are scarcely any more viable.' The second edition of Charles Billard's *Traité des Enfants Nouveau-nés*, edited after his early death by Charles-Prosper Ollivier d'Angers, contained an extensive appendix on viability [40]: 'With Chaussier, one could assume that every infant who dies within the first 24 hours of life should be regarded non-viable irrespective of the cause of death.' Pierre Budin, who directed the Paris special care unit for premature infants, reported somewhat disappointed [41]: 'The special service admitted 395 weaklings during 1895. Of them, 95 were not viable … Of the 16 infants below 1,200 g, only one survived [and none below 1,000 g].' Thomas Morgan Rotch at Harvard wrote in 1896 [42]: 'Very few cases are reported, and none of them appear to be absolutely authentic, where an

infants weighing 1,000 gm or less may be arbitrarily considered previable, since many are biologically unable to support life in an extrauterine environment regardless of the type of resuscitation.' Other authors used the term *previable* to characterize infants of under 28 or 24 weeks' gestation. Alexander Schaffer and Mary Ellen Avery wrote in their textbook of 1971: 'The lower limit of viability is probably about 28 weeks, at which time most infants weigh two pounds, four ounces (1,000 grams)' [44]. San Francisco neonatologist Richard Behrman, in his *Report on Viability*, stated in 1975 [45]: 'In no instance did a reported infant who was both less than 601 grams and of a gestational age of 24 weeks or less survive.'

A few authors refused to give simple answers to the difficult question: The Edinburgh obstetrician John William Ballantyne wrote in 1902 [46]: 'When attempt is made to fix the uterine age at which viability may be said to be acquired, difficulties are at once encountered ... [disturbed developmental process, health of the mother]. It is not possible to fix some date which will account these factors of variability ... the statement cannot be regarded as final, for in ten years it may be possible to make a similar one with respect to the fetus of 6 or even 5 1/2 months. Improvements in the management of premature infants, such as the introduction of the incubator ... have pushed the age of viability back.' And the Munich paediatrician Meinhard von Pfaundler pointed out in 1907 [47]: 'One should refrain from defining a lower limit of viability from body measurements as it is scientifically unsound. It could encourage the withholding of support to an infant believed unviable.' Recently, the Stockholm neonatologist Hugo Lagercrantz proposed [48] that 'an alternative limit of viability could be when a fetus or a preterm infant has developed a brain to achieve a minimum level of consciousness. However, this raises a new question: how to define consciousness?'

Conclusion

The concept of viability may be regarded as a remnant of vitalism, a medical doctrine of Greek origin popularized in 1780 by the Scottish physician John Brown, who interpreted life as excitability [49]. He defined *sthenic* diseases as resulting from excessive stimuli, and *asthenic* diseases from too little stimulus. His doctrine was developed further in France by François Broussais [50], and in Germany by Goethe's physician Johann Christian Hufeland [51]: 'Someone may have a larger amount of vital force than the other, one has strength, the other weakness, depending on strengthening or weakening influences acting upon him.' When reviewing the history of the term viability, the Freiburg historian Eduard Seidler complained in 1967 [52]: 'It seems to be the special fate of "debility of life" (*debilitas vitae*), that despite obstinate fixation in scientific terminology it never attained a precise definition.' Up to the present day, it has never been clarified what is meant by viability, either deliberately or because it is not possible.

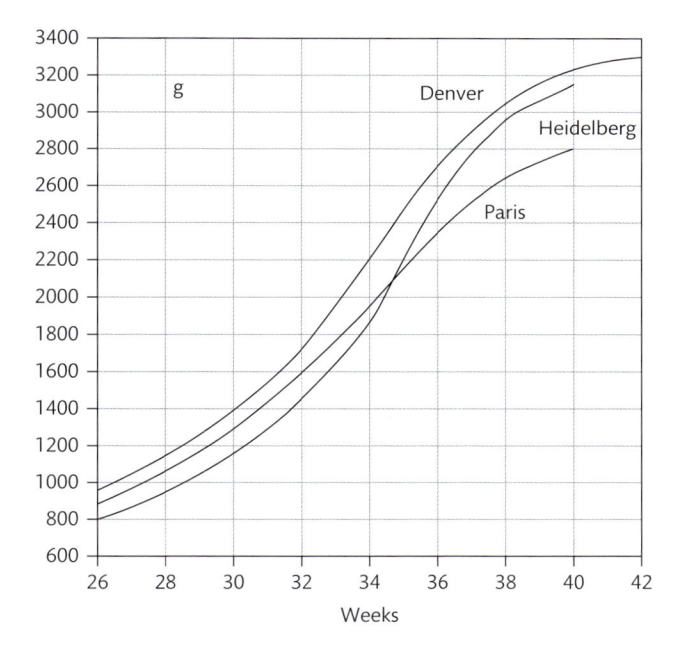

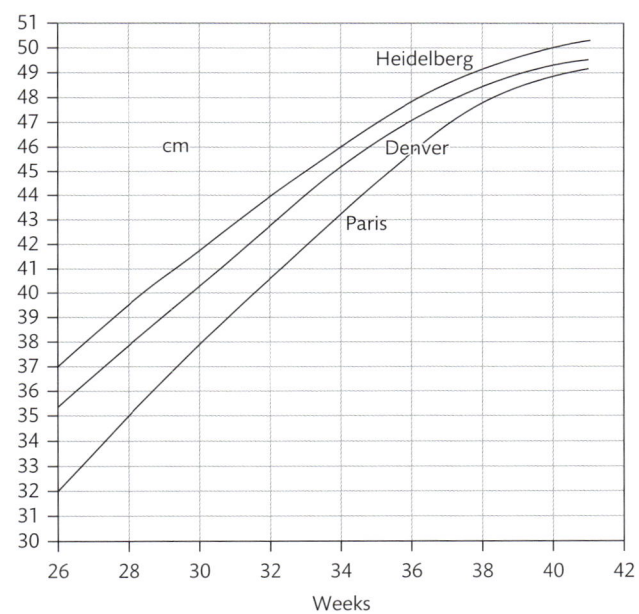

Fig. 3.1.3 Medians of fetal weight (top) and length (bottom) derived from measurements in three different centuries and countries: Lubchenco, Denver 1966 [35, 36]; Naegele, Heidelberg 1843 [34]; Levret, Paris 1747 [33, 57].

infant has survived which was born much before the twenty-seventh or twenty-eighth week of intrauterine life.' The Finnish paediatrician Arvo Ylppö, working in the preterm infants' special care unit in Berlin, wrote in 1919 [5]: 'At the preterm infants' special care unit of the Kaiserin Auguste Victoria Haus, I observed a total of 34 preterm infants with birthweights below 1,000 g. Only three of them survived for several years ... To answer the important question as to whether a preterm infant is viable at all, it is sufficient to know that the lowest limit is a birthweight of 700–800 g.'

In Los Angeles, a controlled study on artificial ventilation was performed in asphyxiated newborn infants in 1958 [43]: 'Premature

REFERENCES

1. Capuron J: Médecine légale, relative à l'art des accouchemens. Paris: Croullebois, 1821: p. 157–8.
2. Silverman WA: Neonatal pediatrics at the century mark. Pediatr Res 1990;**27**:S34–7.

3. Czerny A: Die Pädiatrie meiner Zeit. Berlin: Springer, 1939: p. 65.
4. Pomerance JJ, Ukrainski CT, Ukra T, et al.: Cost of living for infants weighing 1,000 grams or less at birth. Pediatrics 1978;**61**:908–10.
5. Ylppö A: Zur Physiologie, Klinik und zum Schicksal der Frühgeborenen. Z Kinderheilkd 1919;**24**:1–110.
6. Drillien CM: A longitudinal study of the growth and development of prematurely and maturely born children. III. Mental development. Arch Dis Child 1959;**34**:37–45.
7. Reiche A: Fragen des Wachstums und der Lebensaussichten sowie der Pflege und natürlichen Ernährung frühgeborener Kinder. Leipzig: Barth, 1916: p. 1–32.
8. Stewart AL, Turcan DM, Rawlings G, Reynolds EO: Prognosis for infants weighing 1000 g or less at birth. Arch Dis Child 1977;**52**: 97–104.
9. Verloove-Vanhorick SP: Management of the neonate at the limits of viability: the Dutch viewpoint. BJOG 2006;**113** Suppl 3:13–6.
10. Nuffield Council on Bioethics: Critical care decisions in fetal and neonatal medicine: ethical issues. London: Nuffield Council on Bioethics, 2006.
11. Hentschel R, Reiter-Theil S: Treatment of preterm infants at the lower margin of viability—a comparison of guidelines in German speaking countries. Dtsch Ärztebl Int 2008;**105**:47–52.
12. Janvier A, Bauer KL, Lantos JD: Are newborns morally different from older children? Theor Med Bioeth 2007;**28**:413–25.
13. Hippokrates: Über Achtmonatskinder. Berlin: Akademie-Verlag, 1968: p. 83, 89.
14. Hippocrates: Epidemics II, 3:17. Loeb Classical Library 477. Cambridge, MA: Harvard University Press, 1994: Vol. **VII**, p. 63.
15. Haller A: La génération; ou exposition des phénomènes relatifs a cette fonction naturelle. Paris: Doué, 1774: Vol. **2**, p. 438–43.
16. Baskett TF, Nagele F: Naegele's rule: a reappraisal. BJOG 2000;**107**:1433–5.
17. Boerhaave H: Praelectiones academicae in proprias institutiones rei medicae. 2. ed. Amsterdam: Westenius, 1744: Vol. **V**, part 2 (of 6), p. 238, 437.
18. Naegele FC: Erfahrungen und Abhandlungen aus dem Gebiethe der Krankheiten des weiblichen Geschlechtes. Mannheim: Loeffler, 1812: p. 280–1.
19. Denman T: An introduction to the practice of midwifery. Brattleborough, VT: Fessenden, 1807: p. 147.
20. Hess JH: Premature and congenitally disabled infants. London: Churchill, 1923: p. 362.
21. Quetelet A: Über den Menschen und die Entwicklung seiner Fähigkeiten. Stuttgart: Schweizerbart, 1838: p. 355.
22. Fleming JB: Folklore, fact and legend. Ir J Med Sci 1953;6th series:49–63.
23. Bennett M: Scottish customs from the cradle to the grave. Edinburgh: Polygon, 1992.
24. Cone TJ: De pondere infantum recens natorum. The history of weighing the newborn infant. Pediatrics 1961;**28**:490–8.
25. Mauriceau F: Traité des maladies des femmes grosses, et de celles qui sont accouchées (1st ed. 1668). 7. ed. Paris: Compagnie des Libraires, 1740: Vol. **1**, p. 85.
26. Lobb T: A compendium of the practice of physick. London: Buckland, 1747: p. 90.
27. Smellie W: A treatise on the theory and practise of midwifery. London: Sydenham Society, 1878: Vol. **1**, p. 114.
28. Roederer JG: Sermo de pondere et longitudine infantum recens natorum. Comment Soc Reg Scient Gottingae 1753;**3**:410–24.
29. Stein GW: Kurze Beschreibung eines Baromacrometers und eines Cephalometers. Cassel, 1775. In: Stein GW: Kleine Werke zur praktischen Geburtshülfe. Marburg: Academische Buchhandlung, 1789: p. 105–32.
30. Alberti H-J: Maß und Gewicht. Geschichtliche und tabellarische Darstellungen. Berlin: Akademie-Verlag, 1957: p. 229–38, 376–417.
31. Cardarelli F: Encyclopedia of scientific units, weight, and measures. Berlin: Springer, 2005.
32. Zupko RE: Revolution in measurement: western European weights and measures. Philadelphia, PA: American Philosophical Society, 1990.
33. Levret A: L'art des accouchemens, démontré par les principes de physique et de méchanique. 3. ed. Paris: Didot Jeune, 1766: p. 418.
34. Naegele HF-J, Grenser WL: Traité pratique de l'art des accouchements. Paris: Baillière, 1869: p. 67–72.
35. Lubchenco LO, Hansman C, Boyd E: Intrauterine growth in length and head circumference as estimated from live births at gestational ages from 26 to 42 weeks. Pediatrics 1966;**37**:403–8.
36. Lubchenco LO, Hansman C, Dressler M, Boyd E: Intrauterine growth as estimated from liveborn birth-weight data at 24 to 42 weeks of gestation. Pediatrics 1963;**32**:793–800.
37. Aristotle: History of animals. Loeb Classical Library. Cambridge, MA: Harvard University Press, 1991: Vol. **XI**, p. IX (7), 585 a, 12–22, 443.
38. Raulin J: Von Erhaltung der Kinder von dem ersten Augenblick ihres Entstehens an (French ed. 1769). Leipzig: Crusius, 1769: Vol. **1**, p. 391.
39. Stempel CF: De partu debili reficiundo. Dissertatio. Lipsiae: Langenhem, 1754: p. 4–6.
40. Billard CM: Die Krankheiten der Neugeborenen und Säuglinge (1st French ed. 1828). Weimar: Industrie-Comptoir, 1829: p. 31 in Appendix.
41. Budin P: Service des enfants débiles a la maternité. Année 1895. In: Budin P: Femmes en couches et nouveau-nés. Paris: Doin, 1897: p. 389–405.
42. Rotch TM: Pediatrics. The hygienic and medical treatment of children. Edinburgh: Pentland, 1896: Vol. **1**, p. 288.
43. Wilson MG, Roscoe SN: Resuscitation of newborn premature infants. Calif Med 1958;**88**:312–5.
44. Schaffer A, Avery ME: Diseases of the newborn. Philadelphia, PA: Saunders, 1971: p. 23.
45. Behrman RE, Rosen TS: Report on viability and non-viability of the fetus. Washington, DC: Dept. of Health, 1975: p. 12.1–12.116.
46. Ballantyne JW: The problem of the premature infant. BMJ 1902;**1**:1196–200.
47. Pfaundler M: Über die Behandlung der angeborenen Lebensschwäche. Münch Med Wochenschr 1907;**54**:1417–21.
48. Lagercrantz H: The emergence of the mind: a borderline of human viability? Acta Paediatr 2007;**96**:327–8.
49. Brown J: The elements of medicine. London: Johnson, 1788.
50. Broussais FJV: Histoire des phlegmasies, ou inflammations chroniques. Paris: Gabon, 1808.

51. Hufeland CW: Ideen über Pathogenie und Einfluss der Lebenskraft auf die Entstehung und Form der Krankheiten. Jena: Akad. Buchhandlung, 1795: p. 116.
52. Seidler E: Über die 'Lebensschwäche'. Episteme [Milano] 1967;**1**:45–60.
53. Siebold Ed: De paediometro commentarius, quo ad audiendam orationem in dedicando instituto regio obstetrico clinco univesitatis litterariae Berolinensis habendam. Berolini: Typis Reimerianis, 1818.
54. Jacquemet E: Les Maladies de la première enfance. Paris: Baillière, 1892: p. 45.
55. Holt LE: The diseases of infancy and childhood. For the use of students and practitioners of medicine: New York: Appleton, 1898: p. 15.
56. Auvard PVA: Le nouveau-né. Physiologie—hygiène—aillaitement. 5. ed. Paris: Doin, 1905: p. 89–90.
57. Boivin MAV: Mémorial de l'art des accouchements, ou principes fondés sur la pratique de l'hospice de la maternité. 3. ed. Paris: Méquignon, 1824: p. 120–1.

3.2 Surviving against the odds

Introduction: fairy tales and miracle babies

'Miracle births' have been reported over the centuries and the book of records editors keep busy updating the earliest, smallest, or lightest infants each year. Considered dwarfs or miraculous births, preterm infants often resided in fairy tales [1]: '"How dull it is without any children about us; our house is so quiet, and other people's houses so noisy and merry!" "Yes," answered his wife, and sighed, "if we could only have one, and that one ever so little, no bigger than my thumb, we would love him just the same." Then, it came about that the wife was poorly, and seven months later she bore a child; and though all its limbs were perfectly formed, it was no bigger than a thumb. Then the parents said, "He is just what we wished for, and he shall be our own dear child." And because he was so tiny, they called him "Thickasathumb".'

Early survivors

Unreliable gestational age and the unwillingness to measure (see Chapter 3.1) detract from the credibility of early case reports, as does the fact that they were usually reported by the surviving preterm infant's family. In *De animalibus*, the Persian scholar Avicenna wrote around 1000 C.E. [2]: 'There is a credible report about a woman giving birth to a child after six months who lived well.' In his *Generation of Living Creatures*, William Harvey [3] cited a letter from the Alcalá natural philosopher and physician to Philip II, Franciscus Valesius, who 'relates that in his time [1524–1592] a Girle which was borne in the Fifth moneth, did live to enter into the twelfth year of her Age.'

Fortunio Licetus, born in Rapallo, 3 October 1577

Adrien Baillet wrote his encyclopaedia of writers in 1722, albeit 66 years after Licetus' death [4]: 'He was born near the coast of Genova on the 3rd October 1577, at 2 hours after midnight, during a journey his parents made from their small village Recco to Rapallo, where his father [Joseph Licetus] had just established his medical practice. A tiring and rough transport, together with a thunderstorm near Cap Portofino … The father had no doubt that it was an abortion whereas the mother argued that the fruit was not much before its seventh month. This male fetus was not larger than the palm of a hand; his father examined him as a physician and found that he was further developed than an embryo, and transported him to Rapallo alive … To demonstrate his experience in the new practice in Rapallo, he undertook to complete nature's work and to help the infant develop with the same *device* used to raise the chickens in Egypt. He instructed a wet nurse about all she had to do, and had her put his son into a clean oven. He succeeded in raising the child who grew thanks to the uniformity of the ambient warmth precisely monitored with a thermometer.' The *device* was further specified by Nicholas Eloy 1778 [5] as 'a cotton-lined box'. Citing Aristotle in his book *De Monstrorum Caussis*, Licetus alluded to his own immaturity in 1634 [6]: 'Whereas all other animals have a unique duration of pregnancy, only humans have several; and may be born between the seventh (which I often heard from my parents about myself) and the tenth month.' The boy was named Fortunio in reference to his lucky survival, and became a famous philosopher and scientist, author of many books, friend of Galileo, and professor in Padova from 1634 (Fig. 3.2.1, left). He died at the age of 79 years.

Isaac Newton, born in Woolsthorpe, 4 January 1643

In the 'Earlier draft of [John] Conduitt's account of Newton's early life' Robert Iliffe found the following passage [7]: 'He was born upon Christmas day in the year 1642 near 3 months after the death of his father … Sir Isaac Newton told me he had often heard from his mother [Hannah Ayscough] that when he was born he was so little they could have put him into a quart pot & so unlikely to live that two women who were sent to My Lady Packenham at North Witham for some thing for him sate down on a stile by the way & said to one another they need not make haste for the child would certainly be dead before they could get back. He for some time wore a bolster round his neck to keep his head upon his shoulders.' The date refers to the Julian calendar. The Gregorian calendar (1582) corrected for

---

Reproduced with permission from Obladen, M. Historical notes on immaturity. Part 2: Surviving against the odds. *Journal of Perinatal Medicine*, 39:571–577. Copyright © 2011 Walter de Gruyter GmbH, Berlin/Boston.

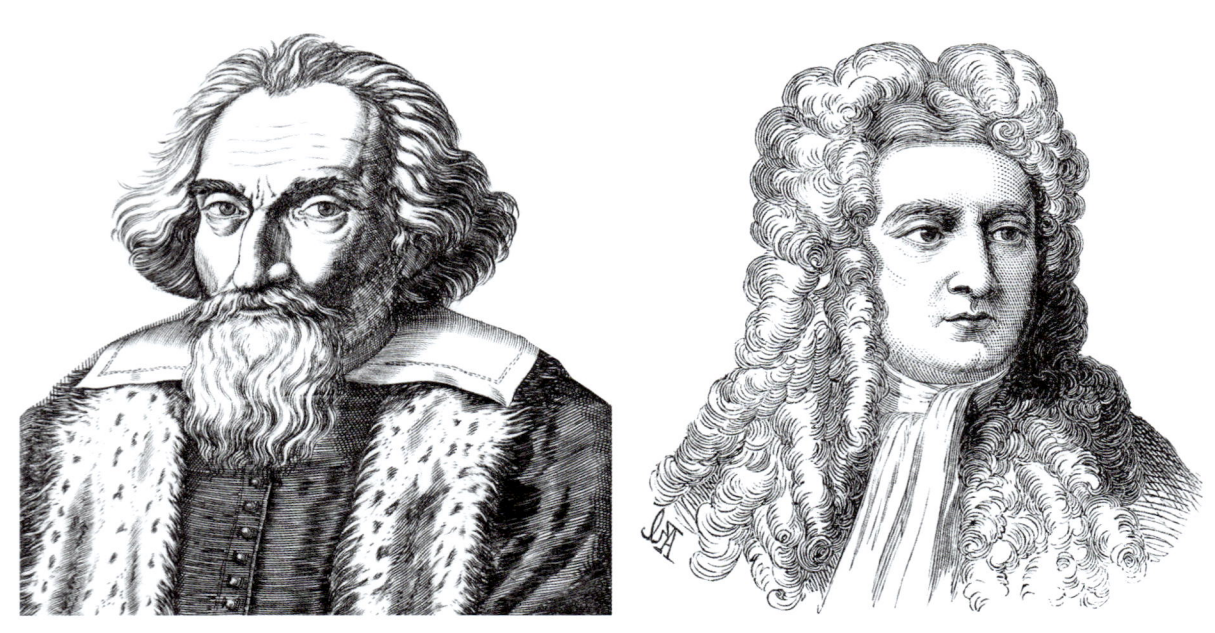

Fig. 3.2.1 Personalities with outstanding intelligence who were immature neonates: left: Fortunio Licetus, 1577–1657, scientist and physician, frontispiece from his book *Litheosphorus* 1640 [6]; right: Sir Isaac Newton, 1643–1727, physicist and mathematician, portrait from Aubrey 1878 [54].

10 intercalated days accumulated since 46 B.C.E., but was not introduced in England until 1752.

Isaac Newton contributed more to the development of physics and mathematics than any other single individual. He detected the laws of gravitational force and of motion, described differential and integral calculus, became professor at Cambridge from 1669 (Fig. 3.2.1, right), was knighted in 1705, and died at the age of 84 years.

Scientific case descriptions

The list of famous immature survivors could be extended, but it should not conceal the fact that nearly all infants with extremely low birthweight did not survive. In the absence of sound definitions, researchers used length of gestation or birthweight as a surrogate for *viability*, and the Moscow Foundling Hospital had the largest numbers: among 121,625 neonates admitted between 1862 and 1880, 6036 were below 2500 g (at that time the definition of prematurity), 41 were under 1000 g, none of which survived, prompting the physician-in-chief, Nikolaus Th. Miller, to note: 'such a degree of immaturity can be called non-viable' [8]. Some of the smallest premature infants who were 'saved' have been compiled by Ahlfeld, 1875 [9], Hess, 1911 [10], and Peiper, 1937 [11], but their perinatal data usually are incomplete and lacking follow-up examinations. The frequently cited patients of Rodman, 1815 [12], Richard de Nancy, 1839 [13], Tait, 1840 [14], Cullingworth, 1878 [15], Oberwarth, 1904 [16], and Hess, 1911 [10] survived the neonatal period, but died after a few months, usually from infection or failure to thrive. The surviving infants of Reiche, 1916 [17] and Ylppö, 1919 [18] did not develop normally. Table 3.2.1 describes several infants born weighing under 1000g before World War II, about whom follow-up is available and the original source known.

Survival statistics and their pitfalls

Besides the extreme cases, the limit of viability, and its change over time, can be appreciated from the birthweights and gestational ages at which half of the infants survived, similar to the LD_{50} in pharmacology. Fig. 3.2.2 illustrates how median survival weight decreased over the last 130 years. In Japan, half of the infants survived who were born weighing 500 g or born at 23 gestational weeks during the years 2003–2004 [36]. Survival statistics of immature infants, however, remained of questionable value, as they depended on the definition of abortion, stillbirth, and live birth, which were not at all comparable across countries. The smallest infants who died minutes after being born were and are often called 'stillbirths' by health professionals who considered them previable; hypothermia and delayed onset of (intensive) care were not infrequent.

When infant mortality declined after the World War I, it became apparent that many countries had found ways to doctor the survival figures of premature infants. In 1925, the League of Nations proposed international recommendations for the registration of births (live births and stillbirths) and deaths [37]. The committee used the presence of breathing to define a live birth, and set a minimum gestational duration of 28 weeks as a criterion for viability, 'having in mind the very great difficulty of rearing an infant born after a shorter period of gestation'. Mary Crosse, who set up the Birmingham preterm baby unit in 1931, wrote in her book (first ed. 1945) [38]: 'It is necessary to know if *all* infants are included in the records even if (1) they are moribund at birth or on admission, (2) they are suffering from a congenital deformity incompatible with life, (3) the birth weight is below 2 lb. (900 g), or (4) the maturity is less than 28 weeks.' Few personalities paved the preterm infant's way to public health recognition as successfully as Ethel Dunham, director at the Washington Children's Bureau from 1935. In her manual she clearly demanded [39]: 'Include in statistics all liveborn infants, regardless of gestation period. No exclusions should be made on the basis of "nonviability."

Table 3.2.1 Several surviving extremely low birthweight infants with reliable perinatal measurements and normal development at follow-up

First author Publication year	Place and date of birth	Sex Gest. age	Weight (g) Length (cm)	Remarks on thermal care and nutrition	Follow-up duration	Refs.
d'Outrepont 1822	Würzburg 24.04.1806	M 27 wks	841# 37	# day 2; placenta praevia, breech, cotton-filled basket; spoon-fed mixed milk, water, sugar, flour	11 y	[19, 20]
Annan 1848	Kinross, Scotland 26.01.1848	F 23 wks	660* ca. 33	* day 7; cotton wool, flannel, earthenware warmed bottle; cream, water and sherry wine	3 mo	[21]
Barker 1851	Dumfries, Scotland 14.05.1847	F 26 wks	454 28	Laid in a nail box set on the kitchen fender before the fire	4 1/2 y	[22]
Villemin 1895	Paris 14.04.1892	F 24–26 wks	950 38?	Arsonval incubator, spoon-fed wetnurse's milk; artificial ventilation for apnoeas on day 13	31 mo	[23]
Mansell 1902	Hastings 25.09.1890	F 6 1/2 mo	510 –	No incubator, swaddled in cotton wool, anointed with cod-liver oil	11 y	[24]
Shepherd 1902	Launcester 19.12.1898	F 6 1/2 mo	900 –	Wrapped in cotton wool, no incubator but placed in a box inside the fender	3 y	[25]
Maygrier 1907	Paris 03.11.1905	F 30 wks	970*, 840* –	* day 5; incubator for 3 months; spoon fed with breast milk	18 mo	[26]
Pfaundler 1907	Graz, Austria 12.11.1902	? 6 mo	860 35.5	Stayed 4 years in foundling hospital; body weight 4 kg at 1 year of age	4 1/2 y	[27]
Mayerhofer 1913 Huber 1921	Vienna 19.06.1913	F 6 mo	790° 31	° day 10; warming tub for 2 months; breast milk by gavage; rickets; discharged home 1 year old	8 y	[28, 29]
Pulford 1928	Woodland, Cal. 12.04.1925	F 217 d	680 36*	* at 1 month; cotton jacket, incubator, breast milk and dextro-maltose by medicine dripper	3 y	[30]
Fischer Bán 1931	Budapest 18.11.1928	F, twin 209 d	600 33	540 g on day 4; cotton padding, thermophor, hot-water bottles replaced every 2–3 hours	2 y	[31, 32]
Hoffman 1938	Chicago 19.08.1935	F 191 d	735*, 595* 30	* on day 8; oxygen incubator bed; breast milk and whisky by dropper; intramuscular blood injections	21 mo	[33]
Pilch 1935	Freiburg 1928	M –	800 34	6 mo in hospital, high-caloric gavage feeding, rickets, inguinal hernia operated	6 y	[34]
Monro 1939	North Sydney, Can 06.06.1937	M 32 wks?	397* –	In oven during night, fed with lactogen, corn syrup, and brandy by dripper	12 mo	[35]

*, at birth; °, at admission; #, at other date as indicated; +, lowest; F, female; M, male; mo, months; wks, weeks; y, years.

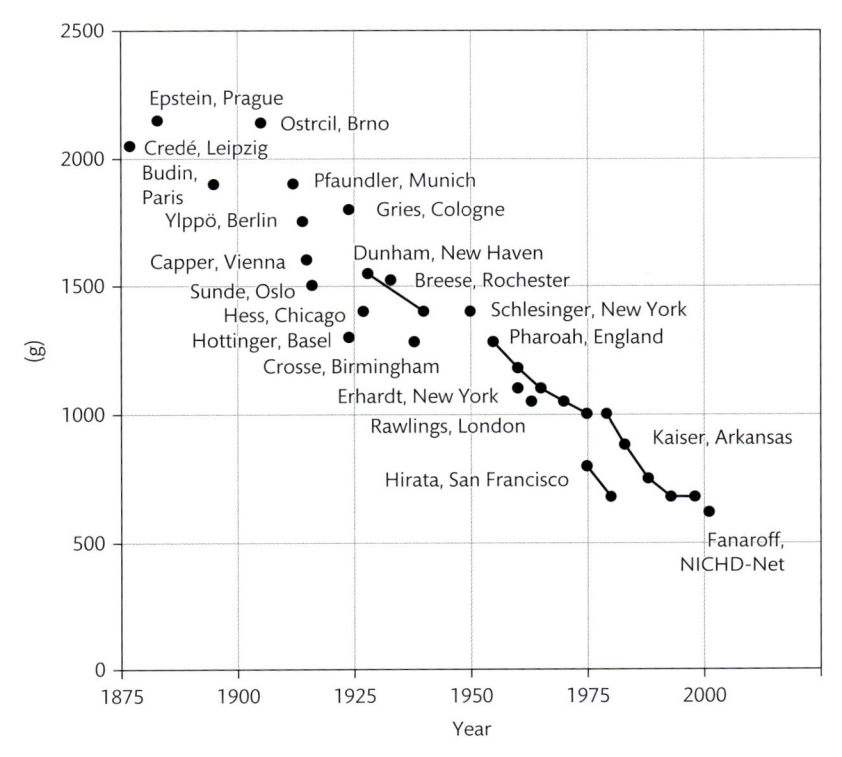

Fig. 3.2.2 Birthweight-specific survival since the begin of institutional medical care of preterm infants: mean birth weight, at which half of the infants survived for at least 28 days or up to discharge home in selected centres. Data are extrapolated or averaged from studies which usually covered several years. NICHD-Net, Neonatal Research Network of the National Institute of Child Health and Human Development.

Arbitrary exclusions should not be made on the basis of low birth weight or birth length, gestation period, or duration of life.'

In 1950, the World Health Organization (WHO) recommended the 'any sign of life' definition of livebirth, which included breathing, a heartbeat, cord pulsation, or movements. These signs were retained in the 1975 revision, and the 'capacity for the fetus to survive independently of its mother' was added as a viability criterion. That definition was then completed by a comment that restricted viability to a minimum gestation of 28 weeks. To confuse things even further, the WHO definitions of 1993 requested the registration of all births, live born or stillborn, weighing 500 g (22 complete weeks) or more, but only in national, not international statistics, where the viability criteria of 1000 g and 28 weeks persisted [40]. Countries were reluctant to change their attitude towards immature infants, and some never adopted WHO definitions. Gourbin reported significant differences among 27 European countries as late as 1991 [37]. Remarkably, many immature or extremely low birthweight infants were not registered in national and local statistics.

question concerns advantages to him when born.' The 13th-century German law book *Sachsenspiegel* [Saxon mirror] regarded a newborn infant as liveborn and entitled to inherit his father's fortune (Fig. 3.2.3), 'if his voice can be heard in all four corners of the house', which excluded stillborn and immature infants from heritage [43]. In Britain, the judge Henry Swinburne from York specified in 1590 [44]: 'Crying is not an only proof of life, since it may be proved by motion, breathing, and such like.' The French civil code (1804) set in article 314 the briefest period after which life may be sustained at 180 days [45], but to determine the beginning of pregnancy stayed notoriously difficult. In the US, the courts have repeatedly and recently tried to regulate decisions in the delivery room, that is, the Baby Doe Rehabilitation Act 1973 and the Born-Alive Infant Protection Act (BAIPA) 2002 [46]. The latter defined that a fetus must be considered viable when *potentially* able to live outside its mother's womb, albeit with artificial aid. Given the vagueness of this definition, the legislation did not markedly alleviate parents' or doctors' difficulty in identifying appropriate limits of treatment.

Legislation

Political leaders have attempted to define viability since ancient times. Plutarch (46–120 c.e.) recounted the Sparta scenario [41]: 'It was not left to the father to rear what children he pleased, but he was obliged to carry the child to a place called *Lesche*, to be examined by the most ancient men of the tribe, who were assembled there. If it was strong and well proportioned, they gave orders for its education, and assigned it one of the nine thousand shares of land. But if it was weakly and deformed, they ordered it to be thrown into the place called *Apothetae*, which is a deep cavern near the mountain *Taygetos*; concluding that its life could be no advantage either to itself or to the public, since nature had not given it at first any strength or goodness of constitution.'

In Rome, *debilitas vitae* was likewise rejected until Christianization. The Justinian enactments (529–564 c.e.) put an end to the *patria potestas* [father's right to kill his offspring], and ruled [42]: 'The fetus in the womb is deemed to be fully a human being, whenever the

Ethical recommendations

In the absence of scientific definitions, ethical recommendations on the obligatory or optional treatment of immature infants came about by consensus conferences. At the border of viability, physicians' behaviour has been shown to vary widely [47]. This fact did not change when different recommendations were issued and re-issued in European countries. Many developed countries currently consider intensive care justified at 25 weeks or more, comfort care at up to 22 weeks, and an individual approach consistent with parental wishes at 23–24 weeks, the 'grey zone' or 'window of uncertainty'. Marked differences exist among countries, as Maria Pignotti reported [48]. The 'window' was set at 22–23 completed weeks in Japan and Germany, 23–24 weeks in the UK, the US, and Canada, and 24–26 weeks in France, the Netherlands, and Switzerland. Pignotti's paper paved the way towards a change from gestation-dependent towards individual estimation of an infant's viability. Instead of a strictly defined window, the concept of *provisional* intensive care offers parents and

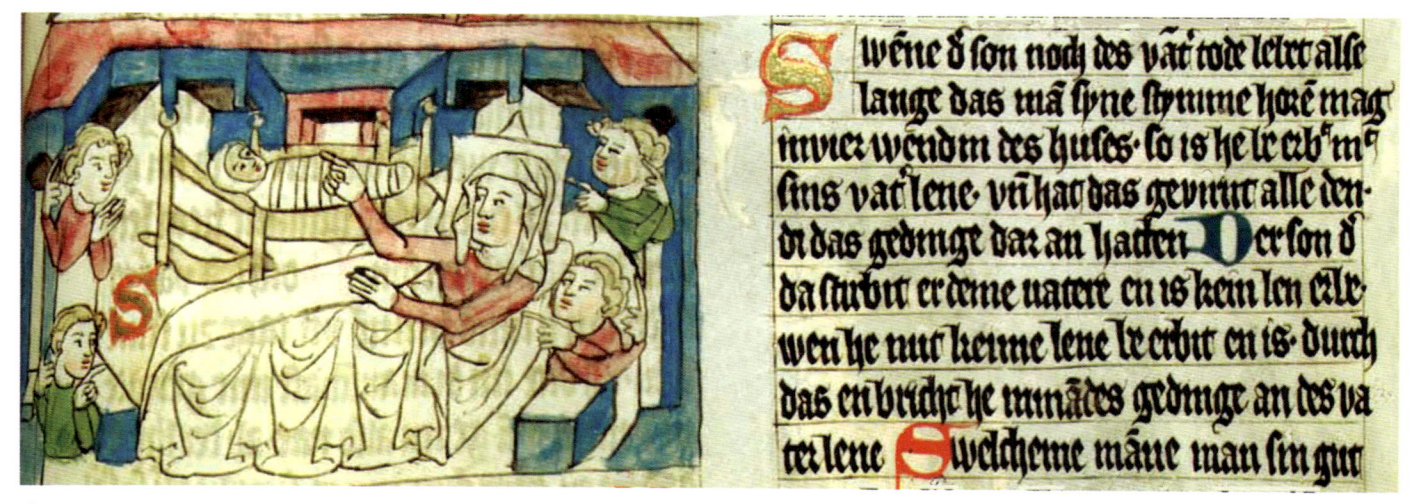

Fig. 3.2.3 Detail from the Medieval lawbook *Sachsenspiegel* (Saxon's Mirror, ca. 1234 c.e.) illustrating that the baby's voice must be hearable in all four house corners to consider it liveborn [43].

physicians the option to withdraw ineffective or futile intensive care when necessary, which permits each infant's individual problems and suffering to be considered. In 2008, Tyson and colleagues [49] published a prospective study of 4446 infants born at 22–25 weeks' gestation in the Neonatal Research Network of the National Institute of Child Health and Human Development with neurodevelopmental follow-up at 18–22 months. They found that antenatal corticosteroids, female sex, singleton birth, and higher birthweight (per each 100 g increment) were each associated with reduction in the risk of death and the risk of any neurodevelopmental impairment equivalent to a 1-week increase in gestational age. Despite the fact that the value of neonatal intensive care has undergone greater scrutiny, and has been found far more cost-effective than adult intensive care, both health professionals and the public felt less obliged to treat the preterm baby [50]. Like assisted reproduction and abortion, the premature infant's survival continued to be the subject of emotional debate and was burdened by the competition for resources.

Conclusion

The viability concept may have had important legal, medical, and ethical implications. Unfortunately, most definitions suffered from inaccuracies: extrinsic availability of specialized care, conditions of survival (natural versus artificial support), and duration of survival were usually not specified, but greatly influenced the definition of viability, as Fost reported [51]. Instead of assessing each newborn's individual prognosis, and ignoring its sex, diseases, and particular reason for premature delivery, several recommendations still use gestational age alone as a criterium for initiating or withholding resuscitation. As John Ballantyne correctly stated in 1902 [52], this largely neglects the infant's specific chances and threats. As in other areas of medicine, in which palliative care must be chosen when intensive care becomes futile, perinatal medicine has to come of age and to stop seeking simple solutions. 'Not everything that counts can be counted; not everything that can be counted counts' [53]. This sentence was posted in the Princeton office of Albert Einstein, who is believed to have been born preterm himself.

REFERENCES

1. Grimm J, Grimm W: Thickasathumb. In: Selected tales. Translated by: David Luke. London: Penguin, 1982: p. 323–8.
2. Avicenna: De animalibus. Per Michaelem Scotum de arabico in latinum translatus: Venetiis: de Gregoriis, [1500]: fol. 24v.
3. Harvey W: Anatomical exercitations, concerning the generation of living creatures. Gryphon Editions, New York, 1991; London: Pulley, 1653: p. 477.
4. Baillet A: Jugemens des savans sur les principaux ouvrages des auteurs. Paris: Moette & Co, 1722: Vol. **6**, p. 135–8.
5. Eloy NFJ: Dictionnaire historique de la Médecine ancienne et moderne ou mémoires disposés en ordre alphabetique. Mons: Hoyois, 1778: Vol. **III**, p. 70–2.
6. Licetus F: Litheosphorus, sive de lapide Bononiense lucem in se conceptum. Utini: Schiratus, 1640: Frontispiece.
7. Iliffe R, Keynes M, Higgitt R: Early biographies of Isaac Newton, 1660–1885. Earlier draft of [John] Conduitt's account of Newton's early life. London: Pickering, 2005: Ms 130.3. pp 3r, 9v.
8. Miller NTh: Die Frühgeborenen und die Eigenthümlichkeiten ihrer Krankheiten. Jahrb Kinderheilk 1886;**25**:179–94.
9. Ahlfeld F: Über unzeitig oder sehr frühzeitig geborene Früchte, die am Leben blieben. Arch Gynäk 1875;**8**:194–205.
10. Hess JH: A study of the caloric needs of premature infants. Am J Dis Child 1911;**2**:302–14.
11. Peiper A: Unreife und Lebensschwäche. Leipzig: Thieme, 1937: p. 81.
12. Rodman J: Case of a child between the fourth and fifth month, and brought up. Edinb Med Surg J 1815;**11**:455–8.
13. Richard de Nancy CJ: Traité pratique des maladies des enfants. Paris: Baillière, 1839: p. 127.
14. Tait W: Birth of a living child on the 179th day. Lancet 1842;**38**:119–20.
15. Cullingworth CJ: Case illustrating the viability of extremely small premature children. Obst J Gt Brit 1878;**63**:163.
16. Oberwarth E: Über eine selten kleine, am Leben gebliebene Frühgeburt. Jahrb Kinderheilk 1904;**60**:377–82.
17. Reiche A: Das Wachstum der Frühgeburten in den ersten Lebensmonaten. I. Mitteilung. Zeitschr Kinderheilk 1915;**12**:369–401.
18. Ylppö A: Zur Physiologie, Klinik und zum Schicksal der Frühgeborenen. Zeitschr Kinderheilk 1919;**24**:1–110.
19. d'Outrepont J: Über die Erhaltung einer Frucht, welche im sechsten Monate der Schwangerschaft geboren wurde. Bamberg: Goebhardt, 1822: Vol. **1**, p. 168–94.
20. Ulsamer A: De partu praematuro generatim et nonnulla de eo arte legitima procurando. Wircebugi: Inaug. Diss., 1820: p. 44.
21. Annan R: Case of a child born betwixt the end of the sixth and the middle of the seventh month and brought up. Med Times 1848;**18**:109–10.
22. Barker WTT: Child born in the beginning of the sixth month, and reared. Am J Med Sci 1851;**41**:257.
23. Villemin: Observation d'un enfant né avant terme. Rev Mens Mal Enf Paris 1895;**13**:22–7.
24. Mansell HR: Survival of a premature child weighing 18 oz. BMJ 1902;**1**:773.
25. Shepherd ThW: Survival of a preterm child weighing less than two pounds. BMJ 1902;**1**:1264.
26. Maygrier C, Schwaab A: Histoire d'un petit prématuré, du poids de 840 grammes. Bull Soc Obst Paris 1907;**10**:216–20.
27. Pfaundler M: Über die Behandlung der angeborenen Lebensschwäche. Münch Med Wochenschr 1907;**54**:1417–21.
28. Mayerhofer E, Roth F: Klinische Beobachtungen über die kalorische Betrachtungsweise der Säuglingsernährung. Zeitschr Kinderheilk 1914;**11**:117–32.
29. Huber O: Ein nunmehr 8 Jahre altes mit einem Geburtsgewicht von 790g frühgeborenes Mädchen. Zeitschr Kinderheilk 1921;**30**:281–90.
30. Pulford DS, Blevins WJ: Premature infant, birth weight 680 grams, with survival. Am J Dis Child 1928;**36**:797–8.
31. Fischer-Bán H: Die unterste Grenze der Lebensfähigkeit Frühgeborener. Klin Wochenschr 1931;**10**:1–11.
32. Temesvary R: Ein am Leben erhaltenes Kind von 600 g Geburtsgewicht. Zentralbl Gynäk 1931;1319–21.
33. Hoffman SJ, Greenhill JP, Lundeen EC: A premature infant weighing 735 grams and surviving. JAMA 1938;**110**:283–5.
34. Pilch D: Schicksal der Frühgeburten von 2000 g und darunter. Freiburg: Inaug. Diss., 1935: p. 7, tab. 6.
35. Monro JS: A premature infant weighing less than one pound at birth who survived and developed normally. Can Med Assoc J 1939;**40**:69–70.

36. Nishida H, Sakuma I: Limit of viability in Japan: ethical consideration. J Perinat Med 2009;37:457–60.
37. Gourbin G, Masuy-Stroobant G: Registration of vital data: are live births and stillbirths comparable all over Europe? Bull World Health Organ 1995;73:449–60.
38. Crosse VM: The premature baby. 5. ed. London: Churchill, 1961: p. 250.
39. Dunham EC: Premature infants. Children's Bureau Publication Nr. 325. Washington, DC: Federal Security Agency, 1948: p. 44.
40. World Health Organization: International statistical classification of diseases and related health problems. 10th Revision. Geneva: WHO, 1993: Vol. 2, p. 129–33.
41. Plutarch: Lives of illustrious men. Lycurgus. London: Valpy, 1831: Vol. 1, p. 104–5.
42. Watson A: The digest of Justinian. Book 1, chapter 5: Human status. Philadelphia, PA: University of Pennsylvania Press, 1998: Vol. 1, p. 1.5.7.
43. Eike von Repgow: Die Dresdner Bilderhandschrift des Sachsenspiegels (ca. 1235). Edited by Karl von Amira. Leipzig: Hiersemann, 1902: Folio LXVr.
44. Swinburne H: A briefe treatise of testaments and last willes very profitable to be understood of all the subjects of this Realme of England, etc. London: Windet, 1590.
45. Dervieux F: Sur la viabilité des nouveau-nés. Rev Med Leg 1913;20:1–6.
46. Sayeed SA: Baby Doe redux? The Department of Health and Human Services and the Born-Alive Infants Protection Act of 2002. Pediatrics 2005;116:e576–85.
47. Cuttini M, Nadai M, Kaminski M, et al. End-of-life decisions in neonatal intensive care: physicians' self-reported practices in seven European countries. Lancet 2000;355:2112–8.
48. Pignotti MS, Donzelli G: Perinatal care at the threshold of viability: an international comparison. Pediatrics 2008;121:e193–8.
49. Tyson JE, Parikh NA, Langer J, Green C, Higgins RD: Intensive care for extreme prematurity: moving beyond gestational age. N Engl J Med 2008;358:1672–81.
50. Janvier A, Bauer KL, Lantos JD: Are newborns morally different from older children? Theor Med Bioeth 2007;28:413–25.
51. Fost N, Chudwin D, Wikler D: The limited moral significance of 'fetal viability'. Hastings Cent Rep 1980;10:10–3.
52. Ballantyne JW: The problem of the premature infant. BMJ 1902;1:1196–1200.
53. McKee M: Not everything that counts can be counted; not everything that can be counted counts. BMJ 2004;328:153.
54. Aubrey WSH: The national and domestic history of England. London: Hagger, 1878: Vol. 3, p. 401.

3.3

Respiratory distress
Understanding surfactant deficiency

Introduction

A condition as dramatic and gruesome as respiratory distress syndrome (RDS) became known before the book printing era. Common terms for the disease were debility, weakness, and atelectasis, and it was poorly distinguished from birth asphyxia. By establishing obstetrics as a science in the large maternity hospitals in London and Paris, François Mauriceau [1], William Smellie [2], Joseph Raulin [3], and Jean Louis Baudelocque [4] laid the foundation for effective treatment of the newborn infant. To spot the scientific hallmarks of respiratory distress and surfactant research, it helps to read Julius Comroe's wise chapter 'Premature Science and Immature Lungs' in his 'Retrospectroscope' [5], and Thomas Cone's comprehensive 'History of the Care and Feeding of the Premature Infant' [6].

Respiratory distress

Detailed texts on neonatology originated in hospices for foundlings, mainly in France, after Napoleon mandated such institutions for every county in 1811 [7–9]. The pulmonary anomalies observed in deceased infants were generally termed 'atelectasis' if the lung failed to float at the postmortem examination. Despite this knowledge, an excised lung's 'floating test' was still used to judge whether an infant had lived after birth, and continued to play a sad role in infanticide trials (see Chapter 8.3). Authors who observed premature infants with RDS were amazed by their dramatic suffering and inevitable death. Charles Billard's fundamental 'Traité des Maladies des Enfants Nouveau-Nés et à la Mamelle' [9] provided a detailed and largely correct classification of neonatal lung disorders in 1828. He wrote 18 pages on the cry of infants, and probably alluded to expiratory grunting in 1828 [9]: 'I have noticed twenty [preterm] children with incomplete cry, where the reprise alone was heard with distinctness, while the cry was smothered … it is very probable that the air does not penetrate, has not penetrated, or has penetrated but very slightly into the lungs.'

Leipzig obstetrician Eduard Jörg described the cry of the infant with 'foetal lung' as 'whimpering, hoarse, whistling or squeaking' and interpreted sternal retractions as the gasping for breath in 1835 [10]. In Vienna in 1852, Alois Bednar named RDS 'fetal state of the lung … The tissue of an atelectatic lung contains no air, and does not crepitate. It is meat-like, dense, violet-red, not tearable and sinks in water.' [11]. In New York in 1901, Vanderpoel Adriance noted 'the respiratory center is unstable, the actions of the lung irregular … attacks of cyanosis' [12]. Also Camilla Hahn, in Paris, was impressed by apnoeic spells: 'Life without respiration may persist for some time.' Around 1900, most authors applied continuous oxygen when caring for infants with RDS in open or closed incubators. To quantify RDS severity, clinical scores were developed to determine the extent of tachypnoea, retractions, grunting, cyanosis, and so on [13, 14], but became obsolete with the availability of blood gas analysis.

Pathophysiology of the immature lung

Ideas on the cause of RDS were published by obstetricians in the second half of the 18th century. Joseph Raulin revealed solid understanding of the immature lung in 1768 [3]: 'The countless lung vesicles must fill with air, and must chase it away again. The largest part of the lung's blood vessels, hitherto collapsed, must open and fill with blood, whose circulation is required unless life extinguishes instantly. If the lung vesicles are too weak, without power, or obstructed with phlegm, they do not accept the atmosphere's air, and the blood vessels collapse. Both functions [ventilation and perfusion] become impossible or very imperfect, and the loss of the infant is imminent.'

After the end of the Napoleonic wars, the stage was set for scientific research and major progress in basic sciences and clinical medicine. The French revolution abolished religious restrictions, which for centuries had impeded scientific progress. The ban on postmortem examination, blood testing, and use of chemistry in analytical medicine was lifted. Medicine was reunited with surgery (and thus with obstetrics), which for centuries had made its progress in the twilight of barber shops and field surgeons. In 1828, Paris surgeon Jean-Jacques Joseph Leroy d'Etiolles wrote a treatise, which

Adapted with permission from Obladen, M. History of Surfactant up to 1980. *Biol Neonate*, 87:308–316. Copyright © 2005 S. Karger AG, Basel.

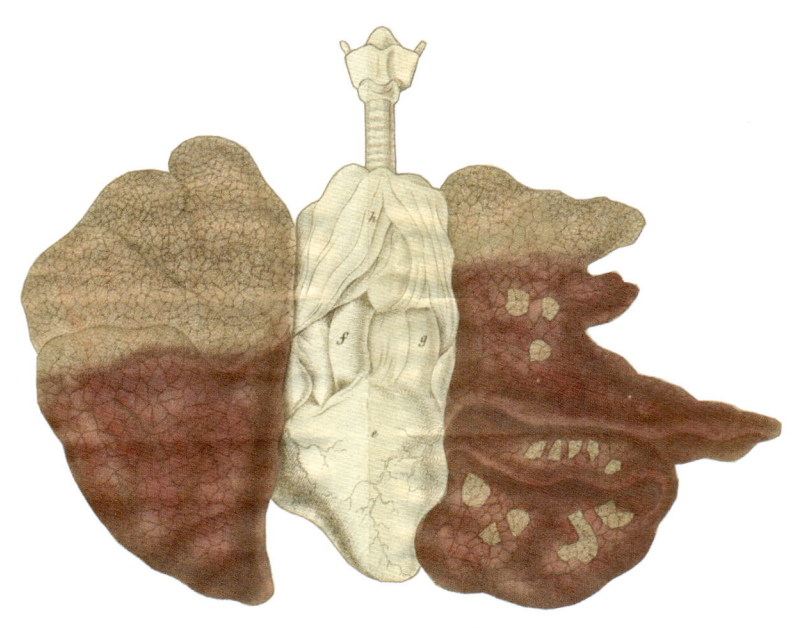

Fig. 3.3.1 Macroscopic view of partially atelectatic lung, depicted by Jörg in 1835 [10].

revealed his understanding of surfactant deficiency [15]. He ventilated the lungs of different living animals, of adults drowned in the Seine river, and of stillborn or deceased neonates, and measured the inflation pressure required to cause pneumothorax. He found that a given pressure was always tolerated by the lungs of stillborn infants, whereas pneumothorax resulted in adult or animal lungs. He concluded: 'The reason may be that the neonate's lung is more compact.'

In 1835, the Leipzig obstetrician Eduard Jörg published an extensive monograph on RDS, *Die Foetuslunge im gebornen Kinde* [10]. The name which he used for the disease, 'fetal lung in the baby who is born', has never been replaced by a better term thereafter. Jörg showed that atelectasis occurred almost exclusively in preterm infants, that birth asphyxia, weakness, and right-to-left shunting contributed to its pathogenesis, and that minimal handling and warming augmented survival (Fig. 3.3.1). He even reported on the small airways' inflammatory response to oxygen administration, a finding today's physicians believe to be a recent discovery.

In 1959, Mary Ellen Avery—at that time a research fellow at the Boston Lying-in Hospital—and Jere Mead published the paper that finally proved that RDS is due to surfactant deficiency [16]. Using a Wilhelmy surface balance, they studied the surface tension of lung extracts from newborn infants who had died of hyaline membrane disease and of infants who died from other causes. In the latter, the mean minimal surface tension was 7.6 dynes/cm, in the RDS infants it was 30.4 dynes/cm at compression in the surface balance. They concluded that 'the disease is associated with the absence or the late appearance of some substances which in the normal subject renders the internal surface capable of attaining low surface tension when lung volume is decreased'.

Pathology of the hyaline membrane

Histologic images of the preterm infant's atelectatic lung were published by Peiser [17] and Ylppö [18] (Fig. 3.3.2). In 1854, Rudolf Virchow described a substance similar to the nerve medulla, present in the alveoli of diseased lungs, staining blue with haematoxylin and termed 'myelin' [19]. Hyaline membranes in the neonatal lung were described by Hochheim in 1903. He believed that they represented aspiration of amniotic fluid contents [20], and as his findings were published in German, hyaline membranes had to be rediscovered by Farber and Sweet, who described 18 cases in 1931, still believing that the membranes were aspirated vernix, therefore calling them 'vernix membrane' [21]. The hyaline membrane, being an end product rather than a cause, shed no light on the pathogenesis, but it did stimulate obscure theories and ineffective therapies. Many clinicians tried to correct pulmonary or systemic hypotension, described by Clement A. Smith to be 'in relation to idiopathic respiratory distress in the newborn' [22]. Others intended to promote fibrinolysis, described as 'a new concept of hyaline membrane disease' by Liebermann in 1959 [23]. In 1956, Gitlin and Craig published a study which associated hyaline membranes with birth asphyxia and showed that hyaline membranes are composed largely of fibrin [24]. They speculated that 'pulmonary hyaline membranes can be produced as the result of: (1) effusion from the pulmonary circulation; or (2) conversion by fibrinogen in the effusion to fibrin'. Still, they continued to regard aspiration of lipid and squamous cells from vernix in the amniotic fluid as pathogenetic variables. The theory that hyaline membranes result from shock, fibrinolysin deficiency, or disseminated intravascular coagulation, persisted for 20 years. Plasminogen infusion, recommended in 1977 by Ambrus and colleagues [25], was believed to alleviate the severity of hyaline membrane disease and overall neonatal mortality.

Oxygen and respiratory support to the neonate

In 1774, the reverend Joseph Priestley discovered oxygen in an attempt to isolate various gases from mercuric oxide in his bathroom

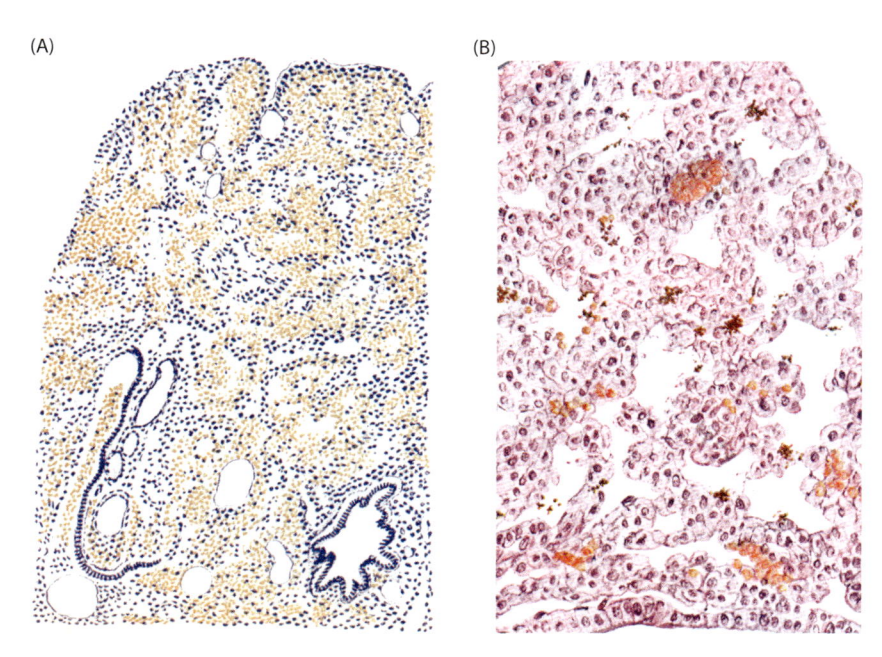

Fig. 3.3.2 Microscopic view of atelectatic lungs in preterm infants: A, near-total atelectasis imbibed with blood, lung of an infant who died on day 3, depicted by Peiser in 1908 [17]; B, partial atelectasis with broad septa, preterm infant of 1050 g who died at 3 hours, depicted by Ylppö in 1919 [18].

in Birmingham [26]. Two years later, the Scottish surgeon John Hunter [27] constructed a bellows-type ventilator with a pressure-limiting valve and suggested using oxygen instead of air. Shortly thereafter, the famous Paris chemist Antoine Lavoisier [28] fully understood Priestley's discovery, gave oxygen its name, and proved that burning is associated with oxygen consumption. His book inspired François Chaussier [29], at that time a young physiologist in Dijon, to construct an apparatus for resuscitating newborn infants with a bag and mask that allowed artificial ventilation with variable inspiratory pressure and oxygen concentration (Fig. 3.3.3). Called to the Paris chair of anatomy and physiology in 1794, Chaussier constructed different curved, silver endotracheal tubes for neonates, which were closed at the end and had oval lateral holes. He became director of the Paris maternity hospital and published many papers on obstetrics and diseases of the neonate from 1805 to 1822. Five years after his retirement, artificial ventilation suffered a major setback when Leroy d'Etiolles [30] discovered that inflating the lung might cause pneumothorax. For exactly 100 years, intermittent positive pressure ventilation made no progress, a fact that halted the development of both anaesthesiology and thoracic surgery. In 1871, the Jena obstetrician Bernhard Schultze [31] observed that right-to-left shunting through the persisting ductus arteriosus may occur in asphyxiated neonates. He believed that abruptly swinging the infant's body would close the duct and facilitate resuscitation (see Chapter 2.2). In 1889, Alexander Graham Bell, the Canadian inventor of the telephone, constructed a body-enclosing ventilator for newborn infants [32]. Bell correctly stated that many preterm infants 'die from inability to expand their lungs sufficiently when they take their first breath. I have no doubt that in many of these cases, lives could be saved by starting the respiration artificially'. His ventilator, however, remained unaccepted. Preterm infants continued to die until in 1929 Drinker and Shaw [33] developed an instrument suitable for long-term ventilation. However, it was not before the report of Donald and Lord [34] in 1953 that artificial ventilation of the neonate became an accepted, although largely unsuccessful, treatment for RDS. Even after Avery and Mead's paper [16] clearly demonstrated that the disease was caused by surfactant deficiency, treatment consisted of oxygen and minimal handling, and the mortality rate exceeded 50% [35]. It took another 10 years until George Gregory, an anaesthesiologist working with the San Francisco group of neonatologists, drew the right conclusions from this disorder's pathophysiology. As grunting was correctly understood as an adaptive mechanism in atelectasis [36], Gregory developed continuous positive airway pressure [37], the first genuinely successful treatment for RDS, which lowered the mortality of this disorder to around 20%. However, in 1973 RDS remained responsible for a quarter of all neonatal deaths [38].

Terminology

Considerable energy was spent during the 1960s discussing the right nomenclature: RDS, with or without idiopathic? Hyaline membrane syndrome, or disease? De and Anderson, in their literature review, listed nine different terms used to describe the same disease in 1953 [39]. Julius Comroe commented this debate sarcastically 'the amount of knowledge of the cause of a disease is inversely proportional to the square of the number of names acquired by the disease' [5].

Conclusion

Not everything has been achieved within the last 5 years, the time interval to that we are educated to restrict the reference list of our publications. Even before nutrition and temperature control became available for preterm infants, remarkable knowledge about the neonatal lung had accumulated through careful clinical and postmortem examination. But effective therapy had to wait for thorough

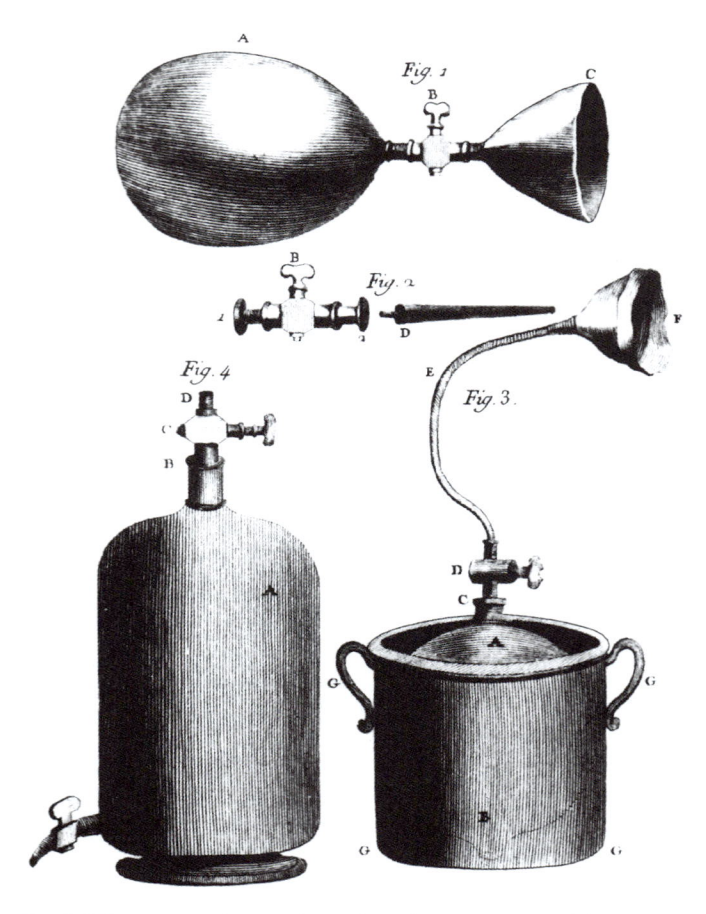

Fig. 3.3.3 François Chaussier's ventilator for neonates, model 1791. Top: mask and bag; centre: adapter for endotracheal tube; bottom left: oxygen tank; bottom right: device for spontaneous breathing with enriched oxygen [29].

understanding of the disease's cause. Also, the latest evidence, based on biochemical and physical studies as well as scientifically controlled trials, is only one point in a continuing process of insight. Research usually leads to better questions rather than final answers.

REFERENCES

1. Mauriceau F: Tractat von Kranckheiten schwangerer und gebärender Weibspersonen (1st French ed. 1668). Basel: Bertsche, 1680.
2. Smellie W: A treatise on the theory and practise of midwifery (1st ed. 1754). London: Sydenham Society, 1878.
3. Raulin J: Von Erhaltung der Kinder (1st French ed. 1768). Leipzig: Crusius, 1769: Vol. **2**, p. 19.
4. Baudelocque JL: L'art des accouchemens (1st French ed. 1781). 2. ed. Paris: Desprez & Méquignon, 1789: Vol. **2**.
5. Comroe JH: Premature science and immature lungs. In: Retrospectroscope: insights into medical discovery: Menlo Park, CA: Von Gehr Press, 1977: p. 140–82.
6. Cone TE: History of the care and feeding of the premature infant. Boston, MA: Little, Brown & Co., 1985.
7. Dugès A: Recherches sur les maladies les plus importantes et les moins connues des enfans nouveau-nés. Paris: Baillière, 1821.
8. Denis P-S: Recherches d'anatomie et de physiologie pathologique sur plusieurs maladies des enfants nouveau-nés. Commercy: Denis, 1826.
9. Billard CM: Die Krankheiten der Neugeborenen und Säuglinge (1st French ed. 1828). Weimar: Industrie-Comptoir, 1829: p. 49.
10. Jörg E: Die Foetuslunge im gebornen Kinde. Grimma: Gebhard, 1835: p. 24–32.
11. Bednar A: Die Krankheiten der Neugeborenen und Säuglinge. Wien: Gerold, 1850: Vol. **3**, p. 67–9.
12. Adriance V: Premature infants. Am J Med Sci 1901;**121**:410–21.
13. Silverman WA, Andersen DH: A controlled clinical trial of effects of water mist on obstructive respiratory signs, death rate, and necropsy findings among preterm infants. Pediatrics 1956;**17**:1–10.
14. Downes JJ, Vidyasagar D, Morrow GM, Boggs TR: Respiratory distress syndrome of newborn infants. Clin Pediatr 1970;**9**:325–31.
15. Leroy d'Etiolles JJ: Second mémoire sur l'asphyxie. J Physiol Exp Path 1828;**8**:97–135.
16. Avery ME, Mead J: surface properties in relation to atelectasis and hyaline membrane disease. Am J Dis Child 1959;**97**:517–23.
17. Peiser J: Über Lungenatelectase. Jahrb Kinderheilk 1908;**67**:589–604.
18. Ylppö A: Pathologisch-anatomische Studien bei Frühgeborenen. Zeitschr Kinderheilk 1919;**20**:212–431.
19. Virchow R: Ueber das ausgebreitete Vorkommen einer dem Nervenmark analogen Substanz in den thierischen Geweben. Arch Pathol Anat 1854;**6**:562.
20. Hochheim K: Ueber einige Befunde in den Lungen von Neugeborenen und die Beziehung derselben zur Aspiration von Fruchtwasser. Centralbl Pathol 1903;**14**:537–8.
21. Farber S, Sweet LK: Amniotic sac contents in the lungs of infants. Am J Dis Child 1931;**42**:1372–83.
22. Smith CA: Circulatory factors in relation to idiopathic respiratory distress (hyaline membrane disease) in the newborn. J Pediatr 1960;**56**:605–11.
23. Liebermann J: Clinical syndromes associated with deficient lung fibrinolytic activity. N Engl J Med 1959;**260**:619–26.
24. Gitlin D, Craig JM: The nature of the hyaline membrane in asphyxia of the newborn. Pediatrics 1956;**17**:64–71.
25. Ambrus CM, Choi TS, Cunnanan E, et al: Prevention of hyaline membrane disease with plasminogen. JAMA 1977;**237**:1837–41.
26. Priestley J: Experiments and observations on different kinds of air. London: Johnson, 1775: Vol. **3**.
27. Hunter J: Proposal for the recovery of people apparently drowned. Phil Trans Lond 1776;**66**:412–25.
28. Lavoisier AL: Traité élémentaire de chimie, présenté dans un ordre nouveau et d'après les découvertes modernes. Paris: Couchet, 1789: Vol. **2**.
29. Chaussier F: Reflexions sur les moyens propres a déterminer la respiration dans les enfants qui naissent sans donner aucune signe de vie. Paris: Histoire de la Société Royale de Médecine, 1780–1781: Vol. **4**, p. 346–54.
30. Leroy d'Etiolles JJ: Recherches sur l'asphyxie. J Physiol Exp Path 1827;**7**:45–65.
31. Schultze BS: Der Scheintod Neugeborener. Jena: Mauke's Verlag (Hermann Dufft), 1871.
32. Stern L, Angeles RD, Outerbridge EW, Beaudry PH: Negative pressure artificial respiration: use in treatment of respiratory failure of the newborn. Can Med Assoc J 1970;**102**:595–601.

33. Drinker P, Shaw LA: An apparatus for the prolonged administration of artificial respiration. I. Design for adults and children. J Clin Invest 1929;7:229–47.
34. Donald I, Lord J: Augmented respiration. Studies in atelectasis neonatorum. Lancet 1953;261:9–17.
35. Usher R: The respiratory distress syndrome of prematurity. Pediatr Clin North Am 1969;8:525–38.
36. Harrison VC, Heese HD, Klein M: The significance of grunting in hyaline membrane disease. Pediatrics 1968;41:549–59.
37. Gregory GA, Kitterman JA, Phibbs RH, Tooley WH, Hamilton WK: Treatment of the idiopathic respiratory distress syndrome with continuous positive airway pressure. N Engl J Med 1971;284:1333–40.
38. Farrell PM, Wood RE: Epidemiology of hyaline membrane disease in the United States. Pediatrics 1976;58:167–76.
39. De TD, Anderson GW: Hyalin-like membranes associated with diseases of the newborn lungs. Obstet Gynecol Surv 1953;8:1–44.

3.4

Holding breath
The development of surfactant substitution

Introduction

The extraordinary stiffness of the deceased preterm infant's lung did not escape the attention of 19th-century researchers, as documented in the reports of Leroy d'Etiolles in 1828 [1] and Jörg in 1835 [2]. A theory of surface forces was elaborated at the end of the 19th century by Lord Rayleigh (John William Strutt), who determined molecular size by preparing monomolecular films [3] and was awarded the Nobel Prize in Physics in 1904. But the entire concept of a film that covers the air–water interface, liquefies during inspiratory spreading, and becomes solid during expiration, thus preventing alveolar collapse, evolved stepwise during the 20th century. The following chapter aims to delineate this development.

Surfactant function and surfactant deficiency

Pulmonary surfactant was detected in 1929 by Kurt von Neergaard, a Swedish physiologist working in Basel. In his paper 'New opinions on a basic principle of breathing mechanics. The retractile force of the lung, dependent on the surface tension in the alveoli' [4], he studied excised pig and dog lungs and measured the pressure–volume curves (Fig. 3.4.1) either with air or with gum arabic and Tyrode solution: 'To eliminate surface tension, the lung was filled with a liquid to remove the effect of the air tissue interfaces.' He concluded 'in all states of expansion, surface tension was responsible for a greater part of total lung recoil than was tissue elasticity' and found that the law of Laplace [5] had to be applied for the pulmonary alveoli to expand and retract. Von Neergaard was well aware of the significance of his findings for the newborn infant: 'The considerable force of surface tension, which later is responsible for the greater part of lung recoil, hampers the lung's initial opening.' The problem was that he published his paper in German and that, for 25 years, no scientists in the evolving field of surfactant research took note of his paper. In 1929, the year in which it appeared, von Neergaard moved to Zurich and began working at the Institute of Physical Therapy. He did not pursue research on lung mechanics or publish any other physiologic paper.

In 1933, Wilson and Farber observed 'cohesion of the moist surfaces in collapsed and airless lungs' of newborn infants [6] and pointed out that 'the initial resistance of the atelectatic lungs to expansion is always present and contributes to the maintenance of atelectasis'. In 1947, the New York pathologist Peter Gruenwald described 'surface tension as a factor in the resistance of neonatal lungs to aeration' [7]. Without knowledge of von Neergaard's work, Gruenwald repeated his experiments and determined the lowest pressure necessary to expand the lungs of stillborn or deceased newborn infants with stained saline solution or air. From the difference in pressure required, he postulated the existence of surface tension at the tissue–air interface: 'The resistance to aeration is due to surface tension which counteracts the entrance of air but has no effect on the aspiration of fluid. Surface active substances reduce the pressure necessary for aeration.' That Gruenwald was Mary Ellen Avery's teacher at Johns Hopkins Hospital may have been important.

Research on chemical warfare

After the end of World War II, research on chemical weapons helped the understanding of pulmonary surfactant to progress dramatically. With the aim of preventing, diagnosing, and treating injuries caused by war gases—notably lung oedema caused by phosgene—military research laboratories were established in the US, Canada, and Great Britain. Supported by Canadian chemical warfare laboratories, Chris Macklin described the lung's 'residual' cells of the lung [8], and measured alveolar size in 1950 [9]. In 1954, he published a paper in which he described 'the pulmonary alveolar mucoid film and the pneumonocytes' [10]. He assumed the presence of an aqueous mucopolysaccharide film on the alveolar wall which maintains 'a constant favourable surface tension': 'There is evidence pointing to the granular pneumonocytes as the originators of the secretion which composes this film.'

At Harvard and with US Army Chemical Center support, Edward Radford wanted to determine alveolar surface area and again filled isolated lungs sequentially with saline and air [11]. His findings

---

Adapted with permission from Obladen, M. History of Surfactant up to 1980. *Biol Neonate*, 87:308–316. Copyright © 2005 S. Karger AG, Basel.

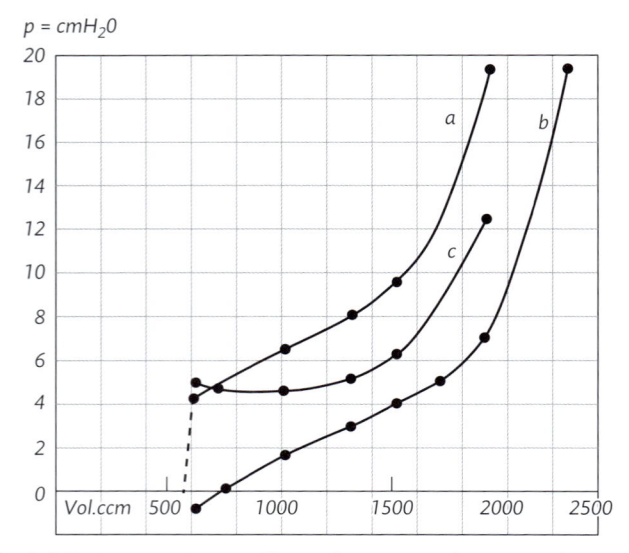

Fig. 3.4.1 Kurt von Neergaard's recoil pressure-volume recordings of isolated porcine lung, published in 1929. a, total lung recoil with air filling; b, tissue elasticity after eliminating surface tension by liquid filling; c, retractile force due to surface tension.

Reproduced from Von Neergaard K. Neue Auffassungen über einen Grundbegriff der Atemmechanik. Die Retraktionskraft der Lunge, abhängig von der Oberflächenspannung in den Alveolen. Z Gesamt Exp Med 1929;66:373–394.

indicated that either the respiratory surface was only one-tenth of that determined microscopically, or that the lung 'consisted of a highly surface active substance', and both conclusions seemed unlikely to Radford.

In 1955, Richard Pattle, employed at the British chemical defence experimental establishment at Porton Down, examined pulmonary oedema foam [12]. He proved that the stable foam bubbles expressed from lung originate from the alveolar lining layer, and speculated that 'absence of the lining substance may sometimes be one of the difficulties with which a premature baby has to contend'. At the same time, John Clements, who worked at the US Army Chemical Center in Edgewood, began to investigate surface tension with a Langmuir trough and Wilhelmy platinum plate [13]. With these devices, he studied surface films from rat, cat, and dog lungs and recognized that surface tension fell from 45 to less than 10 dynes/cm upon compression of the surface to 30% of its area [14]. Shortly after his fundamental paper, Clements left the Army Chemical Center and continued surfactant research at the Cardiovascular Research Institute in San Francisco. Blessed with unlimited curiosity, diligent and systematic workstyle, and a generous personality, John Clements became the unchallenged master in this field.

Surfactant biosynthesis and analysis

Already in 1946, S.J. Thannhauser discovered that the lung contained unusually high amounts of dipalmityl lecithin (now known as dipalmitoylphosphatidylcholine or DPPC) [15], but did not associate his finding with the postulated surface active properties on the alveolar wall. In 1961, Marshall Klaus and colleagues isolated alveolar surfactant from bovine lungs and extracted a phospholipid fraction that exhibited surface active behaviour in the Wilhelmy balance [16]. In 1967, Louis Gluck and his team showed that during lung development, DPPC is secreted into amniotic fluid [17] and in 1972, they developed a practicable test to determine fetal lung maturity: the lecithin/sphingomyelin ratio [18]. Emile Scarpelli, already in 1967, had opened the field of research on fetal pulmonary phospholipid metabolism [19]. In 1975, Mikko Hallman from Helsinki discovered that phosphatidylglycerol contributed to surfactant spreading, and that this lipid is invariably absent in respiratory distress syndrome (RDS) [20].

In papers published in 1972 and 1973, Richard King and John Clements showed that surfactant contains several specific apoproteins [21], and that the major surfactant protein SP-A is glycosylated, interacts with phospholipids, and is responsible for surfactant interaction with the cell surface. The low-molecular-weight hydrophobic surfactant proteins SP-B and SP-C were first identified by Phitzackerley in 1979 [22]. As a site of surfactant storage, Gil and Reiss identified the lamellar bodies of the type II cell [23] and Mary Williams, also a long-time member of the San Francisco group, documented the intra-alveolar transformation of lamellar bodies to tubular myelin [24].

Accelerated lung maturation

In 1968, the New Zealand obstetrician Graham Liggins noted that after infusing ewes with adrenocorticotropin, cortisol, or dexamethasone, premature lambs had unexpectedly mature lungs due to enzyme induction [25]. He concluded that this may be applied to reduce morbidity and mortality from RDS and proceeded to a controlled trial of betamethasone [26], which proved his hypothesis: 'The RDS occurred less often in treated babies.' Antenatal glucocorticoid treatment significantly reduced the risk, severity, and deaths from hyaline membrane disease in infants delivered before 32 weeks. Although the study was published in English in 1972 and was quickly confirmed by other trials, it was not rapidly accepted by the scientific community. The obstetricians' reluctance even increased when a collaborative trial by the National Institute of Health, initiated in 1976 and published in 1981, failed to confirm the beneficial effect of antenatal steroids [27]. This delayed the adoption of Liggins' pioneering discovery in North America for another 10 years, and illustrates how difficult it was for the US to acknowledge progress achieved abroad.

Surfactant substitution

In the report of 1947, in which Gruenwald demonstrated the correlation between surface tension and lung elasticity [7], he used amyl nitrite as an exogenous surfactant to lower the surface tension at the air–water interface and speculated 'the addition of surface active substances to the air or oxygen which is being spontaneously breathed in or introduced by a respirator might aid in relieving the initial atelectasis of newborn infants'. A nebulized detergent mist, available commercially as 'Alevaire', was recommended by Ravenel in 1953 [28] as 'an almost infallible weapon for combating neonatal asphyxia due to the inhalation of amniotic fluid with or without atelectasis'. In 1955, however, Silverman and Andersen published a

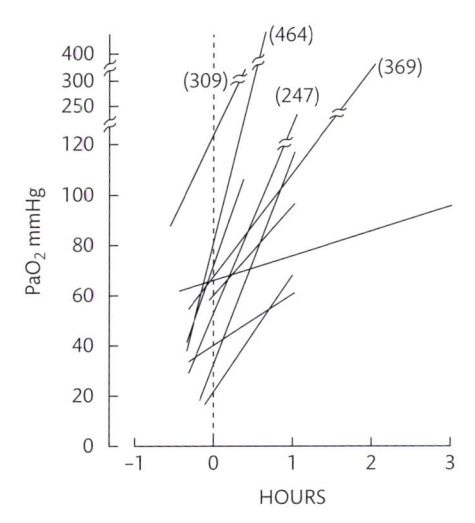

Fig. 3.4.2 Tetsuro Fujiwara's first ten patients with surfactant substitution, published in 1980. Changes of arterial partial pressure of oxygen (PaO$_2$) before and 1–3 h after administration of surfactant extracted from bovine lungs and enriched with phospholipids.
Reproduced with permission from Fujiwara, T., Chida, S., Watabe, Y.J., et al. Artificial surfactant therapy in hyaline membrane disease. *The Lancet*, 315:55–59. Copyright © 1980 Elsevier Ltd.

controlled trial [29] on 'Alevaire', which did not prove any 'therapeutic benefit as judged by death rate and autopsy findings'.

Once Avery and Mead proved that infants who died from hyaline membrane disease lacked pulmonary surfactant [30], and after the major surfactant compound was identified to be DPPC [16], this substance was employed in several clinical trials, usually in nebulized form. Robillard and colleagues [31] and later Shannon and Bunnell [32] treated a few infants, yet their results did not encourage them to pursue these studies. In a more extensive study directed by the Clements Group and performed in Singapore in 1967, Chu and colleagues [33] showed that aerosolized DPPC had no positive effect and might even exert a negative effect on the clinical course of RDS. It thus became clear that besides DPPC other components of natural surfactant were required. Starting in 1972, Enhorning and Robertson used surfactant extracts from adult rabbits to treat premature rabbits, which significantly improved pulmonary mechanics [34]. Forrest Adams and colleagues conducted similar studies in premature lambs in 1978 [35] and from their work, Tetsuro Fujiwara derived the recipe for the exogenous natural surfactant that proved effective in treating newborn infants with RDS [36]. His surfactant was isolated by saline extraction from minced bovine lung and enriched with synthetic lipids. At Akita University in Japan, he treated ten infants with severe RDS requiring ventilator support with a high oxygen concentration. Within 3 h after endotracheal application, arterial partial pressure of oxygen rose from a mean of 45 to 212 mmHg and inspired oxygen could be lowered from 81% to 38% (Fig. 3.4.2).

Multicentre studies and meta-analyses

After Fujiwara's pioneering report, several effective natural surfactants were prepared from calf lung lavage [37], minced bovine and porcine lung [38], and human amniotic fluid [39]. Thanks to carefully controlled multicentre clinical trials, surfactant substitution has become an exceptionally well-studied form of treatment [40–42], while setting high standards for the introduction of new drugs into paediatrics.

Conclusion

The history of surfactant substitution illustrates how dramatically scientific progress evolved from empirical knowledge to scientific observation at the end of the 18th century, then from systematic measurement to the application of basic sciences during the 19th century, and from single experiments to interdisciplinary teamwork in the 20th century. As Julius Comroe pointed out [43], remarkable 'preterm' discoveries that were rejected, ignored, or forgotten after publication, also illustrate how a talented researcher's brilliant idea is not enough to ensure scientific progress: new findings must be communicated at the right time, in the right language, and to the right readers capable of fully understanding their significance in order to enable future progress.

REFERENCES

1. Leroy d'Etiolles JJ: Second mémoire sur l'asphyxie. J Physiol Exp Path 1828;**8**:97–135.
2. Jörg E: Die Foetuslunge im gebornen Kinde. Grimma: Gebhard, 1835: p. 24–32.
3. Lord Rayleigh: On the theory of surface forces, part I and II. Philos Mag 1890;**30**:465–75.
4. Von Neergaard K: Neue Auffassungen über einen Grundbegriff der Atemmechanik. Die Retraktionskraft der Lunge, abhängig von der Oberflächenspannung in den Alveolen. Z Gesamt Exp Med 1929;**66**:373–94.
5. Laplace PS: Traité de mechanique celeste. Paris: Crapalet & Courcier, 1798–1827.
6. Wilson JL, Farber S: Pathogenesis of atelectasis of the newborn. Am J Dis Child 1933;**46**:590–603.
7. Gruenwald P: Surface tension as a factor in the resistance of neonatal lungs to aeration. Am J Obstet Gynecol 1947;**53**:996–1007.
8. Macklin CC: Residual epithelial cells on the pulmonary alveolar wall of mammals. Trans R Soc Can 1946;**40**:93–111.
9. Macklin CC: The alveoli of the mammalian lung. Proc Inst Med 1950;**18**:78–95.
10. Macklin CC: The pulmonary alveolar mucoid film and the pneumonocytes. Lancet 1954;**263**:1099–104.
11. Radford EP: Method for estimating respiratory surface area of mammalian lungs from their physical characteristics. Proc Soc Exp Biol Med 1954;**87**:58–61.
12. Pattle RE: Properties, function, and origin of the alveolar lining layer. Nature 1955;**175**:1125–6.
13. Clements JA: Dependence of pressure-volume characteristics of lungs on intrinsic surface-active material. Am J Physiol 1956;**187**:592.
14. Clements JA: Surface tension of lung extracts. Proc Soc Exp Biol Med 1957;**95**:170–2.
15. Thannhauser SJ, Benotti H, Boncoddo NF: Isolation and properties of hydrolecithin (dipalmityl lecithin) from lung. J Biol Chem 1946;**166**:669–75.

16. Klaus MH, Clements JA, Havel HJ: Composition of surface active material isolated from beef lung. Proc Natl Acad Sci USA 1961;**47**:1858–9.
17. Gluck L, Motoyama EK, Smits HL, Kulovich MV: The biochemical development of surface activity in mammalian lung. Pediatr Res 1967;**1**:237–46.
18. Gluck L, Kulovich MV, Borer C, et al.: Diagnosis of the respiratory distress syndrome by amniocentesis. Am J Obstet Gynecol 1971;**109**:440–5.
19. Scarpelli EM: The lung, tracheal fluid, and lipid metabolism of the fetus. Pediatrics 1967;**40**:951–61.
20. Hallman M, Feldman B, Gluck L: The absence of phosphatidylglycerol in surfactant. Pediatr Res 1975;**9**:396A.
21. King RJ, Clements JA: Surface active materials from dog lung. I. Method of isolation. II. Composition and physiological correlations. III. Thermal analysis. Am J Physiol 1972;**223**:707–14, 715–26, 727–33.
22. Phitzackerley PJ, Town MH, Newman GE: Hydrophobic proteins of lamellated osmiophilic bodies isolated from pig lung. Biochem J 1979;**183**:731–6.
23. Gil J, Reiss OK: Isolation and characterization of lamellar bodies and tubular myelin from rat lung homogenates. J Cell Biol 1973;**58**:152–71.
24. Williams MC: Conversion of lamellar body membranes into tubular myelin in alveoli of fetal rat lungs. J Cell Biol 1977;**72**:260–77.
25. Liggins GC: Premature delivery of foetal lambs infused with glucocorticoids. J Endocrinol 1969;**45**:515–23.
26. Liggins GC, Howie RN: A controlled trial of antepartum glucocorticoid treatment for prevention of the respiratory distress syndrome in premature infants. Pediatrics 1972;**50**:515–25.
27. Collaborative Group on Antenatal Steroid Therapy: Effect of antenatal dexamethasone administration on the prevention of respiratory distress syndrome. Am J Obstet Gynecol 1981;**141**:276–86.
28. Ravenel SF: New technique of humidification in pediatrics. JAMA 1953;**151**:707–11.
29. Silverman WA, Andersen DH: Controlled clinical trial of effects of Alevaire mist on premature infants. JAMA 1955;**157**:707–11.
30. Avery ME, Mead J: Surface properties in relation to atelectasis and hyaline membrane disease. Am J Dis Child 1959;**97**:517–23.
31. Robillard E, Alarie Y, Dagenais-Perusse P, Baril E, Guilbeault A: Microaerosol administration of synthetic beta-gamma-dipalmitoyl-L-alpha-lecithin in the respiratory distress syndrome. Can Med Assoc J 1964;**90**:55–7.
32. Shannon DC, Bunnell JB: Dipalmitoyl lecithin aerosol in RDS. Pediatr Res 1976;**10**:467A.
33. Chu J, Clements JA, Cotton EK, et al.: Neonatal pulmonary ischemia. Pediatrics 1967;**40**:709–82.
34. Enhorning G, Robertson B: Lung expansion in the premature rabbit fetus after tracheal deposition of surfactant. Pediatrics 1972;**50**:55–66.
35. Adams FH, Towers B, Osher AB, Ikegami M, Fujiwara T, Nozaki M: Effects of tracheal instillation of natural surfactant in premature lambs. Pediatr Res 1978;**12**:841–8.
36. Fujiwara T, Chida S, Watabe YJ, Maeta H, Morita T, Abe T: Artificial surfactant therapy in hyaline membrane disease. Lancet 1980;**315**:55–9.
37. Enhorning G, Shennan A, Possmayer F, et al.: Prevention of neonatal respiratory distress syndrome by tracheal instillation of surfactant. Pediatrics 1985;**76**:145–53.
38. Noack G, Berggren P, Curstedt T, et al.: Severe neonatal respiratory distress syndrome treated with the isolated phospholipid fraction of natural surfactant. Acta Paediatr Scand 1987;**76**:697–705.
39. Hallman M, Merritt TA, Jarvenpaa AL, et al.: Exogenous human surfactant for treatment of severe respiratory syndrome. J Pediatr 1985;**106**:963–9.
40. Halliday HL: Overview of clinical trials comparing natural and synthetic surfactants. Biol Neonate 1995;**67** Suppl 1:32–47.
41. Soll RF: Multiple versus single dose natural surfactant extract for severe neonatal respiratory distress syndrome. Cochrane Database Syst Rev 2000;**2**:CD000141.
42. Soll RF, Morley CJ: Prophylactic versus selective use of surfactant in preventing morbidity and mortality in preterm infants. Cochrane Database Syst Rev 2001;**2**:CD000510.
43. Comroe JH: Premature science and immature lungs. In: Retrospectroscope: Insights into medical discovery: Menlo Park, CA: Von Gehr Press, 1977: p. 140–82.

3.5 Anatomy and spontaneous closure of the ductus arteriosus

Introduction

A disposable vessel enabling circulatory transition at birth, the ductus arteriosus has fascinated researchers throughout history.

Anatomy, physiology, and terminology

Galen was wrong on adult and fetal circulation and assumed identical flow towards the fetus in umbilical arteries and vein. By the 2nd century C.E., he was, however, aware of the ductus arteriosus [1]: 'Neither vessel [foramen ovale and ductus arteriosus] is small or the result of an accident; on the contrary, they are very broad and have notable lumens, which could not fail to be recognized not only by anyone having eyes but even by anyone having a sense of touch, provided that he wished to busy himself with dissecting.' And, also in *De Usu Partium* [2]: 'It is right to admire nature here too, because when the viscus [the lung] needed only to grow, she supplied it with pure blood, and when it was changed so that it moved, she made its flesh light as a feather in order that it might be easily dilated and compressed by the thorax. This is the very reason, why a passageway [the foramen ovale] was made connecting the vena cava and the venous artery [v. pulmonalis] in the fetus. Inasmuch as this vessel [the v. pulmonalis], however, serves as a vein for the viscus, it was necessary, I suppose, for the other one [a. pulmonalis] to change into the usefulness of an artery, and therefore nature also connected this one to the great artery [the aorta], but in this case, because there was a space between the vessels, she created another, small, third vessel [the ductus arteriosus] to join the two.'

Pre-Harveyan understanding and terminology of the circulation differed from ours, and for clarification is summarized in Table 3.5.1.

Galen hypothesized that pores in the interventricular septum allowed a small quantity of venous blood to be transferred to the left ventricle. The left ventricle was thought to be the seat of the soul. It was here that the life-giving pneuma was transformed into vital spirit, *pneuma zotikon*, the essential compound of arterial blood [5].

This corresponded with biblical beliefs: 'The Lord God formed man of the dust of the ground, and breathed into his nostrils the breath of life, and man became a living soul' [Gen 2:7] and was further developed in the New Testament: "When he [Jesus] had said this, he breathed on them and saith to them, 'Receive ye the Holy Ghost. Whose soever sins ye remit, they are remitted unto them, and whose soever sins you retain, they are retained' [John 20:22]. Under the influence of St Augustine, the term *pneuma* gradually became identical to the Holy Spirit of the trinity [7] and for a millennium the soul was believed to be enclosed in the heart, as illustrated in 1140 in Hildegard von Bingen's *Liber Scivias* (see Chapter 1.1) [8]. In the emotionally agitated decades between the reformation and the Council of Trent, Galen's misconceptions about circulation became a theological need and were believed in a nearly religious way [9]. Researchers who found contradicting facts in animal experiments had to be cautious or were regarded as heretics. In 1543, Andreas Vesalius described and illustrated the anatomic technique for studying the pulsating heart in living animals and must have seen the blood returning from the lungs. Tabula VI-8 of the *Fabrica* showed the pulmonary veins, but instead of explanatory text provided a figure of the pig experiment [10]. After the 1555 edition of the *Fabrica*, which explicitly denied the interventricular pores [11], Vesalius abandoned the academic world and became principal physician to the emperor Charles V. His death penalty was commuted into a Holy Lands pilgrimage, on which he died after a shipwreck in 1564.

The atria, believed to be sinewy dilatations of the veins, were not known to contract. In 1552, Bartolomeo Eustachi described the valve separating fetal blood flows in the right atrium, but his *Tabulae Anatomicae* remained unpublished in the Vatican library until 1714 [12]. Michael Servetus of Aragon, anatomy fellow student of Vesalius, openly challenged Galen's construct in 1553 [13, 14]: 'Not just air, but blood mixed with air is sent from the lung to the arteria venosa [the pulmonary vein]. Therefore, the mixture occurs in the lungs ... Thus the vital spirit is transfused from the left ventricle into the arteries of the whole body.' The former theologian Servetus understood the far-reaching consequences of his findings. He sent

---

Reproduced with permission from Obladen, M. History of the ductus arteriosus: 1. anatomy and spontaneous closure. *Neonatology*, 99(2):83–89. Copyright © 2011 S. Karger AG, Basel.

Table 3.5.1 Historic terminology of the heart and fetal circulation

Antique era Aristotle, Galen, Augustine, up to 5th century c.e.	Reformation era Vesal, Servetus, Aranzio, Colombo, Fabricius, up to 1600	Modern era From Harvey 1628
Unnamed; transfers blood generated in the liver	Ductus venosus	Ductus venosus
Great vein		Vena cava
Sinewy expansion of the great vein/vena cava	Right auricle	Right atrium
Orifice of the vena cava; passageway right-left	(Vena arteriarum nutrix)	Foramen ovale, transfers fetal blood from right to left atrium
Right ventricle	Right ventricle	Right ventricle
Thick dense vessel, arterial vein	Vena arterialis, tranfers spirited blood in fetus	A. pulmonalis
Branch, third vessel; transfers fetal blood from aorta to A. pulmonalis	Tubulus arteriosus, various assumptions	Ductus arteriosus; transfers fetal blood from A. pulmonalis to aorta
Septum with pores		Septum interventriculare
Thin loose-textured vessel; venous artery	Arteria venosa, pulmonary transit	Venae pulmonales
Sinewy expansion of the venous artery	Various names	Left atrium
Left ventricle, seat of the soul	(Middle ventricle), left ventricle, vapour	Left ventricle
Great artery, great vessel		Aorta
Arteria aspera	Art. aspera, windpipe	Trachea
(Innate) pneuma	(Ambient) spirit	Air (with oxygen from 1772)

Source: Data from [3–6].

handwritten manuscripts of his book to the reformers Calvin and Melanchthon in 1546, thereby denying the existence of trinity. Despite taking refuge in reformed Geneva, he was burnt at the stake in 1553 along with his book.

Vesalius' pupil and successor at Padua, Realdo Colombo, described the pulmonary transit in 1559 [15, 16]. Realizing that the arterial vein was too big merely to afford nourishment to the lung, he declared that the blood moved across the lung and down to the heart once more through the venous artery, which did not carry fuliginous vapours in the opposite direction [6]: 'If one not only if one dissects cadavers, but studies living animals, one will always find the vena pulmonalis filled with blood, which definitely would not occur if it were only created for the sake of pneuma and vapours' [14]. Understanding fetal circulation was hindered by Galen's postulate of flow towards the fetus in all umbilical vessels. The foramen ovale and ductus arteriosus were described by Vesalius' pupil Giulio Cesare Aranzio in 1564 [17], who honestly claimed only to have elaborated Galen's description.

In the same year, the Fallopio-pupil and surgeon Leonardo Botallo pretended to have discovered the foramen ovale ('vena arteriarum nutrix a nullo antea notata') in an appendix to his monograph *De Catarrho* [18]. There is no mention of the ductus arteriosus, also not in the 1641 reedition of Botallo's *De Via Sanguinis* [19, 20]. Seventy-three years after Botallo's death and 32 years after Harvey's groundbreaking work, the Leiden anatomist Johann van Horne re-edited Botallo's *Opera Omnia Medica et Chirurgica*, and added an illustration of the heart (Fig. 3.5.1, bottom) [20, 21]. This figure showed an incorrectly positioned ductus arteriosus ('canalis a pulmonali arteria tendens in aortam'), and the footnote ironically alluded to Botallo's claim: 'Immediately he exclaimed with Archimedes *heureka*, but celebrated the triumph before the victory' [22]. Subsequent writers misunderstood the irony and falsely attributed the figure to Leonardo Botallo, who thus became famous and inadvertently made his way into the Nomina Anatomica at the Basel conference in 1895 [23] and the International Classification of Diseases, 10th Revision (ICD-10) (ICD-10 code Q25.0).

Fabricius ab Aquapendente, a surgeon in Padua and Harvey's teacher, correctly described the ductus arteriosus in his *De Formato Foetu* in 1600 (recte: 1606) [24, 25] (Fig. 3.5.1, top) as 'a branch of the great artery [aorta] to the arterial vein [pulmonary artery]. It appears large in the fetus, but is cord-like after birth … Shortly after the birth of the fetus, the arrangement is changed … both vessels are occluded. For nature takes the little valve [ostiolum] situated on the inside at that right orifice in the vena cava, and glues shut and completely conceals the opening. But she dries up the left arterial branch so that it becomes a cord, without any lumen whatsoever.'

In his fundamental booklet *De Motu Cordis*, William Harvey, a physician in London who was trained in Padua, did not only do away with Galen's physiology in 1628 [26]: 'By Hercules, no such pores can be demonstrated, nor in fact do any such exist', but also firmly established the change from fetal to neonatal circulation: 'Another union is that by the pulmonary artery, and is effected when that vessel divides into two branches after its escape from the heart. It is as if to the two trunks already mentioned a third were superadded, a kind of arterial canal, carried obliquely from the pulmonary artery, to perforate and terminate in the great artery or aorta. So that in the dissection of the embryo, as it were, two aortas, or two roots of the great artery appear springing from the heart. This canal shrinks gradually after birth, and after a time becomes withered, and finally almost removed, like the umbilical vessels.' With oxygen unknown, Harvey's understanding of respiration was limited: 'The right [ventricle] receiving the blood from the auricle, and propelling it by the pulmonary artery, and its continuation, named the ductus arteriosus, into the aorta … the blood is sent through the lungs, in order that it may be tempered by the air that is inspired, and prevented

CHAPTER 3.5 **Anatomy and spontaneous closure of the ductus arteriosus**

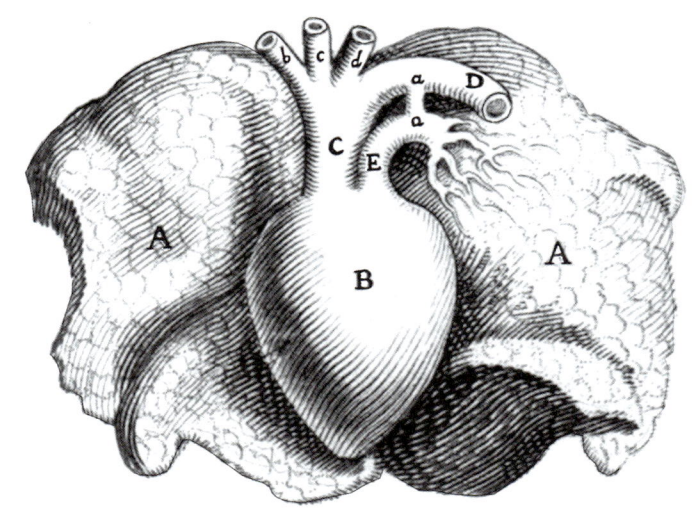

Fig. 3.5.2 Ductus depiction (a–a) by Johann Vesling in *Syntagma Anatomicum* 1651 [27].

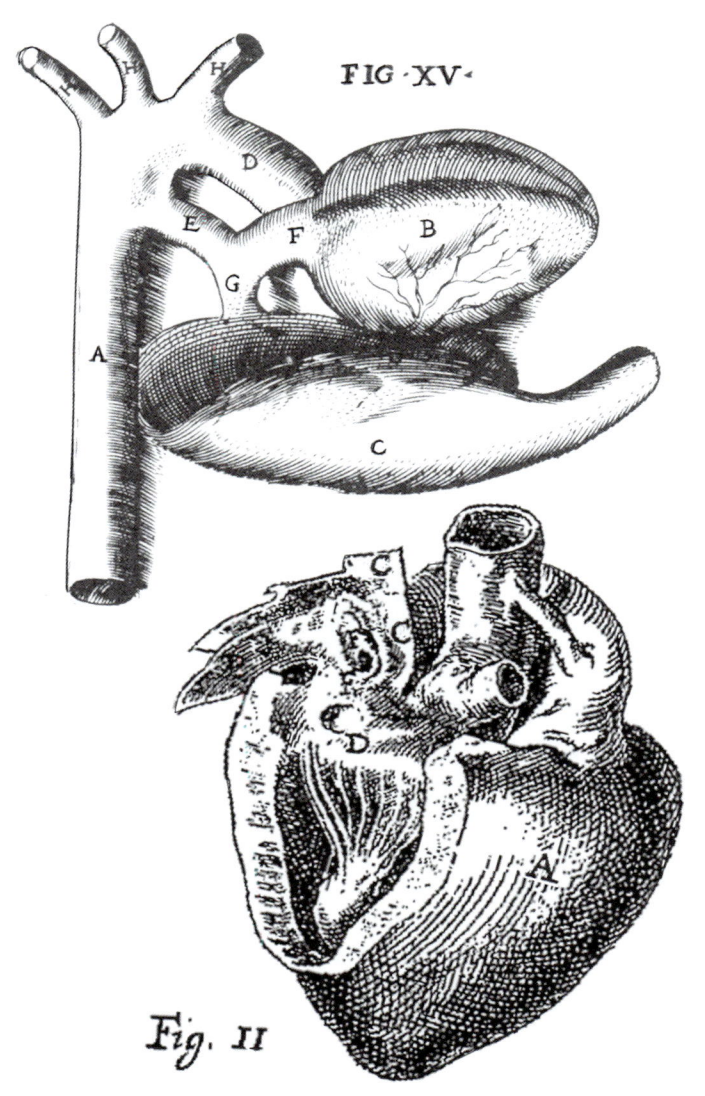

Fig. 3.5.1 Seventeenth-century depictions of the ductus arteriosus. Top: from Fabricius ab Aquapendente in *De Formato Foetu* 1606 [24, 25]. Bottom: from Johan van Horne's addition to Botallo's *Opera Omnia Medica et Chirurgica* 1660 [21].

Mechanical hypotheses explaining spontaneous closure

John Baptist Morgagni, another anatomist in Padua, stated in 1761 [29]: 'But the [umbilical] arteries, when the infant is already born, are tied up together with the vein of that name, and cut off; so that no blood can any longer be carried into them, nor carried back therefrom. And the canaliculus venosus, and the tubulus arteriosus, are afterwards, by degrees, shut up; as the foramen ovale is also at length, if not quite shut up, at least generally diminish'd.'

A surgeon at St Thomas' Hospital, London, William Cheselden, stated in his 'anatomy of the human body' (first ed. 1713): 'The arterial duct shrinks when, after opening of the pulmonary circuit, no blood further flows into it.' Berlin pathologist Rudolf Virchow believed the ductus would close due to thrombus formation [30]; however, Rauchfuß observed thrombosis of the ductus arteriosus in only 4 out of 1400 postmortem infants examined at the St. Petersburg foundling hospital in 1859 [31]. Walkhoff [32] thought that the change in position of the ductus after birth led to kinking, interruption of blood flow, and thrombosis. The Göttingen faculty awarded a prize for his paper, which histologically characterized the ductus tissue and the phases of its closure (Fig. 3.5.3): 'To me it seems these cells transform into connective tissue and elastic fibres... The intima protrusions are highly important and contribute greatly to closure, as they often narrow half of the lumen.'

The Heidelberg pathologist Thoma studied serial sections of human ductuses and in 1882 found [33] 'a complete lack of elastic membranes in the media... and only an elastic layer belonging to the intima'. He believed that decreased flow caused obstruction of the ductus. Fritz Schanz (1889) stated that the aortic end of the ductus was fixed; it was only when breathing began that the ductus was stretched by the attached pericardium and pulmonary arteries [34]. Berlin obstetrician Paul Strassmann [22] wanted to know why 'when the pulmonary artery ceases to provide the ductus with blood, the aorta does not feed the ductus with its blood, being under elevated pressure, and why no flow into the other direction sets in.' He

from boiling up, and so becoming extinguished, or something else of the sort.'

In 1651, anatomist Johann Vesling, also in Padua, transferred Harvey's discovery into his *Syntagma Anatomicum* in 1651 [27], but his depiction of the pulmonary ductal junction and the fetal pulmonary vessels was far from correct (Fig. 3.5.2). In 1774, Albrecht von Haller, a Bernese universal scientist during the Enlightenment, tried to calculate shunt volumes from anatomic measurements [28]: 'I made different experiments of injection into the arteries and measurement of the vessels in hundredths of pouces [1 pouce at that time = 2.71 cm]... The [fetal] ductus arteriosus is of conical shape; at its pulmonary end I measured its diameter to be 5.0 mm, whereas the aorta leaving the heart had 4.3 mm, and the a. pulmonalis 7.3 mm;... therefore, the aorta is much smaller than the a. pulmonalis... and the ductus receives the greater part of the blood which is ejected into the a. pulmonalis.'

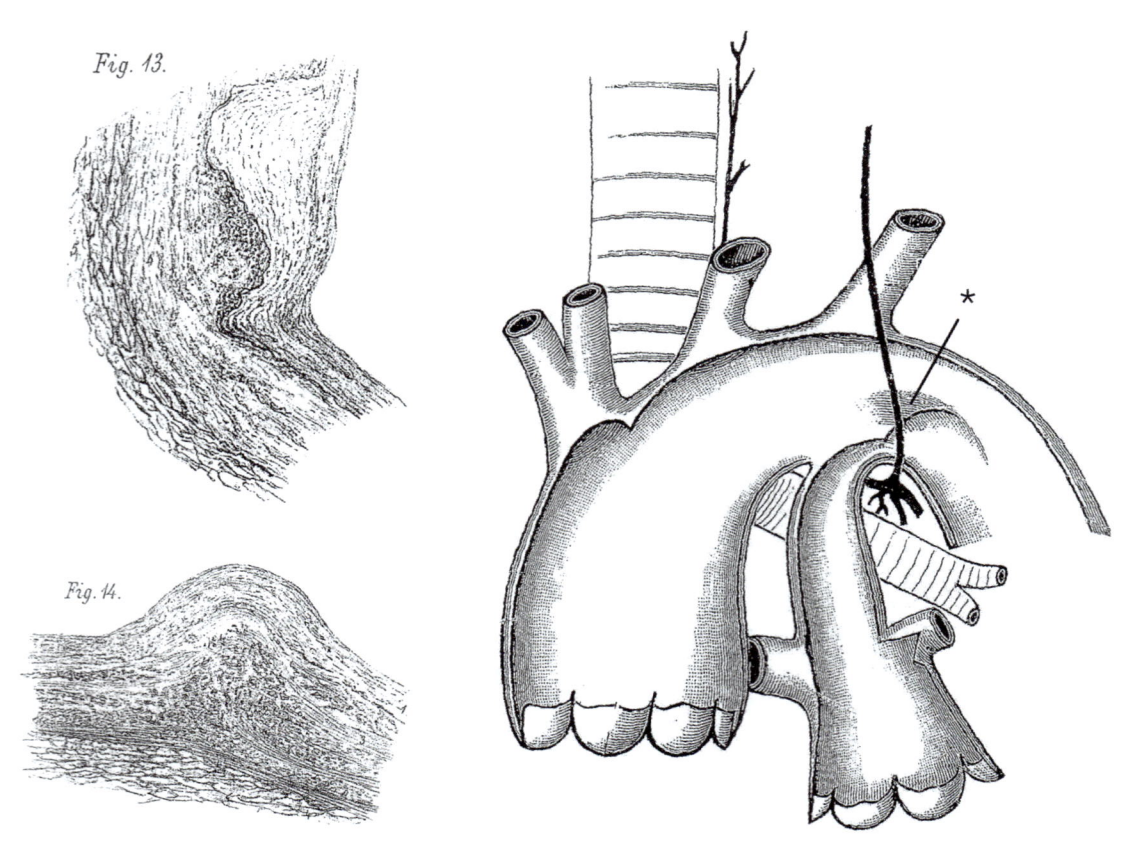

Fig. 3.5.3 Anatomic studies on closure mechanism of the ductus arteriosus. Left: transverse sections from Walkhoff 1869 [32]; fig. 13: ductus art. of 5-day-old infant showing swollen intima and augmented longitudinal media layers; fig. 14: ductus art. of 8-day-old infant showing intima with deposits and proliferated longitudinal media layers. Right: valvular structure (* 'ostium aorticum valvuliforme ductus arteriosi') described by P. Strassmann 1894 [22].

believed that folds at the junction of the ductus and the aorta would act as a valve (Fig. 3.5.3). Kirstein opposed this view in 1910, arguing that the angle at the aortic junction was the principal cause [35]. Linzenmeier also contested Strassmann's view [36], claiming that ductal kinking caused postnatal closure.

Intima cushions

By the end of the 19th century, two phases of ductal closure were clearly distinguished as indicated by the work of Lille anatomist Gérard. His findings, based on 96 postmortem examinations of infants, established [37]: 'The closure of the arterial duct includes: 1. A physiological occlusion effective shortly after birth, rendering the ductus still permeable, but with little or no perfusion. This occlusion follows the onset of breathing. 2. An anatomical obliteration after the first days of life, when the intimal tissue begins to proliferate … In most cases, the histological obliteration is not completed before completion of the second year of life.'

In Chicago, the pathologist Gideon Wells was not content with this description and wrote in 1908 [38]: 'There must be some mechanism which can be relied upon always to perform this occlusion. Any explanation which involves connective tissue proliferation must be inadequate, for the ductus is patent and carrying on its full function up to the moment of delivery, and then is at once occluded when the child begins to breathe; it is necessary to distinguish between the instantaneous *occlusion* of the duct and its subsequent *obliteration*.' Melka [39] assumed that the aorta and pulmonary artery compressed the ductus lying between them. Histological details of ductus closure were clarified by Jager and Wollenman 1942 [40]: 'The intima is peculiar in that there are mounds which project into the lumen. These mounds, which contain fine elastic fibers, smooth muscle and later collagen, are an integral part of the mechanism of closure … The media is loose in structure and is composed of fine, wavy elastic fibers and smooth muscle fibres … Anatomical closure is effected largely by an increase in size and perhaps in number of these intimal mounds, which gradually become infiltrated with collagen … No external elastic lamina is present in the ductus arteriosus.'

Leiden anatomist Adriana Gittenberger-de Groot classified four maturation stages of the ductus arteriosus in 1980, stage II characterized by intimal cushions, stage III by mucoid lakes and cytolytic necrosis in the muscular media, and stage IV by fusion of the intimal cushions [41]. In persistent patency, she found a newly formed subendothelial elastic lamina bordering the lumen.

Endogenous prostaglandins

Prostaglandins were discovered in 1936 by the Stockholm physiologist Ulf von Euler, and their production and biosynthesis were elucidated by the Swedish biochemist Sune Bergstrom. The biochemist John Vane, at the Wellcome Laboratories in Kent, found in 1971 that aspirin and similar compounds prevented prostaglandin biosynthesis [42] and in 1976 that they disappeared from the circulation during pulmonary transit [43]. In 1972, the Auckland paediatricians Elliot and Starling described prostaglandin action on the ductus [44]: 'Prostaglandin F2α can cause the circular constriction of the ductus arteriosus in vitro in the presence or absence of oxygen … Constriction of the ductus is arrested by the addition of the prostaglandin antagonist and subsequent dilation occurs.'

From 1973 onwards, the Toronto group of Coceani and Olley demonstrated [45] that fetal patency of the ductus is an active state maintained by the relaxant action of prostaglandins E1 and E2. This group also found that cyclooxygenase inhibitors such as indomethacin prevent the formation of prostaglandin endoperoxides and, therefore, all endoperoxide derivatives [46]. In 1977, Clyman, Heymann, and Rudolph of the Cardiovascular Research Institute in San Francisco detected that the relaxing effect of prostaglandin E1 on the ductus arteriosus was oxygen dependent [47] and that its sensitivity to prostaglandins continues after birth [48]. *In utero*, circulating endogenous prostaglandins, formed by the action of cyclooxygenases, exert their vasodilatory effect on the ductus arteriosus to maintain its patency. In Chapter 3.6, we will return to the work of these San Franciscan cardiologists.

REFERENCES

1. Galen: On the usefulness of the parts of the body, cap. 6. Ithaca, NY: Cornell University Press, 1968: Vol. **2**, p. 329.
2. Galen: On the usefulness of the parts of the body, cap. 15. Ithaca, NY: Cornell University Press, 1968: Vol. **2**, p. 670.
3. Flourens P: Histoire de la découverte de la circulation du sang. Paris: Baillière, 1854: p. 40–66.
4. Singer C: The discovery of the circulation of the blood. London: Bell, 1922.
5. French RK: The thorax in history. 2. Thorax 1978;**33**:153–66.
6. French RK: The thorax in history. 5. Discovery of the pulmonary transit. Thorax 1978;**33**:555–64.
7. Ratzinger J: The Holy Spirit as communio: concerning the relationship of pneumatology and spirituality in Augustine. Communio 1998;**25**:324–37.
8. Saurma-Jeltsch L: Die Miniaturen im 'Liber Scivias' der Hildegard von Bingen. Wiesbaden: Reichert, 1998: p. 58, fol. 22.
9. Mason S: Religious reform and the pulmonary transit of the blood. Hist Sci 2003;**41**:459–71.
10. Leveling HP: Anatomische Erklärung der Original-Figuren von Andreas Vesal. Ingolstadt: Industriecomptoir, 1800: p. 191, 199.
11. Pagel W: Vesalius and the pulmonary transit of the venous blood. J Hist Med 1964;**19**:327–41.
12. Eustachi B: Tabulae anatomicae. Romae: Gonzaga, 1714.
13. Servetus M: Christianismi restitutio (1553) and other writings. Birmingham: Classics of Medicine Library, 1989: p. 204, 268.
14. Tollin H: Ueber Colombo's Antheil an der Entdeckung des Blutkreislaufs. Virchows Arch 1883;**91**:39–66.
15. Colombo R: De re anatomica libri XV. Venetiis: Bevilaquae, 1559.
16. Tollin H: Matteo Realdo Colombo. Pflügers Arch 1880;**22**:262–90.
17. Aranzio GC: De humano foetu libellus. Bononiae: Rubrius, 1564.
18. Botallo L: De catarrho commentarius … Parisiis: Turrisan, 1564.
19. Bondio MG: Leonardo Botallo, de via sanguinis. Edizione, traduzione ed analisi di un testo ricoperto nel '600. Med Secoli 2005;**17**:663–93.
20. Franklin KJ: Ductus venosus (Arantii) and ductus arteriosus (Botalli). Bull Hist Med 1941;**9**:580–4.
21. Botallo L: Opera omnia medica et chirurgica. Lugduni Batavorum: Gaasbeeck, 1660: p. 76–80, 68–9.
22. Strassmann P: Anatomische und physiologische Untersuchungen über den Blutkreislauf beim Neugeborenen. Arch Gynäk 1894;**45**:393–445.
23. Kopsch F, Knese K-H: Nomina anatomica. Vergleichende Übersicht der Basler, Jenaer und Pariser Nomenklatur. 5. ed. Stuttgart: Thieme, 1957: p. 28.
24. Fabricius Hieronimus ab Aquapendente: Tractatus quatuor. Frankfurt: Zetter, 1624: p. Tab. XVIII, fig. XLI.
25. Adelmann HB: The embryological treatises of Hieronimus Fabricius of Aquapendente. De formatione ovi et pulli. De formato foetu. Ithaca, NY: Cornell University Press, 1942: p. 323.
26. Harvey W: Exercitatio anatomica de motu cordis et sanguinis in animalibus (An anatomical Dissertation upon the Movement of the Heart and Blood in Animals). Francofurti (Canterbury): Fitzeri (Moreton), 1628: p. 18, 39, 41.
27. Vesling J: Syntagma anatomicum publicis dissectionibus, locis plurimis auctum. 2. ed. Patavii: Typis Pauli Frambotti, 1651: p. Cap. 3, tab. II, fig. 3.
28. Haller A: La generation. Paris: Ventes de la Doué, 1774: Vol. **2**, p. 395.
29. Morgagni GB: The seats and causes of diseases investigated by anatomy. London: Millar, 1769: Vol. **2**, p. art. 59.
30. Virchow R: Gesammelte Abhandlungen zur wissenschaftlichen Medizin. Frankfurt: Meidinger, 1856: p. 593.
31. Rauchfuss C: Ueber Thrombose des Ductus arteriosus Botalli. Virchows Arch 1859;**17**:376–397.
32. Walkhoff: Das Gewebe des Ductus arteriosus und die Obliteration desselben. Zeitschr Rat Med 1869;**36**:109–131.
33. Thoma R: Ueber die Abhängigkeit der Bindegewebsneubildung in der Arterienintima von den mechanischen Bedingungen des Blutumlaufes. Virchows Arch 1882;**93**:443–505.
34. Schanz F: Über den mechanischen Verschluss des Ductus arteriosus. Pflügers Arch Ges Physiol 1889;**44**:239–69.
35. Kirstein F: Der Verschluß des Ductus arteriosus (Botalli). Arch Gynäk 1910;**90**:303–34.
36. Linzenmeier G: Verschluß des Ductus arteriosus Botalli nach der Geburt des Kindes. Zeitschr Geburtsh Gynäk 1915;**76**:217–53.
37. Gérard G: De l'obliteration du canal artériel. J Anat Physiol Paris 1900;**36**:323–57.
38. Wells HG: Persistent patency of the ductus arteriosus. Am J Med Soc 1908;**136**:381–400.
39. Melka J: Beiträge zur Kenntnis der Morphologie und Obliteration des Ductus arteriosus Botalli. Anat Anz 1926;**61**:348–61.
40. Jager BV, Wollenman OJ Jr: An anatomical study of the closure of the ductus arteriosus. Am J Path 1942;**18**:595–613.
41. Gittenberger-DeGroot AC, Ertbruggen I van, Moulaert AJMG, Harinck E: The ductus arteriosus in the preterm infant. J Pediatr 1980;**96**:88–93.
42. Vane J: Inhibition of prostaglandin synthesis as a mechanism of action for aspirin-like drugs. Nat New Biol 1971;**231**:232–235.
43. Ferreira SH, Vane JR: Prostaglandins: their disappearance from and release into the circulation. Nature 1967;**216**:868–73.
44. Elliott RB, Starling MB: The effect of prostaglandin F2α in the closure of the ductus arteriosus. Prostaglandins 1972;**2**:399–403.

45. Coceani F, Olley PM: The response of the ductus arteriosus to prostaglandins. Can J Physiol Pharmacol 1973;51:220–5.
46. Coceani F, Olley PM: Role of prostaglandins, prostacyclin, and thromboxanes in the control of prenatal patency and postnatal closure of the ductus arteriosus. Semin Perinat 1980;4:109–13.
47. Clyman RI, Heymann MA, Rudolph AM: Ductus arteriosus responses to prostaglandin E1 at high and low oxygen concentrations. Prostaglandins 1977;13:219–23.
48. Clyman RI, Mauray F, Heymann MA, Rudolph AM: Ductus arteriosus: developmental response to oxygen and indomethacin. Prostaglandins 1978;15:993–8.

3.6

Persisting patency of the ductus arteriosus in the preterm infant

Introduction

Persisting patency of the ductus arteriosus (PDA) could not be detected before pulmonary transit and fetal circulation were clearly established, which was not the case before Harvey, as discussed in Chapter 3.5.

Persisting patency

By 1769, Morgagni knew of both fetal closure and postnatally persisting patency of the fetal connections [1]: 'Some are born, in whom there is an opposite disorder; and those passages, for that reason, [vitiated structure], are not only never wholly shut up; which has been met with by me and others frequently in the foramen ovale; but are not even diminish'd ... Those parts of the umbilical vessels that are in the belly, and the tubulus arteriosus [the ductus] were open.'

Persisting patency along with cardiac malformations was described by Craigie [2] who in 1841 demonstrated that coarctation is frequently combined with PDA. In his 1862 dissertation, Manuel de Almagro—a young Cuban studying in Paris—described isolated persisting PDA [3]: 'Two alterations are found at the same time as the ductus arteriosus persists: First and constantly, a hypertrophy of the heart, mainly of the right-sided cavities; second and more rare, changes of the valves and of the pulmonary vessels.' One of his cases is depicted in Fig. 3.6.1. At the beginning of the 20th century, Lesage, like most authors of paediatric textbooks, was aware of patent ductus associated with other cardiac malformations [4].

Oxygenation and ductus closure

Joseph Bernt, professor of forensic medicine in Vienna, related ductal size to postnatal breathing in 1824. He demonstrated that the aortic end of the ductus constricts when oxygenated blood returns from the lungs [5]. In his 1835 pioneering monograph on the fetal lung in the neonate, the Leipzig obstetrician Eduard Jörg explained ductus closure [6]: 'To close the patent fetal canals, no opportunity will return which is as suitable as the first breaths of the newborn. These must be vigorous because of the relative lack of oxygen ... [In disturbed breathing], nature alone cannot compensate this weakness, because the exciting oxygen is not sufficiently available, ... and the fetal circulation partially persists in the neonate.'

After Jörg, the oxygen hypothesis was ignored and mechanical explanations gained increasing acceptance for the next century. Authors usually regarded patency as a passive and constriction as an active process. As late as 1941, oxygen was rediscovered as modifier of ductal closure, when J. Allen Kennedy and Sam L. Clark investigated guinea pigs in Nashville [7, 8], 'in which the interruption of all known neurological pathways between central nervous system and region of the ductus failed to prevent closure of the ductus following inflation of the lungs with air ... From our experiments it appears that oxygen is a necessary component of the gas mixture since inflation of the lungs with pure nitrogen will not cause closure ... If this seemingly important relationship of oxygen to the mechanism of closure of the ductus is true, it offers a practical indication for treatment of new-born infants, especially those which have difficulty in the oxygenation of their blood.'

This finding corresponded well with epidemiologic studies demonstrating that at high altitudes in Canada, the percentage incidence of PDA was 18 times greater than the average [9]; above 4500 m in Peru the PDA incidence was 30 times greater than at sea level [10]. Eldridge and colleagues measured differences in oxygen saturation in arterialized capillary blood samples from a right neonatal finger and from the toe of either foot [11]. They concluded: 'The ductus arteriosus is the site of a veno-arterial shunt of considerable magnitude which persists in a significant number of infants up to 72 hours of life. A high pulmonary artery pressure is present at birth and persists as long as the veno-arterial shunt exists.'

Born and Dawes [12] showed in preterm lambs that 'the ductus became constricted when the arterial O_2 saturation was raised by exposing the blood to an atmosphere of 100% O_2.' In Los Angeles, Moss and colleagues cannulated both umbilical arteries of 15 healthy term infants [13], placed catheters in their pulmonary artery and

---

Reproduced with permission from Obladen, M. History of the ductus arteriosus: 2. persisting patency in the preterm infant. *Neonatology*, 99(3):163–169. Copyright © 2011 S. Karger AG, Basel.

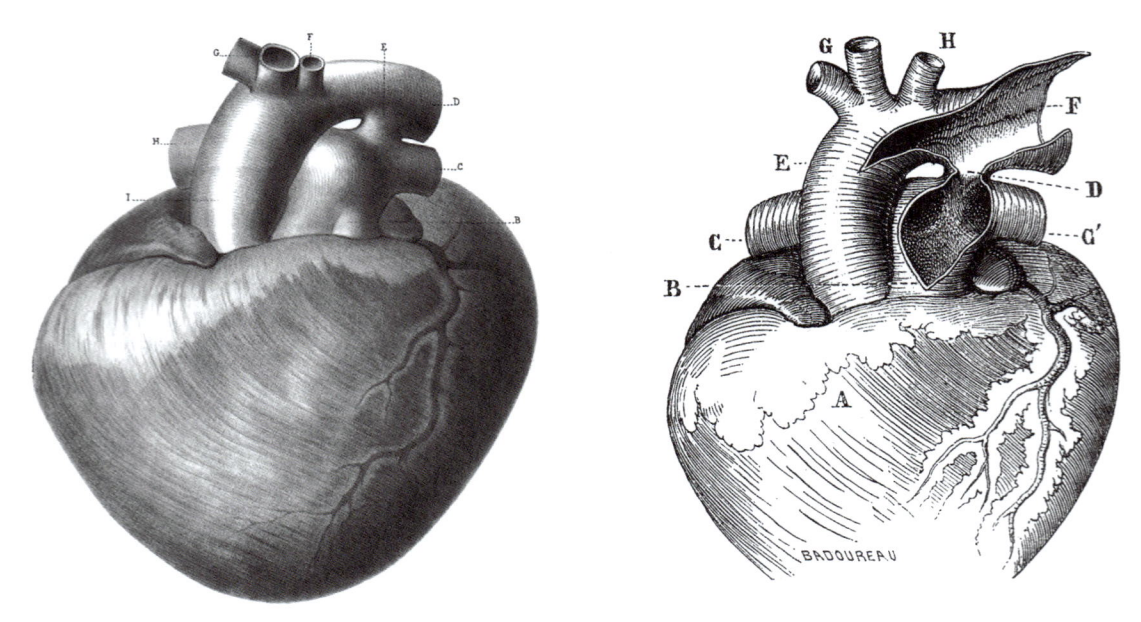

Fig. 3.6.1 Young interns performed fundamental research in the Paris hospitals. Left: persisting PDA in a 19-year-old woman from de Almagro's dissertation 1862 [3]. Right: another view of de Almagro's case as reproduced by Bouchut 1867 [47].

aorta, and changed the inhaled oxygen concentration, confirming Eldridge and Born's findings: hypoxia (13% oxygen in nitrogen) caused the ductus to reopen, whereas 100% oxygen caused the shunt to disappear: 'Since information concerning normal human circulatory adjustments at birth is extremely important, the present investigation was believed justified.' Successful closure of PDA with oxygen was reported [14].

Patency in preterm infants and respiratory distress

Charles Billard determined the age at which the ductus closes by studying deceased neonates (Table 3.6.1) [15]: 'With the greatest attention possible I investigated the changes occurring in the heart, the ductus arteriosus, the ductus venosus, and the umbilical arteries during the first extra-uterine days … The results show that the fetal openings are not obliterated shortly after birth, that the time in which they close is highly variable, and that the foramen ovale and the ductus arteriosus usually are obliterated on day eight or ten … Around and after the time of birth the wall of the ductus augments and develops some kind of concentric hypertrophy, which without diminishing the appearance of the vessel reduces its gauge … Undoubtedly, as long as these transitional phenomena persist, blood oxygenation will be incomplete … However, is it really necessary that the blood of a newborn infant be oxygenated to the same degree than the blood circulating in an adult's arteries?'

Billard did not relate these findings to gestational age and claimed to have largely excluded respiratory causes of death. However, many of the foundlings who died during the first days were most likely premature ('weaklings'). He also depicted the case of a newborn, in whom ductal patency was associated with 'aneurysmatic' dilatation of the ductus (Fig. 3.6.2) [16]: 'Observation 77: October 25, 1826, a three day old male infant was brought to the foundling hospital, and was admitted to the infirmary the next day. His size and constitution were poor, respiration disturbed, face livid, cry suffocated, body temperature natural, his pulse faint, frequent, and easily compressible. This infant remained in the same condition for two days and died on the third without having demonstrated other symptoms than those mentioned … The ductus arteriosus had the shape of a

Table 3.6.1 Patency of fetal anastomoses during the first 8 postnatal days as observed in 138 postmortem examinations by Billard in 1826 [15].

	Day of life					
	1	2	3	4	5	8
Number examined	(18)	22	22	27	29	20
Foramen ovale open	14	15	14	17	13	5
Foramen ovale partly open	2	3	5	8	10	4
Foramen ovale obliterated	2	4	3	2	6	11
Ductus arteriosus open	13	13	15	17	15	3
Ductus arteriosus partly open	4	6	5	7	7	6
Ductus arteriosus obliterated	1	3	2	3	7	11

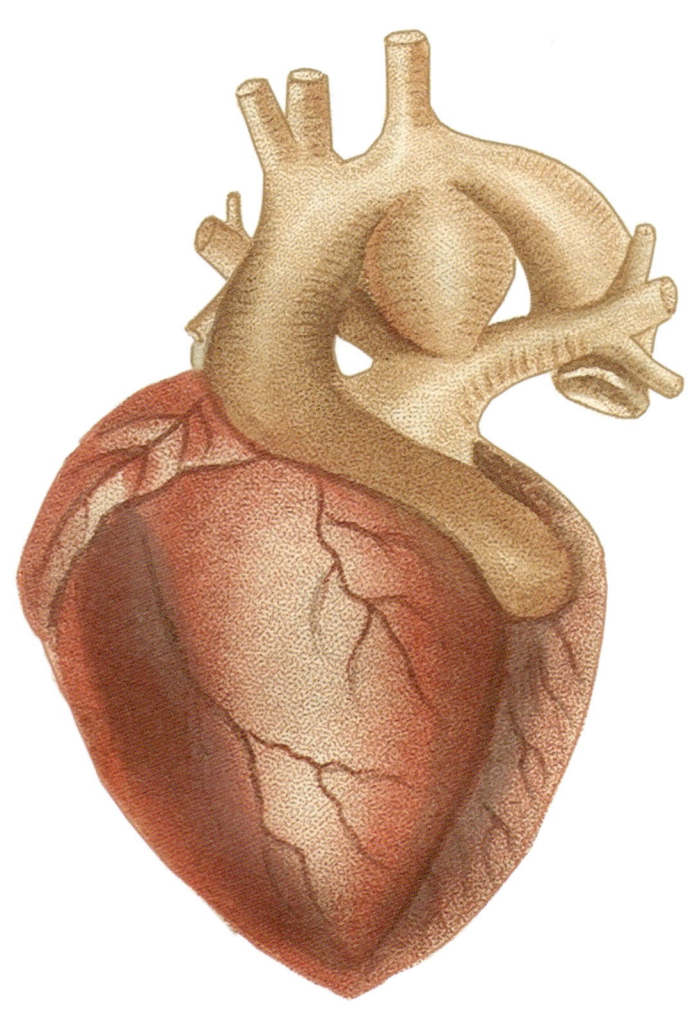

Fig. 3.6.2 Ductus-'aneurysma' in an infant who died on day 3, from Billard's traité 1828 [16].

large cherry stone; its diameter was about 8 mm, the circumference 20 mm. Considered externally, it seemed to join the aorta with a broad opening; but this apparent broadness was only externally, as the tumour's interior was filled with fibrinous clots which were organized into formed layers, as observed in aneurysmatic tumours of adults.'

A.M. Thore, another intern at the Paris foundling hospital, described eight more cases of 'aneurysma-like' ductal patency including their stethoscopic findings—a modern technology in 1842 [17]: 'The boy, born on the 10th of March [1842], is a vigorous well formed infant. On the 10th crepitant rales are heard everywhere around the chest; bronchial breathing and bronchophonia; pulse 150, respiration 50 per minute ... On the 19th a faint sound is heard at the right side of the chest and the humid crepitation on both sides persists ... On the 21st the infant dies ... The ductus arteriosus is one centimeter long, and shows a marked swelling proximal to the aorta; this dilatation, about 6 mm in diameter, contains a clot of a pea's size.'

Carpenter (1894) suggested a direct relationship between PDA and respiratory distress syndrome [18]: 'It may be found in hearts that are otherwise well-formed, and its patent condition arose from the existence of some obstruction at the time of birth, such as atelectasis pulmonum, which passing away left this as a relic of the former mischief. Premature delivery has been likewise assigned as a cause.' Julius Hess, founder of the Chicago special care unit, stated in 1923 [19]: 'The ductus Botalli closes more slowly and later in prematures. On the average blood ceases to pass through after the end of the first or second week of life.' In 1959, the London paediatrician Burnard used auscultation and phonocardiogram to diagnose delayed ductal closure in preterm infants [20]: 'In premature babies the murmur occurred whether there had been asphyxia at birth or not: in them there was a clear connexion with dyspnoea, and the murmur was not heard unless respiratory distress was present. In some prematures the murmur disappeared and then returned if their condition deteriorated. Mature babies who became ill with respiratory embarrassment after birth asphyxia were similar to premature babies in the more ready detection and longer duration of the murmur. There seemed therefore to be some connexion between birth asphyxia or prematurity on the one hand, and the murmur and difficult breathing on the other.'

Abraham Rudolph's group used cardiac catheterization in 1966 and Danilowicz and colleagues showed that the ductus closure is delayed in premature infants [21]. Thibeault and co-workers [22] demonstrated that respiratory distress syndrome predisposes preterm infants to clinically symptomatic PDA. Cotton and colleagues [23] found that PDA increases morbidity and mortality of preterm infants, but also that 'the morbidity among survivors was predominantly related to therapy and not to the underlying physiologic disturbance'.

Surgical intervention

On 26 August 1938, Robert Gross performed the first successful surgical correction of a congenital heart defect. He ligated a PDA in a 7-year-old child in Boston [24]. In 1963, Decanq reported the ligation of a PDA in a 1417 g preterm infant [25]. In San Francisco in 1973, Edmunds and colleagues reported disappointing results among 21 preterm infants following operative closure of the ductus [26]. Surgery was the only treatment for PDA until pharmacological approaches became available in 1976 [27]. Gersony and colleagues [28] compared surgical and pharmacological interventions in a randomized trial. A failed closure rate of 30% was reported in the indomethacin group, whereas more frequent pneumothorax and severe retinopathy was found in the surgical group. Today, PDA surgery in preterm infants is most often a second-line approach for patients in whom pharmacotherapy fails.

Politics and research funding

In the early 1960s, two Americans greatly promoted the treatment of PDA and the development of neonatology as a subspecialty: (1) John F. Kennedy, who started his brief presidency in 1961; and (2) Julius Comroe, director of the newly formed Cardiovascular Research Institute (CVRI) at the University of California, San Francisco, since 1958. Kennedy, unlike most elderly politicians, was a young father with personal concern for neonatal issues: His sister Rosemarie was left handicapped following brain surgery, his firstborn daughter Arabella was stillborn, and his son Patrick was born six weeks preterm and died from respiratory distress syndrome [29]. His sister Eunice Kennedy Shriver motivated the president to establish the National Institute of Child Health and Development (NICHD) in 1962 [30]. Comroe, originally a respiratory physiologist, made the CVRI a world-class research institution within a few years [31]. As a research director, he advocated that neonates were human beings deserving of every research effort. He stimulated the team in the neonatal intensive care unit—George Gregory, Roderic Phibbs, and William Tooley—who published on continuous positive airway pressure in 1971 [32]. Comroe immediately recruited John Severinghaus, who just had developed electrodes to measure pO_2 and pCO_2 [33]. He also brought in John Clements in 1959, who had characterized the properties of alveolar surfactant [34]. And he recruited the whole group of Abraham Rudolph from New York in 1966, pioneers in neonatal cardiology [35] and ductus research [21, 36]. When due to continuous positive airway pressure large numbers of preterm infants survived in San Francisco, Michael Heymann and Abraham Rudolph were at the right place at the right time, and NICHD grant HD 35398 allowed them to study the PDA in preterm infants [26, 37].

Pharmacological intervention

That prostaglandins play an important role in keeping the ductus arteriosus open [38] and that inhibition of prostaglandin synthesis leads to closure of the ductus [39] was shown by Sharpe at the Karolinska Institute and by Coceani in Toronto [40]. In Auckland, the paediatricians Elliott and Starling used prostaglandin E1 to open the ductus of a human infant with pulmonary atresia [41]: 'The infusion was started on the third day of life … With each infusion of PGE1 arterial oxygen saturation rose; two 10 mg doses of indomethacin given rectally between the first and the second infusions of PGE1 may have lowered the arterial saturation … which may have resulted from ductus narrowing.' One year later, two clinical trials with indomethacin were report by William Friedman, San Diego [42], and Michael Heymann, San Francisco [27]: Heyman, in Rudolph's group, observed a dramatic fall in the left atrial/aortic root ratios and concluded: 'Indomethacin produced marked constriction of the ductus arteriosus in 14 of 15 infants, including four who were very immature, whereas aspirin had no effect on the 1200 g infant and an incomplete effect on the 1220 g infant.'

Friedman described the cooperation of the two Californian groups [43]: 'When I received this notification, I called Dr. Abraham Rudolph, who earlier had so willingly taught me chronic instrumentation techniques to access the fetal circulation … and the manuscripts appeared back-to-back in the same issue of the New England Journal of Medicine.' The success story of the CVRI shows how closely heart and lung are connected and has been reported by the protagonists [44–46]. It illustrates how prudently Comroe fostered the scientific cooperation between basic science and the new subspecialties of paediatric cardiology and neonatology.

Conclusion

Due to religious prejudices, the fetal circulation was not understood until after the Reformation. One mechanical theory after the other was offered to explain postnatal contraction. Persisting ductal patency had been observed in the early 19th century, but was only understood after prostaglandins were discovered to play an active role in maintaining ductal patency. With an increasing number of immature infants surviving immediate postnatal adaptation, PDA is likely to gain even more importance. Regarding the mechanisms of ductal closure, more progress has been made during the last three decades than during the previous three centuries. It still remains unclear, however, in which preterm infant and at which postnatal age patency of the ductus is normal, and who will benefit from intervention. These questions can only be answered by randomized controlled trials with long-term endpoints including chronic lung disease, pulmonary hypertension, and neurodevelopmental outcomes.

REFERENCES

1. Morgagni GB: The seats and causes of diseases investigated by anatomy. London: Millar, 1769: Vol. **2**, art. 61, 62.
2. Craigie D: Instance of obliteration of aorta beyond the arch. Edinb Med Surg J 1841;**56**:427–62.
3. De Almagro M: Étude clinique et anatomo-pathologique sur la persistance du canal artériel. Paris: Delahaye, 1862: p. 97, pl. I.
4. Lesage A: Lehrbuch der Krankheiten des Säuglings. Leipzig: Thieme, 1912: p. 544.
5. Bernt J: Über das Verfahren bey unseren Versuchen mit Leichen neugeborner Kinder zur Begründung einer zuverlässigeren Lebensprobe. Med Jahrb Österr Staates N F 1824;274–87.
6. Jörg E: Die Foetuslunge im geborenen Kinde. Grimma: Gebhard, 1835: p. 19.
7. Kennedy JA, Clark SL: Observations on the ductus arteriosus of the guinea pig in relation to its method of closure. Anat Rec 1941;**79**:349–71.
8. Kennedy JA, Clark SL: Observations on the physiological reactions of the ductus arteriosus. Am J Physiol 1942;**136**:140–7.
9. Gardiner JM, Keith JD: Prevalence of heart disease in Toronto children, 1948–1949 Cardiac Registry. Pediatrics 1951;**7**:713–21.
10. Alzamora V, Rotta A, Battilana G, et al.: On the possible influence of great altitudes on the determination of certain cardiovascular anomalies. Pediatrics 1953;**12**:259–62.
11. Eldridge DL, Hultgren HN, Wigmore ME: The physiologic closure of the ductus arteriosus in the newborn infant. J Clin Invest 1955;**34**:987–96.
12. Born GVR, Dawes GS, Mott JC, Rennick BR: The constriction of the ductus arteriosus caused by oxygen and by asphyxia in newborn lambs. J Physiol 1956;**132**:304–42.
13. Moss AJ, Emmanouilides GC, Adams FH, Chuang K: Response of ductus arteriosus and pulmonary and systemic arterial pressure to changes in oxygen environment in newborn infants. Pediatrics 1964;**33**:937–44.
14. Dunn PM, Speidel BD: Use of oxygen to close patent ductus arteriosus in preterm infants. Lancet 1973;**2**:333–4.
15. Billard CM: Traité des maladies des enfants nouveau-nés et a la mamelle. 3. ed. Paris: Baillière, 1837: p. 605–9.
16. Billard CM: Traité des maladies des enfants nouveau-nés et a la mamelle. Paris: Baillière, 1828: obs. 77, atlas pl. VII fig. 1.
17. Thore AM: Mémoire sur les vices de conformation du coeur consistant seulement en une oreillette et un ventricule. Arch Gen Med 1842;**8**:3–30.
18. Carpenter G: Congenital affections of the heart. London: Basel, 1894: p. 42.

19. Hess JH: Premature and congenitally disabled infants. London: Churchill, 1923: p. 38.
20. Burnard ED: The cardiac murmur in relation to symptoms in the newborn. BMJ 1959;**1**:134–8.
21. Danilowicz D, Rudolph AM, Hoffman JIE: Delayed closure of the ductus arteriosus in premature infants. Pediatrics 1966;**37**:74–8.
22. Thibeault DW, Emmanouilides GC, Nelson RJ, et al.: Patent ductus arteriosus complicating the respiratory distress syndrome in preterm infants. J Pediatr 1975;**86**:120–6.
23. Cotton RB, Stahlman MT, Kovar I, Catterton WZ: Medical management of small preterm infants with symptomatic patent ductus arteriosus. J Pediatr 1978;**92**:467–73.
24. Gross RE, Hubbard JP: Surgical ligation of a patent ductus arteriosus. J Am Med Assoc 1939;**112**:729–31.
25. DeCanq HE Jr.: Repair of a patent ductus arteriosus in a 1417 g infant. Am J Dis Child 1963;**106**:402–5.
26. Edmunds LHJ, Gregory GA, Heymann MA, et al.: Surgical closure of the ductus arteriosus in premature infants. Circulation 1973;**48**:856–63.
27. Heymann MA, Rudolph AM, Silverman NH: Closure of the ductus arteriosus in premature infants by inhibition of prostaglandin synthesis. N Engl J Med 1976;**295**:530–3.
28. Gersony WM, Peckham GJ, Ellison RC, et al.: Effects of indomethacin in premature infants with patent ductus arteriosus. J Pediatr 1983;**102**:895–906.
29. Bisiach G: Il Presidente. La lunga storia di una breva vita. Roma: Newton Compton editori, 1990.
30. Cooke RE: The origin of the National Institute of Child Health and Human Development. Pediatrics 1993;**92**:868–71.
31. Kety SS, Forster RE: Julius H. Comroe, Jr.: March 13, 1911–July 31, 1984. Biog Mem Nat Acad Sci 2001;**79**:66–83.
32. Gregory GA, Kitterman JA, Phibbs RH, et al.: Treatment of the idiopathic respiratory-distress syndrome with continuous positive airway pressure. N Engl J Med 1971;**284**:1333–40.
33. Severinghaus JW, Bradley AF: Electrodes for blood pO2 and pCO2 determination. J Appl Physiol 1958;**13**:515–20.
34. Clements JA: Surface tension of lung extracts. Proc Soc Exp Biol Med 1957;**95**:170–2.
35. Rudolph AM, Drorbaugh JE, Auld PAM, et al.: The circulation in the respiratory distress syndrome. Pediatrics 1961;**27**: 551–66.
36. Rudolph AM, Mayer FE, Nadas AS, Gross RE: Patent ductus arteriosus. A clinical and hemodynamic study of 23 patients in the first year of life. Pediatrics 1958;**22**:892–904.
37. Kitterman JA, Edmunds LH, Gregory GA, et al.: Patent ductus arteriosus in premature infants. N Engl J Med 1972;**287**:473–7.
38. Sharpe GL, Larsson KS: Studies on closure of the ductus arteriosus. X. In vivo effects of prostaglandin. Prostaglandins 1975;**9**: 703–19.
39. Sharpe GL, Thalme B, Larsson KS: Studies on closure of the ductus arteriosus. XI. Ductal closure in utero by a prostaglandin synthetase inhibitor. Prostaglandins 1974;**8**:363–8.
40. Coceani F, Olley PM, Bodach E: Lamb ductus arteriosus: effect of prostaglandin synthesis inhibitors on the muscle tone and the response to prostaglandin E2. Prostaglandins 1975;**9**: 299–308.
41. Elliott RB, Starling MB, Neutze JM: Medical manipulation of the ductus arteriosus. Lancet 1975;**1**:140–2.
42. Friedman WF, Hirschklau MJ, Printz MP, Pitlick PT, Kirkpatrick SE: Pharmacologic closure of patent ductus arteriosus in the premature infant. N Engl J Med 1976;**295**:526–9.
43. Friedman WF: A look back: the clinical initiation of pharmacologic closure of patent ductus arteriosus in the preterm infant. NeoReviews 2003;**4**:e259–62.
44. Hoffman J: Abraham Morris Rudolph: an appreciation. Pediatrics 2002;**110**:622–6.
45. Gregory GA: Historical perspectives: continuous positive airway pressure (CPAP). NeoReviews 2004;**5**:e1–4.
46. Silverman N: Cardiologist in the spotlight: Abe Rudolph. Cardiovasc Dis Young Newslett 2001;**4**–7.
47. Bouchut E: Traité pratique des maladies des nouveau-nés et des enfants à la mamelle. Paris: Baillière, 1867: p. 412, fig. 82.

3.7 Intraventricular haemorrhage

Introduction

Intraventricular haemorrhage is a major complication of prematurity and a leading cause of hydrocephalus, disability, and death. There was little information on cerebral bleeding before specialized hospital units for 'weaklings' were established. Without ventilatory assistance, and as preterm infants died soon after birth, the full-blown picture of respiratory distress with prolonged hypoxia and hypercapnia did not develop. Moreover, these infants were considered 'miscarriages', and postmortem examination was seldomly performed. Interest grew in the late 18th century, when male surgeons entered obstetrics, when lying-in hospitals proliferated, and when medical services were established in foundling hospitals. The history of birth injury has been described [1]. This chapter is restricted to brain haemorrhage in premature infants and focuses on the slow shift from mechanical compression to insufficient respiration as its main explanation. It omits periventricular leukomalacia and traumatic haemorrhages such as tentorium which occurs after breech delivery (see Chapter 2.6).

Obstetrics

Court physician Simon Vallambert, one of the early writers on neonatal diseases, considered among the causes of hydrocephalus in 1565 [2] 'the humid constitution of the newborn infant and weakness of its brain ... also the midwife's shaping of the infant's head [see Chapter 5.2] ... At birth the head is compressed, and because the openings and ends of the veins are dilated and stretched, they may open or rupture, and thereby the aqueous blood leaves the veins like sweat.' Royal obstetrician François Mauriceau observed [3]: 'On the 7th may, 1697, I delivered a woman of her first child, a girl, born normally although five weeks preterm. She was very small, even much smaller than expected at this time of gestation. But she seemed vigorous and gave hope for survival. But two months later this hope vanished when an enormous hydrocephalus developed in this infant's head.' Nils Rosenstein devoted 31 pages of his 'Diseases of Children' to hydrocephalus in 1781, but did not mention cerebral haemorrhage as a cause [4]. Edinburgh neurologist Robert Whytt wrote in his monograph on hydrocephalus in 1768 [5]: 'Altho' there has been no original weakness in the brain, yet it may have suffered so much in the time of birth, by the compression of the skull, as afterwards to give rise to a collection of water in its cavities.' Neither professor was affiliated with a foundling hospital, nor did they ever likely see a preterm infant.

Paris obstetrician Joseph Capuron believed the brain to be the main cause of trouble at birth, and classified asphyxia into three groups according to causes [6]: (1) apoplexy = blue asphyxia, resulting from too much blood; (2) asphyxia = white asphyxia, resulting from too little blood; and (3) debility = central apnoea of prematurity; and concluded: 'Debility may be caused by a prolonged delivery.' He cautioned against delayed cord clamping for fear of apoplexy [7] and reported cases of post-haemorrhagic hydrocephalus.

Pathology

As the *in vivo* symptoms of cerebral haemorrhage in the preterm infant are unspecific, lethal cases were usually studied. Charles Billard, who performed hundreds of autopsies at the Paris Foundling Hospital [8], discerned three types of congestion: '1, Injection of the meninges, medulla, and brain is so common in infants at birth, that it has appeared to me more proper to consider it as a natural rather than as a pathological state ... 2, Injection of the cerebral pulp is equally common; it exists under the form of a spotted redness, sometimes colouring deeply the substance of the brain; it usually exists on the lateral parts of the corpora striata ... 3, Lastly, it is possible, but very rare, to find cerebral haemorrhage very circumscribed in the hemisphere.'

In his magnificent atlas of 1829, pathologist Jean Cruveilhier depicted intraventricular haemorrhage in a preterm infant who had died at the Paris Maternité [9] (Fig. 3.7.1) and concluded: 'The cause of apoplexy during birth cannot be determined in most cases. It is not at all the use of the forceps: on the contrary, I am convinced that the forceps prevents many apoplexies ... I regard all apoplexies in newborns as mechanically caused.' At the Vienna Foundling Hospital, Alois Bednar performed autopsies of 53 neonates with brain haemorrhages within 3 years [10]. He classified them as 27 cases of intermeningeal haemorrhage, often surviving for several weeks with some degree of resorption, and 16 cases of intraventricular haemorrhage, of whom nine infants were preterm.

Eugene Bouchut tried to correlate location and cause of the bleeding in 1867 [11]: (1) cerebral congestion, occurring at birth, when delivery was difficult or prolonged; (2) cerebral apoplexy, occurring after birth, in the brain's substance; and (3) meningeal haemorrhage in the subarachnoidal space. Joseph Parrot, director of the Paris Foundling Hospital, identified neonatal brain haemorrhages in five

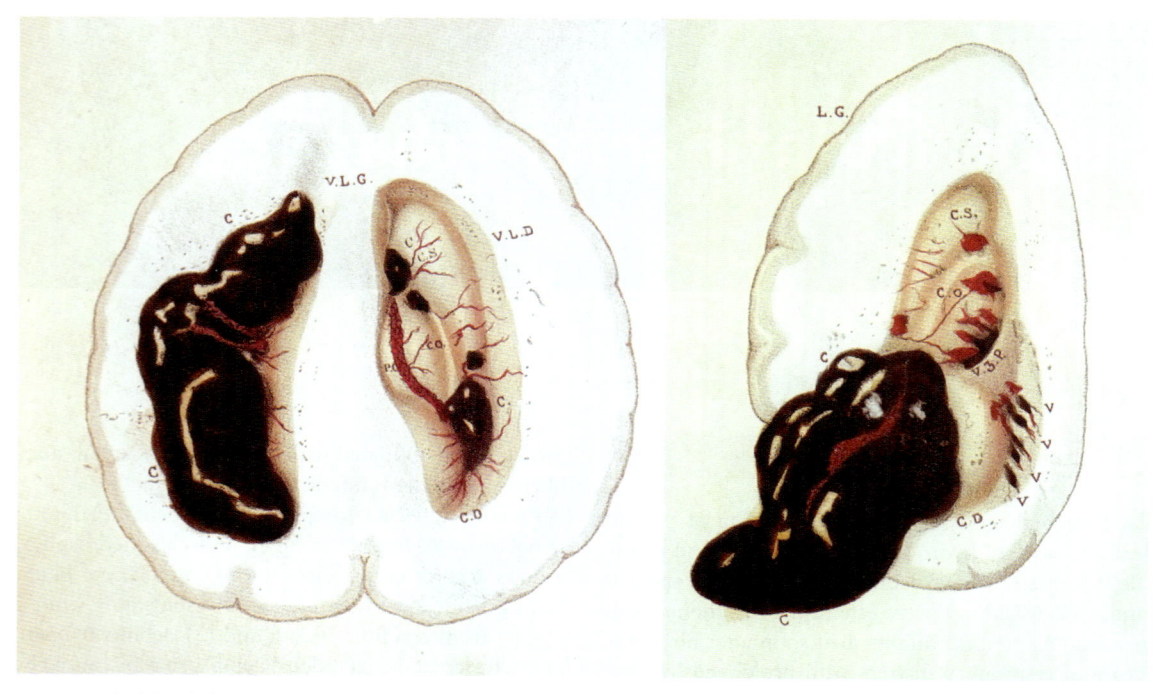

Fig. 3.7.1 Intraventricular blood clots in the brain of an infant of 7 months gestation, depicted by Jean Cruveilhier 1829 [9]. Left: one ventricle is distended by a large coherent clot; the other ventricle contains several small clots. Right: when the clot was moved backwards, the torn veins VVV became visible at the ventricle's base.

locations in 1877 [12]: 'Among 35 infants whom I examined, I found blood 5 times in the arachnoid cavity, … 26 times in the subarachnoid space, … once in the brain tissue, … 5 times in the ventricular cavity, and [most frequently] under the periventricular ependyme (14 times on the right, 12 times on the left side)'. Parrot emphasized that the symptoms were few and unspecific.

At Johns Hopkins University in Baltimore, William Osler observed in 1889 [13]: 'In the cases of birth palsy, which result usually in bilateral hemiplegia or paraplegia, the evidence points strongly to meningeal haemorrhage as one of the chief causes of the disorder.'

Hans Kundrat, pathologist in Vienna, associated intermeningeal bleedings and respiratory distress in 1890 [14]: 'Their lungs are atelectatic, or have returned to their fetal state after hours or days of breathing', but kept the faith of mechanical lesion: 'All hemorrhages must be explained in the same way: by external pressure during the passage through the birth channel, by distorsion, tearing, and rupture of the vessels.' In 1901, Camille Hahn, obstetrician at the Paris Maternité [15], declared bleeding as a disease peculiar to preterm infants and believed it to result from 'compression plus structural immaturity'. In his extensive 'Patho-anatomic studies in preterm infants', Finnish paediatrician Arvo Ylppö, in 1919, discerned multiple small subarachnoidal haemorrhages 'astonishingly regular and frequent' (Fig. 3.7.2) and more extensive bleedings localized around the cerebellum [16] and extensive bleeds filling the lateral ventricles in 'most immature infants below 1000 g birthweight'. In 1898, Victor Wallich reported 55 cases of intracranial haemorrhage in newborns: 'only 6 had birthweight 3,000 g and more; 12 had 2,500–3,000 g and 32 were prematures with birthweight below 2,500 g' [17]. Like Ylppö, Heinrich Finkelstein considered the haemorrhages to result from trauma in 1921 [18]. As late as 1961, Philipp Schwartz, who had performed many autopsies of deceased newborns in Germany and Pennsylvania, insisted [1]: 'Intracerebral hemorrhage from the trunk and radicular zone of the terminal veins are the most important parturitional lesions … they occur only in infants injured during birth.'

For 200 years, mechanical theories were derived from autopsies to explain the origin of cerebral haemorrhages in the preterm infant, and during 19th-century obstetrics, birth trauma was indeed more frequent than today. The idea that postnatal respiratory failure contributed to the dreadful disease, matured slowly. Based on 714 autopsies, Harcke et al. demonstrated in 1972 'hypoxia's role in generating intraventricular hemorrhage and suggested an association with hyaline membrane disease' [19].

Imaging

Up to the 1960s, cerebral haemorrhage of the preterm infant had been the pathologist's domain. This changed dramatically when *in vivo* imaging became available, enabling the occurrence and resorption of the haemorrhage to be observed.

Computerized transaxial tomography was developed in the early 1970s in the United States, the 'EMI-scanner' was immediately used for children [20], and in 1978 Lu-Ann Papile and co-workers in Albuquerque investigated 46 infants weighing less than 1500 g with this technique [21]. They found that about 40% of these infants suffered intraventricular haemorrhages, and identified four grades: (1) subependymal; (2) intraventricular without dilatation; (3) intraventricular with dilatation; and (4) parenchymal haemorrhage. This classification was later adapted to sonography. They also found that grade 1 and 2 bleedings were usually resorbed without sequelae, data confirmed by a larger study in Atlanta in

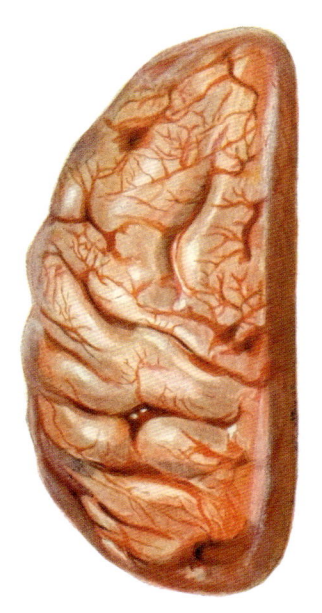

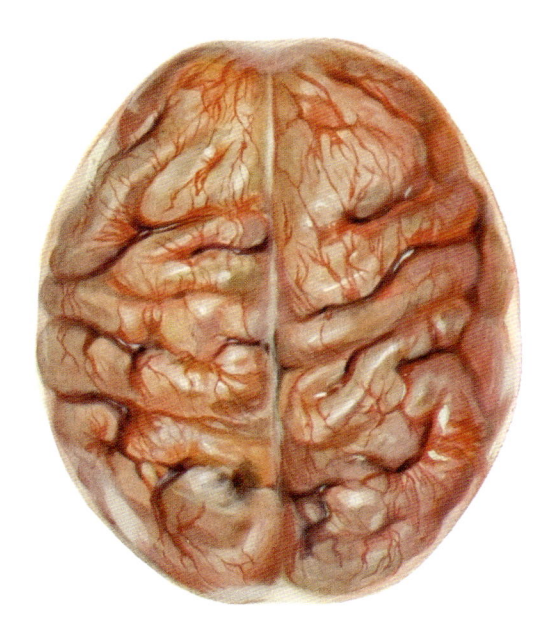

Fig. 3.7.2 Multiple small intermeningeal and subarachnoidal haemorrhages in preterm infants depicted by Arvo Ylppö in 1919 [16]. Left: surface of the left hemisphere of a preterm female infant of 1120 g birthweight who died at 16 days of age from necrotizing enterocolitis. Right: brain surface of a female infant of 1350 g birthweight who died at 34 hours of age from asphyxia.

1980 [22]. Computed tomography rendered obsolete the dangerous older techniques such as myelography, ventriculography, and pneumoencephalography.

A revolution occurred shortly afterwards with ultrasound imaging, spearheaded by Karen Pape, a travelling research fellow from Toronto Children's Hospital, who was at the right place at the right time: with Osmund Reynolds at the University College Hospital, London, she laid the ground for the rapid, bedside, non-invasive detection of intraventricular haemorrhages [23]. Soon the transcranial scan was replaced by views taken through the fontanelle [24], and within few years, sonography became an integral tool in every neonatal intensive care unit with the advantages of rapid bedside examination, no radiation, no need for sedating drugs, and immediate availability of the results. Extensive research in London and elsewhere revealed that preterm infants' cerebral bleeds did not start from the ventricle, but from the germinal layer adjacent to the ventricle [25], and that they occurred during the first 24 hours of life. Magnetic resonance imaging was also developed at the University College Hospital, London, adding functional aspects to the anatomical depiction [26].

Physiology

The preterm infant's cerebral blood flow is not autoregulated but is pressure passive: with rising blood pressure, the cerebral blood flow increases. Based on a wealth of information from *in vivo* imaging, Jonathan Wigglesworth and Karen Pape in 1978 developed a model of pathogenesis of damage to the immature brain [27], in which mechanical factors (head compression, birth trauma, etc.) no longer had an important role. This model remained largely valid until now (Fig. 3.7.3): with respiratory insufficiency, the effects of hypoxia and hypercapnia lead to an increase in cerebral blood flow and breakdown of the blood–brain barrier with resultant haemorrhage. Conversely, hyperventilation with hyperoxia and hypocapnia leads to vasoconstriction and a decrease in perfusion pressure, resulting in ischaemic lesions. With the advent of the Doppler technique, it became possible to measure blood flow velocity in the cerebral arteries [28].

Risk factors identified

In vivo scans revealed haemorrhage incidence in up to 50% of infants with birthweight less than 1500 g, but also the reassuring information, that lower-grade haemorrhages resorb without sequelae. With the Wigglesworth–Pape model and exact timing of the haemorrhages, factors were identified in the 1980s which raised or lowered the preterm infant's risk of suffering a brain haemorrhage. Protective factors were antenatal steroids given to the mother [29, 30], and early substitution of surfactant in the delivery room [31]. Harmful factors independent of gestational age were mainly related to respiratory insufficiency and its management: hypercapnia [32], fluctuating cerebral blood flow [28] or pneumothorax during or following ventilation [33, 34], and prolonged arterial hypotension [35]. Many other conditions occurring between 48 before and 48 h after birth were found to be associated with cerebral haemorrhage, but were usually dependent on gestational age.

From diagnosis to prevention

Since the 1980s, numerous postnatal strategies have been investigated in randomized trials. Beneficial outcomes were proved for antenatal steroids in threatened preterm delivery [36], delayed cord clamping for 30 seconds or more [37], and postnatal indomethacin

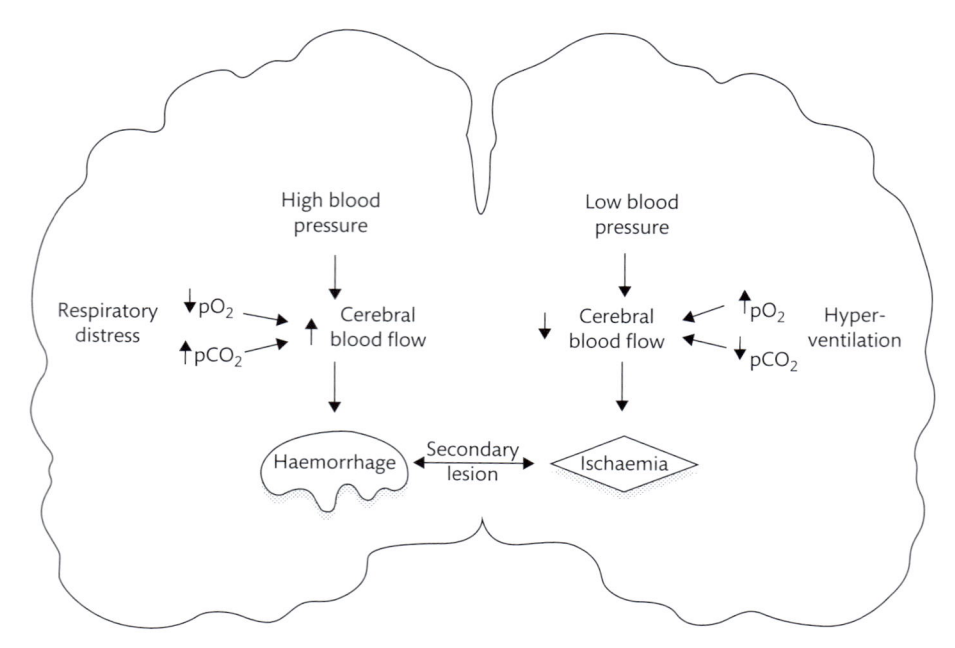

Fig. 3.7.3 Two-part model for the pathogenesis of intraventricular haemorrhage (left) and periventricular leukomalacia (right).
Source: Data from Wigglesworth JS, Pape KE. An integrated model for haemorrhagic and ischaemic lesions in the newborn brain. *Early Human Development* 1978;2:179–199.

[38]. Neonatology came into being in the 1960s with the ability to master artificial ventilation. Thirty years later, it became a major goal of neonatologists to avoid prolonged artificial ventilation, a dream that came true with the triumph of surfactant substitution. In Portland, Maine, the incidence of overall/severe haemorrhage among infants weighing less than 1500 g decreased from 39%/14% in 1980 to 25%/10% in 1987, without planned intervention [39]. Undoubtedly, multiple modifications of neonatal care, and the shortened need for artificial ventilation in the surfactant era had contributed to this progress.

Conclusion

The belief in birth trauma as the predominant cause of cerebral bleeding in preterm infants persisted stubbornly, even once the association with respiratory distress became known. Compression during birth was indeed frequent in the 19th century due to oblique 'rickety' pelvises (Chapter 2.6) and routine forceps deliveries. The latter had been in fashion since the mid-18th century, and functioned as the key that opened the delivery room to male obstetricians. *In vivo* imaging unravelled the complex framework of respiratory insufficiency, hypercapnia, and cerebral blood flow in the aetiology of intraventricular haemorrhage. The greatest benefit of imaging was that it enabled the identification of risk factors for brain haemorrhage in preterm infants, and the development of strategies to avoid these risks. Brain haemorrhage and its consequences contributed to Soranus' 2000-year-old prejudice that preterm infants are not worth rearing [40]. Much progress was achieved when the sonograph entered the neonatal intensive care unit, and severe brain damage in the preterm infant became less frequent, despite the fact that ever more immature infants survived.

REFERENCES

1. Schwartz P: Birth injuries of the newborn: morphology, pathogenesis, clinical pathology and prevention. Basel: Karger, 1961: p. 67.
2. Vallambert S: Cinq livres de la manière de nourrir et gouverner les enfants dès leur naissance. Poitiers: Manefz et Bouchetz, 1565: p. 341.
3. Mauriceau F: Observations sur la grossesse et l'accouchement des femmes. Obs. 78. Paris: Compagnie des Libraires Associes, 1738: Vol. **2**, p. 626.
4. Rosenstein NRv: Anweisung zur Kenntnis und Chur der Kinderkrankheiten (1st Swedish ed. 1764). 4. ed. Göttingen: Dieterich, 1781: p. 590–621.
5. Whytt R: Observations on the dropsy in the brain. Edinburgh: John Balfour, 1768: p. 33.
6. Capuron J: Traité des maladies des enfans, jusqu'à la puberté (1st ed. 1813). 2. ed. Paris: Croullebois, 1820: p. 23.
7. Capuron J: Cours théorique et pratique d'accouchemens. Paris: Croullebois, 1811: p. 273.
8. Billard CM: A treatise of the diseases of infants (1st French ed. 1828). 2. ed. New York: Langley, 1840: p. 473–5.
9. Cruveilhier J: Apoplexie des enfants nouveau-nés. In: Anatomie pathologique du corps humain. Paris: Baillière, 1829–1835: Vol. **1**, p. Livraison 15, plate 1.
10. Bednar A: Die Krankheiten der Neugeborenen und Säuglinge. Wien: Gerold, 1851: Vol. **2**, p. 28–36.
11. Bouchut E: Traité pratique des maladies des nouveau-nés et des enfants a la mamelle. 5. ed. Paris: Baillière, 1867: p. 215–8.
12. Parrot J: Clinique des nouveau-nés: l'Athrepsie. Paris: Masson, 1877: p. 336.
13. Osler W: The cerebral palsies of children. London: Lewis, 1889: p. 89–96.
14. Kundrat: Über die intrameningealen Blutungen Neugeborener. Wien Klin Wochenschr 1890;**46**:887–9.

15. Hahn C: Des prematurés: caracteres, prognostic, traitement. Paris: Steinheil, 1901: p. 69–73.
16. Ylppö A: Pathologisch-anatomische Studien bei Frühgeborenen. Zeitschr Kinderheilk 1919;**20**:212–431.
17. Audebert JL: L'enfant né avant terme. Arch Méd Toulouse 1900;**6**:423.
18. Finkelstein H: Lehrbuch der Säuglingskrankheiten. 2. ed. Berlin: Springer, 1921: p. 121–31.
19. Harcke HT, Naeye RL, Storch A, Blanc WA: Perinatal cerebral intraventricular hemorrhage. J Pediatr 1972;**80**:37–42.
20. Houser W, Smith JB, Gomez MR, Baker HL: Evaluation of intracranial disorders in children by computerized transaxial tomography. Neurology 1975;**25**:607–13.
21. Papile L-A, Burstein J, Burstein R, Koffler H: Incidence and evolution of subependymal and intraventricular hemorrhage. J Pediatr 1978;**92**:529–34.
22. Ahmann PA, Lazzara A, Dykes FD, Brann AW, Schwartz JF: Intraventricular hemorrhage in the high-risk preterm infant. Ann Neurol 1980;**7**:118–24.
23. Pape KE, Blackwell RJ, Cusick G, et al.: Ultrasound detection of brain damage in preterm infants. Lancet 1979;**313**:1261–4.
24. Lipscombe AP, Blackwell RJ, Reynolds EOR, Thorburn RJ, Cusick G, Pape KE: Ultrasound scanning of brain through anterior fontanelle of newborn infants. Lancet 1979;**314**:39.
25. Vohr B, Ment LR: Intraventricular hemorrhage in the preterm infant. Early Hum Dev 1996;**44**:1–16.
26. Cady EB, Dawson MJ, Hope PL, et al.: Non-invasive investigation of cerebral metabolism in newborn infants by phosphorus nuclear magnetic resonance spectroscopy. Lancet 1983;**321**:1059–62.
27. Wigglesworth JS, Pape KE: An integrated model for haemorrhagic and ischaemic lesions in the newborn brain. Early Hum Dev 1978;**2**:179–99.
28. Perlman JM, Volpe JJ: Cerebral blood flow velocity in relation to intraventricular hemorrhage in the premature newborn infant. J Pediatr 1982;**100**:956–9.
29. Clark CE, Clyman RI, Roth RS, Sniderman SH, Lane B, Ballard RA: Risk factor analysis of intraventricular hemorrhage in low-birth-weight infants. J Pediatr 1981;**99**:625–8.
30. Ment LR, Vohr BR, Makuch RW, et al.: Prevention of intraventricular hemorrhage by indomethacin in male preterm infants. J Pediatr 2004;**145**:832–4.
31. Walti H, Paris-Llado J, Egberts J, et al.: Prophylactic administration of porcine-derived lung surfactant is a significant factor in reducing the odds for peri- intraventricular haemorrhage in premature infants. Biol Neonate 2002;**81**:182–7.
32. Cooke RWI: Factors associated with periventricular haemorrhage in very low birthweight infants. Arch Dis Child 1981;**56**:425–31.
33. Hill A, Perlman JM, Volpe JJ: Relationship of pneumothorax to occurrence of intraventricular hemorrhage in the premature newborn. Pediatrics 1982;**69**:144–9.
34. Linder N, Haskin O, Levit O, et al.: Risk factors for intraventricular hemorrhage in very low birth weight premature infants. Pediatrics 2003;**111**:e590–5.
35. Meek JH, Tyszczuk L, Elwell CE, Wyatt JS: Low cerebral blood flow is a risk factor for severe intraventricular haemorrhage. Arch Dis Child Fet Neonat Ed 1999;**81**:F15–8.
36. Roberts D, Brown J, Medley N, Dalziel SR: Antenatal corticosteroids for accelerating fetal lung maturation for women at risk of preterm birth. Cochrane Database Syst Rev 2017;**3**:CD004454.
37. Rabe H, Reynolds G, Diaz-Rossello J: A systematic review and meta-analysis of a brief delay in clamping the umbilical cord of preterm infants. Neonatology 2008;**93**:138–44.
38. Fowlie PW, Davis PG, McGuire W: Prophylactic intravenous indomethacin for preventing mortality and morbidity in preterm infants. Cochrane Database Syst Rev 2010;**3**:CD000174.
39. Philip AGS, Allan WC, Tito AM, Wheeler LR: Intraventricular hemorrhage in preterm infants: declining incidence in the 1980s. Pediatrics 1989;**84**:797–801.
40. Temkin O: Soranus' gynecology. Baltimore, MD: Johns Hopkins Press, 1956: p. 79–80.

PART 4
Multiple birth

4.1 **Unwelcome: the abominable twins** *115*

4.2 **Fertility and fatality: higher-order multiples** *123*

4.3 **Unequal but monozygotic: twin–twin transfusion syndrome** *129*

4.4 **From monster to reversed perfusion: acardiac twins** *137*

INTRODUCTION

The birth of twins was considered an abomination from antiquity until more recent times and at least one twin often was killed. Identical twins were attributed to God's wrath, fraternal twins to maternal adultery. Added to this was the difficulty of breastfeeding two infants, especially among nomadic peoples. Higher-grade multiple births were considered sensational; their incidence increased with the advent of assisted reproduction in the 20th century. Up to the present day, ambiguity towards twin personhood triggered ethical debates and public interest, most frequently concerning conjoined twins. Twin–twin transfusion syndrome results from vascular anastomoses in fused placentas. Twin reversed arterial perfusion results from large arterioarterial and venovenous anastomoses leading to one twin's degeneration: malformed infants without a heart and head have been described since antiquity. Their relation to placental anastomoses was not understood until the mid-19th century.

4.1

Unwelcome
The abominable twins

Introduction

Early societies met multiple births with ambivalence or considered them a bad omen. Babylonian Shumma Izbu (ca. 1500 B.C.E.) prognosticated on tablet I [1]: 'If a woman gives birth to two boys – there will be hard times in the land ... and in the house of their father .... if to two boys feet-first – that house will be scattered ... If she gives birth to two [children] and one [is] a boy, [and] one a girl – there will be dissension in the land.'

The incidence of monozygotic twinning, 0.4% of all deliveries, remained fairly constant around the world. Dizygotic twinning is genetically regulated, aggregated in certain families, and ranges from 0.3% (Japan) to 4% (Nigeria) [2]. In 1964, Milham hypothesized 'that dizygotic twinning in humans may be a visible indicator of excessive maternal gonadotropin activity' [3]. Due to increasing maternal age and assisted reproduction techniques, the incidence of twins recently increased from 1:90 to 1:40, and 70% of all twins in the US now originate from infertility treatment [4].

Usually born preterm and with low weight, after prolonged birth and with an insufficient breast milk supply, twins' chances of surviving were not promising. They also created problems with respect to inheritance and firstborn's rights. Due to their increased mortality, the historic prevalence of twins in populations was lower than today. Their role in history and science was described by Harris [5–7] and Gedda [8]. The present chapter focuses on ambivalence towards twins, and on peculiarities in nomadic and settled peoples. It does not address twin-specific malformations.

Monozygotic twins and divine origin

Monozygotic ('identical') twins develop from a single fertilized ovum that splits. An inscription on the Egyptian granite stela of Suty (Seth) and Hor (Horus), erected during the reign of Amenhotep III (ca. 1360 B.C.E.), suggests ambivalence towards twins and to the confusing character of Seth [9]: 'I am the righteous one, whose abomination is evil ... My brother (who is) like me, with whose ways I am satisfied, went forth with me from the womb on the same day.' The Bible alluded to a celestial twin origin in Mark 3:17: 'And [Christus ordained] James the son of Zebedee, and John the brother of James; and he surnamed them *Boanerges*, which is the sons of thunder.'

In the 5th century B.C.E., Empedocles founded the Greek concept of procreation [10]: '[The embryos] that go to a warm womb become male, those that go to a cool one become female ... Twins and triplets occur because of the excessiveness and division of the sperm.' The Hippocratic Corpus maintained [11]: 'Twins resulting from a single coital act result from splitting the seed, which reaches different uterine cavities [from sheep anatomy, Greek authors assumed bicornuate uterus] ... In the cavity with thick and strong seed a male is created, and in the cavity with humid and weaker seed a female. If strong seed reaches both cavities, two males; if weak seed reaches both cavities, two females are created.' In Aphorismi sectio V, 38 [12] another Hippocratic author stated 'When a woman is pregnant with twins, should either breast become thin, she loses one child. If the right breast becomes thin, she loses the male child; if the left, the female.' Aristotle ascribed procreation to the male seed and assumed that the female only contributed to nourishment for the unborn [13]: 'The material they [men] do emit [semen] is, in the natural course, just sufficient to provide for a single fetation. If ever more of it is supplied, then twins are produced. And hence, also, such creatures seem rather to be monstrosities, because their formation is contrary to the general rule and to what is usual.' Greeks named twin infants *Didyme* or *Didymos*.

In Rome, twins rarely survived, as Pliny reported in 75 C.E. [14]: 'At birth, neither the mother nor more than one of the two children usually lives' and was emphasized by the *cognomen* (additional name) *Geminus*, *Gemellus*, or *Consors* ... A child was named *Vopiscus* if conceived as a twin and retained in the uterus when the other twin perished via abortion. Referring to Hippon and Empedocles, Censorinus (238 C.E.) [15] believed that an excess of seed will split into two parts: 'If both parts implant in warm [uterine] regions, male twins are born; if in cold regions, female; and if in a warm and a cold region, [infants of] different sex are born.'

Dizygotic twins and maternal adultery

Dizygotic ('fraternal') twins result from more than one fertilized egg due to polyovulation. Whereas monozygotic twins gave rise to supernatural explanations, dissimilar twinship was regarded negatively, and associated with impurity, blemish, and adultery: dissimilar twins implied two fathers or divine intervention.

The Hippocratic Corpus contains the book 'On superfetation' [16]: 'Superfetal conception occurs in women when the mouth of the uterus does not close after the first conception.' Confusingly, the Hippocratian term *superfetatio* today means superfecundation: more than one egg is fertilized in one or more coital acts, which in antiquity was understood as the special case of heteropaternal pregnancy. True superfetation, fertilization in subsequent menstrual cycles of a female who is already pregnant, does not occur in humans. In twins differing in sex, weight, or bodily characteristics, superfecundation was assumed, all too familiar from Greek mythology, where it meant maternal adultery. Its prototype was the Homeric Heracles story, recounted by Hesiod (ca. 650 B.C.E.) [17]: Alcmene's beauty impressed Zeus, the greatest of Greek Gods. The very day before her husband Amphitryon returned from war, Zeus seduced Alcmene, impersonating her husband. A night later, Alcmene slept with her husband, and 'being subject in love to a god and to a man exceeding goodly, brought forth twin sons in seven-gated Thebes. Though they were brothers, these were not of one spirit; for one was weaker but the other a far better man, one terrible and strong, the mighty Heracles. She bore him through the embrace of the son of Cronos [Zeus] lord of dark clouds and the other, Iphicles, of Amphitryon the spear-wielder, offspring distinct, this one of union with a mortal man, but that other of union with Zeus, leader of all the gods.' Fig. 4.1.1 shows these unequal twins with their mother and fathers.

Augustinus of Hippo rejected the theory of superfecundation of twins in 410 C.E. [18]: 'Conception results from a single coition, and nature is so powerful that a woman who has conceived cannot conceive again. Therefore twins are procreated in the same moment.' But as late as 1560, Giovanni Savonarola's *Practica* taught that twins were procreated by superfecundation [19]: 'Usually, at the time of impregnation, the uterine mouth closes that even a needle cannot be inserted. But in some women it does not close completely and they may conceive again. In such women the first fetus and also the second is weak. The superimpregnation occurs in slim and hirsute women who are warm-blooded and draw in the sperma more firmly. Twinning occurs when a large quantity of sperma is ejected and separates, so that two embryos develop in different uterine chambers. Our informant reports that in his town Abano [near Padova] a woman brought forth six embryos.'

Heteropaternal superfecundation is rare but evident from Baudelocque's 1789 edition [20] reporting 'the delivery of one black and one white infant by a woman of Guadeloupe who declared to have complied with her slave's approach soon after her husband's embrace'. A similar case was published in 1810 by John Archer from Harford [21]. Heteropaternal superfecundation was proven via human leucocyte antigen-typing by Terasaki in 1978 [22].

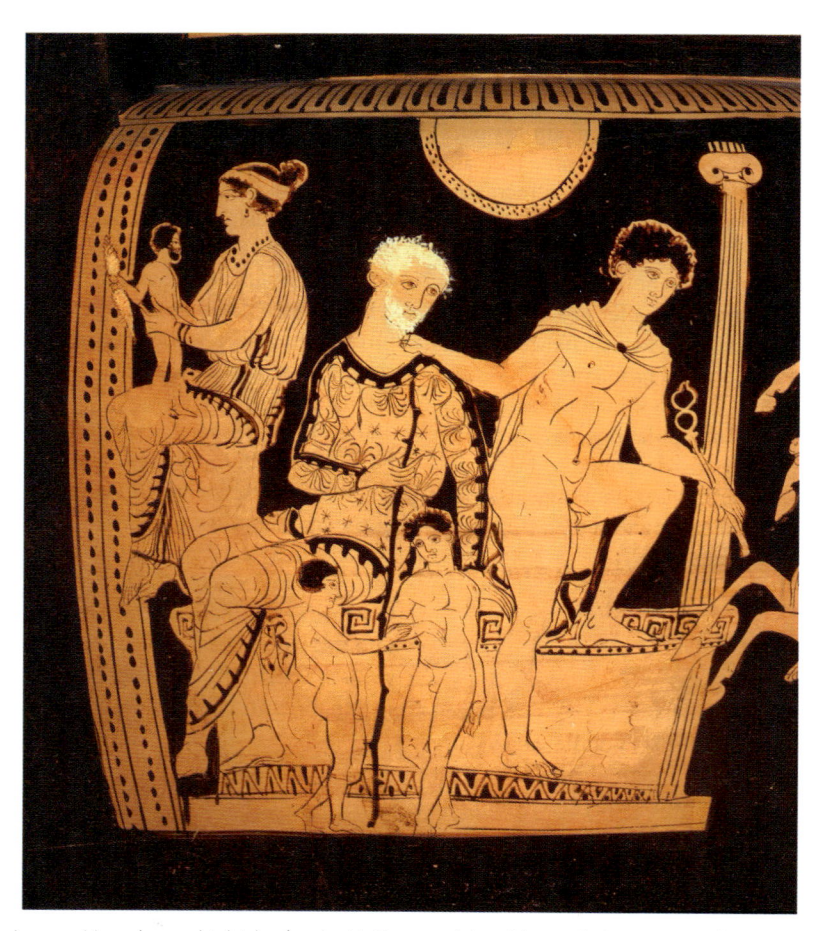

Fig. 4.1.1 Alcmene with her twin sons Heracles and Iphicles (and with Zeus and Amphitryon?), Lucanean column krater, ca. 400 B.C.E. Antikensammlung Berlin, inv. 1969.6.
© Antikensammlung; Staatliche Museen zu Berlin-Preussischer Kulturbesitz. Photo: Johannes Laurentius.

Heavenly twins

Ambivalence towards twins was overcompensated in many cultures through ritual veneration and divination. This occurred in prehistoric times, before Babylonian astrology located the heavenly twins in the Zodiac [23]. In Kisiga (north Babylonia, ca. 1500 B.C.E.), the twin war gods Lugalirra and Meslamtaea were revered [24], as were the *Ashvins* in the Indian Rig-Veda (ca. 1200 B.C.E.), twin deities believed to avert misfortune and blindness [25] and to protect the unborn (hymns 74 and 78):

'O Ashvins, may your car approach, most excellent of cars for speed.
Through many regions may our praise pass onward among mortal men,
May our laudation of you Twain, lovers of meath! be sweet to you.
Fly hitherward, ye wise of heart, like falcons with your winged steeds …
So steer in thee the babe unborn, so may the ten-month babe descend.
So also, ten-month babe, descend together with the after-birth.
The child who hath for ten months' time been lying in his mother's side.
May he come forth alive, unharmed, yea, living from the living dame.'

Equipped with horses and a chariot, the *Ashvins* were predecessors of the Greek *Dioscuri*. These prototypes of twin deities were born by Leda, Castor being the mortal son of Tyndareus and Pollux (Polydeuces) being the immortal son of Zeus. The Greek pantheon was rich in twins: Apollo and Artemis, gods of fine arts and hunting, respectively, begotten by Zeus and Leto; and Amphion and Zethos, founders of Thebes, begotten by Zeus and Antiope. Harris enumerated many twin gods and heroes [6]. Hebrews admired the twin Jacob as the progenitor of the tribes of Israel. The Aztec goddess of fertility and female beauty and patroness of childbirth Xochiquetzal was the twin sister of Xochipilli, god of arms, games, beauty, and flowers. Zuni Indians in western New Mexico revered the twin gods of war Ahayu'da [26].

Abandoned twins

Abandoning unwanted infants was frequent in New Babylonia [7th century B.C.E.], and clay-tablet contracts prove that twin foundlings 'saved from the dog's mouth' were adopted to be enslaved [27]. In European mythologies, twins who survived despite being cast away were venerated as founders of cities or kingdoms. Abandoning by the mother, such as Tyro, Phylonome, Aura, and so on, reveals that giving birth to twins had grim consequences for the Greek mother. Neleus and Pelias, begotten by Poseidon and Tyro, were abandoned, suckled by a mare, and became the founders of Pylos and Iolkos. Romulus and Remus, sons of Mars and the vestal Rhea Silvia, were condemned to be drowned in the Tiber, but were stranded and raised by a she-wolf to become the founders of Rome (Fig. 4.1.2). The Anglo-Saxon divine twins Hengist and Horsa led the invasion of Britain in the 5th century. Twins were frequent among the unloved inhabitants of European foundling homes [28] and the abandonment of twins remained common in the Igbo and Ibo societies of Nigeria [29].

Deceased twins

Early societies were well aware of the increased mortality and morbidity of twins [30], which was mostly due to prematurity, but also

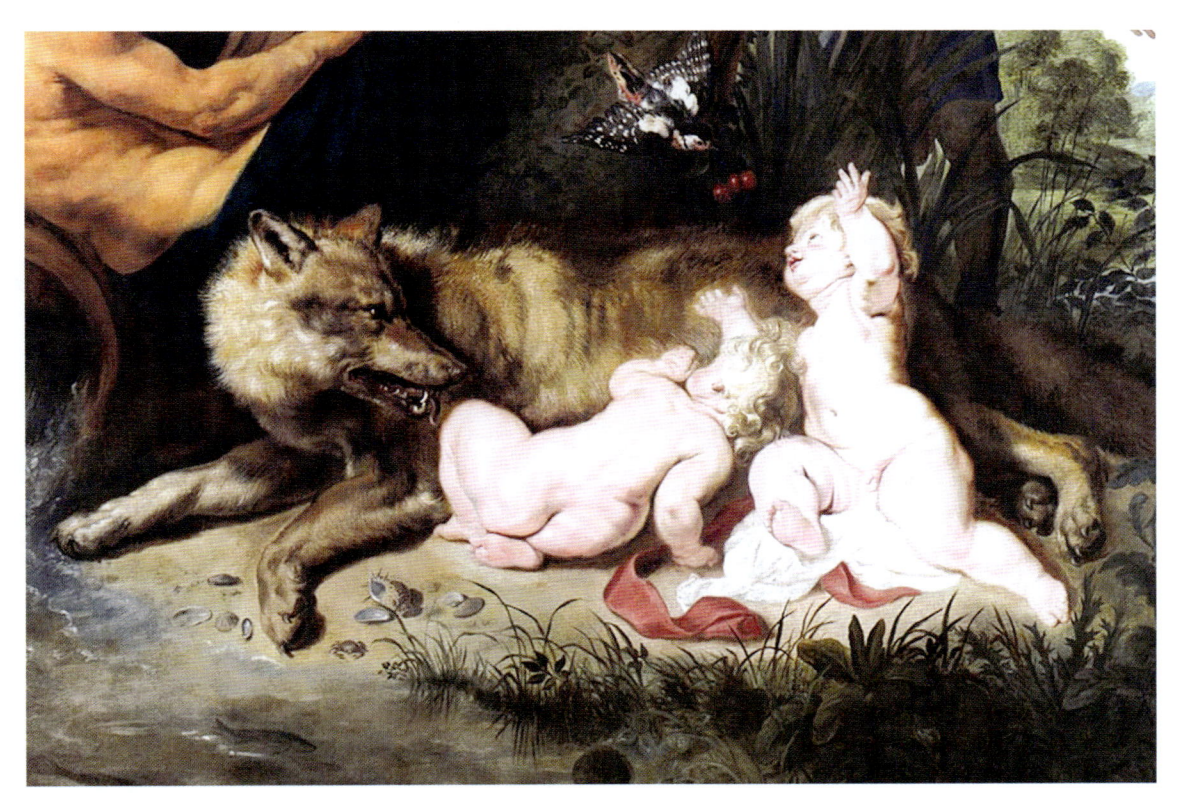

Fig. 4.1.2 Romulus and Remus nursed by the she-wolf. Detail of a painting by Peter Paul Rubens, 1615.
Rome, Pinacoteca Capitolina, with permission.

to a higher rate of congenital malformations [31]. The Northern Japanese Ainu looked upon (rare) twin births with awe and fear, believing that a spirit was the father of one of them; and if one died they identified him as the one with the spirit-father [5]. The natives of Savu (Indonesia) despised twins of opposite sex and killed the female for assumed intrauterine incest. The Kvakiutl of Vancouver Island developed complex rites to console the surviving twin whose sibling died [32].

Twin infanticide

Killing twins has been very common throughout human history, as reviewed by Schapera [33], Granzberg [34], and Ball [35]. As in all infanticide, the underlying cause was insufficient resources. Newborns classified as 'bad birth' were those who, especially in nomadic peoples, could not be successfully reared. Breastfeeding two infants for years was virtually impossible for a woman who was also expected to gather food or work in the fields. The economic perspective of twin infanticide was elaborated upon by Marroquin [36], and Harris described sociocultural justifications [5]. Usually, twins (and their mother) were regarded as unclean. With advancing agriculture, peoples formed settlements and the conditions for raising twins improved. Nevertheless, in rural Finland of 1769–1850, the survival of twins up to age 15 (34% versus 71% in singletons) was so low that

mothers of twins remained less reproductive [37]. Among American natives, twin infanticide was the rule rather than the exception. In 1649, the Archbishop of Lima (Peru), Pedro de Villa Gomez, admonished the vicars in a letter of exhortation to examine 'to what *huaca* [idol] do they [Indians] offer twins, which they call *Chuchu*, and what dead bodies of *Chuchus* they have in their houses' [38]. From an expedition to the Orinoco Indians (Venezuela) in 1800, Alexander von Humboldt listed several reasons for the abomination of multiple birth [39]: 'If the infants are twins, bizarre prejudices and fixed ideas of convention and family honor demand that they be killed. To bring twins into the world means to expose oneself to public ridicule, to resemble rats, opossums, the lowest animals, who bring forth a great number of young at one time. Even more: two infants born during the same delivery cannot belong to the same father.' The Tepehuan of Mexico [40], Birmin-Kuskusmin of Papua New Guinea [41], Australian Aborigines [35], and many other societies killed multiples. As late as 1975, twin infanticide was common among the Ayoreo of Bolivia and Paraguay [42]: named *garaja*, twin birth was considered appropriate for animals but not for humans.

Some African tribes who practised twin infanticide up to the mid-19th century are listed in **Table 4.1.1**. Reports by travellers (often exploiters and racists) and missionaries (often paternalists and racists) must be regarded with caution. Dutch physician Olfert Dapper was not in Africa himself, but evaluated reports of Jesuit missionaries from many African states. Reported from Benin in 1670, he wrote

Table 4.1.1 Abomination of twins or their mothers in pre-industrial Africa up to the middle of the 19th century. Examples of twin infanticide from sub-Saharan cultures, listed from north to south

Peoples/region	Abominated	Religious reasoning	Rituals/counter-measures	Reference
Amhara: Ethiopia	Mother	'The mother of twins, because of what she carries on her back, she dies.'		[34]
Kedjom/Oku: Northeast Cameroun	Both twins, or 'single twin'	Connection with a discontented ancestor, twin has mercurial and mischievous personality, brings misfortune to family	Lifelong medication for twins to render them less vulnerable	[46]
Agotime: Togo, Ghana		'Fetish children', whose properties must be adapted for the community's good	Wooden effigy of deceased twin carried by the mother	[35]
Yoruba/Oyo/Ekiki: Southwest Nigeria	Secondborn or weaker twin 'went to Lagos'	Twins believed to be spiritual beings with great powers, stemming from the thundergod *Orisha* or from infidelity. Today twins are revered	*Ere Ibeji* statuettes, ritually washed, carried by mother until surviving twin matured. At feasts, statuettes were dressed and decorated with cowries, carried during dance	[47–50]
Ibo/Ibibio/Efik: South Nigeria	Both twins and mother	One of twins begotten by devil, impossible to tell which, elicits wrath of earth-god Ani, brings misfortune to family	Twins thrown into bush or river. Mary Slessor campaign 1876; Mary Elms twin house in Onitsha 1910	[36, 51–53]
Ndembu/Tabwa: DR Congo, Zambia	Both twins	Twinship considered animal-like, simultaneously a blessing and misfortune	Wooden effigy given to surviving twin to prevent loneliness. Ritual *Wubwang'u* to remove dangerous contagion	[54–56]
Tshokwe/M'bali: Angola	Both twins	Twinship considered a disaster for the whole country	*Tsilela* statuette of deceased twin to be carried by surviving twin	[57]
Makalanga/Tonga: Zimbabwe	Both twins	Twins considered *malweza* (wretched); if allowed to live, father was believed to die	Twins destroyed and buried in a pot unless born in family with a series of multiple births	[33, 58]
Dobe !Kung: Kalahari, Botswana	Male if opposite, both if same sex	God Prishiboro; no distinction between infanticide and natural death	One twin buried alive immediately after birth	[33, 59]
Tswana: Botswana, South Africa	Female if opposite, weaker if same sex	Twins considered a monstrosity, birth kept hidden by the parents	Strangled at birth, dead twin buried in clothes of surviving twin	[33, 60]
Zulu: South Africa	Smaller twin; mother if she had twins repeatedly	Twins believed to be born to disgraceful family; considered barely human, unpredictable, and deceitful	Suffocation; no name given to surviving twin, who was considered dangerous and never beaten	[33, 61]
Khoikhoi: South Africa	Female twins, or weaker twin	Family too poor to raise female twins	Exposing the twin(s) on the bough of a tree or among the bushes	[44]

[43]: 'No twins are ever found; but they are born there as well as elsewhere, for it is suspected that either of them is choked by the midwife, as giving birth to twins is considered a dishonor in the country, for they firmly believe that one man cannot be the father of two children at the same time.' Peter Kolb, astronomer and meteorologist, lived in Kapstad from 1705 to 1713, reporting that the Khoisan usually spared male twins [44]: 'But if the twins are girls and parents are poor, their Poverty is their Plea for exposing or making away of one of 'em … they carry the babe a considerable distance from the *Kraal*, and look for a Hole in the earth … where they lay the baby alive … if they find not such a Sepulchre presently, they tie the Babe, stretch'd on his back, to a nether Bough of the next Tree, and leave it to starve or be devour'd by Birds or Beasts of Prey' (Fig. 4.1.3). Hugh Crow, captain of a slave trading ship which sailed from Liverpool to Bonny/Nigeria eight times from 1798 to 1808 reported [45]: 'A horrid custom prevails amongst these people in the case of a woman happening to be the mother of more than one child at a birth. Both herself and her offspring are immediately put to death.'

In Nigeria with its many multiples, missionaries established peculiar twin cities and foundling homes to save these infants [51, 52]. A unique art form evolved around twins and their death: the Yoruba carved *Ere-Ibeji* figures that were revered in the house and carried at ritual dances, to escape the revenge of the deceased. The Tabwa produced wooden dolls representing the deceased to console the surviving co-twin (Fig. 4.1.4). The abomination of twins was not always the same in one area: in Uganda, twins were considered a treasured gift from God, and represented great bounty [62]. Parents enjoyed privileges, changed their own names, and named firstborn girls *Babirye*, firstborn boys *Waswa*; secondborn girls were named *Nakato* and boys *Kato*. Fixed names for twins were common in many societies. The Yoruba named the firstborn *Taiwo* and the secondborn *Kehinde*. With the advent of Christian missionaries and legislation by colonial governments, infanticide fell from grace and now twins were revered and the old rites adapted [63].

Twin research

In 1671, Cosme Viardel, court surgeon in Paris, described a difference in the membranes enveloping twins [64]: 'When they are of the same sex, they share the placenta, but each has its own umbilical cord. When they are of different sex, they are always separated by several membranes, ensuring the rules of chastity.' René de Graaf detected the follicle in 1672, but believed it to be the oocyte [65]. Human reproduction remained elusive until the microscope was used by the Estonian researcher Karl-Ernst von Baer who identified the oocyte in 1827 [66]. Francis Galton compared the histories of 35 very similar twin pairs to 20 pairs with sharply contrasting characteristics in 1876 [67] and concluded: 'There is no escape from the conclusion that nature prevails enormously over nurture

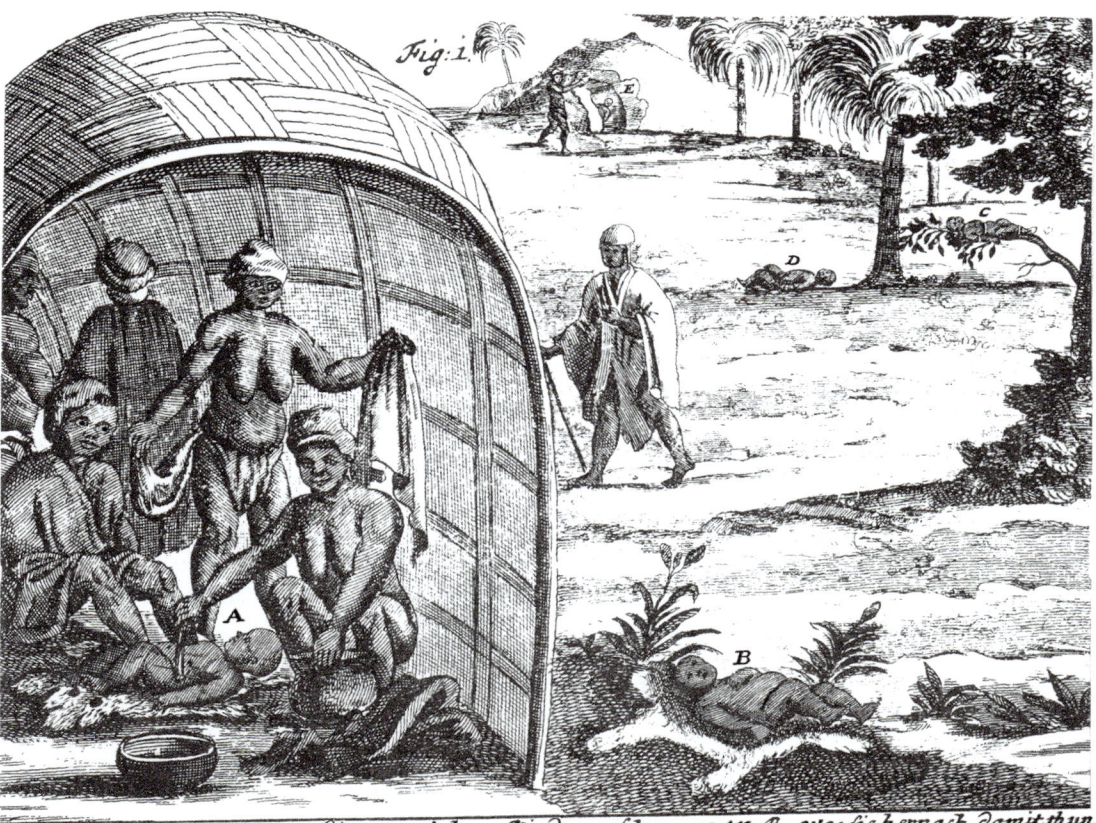

Fig. 4.1.3 Peter Kolb's depiction of Khoisan customs of twin infanticide, 1719 [44]. The baby is washed with cow manure (A) and dried on a pelt (B). Female twins are abandoned, tied to a tree (C), exposed in the field (D), or buried alive (E).

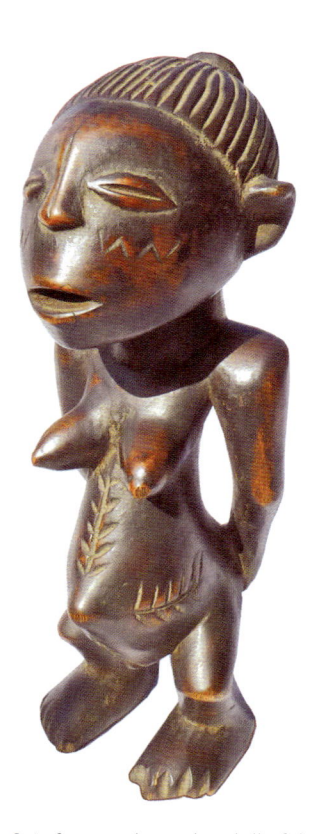

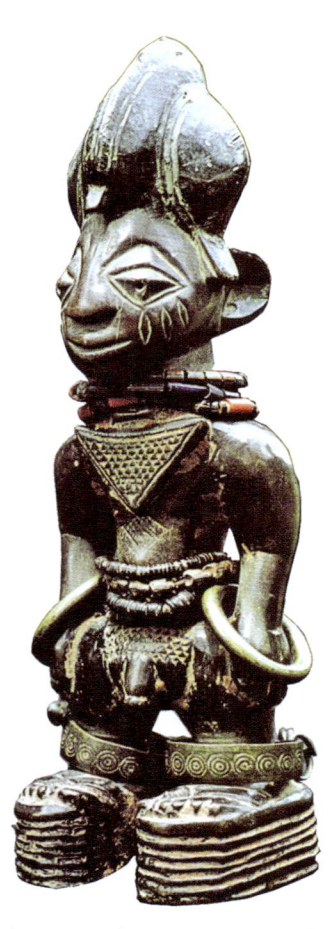

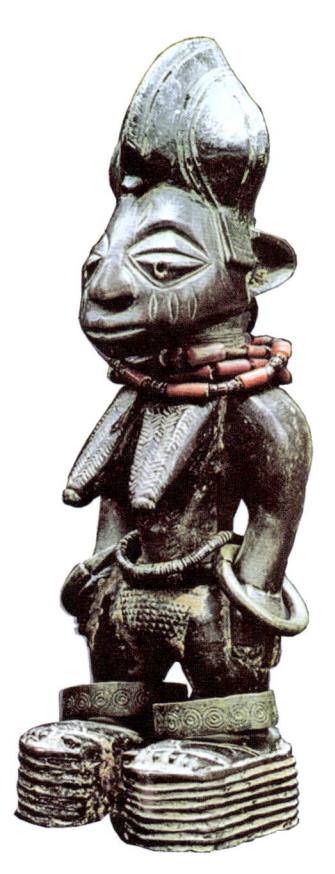

Fig. 4.1.4 Left: carved wooden doll of deceased female twin given to the surviving co-twin by the Tabwa (19th century c.e.), Lake Tanganijka, Democratic Republic of the Congo. Centre and right: Ere Ibeji figures of the Yoruba tribe, Nigeria, made to commemorate deceased twins.

when the differences of nurture do not exceed what is commonly to be found among persons of the same rank and in the same country.' Galton's paper paved the way towards social Darwinism and eugenics in the early 20th century. Among the atrocities committed by German physicians in the concentration camps during the Nazi regime, their experiments with twin children are among the most heinous crimes [68, 69]. The history of modern twin research was reviewed by Benirschke 1973 [70]. Wilhelm Weinberg combined clinical observation with population statistics and demonstrated in 1901 that the dizygotic, but not monozygotic twinning tendency is inherited [71]. In the Birmingham twin survey of 1968, Hugh Cameron studied various methods of zygosity determination in 668 pairs of twins [72]: 35% were known to be dizygotic because they were of different sex, 20% were known to be monozygotic because they had a monochorionic placenta. Of the remaining 45% who underwent genotyping, 37% proved to be dizygotic and 8% monozygotic. Despite more refined blood typing, zygosity determination remained difficult, limiting investigation of the infants' development more exactly.

Conclusion

Representing the exceptional in reproduction, twins were met with ambivalence in many cultures. As the origin of twinning was unknown well into the 19th century, irrational arguments were rooted in taboos: the infants were believed to be unnatural, monstrous, portending evil, conceived under inappropriate circumstances. Heteropaternal superfecundation was assumed, meaning the involvement of two fathers and thus maternal adultery. Parental and societal reactions towards twins reveal a wide spectrum of reactions, extending from rejection and infanticide to ambivalence and acceptance, and even to veneration and deification. Pre-industrial societies in which infants were breastfed and continuously carried by their mother for 2 years could scarcely handle frail infants. From an economic point of view, twins were not killed because they were twins, but because several factors accumulated in them that diminished the chances for survival: twin infanticide was an adaptive strategy that ultimately enhanced reproductive success.

REFERENCES

1. Leichty E: The omen series Summa Izbu. In: A. Leo Oppenheim: Texts from cuneiform sources. Locust Valley, NY: Augustin, 1970: Vol. **4**, p. 39.
2. Nylander PPS: Serum levels of gonadotrophins in relation to multiple pregnancy in Nigeria. J Obstet Gynecol 1973;**80**:651–3.
3. Milham S: Pituitary gonadotrophin and dizygotic twinning. Lancet 1964;**284**:566.

4. Evans MI, Britt DW: Multifetal pregnancy reduction: evolution of the ethical arguments. Semin Reprod Med 2010;**28**:295–302.
5. Harris JR: Boanerges. Cambridge: Cambridge University Press, 1913: p. 161, 169.
6. Harris JR: The cult of the heavenly twins. Cambridge: Cambridge University Press, 1906.
7. Harris JR: The dioscuri in the Christian legends. London: Clay, 1903.
8. Gedda L: Twins in history and science. Springfield, IL: Thomas, 1961.
9. Baines J: Egyptian twins. Orientalia 1985;**54**:461–82.
10. Inwood B: The poem of Empedocles. Toronto: University of Toronto Press, 1992: p. 185.
11. Hippocrates: De natura pueri. Translated and edited by: Anutius Foesius. Francofurti: Wecheli, 1596: p. 205.
12. Hippocrates: Aphorisms. Loeb Classical Library. Cambridge MA: Heinemann/Harvard University Press, 1959: Vol. **4**, p. 167.
13. Aristotle: Generation of animals. Loeb Classical Library. Edited by: G. P. Goold. Cambridge, MA: Harvard University Press, 1942: p. 772 b 1–10.
14. Plinius the Elder: Natural history. Translated by: Philemon Holland. London: Wernerian Club, 1847: Vol. **1**, p. 193–9.
15. Censorinus: Liber de die natali (238 C.E.). Hamburg: Hering, 1614: Vol. **6**, p. 9–10.
16. Hippocrates: De superfetatione. Loeb Classical Library 509. Cambridge MA: Harvard University Press, 1923–2010: Vol. **9**, p. L8, 476–508, 313–54.
17. Hesiod: Shield of Heracles. In: The Homeric hymns and Homerica. Cambridge MA: Heinemann/Harvard University Press, 1914: verse 48–56.
18. Augustinus of Hippo A: De Civitate Dei Liber V. In: Corpus Christianorum Series Latina, Vol. 47. Turnholti: Typographi Brepols, 1955: Vol. **5**, p. 133.
19. Savonarola JM: Practica (de aegritudinibus). Venetiae: Müllerheim, 1560: Vol. Tractatus VI, Fol 264v.
20. Baudelocque JL: L'art des accouchemens. Nouvelle édition. 2. ed. Paris: Desprez & Méquignon, 1789: Vol. **2**, p. 640.
21. Archer J: Facts illustrating a disease peculiar to the female children of Negro Slaves. Medical Repository of Original Essays and Intelligence 1810;**1**:319–23.
22. Terasaki PI, Gjertson D, Bernoco D, et al.: Twins with two different fathers identified by HLA. N Engl J Med 1978;**299**:590–2.
23. Van der Waerden BL: History of the Zodiac. Arch Orientforsch 1952;**16**:216–30.
24. Lambert WG: Lugalirra and Meslamtaea. In: Reallexikon der Assyriologie und vorderasiatischen Archäologie. Berlin: de Gruyter, 1990: Vol. **7**, p. 143–5.
25. Griffith RTH: The hymns of the Rigveda. 5. ed. Varanasi: Chowkhamba Sanskrit Series Office, 1971: Vol. **1**, p. 542–5.
26. Merrill WL, Ladd EJ, Ferguson TJ: The return of the Ahayu'da. Curr Anthropol 1993;**34**:523–67.
27. Wunsch C: Findelkinder und Adoption nach neubabylonischen Quellen. Arch Orientforsch 2001;**50**:174–244.
28. Gaillard AH: Recherches administratives, statistiques et morales sur les enfants trouvés. Paris: Leclerc, 1837.
29. Ilogu E: Christianity and Igbo culture. Leiden: Brill, 1974: p. 63–4.
30. Yerushalmy J, Sheerer SE: Studies on twins. II. On the early mortality of like-sexed and unlike-sexed twins. Hum Biol 1940;**12**:247–63.
31. Layde PM, Erickson JD, Falek A, McCarthy BJ: Congenital malformations in twins. Am J Hum Gen 1980;**32**:69–78.
32. Sternberg L: Der antike Zwillingskult im Lichte der Ethnologie. Zeitschr Ethnol 1929;**61**:152–200.
33. Schapera J: Customs relating to twins in South Africa. J Roy Afr Soc 1927;**26**:117–37.
34. Granzberg G: Twin infanticide. Ethos 1973;**1**:405–12.
35. Ball HL, Hill CM: Reevaluating 'twin infanticide'. Curr Anthropol 1996;**37**:856–63.
36. Marroquin A, Haight C: Twin-killing in some traditional societies. J Bioecon 2017;**19**:261–79.
37. Haukioja E, Lemmetyinen R, Pikkola M: Why are twins so rare in Homo sapiens? Am Nat 1989;**133**:572–7.
38. Rivero ME, Tschudi JJ: Peruvian antiquities. New York: Putnam, 1853: p. 173–7.
39. Humboldt A: Voyage aux régions équinoxiales du nouveau continent. Paris: Maze, 1819: Vol. **2**, p. 305.
40. Hill CM, Ball HL: Abnormal births and other 'ill omens'. Hum Nat 1996;**7**:381–401.
41. Brewis AA: Anthropological perspectives on infanticide. Arizona Anthropol 1992;**8**:103–19.
42. Pérez Diez AA, Salzano FM: Evolutionary implications of the ethnography and demography of Ayoreo Indians. J Hum Evol 1978;**7**:253–68.
43. Dapper O: Umbständliche und Eigentliche Beschreibung von Africa, und denen dazu gehörigen Königreichen und Landschaften. Amsterdam: Meurs, 1670: p. 488.
44. Kolb P: Vollständige Beschreibung des Africanischen Vorgebürges der Guten Hoffnung. Nürnberg: Monath, 1719: p. 442–7.
45. Crow H: Descriptive sketches of the western coast of Africa, particularly of Bonny. London: Longman, 1830: p. 238–9.
46. Diduk S: Twins, ancestors and socio-economic change in Kedjom society. Man 1993;**28**:551–71.
47. Leroy F, Olaleye-Oruene T, Koeppen-Schomerus G, Bryan E: Yoruba customs and beliefs pertaining to twins. Twin Res 2002;**5**:132–6.
48. Thompson RF: Black gods and kings. Bloomington, IN: UCLA, Indiana University Press, 1971.
49. Oruene TO: Cultic powers of Yoruba twins. Acta Genet Med Gemellol 1983;**32**:221–8.
50. Houlberg M: Ibeji images of the Yoruba. Afr Arts 1973;**7**:20–7, 91–2.
51. Bastian M: The demon superstition: abominable twins and mission culture in Onitsha history. Ethnology 2001;**40**:13–27.
52. Buchan J: The expendable Mary Slessor. 1. ed. Edinburgh: St Andrew Press, 1980: p. 65, 76.
53. Talbot PA: Women's mysteries of a primitive people. 1. ed. London: Cass, 1968: p. 23–38.
54. Corney G: Mythology and customs associated with twins. In: MacGillivray I: Human multiple reproduction. London: Saunders, 1975: p. 1–15.
55. Turner VW: Paradoxes of twinship in Ndembu ritual. In: Turner VW: The ritual process: structure and anti-structure. London: Routledge & Kegan Paul, 1969: p. 44–93.
56. Hartland ES: Twins. In: Hastings J: Encyclopaedia of religion and ethics. Edinburgh: Clark, 1921: Vol. **12**, p. 491.

57. Delaunay V: Improving knowledge on child abandonment and care in Africa. Afr Popul Stud 2011;**25**:73–94.
58. Colson E: Marriage and the family among the Plateau Tonga of Northern Rhodesia. Manchester: Manchester University Press, 1958: p. 160–5.
59. Howell N: Demography of the Dobe !Kung. New York: Academic Press, 1979: p. 120.
60. Comaroff J, Comaroff J: Of revelation and revolution. Chicago, IL: University of Chicago Press, 1991: Vol. **1**, p. 144–5.
61. Kuper A: South Africa and the anthropologist. London: Routledge and Kegan Paul, 1987: p. 191.
62. Salter Ainsworth MD: Infancy in Uganda. Baltimore, MD: Johns Hopkins Press, 1967: p. 154.
63. Ekpunobi E, Ezeaku I: Socio-philosophical perspective of African traditional religion. Enugu: New Age Publishers, 1990.
64. Viardel C: Anmerckungen von der weiblichen Geburt (1st French ed. 1671). Franckfurt: Zubrodt, 1676: p. 20.
65. Graaf Rd: De mulierum organis generationi inservientibus. Lugduni Batavorum: Off. Hackiana, 1672: p. cap. 12.
66. von Baer KE: De ovi mammalium et hominis genesi. Leipzig: Voss, 1827: p. 39–40.
67. Galton F: The history of twins as a criterion of the relative powers of nature and nurture. J Anthrop Inst Great Brit 1876;**5**: 391–406.
68. Müller-Hill B: The blood from Auschwitz and the silence of the scholars. Hist Phil Life Sci 1999;**21**:331–65.
69. Segal NL: The twin children of Auschwitz-Birkenau: conference on Nazi medicine. Twin Res Hum Genet 2013;**16**:751–4.
70. Benirschke K, Kim CK: Multiple pregnancy. N Engl J Med 1973;**288**:1276–84; 1329–36.
71. Weinberg W: Beiträge zur Physiologie und Pathologie der Mehrlingsgeburten beim Menschen. Pflügers Arch Physiol 1901;**88**:346–430.
72. Cameron AH: The Birmingham twin survey. Proc R Soc Med 1968;**61**:229–34.

4.2 Fertility and fatality
Higher-order multiples

Introduction

Higher-grade multiples are defined as three or more infants in a single pregnancy. Today well known to every neonatologist, they were rare for most of human history and most infants died, usually due to prematurity or birth asphyxia. The topic was reviewed by Gould and Pyle [1] and a catalogue of quadruplets was published by Clay [2]. The aim of this chapter is to explain the recent increase in both the frequency and survival rate of higher-order multiples in countries with advanced health systems, and to shed light on the problems therein.

Frequency

Mathematical models to determine the rate of multiples were developed by Veith in 1855 [3] and Wappäus in 1859 [4], but were frequently ascribed to the Leipzig pathologist Dionys Hellin, who published his hypothesis in 1895 [5]: when twins occurred once in 89 births, then triplets occurred once in 89^2 and quadruplets once in 89^3 births. More reliable algorithms were developed by Zeleny in 1921 [6] and Guttmacher in 1953 [7], but could not heal the difficulty that polyzygosity, not monozygosity, is genetically regulated and age dependent. In addition to genetic regulation, nutritionally stimulated ovulation (by eating yams roots) has been suggested to explain Nigeria's high rate of multiples [8]. Even before the boom in reproductive medicine, the rate of triplets increased from 0.9 per 10,000 in 1970 to 4.5 per 10,000 in 1990 in the Netherlands [9], for the most part due to increasing maternal age. In England and Wales, the triplet rate rose from 1.02 to 2.28 per 10,000, and the quadruplet rate from 0.018 to 0.17 per 10,000 [2]. With advancing childbearing age and more frequent infertility treatments, the incidence of triplets and higher-order births in the US increased fivefold from 3.7 per 10,000 live births in 1980 to 19.4 per 10,000 live births in 1998 [10, 11].

Antique descriptions and thoughts on causes

In Babylonia, higher-grade multiples were considered a bad omen, as specified in the Shumma Izbu (ca. 1500 B.C.E.) [12]: 'If a woman gives birth to triplets—the owner of the house will die ... If ... to four boys and they live—an enemy will surround and seize the city ... If ... to four boys, and they die—an enemy will surround the city, but will not seize it ... If ... to four [children], two boys [and] two girls—ravaging by the enemy; hard times will seize the land.'

Aristotle believed fertility was greater in warm climates [13]: 'For although women mostly, and among most peoples, bear single children, frequently and in many places they have twins, as indeed in Egypt. They even bear three or four, especially in certain places as we have said before. The greatest number at a birth is five: This has already been seen to happen in several cases.'

Graeco-Roman authors assumed heteropaternal superfecundation as the cause of multiple pregnancy, which always implied maternal adultery [14]. The elder Pliny [24–79 C.E.] explained that higher-grade multiples were disliked [15]: 'About the latter end of the Reign of Divus Augustus, a Woman at Ostia named Fausta, of ordinary Rank, was delivered of two Boys and as many Girls; but this was a Portent beyond doubt of the Famine that ensued.'

Polyovulation: child-rich mothers

Multiple births clustered in certain women and numerous children usually meant lifelong poverty. A quadruplet birth was depicted in 1450 by a south-German painter (Fig. 4.2.1). The saint intervening in this picture suggests that the quadruplets may have survived. Long lists of higher-grade multiples began to be published when the printing press became available. Some of the better documented cases are described as follows.

In 1498, the council of Bönnigheim (near Heilbronn) drafted a document testifying that Barbara Schmotzer brought forth 53 infants in 29 pregnancies within 30 years [16]. Among them were five times twins, four times triplets, once sixtuplets, and once septuplets. None of them survived over 7 years. An altarpiece in the St. Cyriak church (Fig. 4.2.2) illustrates the case: 'Barbara Schmotzer, housewife of Adam Stratzmann, with her 15 daughters, and Adam Stratzmann with his 38 legitimate sons.' The inscription continues: 'Walk about all lands and kingdoms and read all histories: Among all miraculous women you will not find any who bore as many infants ... We will hardly see such a woman again.' Several sources concerning Barbara Schmotzer's births were compiled by Holländer [17] and Lauritzen [18].

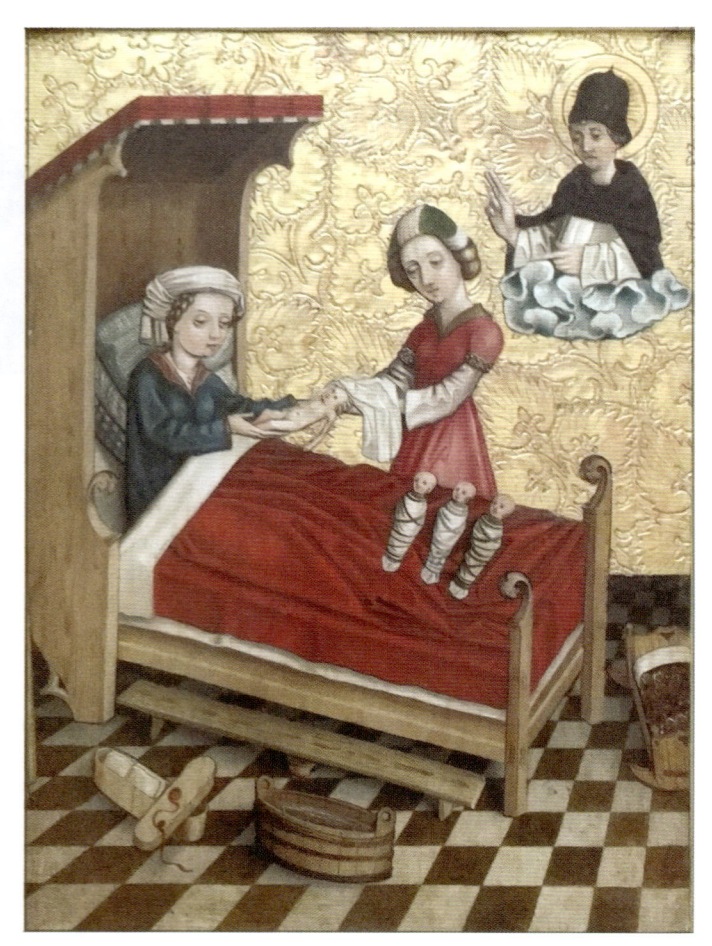

Fig. 4.2.1 Quadruplets of Lichtenstein 1450, with the intervention of a saint.
Lichtenstein Castle, Herzog von Urach, with permission.

a quintuplet birth in the *Philosophical Transactions* [24]: 'Margaret Waddington, a poor woman of the township of Lower Darwin in Lancashire ... at the end of the first month, she became lame, complained of considerable pains in her loins, and the enlargement of her body was so remarkably rapid, that she was judged by her neighbors to be almost half gone with child ... By the 24th of April, 1786, when being supposed to have arrived at the twentieth week she was seized with labor pains ... the five children were all females, their length ranging from 20 to 23 cm ... All five died within a short time.'

On 21 September 1836, the birth of triplets was recorded at 29 weeks' gestation in the Lying-In Hospital of St. Petersburg [25]. The girls weighed 1220, 1100, and 856 g, and died at 5–8 hours of age. But their treatment is remarkable as modern equipment has been employed: the birth was monitored by stethoscope, invented in Paris 15 years before, the infants were cared for in a heated incubator called 'Rühl-cradle,' invented 7 years before, and placental perfusion was studied with dyed solutions.

In 1919, Charles Davenport reported the case of a woman from Cleveland, who in ten pregnancies from 1902 to 1913 had 30 infants: three times twins, four times triplets, and three times quadruplets, and concluded 'the tendency to multiple births is hereditary' [26]. In 1926, Kristine Bonnevie published a pedigree study about 12,034 births (466 of them twins) in remote Norway and developed the theory of a single recessive factor responsible for dizygotic twinning [27]. Among her cases was a woman who delivered eight pairs of twins, with no multiples in the pedigree, 'the first appearance of an anomaly in the ovary causing double ovulations'. In 1938, Greulich described a woman who had six consecutive pairs of fraternal twins and concluded 'the presence of polyovular follicles would suggest that the observed twinning is attributable to some ovarian peculiarity and is therefore an exclusively maternal attribute' [28]. Polyovulation seems to result from overproduction of gonadotropins [29]. Its molecular basis has not been clarified.

Spontaneous and surviving cases

Before reproductive medicine and neonatology evolved, higher-grade multiples rarely survived the first year of life. Those who did were celebrated in newspapers or broadsheets. The following are some famous examples.

A set of quadruplets who survived the first year of life were born to the clothworker Sch. in Crimmitzschau (Saxony) in May 1847. Birth weight and gestational age are unknown, the placentas were fused [30]. In Switzerland, the tetrazygotic Gehri quadruplets, two boys and two girls, were born in September 1880 with birthweights between 1330 and 2080 g [31]. They all survived and developed normally; when they were 60 years old, Otto Schlaginhaufen did extensive genealogical and anthropometrical research on them and their family [32] and detected an accumulation of 15 twin births among 82 births. In October 1929, the Perricone quadruplets were born in Beaumont (Texas), with birth weights ranging from 1135 to 1590 g. Dermatoglyphic studies proved they were tetrazygotic [33]. Their childhood development was normal.

In May 1934, the Dionne quintuplets, the most famous of all multiples, were born in rural Callander, Ontario, at 32 weeks of gestation. Their combined weight on the second day of life was 6067 g, giving an average birth weight of 1200 g. On day 3, incubators were

In 1507, Francesco Pico della Mirandola described Antonia from Modena, who 'brought forth a total of 40 infants until she was forty years of age, often triplets or quadruplets in one birth' [19]. The same author published another famous case [19]: 'A German woman named Dorothea [Kristels Losels from Rotenpuch, Tyrolia] gave birth to 20 children in two deliveries, once 9 and once 11. The locals told me (as I saw her myself neither during pregnancy nor at birth) that she carried the heavy weight of her belly, hanging down to her knees, with the help of a girdle fixed at her neck and shoulders. I am not telling stories but have serious witnesses, also from Italy.' The same birth was reported more extensively in Deichsler's Nuremberg Chronicle for 1488–1506 [20], and was cited and retrospectively illustrated by Conrad Lycosthenes in 1557 [21] and by Ambroise Paré in 1573 (**Fig. 4.2.3**). Ambroise Paré reported from Seaux 'a familie and noble hous ... the wife of the Lord of Maldemeure, the first year shee was married brought forth twins, the second year shee had three children, the third year four, the fourth year five, the fifth year six, and of that birth shee died' [22].

The septuplets of Hameln were born to Anna Breyers on 9 January 1600 and are commemorated on a famous epitaph. In 1656, Pierre Borel described the birth of octuplets by the noblewoman D. Darre from Castres (Tarn), and of surviving quadruplets by a Mrs Fricov from Bédarieux (Hérault) [23]. In 1787, Maxwell Gartshore published

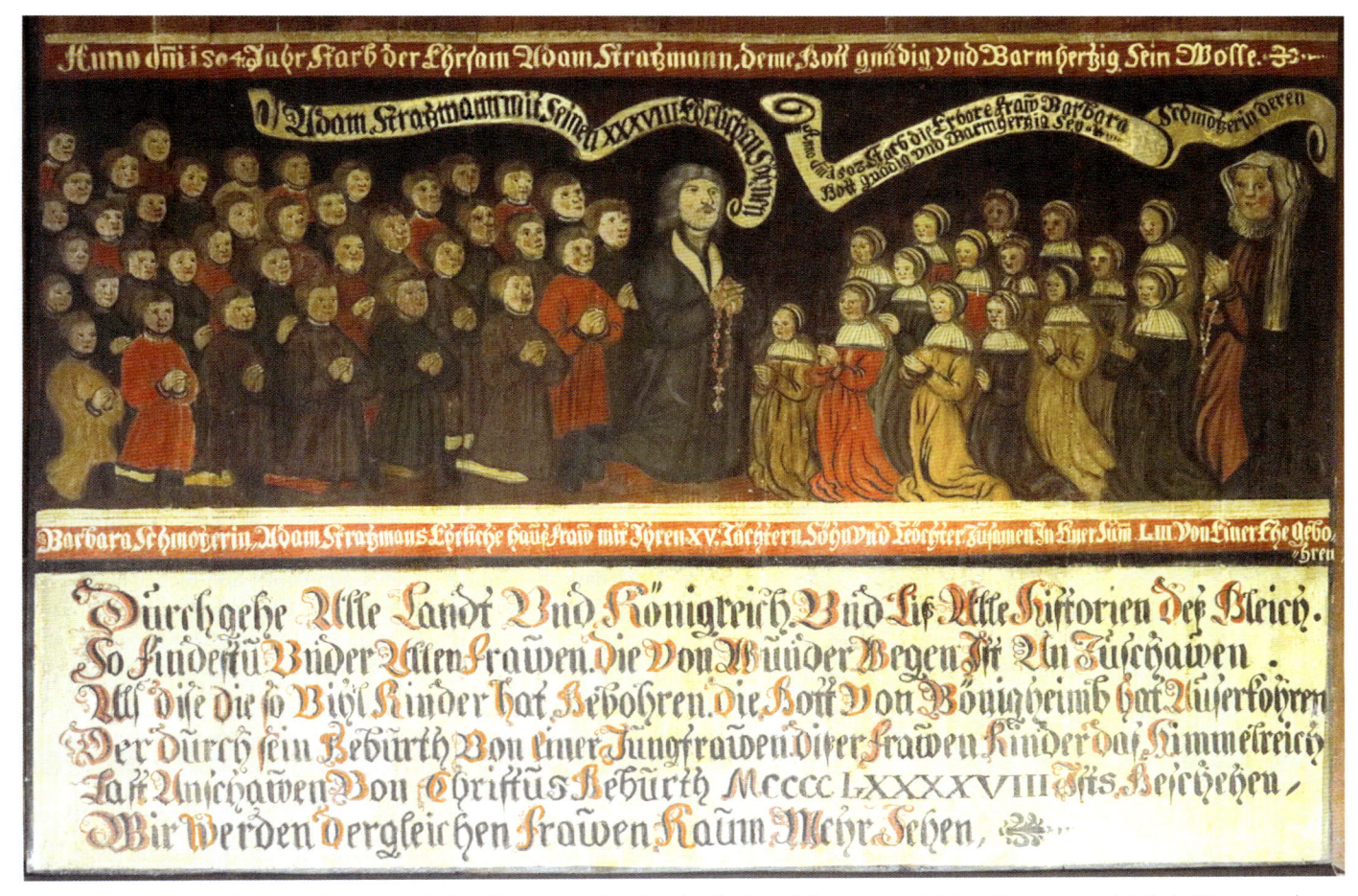

Fig. 4.2.2 Altarpiece of 1505 in the St. Cyriak church, Bönnigheim, showing Barbara Schmotzer and Adam Stratzmann with their 38 sons and 15 daughters [18]. The infants, none of whom reached age 7 years and of whom 19 were not even baptized, are depicted as if they were adults. See text for details.

Evangelische Gemeinde Bönnigheim, with permission.

brought from Chicago, as were cylinders with 95% oxygen and 5% carbon dioxide, at that time the usual tools in caring for preterm infants [34]. Their obstetrician Alan Roy Dafoe wrote [35]: 'The publicity in connection with the case has been a serious problem.' This, however, did not hinder him from accepting guardianship for the five girls and from taking advantage of their publicity to establish the 'Dafoe Hospital and Nursery' when the government declared the children wards of the state, taking the guardianship away from the parents for 9 years. Meanwhile, the 'hospital' was transformed to 'Quintland', a kind of circus where the girls were exposed to the gawping public. Films were produced in Hollywood, and dozens of researchers studied the quintuplets, as they were monozygotic. In 1997, the surviving three sisters wrote in an open letter [36] to the parents of the McCoughey septuplets: 'Multiple births should not be confused with entertainment, nor should they be an opportunity to sell products … Our lives have been ruined by the exploitation we suffered … We were displayed as a curiosity three times a day for millions of tourists.'

In July 1944, the Diligenti quintuplets were born in Buenos Aires, Argentina, at 40 weeks' gestation, three girls and two boys whose birthweight ranged from 1150 to 1500 g. The infants were 'wrapped in cotton wool and kept warm with stove heat and hot water bags. Incubator, oxygen, and carbon dioxide were never used' [37]. These quintuplets grew up normally and healthy, and their father managed to shield them from the circus-like publicity the Dionne girls had experienced 9 years earlier.

In July 1963, the Fischer quintuplets were born at 32 weeks' gestation in Aberdeen, South Dakota. Four girls and one boy, with birth weight ranging from 1020 to 1590 g, the infants were cared for in incubators and survived without complications [38].

Understanding ovulation

Endocrine functions were not understood before the 20th century. Galen (200 C.E.) believed the pituitary gland acted as a funnel leading mucus produced by the brain into the nose [39]. As late as 1665, Conrad Schneider found that such secretions are produced by the nasal mucosa [40] but still in 1842, François Magendie believed the pituitary to be a sort of lymph gland interposed in the fluid pathway: 'The hydrocephalus is frequently caused by the pituitary gland' [41]. In 1672, René de Graaf described the follicle and is believed to have identified the ovum [42]. That, however, was detected by Estonian (then Russian) scientist Karl Ernst von Baer in

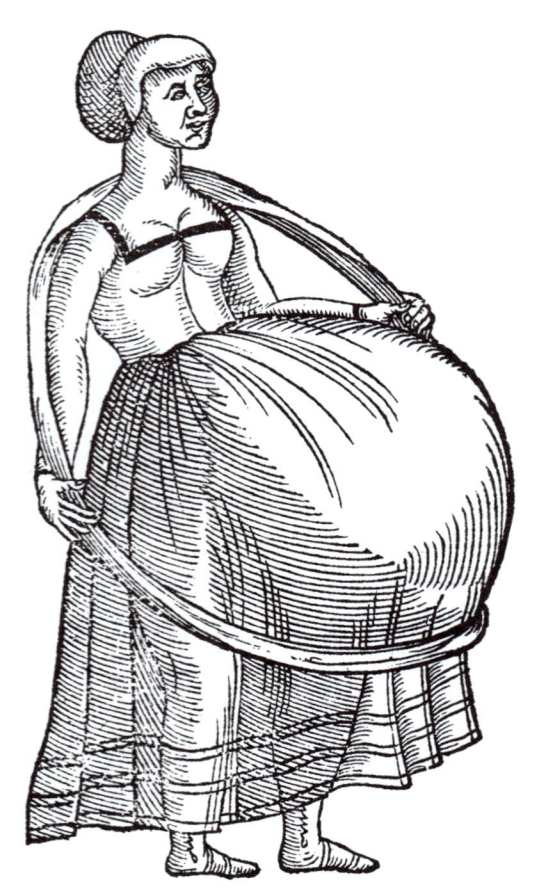

Fig. 4.2.3 'Dorothy great with many chylde.' Pico de la Mirandola's case of 1499 [19], illustrated by Ambroise Paré in 1573 [22]. See text for details.

1827 [43]. Pituitary gonadotropin was described by Philip Smith in 1926 [44], and in 1928 Zondek and Aschheim discovered that it is the pituitary hormone that stimulates the ovarian follicle [45].

Side effect of assisted reproduction techniques

In 1944, Rock and Menkin succeeded in fertilizing human eggs *in vitro* [46]. Louise Brown, the first baby born through *in vitro* fertilization, was born in July 1978 [47]. Intracytoplasmic sperm injection followed in 1992. In 2010, after 4 million infants were born following *in vitro* fertilization, Robert Edwards was awarded the Nobel Prize in Physiology or Medicine; his co-worker Patrick Steptoe had died in 1988. From 1958, Carl Axel Gemzell of Uppsala treated infertile women with gonadotropin obtained from cadaver hypophyses and reported in 1966 that of 43 women delivered, 14 had twins and nine triplets or more [48]. In 1964 Milham hypothesized [29] that dizygotic twinning might result from excess maternal gonadotropin activity. In 1966, Liggins and Ibbertson reported a 'successful quintuplet pregnancy following treatment with human pituitary gonadotrophin' [49] and in the era of neonatal intensive care, higher-grade multiples who all survived became more frequent. In 1974, Gutowitz reported on the surviving Rosenkowitz sextuplets from Kapstadt after treatment with human gonadotropin [50]. In 1997, Suvalsky and colleagues reported the survival of the McCaughey septuplets from Des Moines, Iowa [51], after treatment with Metrodin. In January 2009 the Suleman octuplets were born in Bellflower, California, result of a transfer of 12 embryos to an unmarried mother who already had six children born through *in vitro* fertilization. The case made international headlines and raised multiple ethical questions later detailed by Rosenthal [52]. The gynaecologist Kamrava, who had sequentially implanted 59 embryos in that woman, lost his licence. The Suleman case marked the limit of acceptance by society, even in the US, and revealed that ethical issues in reproductive medicine must be legally regulated. High-grade multiples are burdened with all the problems of preterm infants—surfactant deficiency, brain haemorrhage, necrotizing enterocolitis, retinopathy, and their sequelae. Moreover, they often suffer malformations: after an evaluation of Australian registries in 2002, Michèle Hansen and colleagues reported [53] that '8.6 % of infants conceived via intracytoplasmatic sperm injection, and 9.0 % of those conceived through in vitro fertilization had a major birth defect diagnosed by one year of age, as compared with 4.2 % naturally conceived infants'. Nowadays the number of fetuses in triplet and higher-order pregnancies is usually reduced operatively [54], with better neonatal outcomes in terms of immaturity, morbidity, and neurodevelopmental disability, but with a 7% risk of pregnancy loss [55].

Conclusion

The Dionne and Suleman multiples illustrate a remarkable phenomenon not unusual in higher-grade multiples and in conjoined twins: they were considered public property. Physicians compromised medical confidentiality; the press hastened to sell the sensation, courts stepped in to take away custody, and governments and researchers dared to exploit the infants. The recent surge in multiple births sheds light on a changing view of human reproduction: children are no longer accepted as a gracious gift bestowed by God or fortune, but as a guaranteed right to be provided by medicine. With this perspective, it will become even harder for disabled infants to be accepted by their parents.

REFERENCES

1. Gould GM, Pyle WL: Anomalies and curiosities of medicine. Philadelphia, PA: Saunders, 1901: p. 144–60.
2. Clay MM: Quadruplets and higher multiple births. Oxford: Blackwell/Lippincott, 1989: p. 16.
3. Veith G: Beiträge zur geburtshülflichen Statistik. Monatsschr Geburtsk Frauenkrank 1855;**6**:101–32.
4. Wappäus JE: Allgemeine Bevölkerungsstatistik. Leipzig: Hinrich, 1859–1861: Vol. **1 and 2**.
5. Hellin D: Die Ursache der Multiparität der uniparen Tiere überhaupt und der Zwillingsschwangerschaft beim Menschen insbesondere. München: Seitz & Schauer, 1895.
6. Zeleny C: The relative number of twins and triplets. Science 1921;**53**:262–3.
7. Guttmacher AF: The incidence of multiple births in man and some of the other unipara. Obstet Gynecol 1953;**2**:22–35.
8. Hardman R: Pharmaceutical products from plant steroids. Trop Sci 1969;**11**:196–228.

9. Keith LG, Papiernik E, Keith DM, Luke B: Multiple pregnancy. New York: Parthenon, 1995: p. 151.
10. Russell RB, Petrini JR, Damus K, et al.: The changing epidemiology of multiple births in the United States. Obstet Gynecol 2003;**101**:129–35.
11. Elliott JP: High-order multiple gestations. Semin Perinatol 2005;**29**:305–11.
12. Leichty E: The omen series Summa Izbu. In: Texts from cuneiform sources. Locust Valley, NY: Augustin, 1970: Vol. **4**, p. 39.
13. Aristotle: History of animals. Loeb Classical Library 439. Cambridge, MA: Harvard University Press, 1991: Vol. **XI**, p. IX (7), 584 b, 26–34.
14. Dasen V: Multiple births in Graeco-Roman antiquity. Oxf J Archaeol 1997;**16**:49–63.
15. Plinius the Elder: Natural history. Translated by: Philemon Holland. London: Wernerian Club, 1847: Vol. **1**, p. 187, 192–9.
16. Deumling F: Protocol of Barbara Stratzmann's testimony. Hornberg: Schloßbibliothek, 1498: Inv. Nr. 78.
17. Holländer E: Wunder, Wundergeburt und Wundergestalt in Einblattdrucken. Stuttgart: Enke, 1921: p. 242–6.
18. Lauritzen C, Göretzlehner G: Die kinderreichste Frau Deutschlands. J Fertil Reprod 1999;**9**:22–33.
19. Pico della Mirandola JF: Hymni heroici tres. Mediolani: Minutianus, 1507: Fol. 25r.
20. Deichsler H: Die Chroniken der deutschen Städte vom 14. bis ins 16. Jahrhundert. Leipzig: Hirzel, 1874: Vol. **11**, p. 626–8.
21. Lycosthenes C: Wunderwerck oder Gottes unergründliches Vorbilden. Basel: Henrichus Petri, 1557: p. 10, 462.
22. Paré A: On monsters and marvels (1st ed. 1573). Chicago, IL: The University of Chicago Press, 1982: p. 23–5.
23. Borel P: Historiarum et observationum medicophysicarum centuriae IV. Paris: Jillaine & Dupuis, 1656: Cent. II, p. 143.
24. Garthshore M: A remarkable case of numerous births. Phil Trans Roy Soc Lond 1787;**77**:344–58.
25. Goedechen A: Drillinge. Zeitschr Ges Med 1840;**14**:536–46.
26. Davenport CB: A strain producing multiple births. J Hered 1919;**10**:382–4.
27. Bonnevie K, Sverdrup A: Hereditary predispositions to dizygotic twin-births in Norwegian peasant families. J Genet 1926;**16**:125–88.
28. Greulich WW: The birth of six pairs of fraternal twins to the same parents. JAMA 1938;**110**:559–63.
29. Milham S: Pituitary gonadotrophin and dizygotic twinning. Lancet 1964;**284**:566.
30. Leopold G: Eine Vierlingsgeburt. Arch Gynäkol 1871;**2**:285–8.
31. Glaser D: Ein Fall von Vierlingsgeburt. Corr Blatt Schweizer Ärzte 1881;**11**:302.
32. Schlaginhaufen O: Die Vierlingsgeschwister Gehri und ihr Verwandschaftskreis. Arch Julius Klaus Stift Vererbungsforsch Sozialanthropol Rassenhyg 1940;**15**:309–99.
33. Gardner IC, Newman HH: The alphabetical Perricone quadruplets. J Hered 1940;**31**:307–14.
34. Dafoe AR: The survival of the Dionne quintuplets. Am J Obstet Gynecol 1940;**39**:159–64.
35. Dafoe AR: The Dionne quintuplets. JAMA 1934;**103**:673–7.
36. Dionne A, Dionne C, Dionne Y: Advice from the Dionne quintuplets. Time Magazine 1997;1 December.
37. Beruti JA: Birth of the Argentine quintuplets. Semana Méd 1944;**51**:689–97.
38. Berbos JN, King BF, Janusz A: Quintuple pregnancy. Report of a case. JAMA 1964;**188**:813–6.
39. Galen: On the usefulness of the parts of the body. Ithaca, NY: Cornell University Press, 1968: Vol. **2**, p. 424–61.
40. Schneider CV: Liber primus de catarrhis. Wittenberg: Mevius, 1660: p. 149–53.
41. Magendie F: Recherches physiologiques et cliniques sur le liquide céphalo-rachidien ou cérébro-spinal. Paris: Méquignon, 1842: p. 77.
42. Graaf Rd: De mulierum organis generationi inservientibus. Lugduni Batavorum: Off. Hackiana, 1672: p. cap. 12.
43. von Baer KE: De ovi mammalium et hominis genesi. Leipzig: Voss, 1827: p. 39–40.
44. Smith PE: Hastening the development of the female genital system by daily homoplastic pituitary transplants. Proc Soc Exp Biol Med 1926;**24**:131–2.
45. Zondek B, Aschheim S: Das Hormon des Hypophysenvorderlappens. Klin Wochenschr 1928;**7**:831–5.
46. Rock J, Menkin MF: In vitro fertilization and cleavage of human ovarian eggs. Science 1944;**100**:105–7.
47. Steptoe PC, Edwards RG: Birth after reimplantation of a human embryo. Lancet 1978;**312**:366.
48. Gemzell CA, Roos P: Pregnancies following treatment with human gonadotropins with special reference to the problem of multiple births. Am J Obstet Gynecol 1966;**94**:490–6.
49. Liggins GC, Ibbertson HK: A successful quintuplet pregnancy following treatment with human pituitary gonadotrophin. Lancet 1966;**1**:114–7.
50. Gutowitz HE, Baillie P, Harrison V, Zieff S: Sextuplet gestation. A case report. S Afr Med J 1974;**48**:1449–52.
51. Suvalsky SD, Benda JA, Hansen K, et al.: Septuplet placenta: a case report. Am J Obstet Gynecol 2005;**192**:2076–81.
52. Rosenthal MS: The Suleman octuplet case: an analysis of multiple ethical issues. Women's Health Issues 2010;**20**:260–5.
53. Hansen M, Kurinczuk JJ, Bower C, Webb S: The risk of major birth defects after intracytoplasmatic sperm injection and in vitro fertilization. N Engl J Med 2002;**346**:725–30.
54. ACOG Committee on Ethics: Multifetal pregnancy reduction. Obstet Gynecol 2017;**130**:670–1.
55. Cihangir Yilanlioglu N, Semiz A, Arisoy R, et al.: The outcome of the multiple pregnancy reduction procedures in a single centre. Eur J Obstet Gynecol Reprod Biol 2018;**230**:22–7.

4.3

Unequal but monozygotic
Twin–twin transfusion syndrome

Introduction

The birth of twins was considered disreputable since the time of Aristotle [1] and twins were killed in several cultures [2, 3]. Archaic beliefs about superfecundation and maternal adultery, but also the high mortality of mother and infants and difficulty of raising twins (especially among nomads) may have contributed to this negative image.

Unequal twins, a bad omen

Rebecca and Isaac's sons may have suffered from acute twin–twin transfusion syndrome (TTTS), or they may have been dizygotic with one of them affected by hypertrichosis [Genesis 25: 23–6]: 'And the Lord said unto her [Rebecca], Two nations are in thy womb, and two manner of people shall be separated from thy bowels; and the one people shall be stronger than the other people; and the elder shall serve the younger. And when her days to be delivered were fulfilled, behold, there were twins in her womb. And the first came out red, all over like a hairy garment, and they called his name Esau. And after that came his brother out, and his hand took hold on Esau's heel, and his name was called Jacob.' 'Holding the heel' of the first twin indicated birth of the second from the breech position (Fig. 4.3.1), a mode of delivery not likely to be survived in antiquity.

Chronic TTTS may lead to fetal hydrops in either twin. Louise Bourgeois was cited by Graetzer [4] and Ballantyne [5] as having published on TTTS in 1609. However, the hydropic twin noted in her observation 43 was female and the normal twin was male, making TTTS unlikely [6]. A 1617 painting in the Muiderslot, Netherlands, shows a pale and a red-faced swaddled twin (Fig. 4.3.2A). As Berger and colleagues found out [7], the boys were the children of Amsterdam mayor Jacob de Graeff. They were probably liveborn as suggested by their opened eyes, deceased shortly after death, and were portrayed postmortem, a common practice among the nobility in the 17th century.

To tie or not to tie

Before the stethoscope and ultrasound uncovered most of childbirth's mysteries, twins always had to be expected. Uncertainty about the need for ligating the placental end of the cord in twin deliveries led to a vivid controversy among obstetricians.

An unusual type of vascular anastomosis was described in 1687 by Cornelis Stalpart van der Wiel, physician at the Hague [8] (Fig. 4.3.3, top): 'The midwife informed me, that she delivered twins in another part of the Hague [Speuy, in the community of Cabel, on 18 February 1677], each enclosed in a separate membrane, who used altogether three navel-strings, as shown in figure 1 of plate six. Each fruit had its own placenta, both of which were separated but close to each other, and were fixed, one in the uterine fundus and one laterally … The third cord and the common umbilical vessels showed gyrations and nodes as usually seen in the newly born.' He concluded: 'It could also be, that blood transits from one vessel into the other, and what undoubtedly happened in our case, that all the blood contained in placenta and cord of one [twin] was transfused to the other. This communication of the placental blood doubtless makes twins more similar in temper and other peculiarities'.

Paris royal accoucheur François Mauriceau denied the existence of interfetal anastomoses in his 1668 traité [9] (Fig. 4.3.3, bottom): '[Multiples] born from the same conception usually have one after-birth equipped with as many umbilical cords as there are infants; however they are, by their peculiar membranes, completely separated from each other. Within separated amniotic sacs each infant is contained with its waters.' He did not change his mind when he discovered frequent infant morbidity in 14 sets of twins with fused placentae. In observation 540, Mauriceau recorded [10]: 'On September 13, 1688, I delivered a woman at eight and a half months in her first pregnancy of two girls who had only one after-birth which they shared. The first of these girls came naturally and adapted very well; but the second passed a hand with the head, and was so weak when she came into the world, that she expired an hour later, even though she had not suffered any violence during the

---

Reproduced with permission from Obladen, M. Unequal but monozygous: a history of twin-twin transfusion syndrome. *Journal of Perinatal Medicine*, 38(2):121–128. Copyright © 2010 Walter de Gruyter GmbH, Berlin/Boston.

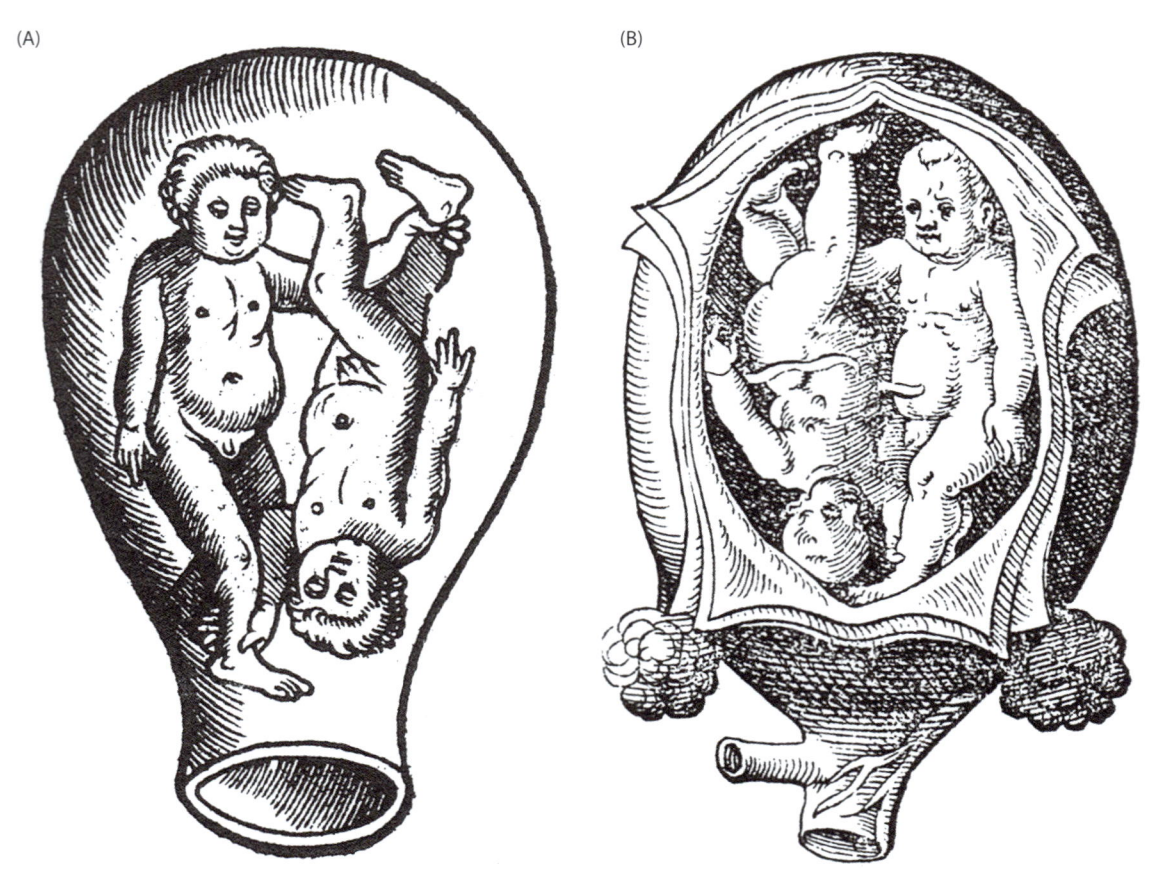

Fig. 4.3.1 Inverted twins in early obstetric texts: A, Roesslin 1513 [33]; B, Rueff 1587 [34], both showing one twin in the breech position ('holding the heel').

operation I performed to make room for nature to expel this second infant … without much pain to the mother. Her legs and feet were swollen during the last months of her pregnancy, which is common in all women who are carrying several infants, which they always deliver fifteen days or three weeks before the end of the ninth month, because the great distension of their womb prevents them bearing the infants for nine entire months.'

In 1752, William Smellie used the technique of injection to solve the controversy regarding the ligation of the firstborn twin's cord [11]: 'Yet, by an instance that lately fell under my observation, it appears that sometimes twins have but one placenta in common. Whether or not there were two sets of membranes, I could not discover, because they had been tor[n] off by the gentleman who delivered the woman; but when the artery in one of the navel-strings was injected, the matter flowed out at one of the vessels belonging to the other; and the communication between them is still visible, though they are separated at the distance of three or four inches.'

Royal accoucheur André Levret was aware that inter-fetal vessel connections may occur in monochorionic twins, writing in 1766 [12]: 'On first glance one would assume that it is only one placenta, but in reality there are two, however, with communicating great vessels in the placentae themselves.' His successor Jean Louis Baudelocque assumed a rather inconsistent position in his 'L'Art des Accouchemens' [13]: 'The placenta should be delivered after the last infant's birth, except when nature forces us to proceed differently and the first infant's placenta obstructs the exit towards the vagina. Some have recommended it may not be useless, while waiting, to ligate the cord which descends from this mass: But it must be untied at the moment of delivery, to allow for emptying of the common afterbirth and thereby facilitate its exit.' Claude François Lallemand observed acute TTTS in 1816 [14, 15]: 'After several hours of labour, a living fetus came out, [resembling] seven to eight months. The umbilical cord was cut and tied at the infant's end. Monsieur Patissier, who had the placental end in his fingers, noticed that it spilled more blood than usual, which prompted him to examine the matter more closely. All who were present were convinced that the expelled blood sprayed over a rather long distance, just like after amputation of a small artery … Twins … The two placentae were fused to one common mass, but the membranes were adjoined: One cord entered the center of the fetal surface and the other the circumference. We did not try to inject the placenta because a portion of it was torn off; but it was evident that the two fetuses were not only connected during their development, but that this was done by large vessels.' The discussion on double cord clamping continued throughout the 19th century.

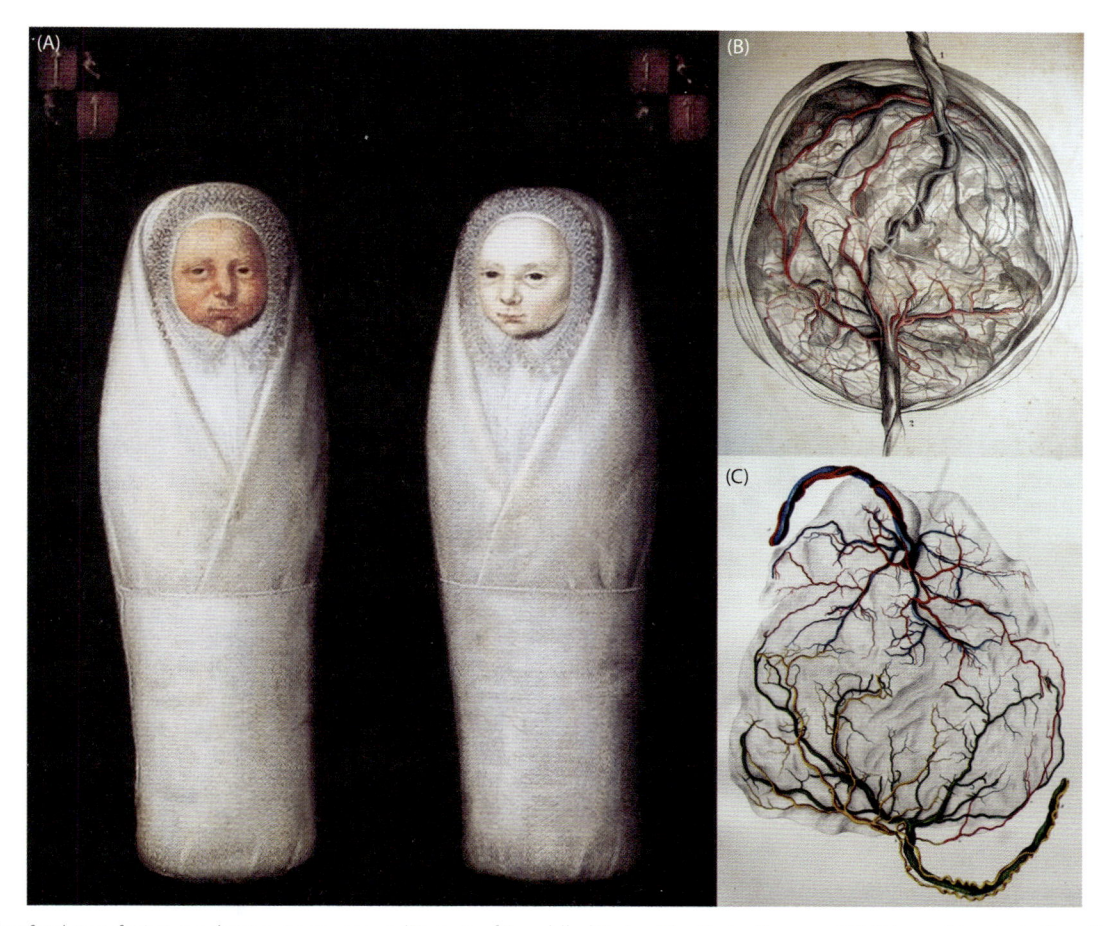

Fig. 4.3.2 A, fetofetal transfusion syndrome. Anonymous: 'Portrait of Swaddled Twins: The Early-Deceased Children of Jacob de Graeff and Aeltge Boelens', ca. 1617. Oil on panel. Amsterdam, Rijksmuseum. B and C, placental anastomoses shown with injection technique; B, by C. Hueter 1845 [21] and C, by J. Hyrtl 1870 [22].
A: Amsterdam, Rijksmuseum, on loan to Rijksmuseum Muiderslot, with permission.

Placental anastomoses injected and classified

The Göttingen obstetrician Friedrich Benjamin Osiander reported on the birth of twins on 25 December 1781 in Cassel [16]: 'Both infants, of male gender, lived; the afterbirth was fused. The cords inserted opposite to each other at the placental edge ... Soemmerring injected red and green dyes into the afterbirth [vessels]. It became evident that not only the two parts of the twin placenta were fused, but also that both the arteries and veins of one part were connected with those of the other via the strongest branches; it is astonishing that there was no fatal bleeding in the second infant from the maternal part of the first infant's cord.' The controversy over double cord ligation prompted Louis-Xavier Lebaube to publish a dissertation on five cases of TTTS in 1817 [17]: 'On December 18, 1815, a 28-year-old woman in labor presented to the service of Dr. Le Breton ... gave birth to a male infant of small size, but nonetheless living. The umbilical cord was cut and ligated immediately; but its maternal end, from which but little blood drained, was not ligated ... The two placentae were completely fused; the membranes distinct; there were two umbilical cords, the larger of which inserted into the center and the other into the circumference of the fused mass. Mr. Le Breton, desiring to know if there was a vascular connection between the two placentae, asked Mr. Breschet [surgeon at the Hotel-Dieu] to perform an injection. The liquid injected into the umbilical vein of the larger cord penetrated at the first push of the syringe into all areas of the fused mass.' Alexander Lebreton described the postmortem findings from the same secondborn infant [18]: 'It was in a state I call syncope, of black, yellow, and violet color, which is especially rare at the soles of the feet ... Dry friction was applied to the skin ... mouth inflation into the chest followed, thereafter with a bellows ... All measures were in vain ... After 12 hours I opened the infant and found all cardiac cavities filled with blood. The venous and arterial systems abounded with very dark blood; the lungs revealed the same dark blue color.'

Jean Louis Brachet, a physician from Lyon not to be confused with Breschet, also used the injection technique to study placental anastomoses [19]: 'The 13th of December, 1821, Madame Debrall, after a stormy pregnancy ... Given that this [first born] girl was very weak, I performed the rescue measures myself ... After six to eight minutes, I [returned to the woman and] found the umbilical cord retracted and some clots formed before the genital organs ... The second infant, also of female gender, was exsanguinated and lifeless, even though it had shown some activity when labor began. All resuscitation efforts were futile ... The two cords were inserted close

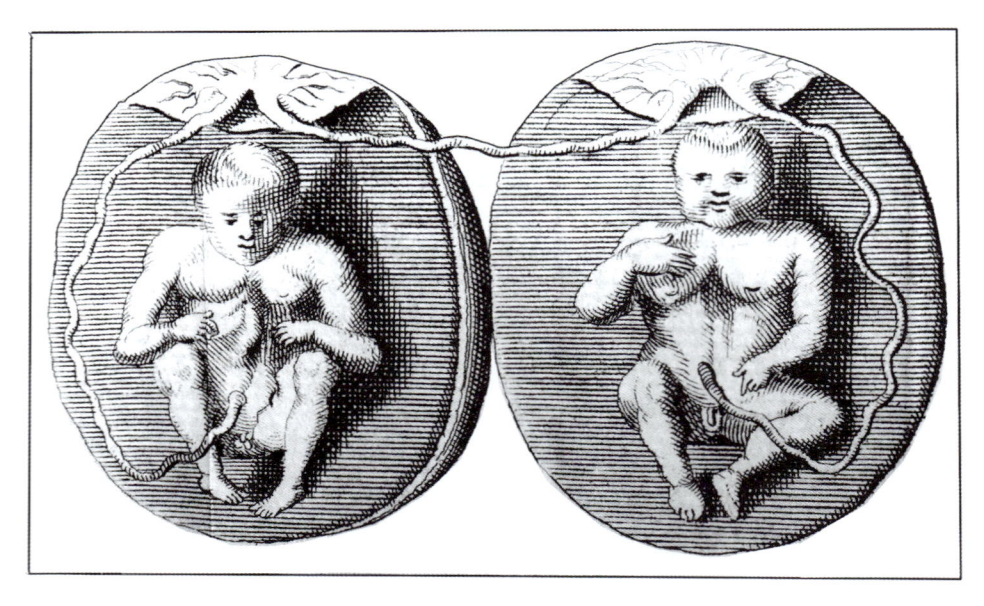

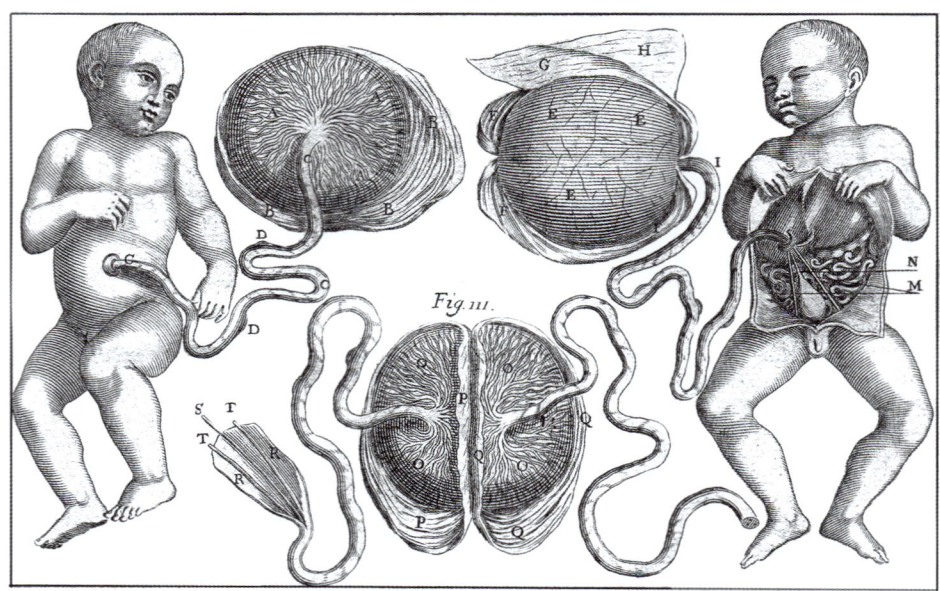

Fig. 4.3.3 Placenta vasculature in twins. Top: anastomosis as described by C. Stalpart van der Wiel in 1682 [8]. Bottom: separated circulations as described by F. Mauriceau 1668 [9].

to each other near the center of the afterbirth. With a small silver syringe I injected water into the umbilical vein of one cord; the common tissue enlarged and soon reddish water returned from the second cord. I injected wine to follow the vessel's course and it was obvious that several rather voluminous vessels communicated via multiple anastomoses on the placenta's fetal surface.'

In 1833, D. Guillemot compiled several cases from the literature and added a description of a compressed hypotrophic girl (stuck twin) followed by the birth of a very large (hydropic) infant [20]: 'The two placentae were united and showed no other trace of separation but some small shreds of membranes on the part of the compressed fetus. The arrangement of vessels revealed an umbilical vein of each cord split off a branch that anastomosed both vessels near their insertion into the placenta.' Carl Hueter, an obstetrician from Marburg, published injection studies of fused monochorionic placentae in his 1845 monograph [21]. He described a TTTS case in which a dead firstborn boy with oligohydramnios (diminished amniotic fluid) was followed by a living boy with polyhydramnios (excess amniotic fluid). Fig. 4.3.2B shows the fetal surface of the placenta, the arteries of the secondborn twin are injected with red, and the veins of the firstborn infant with blue matter. Multiple anastomoses are visible. Vienna pathologist Josef Hyrtl perfected the technique of placental injection [22] and initiated a large collection of twin placentas (Fig. 4.3.2C). In 1882, W. Nieberding described a potential relationship between fetal hydrops and hydramnios in twins, assuming that a hydropic twin may be accompanied by an oligohydramnic sibling [23].

No researcher studied placental anastomoses as extensively as the Rostock obstetrician Friedrich Schatz. From 1875 to 1910, he published a series of 14 scholarly papers totalling 726 pages devoted to

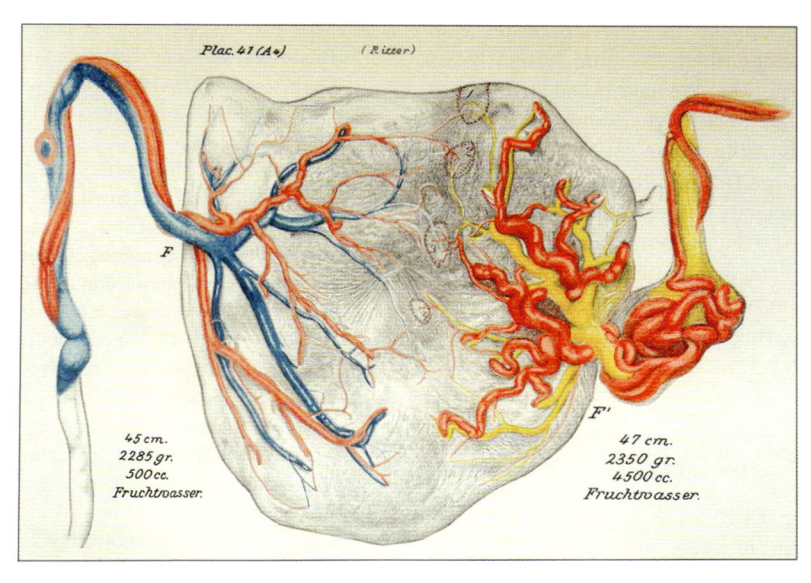

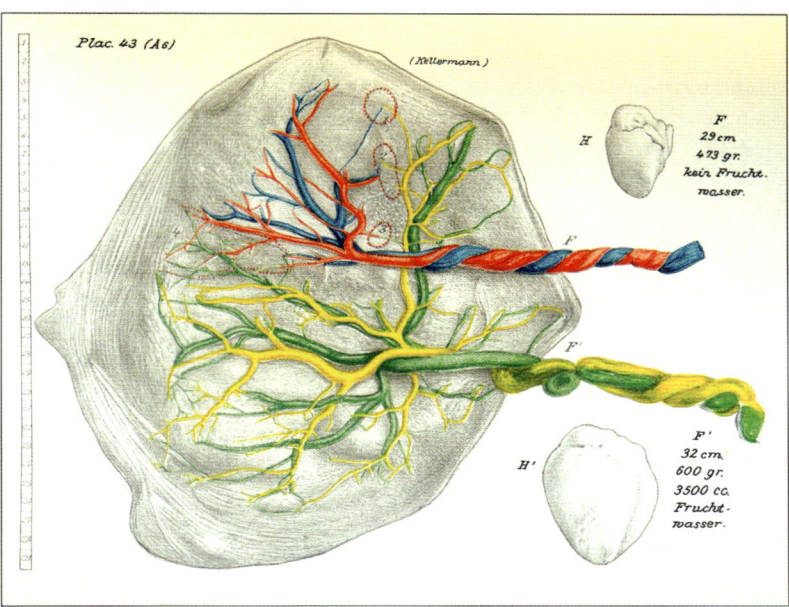

Fig. 4.3.4 Placental anastomoses and twin–twin transfusion syndrome, examined by injecting dyes by F. Schatz 1898 [25]. Top: case Ritter (placenta 41), showing oligohydramnios (500 mL) in the donor twin F and polyhydramnios (4500 mL) in the recipient twin F'; Bottom: case Kellermann (placenta 43) showing microcardia and anhydramnios in the donor and cardiomegaly as well as polyhydramnios (3500 mL) in the recipient.

various types of anastomoses. A systematic table of contents of most of his works appeared in 1900 [24], and two examples of his skilfully injected placentae are depicted in Fig. 4.3.4 [25]. Schatz used the term 'chorioangiopagous vessels' to denote the connecting anastomoses arising during placental vessel development and suggested a complex system of aberrations. He described a host of adverse outcomes suggesting that the type of anastomoses greatly influenced the resulting pathology depending on how long and how much blood flowed through the anastomoses: the spectrum included (1) microcardia/oligohydramnios due to anaemia in the donor (Fig. 4.3.4, top); (2) cardiomegaly/polyhydramnios due to volume overload in the recipient (Fig. 4.3.4, bottom); (3) unequal weight and organ size; (4) hydrops fetalis in either twin; and (5) acardiac twinning with reversed perfusion (see Chapter 4.4). Through the combined use of X-rays, coloured celloidin injection, and corrosion technique, Basel obstetrician Wenner defined six different forms of interfetal anastomoses in 1947 [26]. In 1961, Boston pathologist Kurt Benirschke studied 250 placentae of twins prospectively and found vascular anastomoses in all cases of monochorionicity [27].

Prenatal diagnosis by sonography

In the era of ultrasound, twin pregnancies were usually diagnosed early. TTTS was suspected if there was retarded or discordant fetal growth and abnormal blood flow velocity. However, the mortality and morbidity of infants with this disorder remained high, the recipient being more affected by acute volume overload and the donor endangered by chronic hypoperfusion. In 1999, an obstetrician from Tampa, Ruben Quintero, described a staging system based on serial ultrasound examination [28]: 'We have noted an apparent time sequence of events as follows: (1) Polyhydramnios of the recipient and/or oligohydramnios of the donor. (2) Nonvisualization of the bladder in the donor twin. (3) Critically abnormal Doppler studies as absent end-diastolic velocity in the umbilical artery of the donor and/or reversed flow in the ductus venosus of the recipient. (4) Hydrops in either twin. (5) Fetal demise of either or both twins.' This system allowed comparison of TTTS outcomes and different treatment modalities, thereby paving the way for planned antenatal approaches in specialized centres.

Prenatal intervention

Two different interventions for TTTS were proposed: serial amniocentesis and vessel obliteration using laser technique. Serial amnioreduction was performed by Mahony 1990 in Seattle, resulting in the survival of 11 out of 16 fetuses [29]: 'This is significantly improved compared with a fetal survival rate of 20% among the five preceding pregnancies managed without serial amniocenteses.' In 1991 in Phoenix, Elliott and colleagues restored amniotic fluid volume to normal levels in both sacs by aggressive therapeutic amniocentesis [30]. Fetal hydrops resolved in three of five fetuses and perinatal survival was 79%. The laser technique required highly specialized centres, it was not readily adopted. In 1999, Hecher and colleagues conducted a non-randomized study comparing two centres. Their findings suggested that endoscopic laser coagulation of placental vascular anastomoses may be more effective than serial amniocenteses [31], but some uncertainty remained until the Eurofoetus Consortium performed a randomized controlled trial in severe TTTS, comparing serial amnioreduction with selective fetoscopic laser coagulation of the communicating vessels at mid-gestation. The study, published by Marie-Victoire Senat and co-workers in 2004 [32], established the current treatment standard: 'The trial was concluded early, after 72 women had been assigned to the laser group and 70 to the amnioreduction group, because a planned interim analysis demonstrated a significant benefit in the laser group … higher survival rates and lower rates of neurologic complications at 6 months of age.'

Conclusion

Despite progress in teratology and prenatal diagnosis, TTTS will remain a serious threat to monozygotic twin gestations. Given our lack of knowledge on what causes the twins' blood vessels to connect within the placenta, no primary prevention can be expected until these mechanisms are better understood.

REFERENCES

1. Aristotle: History of animals. Loeb Classical Library 439. Cambridge, MA: Harvard University Press, 1991: Vol. **XI**, p. IX (7), 584 b, 26–34.
2. Ploss H: Auffassung und Behandlung der Zwillinge. In: Das Kind in Brauch und Sitte der Völker. 3. ed. Leipzig: Grieben, 1911: Vol. **1**, p. 145–59.
3. Seler E: Codex Borgia. Eine altmexikanische Bilderschrift der Bibliothek der Congregatio de Propaganda Fide. Berlin: v. Gerbrunger, 1904–1906: Vol. **2**, p. 186, fig. 169.
4. Graetzer J: Die Krankheiten des Foetus. Breslau: Aderholz, 1837: p. 113.
5. Ballantyne JW: The diseases and deformities of the foetus. Edinburgh: Olver and Boyd, 1892: Vol. **1**, p. 167.
6. Bourgeois L: Observations diverses sur la sterilité, perte de fruits, foecondité, accouchments, et maladies de femmes, et enfants nouveaux-naiz. Paris: Dehoury, 1609: p. 112.
7. Berger HM, de Waard F, Molenaar Y: A case of twin-to-twin transfusion in 1617. Lancet 2000;**356**:847–8.
8. Stalpart van der Wiel Co: Observationum rariorum medic. anatomic. chirurgicarum centuria prior, accedit de nutritione foetus exercitatio. Lugduni Batavorum: Peter van der Aa, 1687: Vol. **1**, p. 329–31.
9. Mauriceau F: Tractat von Kranckheiten schwangerer und gebärender Weibspersonen (1st French ed. 1668). Basel: Bertsche, 1680: p. 148.
10. Mauriceau F: Observations sur la grossesse et l'accouchement des femmes. Paris: Compagnie des Libraires, 1738: Vol. **2**, p. 448.
11. Smellie W: A treatise on the theory and practise of midwifery (1878 ed.). London: Sydenham Society, 1752: Vol. **1**, p. 116.
12. Levret A: L'art des accouchemens. 3. ed. Paris: Didot Jeune, 1766: p. 70.
13. Baudelocque JL: L'art des accouchemens. Nouvelle édition. 2. ed. Paris: Desprez & Méquignon, 1789: Vol. **2**, p. 640.
14. Lallemand C-F: Placenta: communication libre des vaisseaux. In: Dictionnaire des sciences médicales. Paris: Pancoucke, 1816: Vol. **42**, p. 524–6.
15. Lallemand C-F: Observations pathologiques propres a éclairer certains points de physiologie. Paris: Didot Jeune, 1818.
16. Osiander FB: Beobachtungen, Abhandlungen und Nachrichten, welche vorzüglich Krankheiten der Frauenzimmer und Kinder und die Entbindungswissenschaften betreffen. Tübingen: Cotta, 1787: p. 188–94.
17. Lebaube L-X: Dissertation sur la délivrance en général, et sur la ligature du cordon ombilical dans le cas de grossesse composée. Paris: Didot Jeune, 1817: p. 41.
18. Lebreton A: Untersuchungen über die Ursachen und die Behandlung mehrerer Krankheiten des Neugeborenen. Leipzig: Industrie-Comptoir, 1820: p. 75.
19. Brachet JL: Mémoire sur la communication vasculaire des placenta, dans le cas de grossesse multiple. J Gen Med Chir Pharm 1822;**49**, 18 de la 2e série:3–22.
20. Guillemot DMP: De la gestation des jumeaux. Arch Gen Med 1833;IIe série, T. **1**:55–87.
21. Hueter CC: Der einfache Mutterkuchen der Zwillinge. Marburg: Elwert, 1845: p. 10–4.
22. Hyrtl J: Die Blutgefässe der menschlichen Nachgeburt in normalen und abnormen Verhältnissen. Wien: Braumüller, 1870: p. 134–9, plate 18.
23. Nieberding W: Zur Kenntniss der Genese des Hydramnion. Arch Gynäk 1882;**20**:310–6.
24. Schatz F: Die Gefäßverbindungen der Plazentakreisläufe eineiiger Zwillinge, ihre Entwickelung und ihre Folgen. Inhaltsverzeichnis. Arch Gynäk 1900;**60**:559–84.
25. Schatz F: Die Gefäßverbindungen der Plazentakreisläufe eineiiger Zwillinge, ihre Entwickelung und ihre Folgen. III. Die Acardii. Arch Gynäk 1898;**55**:485–607.
26. Wenner R: Über den plazentaren Blutkreislauf bei eineiigen Zwillingen. Schweiz Med Wochenschr 1947;**47**:140–1.
27. Benirschke K: Accurate recording of twin placentation. Obstet Gynecol 1961;**18**:334–47.

28. Quintero RA, Morales WJ, Allen MH, et al.: Staging of twin-twin transfusion syndrome. J Perinatol 1999;**19**:550–5.
29. Mahony BS, Petty CN, Nyberg DA, et al.: The 'stuck twin' phenomenon. Am J Obstet Gynecol 1990;**163**:1513–22.
30. Elliott JP, Urig MA, Clewell WH: Aggressive therapeutic amniocentesis for treatment of twin-twin transfusion syndrome. Obstet Gynecol 1991;**77**:537–40.
31. Hecher K, Plath H, Bregenzer T, Hansmann M, Hackeloer BJ: Endoscopic laser surgery versus serial amniocenteses in the treatment of severe twin-twin transfusion syndrome. Am J Obstet Gynecol 1999;**180**:717–24.
32. Senat MV, Deprest J, Boulvain M, et al.: Endoscopic laser surgery versus serial amnioreduction for severe twin-to-twin transfusion syndrome. N Engl J Med 2004;**351**:136–44.
33. Rößlin E: Der Swangern Frauwen und hebammen Rosegarten. Straßburg: Flach, 1513: p. 36.
34. Rueff J: De conceptu, et generatione hominis. Frankfurt: Feyerabend, 1587: p. 34v.

4.4
From monster to reversed perfusion
Acardiac twins

Introduction

A malformation as frightening as acardius–acranius (absence of head and heart) did not escape the interest of antique historians. Roman writers adopted the Greek habit of imagining the stillborn or moribund malformed neonate as a living adult, and incorporated the malformation into their mythology. In the case of acranic individuals even a mystical population in a remote area was imagined.

Antique enigmatic people and medieval monsters

In the 5th century B.C.E, Herodotus speculated [1]: 'In that country [North Africa near the Red Sea coast] are large snakes and lions, and elephants and bears and asps, horned asses and dog-headed [kynekephaloi] and headless [akephaloi] men with eyes in their chests, as the Libyans say, and the wild men and women besides many other creatures not fabulous.' Pliny the Elder, who lived from 24 to 79 C.E., located the enigmatic people in Ethiopia [2]: 'The Blemmyes are reported to have no heads, their mouth and eyes being attached to their chests.'

This combination of poor observation, superstition, and ignorance persisted throughout the Middle Ages and was repeated by the Dominican Thomas of Cantimpré in 1263 [3] and depicted by Nuremberg encyclopaedist Hartmann Schedel in 1493 [4] and by Conrad Lycosthenes in 1557 [5] (Fig. 4.4.1A, B). The term 'mooncalf', coined in the 16th century to denote severe malformation, became popular through treatises by Luther and Melanchthon and by its use in Shakespeare's *The Tempest* [6]. The term 'headless monster' was used in scientific publications.

God's wrath, imagination, and the baptism dilemma

The 'headless monster' was always accompanied by a normally shaped infant (the 'pump twin'). This was illustrated in printed leaflets, the popular press in the Renaissance [7] (Fig. 4.4.1, right): 'On the fourth of December, 1551, the Friday after St. Andrew's day, three children were born in the new hospital at Breslau named All Saints', to a butcher's wife named Ursula Walter Hosperg. One was a small boy who died soon after baptism. The other two were girls and one was imperfect [immature] and stillborn. The third, which is depicted here had a wondrously strange and frightening shape. For it had neither head nor hands nor arms, only the trunk and the feet could be discerned. But it was imperfect [immature] and stillborn. – Because such frightening miracles and monsters are usually a sign of God's wrath, all Christian souls should sigh and pray to God, our dear Lord Jesus Christ's eternal father, to avert his punishment and anger.' Observation blended with fantasy readily in this century of superstition and pietism [8]: 'Around Christmas of 1569 Caspar Hugen's wife, from Matzingen/Thurgau, gave birth to two infants in one delivery. One revealed no defect or blemish, while the other had no head. Instead of a head it had a great black hole out of which it cried; it also had two goose feet and expired after emitting one or two cries.'

On 6 April 1701, anatomist Alexis Littre reported to the Paris faculty on an acranic and two anencephalic fetuses and pondered about the brain's function as assumed since Aristotle [9]: 'The first two male fetuses, of seven and eight months gestation, were both large and fat [hydropic]. That of seven months had neither head nor neck, and the upper part of the trunk was covered with skin... This observation sheds doubt on the purpose ascribed to the brain or at least to make it suspect, that the spirits which its glands separate from the blood are as necessary as assumed for movement, nutrition, and other functions of the body... The larger a human's brain, the more the functions of his soul are perfect, and the more he is able to carry them out.' Highly relevant in theological terms and in contrast to St. Augustine, newborns without a head forced the catholic church to localize the infant's soul in the head: the inquisitor Cangiamila, in addition to theology a graduate in medicine and law, was appointed to rule on baptism and decreed (1st ed. 1745) [10]: 'Therefore the acranius, how many relicts of the human body he might have, should under no circumstances be

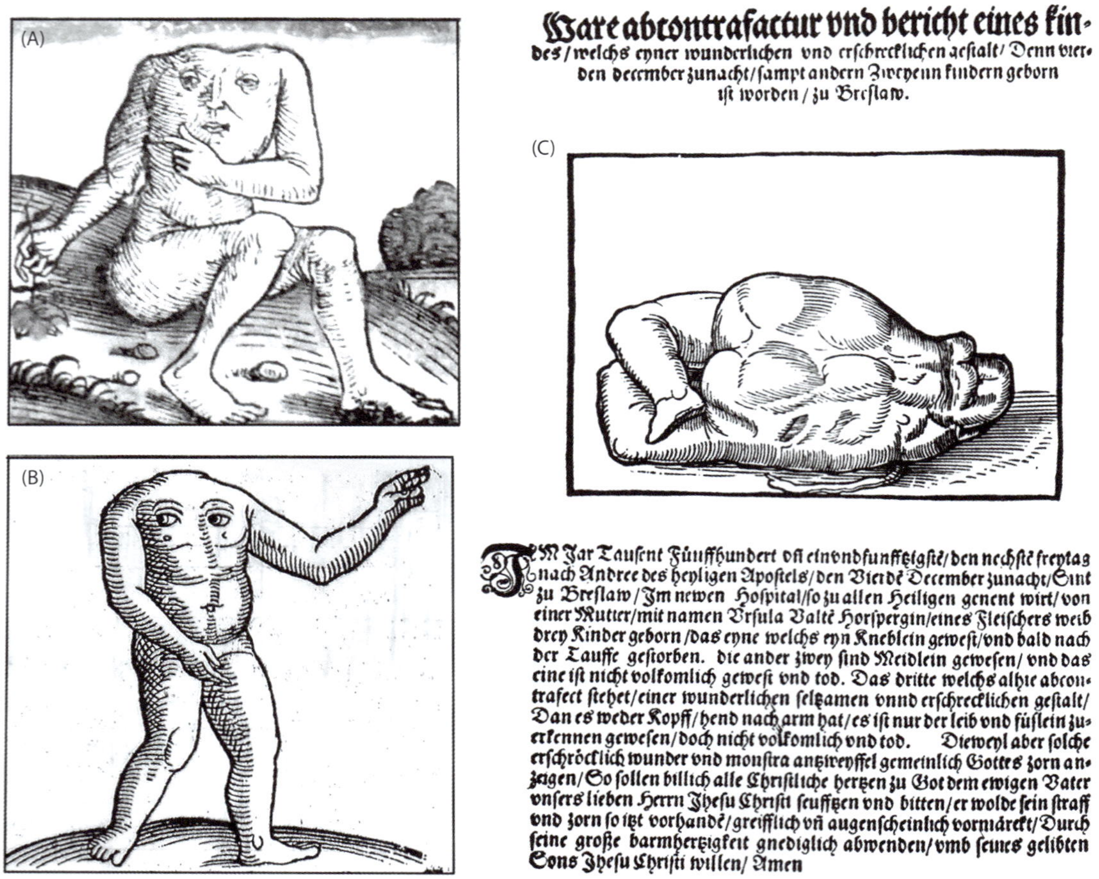

Fig. 4.4.1 Pre-scientific accounts of acranius as a moral warning. A, 'Headless blemmye' from Schedel's Weltchronik 1493 [4]; B, 'Brustbutzen' from Lycosthenes' marvellous wonders 1557 [5]; Right: 'Frightening prodigy' from a Breslau leaflet 1551, see text for details [7].

baptised: because the head is missing, undoubtedly the primary seat of soul and reason.'

A twin-specific disorder with abnormal umbilical vessels

Mauriceau, the man who established obstetrics as a science, wrote in his traité (1st ed. 1668) [11]: 'The moon-calves are nourished in the womb, to which they nearly always adhere at some place, and are maintained by the blood of which they are perfused like plants watered from the earth. Besides the moon-calf there is often another infant, from which it may be separated.' In 1720, Parisian surgeon Jean Mery reported to the Académie des Sciences [12]: 'Marie Guerlin, aged 30 years and pregnant for 6 months, delivered two little girls on September 10 of last year. Nothing was missing from the perfect firstborn infant's body, it lived for half an hour. But the dead [secondborn] had a severely deformed trunk whose upper part ended with the first dorsal vertebra. This trunk had no head, neck, scapula, clavicula, nor arms … The two little girls shared but one placenta whose membranes formed one pouch enclosing them both, which is very rare. Of this fused placenta sorted but one cord, which in the middle of its length divided in two which separately ended at their navels … Having opened the body, we found … neither lungs nor heart, but in front of the spine there were two vessels in addition to those already described.' Mery ordered drawings to be made during the dissection by Mr. Châtillon, dessinateur de l'Académie; however, these depictions could not be located.

In 1789, the Sommerfeld physician Kähler associated the acardiac malformation with abnormal umbilical vessels in one of triplets [13]: 'The midwife [after delivering two stillborn infants at 7 months' gestation in June 1777] found that something was left in the uterus, which did not feel like a properly shaped fruit … It was larger and heavier than the twins, with imperfect genitalia, cleft lip, and a bundle of empty and thin vessels around the umbilicus … The skull contained a rudimentary and imperfect brain, the chest abnormal remnants of the lung. The eyes, heart with its large vessels, the trachea and esophagus were entirely absent: Likewise all abdominal viscera lacked except small intestines, which by size and position were abnormal. Lacking a good artist, I could only obtain a rough drawing [Fig. 4.4.2A].' In 1812, the Halle anatomist Johann Friedrich Meckel (Junior) compiled over 50 cases of acrania from the world literature and included four of his own [14], stating that the disorder is specific for twin gestation, but could not explain its pathogenesis. That was ultimately achieved by his nephew and foster son Heinrich Meckel, 38 years later [15]. In June of 1826, Etienne Geoffroy St. Hilaire verbally accosted a colleague of his in the Paris faculty, sarcastically remarking [16]: 'Mr. Moreau gave me the honor of informing me that he will present a human monster born this morning, a complete acephalus. Will you also present, I answered, his firstborn twin and

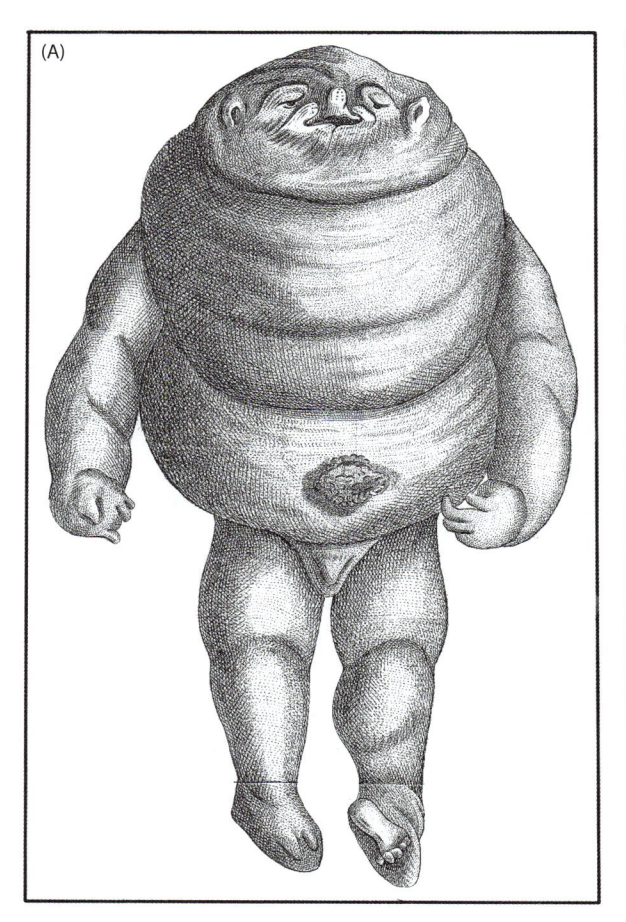

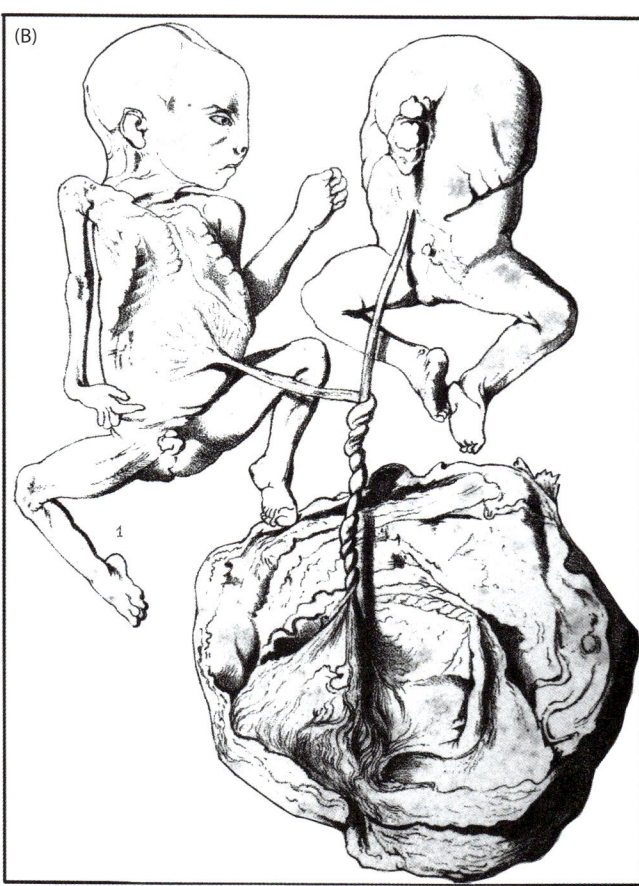

Fig. 4.4.2 A, hydropic acardius anceps 'larger and heavier than the accompanying twins', described by Kähler in 1777 [13], B, Acardius acranius with twisted cord depicted by Ahlfeld in 1882 to 'illustrate the connection between the acardius and his twin brother in the placenta' [46].

the placenta in common between the two individuals? … The presence of a twin is necessarily linked with development of an acephalic monster … Mr. Moreau was stricken by the unequal distribution [of the amniotic fluid] in the two pouches; abundant to the excess in the pouch containing the regular fetus, and scarce or nearly absent in that of the monstrous fetus.' Geoffroy proceeded to mock Winslow and the common belief of maternal imagination as cause of malformation, and the frequent use of the scaffold: 'Sulsman notified Winslow that on the 14th of April 1726, a human monster without a head was born in Strasbourg. Winslow invited him to publish this observation in the Journal des Savans. Searching for the cause in reasons other than the existence of a co-twin … he conducted the following remarkable conversation with the mother: Did you witness any execution during your pregnancy? – No, not at all. – Nevertheless, to give birth to an infant without a head, you must have watched a criminal being decapitated, or at least have seen the neck of a hanged man dislocated.'

Reversed perfusion: aetiology and classification

Extensive reports on acardiacs were published by Tiedemann in 1813 [17], Béclard in 1817 [18], Vrolik in 1834 [19], and Otto in 1841 [20]. They classified different variants of the malformation and helped to distinguish it from anencephaly. They interpreted it as a sign of arrested development and did not attempt an adequate explanation of its cause. In 1836, Thomas Hodgkin and Astley Cooper of Guys Hospital described anastomoses on the placental surface and concluded [21]: 'The heart [of the normal fetus] impelled the blood into the arteries of the placenta and funis.' Heinrich Meckel von Hemsbach understood in 1850 that the acardiac twin must be kept alive by the pump twin [15]: 'In fruits, whose own circulation is impossible due to a malformed heart, a meagre life is supported by the other fetus, while general hydrops of the acephalus results from circulatory failure.'

In his thoughtful booklet, the anatomist Friedrich Claudius from Kiel [22] denied that the acardiac twin's malformation is primary and linked the problem exclusively to fetal circulation: 'Certain appending or turned-out skin parts occur where organs declined; at the site of the head, the tips of the extremities, the ventral surface of the trunk, never the dorsal. Sometimes a small retraction is found instead of an appendix … One umbilical artery of the healthy [twin] branches over half of the placenta, the other proceeds towards the second insertion, bends from the surface and enters the umbilical cord of the acardiac; the umbilical vein divides into two larger branches, which accompany both arteries; one of them proceeds towards the second insertion and becomes the acardiac's umbilical vein … In the acardiac's umbilical artery the blood therefore flows backwards, from the placenta into the body; the flow splits at the hypogastric division,

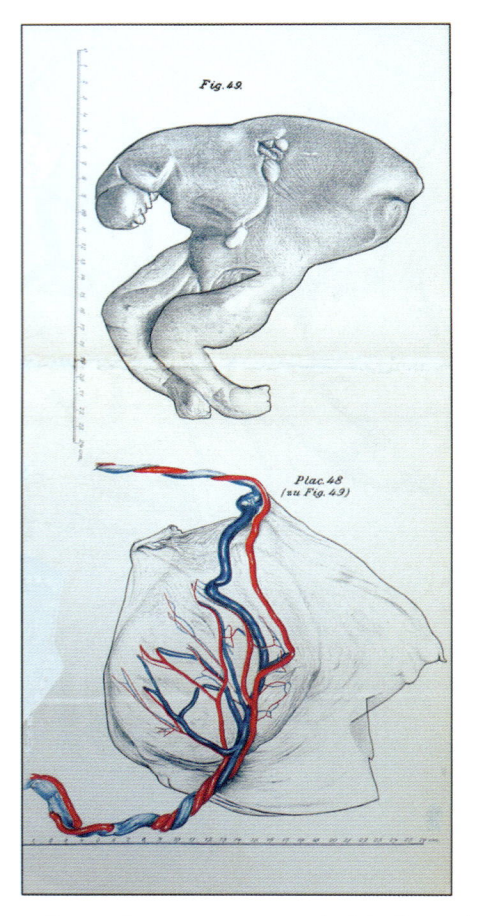

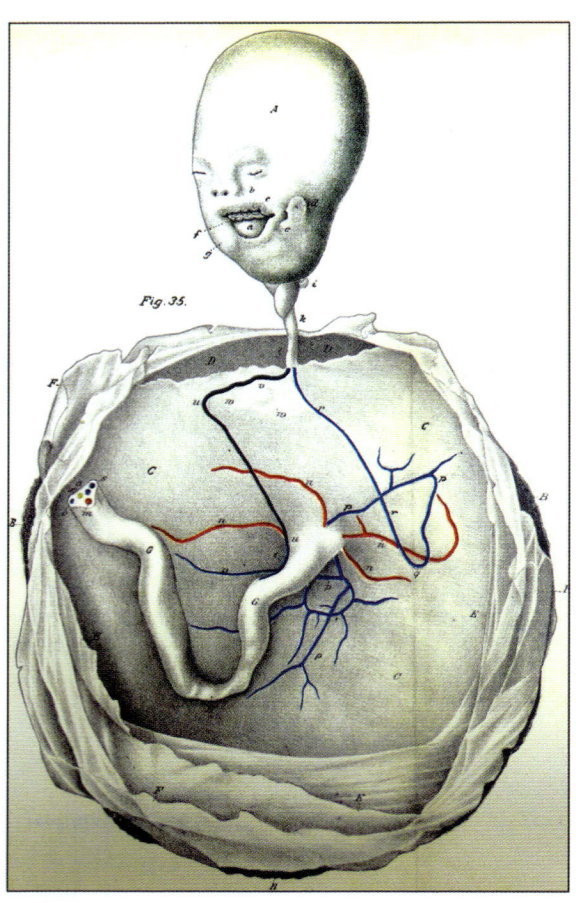

Fig. 4.4.3 Schatz studies on placenta anastomoses by injection technique, 1899 [23]. Left: acardius acranius; right: acardius acormus.

one half descends the legs, the other half up towards the a. iliaca communis, the aorta likewise receives a current in the wrong direction, from bottom to top.'

Friedrich Schatz, whose extensive work on placental anastomoses is acknowledged in Chapter 4.3, advanced Claudius' theory by postulating the gradual taking over of both circulations by the stronger, better placed, and better nourished individual. This process subsequently led to the degeneration of the weaker fetus. He showed that interplacental anastomoses (Fig. 4.4.3) in acardia are arterioarterial and venovenous, in contrast to arteriovenous anastomoses in twin–twin transfusion syndrome. Schatz postulated a 'third circulation' in the placenta [23].

Das [24] classified four variants in 1902 (Fig. 4.4.4), according to the development of allantois and placenta, a classification that is still valid today:

'1. *Acardius anceps* is the least atrophied form, characterized by absence or non-development of face, the extreme anterior part of the body. There are rudiments of cranial bones and of the brain. More or less perfect trunk and extremities [Fig. 4.4.2A].
2. *Acardius acephalus* is the most common species. Head wanting, or very rudimentary. Intestines and abdominal organs rudimentary, and the organs above the diaphragm represented by the merest trace. Shoulder girdle undeveloped [Fig. 4.4.2B].
3. *Acardius amorphus*, least developed form. Little more than a lump of connective tissue, covered by oedematous skin. There may be some rudiments of visceral tissue.
4. *Acardius acormus*, rarest. Head alone present, but never fully developed [Fig. 4.4.3, right].'

Elusive pathogenesis

Two hypotheses on pathogenesis persisted: (1) Meckel's theory, that the heart fails to develop or is arrested during development, while the acardiac fetus is maintained by the pump twin as recently supported by Napolitani [25]. (2) The theory of Claudius assumed that the heart develops and then degenerates when reversed flow triggers thrombosis. This theory was supported by Fujikura and Wellings [26]. Van Allen and colleagues proposed the term 'twin reversed arterial perfusion' (TRAP sequence) in 1983 to name this disorder [27]. However, it still seems plausible that both mechanisms are at work given that a purely circulatory explanation has several shortcomings: (1) when chromosomal analysis became possible, Rashad and Kerr in 1966 [28] and Turpin in 1967 [29] described gross karyotype anomalies in acardiac twins, and systematic karyotyping revealed chromosomal anomalies in a third of acardiacs [30]. (2) As Benirschke and colleagues pointed out [31], acardiac twins frequently have heterogeneous, but typical patterns of human

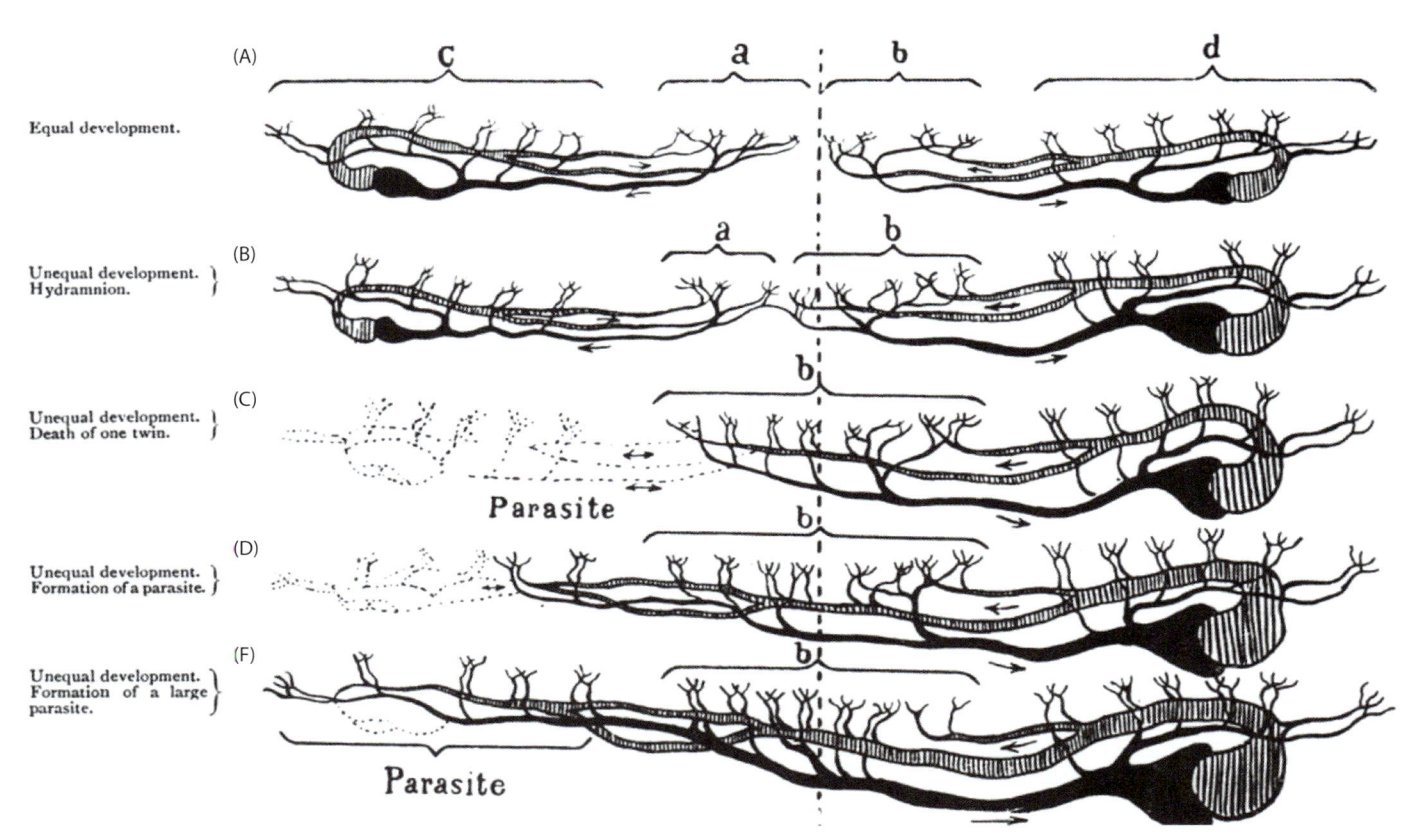

Fig. 4.4.4 Equal and unequal development in twins from one ovum, as classified by Das in 1902 [24]. a and b, placental circulations; c and d, simplified heart and circulatory apparatuses.

malformation such as cleft lip or omphalocele, anomalies difficult to attribute to degeneration alone. (3) Genotyping studies showed that human acardiac twinning including placental anastomosis is not, as was believed earlier, restricted to monochorionic placentas, but may occur in dichorionic monozygotic twins [32] or in triploidy arising from fertilization of a polar body of the normal twin [33]. On the other hand, evidence from experimental animals revealed that correct folding of the cardiac tube depends on normal blood flows and pressures [34]. The cause of the formation of large anastomoses in the placentae of some twins, with or without primary malformation, remains poorly understood.

Antenatal diagnosis and treatment

Gillim and colleagues [35] calculated the prevalence of TRAP as 1% of monozygotic twins (1 in 35,000 deliveries). Analysing 184 cases of acardia published from 1960 to 1991, Healey identified a perinatal mortality of 35% for the pump twin [36]. The principal problems were congestive cardiac failure, polyhydramnios, and preterm labour. When ultrasound revolutionized prenatal diagnostics in the 1960s, effective management and interventions became possible to save the pump twin. Lehr and DiRe described the prenatal ultrasound appearance of an acardiac twin in 1978 [37], and Pretorius and colleagues, in San Diego, documented the reversed arterial perfusion pattern with colour Doppler ultrasound in 1988 [38]. The obstetrician Lawrence Platt in Los Angeles described antenatal diagnosis with ultrasound in 1983 [39]: 'It is believed that these fetuses often develop congestive heart failure because of the cardiovascular demands placed on the normal twin. If this hypothesis is correct, then the proposed surgical procedure of clamping the cord of the acardiac fetus, either by exteriorizing the cord of the fetus and clamping it or by using a small operating laparoscope with a clip holder and clip, should prove useful.'

In 1989, Robie and colleagues selectively delivered a 710 g acardiac twin at 22 weeks by sectio parva, with subsequent delivery of a surviving 2130 g pump twin at 33 weeks [40]. Percutaneous cord occlusion was described by Porreco and co-workers [41]. In 1994, Quintero and colleagues reported successful fetoscopic ligation of the umbilical cord [42]. In 1987, Seeds and co-workers described an unsuccessful attempt to obliterate the vessels within the acardiac twin via laser [43], a technique successfully used by Sepulveda and colleagues in 1995 [44]. Using radiofrequency ablation to block the acardiac twins' circulation, Tsao and co-workers reported 12 out of 13 pump twins surviving from 1998 to 2001 [45].

Conclusion

TRAP will remain a rare event. Thanks to better understanding of its pathogenesis, it has lost its mythical associations, and prenatal diagnosis and interventions have increased the chances of pump twin survival. However, large gaps remain in the understanding. Only better insight into the cause of anastomosis formation within the placenta will open a door towards preventing this most severe human malformation.

REFERENCES

1. Herodotus: The histories. New York: Pantheon, 2007: Vol. **I**, p. 302–12.
2. Pliny the Elder: Natural history. Loeb Classical Library. Cambridge, MA: Harvard University Press, 1952: p. lib 5, cap. 8, p. 46.
3. Cantimpratensis T: Liber de natura rerum. Berlin: De Gruyter, 1973: p. 99.
4. Schedel H: Weltchronik. Kolorierte Gesamtausgabe von 1493. Nürnberg: Koberger, 1493: p. XII recto.
5. Lycosthenes C: Wunderwerck oder Gottes unergründliches Vorbilden. Basel: Henrichus Petri, 1557: p. 10, 462.
6. Smith P: The mooncalf. Modern Philology 1814;**11**:355–61.
7. Holländer E: Wunder, Wundergeburt und Wundergestalt in Einblattdrucken. Stuttgart: Enke, 1921: p. 242–6.
8. Sonderegger A: Missgeburten und Wundergestalten in Einblattdrucken und Handzeichnungen des 16. Jahrhunderts. Zürich: Orell Füssli, 1927: p. 123.
9. Littre Ad: Observations sur un foetus humain monstrueux. Mem Acad R Sci Paris 1701;120–9.
10. Cangiamila FE: Embryologia sacra sive de officio sacerdotum, medicorum, et aliorum circa aeternam parvulorum in utero existentium salutem. 3. ed. Augustae Vindelicorum: Mauracher, 1765: p. 489.
11. Mauriceau F: Traité des maladies des femmes grosses, et de celles qui sont accouchées (1st ed. 1668). 7. ed. Paris: Compagnie des Libraires, 1740: Vol. **1**, p. 114.
12. Méry J: Observations faites sur un foetus humain monstrueux. Hist Acad Sci Paris 1720; Mémoires de mathematique et de physique:9–17.
13. Kähler D: Geschichte einer Zwillings-Geburt mit einer Mißgeburt verbunden. Starks Archiv für die Geburtshülfe, Frauenzimmer- und neugebohrner Kinder-Krankheiten 1789;**2**:58–62.
14. Meckel JF: Handbuch der pathologischen Anatomie. Leipzig: Reclam, 1812: Vol. **1**. p. 140–260.
15. Meckel von Hemsbach H: Ueber die Verhältnisse des Geschlechts, der Lebensfähigkeit und der Eihäute bei einfachen und Mehrgeburten. Arch Anat Physiol Wiss Med 1850;234–72, Tafel 7 mit 14 fig.
16. Geoffroy Saint Hilaire E: Sur quelques conditions générales de l'Acéphalie complète. Revue médicale française et étrangère et journal de clinique de l'Hôtel-Dieu 1826;**3**:36–51.
17. Tiedemann F: Anatomie der kopflosen Mißgeburten. Landshut: Thomann, 1813: p. 84.
18. Béclard PA: Mémoire sur les foetus acéphales. Bulletin de la Faculté de médecine de Paris 1817;**5**:488–517.
19. Vrolik G: Mémoires sur quelques sujets intéressans d'anatomie et de physiologie. Utrecht: van der Post, 1834: p. 25–63.
20. Otto AW: Monstrorum sexcentorum descriptio anatomica. Breslau: Hirt, 1841: p. 4–5.
21. Hodgkin T, Cooper A: The history of an unusually formed placenta and imperfect fetus. Guys Hosp Rep 1836;**I**:218–41.
22. Claudius FM: Die Entwicklung der herzlosen Missgeburten. Kiel: Schwers, 1859: p. 7, 23.
23. Schatz F: Die Gefäßverbindungen der Plazentakreisläufe eineiiger Zwillinge, ihre Entwickelung und ihre Folgen. III. Die Acardii und ihre Verwandten; zweite Fortsetzung. Arch Gynäk 1899;**58**:1–82.
24. Das K: Acardiacus anceps. J Obstet Gynaecol Br Emp 1902;**2**:341–55.
25. Napolitani FH, Schreiber I: The acardiac monster. Am J Obstet Gynecol 1960;**80**:582–9.
26. Fujikura T, Wellings SR: A teratoma-like mass on the placenta of a malformed infant. Am J Obstet Gynecol 1964;**89**:824–5.
27. Van Allen MI, Smith DW, Shepard TH: Twin reversed arterial perfusion (TRAP) sequence. Semin Perinatol 1983;**7**:285–93.
28. Rashad MN, Kerr MG: Observations on the so-called holoacardius amorphus. J Anat 1966;**100**:425–6.
29. Turpin R, Bocquet L, Grasset J: Etude d'un couple monozygote: fille normale—monstre acardique feminin. Ann Genet (Paris) 1967;**10**:107–13.
30. Kaplan C, Benirschke K: The acardiac anomaly. Acta Genet Med Gemellol 1979;**28**:51–9.
31. Benirschke K, Des Roches Harper V: The acardiac anomaly. Teratology 1977;**15**:311–6.
32. French CA, Bieber FR, Bing DH, Genest DR: Twins, placentas, and genetics. Hum Pathol 1998;**29**:1028–31.
33. Bieber FR, Nance WE, Morton CC, et al.: Genetic studies of an acardiac monster. Science 1981;**213**:775–7.
34. Rychter L: Experimental morphology of the aortic arches and heart loop in chicken. Adv Morphol 1962;**2**:333–71.
35. Gillim DL, Hendricks CH: Holocardius. Obstet Gynecol 1953;**2**:647–53.
36. Healey MG: Acardia: Predictive risk factors for the co-twin's survival. Teratology 1994;**50**:205–13.
37. Lehr C, DiRe J: Rare occurrence of a holoacardius acephalic monster. J Clin Ultrasound 1978;**6**:259–61.
38. Pretorius DH, Leopold GR, Moore TR, et al.: Acardiac twin. J Ultrasound Med 1988;**7**:413–6.
39. Platt LD, DeVore GR, Bieniarz A, Benner P, Rao R: Antenatal diagnosis of acephalus acardia. Am J Obstet Gynecol 1983;**146**:857–9.
40. Robie GF, Payne GG, Morgan MA: Selective delivery of an acardiac, acephalic twin. N Engl J Med 1989;**320**:512–3.
41. Porreco RP, Barton SM, Haverkamp AD: Occlusion of umbilical artery in acardiac, acephalic twin. Lancet 1991;**337**:326–7.
42. Quintero RA, Reich H, Puder KS, et al.: Brief report: umbilical-cord ligation of an acardiac twin by fetoscopy at 19 weeks of gestation. N Engl J Med 1994;**330**:469–71.
43. Seeds JW, Herbert WN, Richards DS: Prenatal sonographic diagnosis and management of a twin pregnancy with placenta previa and hemicardia. Am J Perinatol 1987;**4**:313–6.
44. Sepulveda W, Bower S, Hassan J, Fisk NM: Ablation of acardiac twin by alcohol injection into the intra-abdominal umbilical artery. Obstet Gynecol 1995;**86**:680–1.
45. Tsao KJ, Feldstein VA, Albanese CT, et al.: Selective reduction of acardiac twin by radiofrequency ablation. Am J Obstet Gynecol 2002;**187**:635–40.
46. Ahlfeld F: Die Missbildungen des Menschen. Atlas. Leipzig: Grunow, 1882: Vol. **1**, p. 36–47, plate IV, fig. 1.

PART 5
Odd shape

5.1 Cats, frogs, and snakes: concepts of neural tube defects *145*

5.2 In God's image? The tradition of infant head shaping *155*

5.3 Lame from birth: concepts of cerebral palsy *165*

5.4 Possessed by evil spirits: seizures in infancy *173*

5.5 Birthmark and blemish: the doctrine of maternal imagination *183*

5.6 Cast aside: infants with Down's syndrome *191*

5.7 Crooked limbs: the thalidomide catastrophe *197*

5.8 A wretched condition: cleft urinary bladder *205*

INTRODUCTION

Malformations have been attributed to supranatural causes since antiquity. In severely malformed infants, called monsters, mothers were blamed, and coition at the wrong time, in the wrong way, with the wrong partner, or sodomy was suspected. Malformed infants were ostracized from society, and despised in many cultures. Severely malformed infants were usually killed at birth. From the 16th century, maternal imagination was made responsible for fetal impairments, making the birth of a malformed infant a misfortune rather than a crime. The impact of folate deficiency was understood only recently. Intentional modification of the infant's head shape was a common practice in many cultures, for aesthetic reasons, alleged health benefits, or ethnic or social identification. Tight swaddling was believed to prevent cerebral palsy. Seizures in infancy were considered to be of supranatural origin and dealt with by incantations and exorcising rituals. Coral amulets were believed to be protective. Surgical interventions for cleft bladder were developed in the 18th century.

5.1

Cats, frogs, and snakes
Concepts of neural tube defects

Introduction

With a prevalence of around 1:1000 pregnancies, neural tube defects are the second most common serious birth defect, and their aetiology is poorly understood. Observers of all eras did not miss opportunities to describe them, leaving an abundance of information. **Fig. 5.1.1** (from the school of Hans Baldung Grien around 1506), entitled *Young Woman with the Death*, has been interpreted as *Eve and Blind Cupid* [1]. However, the shape of the baby's head suggests that an anencephalic (brainless) infant is being represented, the bandage sparing the viewer the dreadful appearance of the malformation, the death figure alluding to the hopeless prognosis, and the mother's face without guilt.

An Egyptian prodigy sold in Paris

Following Napoleon's Egyptian Campaign (1798–1801), researchers and adventurers from all over Europe discovered and plundered four millennia of culture and artefacts in the Nile Valley. Joseph Passalacqua, amateur archaeologist from Trieste and later director of Berlin's Egyptian Museum, offered 1598 pieces collected in Thebes and Hermopolis in a sales exhibition in Paris in 1826. Item no. 364 was a mummified creature with an earthenware baboon amulet attached, classified among the *holy animals* but named 'human monster' [2]. It was identified by Etienne Geoffroy Saint-Hilaire, Paris professor of zoology and former scientific member of the Egypt expedition, who presented it to the Academy on 9 January 1826 [3]: 'A human monster embalmed three thousand years ago. None of the other features is missing which make an anencephalic perfectly specific in its form and rigorously determinable. The mummy had been positioned sitting up, its feet joined, and its hands resting on its knees. Mr. Passalacqua presented it as a monkey whose species he wanted to know.' Obviously, the malformed infant had been mistaken for the baboon-headed god *Hapy* and was embalmed before being solemnly buried at the Hermopolis necropole. Geoffroy Saint-Hilaire had studied and classified cerebral malformations and reported from Greece: 'Exceptional childbirth generated sinister presages, obliging [the mothers] to ritual baths and general purifications: This occurred when they had born creatures characterized as monkeys or elephants due to the shape of their heads... which I previously characterized as *anencéphales* and *rhinencéphales* (the latter born with a trunk and single eye)' (see Chapter 5.5).

Miswatching and imagination

The term *cat*- or *monkey*-head denoted a missing skull-cap with bulging temples and low-positioned ears; *frog*- or *toad*- head referred to a missing orbital roof with bulging eyes; and *open back*, *tail*, or *snake* meant various forms of spina bifida. Soranus of Ephesus, practising in Rome in the 2nd century C.E., wrote in his *Gynecology* [4]: 'What is one to say concerning the fact that various states of the soul also produce certain changes in the mold of the fetus? For instance, some women, seeing monkeys during intercourse, have borne children resembling monkeys.'

Superstitions based on the birth of animal-headed infants were to persist for 1500 years (see Chapter 5.5). It is unlikely that the artists who made the woodcuts of **Fig. 5.1.2** had actually seen such malformed infants. Pseudo-Albertus Magnus wrote in his widely distributed book *Women's Secrets* (ed. 1508) [5]: 'A woman once gave birth to a toad, and the cause of this was simply that at the moment of ejaculation the seed was infected and badly disposed by the lightening, because the vapor of lightening is sometimes poisonous.'

Conrad Wolffhart, a Basel historian, published a macabre chronicle of prodigies under the name Lycosthenes [6] in which he depicted various neural tube defects: 'On the 27th of August [1555] a horrible monstrous girl was born in Strasbourg. The top of her head was open, she had a wide mouth, oxen eyes, and a hawk's nose' (**Fig. 5.1.2A**); 'In September 1494 a woman of Krakow [living] in Holy Spirit's lane gave birth to a dead child with a live snake attached to its back which was gnawing continuously on it' (**Fig. 5.1.2B**). Describing an occipital brain hernia, Thomas Bartholin explained its increased incidence among the poor by miswatching in 1661 [7]: 'I believe that the imagination marks the monsters. Frequently the prosperous

PART 5 Odd shape

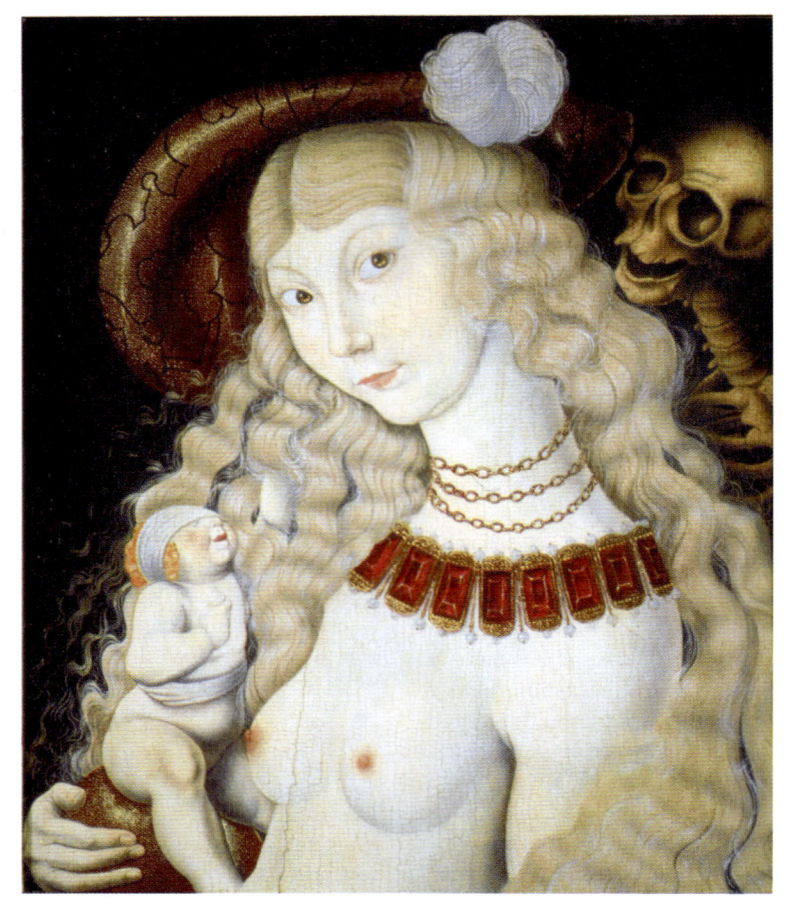

Fig. 5.1.1 Hans Baldung Grien, ca. 1506: 'Young woman and death'; oil on wood. Brussels, Royal Museum of Fine Arts of Belgium, Inv. Nr. 8756.
© Royal Museums of Fine Arts of Belgium, Brussels/photo: J. Geleyns – Art Photography.

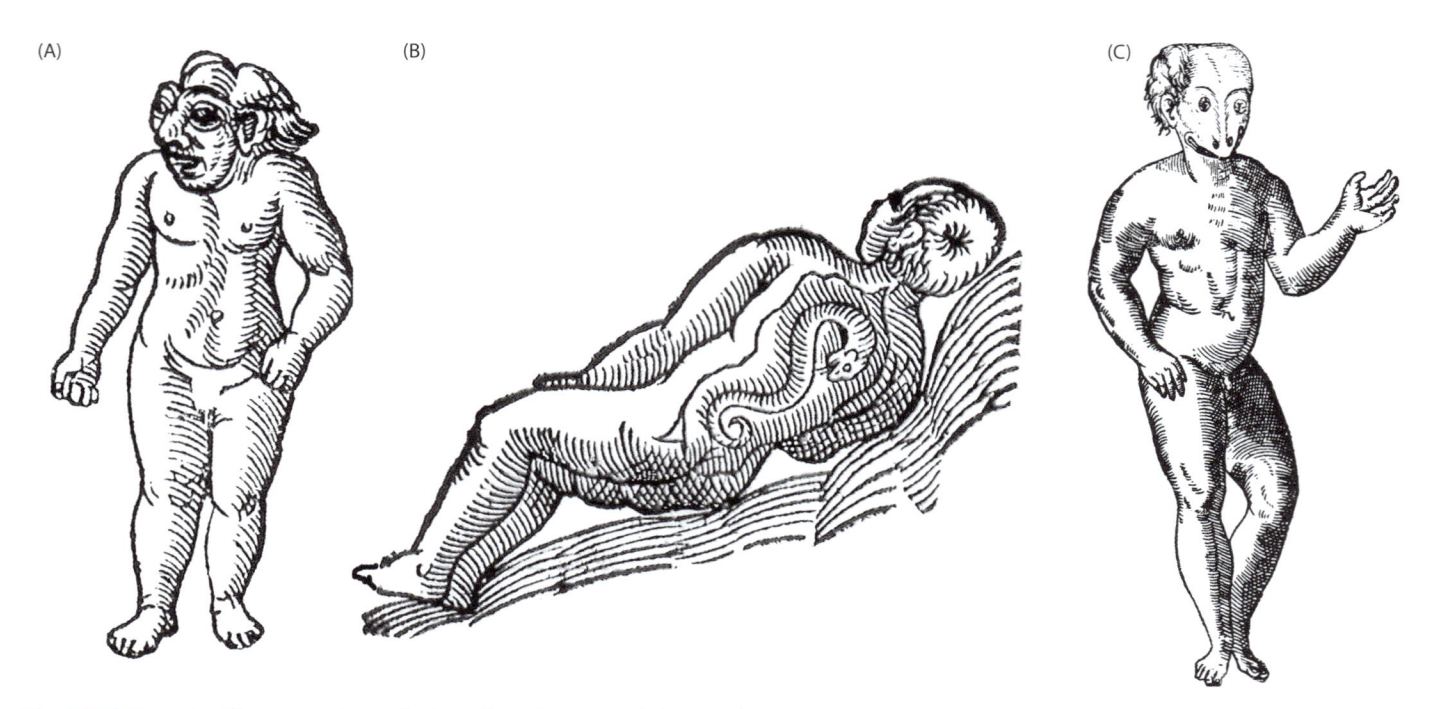

(A)   (B)   (C)

Fig. 5.1.2 Pre-scientific reports of neural tube defects: A, anencephaly: B, rachischisis interpreted as snake by Lycosthenes in 1557 [6]; C, frog-faced child depicted by Paré in 1575 [8]. See text for details.

women wear pendulous plaits and precious caps; which poor pregnant women observe enviously, and these may easily impress their form onto the head of the foetus.' The Paris surgeon Ambroise Paré reported the following case in 1573 [8]: '[Esme Petit, the father] figured that, his wife having a fever, one of her neighbor ladies advised her, in order to cure her fever, to take a live frog in her hand and to hold it until said frog should die. That night she went to bed with her husband, still having said frog in her hand; her husband and she embraced and she conceived; and by the power of her imagination, this monster had thus been produced' (Fig. 5.1.2C).

Imagination was also held responsible by the queen's surgeon Cosme Viardel [9] for an infant with 'a head very much similar to a fox head … The mother had gone to a puppet theatre in Saint Germain where she eagerly watched a puppet drummer with a fox's head; which she enjoyed so much that she crossed the *Pont Neuf* several times to satisfy her desire to observe the puppet extensively.'

The obstetrician William Smellie saw in London 'a child born, in which all the upper part of the skull was wanting' [10] and explained: 'Upon the ninth of April, 1747, when she was near two months gone with child, she was grievously frightened with thinking on Lord Lovat, who was that day to be beheaded. Her husband was gone to see the execution amongst the crowd on Tower Hill; and when the news came to her hearing, that a scaffolding was fallen down, by which accident many people were hurt, and some killed on the spot, she immediately feared that her husband might be of the number, and was greatly affected.' As late as 1899 the Berlin sexologist Ivan Bloch [11] reported a case where 'the husband returned from fishing with a frog on the fish-hook whose head was nibbled away by the fish … [the pregnant woman] was so frightened that she fainted. The infant delivered at term bore a head similar in all details to a frog's head.'

As early as 1716, Eustache Marcot, professor in Montpellier, doubted the role of imagination [12]: 'I ask what is this link and this close communication supposed between the mother's imagination and that of the fetus?' Other 18th century researchers who opposed the traditional idea of imagination were Albrecht von Haller and William Cooper [13]: 'The usually assigned cause of the mother's imagination is by no means equal to the manifold effects produced. And on the other hand, this injurious doctrine is pregnant with continual mischief to society. It frequently makes women very unhappy.' Likewise, Isidore Geoffroy Saint-Hilaire rejected the idea in his monumental *Histoire Générale* [14]: 'It is against all scientific data and reason to believe that an observed object feared or desired by the mother could ever, so to speak, paint itself onto the body of the infant she is carrying in her womb.'

Procreation by animals and devils

Human dignity was denied to severely malformed infants since antiquity, and the Roman *law of twelve tables* (450 B.C.E.) demanded: 'A dreadfully deformed child should be quickly killed' [15]. Superstition and religious passion characterized the 16th century. Among 13 causes of malformation, Ambroise Paré listed hereditary conditions and the womb's narrowness, but also imagination, God's glory, God's wrath, and demons and devils [8]. In 1275, three centuries prior to Europe's witch-craze, a woman named Angela de la Barthe was burned in Toulouse because she had given birth to a monster with a wolf's head and a serpent's tail. During the trial, she confessed [16], 'that she had had sexual intercourse with the devil in person and, since this monster, her own child, had fed on the flesh of children, she had been forced to kill other children'.

The question as to how the devil could create malformations was hard to answer. Not only printed leaflets had simple answers [17]: 'We Christians know that those deformations result from sinning and that Satan seeks manifold opportunities to stigmatize the magnificent works of natural childbirth.' Even the learned Paracelsus wrote in 1537 [18]: 'Thus the devil marks his infants by the mother's imagination, which she has due to evil lust, evil desire, and evil thoughts during conception … None of them is blessed, as they are not in God's image.' Before being charged in 1536, Anne Boleyn had supposedly given birth to a deformed boy who according to historian Retha Warnicke, Henry VIII saw as a sign of witchcraft and doomed marriage [19]. Marcot in 1716 mentioned the child as having been anencephalic [12] but the evidence is weak. Among many anencephalic infants in Zurich's Wick collection, a boy is described born on 8 August 1566 near Schmalkalden, in whom 'the mother was not frightened and also did not long for something according to pregnant women's habit … Without doubt God punishes with that [malformation] the world's exaggerated splendor and arrogance, which increase daily' [20]. Toads were the animals most associated with poison and witchcraft, and Jean Bodin, French philosopher and lawyer, noted in 1591 [21]: 'And while I am writing this, I am admonished that near the city of Laon, a woman conceived from a toad which the midwife and other women who attended the delivery frightfully, have testified; they brought the toad to the town hall; where many saw it and noticed that it did not resemble other toads.' Martin Schurig compiled over a dozen malformed infants published before 1732 to have been procreated by toads or frogs [22] and Ernest Martin in 1880 claimed Bartholin reported a woman who was burned having born a *cat-head* '*ob lasciviorum cum fele jocum*' [23]. The superstition was even exported to America: in the charge against Boston Quaker Mary Dyer the fact played a role that she had given birth to an anencephalic girl on 17 October 1637 [24]. Whereas malformed infants were frequently killed, the prosecution of women who had given birth to a child with neural tube seldom occurred.

Embryogenesis and neural tube

Fabricius ab Aquapendente anticipated the formation of the neural tube in 1612 [25]: 'If the spine, like a keel, is produced before other structures, it was a prime necessity that the spinal cord, too, should first be placed inside. But if the spinal cord must be formed before the spine and included within it, it was certainly fitting that the brain, which is the commencement of the spinal cord, should be fashioned earlier.' The microscope had been available since 1590; but to study embryogenesis, it was Marcello Malpighi in Bologna who used it extensively in 1672 [26]. Even if not mentioned explicitly in his text, Malpighi depicted a chicken embryo after 38 hours of incubation, which shows the neural tube and forebrain, midbrain, and hindbrain (Fig. 5.1.3A). In his 1759 dissertation *Theoria Generationis*, Caspar Friedrich Wolff explained the formation of the nervous system, providing a precise drawing of the neural tube

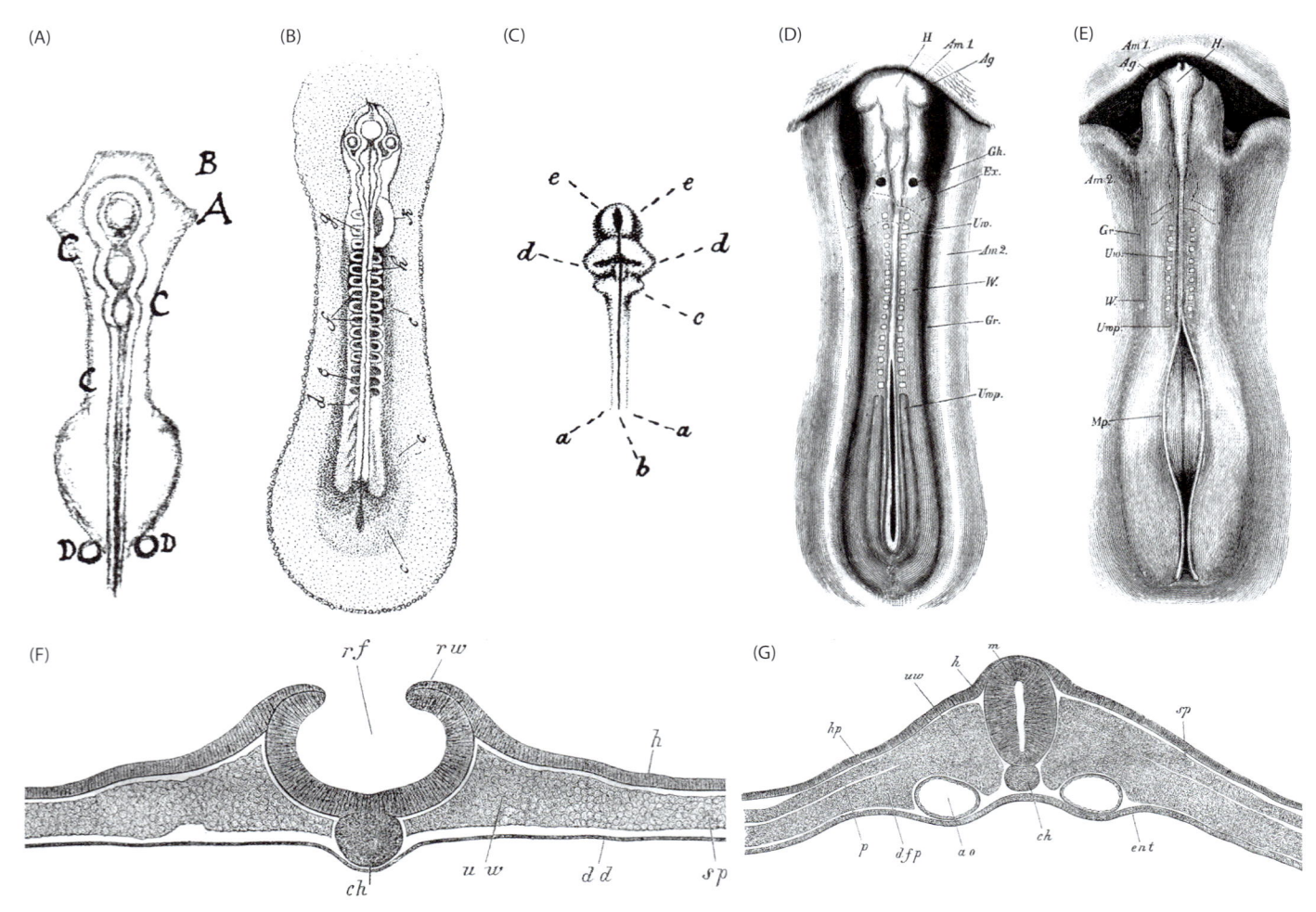

Fig. 5.1.3 Embryologic studies on neural tube closure: A: Malpighi's illustration of a 38-hour-old chicken embryo, 1672 [26]; B, chicken embryo after 36 hours of incubation, from Wolff's dissertation, 1759 [27]. C, Human embryo of the seventh week, from Tiedemann, 1816 [28]; D and E, chicken embryos, second day of breeding, from His [30]; F and G, transverse sections from chicken embryos on the end of the first and on the second day, from Kölliker 1861 [29].

(Fig. 5.1.3B) [27]. Friedrich Tiedemann described and depicted the neural tube in the human embryo (Fig. 5.1.3C) [28]. Malpighi and Wolff initiated the great debate in embryology—the controversy over whether the organs of the embryo are formed *de novo* at each generation (epigenesis), or whether the organs are already present, but in miniature form (preformation), within the egg (ovoists) or sperm (animalculists).

The anatomist Albert Kölliker had access to a high-quality microscope in Würzburg, demonstrating neural tube closure in 1861 on a cellular basis (Fig. 5.1.3F, G) [29]. Basel anatomist Wilhelm His assumed in 1874 [30] that the epidermis lateral to the neural plate expands actively and in doing so compresses the neural plate, making it change shape and buckle (Fig. 5.1.3D, E). He studied bending of sheets of many materials, including metal, clay, paper, cardboard, and complex laminates, in an effort to understand how lateral compression due to cell division leads to neural tube rolling and closure [31]. Otto Glaser, a biologist at Michigan University [32], proposed in 1916 that the rolling up of the neural plate into a tube was due to a greater uptake of water by the basal ends of the neural plate cells than at their apical ends. The resultant pressure and swelling would produce bottle-shaped cells of increased volume. Freiburg zoologists Hans Spemann and Hilde Mangold described in 1924 that the dorsal blastopore lip induces formation of the neural plate when transplanted to another embryo [33]. The last few decades have brought forth a host of genes responsible for the primary and secondary closure of different neural tube sites [34].

Teratology, genetics, and disruption

Like other *monsters*, neural tube defects were disenchanted when in the 18th century systematic collections were gathered by anatomists and the specimens, preserved in spirit, and passed from father to son enabled systematic study. Impressive collections were amassed by the families Geoffroy Saint-Hilaire in Paris, Vrolik in Amsterdam, and Meckel in Halle. Describing a case in Montpellier, Eustache Marcot pondered in 1716 [12]: 'This opening announces a hydrocephalic accumulation of waters in the brain ventricles, which when enlarged compressed the brain substance.' After describing eight anencephalic fetuses, Padovan anatomist Giambattista

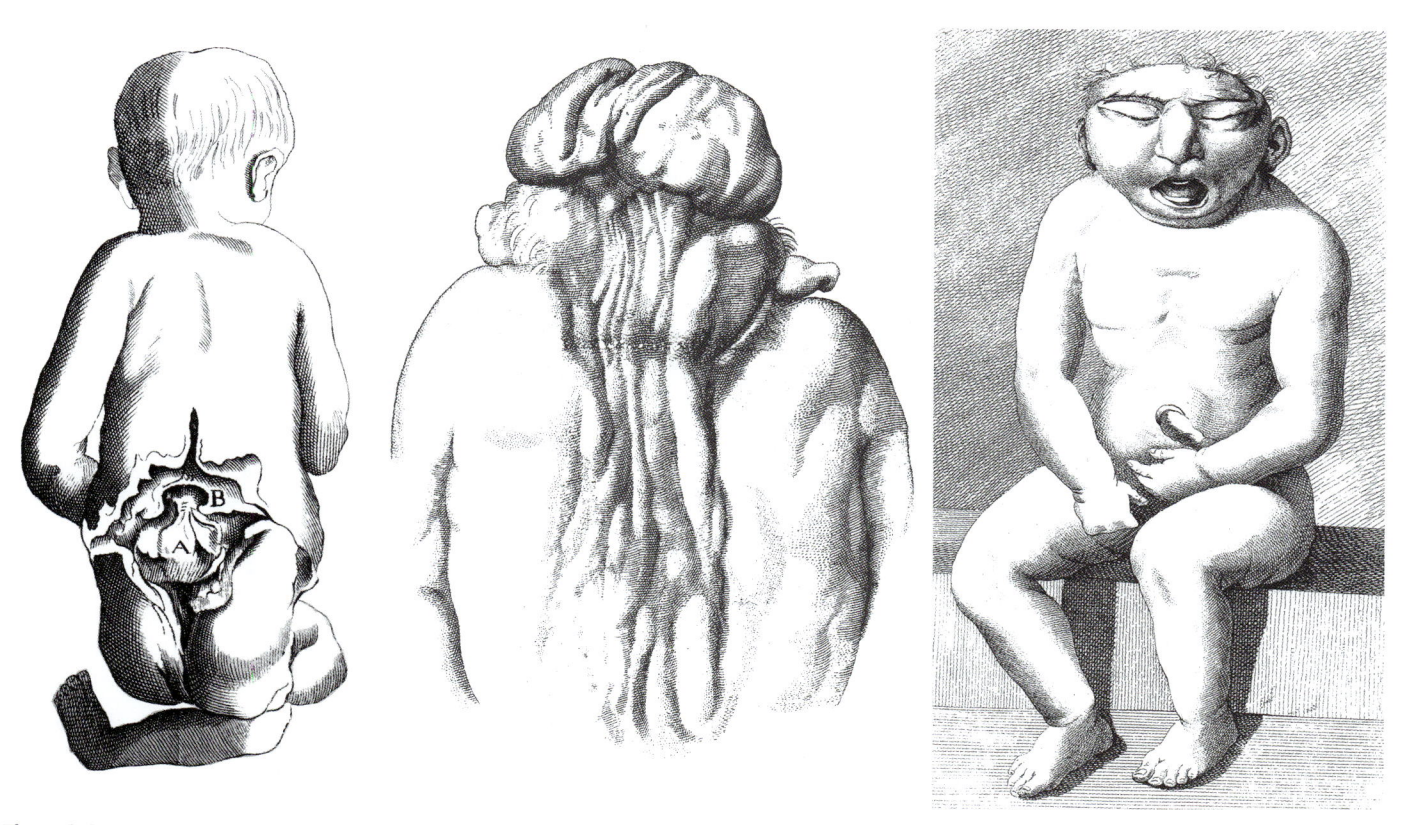

Fig. 5.1.4 Pioneer works on neural tube defects. Left: ruptured meningocele from Stalpart van der Wiel, 1682 [68]; centre: craniorachischisis from Denys, 1733 [69]; right: anencephalus published by Soemmerring, 1791 [36].

Morgagni suspected mechanical disruption in 1769: 'You perceive, that in this case, the cerebrum, medulla oblongata, and the greatest part of the cerebellum, were destroy'd by the hydrocephalus, the water of which had not yet universally flow'd out.' But, after another three case descriptions, he added [35]: 'What is then the case? ... I shall readily accuse chance if you please; but in some of the examples I shall rather accuse something else, which I confess I do not understand.'

Samuel Thomas Soemmerring, describing the anencephalics of the Kassel collection in 1791 [36] found it 'remarkable that most malformations of this type are female, as Morgagni noted correctly. One finds the absence of the brain associated with faults of the spine and spinal cord – "spina bifida" ... Even with malformations nature generally follows a specific order, determined sequence, and uniform pattern' (**Fig. 5.1.4**). Syndromally combined occipital encephalocele with polycystic kidneys and hexadactyly recurring in the same family was described by the Halle pathologist Johann Friedrich Meckel (the younger) in 1822 [37]. Present in virtually all neural tube defects, the herniation of cerebellar parts and the fourth ventricle through the enlarged foramen magnum, with subsequent hydrocephalus, was described by Ollivier d'Angers in 1824 [38] and rediscovered by Chiari, Cleland, and Arnold. The current view, indebted to Recklinghausen in 1886, is that anencephaly develops because the medulla plate remains open [39, 40]. During the 19th century, various neural tube defects were scientifically classified (**Fig. 5.1.5**) and the association with animals vanished. Identified teratogens include radiation, maternal hyperthermia, viral infections, and valproate. Timing for the latest occurrence is 20–22 days for craniorachischisis, 24 days for anencephaly, and 26 days for myelomeningocele [41]. A theory that neural tube overdistension is responsible for the dysraphic conditions was propagated by James Gardner in 1980 [42] and may explain parts of the amnion rupture sequence.

From epidemiology to folic acid deficiency

In addition to genetics, environmental interaction in causation was observed early and a nutritional hypothesis formulated by Meissner in 1844 [43]: 'The mother's poor nutrition and cachexia definitely exert an influence, especially a scrofulous and rachitic disposition: This can be the only explanation why a mother may repeatedly give birth to infants with this malformation [spina bifida].' Neural tube defects were more frequent in the lower class, and showed considerable seasonal variation [44]. In 1963, David Hewitt ascribed an incidence gradient across the US to 'differences in the average degree of inbreeding' [45]. Regional prevalence varied remarkably (**Fig. 5.1.6**), which according to Paris geneticist Jean Frézal in 1964 [46], 'implies the necessary intervention of environmental agents, deleterious or favorable, to explain the occurrence of the malformation in the predisposed child ... it seems very remarkable that folic acid deficiency as well as other teratogens in pregnant animals provoke a series of defects comparable with anencephaly'.

Epidemiologic studies accumulated in the British Isles, which were most seriously tormented by neural tube defects (**Fig. 5.1.6**) [47]. In addition, epidemics were recorded in England and the US during the Depression from 1929 to 1932 [48] and in post-war

PART 5 Odd shape

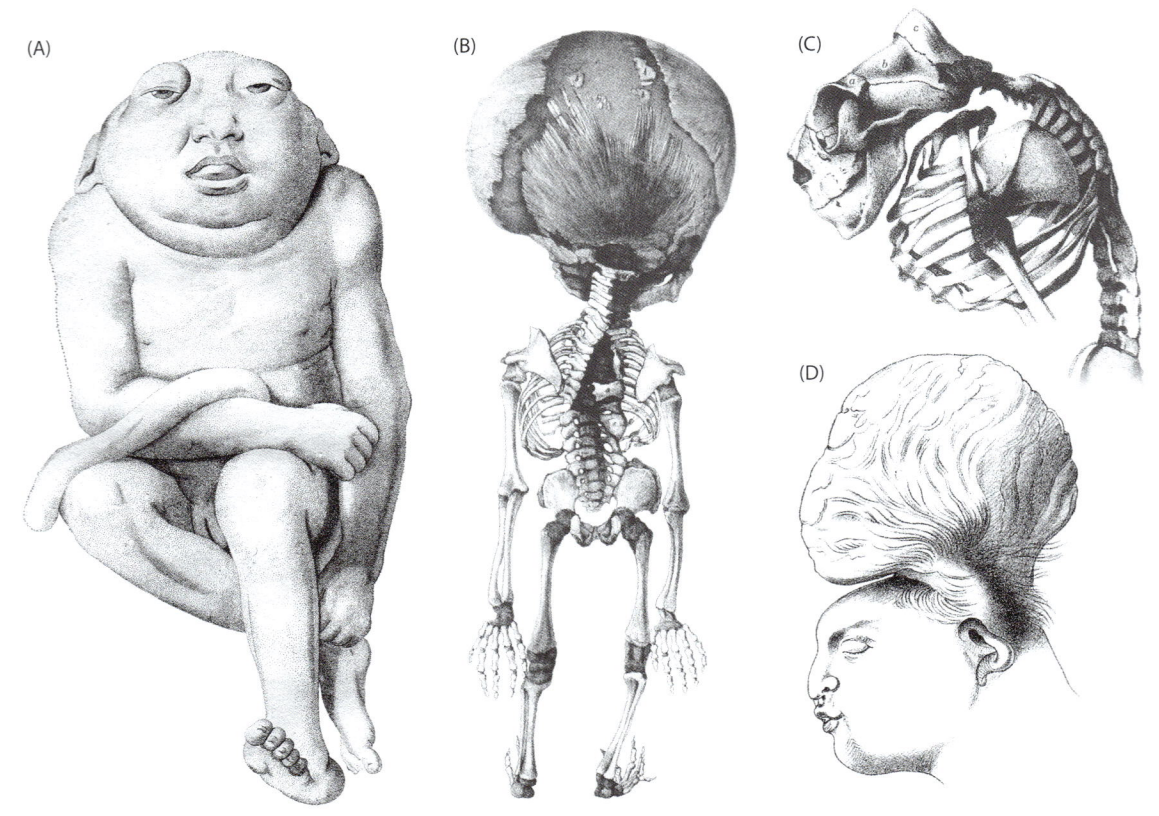

Fig. 5.1.5 Research in the 19th century: A, anencephalus ('Frog-head') from Busch 1817; B, spina bifida with hydrocephalus and C, anencephalus ('Cat-head'), both from Vrolik 1844 [70]; D, occipital encephalocele from Ahlfeld 1882 [71].

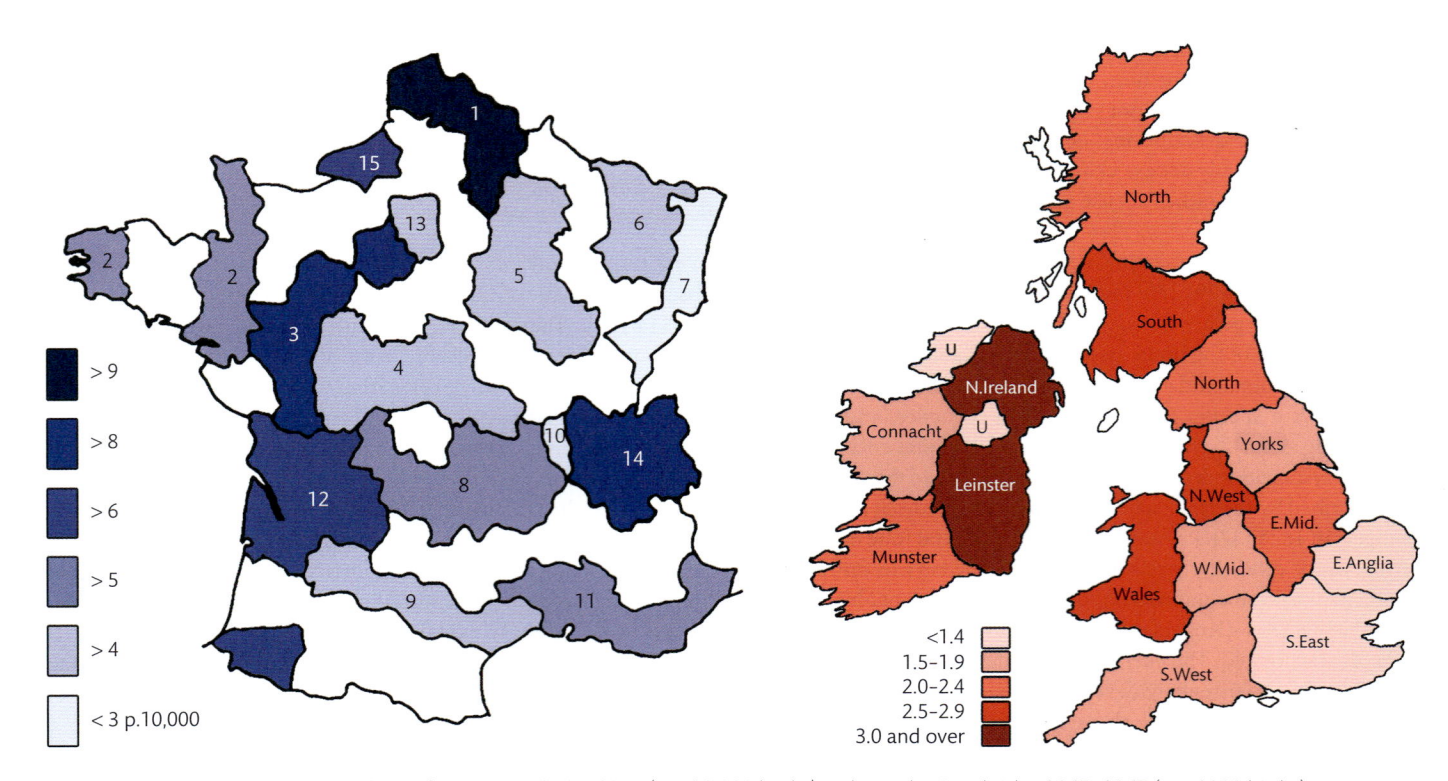

Fig. 5.1.6 Incidence of anencephalus. Left: in France 1945–1955 (per 10,000 births); right: in the British Isles 1965–1967 (per 1000 births).
Source: Data from Frézal, J., Kelley, J., Guillemot, M.L., Lamy, M. Anencephaly in France. *Am J Human Genetics* 1964;16:336–350; Data from Elwood, J.H. Anencephalus in the British Isles. *Develop Med Child Neurol* 1970;12:582–595.

Germany [49]. Regional and seasonal variations in the incidence of anencephaly casted suspicion on environmental determinants. The suspicion fell on white bread, cereals, canned peas, and cured meats as 'toxins' and on cheese, meat, and apples as 'protective' [50]. A study of the traditional British beverage led Oxford epidemiologist Jean Fedrick 1974 to the conclusion [51]: 'Women who had given birth to anencephalic stillbirths were significantly more likely to drink 3 or more cups of tea per day, but only if they resided in high or medium incidence areas.' When James Renwick proposed the potato-hypothesis in 1972 [52], a controlled trial in high-risk pregnancies was performed in Belfast, which failed to show a benefit when potato consumption was avoided [53].

Folic acid entered the stage when Lucy Wills, a London haematologist doing research in India in the late 1920s, found the yeast extract Marmite effective in preventing macrocytic anaemia in pregnancy [54]. The vitamin received its name after being isolated from spinach leaves [55], was synthesized in 1945 [56], and was used to treat megaloblastic anaemias of all types. Shortly thereafter, the anti-folates aminopterin and methotrexate were developed to treat leukaemias and other malignancies [57]. But the teratogenic principle remained elusive. The breakthrough occurred in Liverpool, where paediatrician Richard Smithells set up a registry of congenital malformations in 1959 [58]. In the same city, gynaecologist Bryan Hibbard studied pregnant women 'of social classes four and five … living in overcrowded conditions in old back-to-back houses … unemployed … dietary standards generally poor' in 1961, and found 'defective folic acid metabolism in one of ten pregnancies … It is probable that defective folic acid metabolism is responsible for a certain number of abortions and foetal malformations' [59]. Folic acid metabolism and its role in neural tube closure were thereafter intensely studied and are shown in Fig. 5.1.7. Low folate leads to elevated homocysteine. Both low maternal folate intake and disturbed metabolism may diminish methylenetetrahydrofolate reductase activity [60]. Neural tube defects are associated with autoantibodies to the folate receptor [61] and with polymorphisms of methylenetetrahydrofolate reductase associated with hyperhomocysteinaemia. It remains unclear whether direct toxicity of homocysteine or insufficient methylation of crucial metabolites is the causative mechanism. Wang and colleagues in 2010 found diminished methylation of genomic DNA and interspersed nucleotides of aborted fetuses with cephalic malformations [62] suggesting 'that disturbed one-carbon unit metabolism could have a deleterious effect on DNA methylation during pregnancy'. The presence of a highly methylated second X chromosome in all cells may also explain the higher incidence of neural tube defects in female fetuses [63].

Nutritional prevention, success, and failure

Smithells and colleagues performed a controlled trial in five British centres in 1980 with a multivitamin preparation containing 0.35 mg folic acid per day in women who had already given birth to infants with neural tube defects [64]: 'One of 178 infants/fetuses of fully supplemented mothers (0.6%) had a neural tube defect, compared with 13 of 260 infants/fetuses of unsupplemented mothers.' A large trial by the Medical Research Council demonstrated that 75% of neural tube defects could be prevented by folate supplementation [65], and a Hungarian trial showed that periconceptional vitamin supplementation including 0.8 mg of folic acid per day was beneficial for women who had not given birth to a malformed infant before: the incidence of all malformation was reduced from 23 to 13 per 1000, and no neural tube defects occurred in the supplemented group of 2052 deliveries [66]. Meta-analyses showed an odds ratio of 0.21 (0.12–0.36) for recurrence and of 0.58 (0.41–0.74) for occurrence of neural tube defects [61]. Consequently, most governments recommend folate supplementation during pregnancy. However, as

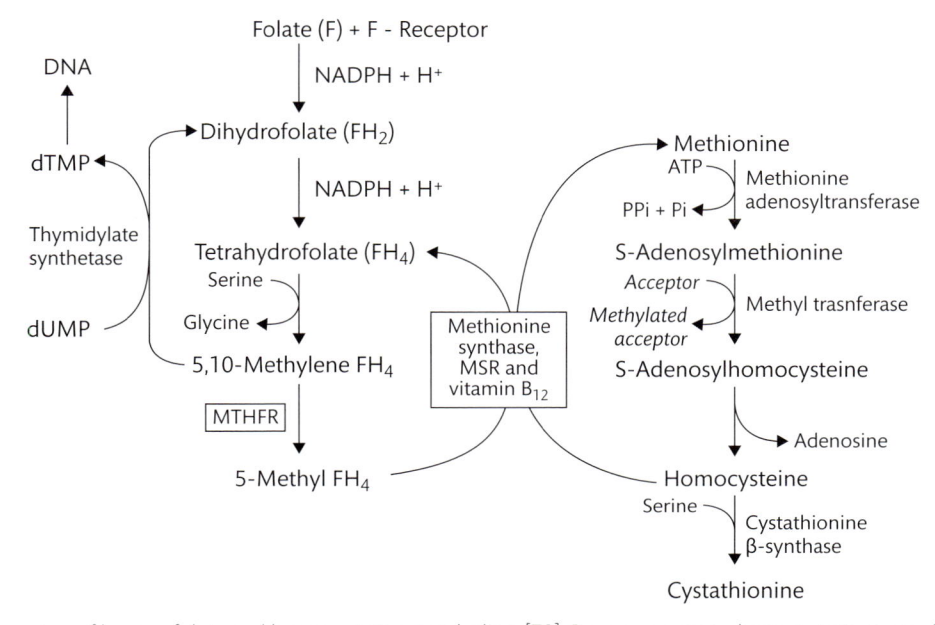

Fig. 5.1.7 Simplified overview of human folate and homocysteine metabolism [72]. Boxes: enzymes whose mutations may lead to neural tube defects. MSR, methionine synthase reductase; MTHFR, methylene tetrahydrofolate reductase.
Source: Data from Zetterberg, H. Methylenetetrahydrofolate reductase and transcobalamin genetic polymorphisms in human spontaneous abortion. *Reprod Biol Endocrinol*. 2004;2:1–8.

half of all pregnancies occur unplanned and most women do not realize that they must take folic acid *before* becoming pregnant, it is no wonder that most recommendations have failed to reduce the prevalence of neural tube defects. Some countries, among them the US, Canada, Australia, and Chile, proceeded to supplement staple foods such as wheat, cereals, or bread, which reduced the prevalence of neural tube defects by 30–70%. Most European countries, despite notoriously low folate intakes, opted not to fortify foods, maintaining high rates of neural tube defects [67] and leaving the problem to the gynaecologists, who terminate most of these pregnancies following prenatal diagnosis. The public debate has included objections by health professionals as well as irrational fears all too familiar from discussions about iodine to prevent goitre or vitamin D to prevent rickets.

Conclusion: problems unsolved

Despite extensive research, neural tube defects continue to challenge us by their complex pathogenesis and difficult prevention and treatment. They display features of genetic disease, vitamin deficiency, embryotoxicity, and mechanical disruption. Theoretically speaking, two-thirds could be prevented by the periconceptional intake of folic acid. The failure to standardize the intake of this vitamin during the critical phase of neural tube closure reveals the limits of public health education.

REFERENCES

1. Panofsky E: Studies in iconology. New York: Harper & Row, 1972: p. 95–129.
2. Passalacqua J: Catalogue raisonné et historique des antiquités découvertes en Égypte. Paris: Galerie d'Antiquités Égyptiennes, 1826: p. 21, 148.
3. Geoffroy Saint-Hilaire É: Communication faite a l'Académie Royale des Sciences, dans sa séance du 9 janvier 1826. Arch Gen Med 1826;série **1**:124–6.
4. Temkin O: Soranus' Gynecology. Baltimore, MD: The Johns Hopkins Press, 1956: Book II, p. 107, 113–22.
5. Lemay HR: Women's secrets. New York: State University of New York Press, 1992: p. 105.
6. Lycosthenes C: Wunderwerck oder Gottes unergründliches Vorbilden. Basel: Petrus, 1557: p. 359, 509.
7. Bartholin T: Historiarum anatomicarum rariorum Centuria V–VI. Hafniae: Hauboldt, 1661: p. 357.
8. Paré A: On monsters and marvels (Paris, 1573). Chicago, IL: University of Chicago Press, 1982: p. 42, fig. 28.
9. Viardel C: Anmerckungen von der weiblichen Geburt (1st French ed. 1671). Franckfurt: Zubrodt, 1676: p. 140.
10. Smellie W: A treatise on the theory and practise of midwifery (London, 1752). London: New Sydenham Society, 1876: Vol. **3**, case 422, p. 215.
11. Welsenburg Gv: Das Versehen der Frauen in Vergangenheit und Gegenwart. Leipzig: Barsdorf, 1899: p. 151.
12. Marcot E: Mémoire sur un enfant monstrueux. Hist Acad Roy Soc Sci Paris 1716;**329**, 342.
13. Cooper W: An account of an extraordinary acephalous birth. Phil Trans 1775;**65**:311–21.
14. Geoffroy Saint-Hilaire I: Histoire générale et particulière des anomalies de l'organisation chez l'homme et les animaux. Paris: Baillière, 1832: Vol. **3**, p. 391.
15. Scott SP: The civil law: Including the twelve tables, the institutes of Gaius … Cincinnati: Central Trust, 1932: Vol. **1**, p. Art.1.
16. Lewinsohn R: A history of sexual customs. New York: Longmans, 1958: p. 129.
17. Holländer E: Wunder, Wundergeburt und Wundergestalt in Einblattdrucken des fünfzehnten bis achtzehnten Jahhunderts. Stuttgart: Enke, 1921: p. 321.
18. Paracelsus: De natura rerum (Villach 1537). München: Oldenbourg, 1928: Vol. **11**, p. 316.
19. Warnicke RM: The fall of Anne Boleyn revisited. Engl Hist Rev 1993;**108**:653–65.
20. Sonderegger A: Missgeburten und Wundergestalten in Einblattdrucken und Handzeichnungen des 16. Jahrhunderts. Zürich: Orell Füssli, 1927: p. 70.
21. Bodin J: Vom ausgelasnen wütigen Teuffelsheer. Graz: Akademische Druck- und Verlagsanstalt, 1973: p. 141.
22. Schurig M: Embryologia historico-medica. Dresden & Leipzig: Hekel, 1732: p. 657–62.
23. Martin E: Histoire des monstres depuis l'antiquité jusqu' a nos jours (orig. ed. 1880.) Grenoble: Millon, 2002: p. 84.
24. Winthrop J: The history of New England (Winthrop's journal 1630–1649). New York: Scribner, 1908: p. 19.
25. Adelmann HB: The embryological treatises of Hieronimus Fabricius of Aquapendente. Ithaca, NY: Cornell University Press, 1942: Vol. **1**, p. 201.
26. Adelmann HB: Marcello Malpighi and the evolution of Embryology. **5** vols. New York: Cornell, 1966: p. 951; plate II, fig. 11.
27. Wolff CF: Theorie von der Generation in zwei Abhandlungen erklärt und bewiesen (Theoria Generationis, 1759). Hildesheim: Olms, 1966: p. Tab. II, fig. 5.
28. Tiedemann F: Anatomie und Bildungsgeschichte des Gehirns im Foetus des Menschen. Nürnberg: Stein, 1816: p. Tab. I, fig. 3.
29. Kölliker A: Entwicklungsgeschichte des Menschen und der höheren Tiere. Leipzig: Engelmann, 1861: p. 46–51.
30. His W: Unsere Körperform und das physiologische Problem ihrer Enstehung. Leipzig: Vogel, 1874: p. 12.
31. His W: Über mechanische Grundvorgänge thierischer Formbildung. Arch Anat Physiol Wiss Med Anat Abth **1894**: 1–80.
32. Glaser OC: The theory of autonomous folding in embryogenesis. Science 1916;**44**:505–9.
33. Spemann H, Mangold H: Über Induktion von Embryonalanlagen durch Implantation artfremder Organisatoren. [Roux Arch] Dev Genes Evol 1924;**100**:599–638.
34. Copp AJ, Greene ND, Murdoch JN: The genetic basis of mammalian neurulation. Nat Rev Genet 2003;**4**:784–93.
35. Morgagni GB: The seats and causes of diseases investigated by anatomy. London: Millar, Cadell, Johnson and Payne, 1769: Letter XLVIII, art. 54.
36. Soemmerring ST: Abbildungen und Beschreibungen einiger Misgeburten. Mainz: Kurfürstl. Universitätsbuchhandlung, 1791: Tab. I.
37. Meckel JF: Beschreibung zweier durch sehr ähnliche Bildungsabweichung entstellter Geschwister. Dtsch Arch Physiol 1822;**7**:99–176.
38. Ollivier (d'Angers) CP: De la moelle épinière et de ses maladies. 2. ed. Paris: Crevot, 1824: Vol. **1**, p. 123, plate I.

39. Recklinghausen Fv: Untersuchungen über die Spina Bifida. [Teil 3]. Arch Path Anat Physiol Klin Med 1886;**105**:373–455.
40. Recklinghausen Fv: Untersuchungen über die Spina Bifida. [Teil 2]. Arch Path Anat Physiol Klin Med 1886;**105**:296–330.
41. Lemire RJ, Loeser JD, Leech RW, Alvord EC: Normal and abnormal development of the human nervous system. Hagerstown, MD: Harper & Row, 1975.
42. Gardner WJ, Breuer AC: Anomalies of heart, spleen, kidneys, gut, and limbs may result from an overdistended neural tube: a hypothesis. Pediatrics 1980;**65**:508–14.
43. Meissner FL: Die Kinderkrankheiten nach den neusten Ansichten und Erfahrungen. 3. ed. Leipzig: Fest, 1844: Vol. **1**, p. 303.
44. Edwards JH: Congenital malformations of the central nervous system in Scotland. Brit J Prev Soc Med 1958;**12**:115–30.
45. Hewitt D: Geographical variations in the mortality attributed to spina bifida and other congenital malformations. Br J Prev Soc Med 1963;**17**:13–22.
46. Frezal J, Kelley J, Guillemot ML, Lamy M: Anencephaly in France. Am J Hum Genet 1964;**16**:336–50.
47. Elwood JH: Anencephalus in the British Isles. Develop Med Child Neurol 1970;**12**:582–95.
48. MacMahon B, Yen S: Unrecognised epidemic of anencephaly and spina bifida. Lancet 1971;**1**:31–3.
49. Leck I: Causation of neural tube defects: clues from epidemiology. Br Med Bull 1974;**30**:158–63.
50. Knox EG: Anencephalus and dietary intakes. Br J Prev Soc Med 1972;**26**:219–23.
51. Fedrick J: Anencephalus and maternal tea drinking. Proc R Soc Med 1974;**67**:356–60.
52. Renwick JH: Hypothesis: anencephaly and spina bifida are usually preventable by avoidance of a specific but unidentified substance present in certain potato tubers. Br J Prev Soc Med 1972;**26**:67–88.
53. Nevin NC, Merrett JD: Potato avoidance during pregnancy in women with a previous infant with either anencephaly and/or spina bifida. Br J Prev Soc Med 1975;**29**:111–5.
54. Wills L: Treatment of "pernicious anaemia of pregnancy" and "tropical anaemia" with special reference to yeast extract as a curative agent. BMJ 1931;**1**:1059–64.
55. Mitchell HK, Snell EE, Williams RJ: The concentration of "folic acid". J Am Chem Soc 1941;**63**:2284.
56. Angier RB, Boothe JH, Hutchings BL, et al.: Synthesis of a compound identical with the L. Casei factor isolated from liver. Science 1945;**102**:227–8.
57. Farber S, Diamond LK: Temporary remissions in acute leukemia in children produced by folic acid antagonist, 4-aminopteroyl-glutamic acid. N Engl J Med 1948;**238**:787–93.
58. Smithells RW: The Liverpool congenital abnormalities registry. Dev Med Child Neurol 1962;**4**:320–4.
59. Hibbard BM: The role of folic acid in pregnancy. J Obstet Gynaecol Br Commonw 1964;**71**:529–42.
60. Blom HJ, Shaw GM, den Heijer M, Finnell RH: Neural tube defects and folate: case far from closed. Nat Rev Neurosci 2006;**7**: 724–31.
61. Blom HJ: Folic acid, methylation and neural tube closure in humans. Birth Defects Res A Clin Mol Teratol 2009;**85**:295–302.
62. Wang L, Wang F, Guan J, et al.: Relation between hypomethylation of long interspersed nucleotide elements and risk of neural tube defects. Am J Clin Nutr 2010;**91**:1359–67.
63. Gelineau-van Waes J, Finnell RH: Genetics of neural tube defects. Semin Pediatr Neurol 2001;**8**:160–4.
64. Smithells RW, Sheppard S, Schorah CJ, et al.: Possible prevention of neural-tube defects by periconceptional vitamin supplementation. Lancet 1980;**1**:339–40.
65. MRC Vitamin Study Research Group: Prevention of neural tube defects. Lancet 1991;**338**:131–7.
66. Czeizel AE, Dudas I: Prevention of the first occurrence of neural-tube defects by periconceptional vitamin supplementation. N Engl J Med 1992;**327**:1832–5.
67. Busby A, Abramsky L, Dolk H, et al.: Preventing neural tube defects in Europe: a missed opportunity. Reprod Toxicol 2005;**20**: 393–402.
68. Stalpart van der Wiel C: Observationum rariorum medic. anatomic. chirurgicarum centuria prior. Leidae: apud Johannem a Kerkhem, 1727: Vol. **2**, p. 369, tab. 9.
69. Denys J: Verhandelingen over het ampt der vroed-meesters, en vroed-vrouwen. Leyden: Wishoff, Juriaan, 1733: fig. 2.
70. Vrolik W: Tabulae ad illustrandam embryogenesin hominis et mammalium. Amsterdam: Londonck, 1844–1849: p. tab. 39, 43.
71. Ahlfeld F: Die Missbildungen des Menschen. Atlas. Leipzig: Grunow, 1882: Vol. **1**, plate 43.

5.2

In God's image?
The tradition of infant head shaping

Introduction

Instead of admiring nature's work and the beauty of an infant's head, humans of all cultures have sought to improve it. As the rapidly growing neonatal skull is malleable due to open sutures, compression during the first months of life results in a deviant head shape. Various shapes were fashionable in different eras and regions, and different shapes were sometimes in use in the same region at the same time. Frequent practices were repeated uniform hand massage, anterior–posterior compression by plates or pads, and circumferential binding of the vault with textiles or wooden boards.

Prehistoric peoples

Before being forced into extinction by his cleverer contemporary, *Homo neanderthalensis* deformed his offspring's skulls around 45,000 B.C.E., as evident in the Shanidar 1 man in Iraq [1]. The Neanderthals' crania fuelled the debate, if they were to be considered *Homo sapiens* at all [2]. Peking men shaped the head in 30,000 B.C.E. [3], as did Palaeolithic *Homo sapiens*, prior to domesticating plants, taming animals, and melting metals: the mother's hand probably modified neonatal skulls, as shown in the Australian Nacurrie [4]. During the Neolithic period, head shaping was widespread in the Middle East [5, 6], and in the Andean regions of present-day Peru and Chile [7, 8] (Fig. 5.2.1). The absence of written history prohibits speculation regarding the motives for this practice.

Antique cultures

In the Nile valley, head shaping was uncommon during the 18th dynasty (1350 B.C.E.). As modified skulls are rare among Egyptian mummies, there is doubt that Akhenaton and his daughters (Fig. 5.2.2) had deformed skulls, their head shape being a manneristic symbol, or symptom of acromegaly [9]; the girls may be shown wearing a lateral hair plait with a clasp and not a circumferential bandage [10]. The Hippocratic book *De Aere, Aquis et Locis* recounted in the 5th century B.C.E. [11]: 'Now I will treat of those [living near the Maeotian Lake] and, first, concerning the Macrocephali. There is no other race of men which have heads in the least resembling theirs. At first, usage was the principal cause of the length of their head, but now nature cooperates with usage. They think those the most noble who have the longest heads. It is thus with regard to the usage: immediately after the child is born, and while its head is still tender, they fashion it with their hands, and constrain it to assume a lengthened shape by applying bandages and other suitable contrivances whereby the spherical form of the head is destroyed, and it is made to increase in length.' The ancient Maeotian lake is now called the Sea of Azov, and in Crimea and north of the Caucasus, antique skulls were indeed found which had been deformed by bands [12]. The obstetrician Soranus of Ephesus warned in 115 C.E. [13]: 'Then one must lay the newborn down, but not on something hard and resistant as do the Thracians and Macedonians who tie down the newborn on a level board, so that the part around the neck and the back of the head may be flattened.'

In pre-Columbian America, head shaping was extensively practised, especially among the literate elite. Olmecs [14] and Maya [15] regarded a longitudinal head as proof of noble birth and maximum beauty, especially in males [16]. In the Peruvian Paracas culture, Virchow described 'large cemeteries where one must go to great lengths to find a single normally shaped skull' [17]. The Incas used various types of shaping to distinguish between coexisting sociocultural groups [18]. The Merovingians, a Salian Frankish dynasty inhabiting ancient Gaul from the 5th to the 8th century C.E., used circular head binding to produce longheads [19].

Early modern age

On Friday, 12 October 1492, Christopher Columbus landed on 'a small island, one of the Lucayos, called in the Indian language Guanahani'. The next day, he recorded in his diary [20]: 'At daybreak great multitudes of men came to the shore, all young and of fine shapes, very handsome; their hair not curled but straight and coarse like horsehair, and all with foreheads and heads much broader than any people I had hitherto seen; their eyes were large and very beautiful.'

PART 5 Odd shape

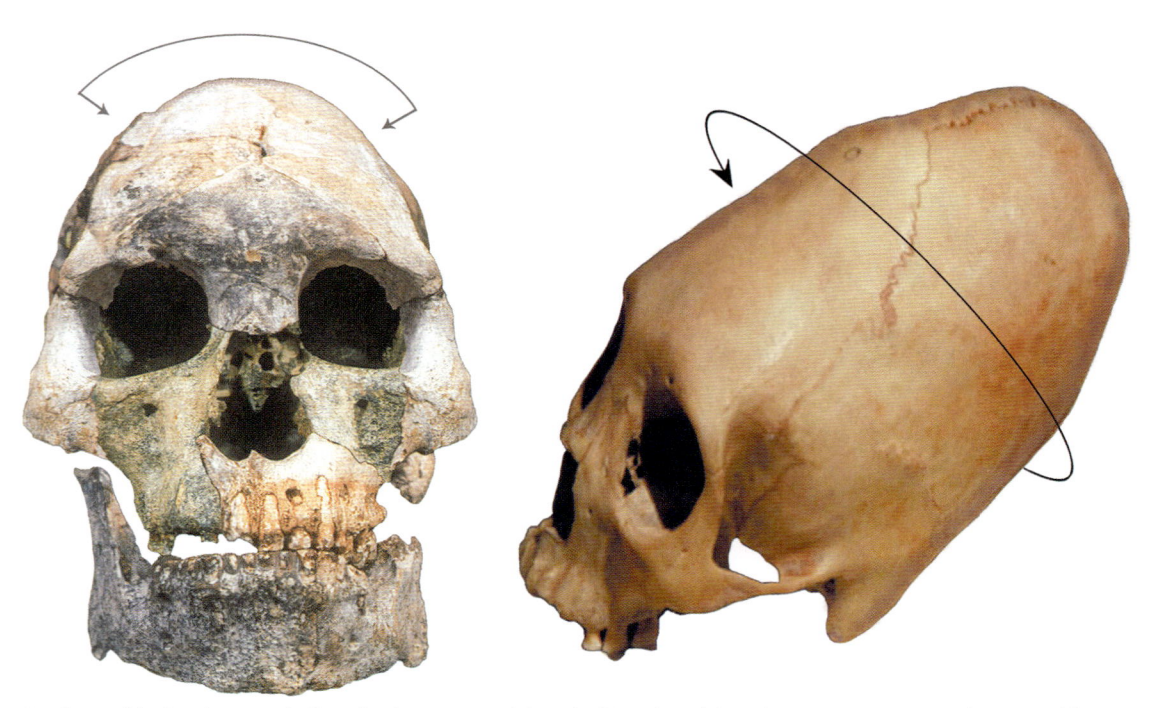

Fig. 5.2.1 Artificially modified prehistoric skulls. Left: Pleistocene adult male (9000 b.c.e.) found near Nacurrie, Australia. Frontal flattening and high parietal curve due to postnatal compression [4]. Right: annular type in a Neolithic Central Andean longhead resulted from circular binding (600 b.c.e.); found in the Paracas region, modified from an exponate in the Museo Regional de Ica, Peru.
Source: Data from Brown, P. Nacurrie 1: Mark of ancient Java, or a caring mother's hands, in terminal Pleistocene Australia? *J Hum Evol* 2010;59:168–87.

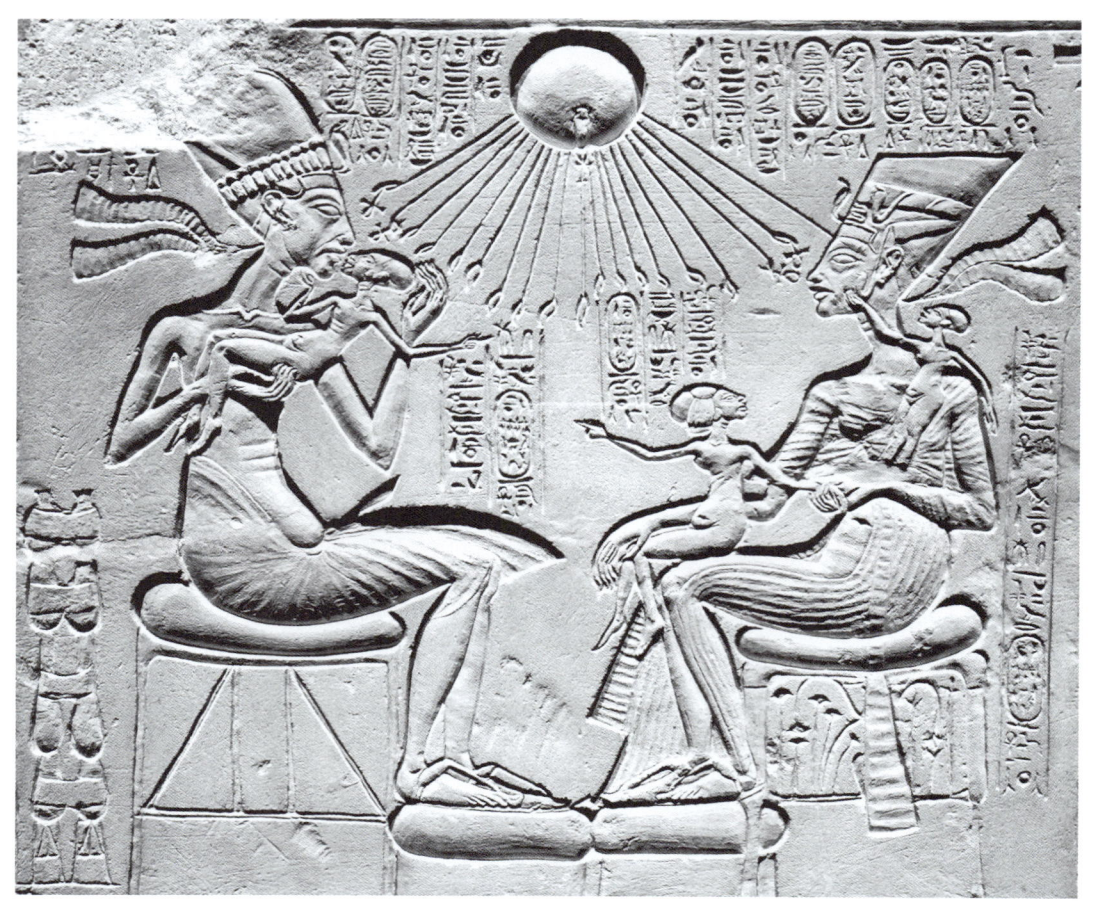

Fig. 5.2.2 Egypt, Amarna culture, 18th dynasty (1350 b.c.e.): Pharaoh Akhenaton (left), Queen Nefertiti (right), and three of their daughters worshiping the sun-god Aton [58].

The few Aztecs, Maya, and Incas who survived the *conquista* and the smallpox, continued to modify their infants' skulls. Pavia professor Girolamo Cardano described the American Indian techniques of head shaping in 1558 and listed among the areas of use Chicora (Pennsylvania), Cuba, Mexico, Cumaná (Venezuela), Porto Velho (Brazil), and Peru [21]. During the third Mexican Council held in Lima on 17 July 1585, the church decided to ban and punish head shaping [22]: 'The Indians should not deform their infants' heads with devices: We wish to exstirpate this abusive and superstitious practice, by which the Indians everywhere deform their infants' heads and which they call themselves *caito*, *oma*, *opalta*; as well as certain fashions of designing, shaving, and extracting the head hair with unguents, which are superstitions worthy of remedy. Therefore we decide and decree that any Indian who does such activity, if he is a chief or *cacique*, or an aristocrat, must serve in the church close to his residence for ten days for the first vice, and for twenty days for the second. And for the third vice he shall be reported and presented to the province vicar. A commoner shall suffer twenty strokes for the first vice, twice that many for the second, and for the third, he shall be informed upon and presented to the vicar mentioned.' The ecclesiastical ban was unsuccessful, as travellers and scientists described or depicted the custom extensively well into the 19th century [23, 24]; they also collected skulls, many of which ended in the *Crania Americana* collection in Philadelphia. Influenced by Gall's *Phrenology*, Samuel George Morton linked skull shape with intelligence and character traits. His ideas evolved into bizarre theories of human races, which should have expired 20 years later with Darwin's book. Morton derived a classification of skull shapes from craniometric measurements, even though he was aware of artificial head shaping [25]: 'The Wallamet Indians place the infant, soon after birth, upon a board, to the edges of which are attached little loops of hempen cord or leather, and other similar cords are passed across and back, in a zigzag manner, through these loops, enclosing the child and binding it firmly down. To the upper edge of this board, in which is a depression to receive the back part of the head, another smaller one is attached by hinges of leather, and made to lie obliquely upon the forehead; the force of the pressure being regulated by several strings attached to its edge, which are passed through holes in the board upon which the infant is lying, and secured there.'

Toronto painter Paul Kane spent 4 years travelling among the American Indians in the Northwest, describing and depicting their lives [24]: 'The Chinooks and Cowlitz carry the custom of flattening the head to a greater extent than any other of the Flathead tribes ... The Indian mothers all carry their infants strapped to a piece of board covered with moss or loose fibres of cedar bark, and in order to flatten the head they place a pad on the infant's forehead, on the top of which is laid a piece of smooth bark, bound on by a leathern band passing through holes in the board on either side, and kept tightly pressed across the front of the head, a sort of pillow of grass or cedar fibres being placed under the back of the neck to support it. This process commences with the birth of the infant, and is continued for eight to twelve months, by which time the head has lost its natural shape, and acquired that of a wedge: the front of the skull flat and higher at the crown, giving it a most unnatural appearance [Fig. 5.2.3, left] ... I have never heard the infants crying or moaning, although I have seen the eyes seemingly starting out of the sockets from the great pressure ... This unnatural operation does

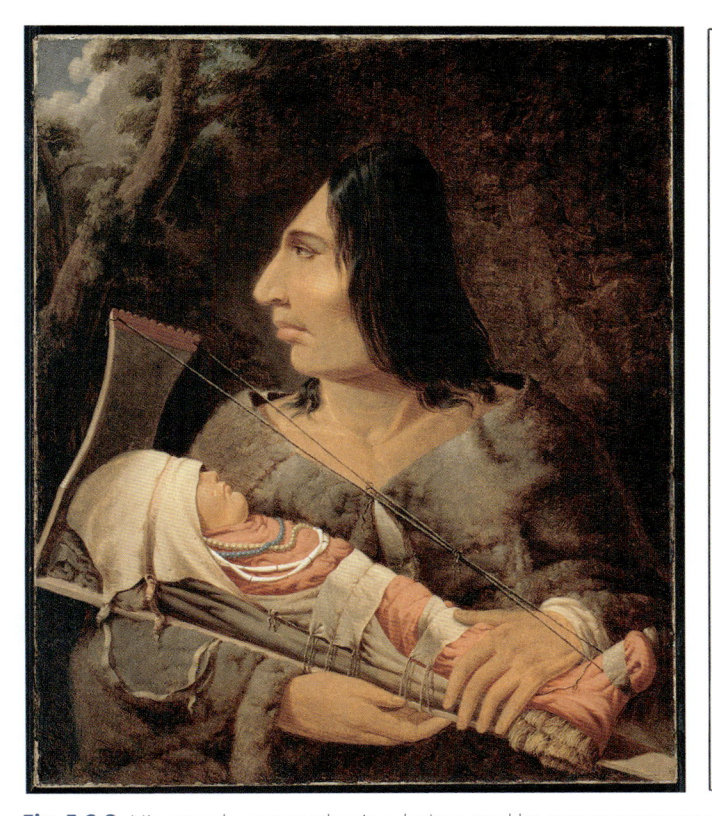

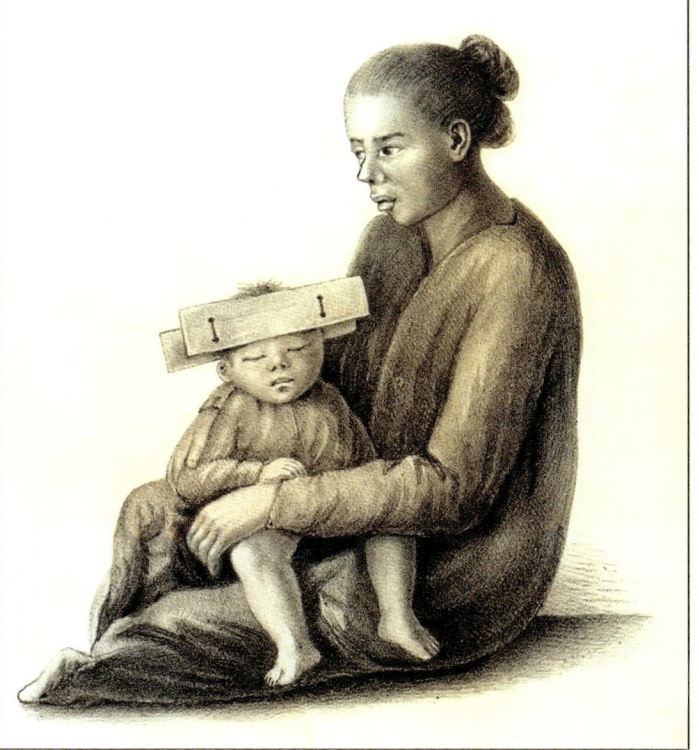

Fig. 5.2.3 Nineteenth-century shaping devices used by contemporaneous natives. Left: Caw Wacham, Chinook Indians, northwestern US. Right: Northern Sulawesi, Indonesia; from Riedel 1871 [27].
Left, Paul Kane, Mallow, Ireland, 1810—Toronto 1871, Caw-Wacham, About 1848, oil on canvas, 75.7 × 63.2 cm, The Montreal Museum of Fine Arts, Purchase, William Gilman Cheney Bequest, Photo MMFA, Christine Guest.

not, however, seem to injure the health, the mortality amongst the Flathead children not being perceptibly greater than amongst other Indian tribes; nor does it seem to injure their intellect. On the contrary, the Flatheads are generally considered fully as intelligent as the surrounding tribes, who allow their heads to preserve their natural shape, and it is from amongst the round heads that the Flatheads take their slaves, looking with contempt even upon the white for having round heads, the flat head being considered as the distinguishing mark of freedom.'

Initially, cradleboards may have enabled breastfeeding mothers to work outside their homes. Their shaping effects could be a secondary motive, derived, like other initiation rituals, from the idea of the neonate's unfinished self. Californian historian Hubert Bancroft wrote in 1875 in his monumental *Native Races* [16]: 'The [Nootka] flattening process begins immediately after birth, and is continued until the child can walk … Observers generally agree that little or no harm is done to the brain by this infliction, the traces of which to a great extent disappear later in life … In Nicaragua, the compressed forehead was the sign of noble blood and the highest type of beauty; and besides that the head was thus better adapted to the carrying of burdens. In Yucatán, according to Landa, the same custom obtained. Four or five days after birth the child was laid with the face down on a bed and the head was compressed between two pieces of wood, one on the forehead and the other on the back of the head, the boards being kept in place for several days until the desired cranial conformation was effected.'

On the Antilles, the Caribbeans did not use cradleboards but rather small plates tightly fixed to the front to flatten the forehead [26]. Johann Riedel reported a similar technique from Sulawesi in 1871 [27]: 'The skull is encircled with beaten bark of the *Lahendang* tree [*Sponia* sp.], later with calico or denim, and is clamped between two boards as shown in [Fig. 5.2.3, right]. The skulls thereby acquire unusual breadth, which is considered a peculiar beauty trait. The child usually remains wedged between the boards for four to five months.' Munich anatomist Nikolaus Rüdinger discerned four types of modification in America [28], whereas Geneva physician Louis André Gosse classified 16 types of artificial deformation worldwide in 1855, showing that it was not limited to native tribes, but also widely used among the well-educated *bourgeois* in France and Switzerland (Fig. 5.2.4) [26].

In 1851, Rivero and Tschudy described occipital sutural bones in Peruvian crania and termed them *Inca* bones [29], starting a long debate on their hereditary or mechanical origin. In 1897, Dorsey claimed that wormian bones in the coronary suture of artificially deformed Kwakiutl skulls represent stopgaps in response to stress [30]. Recent studies confirmed that culturally deformed skulls exhibit lambdoid ossicles and occipito-mastoid wormian bones significantly more often [31].

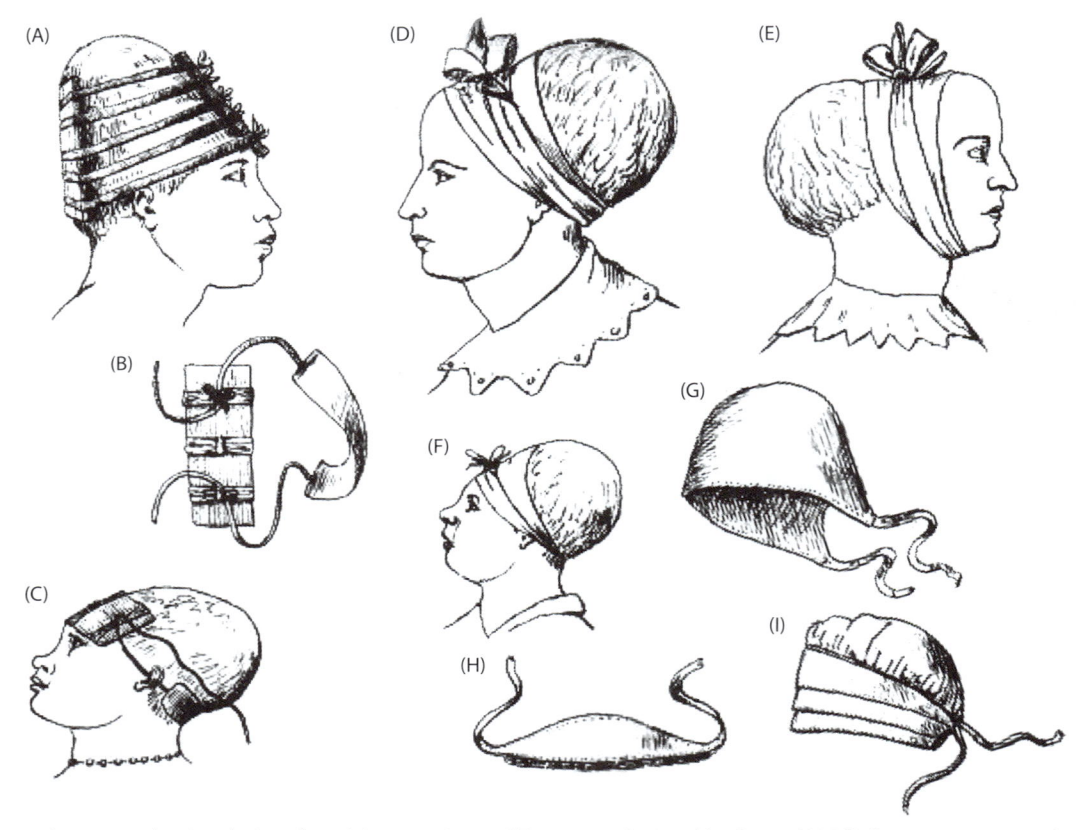

Fig. 5.2.4 Nineteenth-century shaping devices from Mesoamerica and Europe, as depicted by Gosse 1855 [26]: A, Peruvian cuneiform head with tablets tightened daily for 5 years. B and C, Caribbean cotton-padded plank, tightly fixed with a ribbon to flatten the forehead. D, annular shape from band compression used in girls in the lower Seine region. E, bilobed head achieved by fontanelle compression, Dépt. Deux-Sèvres. F, head presser called *fronteau*, used in the Geneva region. G–I, bonnet named *béguin* and headbands for frontal flattening, Dépt. Haute Garonne.

Spontaneous moulding before delivery

The term *moulding* today denotes a non-intentional change in the fetal cranial bone relationship during delivery. It occurs in every vaginal birth to a certain degree and can be viewed as an evolutionary adaptation to the narrow birth canal which resulted from the upright gait. In 1672, when rickets frequently constricted the maternal pelvis, Derby *accoucheur* Percival Willughby observed [32]: 'A great person in Ireland, having the bones of the genital parts ovally, by infirmity, pressed together, after the loss of severall children, drawn from her body by the chirurgions … I espied in the child's forhead a long dawk, deeply dented, even to her nose; whereupon I conjectured that, through this woman's hard, long labour, also by the dawk in the child's forehead, that the ill conformation of the [pelvical] bones was the cause of her sufferings.'

Midwifes and obstetricians often believed the infant endangered by moulding, as Johann Storch, who in 1751 feared 'dullness … if the infant's head is compressed and disfigured during delivery' [33]. Göttingen obstetrician Johann Georg Roederer described lethal wedging of the fetal head in oblique position and constricted pelvis in 1793 [34]. Johann Peter Frank, Director of the Vienna General Hospital, wrote in 1794 [35]: 'In severe cases the parietal bones slide over the frontal or occipital bone, which most often leads to severe bruising of these parts, lacerates the fibers and vessels, and compresses the brain … In less severe cases and vigorous children, gentle and smooth manual pressing suffices to gradually restore head shape. But one should beware of careless or heavy pressure onto the head, which causes future stupidity.' In 1890, Edinburgh obstetrician John Ballantyne explained that moulding is a normal process (Fig. 5.2.7C) [36]: 'During labour the frontal bone is somewhat depressed under the margins of the parietal bones, the tip of the occiput is also depressed below the parietals, and the parietal bone, which lies anteriorly in the pelvis, slightly overrides that which lies next to the sacrum.'

Head shaping by midwives

In contrast to mild, long-term modification, rapid one-time shaping was a dangerous, but standard approach to overlapping sutures since advocated by Soran in the 2nd century C.E. [13]: 'Afterwards, she should first, by rotatory movements with each hand, massage the little head round and round. Secondly, with her hands facing each other she should somehow mould it, now with one hand placed against the back of the head and the other against the forehead, now with one against the top of the head and the other under the chin. And she should dexterously bring the skull into good proportions, so that it may become neither too lengthy nor pointed.'

Padovan professor Paulus Bagellardus repeated Soran's advice in his *Little Book on the Diseases of Children* in 1472 [37]: 'Then having tied the umbilicus, the midwife should lay the infant in a basin or mostellum [pot?] or some similar vessel filled with sweet water, comfortably warm, not stinging nor cold, or salty, according to the custom of the Greeks. And she should introduce the infant into this water or bath, its head elevated with her left hand, while with her right hand she should shape its head, its sightless eyes, clean its nostrils, open its mouth, rub its jaws, shape its arms and its hands and everything.'

Details of Soran's grip must have impressed the painters of Albrecht Dürer's entourage who integrated them into altarpieces showing Mary's birth in the early 16th century (Fig. 5.2.5). Walter Ryff, re-editing Rösslin's *Rosengarten* in 1561, advised the midwife [38]: 'With the right hand she should form the orbital rim, and squeeze the head into the right shape.' Midwives who overdid head shaping were warned by Basel surgeon Felix Würtz in 1563 [37]: 'A tender Child must not be handled rudely; laying the Child in a Cradle purposely made, whereby the Childs head may be framed round: this kind of lying hurteth the Childs memory very much, or it causes melancholly dreams, or other simptoms, which afterward are not reduced so easily.'

The Passau midwives rule of 1595 demanded [39]: 'During the bath she should lift the infant's head with her left hand. With her right she should form the eyebrows … She should press the head gently into the right form and roundness … After that she should use smooth and warmed towels to dry the infant … and apply a bonnet or hood over the head to maintain its roundness and to prevent a pointed, bulky, or awkward shape.' Royal midwife Louise Bourgeois alluded to controversies on head shaping in 1609 [40]: 'One hand upon the os frontale, the other upon the os [parietale], compressing gently what moved during labor, but not shifting the bones against each other: It is a bad habit to clench the infants' head, as is binding which gives them the long head one can observe in the Paris infants.' Johann Muralt, city physician of Zurich, published a textbook on midwifery [41] which reveals that head shaping was not the exception but the rule in 1697: 'As soon as the midwife has the child on her lap, she should observe it everywhere to make sure it is well formed … hold its head with a scarlet rag and cap, and give it its round shape.' Head shaping still was imposed in the midwives' rules of Sachsen-Altenburg 1705, Oldenburg 1738, and Regensburg 1779.

Another grip that Soranus taught midwives targeted the nose [13]: 'With the thumbs, she should shape the nose, raising it if flat, pressing it if aquiline. And in a case of an aquiline nose she should not correct it at the top of the curve, but where it is prominent around the tip, and should draw forward the raised alae of the nose.' Giotto's fresco in the marvellous Scrovegni chapel suggests that this grip was still used in Padova in 1305 (Fig. 5.2.6).

Attitudes shifted around 1780, and head shaping gradually fell from grace [42]: the manoeuvre was prohibited in the midwives' rule of Isenburg 1782: 'The nonsense of compressing the infant's head is strictly forbidden to the midwives' and similar interdictions crept into the rules of Freiberg 1785, Zittau 1792, and Baden 1795: 'Under no circumstances may she straighten the crooked or pointed head of an infant.' Despite the ban, postnatal head shaping persisted for another century under the pretext of the 'necessary' bath. As late as 1824, the Leipzig obstetrician Friedrich Ludwig Meissner complained [43]: 'To give the head a better form, stupid and cheeky midwives thoughtlessly often squeeze the head violently, thereby causing the infant's death … As such brute head squeezing is entirely useless, and nature compensates all irregularities more gently and better, one should never allow anyone to assault the infant's molded head.' Midwives' rough head shaping and the warnings in the textbooks disappeared during the 20th century, but persist in the German idiom *den Kopf zurechtrücken* (to reproach sharply).

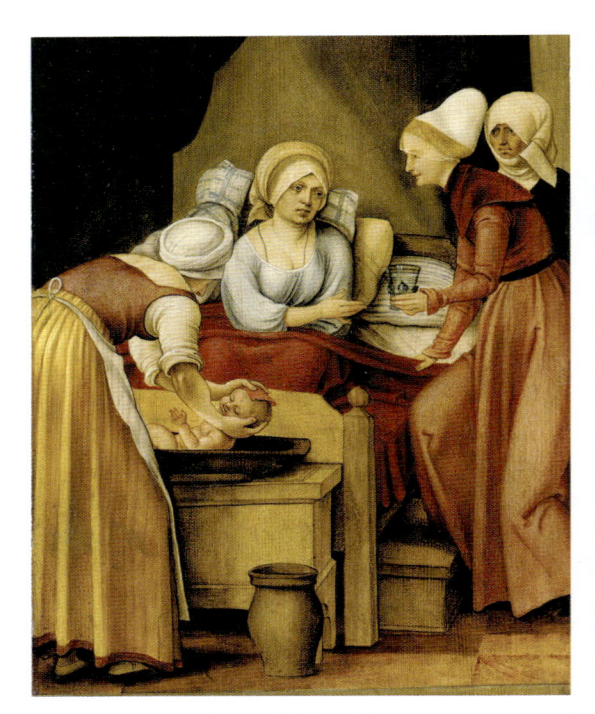

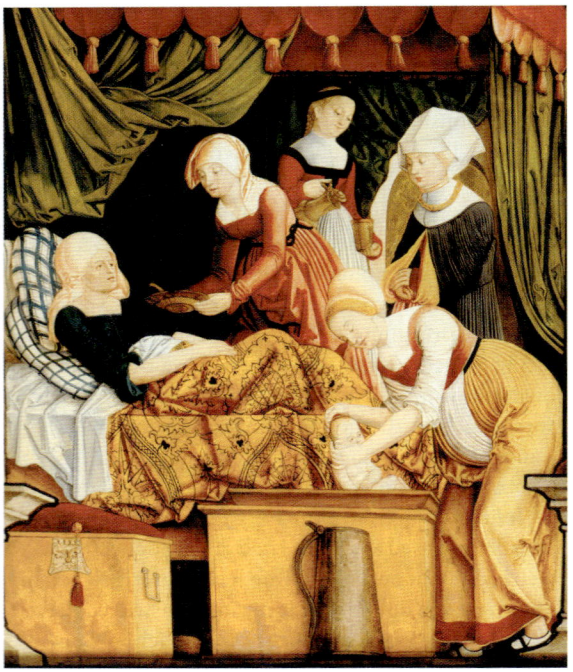

Fig. 5.2.5 Artists' observations of midwife's head shaping in two Nuremberg altarpieces showing Mary's birth. Left: by Hans Suess von Kulmbach 1510/1511, Museum der Bildenden Künste; right: by Barthel Beham 1522/1524, Germanisches Nationalmuseum.
Left, Museum der Bildenden Künste, Leipzig. Inv.-Nr. G52/1, with permission. Right, by Barthel Beham 1522/24, Germanisches Nationalmuseum, Nürnberg, Leihgabe Protestantische Kirchenverwaltung, with permission.

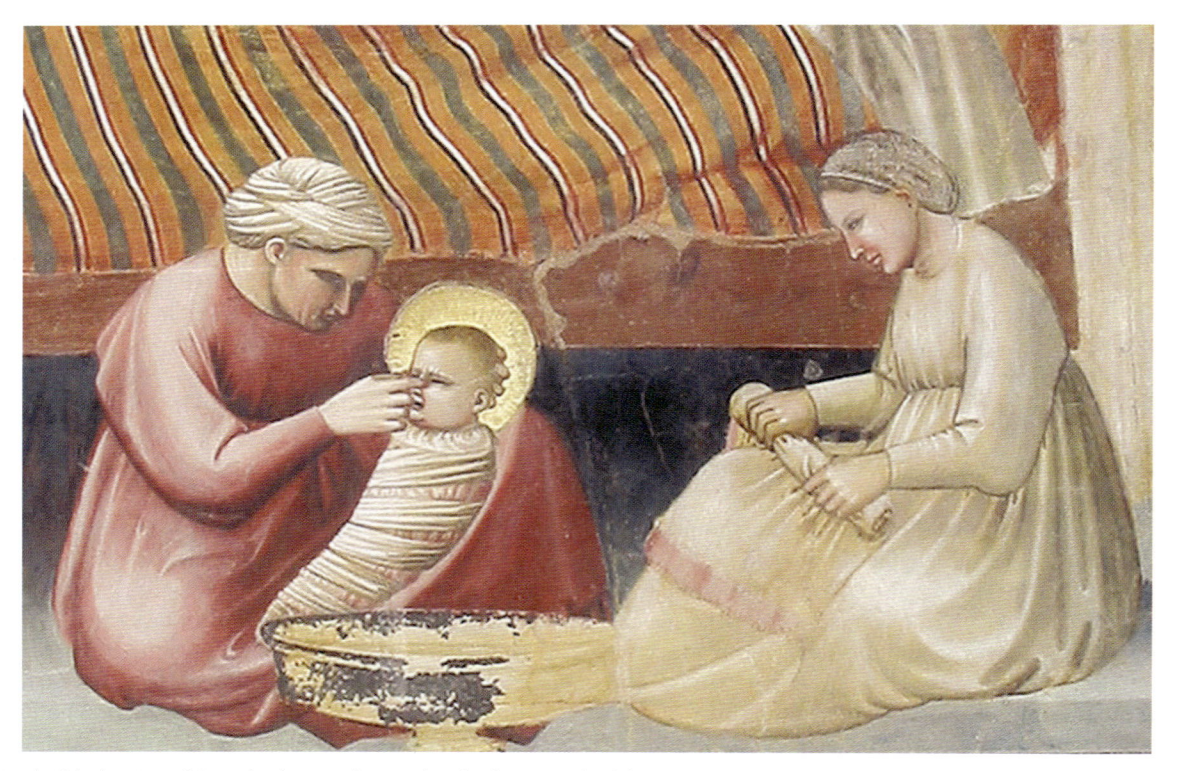

Fig. 5.2.6 Midwife's shaping of the infant's nose depicted in the fresco *Birth of the Virgin* by Giotto di Bondone in 1305. See text for details.
Padova, Scrovegni Chapel, north wall, with permission by Commune di Padova, Assessorato alla Cultura.

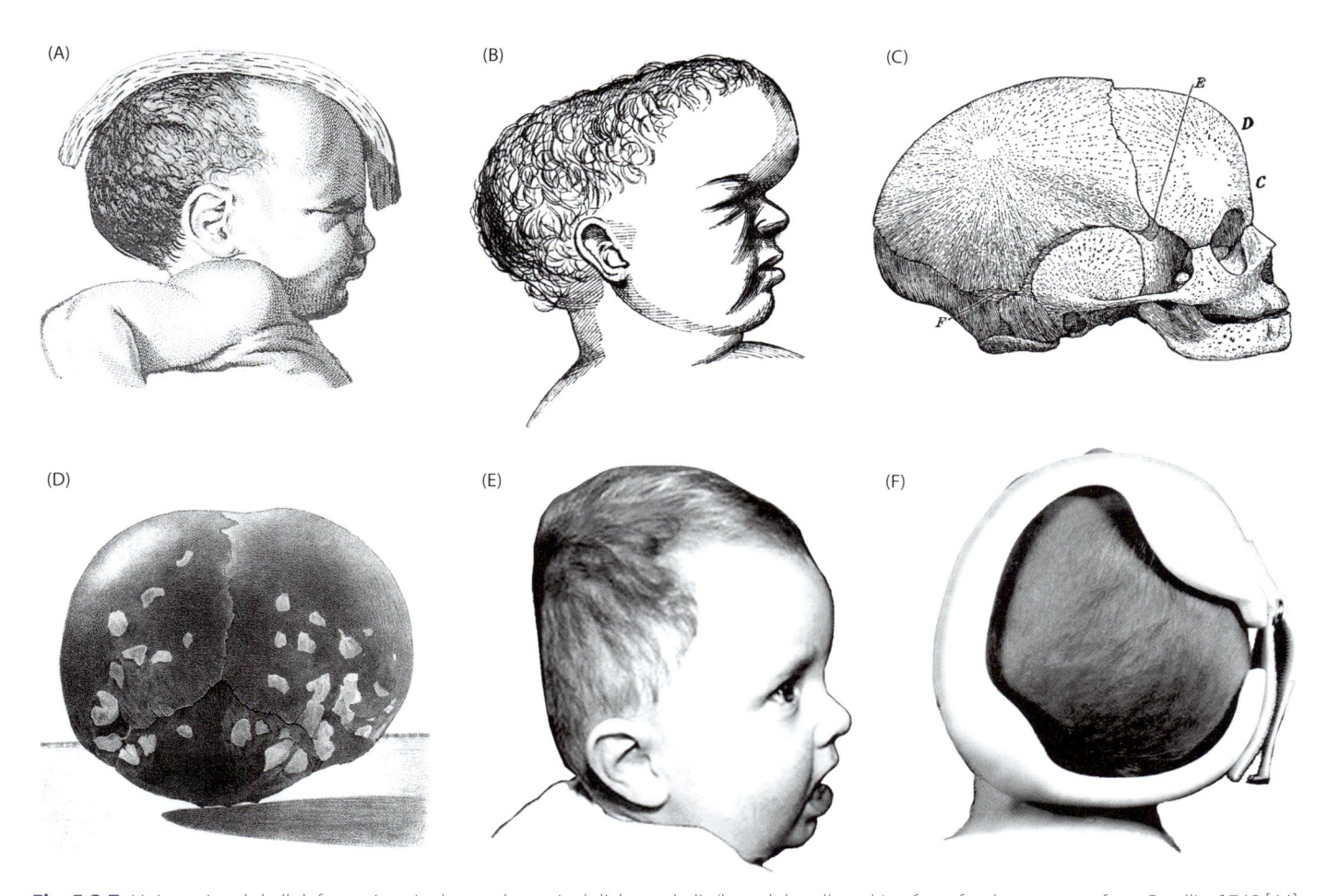

Fig. 5.2.7 Unintentional skull deformations in the newborn: A, dolichocephalic 'breech head' resulting from fundus pressure, from Smellie, 1748 [44]; B, prominent forehead resulting from brow positioning as depicted by Swayne, 1867 [45]; C, os parietale overlapping os frontale as depicted by Pope, 1913 [59]; D, severe occipital craniotabes in a 6-month-old rachitic twin, from Elsässer, 1843 [48]; E, positional brachycephalus modified from [53]. F, helmet proposed to correct positional plagiocephaly.
Source: Data from Littlefield, T. R. Cranial remodeling devices: treatment of deformational plagiocephaly and postsurgical applications. *Semin Pediatr Neurol* 2004;11:268–77.

Unintended skull deformation after birth

Craniosynostosis (early closure of skull sutures) affects 1 in 2000 infants and may deform the skull permanently. Fetal position greatly, but reversibly influences neonatal head shape. The dolichocephalic *breech head*, depicted by Smellie in 1748 [44] and the *brow head*, described by Swayne in 1867 [45] have been rediscovered [46, 47]. Craniotabes (soft occipital bone) resulting from rickets was described by Elsässer [48]. Prematurity led to bitemporal flattening [49], especially with lateral positioning during long-term ventilation and when combined with osteopenia of prematurity [50]. Some of these conditions are depicted in **Fig. 5.2.7**.

Present practice

In 1998, Ellen FitzSimmons found head shaping prevalent among various ethnic groups among adults in Chicago and New York; motives including the wish to enhance beauty, health, or intelligence [51]. Since the Back to Sleep campaign of 1992 [52], sudden infant death has become rare, but positional brachycephalus resurged [53]. Fashion is subject to change, and occipital flattening, a regional aesthetic ideal for millennia, has gradually lost esteem and is now considered a disease ('positional plagiocephaly', International Classification of Diseases, Tenth Revision code Q67.3). Anomalous head shape has been attested to every fourth infant [54]. Expensive helmets were developed and promoted under the name orthotic devices (**Fig. 5.2.7F**), and surgical treatments, originally developed for craniosynostosis, were proposed for positional deformations. Formerly in the domain of the midwife or mother, postnatal infant head shaping is now widely practised by cranial therapists. Congresses are held and handbooks written on the topic [55]. Lawsuits have been filed to decide whether health insurers must cover the treatment [56]. Positional plagiocephaly is usually spontaneously reversible within 5 years [57].

Conclusion

Motives for head shaping remain difficult to understand, and scientific evidence of any benefit is lacking. However, concern is unwarranted that a practice that existed since the origin of mankind will disappear from earth. As Rudolf Virchow rightly stated in 1892 [17]: 'Once we understand that headshaping has spread so widely over the earth, we must bow to the assumption that a certain conformity of the human mind brought about these customs in various places. This does not allow us to deduce peoples' origins or prehistoric migration.'

REFERENCES

1. Trinkaus E: Artificial cranial deformation in the Shanidar-1 and Shanidar-5 Neanderthals. Curr Anthropol 1982;**23**:198–9.
2. Drell JRR: Neanderthals: a history of interpretation. Oxf J Archaeol 2000;**19**:1–24.
3. Weidenreich F: On the earliest representatives of modern mankind recovered on the soil of East Asia. Bull Nat Hist Soc Peking 1939;**13**:161–74.
4. Brown P: Nacurrie 1: mark of ancient Java, or a caring mother's hands, in terminal Pleistocene Australia? J Hum Evol 2010;**59**:168–87.
5. Arensburg B, Hershkovitz I: Cranial deformation and trephination in the Middle East. Bull Mém Soc Anthrop Paris 1988;**5**, série XIV:139–50.
6. Ozbek M: Cranial deformation in a subadult sample from Degirmentepe (Chalcolithic, Turkey). Am J Phys Anthropol 2001;**115**:238–44.
7. Rhode MP, Arriaza BT: Influence of cranial deformation on facial morphology among prehistoric South Central Andean populations. Am J Phys Anthropol 2006;**130**:462–70.
8. Schijman E: Artificial cranial deformation in newborns in the pre-Columbian Andes. Childs Nerv Syst 2005;**21**:945–50.
9. Snorrason E: Cranial deformation in the reign of Akhnaton. Bull Hist Med 1946;**20**:601–10.
10. Gerhard K: Waren die Köpfchen der Echnaton-Töchter künstlich deformiert? Z Ägypt Sprache Altert Kd 1967;**94**:50–62.
11. Hippocrates: Airs, waters, and places. In: The genuine works of Hippocrates. London: Sydenham Society, 1849: Vol. **1**, p. 207–8.
12. v. Baer KE: Die Makrocephalen im Boden der Krym und Österreichs. Mémoires de l'Académie Impériale des Sciences de St. Petersbourg 1860;Série **7**:6–86.
13. Temkin O: Soranus' Gynecology. Baltimore, MD: The Johns Hopkins Press, 1956: p. 87, 106–8.
14. Lekovic GP, Baker B, Lekovic JM, Preul MC: New World cranial deformation practices: historical implications. Neurosurgery 2007;**60**:1137–46; discussion 1146–7.
15. Romero-Vargas S, Ruiz-Sandoval JL, Sotomayor-Gonzalez A, et al.: A look at Mayan artificial cranial deformation practices. Neurosurg Focus 2010;**29**:E2, 1–5.
16. Bancroft HH: The native races of the Pacific States of North America. Leipzig: Brockhaus, 1875: Vol. **1**, p. 180, 731.
17. Virchow R: Crania Ethnica Americana. Zeitschr Ethnol 1892;**24**:5, 20.
18. Gerszten PC: An investigation into the practice of cranial deformation among the pre-Columbian peoples of northern Chile. Int J Osteoarchaeol 1993;**3**:87–98.
19. Ménard J: Étude craniologique et odontologique de Mérovingiens adultes du Vexin Francais. Bull Mém Soc Anthrop Paris, Série XIII 1977;**4**:229–43.
20. Columbus C, LasCasas B: Personal narrative of the first voyage of Columbus. Samuel Kettell: Boston, MA: T.B. Wait and Son, 1827: p. 37.
21. Cardano G: De rerum varietate libri XVII. Avinione: Vincent, 1557: p. 31, 414.
22. Sáenz de Aguirre J: Synodus III. dioecesana Limensis celebrata in oppido sancti Dominici de Yungay die 17. Julii, anno 1585. In: Collectio maxima conciliorum omnium Hispaniae et Novi Orbis. Romae: Fulganus, 1755: Vol. **6**, p. 204.
23. Catlin G: Die Indianer Nord-Amerikas und die während eines achtjährigen Aufenthalts unter den wildesten ihrer Stämme erlebten Abenteuer und Schicksale. Brussels: Muquardt, 1851: Vol. **1 and 2**.
24. Kane P: Wanderings of an artist among the Indians of North America. London: Longman Brown, 1859: p. 180–1.
25. Morton SG: Crania Americana. Philadelphia, PA: Penington, 1839: p. 204.
26. Gosse L-A: Essai sur les déformations artificielles du crâne. Paris: J.B. Baillière, 1855: p. 23, 43, 64, plates 5 and 6.
27. Riedel JGF: Über künstliche Verbildung des Kopfes. Zeitschr Ethnol 1871;**3**:110–1, plate p. 574.
28. Rüdinger N: Ueber die willkürliche Verunstaltung des menschlichen Körpers. Corr Bl Dt Ges Anthropol 1874;**28**.3.
29. Rivero y Ustariz ME, Tschudy JJv: Peruvian antiquities. Vienna: Müller, 1851.
30. Dorsey GA: Wormian bones in artificially deformed Kwakiutl crania. Am Anthrop 1897;**10**:169–73.
31. O'Loughlin VD: Effects of different kinds of cranial deformation on the incidence of wormian bones. Am J Phys Anthropol 2004;**123**:146–55.
32. Willughby P: Observations on midwifery [1672]. Wakefield, Yorkshire: S.R. Publishers, 1972: p. 239–40.
33. Storch J: Theoretische und practische Abhandlung von Kinder-Kranckheiten. Eisenach: Grießbach, 1751: Vol. **4**. p. 217.
34. Roederer JG: Anfangsgründe der Geburtshülfe. Jena: Akademische Buchhandlung, 1793: p. 262, §430.
35. Frank JP: Abhandlungen über die gesunde Kindererziehung nach medizinischen und physikalischen Grundsätzen. 2. ed. Leipzig: von J. G. von Gruber: 1803: p. 13.
36. Ballantyne JW: The head of the infant at birth. Edinb Med J 1890;**36**:97–111, 429–40.
37. Ruhräh J: Pediatrics of the past. New York: Hoeber, 1925: p. 34, 203.
38. Ryff WH: Schwangerer Frawen Rosengarten. Frankfurt: Egenolff, 1561: p. 99.
39. Burckhard G: Die deutschen Hebammenordnungen von ihren ersten Anfängen bis auf die Neuzeit. Leipzig: Engelmann, 1912: Vol. **1**, p. 122, 247.
40. Bourgeois L: Observations Diverses sur la Sterilité, Perte de Fruits, Foecondité, Accouchments, et Maladies de Femmes, et Enfants Nouveaux-naiz. Paris: Dehoury, 1609: p. 96.
41. Muralt J: Kinder- und Hebammenbüchlein. Basel: König, 1697: p. 39.
42. Nöth A: Die Hebammenordnungen des XVIII. Jahrhunderts. Bottrop: Postberg, 1931: p. 57, 130, 161.
43. Meissner FL: Ueber die physische Erziehung der Kinder in den ersten Lebensjahren. Leipzig: Hartmann, 1824: p. 14–15.
44. Smellie W: Tabulae anatomicae. Anatomische Tafeln zur Hebammenkunst. Nürnberg: Seligman, 1758: p. 99, plate 33.
45. Swayne JG: Changes in the shape of the foetal head produced by labour. BMJ 1867;**1**:768–9.
46. Haberkern CM, Smith DW, Jones KL: The 'breech head' and its relevance. Am J Dis Child 1979;**133**:154–6.
47. Sunderland R: Fetal position and skull shape. Br J Obstet Gynaecol 1981;**88**:246–9.

48. Elsässer CL: Der weiche Hinterkopf. Stuttgart und Tübingen: Cotta, 1843: p. 91, plate II.
49. Baum JD, Searls D: Head shape and size of pre-term low-birthweight infants. Dev Med Child Neurol 1971;**13**:576–81.
50. Steichen JJ, Gratton TL, Tsang RC: Osteopenia of prematurity: the cause and possible treatment. J Pediatr 1980;**96**:528–34.
51. FitzSimmons E, Prost JH, Peniston S: Infant head molding: a cultural practice. Arch Fam Med 1998;**7**:88–90.
52. American Academy of Pediatrics: Positioning and SIDS. Pediatrics 1992;**89**:1120–6.
53. Graham JM Jr, Kreutzman J, Earl Deal: Deformational brachycephaly in supine-sleeping infants. J Pediatr 2005;**146**:253–7.
54. Peitsch WK, Keefer CH, LaBrie RA, Mulliken JB: Incidence of cranial asymmetry in healthy newborns. Pediatrics 2002;**110**:e72.
55. Dobson J: Baby beautiful: a handbook of baby head shaping. Carson City, NV: Heirs Press, 1994.
56. Sozialgericht Aachen: Behandlung einer Schädelasymmetrie (Plagiocephalie) mittels einer Kopforthese. 18/11/2010, S 2 KR 151/10.
57. Hutchison BL, Stewart AW, Mitchell EA: Deformational plagiocephaly. Arch Dis Child 2011;**96**:85–90.
58. Schaefer H: Ägyptische Kunst. In: Kunstgeschichte in Bildern. Vol. **1**: Das Altertum. Leipzig: Seemann, 1912: p. 19.
59. Pope AE: Anatomy and physiology for nurses. New York: Putnam's Sons, 1913: p. 53.
60. Littlefield TR: Cranial remodeling devices: treatment of deformational plagiocephaly and postsurgical applications. Semin Pediatr Neurol 2004;**11**:268–77.

5.3

Lame from birth
Concepts of cerebral palsy

Introduction

The brain's anatomy, physiology, and disorders were and remain incompletely understood. As long as the central nervous system had not been described and no distinction was made between nerves and tendons, neurology had no chance to develop. The Hippocratic writers (5th century B.C.E.) regarded the brain as a mucous gland with the task 'of cleaning the blood, be it in the uterus or after birth ... The secreted cold phlegm descends toward the lung or heart and cools the blood' [1]. Lack of knowledge gave way to superstition.

Magic and God's wrath

Deformations have been attributed to supernatural causes since antiquity. Four-thousand-year-old Sumeran, Chaldean, and Babylonian incantations against the evil eye were translated from the cuneiform writings found in the Niniveh library [2]. Pregnant women and neonates were, and still are, believed to be particularly vulnerable to the evil eye, and mothers hid their neonates from the gaze of strangers and tried to protect themselves with amulets. Perinatal spastic hemiplegia caused the Greek blacksmith god, Hephaistos, to be mocked by the other Olympians [3]. Hephaistos' mythologic character evolved into the flute-playing Pan and medieval horned devil, both identified by goats' legs or clubfeet. Greek society blamed dreadful political crises on a 'scapegoat'. The victim, usually ugly and deformed, suffered ritual expulsion or execution [4]. Spastic palsy and other disorders disabling the limbs (clubfoot, rickets, gout, rheumatism) were not well differentiated, perinatal origins were implied in the designation 'lame from mother's womb' [Acts 14:8–10]. When lame, Jews were forbidden from approaching the altar [Leviticus 21:18–21], because to be 'halted' was regarded as God's punishment [Micah 4:6–7]. In the New Testament, the 'halted' camped outside the city walls, bathing in the Bethesda pool [John 5:2–3].

Inadequate swaddling

Plato (4th century B.C.E.) was convinced that proper swaddling prevented limb deformities and ironically proposed a law [5]: 'Do you wish us to go ahead despite the laughter and set forth laws to the effect that a pregnant woman must go for walks, and that when the child is born she must mold it like wax so long as it remains moist, swaddling it in clothes until it is two years old?' Tight swaddling became the rule despite Plato's irony, as shown in Attic tombstones preserved from 700–300 B.C.E. (Fig. 5.3.1) [6] and was reinforced in Soranus' *Gynecology* (2nd century C.E.) [7]: 'Since in our opinion, however, the swaddling clothes serve to give firmness and an undistorted figure, we deem it right to loosen them when the body has already become reasonably firm and when there is no longer fear of any of its parts being distorted.' François Mauriceau, accoucheur in Paris, taught in 1668 [8]: 'Its arms and legs should be extended and bound straight at the side of the body ... It should be swaddled to give the small body a straight shape, which is the most decent and suitable for the human, and to accustom it to stand on its feet.' The cruel habit of tight swaddling persisted in many regions into present times.

Changeling, murder, and abandon

The 16th century, with its wars, plagues, witch trials, and paucity of books, was fertile soil for relying on superstition to explain malformations and deformities, believed to result from intercourse between witch and devil or as changelings taking the place of healthy children (Fig. 5.3.2). Together with mental retardation and an enlarged head (undifferentiated from hydrocephalus, hypothyroidism, or metabolic disease), they were called 'killcrops' and destroyed, and Martin Luther proposed they be drowned [9]: 'The devil replaces legitimate children with changelings and killcrops to plague mankind. He often pulls certain girls into the water, impregnates them, and keeps them with him until

---

Adapted with permission from Obladen, M. Lame from birth: early concepts of cerebral palsy. *Journal of Child Neurology*, 26(2):248–256. Copyright © 2011, © SAGE Publications.

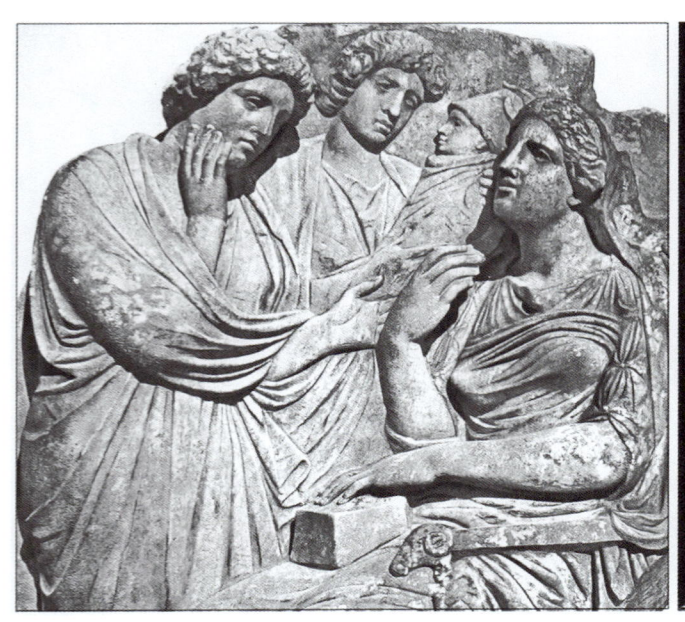

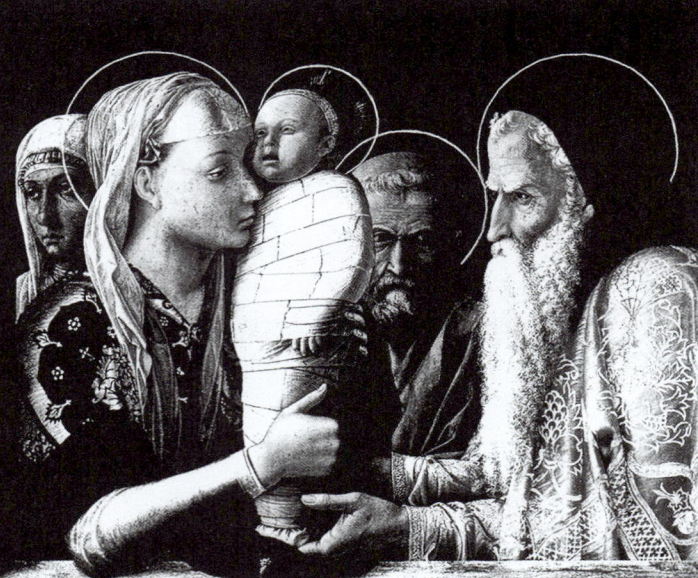

Fig. 5.3.1 Tight swaddling of the neonate was believed to prevent extremity deformation. Left: Attic tombstone from the 5th century b.c.e. [6]; right: painting by Mantegna 1465 [50].

they deliver their children; he then places those children in cradles, taking the legitimate children away.' Luther's proposal to kill these infants was taken up by Werner Catel, the Leipzig paediatrician who helped organize the murder of disabled children in Nazi Germany (see Chapter 8.4). Thomas Phaer alluded to social problems of the Tudor era in his *Boke of Chyldren* published in 1545: 'Of the stifnes or starckenes: Sometime it happeneth that the lymmes are starke, and can not well come together without the greater peyne which thing procedeth many tymes of cold, as when the chylde is found in the frost, or in the strete, cast away by a wicked mother.'

Maternal miswatching

Analogous to congenital malformations, the occurrence of spastic deformities was related to maternal impressions during intercourse or pregnancy, called 'miswatching'. As adults with cerebral palsies were usually dependent on public alms, medieval cities passed beggars' laws, such as in the Bavarian city of Regensburg in 1514 [10]: 'Who has an affliction that might dread or horrify pregnant women, should be separated from the other [beggars] and should decently cover and hide his deformity by threat of punishment from the beggars' master.' As late as 1731, the Erfurt obstetrician Jacob Kornmann recommended in his textbook [11]: 'A pregnant woman should caution not to watch an evildoer be executed, either by the sword or otherwise. Nor should she observe cattle being slaughtered, as this may harm her fruit.'

Midwife's negligence

Felix Würtz, a surgeon in Zurich, distinguishing connatal and postnatally developing palsies [12], described spastic diplegia in 1563: 'Some children are born with crooked feet, placed and pressed upon each other, so that they are forced to walk on their ankles, and are lame from mother's womb. It is thought that this is caused by fright, strange sights, or carelessness for which the nurse should be held responsible.' Since Sydenham [13], who ascribed a multitude of disorders to difficult dentition, many authors associated this normal process with convulsions. Osler explicitly mentioned teething as the cause of convulsions in 1889 in at least four cases of infantile hemiplegia [14].

Brain maturation and periventricular leukomalacia

Modern embryology began with Hieronymus Fabricius ab Aquapendente, from 1565 to 1613 joint chair of anatomy and surgery in Padua, and his student William Harvey, from London. Fabricius referred to Galen when denying the fetal brain a function [15]: 'But the brain does not perform a public function … it is not at all necessary for the fetus to see, hear, taste, or smell, nor must it use its feet or hands; similarly it needs no sense of touch, and no imagination, thought, or memory.' Harvey specified the development of the fetal brain, stating: 'Now in the fourth moneth, … the large and fluid braine resembled cheese-curd, and was embroidered with larger veines' [16]

Giovanni Battista Morgagni, likewise an anatomist in Padova, mentioned in his monumental *Seats and Causes of Diseases* that large parts of the neonatal brain can liquefy [17]. Charles Prosper Ollivier, familiar with disorders at the Paris Foundling Hospital, wrote in 1827 [18]: 'The brain of the new-born child is often found softened and destroyed without any symptoms having permitted the practitioner to suspect it during life.' As a distinct disorder, Alois Bednar, director of the Vienna Foundling Hospital, described leukomalacia in 1851 [19]: 'Even though edema and white softening may be widespread,

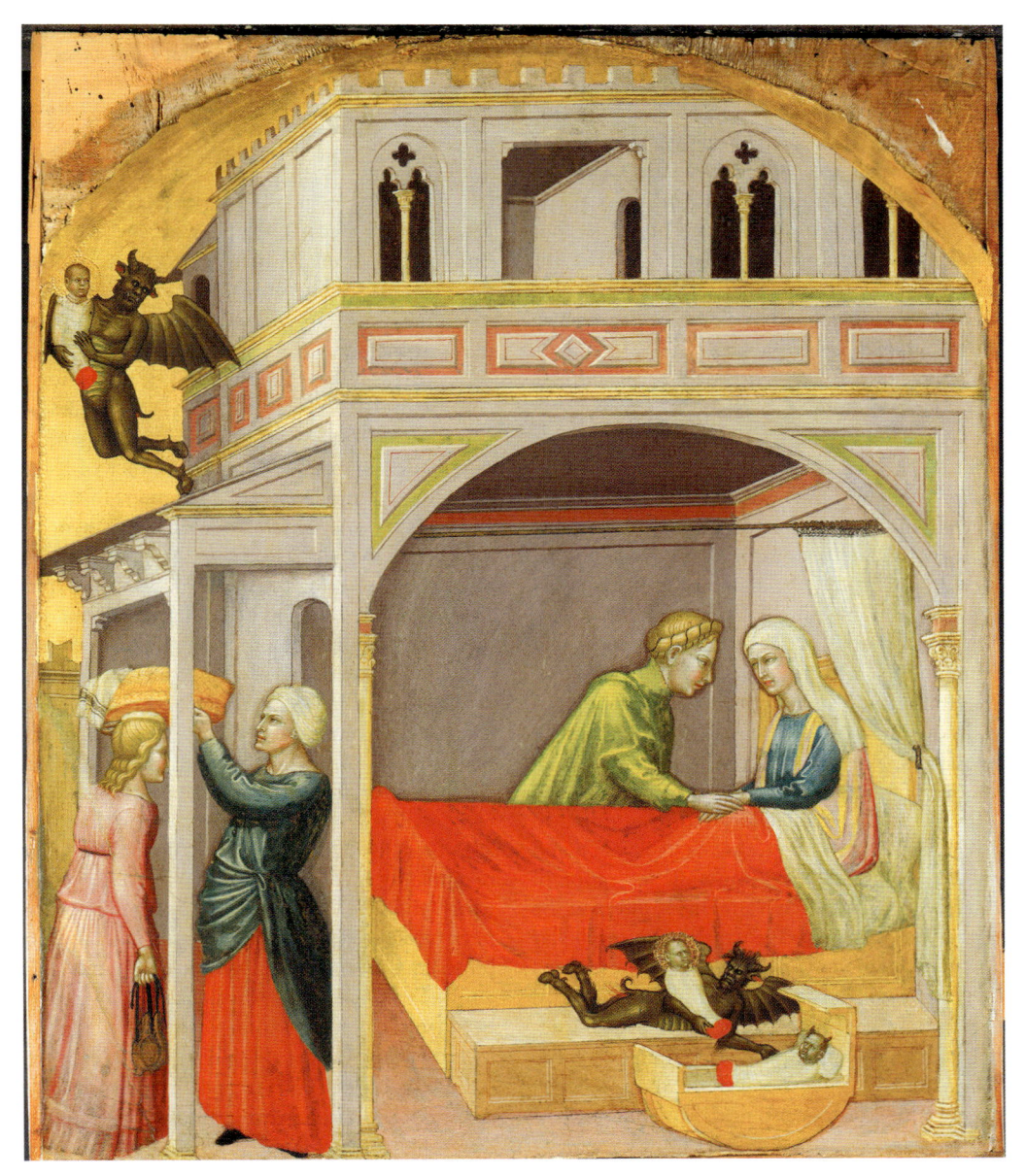

Fig. 5.3.2 Exchange and abduction of the newly born St Stephanus. Part of an altarpiece by Martino di Bartolomeo, early 15th century. © Städel-Museum Frankfurt/M, U. Edelmann, Artothek.

they usually occupy parts adjacent to the lateral ventricles, or they are more obvious there than in the remaining marrow.'

Prematurity

Infantile cerebral palsy was described in 1801 by the London surgeon and male midwife Michael Underwood [20]: '[Palsy of the lower extremities] is not a common disorder any where, I believe, and seems to occur seldomer in London than in other parts of this kingdom… it seems to arise from debility [prematurity], and usually attacks children previously reduced by fever; seldom those under one, or more than four or five years old … so that the first thing observed is a debility of the lower extremities, which gradually become more infirm, and after a few weeks are unable to support the body.'

The Leipzig obstetrician Johann Christian Gottfried Jörg wrote in 1826 [21]: 'This weakness remains most expressed in the muscles and may persist until puberty or longer. It hinders the children in their early life both in using their extremities and in supporting head and trunk, and therefore frequently leads to deformed spine and legs … I also observed that children born prematurely were prone to brain dropsy and sometimes were foolish when their mind was about to develop. Prematurity therefore is always unfavourable for the child and leads into manifold and great dangers.' In 1894, the pathologist Edouard Brissaud proposed disturbed brain differentiation due to immaturity as main cause of spastic palsy [22]: 'What takes the pyramidal tract three weeks to grow in the fetus, will be attained within three years, or never, in postnatal life of the infant born prematurely, and thence arises spastic paralysis.' Developmental follow-up studies seemed to confirm this theory: Maria Comberg found two children with 'Little's disease' and 30 with 'pronounced nervousness' among 81 preterm infants surviving in Berlin's Kaiserin Auguste Victoria Haus in 1919–1922, concluding 'The term *neuropathy* is so poorly defined and depends so much of the surrounding social conditions, that no further statistics can be based upon it' [23]. Aaron Capper studied 103 prematures who survived in Vienna in 1911–1926 and published follow-up results at 2–15 years of age in Philadelphia [24]: 'Of 51 children investigated at school age, four had Little's disease associated with idiocy or imbecility ... The fate of immature children is not enviable; almost half of them die during the first year of life. Of those that remain alive, the majority are physically as well as mentally underdeveloped.'

Birth trauma

The Scottish obstetrician William Smellie correlated birth mechanics with brain damage in his *Midwifery* in 1752 [25]: 'In lingering labours, when the head of the child hath been in the pelvis, so that the bones ride over one another and the shape is preternaturally lengthened, the brain is frequently so much compressed that violent convulsions ensue before or soon after delivery to the danger and oft-times the destruction of the child.' The Paris obstetrician Joseph Capuron confirmed in 1820 [26]: 'The practitioners frequently observe neonates struck by apoplexy or asphyxia and sometimes in an alarming degree of weakness. Not seldom, especially after difficult and protracted labour, the infant is born with contusions, dislocated limbs, or fractures.' He distinguished *apoplexy* (corresponding to 'blue asphyxia'), *asphyxia* (corresponding to 'white asphyxia'), and *debility* (central apnoea of the premature). Traumatic laceration of the tentorium was described by Prosper Sylvain Denis, intern at the Paris Foundling Hospital in 1826 [27]: 'Principally, the cerebellar tentorium is the seat of this pathology, which results from forced distension of the wrapping fold, for instance due to pulling the head during delivery.' In 1885, New York neurologist Sarah McNutt described a child with difficult birth, convulsions, and 'double infantile spastic hemiplegia' [28]. After death at the age of 2 years, autopsy revealed cerebral atrophy with sclerosis and nearly total absence of ganglia. In light of other cases, she concluded that spastic palsies were caused by meningeal haemorrhages [29], an explanation also supported by William Gowers [30] and generally accepted up to the works of Sigmund Freud.

William Osler, professor of clinical medicine in Philadelphia, used the term *cerebral palsy* in 1889 to describe 120 children with hemiplegia and another 20 with diplegia [14]: 'We have then in the spastic diplegia, and in a few cases of hemiplegia – the true birth palsies – information which enables us to assign haemorrhage an important role ... Infantile hemiplegia is probably the result of a variety of different processes, of which the most important are: Haemorrhage during a paroxysm of whooping cough; post-febrile processes, encephalitis; and thrombosis of the cerebral veins.' Philip Schwartz, pathologist in Frankfurt (later in Warren, Pennsylvania) held mechanic trauma as the main cause of perinatal brain damage still in 1961 [31] and demanded: 'Legal guarantees for motherhood, and legal guarantees for the conservation and development of human life, are the two leading principles which must form the basis of the fight against neonatal losses and the pernicious outcome of parturitional injuries in general.' In medical malpractice claims closed in the US from 1995 to 2004, 19% of the plaintiffs were neonates, with perinatal brain injury and its sequelae being a common motive for the suits [32].

Birth asphyxia and hypoxia

Opinions on perinatal brain damage are still influenced by the London physician William John Little, founder of modern orthopaedics and sufferer from a clubfoot himself. He began to study medicine at age 16 years, and was admitted to the Royal College of Surgeons at age 22 years. In 1843, *The Lancet* accorded Little a series of 18 illustrated articles [33], the eighth of which described contractures of cerebral origin (Fig. 5.3.3), discussing several aetiologies: 'The lesion [in the central organ] is, in most cases, inflammation, chronic or acute, in either of its stages of congestion, effusion, or ramollissement ... In many instances, the spasmodic affection is produced at the moment of birth, or within a few hours or days of that event ... The individuals were born in a state of asphyxia, resuscitation having been obtained, at the expiration of two hours.' In 1845, Little obtained a Royal grant to build an orthopaedic hospital, and gave an influential lecture for the Society of Obstetrics in 1861 [34], in which he presented 63 cases of cerebral palsy, with access to the perinatal history in 47; he attributed 'spastic rigidity' to certain 'moments' at delivery: 'The forms of abnormal parturition which I have observed to precede certain mental and physical derangements of the infant consisted of difficult labours, i.e. unnatural presentations, tedious labours from rigidity of maternal passages or apertures, instrumental labours, labours in which turning was had recourse to, breech presentations, premature labours, and cases in which the umbilical cord had been entangled around the infant's neck or had fallen down before the head ... I may remark, that asphyxia neonatorum, from whatever amount of disturbance in separation of the foetus from the uterus it may have resulted, is, as might be surmised, very apt to be accompanied with, or to be succeeded by, convulsions at variable periods after birth.' His conclusions were limited by his study's retrospective design, an absent definition for asphyxia, and the lack of postmortem brain studies. Little's findings were challenged by Sigmund Freud, an experienced neuropathologist and later founder of psychoanalysis, who had worked in a neurological children's ward in Vienna. In 1897, Freud published an extensive monograph compiling 270 cases of cerebral palsy and 63 of his own postmortem examinations [35], he found 'Little's moments' in only half of the cases and concluded: 'Premature, precipitate and difficult birth and asphyxia neonatorum are not causal factors for diplegia: they are only associated symptoms of deeper lying influences which have dominated the development of the fetus.' Freud emphasized the difference between spastic hemiplegia and clubfoot and called attention to the misnomer of Ribeira's famous painting in the Louvre.

As every fetus develops at remarkably low oxygenation, it is difficult to comprehend how the concept of perinatal *hypoxia* came to be. In 1942, Harvard physiologist Clement A. Smith showed that it can take up to 2–3 h after birth to reach the oxygen saturation of an adult [36]. In 1953, the New York anaesthetist Virginia Apgar rightly bemoaned the poor quality of neonatal resuscitation studies and proposed a score to assess the chance for survival and guide

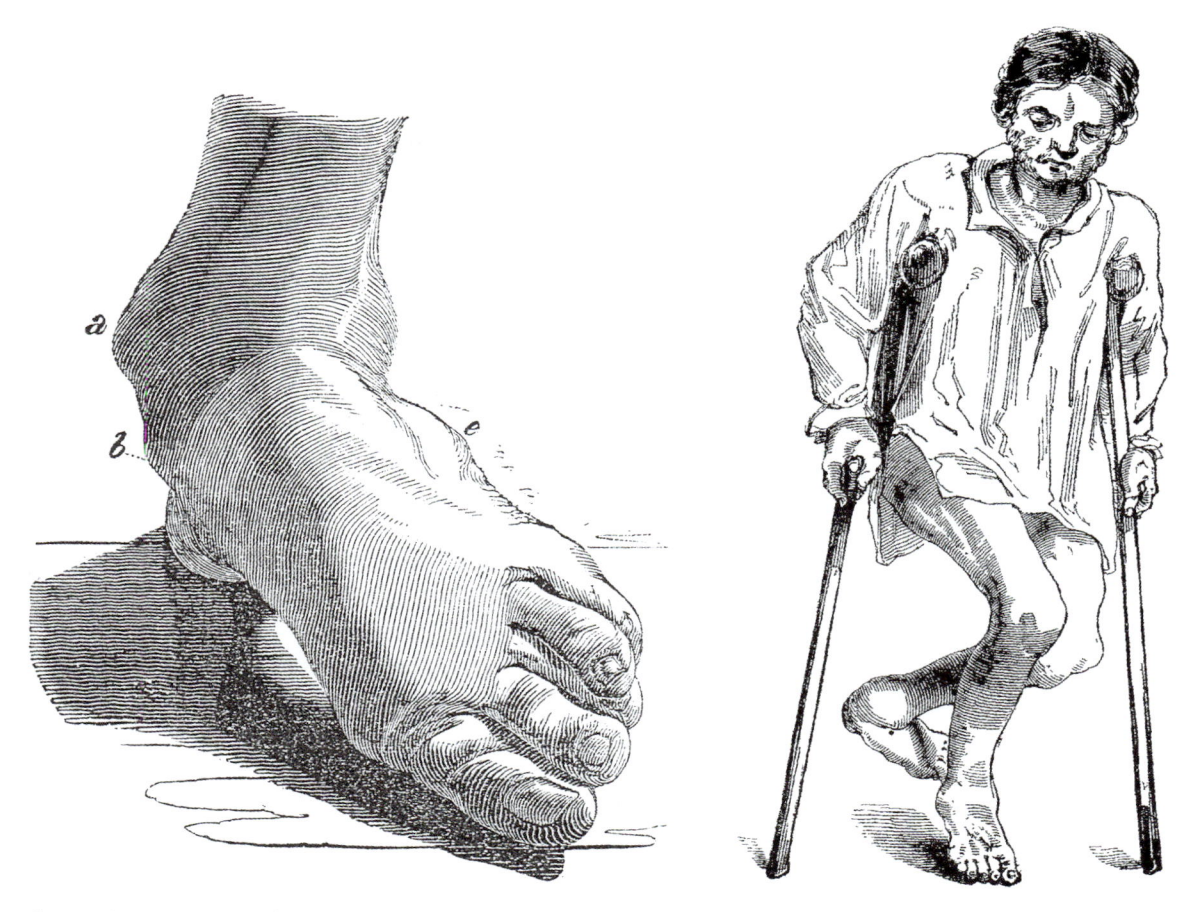

Fig. 5.3.3 William Little, spastic palsies from the 1843 lectures 8 and 9. Left: talipes calcaneo-valgus due to paresis of gastrocnemius and anterior tibial muscles; right: spastic flexor and adductor contractures of both thighs [33].

resuscitation [37]. In 1955, Apgar also published a follow-up study of 215 asphyctic infants, reporting 'no significant correlation between I.Q. [at 4 years] and oxygen content or saturation at any time during the first 3 hours of life' [38]. Unintended and without controlled studies, Apgar paved the way for oxygen in delivery rooms and promoted the belief in brain damage caused by lack of oxygen (see Chapter 2.3).

Inflammation and apoptosis

To periventricular leukomalacia, the Berlin pathologist Rudolf Virchow added a microscopic description in 1867 [39]: 'When in certain sites the granulated fat-spheres accumulate, it leads to a white or grayish white non-transparent spot or focal point recognizable with the naked eye. There are cases where it is larger and may reach a diameter of 1/4 or 1/2 inch ... For the time being I estimate the process to be active or irritative, with other words an *encephalitis* or *myelitis* in the *interstitium*'. One year later he published a figure (**Fig. 5.3.4**) of the lesion now termed *interstitial encephalitis* and concluded [40]: 'Certainly nobody will deny the inflammatory character of the yellow or grey-whitish lesions.'

Joseph Marie Jules Parrot, who had run the Paris Foundling Hospital since 1867, coined the term *athrepsia* which included diminished supply and ischaemia, and to which he subsumed the postasphyctic lesions in the brain [41]. He rejected Virchow's idea of an inflammatory process, discerning diffuse and focal fat accumulation, and called the process *acute white leucomalacia*, emphasizing its location 'nearly exclusively besides the lateral ventricles, especially in their dorsal aspect' (**Fig. 5.3.5**).

The pathogenesis of periventricular leukomalacia was further elucidated in 1976 by Alan Leviton and colleagues from Boston Children's Hospital who showed again what Virchow had posited 109 years earlier: that astrocytosis and amphophilic globuli within the white matter are associated with inflammatory processes in the perinatal period [42]. They hypothesized that bacterial endotoxins disturb marrow development. Together with Karin Nelson, Leviton pointed out that neonatal neuronal lesions correlate very weakly with obstetric complications, fetal distress, and biochemical markers of perinatal asphyxia, and that most infants survive severe birth asphyxia without neurological sequelae [43]. In 1981, Karin Nelson and Jonas Ellenberg compared the Apgar score at delivery with neurodevelopmental follow-up status at age 7 years in 49,000 children [44]. They found a remarkably weak association, even in a degree of asphyxia that not half of the infants survived. In 1994, the Iowa obstetrician Fritz Beller called 'the cerebral palsy story ... a catastrophic misunderstanding' [45]. Recent experimental data suggest, that caspase-mediated interaction of *hyperoxia* and inflammatory

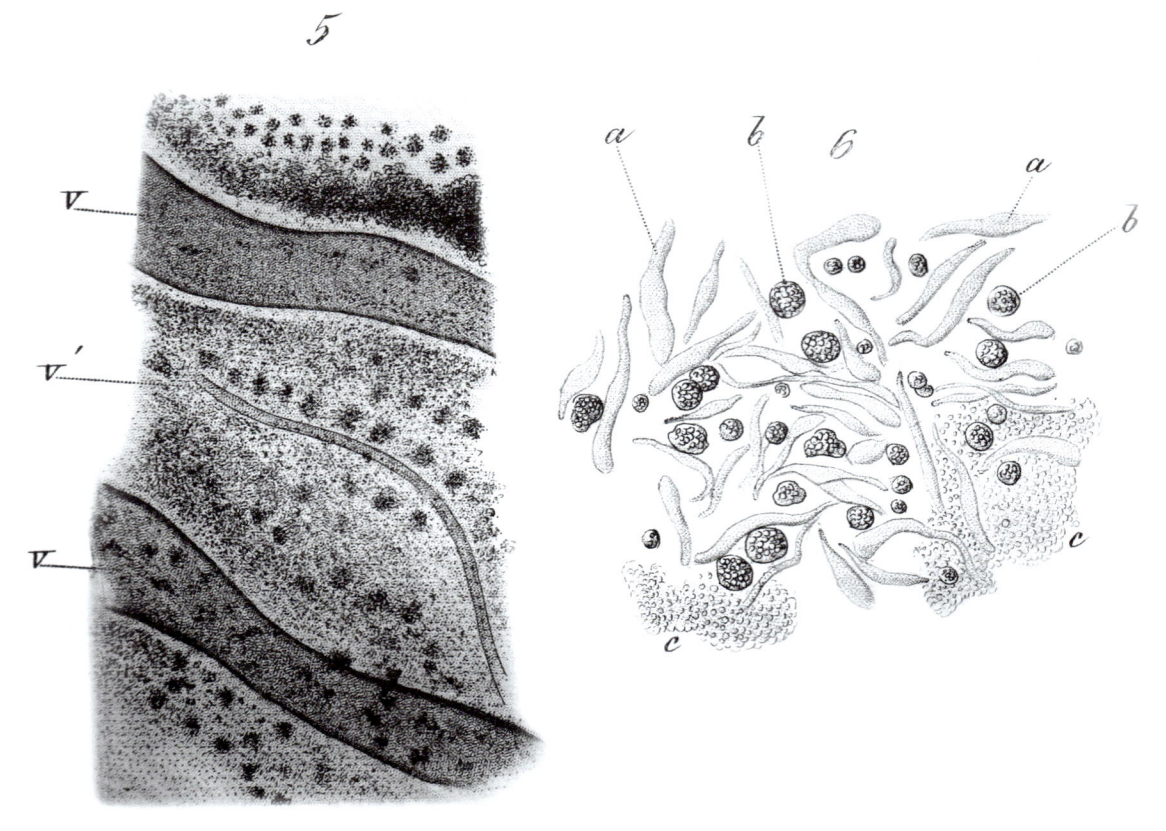

Fig. 5.3.4 Rudolf Virchow, 'interstitial encephalitis', 1868. Left: fatty degeneration of the brain with normal (v′) and dilated (v) vessels; right: higher enlargement; a, spindle- or club-shaped nerve fibres; b, granulated spheres; c, finely granulated matrix [40].

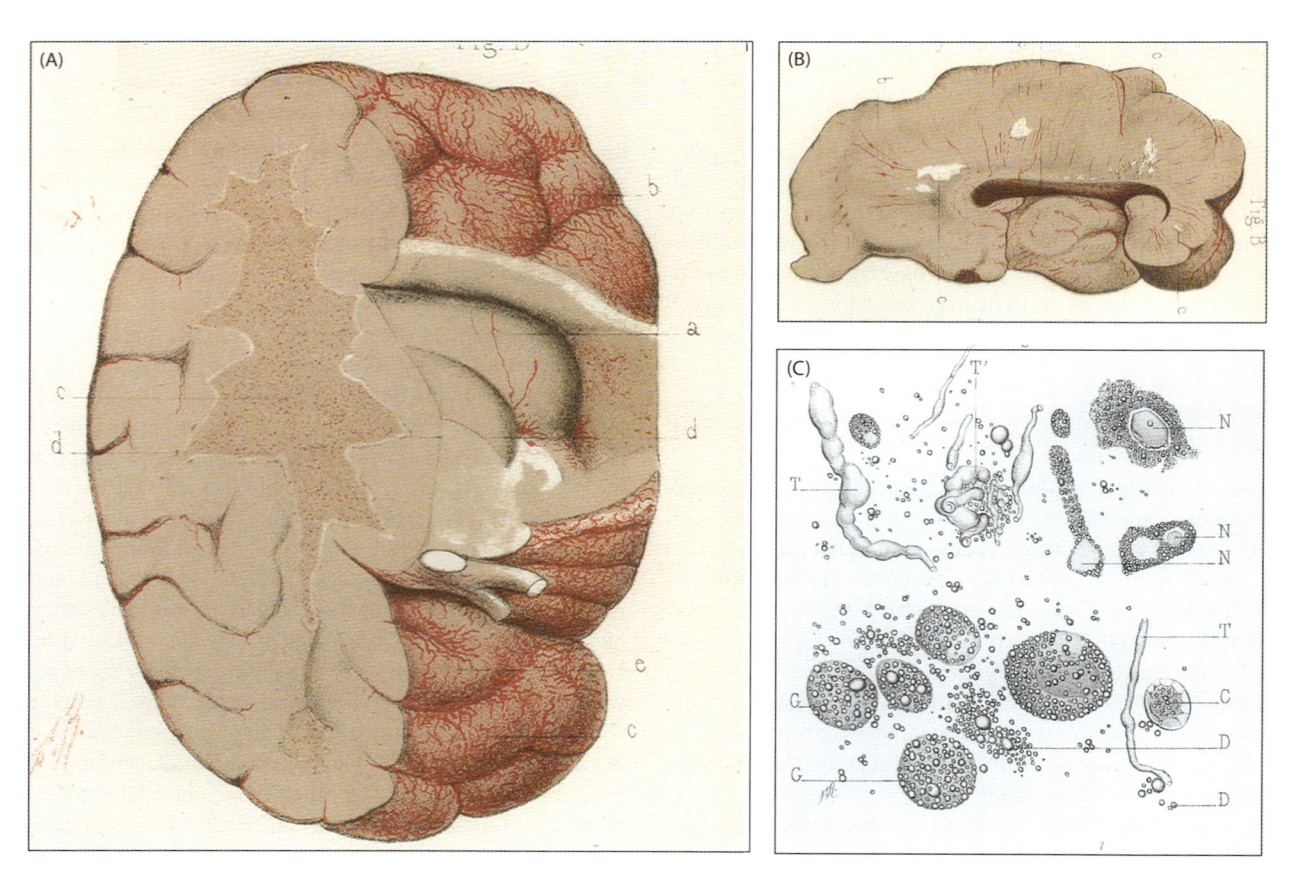

Fig. 5.3.5 Joseph Parrot, 'athrepsie', acute white softening of the brain, 1877, plates IV and IX: A, central diffuse; B, periventricular focal steatosis and malacia; C, microscopy ×600. Elements forming the opaque spots of the steatosis: G, granulated bodies; C, degenerated neuroglia; D, fat globules; T, degenerated nerve tubes [41].

cytokines activates apoptosis and could be a major pathway for damage to the immature brain [46]. Premyelinating oligodendrocytes are the target of free radical injury [47]. A strict definition of *asphyxia* was agreed upon in 1999 [48] and the uncritical use of the Apgar score abandoned [49].

Conclusion

Children and, even more so, adults with cerebral palsy have been excluded and despised in many cultures. Longer than with other disorders, scapegoats of all sorts replaced the scientific search for causative mechanisms. Blame was placed on God's wrath, witchcraft and magic, the expectant mother's 'imagination', the midwife's negligence, and teething. In more recent times, prematurity, asphyxia, hypoxia, ischaemia, traumatic haemorrhage, and inflammation were held responsible. Although a causal relation with giving birth has never been established and appears unlikely, the search for someone or something to blame for perinatal brain damage has remained common.

REFERENCES

1. Hippocrates: Opera Omnia. De la maladie sacrée. Edited by: E. Littré. Amsterdam: Hakkert, 1962: Vol. **6**, p. 364–75.
2. Lenormant F: Les sciences occultes en Asie; la magie chez les Chaldéens et les origines accadiennes. Paris: Maisonneuve, 1874.
3. Homer: Ilias. Tübingen: Cotta, 1806: p. 590–9.
4. Garland R: The eye of the beholder: deformity and disability in the Graeco-Roman world: Ithaca, NY: Cornell University Press, 1995: p. 23.
5. Plato: The laws. Chicago, IL: University of Chicago Press, 1980: Book VII, 789e, p. 177.
6. Conze A: Die attischen Grabreliefs. Berlin: de Gruyter, 1911–1922: Vol. **1**, p. Nr. 306/plate LXXIII.
7. Temkin O: Soranus' Gynecology. Baltimore, MD: The Johns Hopkins Press, 1956: Vol. **II**, p. 107, 113–22.
8. Mauriceau F: Traité des maladies des femmes grosses, et de celles qui sont accouchées (1st ed. 1668). 7. ed. Paris: Compagnie des Libraires, 1740: Vol. **3**, p. 472.
9. Luther M: Tischreden. Weimarer kritische Gesamtausgabe. Weimar: Böhlau, 1883–2009: p. tabletalk note of 20 April 1539.
10. Gemeiner CT: Regensburger Bettelordnung von 1514. In: Regensburgische Chronik. Regensburg: 1801–1824: Vol. **4**, p. 249.
11. Kornmann LJM: Höchstnöthiger Unterricht von der Geburth des Menschen. Erfurth: Zimmer, 1731: p. 23.
12. Würtz F: Ein schön nützliches Kinder-Büchlein. Basel: Sebastian Henricpetri, 1563: p. 78.
13. Sydenham T: Opera medica. Geneva: Fratres de Tournes, 1736: Vol. vol. **4**, p. 122.
14. Osler W: The cerebral palsies of children. London: Lewis, 1889: p. 91, 96.
15. Adelmann HB: The embryological treatises of Hieronimus Fabricius of Aquapendente. Ithaca, NY: Cornell University Press, 1942: Vol. **1**, p. 201.
16. Harvey W: Anatomical exercitations, concerning the generation of living creatures. London: Pulley, 1653: p. 337.
17. Morgagni GB: The seats and causes of diseases investigated by anatomy. London: Millar, 1769: p. Letter XLVIII, art. 54.
18. Ollivier (d'Angers) CP: De la moelle épinière et de ses maladies. 2. ed. Paris: Crevot, 1824: Vol. **1**, p. 123, plate I.
19. Bednar A: Die Krankheiten der Neugeborenen und Säuglinge. Wien: Gerold, 1851: Vol. **2**, p. 65.
20. Underwood M: A treatise on the disorders of childhood, and management of infants from the birth. 2. ed. London: Matthews, 1801: Vol. **2**, p. 89–90.
21. Jörg JCG: Handbuch zum Erkennen und Heilen der Kinderkrankheiten. Leipzig: Knobloch, 1826: p. 369.
22. Brissaud E: Maladie de Little et tabes spasmodique. Sem Méd Paris 1894;**14**:89–92.
23. Comberg M: Über Schicksal und Entwicklung von Frühgeborenen. Zeitschr Kinderheilk 1927;**43**:462–82.
24. Capper A: The fate and development of the immature and of the premature child. Am J Dis Child 1928;**35**:262–88, 443–91.
25. Smellie W: A treatise on the theory and practise of midwifery (London 1752). London: Sydenham Society, 1876: Vol. **3**, case 422, p. 215.
26. Capuron J: Traité des maladies des enfans, jusqu`a la puberté. 2. ed. Paris: Croullebois, 1820: p. 464.
27. Denis P-S: Recherches d'anatomie et de physiologie pathologique sur plusieurs maladies des enfants nouveau-nés. Commercy: Denis, 1826: p. 392.
28. McNutt SJ: Double infantile spastic hemiplegia. Am J Med Sci 1885;**89**:58–79.
29. McNutt SJ: Seven cases of infantile spastic hemiplegia. Arch Pediat 1885;**2**:20.
30. Gowers WR: Epilepsy and other chronic convulsive diseases. London: Churchill, 1881.
31. Schwartz P: Birth injuries of the newborn. Basel: Karger, 1961: p. 98.
32. Studdert DM, Mello MM, Gawande AA, et al.: Claims, errors, and compensation payments in medical malpractice litigation. N Engl J Med 2006;**354**:2024–33.
33. Little WJ: Course of [18] lectures on deformities of the human frame. Lancet 1843–1844;**41**:Lecture 8: 318–22; Lecture 9: 350–3.
34. Little WJ: On the influence of abnormal parturition, difficult labours, premature birth and asphyxia neonatorum on the mental and physical condition of the child, especially in relation to deformities. Trans Obstet Soc Lond 1861–1862;**3**:293–344.
35. Freud S: Die infantile Cerebrallähmung. In: Nothnagel H: Specielle Pathologie und Therapie. Wien: Hölder, 1897: Vol. **9**.
36. Smith CA, Kaplan E: Adjustment of blood oxygen levels in neonatal life. Am J Dis Child 1942;**64**:843–59.
37. Apgar V: A proposal for a new method of evaluation of the newborn infant. Curr Res Anesth Analg 1953;**32**:260–7.
38. Apgar V, Girdany BR, McIntosh R, Taylor HC Jr: Neonatal anoxia. I. A study of the relation of oxygenation at birth to intellectual development. Pediatrics 1955;**15**:653–62.
39. Virchow R: Zur pathologischen Anatomie des Gehirns. 1. Congenitale Encephalitis und Myelitis. Virchows Arch 1867;**38**:129–42.
40. Virchow R: Über interstitielle Encephalitis. Virchows Arch 1868;**44**:472–6.
41. Parrot J: Clinique des Nouveau-Nés: l'Athrepsie. Paris: Masson, 1877: p. 298–345, pl. IV, IX.
42. Leviton A, Gilles F, Neff R, Yaney P: Multivariate analysis of risk of perinatal telencephalic leucoencephalopathy. Am J Epidemiol 1976;**104**:621–6.
43. Nelson KB, Leviton A: How much of neonatal encephalopathy is due to birth asphyxia? Am J Dis Child 1991;**145**:1325–31.

44. Nelson KB, Ellenberg JH: Apgar scores as predictors of chronic neurologic disability. Pediatrics 1981;**68**:36–44.
45. Beller FK: The cerebral palsy story: a catastrophic misunderstanding in obstetrics. Obstet Gynecol Surv 1995;**50**:83.
46. Felderhoff-Mueser U, Sifringer M, Polley O, et al.: Caspase-1-processed interleukins in hyperoxia-induced cell death in the developing brain. Ann Neurol 2005;**57**:50–9.
47. Folkerth RD: Neuropathologic substrate of cerebral palsy. J Child Neurol 2005;**20**:940–9.
48. MacLennan A: A template for defining a causal relation between acute intrapartum events and cerebral palsy: international consensus statement. BMJ 1999;**319**:1054–9.
49. Committee on Obstetric Practice, American College of Obstetricians and Gynecologists: Inappropriate use of the terms fetal distress and birth asphyxia. Obstet Gynecol 2005;**106**:1469–70.
50. Knapp F: Andrea Mantegna. Des Meisters Gemälde und Kupferstiche. Stuttgart: Deutsche Verlagsanstalt, 1910: p. 159.

5.4

Possessed by evil spirits
Seizures in infancy

Introduction: a supranatural disease

Already in the 5th century B.C.E., authors of the *Corpus Hippocraticum* opposed the superstition associated with epilepsy in the book *De Morbo Sacro* [1]: 'This disease is in my opinion no more divine than any other disease; it has its own nature and cause ... the cause of this affection is in the brain.' The brain was considered a mucous gland required 'to purge the blood, both in the fetus and after birth. The cold phlegm which it secretes descends to lung and heart and cools the blood ... Very young infants affected with seizures mostly die, when the flow of phlegm is considerable and the wind blows from south. Their narrow veins cannot collect the abundant and thick pituitary secretion, the blood cools and coagulates, and death follows.' As late as 1660, Konrad Schneider [2] realized that nasal secretions do not originate from the pituitary, but from mucous membranes. In older children and adults, epilepsy was attributed to bile accumulation, 'and they are not killed by the convulsions, nor do these cause contortions [spasms]'. The *Prognostics* [3] described symptomatic seizures as 'if acute fever be present, and the belly be constipated, if they cannot sleep, are agitated, and moan, and change colour, and become green, livid, or ruddy. These complaints occur most readily to children which are very young.'

Avicenna (11th century C.E.) discerned moist and dry forms, attributing the former to hydrocephalus and the latter to teething [4]: 'Convulsions during dentition are generally due to fermentative changes in the digestion, added by nervousness, especially if the baby is over-fat and humid in constitution.' Historical aspects of epilepsy have been elaborated upon extensively [5–7], but seizures in neonates and young infants have been largely neglected in these histories.

Classification

Complex, inconsistent, and frequently changing terminology signals that a disease is incompletely understood. Antoine Josat [8] wrote in 1856: 'I was struck by the amazing number of denominations the disease has been given.' *Mater puerorum* [the mother in children] was a term coined by Rhazes [9] who practised during the 10th century C.E. in Baghdad. It described neonatal convulsions or pavor nocturnus and was clearly discerned from epilepsy. Paulus Bagellardus [10] distinguished in 1472 '*epilepsy* from birth, which is not to be cured ... and *convulsions*, resulting from repletion (in the fleshy) or from inanition (in dehydrated infants)'. Cornelius Roelans of Mecheln [11] classified infant convulsions in no fewer than six different types in 1485: *pavor nocturnus*, terrible dreams or nightmares; *mother in children*, identical to epilepsy and occurring in infants and older children; *relaxation of nerves*, probably atonic seizures; *spasm*, preferring the head and mouth; *alcuzen*, rigid extension identical to tetanus; and *spasm and tetanus from inanition*, or dehydration, which also comprised febrile convulsions. In 1545, Thomas Phaire of Kilgerran [12] distinguished *The Fallyng Euill* (identical to epilepsy and also occurring in older children) and *Crampe* (identical to spasms). Simon Vallambert of Orleans [13] discerned *convulsion proportionnée* (clonic), *rigueur* (tonic), *convulsion non proportionnée* (possibly myoclonic), and *relaxation* (atonic) in 1565. His term for spasm was *prostotonos*. Hieronymus Mercuriale of Padova distinguished two diseases in 1584 [14]: the *falling evil* revealed by generalized movements and caused by inheritance, hydrocephalus, and teething; and the *dangerous convulsion* limited to certain limbs, frequently lethal within the first week of life, and attributed to the nurse's bad milk (see Chapter 6.1).

Table 5.4.1 represents an attempt to match several terms used in the 18th and 19th centuries to describe seizures in infancy with modern semiotics. Predisposition should not be understood as causality, as the seizure type is not disease specific in infancy. It is not the aim of the present chapter to describe the causes of infantile seizures, which include practically every type of metabolic disturbance and encephalopathy occurring perinatally and during infancy. As it mainly distinguishes between partial and generalized seizures, the classification system of the International League Against Epilepsy has not proven useful in infancy [15]. Seizures in this age group are usually classified according to Volpe [16] and Nordli [17]. The term epilepsy usually describes chronic seizure disorders, and has rarely been used during the first year of life. The term *grand mal* describes generalized tonic–clonic seizures, which are very rare during the

---

Adapted with permission from Obladen, M. Possessed by evil spirits: a history of seizures in infancy. *Journal of Child Neurology*, 29(7):990–1001. Copyright © 2014, © SAGE Publications.

PART 5 Odd shape

Table 5.4.1 Typical seizure types of newborns and young infants and their terminology during the 18th and 19th centuries

Seizure type	Subtle	Clonic	Tonic	Myoclonic	Infantile spasm	Atonic	References
Synonyms in contemporary use	Fit, automatism				Jack knife seizure, Blitz-Nick-Salaam	Astatic	
Characteristics	Eye deviation with or without jerking, eyelid flutter, tonic limb posturing, oral-buccal movement	Rhythmic, usually slow (1–3/s) movements, focal or generalized, involving face, limbs, neck or trunk	Generalized, rarely focal sustained stiffening of limbs or asymmetric posturing of trunk and/or neck	Rhythmic, rapid jerks with particular predilection for flexor muscle groups	Brief contraction involving muscles of the neck, trunk, and extremities, usually bilaterally and symmetrically, often in clusters	Sudden loss of muscle tone and posture, most often as head drop. Sometimes combined with myoclonic jerks	[16] [19] [20] [21]
Typical age at onset; typical predisposition	First week; prematurity	Term, first day; hypoxia, ischaemia	First day; haemorrhage	Second week; metabolic	3–5 months; fetal brain lesion	Rare in young infants	[22] [23]
Stahl, Berlin 1718 Kornmann, Erfurt 1731	–	Zucken	–	Krampff	Böses Wesen, schwere Noth	–	[24]
Harris, London 1736, 1742	–	Convulsive fits	–	–	Grievous convulsions	Epilepsia?	[25] [26]
Rosén, Uppsala 1781	–	Convulsion, zuckung	Tetanus, opisthotonus	–	Hiärtsprång, jammer	–	[27]
Armstrong, London 1783 Underwood, London 1784	Inward fits	Symptomatic convulsion, hiccup	Idiopathic convulsion = due to brain disease or hydrocephalus		Hectic fever, paroxysm of dentition	–	[28] [29]
Baumes, Montpellier 1805	Convulsion	Clonisme, hoquet	Tonisme, trisme	Eclampsie	Paroxysme spasmodique	–	[30]
Henke, Erlangen 1821	Innere Krämpfe, Schäuerchen	Gefraisch, Kopf- Fraisen	Starrkrampf, trismus, tetanus	Gichter, Fraisen	Schlagender Jammer	–	[31]
Jahn, Meiningen 1803 Jörg, Leipzig 1826	Stiller innerer Jammer	Krämpfe, Gichter, convulsiones	Starrsucht, trismus	Gichter, eclampsia	Jammer	Delirium	[32] [33]
Wendt, Breslau 1826	Risus sardonicus	Allgemeiner Krampf, convulsio	Starrkrampf, trismus	Ecclampsia	Emprosthotonus	Betäubung, stupor	[34]
Rotch, Boston 1896 Holt, New York 1898	Convulsive twitching	Clonic convulsions	Tonic, tetanus, opisthotonus	Reflex convulsions	Spasmodic attacks	–	[35] [36]
Henoch, Berlin 1895 Zipperling, Graz 1913	Stäupchen	Konvulsionen	Starre, trismus	Eclampsia infantilis	Nickkrampf, spasmus nutans	Apathie	[37] [38]

Classification is based on observation of the infant, published by Volpe [16, 19], Mizrahi and Kellaway [20], and Nordli [21]. Historic sources include conditions with which some seizure types were frequently confused (e.g. tonic seizures and tetanus).

first year of life. The incidence rate of neonatal seizures is 2.6 per 1000 live births and 11.1 in preterm neonates [18].

Evil spirits and witchcraft

Despite the warning in the *Corpus Hippocraticum* [1], invisible evil powers continuously at work have been part of virtually all religious beliefs since prehistoric times [39]. Babylonic cuneiform tablets (17th century B.C.E.) described a grim prognosis for seizures in neonates [40]: 'If the baby, two, three days having passed after it is born, does not accept the milk, *miqtu* is falling upon him, time and again: The disease's name is Hand of the Goddess [Ishtar], the Snatcher – he will die.' In many cultures, including all Mediterranean nations, seizures in babies were attributed to the *evil eye*, also called *fascination* or *overlooking*. The gospel [Mark 1:26] equated seizures with *unclean spirits*: 'When the unclean spirit had torn him, and cried with a loud voice, he came out of him.' Christians believed the neonate to be especially subject to diabolical powers (**Fig. 5.4.1**, left), and starting in 215 C.E., exorcism became part of the baptismal rite [41]. Martin Luther retained exorcism in his *Taufbüchlein* of 1526 [42]: 'Depart thou unclean spirit, and make room for the Holy Spirit.' This caused bitter controversy with the Calvinists throughout the 16th century [43]. The Catholic baptismal rite still contains a short exorcism to the present day. The *malleus maleficarum* (hammer of witches) [44] of the Dominicans Heinrich Kramer and Jakob Sprenger claimed in 1487: 'For we have often found that certain people have been visited with epilepsy or the falling sickness by means of eggs which have been buried with dead bodies, especially the dead bodies of witches, together with other ceremonies of which we cannot speak, particularly when these eggs have been given to a person either in food or drink.'

A few years later in his painting of St Anthony's temptation, Hieronymus Bosch depicted a witch casting a spell on a swaddled baby, who is also being gazed upon by a knight, illustrating the *malocchio* of the *jettatore dei bambini* (**Fig. 5.4.1**, right). The infant is not shown having a seizure, but this feared consequence of bewitching may occur later. In 1603, the Jesuit Martin Del-Rio published the six-volume *Disquisition in Magic*, which ascribed the calamities of mortals to evil spirits [45]: 'Fascination is a power

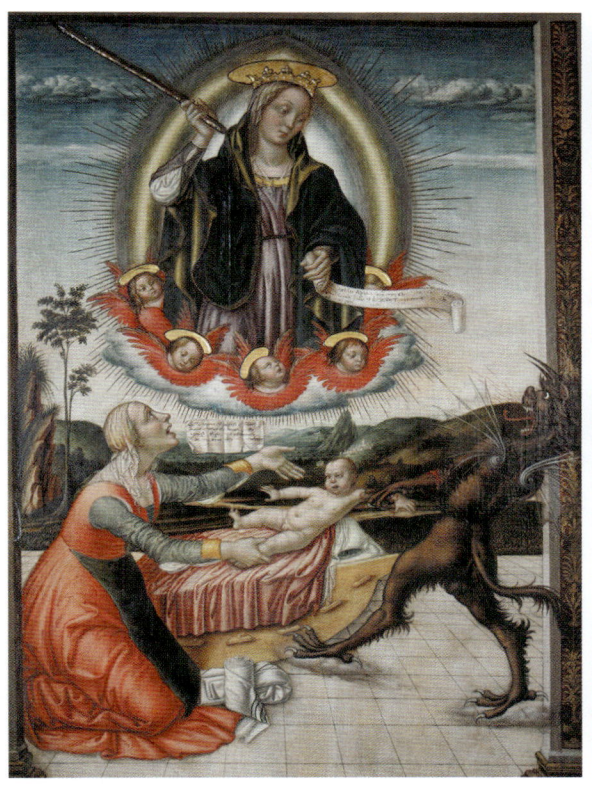

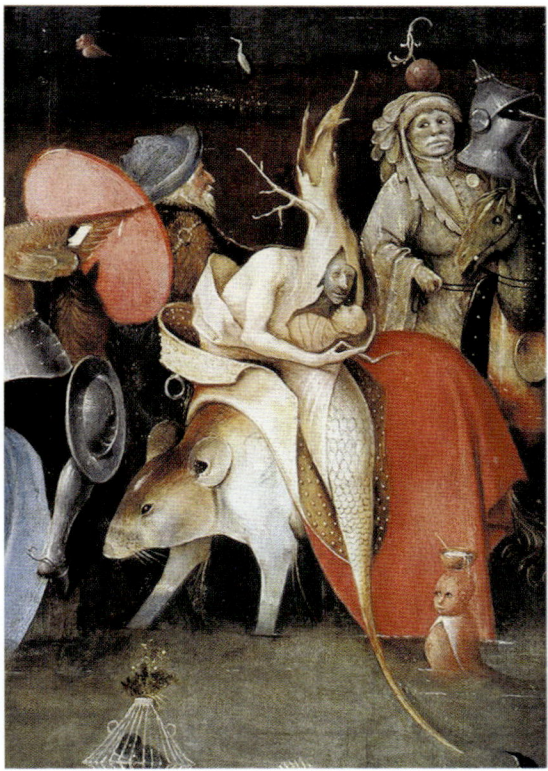

Fig. 5.4.1 Ideas on the pathogenesis of seizures in infancy in the 15th century. Left: the devil tries to snatch away an infant from its mother. The infant is depicted with rolled up eyes and splayed fingers and toes. Right: a sorcerer (*strega*) bewitches and a soldier (*jettatore*) casts an evil eye onto a swaddled infant. Detail of the *Triptych of Temptation of St. Anthony* by Hieronymus Bosch, ca. 1505.
Left: Madonna del soccorso by Niccolo Alunno, ca. 1480: Rome, Galleria Colonna, with permission. Right: Lisbon, Museu Nacional de Arte Antiga, © DGPC/ADF Luisa Oliveira, 2011, with permission.

derived by contact with the devil, who, when the fascinator looks at another with evil intent, or praises by means known to himself, infects with evil the person at whom he looks.' A contagious nature was attributed to convulsions. As late as 1751, the four-volume paediatric textbook of Johann Storch [46] contained 60 pages on diseases resulting from sorcery, among them 'epilepsiam, spasmos, convulsiones, ecstasin'.

Maternal imagination

Fabricius Hildanus [47] described a case he observed in Cologne in 1599, where 'a young honest pregnant woman walked in the street, when an epileptic fell to the ground close to her, cried out, and threw about his limbs, upon which the woman was much frightened. Her term fulfilled, she was happily delivered of a son, who, shortly thereafter, was seized by frequent convulsions, which carried him off before he was a year old.' This description started a discussion on maternal imagination as a cause of convulsions in infancy which lasted well into the 18th century [48–50].

Protective gods and patron saints

In the antique pantheon, specific gods were believed to protect infants from diseases. In India, Lord Shiva Nataraja, the cosmic dancer, personified the fight against the evil [51]: his right foot is crushing Apasmara Purusha, the demon of ignorance, the embodiment of evil, depicted as a dwarf or a baby with twisted hands (**Fig. 5.4.2**). In traditional Hindu medicine, *apasmara* is the term for epilepsy [52]. Christians defined various patron saints to combat *unclean spirits*. For St Valentine alone, Kluge and Kudernatsch [53] collected 341 illustrations and sculptures from eight centuries showing the bishop exorcising epileptics (**Fig. 5.4.3**). St Valentine's skull was venerated as a relic in Rouffach, Alsace [54], since 1181, where people with epilepsy made pilgrimages for a cure and a hospice was established in 1507. This hospice remained active until the French Revolution put an end to the priory in 1789 [55].

Dentition and infant mortality

The work *on dentition* in the *Corpus Hippocraticum* reveals strong views [56]: 'Those who during teething frequently defecate are less subject to seizures than those who are constipated … Not all infants die who are affected by seizures during dentition; many also escape alive.' London surgeon Walter Harris [26] noted in 1742: 'Of all the disorders which threaten the lives of Infants, there is none that is wont to produce so many grievous Symptoms as a *difficult* and laborious *Breeding of Teeth* … The physician therefore ought to take care that the *Incision* be always made with a proper instrument, whether it be a *Penknife*, or any other knife that has a thick Back.'

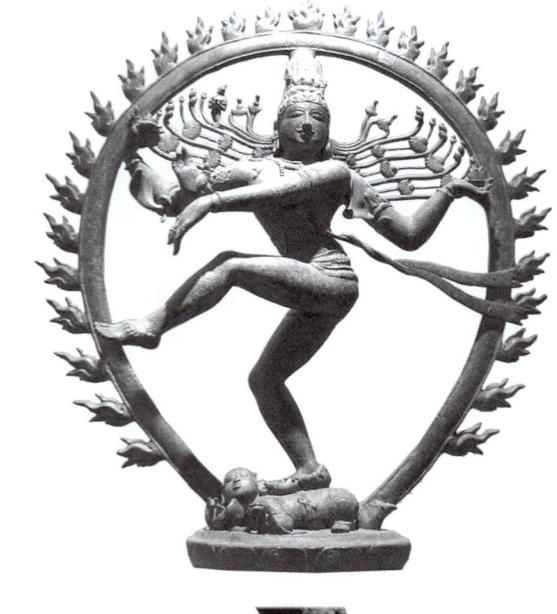

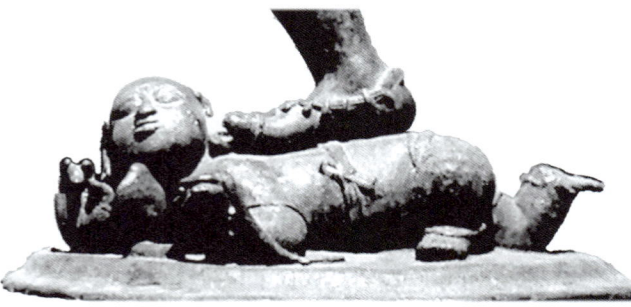

Fig. 5.4.2 The healing Hindu God Shiva Nataraja dancing on the body of the evil spirit Apasmara, the demon of ignorance. Bottom: detail showing Apasmara as an infant with twisted hands and feet. Modified from a bronze sculpture of the 11th century c.e., Paris, Musée Guimet.

George Armstrong, who instituted the London Dispensary of the Infant Poor in 1769, wrote [28]: 'As to the convulsions in which most of the diseases of children terminate before they die, they are so well known to every body, that it would be needless to describe them. I take them in general to be owing to a *stimulus* communicated to the nerves, either by the acrimony of the bowels, or by an inflammation in those parts, or in the gums at the time of teething, unless where the brain is primarily affected … Teething, in the same manner as was observed on convulsions, is said to carry off a much greater number of children than it actually does; for almost all children that die while they are about teeth, are said to die of teething.' Cutting the gums remained widespread to prevent and treat seizures in infancy, as described by Robert Todd [57] from London in 1842: 'Mr Pincott, the excellent resident assistant, having found the gums swollen, scarified them freely … however, [this] was not followed by any improvement in the symptoms; the child was then immersed in a warm bath for ten minutes … half an hour afterwards, with the view of removing any irritating matter which might have accumulated in the bowels, an enema was administered … but without good effect. Cold sponging of the head was next tried, and two leeches were applied to the right temple … five hours from the commencement of the fit … applying ice along the back of the neck and spine, with a view of calming, by the sedative agency of cold, the irritable state of that portion of the cerebro-spinal axis.'

During the years 1805–1815, every fifth infant born in Bern, Switzerland, failed to survive the first year of life [58] and in 75% of them the assumed cause of death was classified as 'cramps'. This category included the denominations 'tetanus, convulsions, gichteren, and epilepsy'. The high prevalence of rickets associated with tetanic clonus may have contributed to this figure, and 'difficult teething' probably was scurvy in most cases (see Chapter 7.6).

Irritation of the gut

Nils Rosén von Rosenstein [59], professor in Uppsala, wrote in *Diseases of Children* (first ed. 1764): 'Meconium will cause epilepsy, if not sufficiently carried off, by growing acrid in the body, and by irritating the intestines … Children will also get this disease by sucking a nurse at the time her menses are upon her … worms commonly cause the epilepsy by violent fits, and frequent returns.' And Underwood pointed out in 1784 [29]: 'A very common cause of convulsions is worms.' In 1780, the Paris Medical Faculty offered a scientific price for 'exposure of the different types of seizures in infants, their causes, diagnosis, prognosis and treatment'. The prize winner Jean Baptiste Baumes published a 513-page treatise. He added to the usually assumed causes *acrimonie*, a metabolic anomaly attributed to spoiled milk and enteritis, and now understood as metabolic acidosis [30]: 'In mid-January 1778 I was called to a 24-hour-old infant who had passed but a tiny quantity of meconium. It had repeatedly been given sugared wine and olive oil, but without success. The infant had heavy eclamptic attacks … The extended habit [to discard the colostrum and] to give, as first nourishment, the aged milk of a wet-nurse, frequently evokes convulsions, as it causes meconium retention.' *Unwholesome* milk meant blaming the mother or the nurse for seizures, as London obstetrician Charles Routh [60] did in 1879: 'Evidence that the mother's milk does not agree with the child: it may produce diarrhea, insomnia, it may be convulsions. This is more especially the case in very impressionable women.' Very common before the advent of sound hygiene, intestinal worms remained—after teething—the second most frequently claimed cause of convulsions in paediatric textbooks from New York to Moscow up to the beginning of the 20th century [36, 61].

Inheritance

Thomas Phaire [12] maintained traditional views in his *Boke of Children*, first published in 1545: 'Lytle chyldren are oftentimes afflicted, with this greuouse syckenes [grievous sickness], sometyme by nature receyued of the parents, and then it is impossible, or difficile to cure, sometyme by euyll and vnholsome diet, wherby there is engendred many colde and moyst humours in the brayne.' Walter Harris [26] observed in 1742 that 'some families have untimely lost several of their Children, one after another, by a sort of hereditary Convulsions'. The Weimar Court obstetrician Johann Bernstein [62] wrote in 1797: 'Among the causes of neonatal convulsions are counted faulty constitution, bad air, abuse of food … Of special importance is the transmission of convulsions from father or mother to the child.'

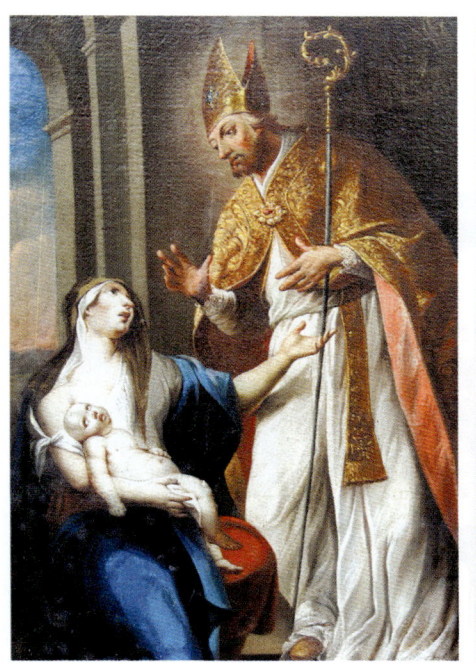

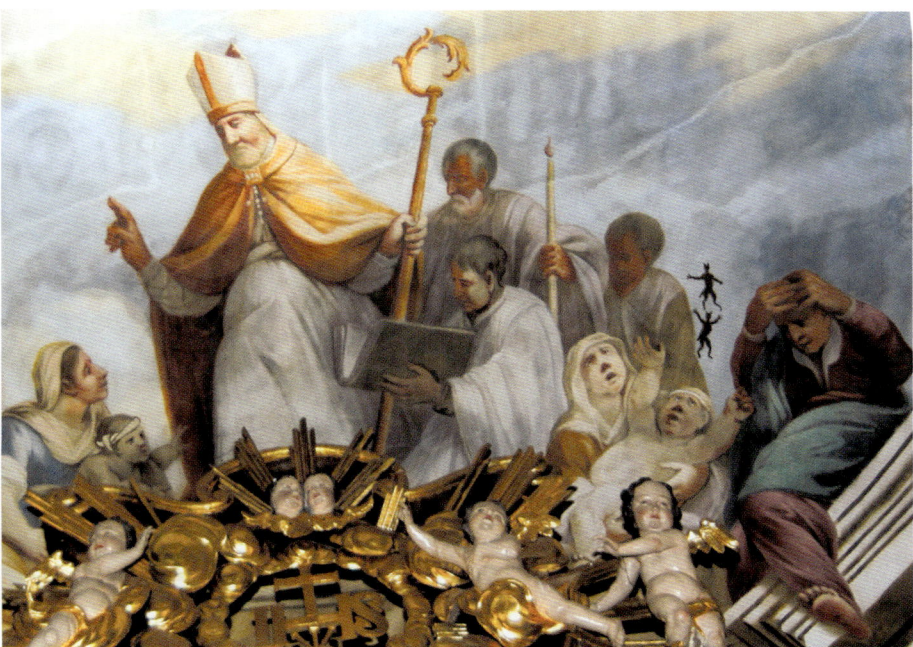

Fig. 5.4.3 St Valentine exorcising evil spirits from infants whose convulsions are depicted with remarkable precision. Left: atonic seizure; right: spasms in two infants wearing head protectors; two black demons are shown leaving one of the infants.
Left: Atonic seizure; unknown artist, early 18th century, St. Michael's Church, Röhrnbach, with permission. Right: Giovanni Marchini 1740, Valentine chapel, Unterleiterbach. Marktgemeinde Zapfendorf, with permission.

Perinatal brain injury

A difficult delivery and convulsions were correlated by the Scottish obstetrician William Smellie in 1752 [63]: 'In lingering labours, when the head of the child hath been in the pelvis, so that the bones ride over one another and the shape is preternaturally lengthened, the brain is frequently so much compressed that violent convulsions ensue before or soon after delivery to the danger and ofttimes the destruction of the child.' Of 176 neonates with convulsions, Peterman [64] considered birth injury in 69% and acute infection in 10% as the most frequent causes in 1946. As late as 1948, Nielsen and Butler, who studied 992 cases of epilepsy, believed that 3 min of birth asphyxia could later cause epilepsy [65]. In the pre-ultrasound era, W.S. Craig [66] at the Edinburgh Simpson Memorial Hospital found intracranial haemorrhages in 97 of 158 infants who had seizures and died within the first 10 days of life; in 216 survivors of the same condition, a firm diagnosis was made in only 26.

Syndromes with infantile spasms

In January 1841, the surgeon William James West of Tunbridge appealed for help for his son James Edwin in a letter to *The Lancet*, thereby providing the classic description of infantile spasm, now termed *West syndrome* [67]: '[When] he was four months old, I first observed slight *bobbings* of the head forward, which I then regarded as a trick, but were, in fact, the first indications of disease; for these *bobbings* increased in frequency, and at length became so frequent and powerful, as to cause a complete heaving of the head forward toward his knees, and then immediately relaxing into the upright position, something similar to the attacks of emprosthotonos ... He neither possesses the intellectual vivacity or the power of moving his limbs, of a child of his age ... The view I took of it was that, most probably, it depended on some irritation of the nervous system from teething ... treatment of leeches and cold applications to the head, repeated calomel purgatives, and the usual antiphlogistic treatment; the gums were lanced, and the child frequently put into warm baths ... Finding no benefit from all that had been done, I took the child to London, and had a consultation with Sir Charles Clarke ... who, from the peculiar bowing of the head, called it the "salaam convulsion".' Other age-related epileptic brain diseases involving spasms include Ohtahara syndrome, Aicardi syndrome, Down's syndrome, and Lennox Gastaut syndrome, all associated with structural lesions in the cortex and severe intellectual disability.

Electroencephalography

Fifty-six years before the advent of electroencephalography, John Hughlings Jackson [68] defined in 1873: 'Epilepsy is the name for occasional, sudden, excessive, rapid and local discharges of the gray matter.' After the electroencephalogram (EEG) was described by Hans Berger [69] in 1929, neurophysiology laboratories were established in many countries. In Boston from 1934, Frederic and Erna Gibbs together with William Lennox used the EEG to classify epileptic seizures [70]. In 1945, the Gibbs went to Chicago and developed with Percival Bailey a technique for temporal lobectomy [71]. In 1952, they described in the second volume of their *Atlas of Encephalography* 'an exceedingly abnormal interseizure EEG commonly encountered in infants with a clinical history of

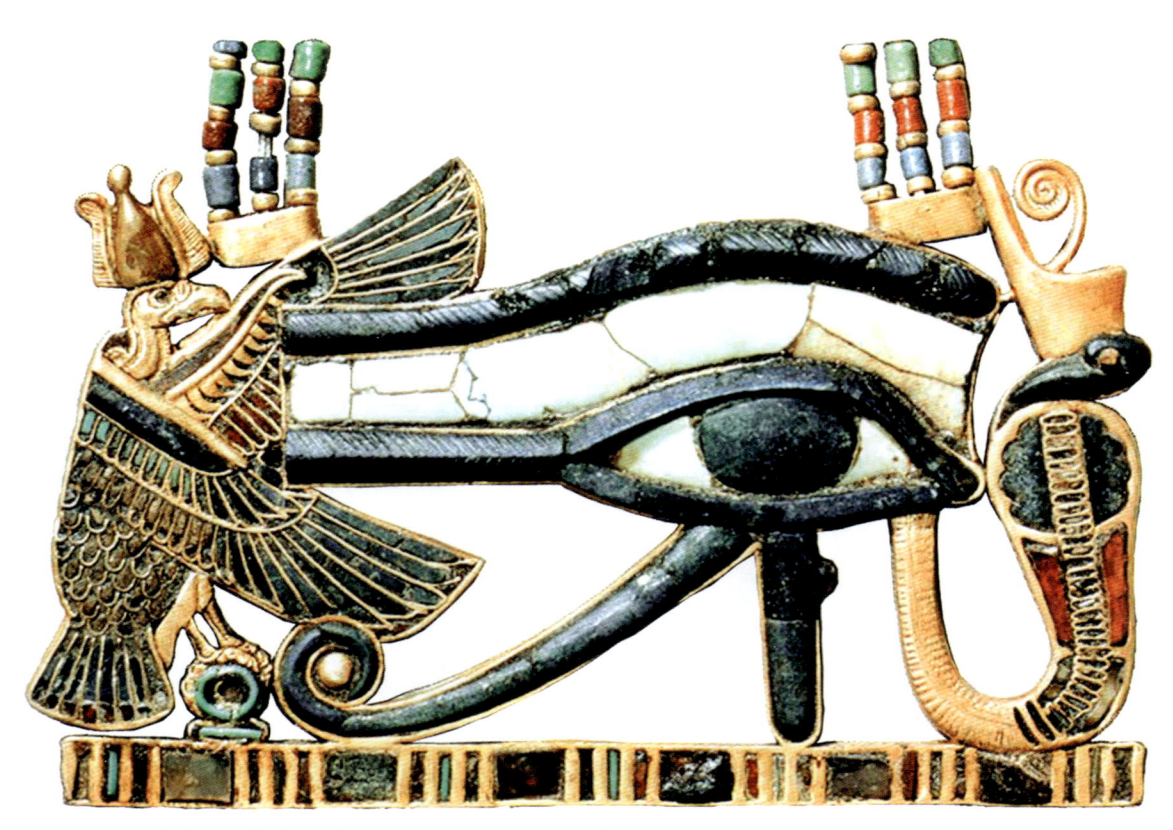

Fig. 5.4.4 Antique emblem (*Udjat Eye*) believed to protect against seizures. The sacred eye of Horus is surrounded by royal insignia. Modified from a gold and glass pectoral amulet in the tomb of Tutankhamun near Luxor, 13th century b.c.e.

spasms' and called it *hypsarhythmia* [72]. Electroencephalography revolutionized the diagnosis of seizure disorders and today guides anticonvulsive treatment.

Protective amulets and the evolution of treatment for seizures in infancy

In the absence of effective treatment and believing in supranatural origin, amulets and charms evolved in all cultures to prevent or treat infant convulsions [73]. Egyptian medicine very likely associated seizures with direct divine intervention, demoniacal possession, and the lunar cycle [74]. The *udjat* (sacred eye of Horus) is ubiquitously encountered in Egypt and was worn as a pectoral amulet and buried with its bearer. In use from the Old Kingdom (2500 B.C.E.) and produced until the Roman Period (50 B.C.E.), its forms were many, and its assumed protection was not specifically directed against seizures [75]. Both the *injured* (left) lunar eye (plucked out by Horus' rival Seth and restored by the lunar deity Thoth) and the *sound* (right) solar eye were used as amulets of protection. Fig. 5.4.4 shows an example from Tutankhamun's grave. In the Roman Empire, house amulets or images acting against the evil eye were fixed to the wall or floor. The famous Antioch mosaic shows the evil eye surrounded by protectors: a centipede, dog, snake, scorpion, sword, trident, bird, cat, a priapic dwarf carrying a dowsing rod, and the words *KAI CY* (and you).

Coral was esteemed as a powerful anticonvulsant for 1200 years. Alexander of Tralles (6th century C.E.) recommended [76] 'to collect coral and peony when the moon shrinks, wrap it into cloth, and hang it around the neck'. Medieval and Renaissance paintings from all over Europe display coral amulets around the Christ Child's neck (Fig. 5.4.5). Paracelsus, a famous Swiss physician and alchemist, recommended [77] in 1530 'coral subtly ground and extracted with alcohol until all redness disappeared … very helpful for *caducis*', and Thomas Phaire [12] recommended in 1545: 'There be diuers things that are good to procure an easy breeding of teeth … the first cast toath of a colte, set in silver and borne, or redde coralle in lyke manner, hanged about the necke … the coral by consent of all authors … helpeth the chyldren of the falling euill.' Even Thomas Willis, who in 1664 described the arterial circle and distinguished tetanus and seizures, did not hesitate to prescribe amulets [78]: 'It is usual to pour into the Mouth of an Infant newly Born, as soon as it begins to Breath, some Anticonvulsive Medicine … On the third or fourth Day after it is born, let an Issue be made in the Nucha, then let a little Blood be drawn from the Jugular Veins by Leeches … let a Periapt of the Roots and Seeds of the greater Peony with a little addition of Elks-beef be hung about the Neck … red Coral prepar'd.'

The *Anodyne* necklace, advertised and sold in Britain during the 18th century 'for convulsions and difficult breeding of teeth', also contained peony root, among other ingredients [79]. Its use was widespread and Michael Underwood complained in 1801 [80]: 'I am almost ashamed of noticing among [the charms and amulets] that very common one, anodyne necklace. It is impossible that a bit of dried bone hung around the neck can remove convulsions.' In Bavaria and Austria, infants with seizures wore necklaces called *Fraisenkette* (Fig. 5.4.6A) well into the 20th century. It united multiple amulets

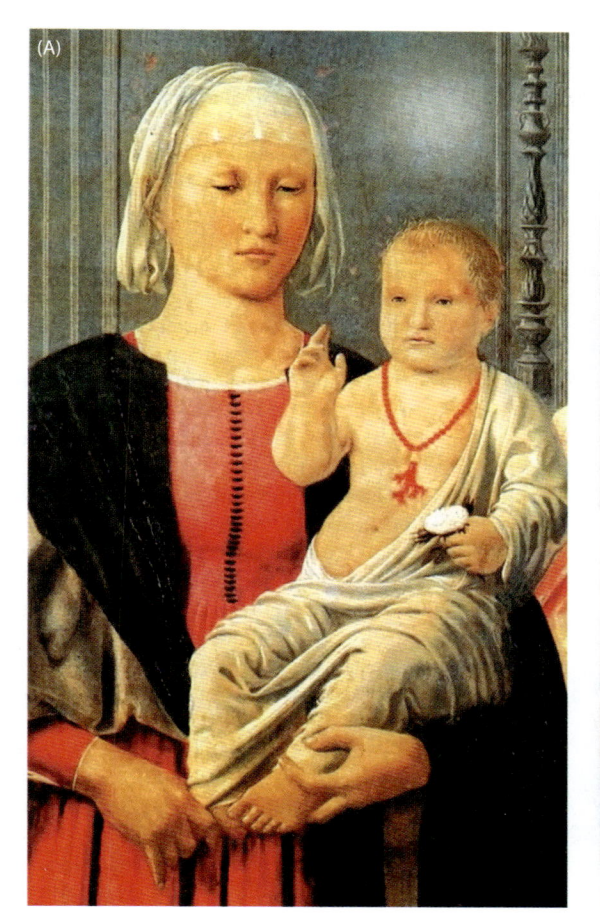

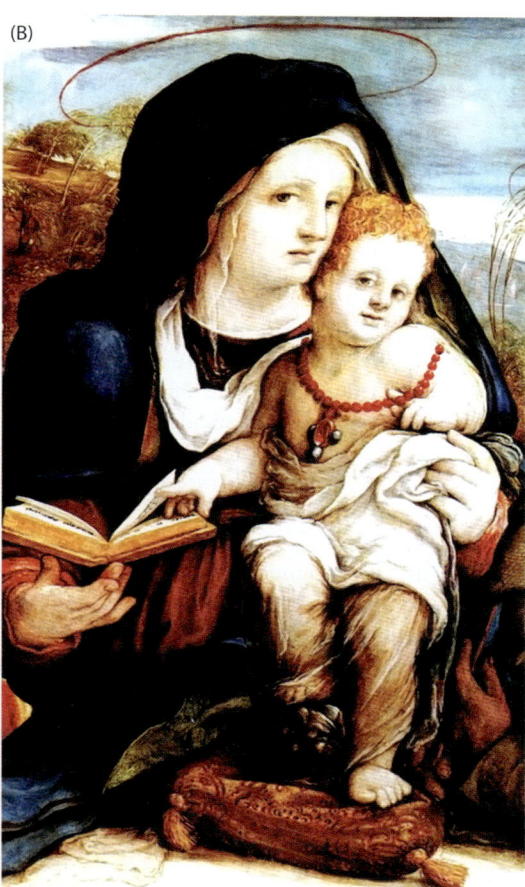

Fig. 5.4.5 A and B, details of coral chains and amulets in Christian sacral paintings from the 15th and 16th centuries believed to protect the infant from the evil eye, especially from convulsions.
A, Piero della Francesca ca.1470: Urbino, Galleria Nazionale delle Marche, with permission. B, Amico Aspertini, 1520: Cardiff, National Museum of Wales, with permission.

and charms, among them a wolf's tooth, a crystal, and printed or written prayers (*Agathazettel*). Influenced by Mesmer's animal magnetism, Victor Burq [81] developed *metallothérapie* for convulsions in infancy using necklaces with various metal plates (**Fig. 5.4.6B**), a method which survives in alternative medicine. Today, 11% of the infants admitted to a tertiary centre in Nigeria are wearing amulet necklaces [82].

Early drugs

In 117 C.E., Soranus, an influential obstetrician teaching in Rome, recommended [83]: 'From the fifth month on one should persistently rub the gums during the bath with an anointed finger and soften them with chicken fat. And the brain of an hare acts the same way.' Most

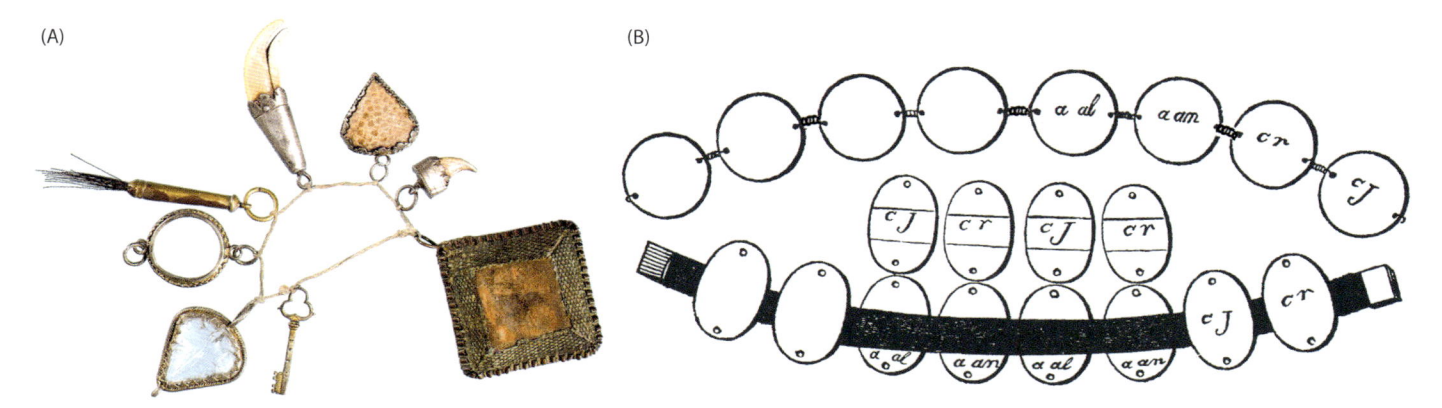

Fig. 5.4.6 Protective amulet necklaces of the 19th century. A, *Fraisenkette* from Graz. Inv.-Nr. 6.975; B, chain used for metallotherapy in France; aal, German steel; aan, English steel; cj, brass; cr, copper; from Victor Burq 1853 [81].
© Universalmuseum Joanneum, Graz, Austria, with permission.

of Soranus' proposals were followed slavishly for 1500 years. Famous paediatric texts that propagated smearing the gums with hare's brain were published by Aetius of Armida [84] (550 C.E.), Paulus Aegineta [85] (640 C.E.), Rhazes [9] (900 C.E.), Heinrich Louffenberg [86] (1434), Bartholomäus Metlinger [87] (1473), Thomas Phaire [12] (1545), Simon de Vallambert [13] (1565), Hieronymus Mercuriale [14] (1584), Robert Pemell [88] (1653), Nils Rosén [59] (1776), and many others.

Originally used for snakebites, *tyriaca* (theriac) evolved into a universal antidote and was recommended by Galen (ca. 200 C.E.) to treat almost every complaint, especially brain disorders [89]. Theriac's initial 64 ingredients, which included rare animal extracts, were augmented up to 100, making the drug expensive. Peony seed or root, taken orally and as a necklace, remained the standard anticonvulsive for the poor. Both drugs were prescribed for 1500 years. Effective anticonvulsants were detected a century before their action was understood, namely the enhancement of GABAergic neurotransmission. As elaborated by Klitgaard [90], most of them were discovered by serendipity. Thanks to modern anticonvulsants, today there are few progressive and degenerative brain diseases in infancy for which seizure control cannot be achieved.

Conclusion

Ignorance about the brain's function, especially its electrical activity, was the main reason for the long-standing superstitious belief in 'possession' as an explanation for seizures in infants. The lack of a convincing theory encouraged supranatural explanations for the threatening symptoms. Inconsistent and frequently changing classifications, also an expression of inadequate understanding, delayed a systematic approach and effective treatment. Elucidation of the brain's cortical structure, electrical activity, and neurotransmission transformed the 'sacred' to a 'normal' disease. In the 20th century, effective anticonvulsive treatment made life with seizures easier for all age groups. In addition, seizures in infancy were finally demystified as postulated in the *Corpus Hippocraticum*.

REFERENCES

1. Hippocrates: Opera omnia. De la maladie sacrée. Edited by: E. Littré. Amsterdam: Hakkert, 1962: Vol. **6**, p. 364–75.
2. Schneider CV: Liber primus de catarrhis. Wittebergae: Mevius, 1660: p. 149–53.
3. Hippocrates: Prognostics. In: The genuine works. London: Sydenham Society, 1849: Vol. **1**, p. 24.
4. Gruner OC: A treatise on the canon of medicine of Avicenna, incorporating a translation of the first book. London: Luzac & Co., 1930: p. §§ 711–9.
5. Baumann ED: De Heilige Ziekte. Rotterdam: Nijgh & Van Ditmar, 1923.
6. Von Storch TC: An essay on the history of epilepsy. Ann Med Hist New Series 1930;**2**:614–50.
7. Goedhart G, van der Wal MF, van Eijsden M, Bonsel GJ: Maternal vitamin B-12 and folate status during pregnancy and excessive infant crying. Early Hum Dev 2011;**87**:309–14.
8. Josat A: Recherches historiques sur l'epilepsie. Paris: Baillière, 1856.
9. Radbill SX: The first treatise on Pediatrics: booklet on the ailments of children and their care. Arch Pediatr 1971;**122**:369–76.
10. Bagellardus P: Libellus de egritudinibus infantium. Padova: Valdezocchio, 1472: p. 13, 16.
11. Brüning H: Cornelius Roelans von Mechelm "Das Buch der Kinderkrankheiten" (Löwen ca. 1485). Rostock: Universität Rostock, 1953–1954: p. 17–109.
12. Phaire T: The boke of children, 1553. Edinburgh: Livingstone, 1955: p. 28–38.
13. Vallambert Sd: Cinq livres de la manière de nourrir et gouverner les enfants dès leur naissance. Reprint Droz, Genève 2005. ed. Poitiers: Manefz et Bouchetz, 1565: p. 312–8.
14. Mercuriale G: De puerorum morbis tractatus locupletissimi. Frankfurt: Wechelius, 1584: p. 200–22, 324.
15. Hsieh DT, Walker JM, Pearl PL: Infantile seizures. Curr Neurol Neurosci Rep 2008;**8**:139–44.
16. Volpe JJ: Neonatal seizures: current concepts and revised classification. Pediatrics 1989;**84**:422–8.
17. Nordli DR, De Vivo DC: Classification of infantile seizures. J Child Neurol 2002;**17 Suppl 3**:S3–8.
18. Ronen GM, Penney S, Andrews W: The epidemiology of clinical neonatal seizures in Newfoundland. J Pediatr 1999;**134**:71–5.
19. Volpe JJ: Neonatal seizures. N Engl J Med 1973;**289**:413–6.
20. Mizrahi EM, Kellaway P: Characterization and classification of neonatal seizures. Neurology 1987;**37**:1837–44.
21. Nordli DR Jr, Bazil CW, Scheuer ML, Pedley TA: Recognition and classification of seizures in infants. Epilepsia 1997;**38**:553–60.
22. Wong M, Trevathan E: Infantile spasms. Pediatr Neurol 2001;**24**:89–98.
23. Holden KR, Mellits ED, Freeman JM: Neonatal seizures. I. Correlation of prenatal and perinatal events with outcomes. Pediatrics 1982;**70**:165–76.
24. Stahl GE: Kurtze Untersuchung der Kranckheiten, welche bey dem kindlichen Alter des Menschen fürnemlich vorzukommen pflegen. Leipzig: Eysseln, 1718: p. 72–7.
25. Harris G: De morbis acutis infantum. 4. ed. Amsterdam: Janssonio-Waesbergios, 1736: p. 157–62.
26. Harris W: A treatise of the acute diseases of infants (1st ed. 1689). London: Astley, 1742: p. 74, 91–106.
27. Rosen von Rosenstein N: Anweisung zur Kenntnis und Chur der Kinderkrankheiten (1st Swedish ed. 1764). 4. ed. Göttingen: Dieterich, 1781: p. 47–55, 64.
28. Armstrong G: An account of the diseases most incident to children (1st ed. 1767). 2. ed. London: Cadell, 1783: p. 48–52, 75–81.
29. Underwood M: A treatise on the diseases of children. London: Mathews, 1784: p. 26, 82–5.
30. Baumes JBT: Traité des convulsions dans l'enfance, de leurs causes, et de leur traitement. 2. ed. Paris: Méquinon, 1805: p. 136.
31. Henke A: Handbuch zur Erkenntniß und Heilung der Kinderkrankheiten. 3 (1st. ed. 1809). Frankfurt: Wilmans, 1821: Vol. **1**, p. 215.
32. Jahn F: Neues System der Kinderkrankheiten. Arnstadt: Langbein & Klüger, 1803: p. 130.
33. Jörg JCG: Handbuch zum Erkennen und Heilen der Kinderkrankheiten. Leipzig: Knobloch, 1826: p. 369.
34. Wendt J: Die Kinderkrankheiten systematisch dargestellt. 2. ed. Breslau und Leipzig: Korn, 1826: p. 151.
35. Rotch TM: Pediatrics. The hygienic and medical treatment of children. Edinburgh and London: Pentland, 1896: p. 754–9.
36. Holt LE: The diseases of infancy and childhood. New York: Appleton &Co, 1898: p. 399.

37. Henoch E: Vorlesungen über Kinderkrankheiten. 8. ed. Berlin: Hirschwald, 1895: p. 172.
38. Zipperling W: Über eine besondere Form motorischer Reizzustände bei Neugeborenen (sog. "Stäupchen"). Zschr Kinderheilk 1913;**5**:31–40.
39. Elworthy FT: The evil eye. An account of this ancient and wide spread superstition. London: Murray, 1895.
40. Stol M: Epilepsy in Babylonia. Groningen: Styx Publications, 1993: p. 10.
41. Leeper EA: From Alexandria to Rome: the Valentinian connection to the incorporation of exorcism as a prebaptismal rite. Vigiliae Christianae 1990;**44**:6–24.
42. Luther M: Das Taufbüchlein aufs Neue zugerichtet (1526). Weimarer kritische Gesamtausgabe. Weimar: Böhlau, 1883–2009: Vol. **19**, p. 539–41.
43. Nischan B: The exorcism controversy and baptism in the late reformation. Sixt Century J 1987;**18**:31–52.
44. Kramer H, Sprenger J: Malleus maleficarum, or: The hammer of witches (1487). London: Rodker, 1928: p. 219.
45. Del-Rio M: Disquisitionum magicarum libri sex in tres tomos partiti. Moguntiae: Johann Albinus, 1603: p. 386, 415.
46. Storch J: Theoretische und practische Abhandlung von Kinder-Kranckheiten. Eisenach: Grießbach, 1751: Vol. **4**, p. 228–94.
47. Fabricius von Hilden W: Observationum et curationum chirurgicarum centuria tertia (1st ed. 1614). Frankfurt: Dufour, 1682: p. 191.
48. Boerhaave H: Praelectiones academicae de morbis nervorum. Venetiis: Typographia Remondiniana, 1762: Vol. **1**, p. 316.
49. Blondel J: Dissertation physique sur la force de l'imagination des femmes enceintes sur le fetus. Leyden: Langerak & Lucht, 1737: p. 130.
50. Turner D: De morbis cutaneis. A treatise of diseases incident to the skin. 4. ed. London: Walthoe, 1731: p. 174.
51. Mittal S, Thursby G: The Hindu world. New York: Routledge, 2004: p. 119–39.
52. Manyam BV: Epilepsy in ancient India. Epilepsia 1992;**33**:473–5.
53. Kluger G, Kudernatsch V: St. Valentine—patron saint of epilepsy: illustrating the semiology of seizures over the course of six centuries. Epilepsy Behav 2009;**14**:219–25.
54. Adam P: Hopitaux specialisés pour d'autres maladies graves: Epilepsie, feu de St. Antoine, Syphilis. In: Adam P: Charité et assistance en Alsace au Moyen Age. Strasbourg: Librairie Istra, 1982: p. 196–213.
55. Sudhoff K: Ein spätmittelalterliches Epileptikerheim zu Rufach im Oberelsass. Arch Gesch Med 1913;**6**:449–55.
56. Hippocrates: Opera omnia: de la dentition. Reprint of ed. 1853. Edited by: E. Littré. Amsterdam: Hakkert, 1982: Vol. **8**, p. 545–9.
57. Todd RB: Convulsions consequent upon dentition, treated by the application of ice to the spine. Boston Med Surg J 1842;**26**:295–8.
58. Ruttimann D, Loesch S: Mortality and morbidity in the city of Bern, Switzerland, 1805–1815. Homo 2012;**63**:50–66.
59. Rosén von Rosenstein N: The diseases of children, and their remedies. London: Cadell, 1776: p. 32–8.
60. Routh CHF: Infant feeding and its influence on life. 3. ed. New York: Wood, 1879: p. 31–3, 104, 117.
61. Filatow N: Kurzes Lehrbuch der Kinderkrankheiten. Wien: Sáfár, 1897: p. 95.
62. Bernstein JG: Praktisches Handbuch der Geburtshülfe. 2. ed. Leipzig: Schwickert, 1797: p. 81.
63. Smellie W: A treatise on the theory and practise of midwifery (1752). London: Sydenham Society, 1878: Vol. **1**, p. 228.
64. Peterman MG: Convulsions in childhood. Twenty year study of 2,500 cases. Am J Dis Child 1946;**72**:399–410.
65. Nielsen JM, Butler FO: Birth primacy and idiopathic epilepsy. Bull Los Angeles Neurol Soc 1948;**13**:176.
66. Craig WS: Convulsive movements occurring in the first 10 days of life. Arch Dis Child 1960;**35**:336–44.
67. West WJ: On a peculiar form of infantile convulsions. Lancet 1841;**35**:724–5.
68. Jackson JH: On the anatomical, physiological and pathological investigation of epilepsies. West Riding Lunatic Asylum Med Rep 1873;**3**:315–39.
69. Berger H: Über das Elektrenkephalogramm des Menschen. Arch Psychiatr Nervenkr 1929;**87**:527–70.
70. Gibbs FA, Lennox WG, Gibbs E: The electro-encephalogram in diagnosis and in localization of epileptic seizures. Arch Neurol Psychiatry 1936;**36**:1225–35.
71. Bailey P, Gibbs FA: The surgical treatment of psychomotor epilepsy. J Am Med Assoc 1951;**145**:365–70.
72. Gibbs FA, Gibbs EL: Infantile spasms. In: Atlas of encephalography. Reading, MA: Addison-Wesley, 1952: Vol. **2**, p. 24–30.
73. Seligmann S: Der böse Blick und Verwandtes. Berlin: Barsdorf, 1910.
74. Shanks RA: The historical background of convulsions in childhood. Arch Dis Child 1948;**23**:281–9.
75. Andrews C: Amulets of ancient Egypt. London: British Museum Press, 1994: p. 43.
76. Puschmann T: Alexander von Tralles. Original-Text und Übersetzung. Wien: Braumüller, 1878: Vol. **1**, p. 566.
77. Paracelsus TvH: Von den hinfallenden Siechtagen (De Caducis 1530). Edited by: Karl Sudhoff. München: Barth, 1924: Vol. **8**.
78. Willis T: The London practice of Physick. London: Basset, 1685: p. 250–5.
79. Doherty F: The anodyne necklace: a quack remedy and its promotion. Med Hist 1990;**34**:268–93.
80. Underwood M: A treatise on the disorders of childhood, and management of infants from the birth. 2. ed. London: Matthews, 1801: Vol. **1**, p. 172.
81. Burq V: Métallothérapie. Paris: Baillière, 1853: p. 46.
82. Adeboye MA, Adegboye OA, Abdulkarim AA, et al.: Amulets, bands and other traditional applications seen among emergency and neonatal pediatric admissions in a tertiary centre, Nigeria. Oman Med J 2011;**26**:337–41.
83. Temkin O: Soranus' Gynecology. Baltimore, MD: The Johns Hopkins Press, 1956: Vol. **II**, p. 107, 113–22.
84. Wegscheider M: Geburtshilfe und Gynäkologie bei Aetios von Amida. Berlin: Springer, 1901.
85. Paulus Aegineta: The seven books. translated from the Greek, with a commentary by Francis Adams: London: Sydenham Society, 1844: Vol. **1**, p. 13.
86. Louffenberg H: Die Versehung des Leibs—regimen sanitatis. Augspurg: Ratdolt, 1491.
87. Metlinger B: Regiment der jungen Kinder. Augsburg: Zainer, 1473: Vol. cap. 3, Folio 31.
88. Pemell R: De morbis puerorum or, a treatise of the diseases of children. London: Legatt, 1653.
89. Galen: Libellus de theriaca ad Pisonem. Interprete et commentatore: Joannes Iuvenes. Antverpiae: Apud Ioannem Bellerum, 1575: p. 132–8.
90. Klitgaard H: Antiepileptic drug discovery: lessons from the past and future challenges. Acta Neurol Scand Suppl 2005;**181**: 68–72.

5.5

Birthmark and blemish
The doctrine of maternal imagination

Introduction

Without selection via prenatal diagnostics, 1 in 50 neonates was born with a major malformation [1], and surgical correction was usually unavailable. Although many malformed infants died spontaneously or were killed after birth, most birth defects were widely known, and numerous theories were promulgated to explain the causation of 'monsters', most of which blamed the mother. Ambroise Paré's menu of 1573 included [2]: '(1) the glorie of God; (2) His punishment; (3) abundance of seed; (4) too little quantity of seed; (5) imagination; (6) narrowness of the womb; (7) disorderly posture of the child; (8) a fall or stroke against the mother's belly; (9) heredity or affects by other accidents; (10) confused mingling of seed; (11) the devil's craft and wickedness.'

Widespread and obstinate was the belief in maternal imagination (*mental impressions, fantasies, miswatching*) that compromised fetal development or shape. The history of this doctrine was addressed by Preuss [3] and Kahn [4] from an ethnological perspective, and by Ballantyne in his thoughtful history of teratogenesis [5]. Concentrating on skin malformations, this chapter delineates the origins of the imagination doctrine, investigates its changes, and explains its persistence for millennia. Its focus is not folkloric, but rather the scientific debate on imagination.

Antique explanations

Since antiquity, animals were associated with human malformations, such as hares with cleft lip or frogs with anencephaly (see Chapter 5.1). The Chinese silk manuscript *Taichan Shu* (before 188 B.C.E.) ordered [6]: 'During [the 3rd month, the fetus] does not yet have a fixed configuration, and, if exposed to things, it transforms. For this reason lords, sires and great men must not employ dwarves. Do not observe monkeys.' Soranus (2nd century C.E.) attributed a forming capacity of *both* parents' fantasy unto the fetus [7]: 'Intercourse shall [not] be practised when the body is heavy in indigestion and drunkenness ... Some women, seeing monkeys during intercourse have borne children resembling monkeys.' Galen (2nd century C.E.) explained the origin of malformations [8]: 'Whenever some little thing goes wrong while [the embryo] is formed ..., first untimely intercourse of the male with the female and later the regimen of the pregnant woman are to blame.' Galen also explained imagination [9]: 'An ugly man wanted to beget a beautiful child and had an image of an elegant infant painted on a board, telling his wife to look at it during coition ... I believe the strength of vision transmits resemblance by the mind and not by means of particles.' Byzantine court physician Aetius of Amida (ca. 550 C.E.) cautioned [10]: 'In early pregnancy women must be protected from fear, sadness, and all strong agitation of the mind.' Avicenna (11th century C.E.) believed [11]: 'The parents' state of mind affects the body of the offspring; as for instance, phantasies. As a rule, it is some natural object which impresses the body. For instance, some image of a boy pictured by both parents at the time of conception may be realized in the infant when born ... seen by the mother whilst the seminal fluid was flowing into her at coitus, or by the father at the time of this flow.' The Salernitan *Trotula* text (12th century C.E.) proposed unfulfilled desire [12]: 'When a woman is in early pregnancy, care ought to be taken that nothing is named in front of her which she is not able to obtain, because if she sets her mind on it and it is not given to her, this occasions miscarriage.'

The elephant head

Ganesha, the elephant-headed god of the beginning and remover of obstacles, is a devoutly worshipped deity in the Hindu pantheon. Various explanations exist why he has an elephant head. His procreation by Shiva was described in the Suprabhedagama (6th century B.C.E.) [13]: 'I, in company with Parvati once retired to the forest on the slopes of the Himalaya, when we saw a female elephant making herself happy with a male elephant. This exited our passion and we decided to enjoy ourselves in the form of elephants. I became a male elephant and Parvati, a female elephant and we pleased ourselves; as a result you were born with the face of an elephant.'

Remarkable and more difficult to explain is the imagination of elephants in regions where such animals never existed (**Fig. 5.5.1**). Among the portents of Scipio's departure for the Punic war (218 B.C.E.), Livius reported [14]: '[At Sinuessa] a boy was born with an elephant's head.' And Plinius (75 C.E.) recounted [15]: '[The Greek princess] Alcippe was delivered of an Elephant, and that certainly

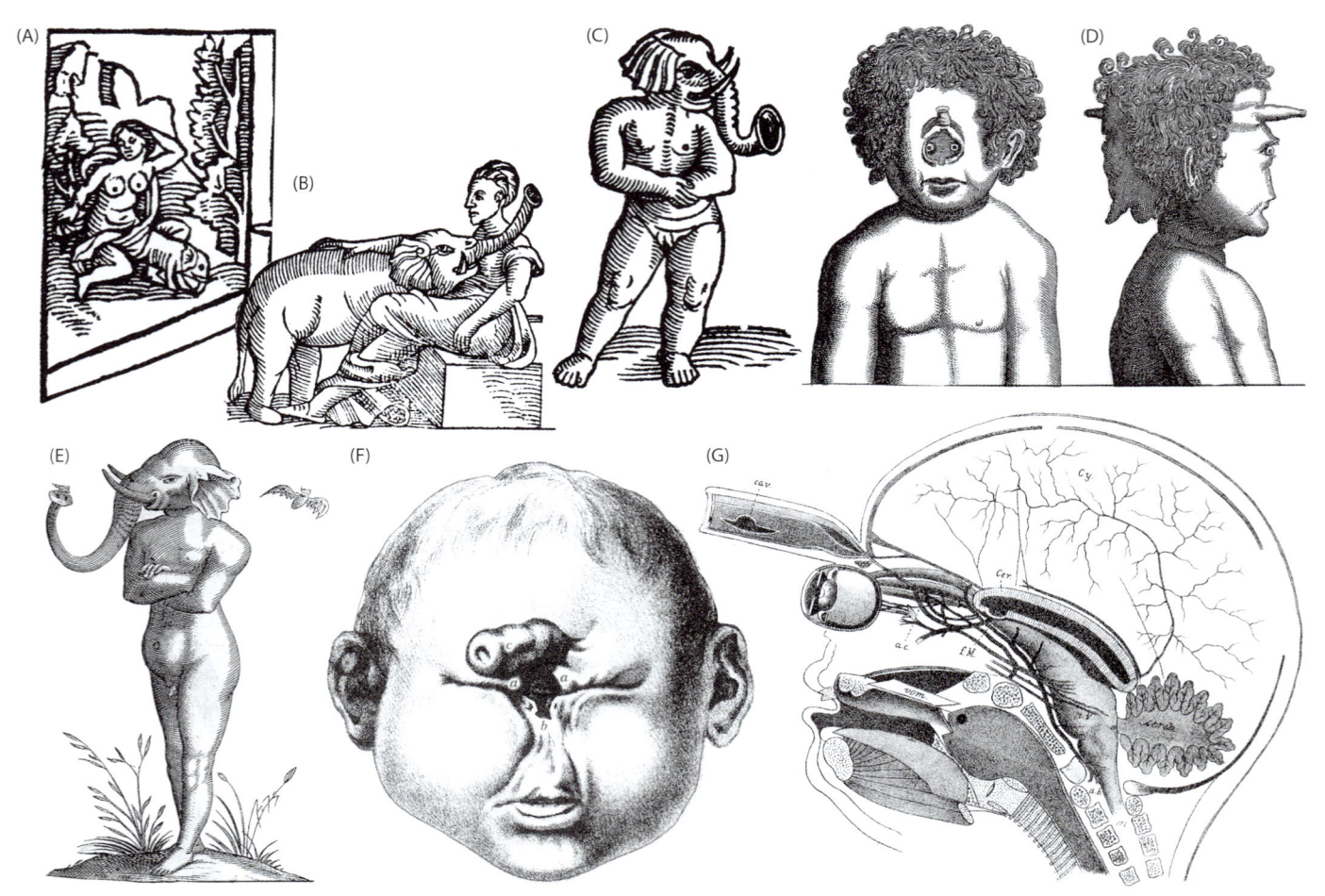

Fig. 5.5.1 Infants born by human females and reported to resemble elephants: A, Greek mythology, Alcippe giving birth to an elephant, depicted by Jean DuPré 1534 [63]; B, Alcippe with her elephant child, depicted by Conrad Lycosthenes, 1557 [64]; C, infant with elephant head, reported by Livius [14], depicted by Lycosthenes in 1557; D, infant with cyclopia and proboscis, and E, infant with elephant head, depicted by Fortunio Licetus, 1665 [16]; F, infant with holoprosencephaly and proboscis, depicted by Willem Vrolik, 1849 [18]; G, infant with cyclopia and proboscis, sagittal view by Friedrich Ahlfeld 1882 [52]. cer, rudimentary forebrain.

was a monstrous Token.' 'Elephant heads' probably were cases of holoprosencephaly, frequently due to trisomy 13, whereby the forebrain fails to develop into two hemispheres and a frontal *proboscis* (trunk) replaces the nose. Early pictures of malformations were delineated from tales, as the artists had not seen the infant. Liceti's *De Monstris* of 1665 depicted both a fabulous elephant head and a case of cyclopia (single-eyedness) and proboscis [16]. Thomas Bartholin described the syndrome in 1657 [17]: 'I deem it a monster and a game of nature.' In 1844, Willem Vrolik correctly associated proboscis and cyclopia [18]. Johann Kundrat named it arhinencephaly in 1882 [19]. In 1880, Ahlfeld exhibited [20] most of a skull filled by a cyst instead of a forebrain.

Bear child, marine monster, 'white negro': skin disease

Visual transmission was believed to cause systemic skin diseases. The correlation with maternal imagination was sometimes unclear or inconsistent. *Congenital generalized hypertrichosis* leads to excessive hair growth. Conrad Lycosthenes described a famous case [21]: '[In 1282] a Noble woman that was the Popes necessarie, brought forth a hearie Boye, hauing hands and faete like a Beare, with whiche monstrous byrth the Pope being sore troubled, commanded all the Images of Beares whiche by chaunce were in her house to be put out, for a manifest argument of imagination conceyued by her in conception' (Fig. 5.5.2, left). The traumatic paintings were not there *by chaunce*: the French pope Martin IV, accessing the Holy Chair in 1281, was unwelcome in Italy and had reason to remove the ubiquitous coat of arms of his predecessor Nicholas III from the powerful Orsini family, which displayed two bears. In 1580, Michel de Montaigne recounted a case of 1354 [22]: 'Presented to Charles the Emperor a girl from Pisa, all over rough and covered with hair, whom her mother said to be so conceived by reason of a picture of St. John the Baptist [with long hair and beard], that hung within the curtains of her bed.'

Ichthyosis vulgaris leads to thickened skin. A broadside illustrates a child born around 1670 (Fig. 5.5.2, right) [23]: 'Elizabeth Risiana, having observed turtles and angel sharks at the coast... gave birth to a boy resembling these animals... a blackish and indured skin with

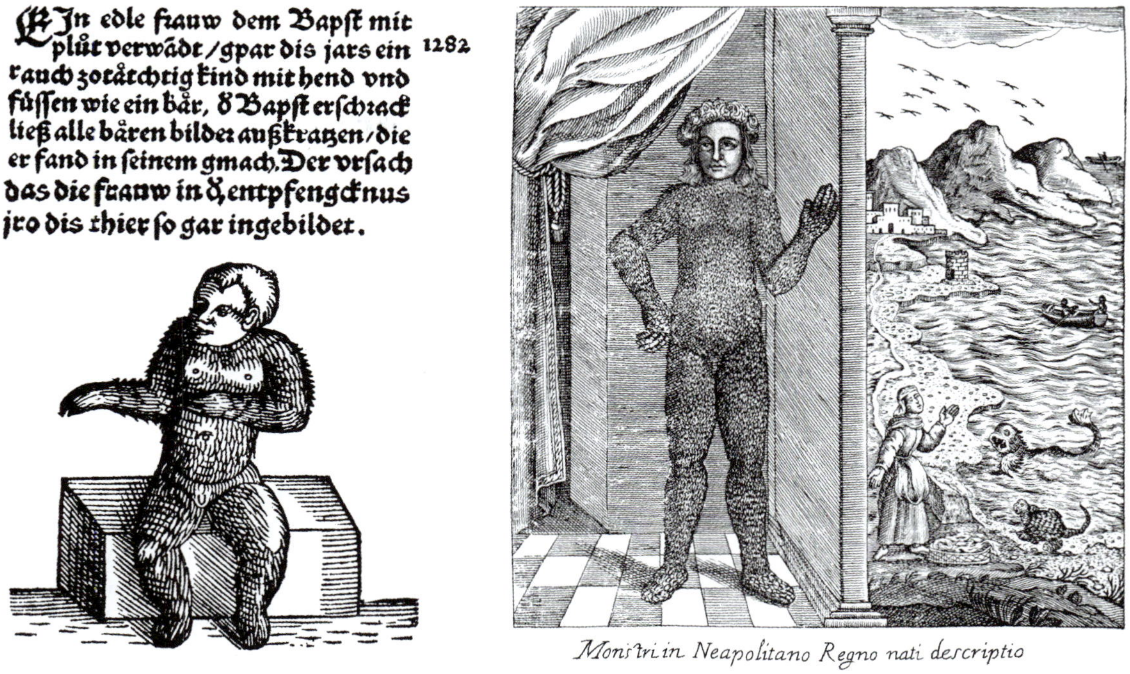

Fig. 5.5.2 Systemic skin disorders attributed to maternal imagination. Left: hypertrichosis: bear infant of 1282, described by Conrad Lycosthenes 1557 [64]; Right: ichthyosis, 'Fish-monster of Naples', broadside published around 1680 [23]. See text for details.

scales.' Called the 'fish monster of Naples,' the boy was displayed on markets and became a European celebrity. Anthony Leeuwenhoek examined him at about 10 years of age in 1683 [24]: 'Much different from the Report. For there appeared to my naked Eye and Microscope, no part of the Body which I could say was covered with *Fish Scales*, but rather with a thick Callus, and more especially within the hands and under the feet.'

Albinism due to tyrosinase deficiency is frequent in central Africa. In the 3rd century C.E., Heliodorus described the queen Persina, who wrote to her daughter [25]: 'But thou wert born white, which colour is strange among the Ethiopians. I knew the reason, that it was because, while my husband [Hydaspes] had to do with me, I was looking at the picture of Andromeda brought down by Perseus naked from the rock, and so by mishap engendered presently a thing like to her. Being certain that thy colour would procure me to be accused of adultery, I determined to [abandon you] which was far to be preferred to present death or to be called a bastard.' Capuchin friar Cavazzi conveyed from a 1654 mission to Congo [26]: 'Those are called *Ndumbdù* who are born from black people, are rather white in color, with yellow frizzy hair, a stupid face, and unable to tolerate the sun's light.' In 1765, James Parsons published a series of 'white negroes' born to black slaves in Virginia and assumed heredity [27]: 'My father was a white man, though my grandfather and grandmother were as black as you and myself; and although we came from a place where no white people ever were seen, yet there was always a white child in every family related to us.' Robert McCrackin reported in 1937 [28] that various African tribes linked albinism to maternal impression, adultery, or another parental sin, and that the Basa tribe, in French Cameroon, 'only rarely permitted [albinos] to survive, so keenly are they held in disrepute'. Ostracizing children with albinism remains a major public health problem in Africa to the present day [29].

Birthmarks and blemishes: 16th-century doctrines

The doctrine of imagination changed during the late Middle Ages. Rather than untimely, satanic, or bestial intercourse, imagination now explained deformities, making their birth a misfortune rather than a crime. The common denominator remained blaming the mother. Only maternal, no longer paternal, imagination was considered to deform the fetus, whose alleged vulnerability extended over the entire gestation. This may reflect a change in the presumed susceptible period from conception to gestation. In Islamic medicine, Muhamad Al-Balawi attributed a *vis imaginativa* to causing malformations, birthmarks, and undesired infant character in 965 C.E. [30]. Scientists were hardly able to reconcile various superstitions by one theory of transmission: fantasy, gazing, longing, dream, fright, and horror.

Konrad von Megenberg wrote in 1349 [31]: 'The infant in the mother's womb befits according to the pregnant woman's craving, therefore she should watch no ugly thing, but nice people and beautiful pictures, especially in early pregnancy.' In Naples, Giambattista della Porta explained the action of unfulfilled desires in 1560 [32]: 'When pregnant women ardently desire something, their blood moves and modifies the internal spirits. In this excitation the image of the desired object is impressed into the soft fetal tissue.' Other scientists doubted imagination, at least in later pregnancy, as did Ambroise Paré in 1573 [33]: 'Manie from their birth have spots or marks, which the common people of France call *signes*, that is, marks or signs. Som of these are plain and equal with the skin, others are raised up in little tumors, and like unto warts, som have hairs upon them, manie times they are smooth, black or pale; yet for the most part red. When they rise in the face, they spread abroad there on manie times with great deformitie. Manie think the caus thereof to be a certain portion of the menstrual matter cleaving to the sides of the womb … When the chylde is formed, no imagination is able to leave the impression anie thing in it.' It seems that Paré foresaw by 433 years the present debate on the origin of haemangiomas from fetal placental endothel [34]. In 1578, pregnant women aware of but unable to satisfy their wish were advised 'to touch their backside … that no mark affects the infant's face, nose, eye, mouth, or neck' [35]. Lutheran theologian Christopher Irenäus taught in 1584 [36]: 'Imagination and phantasy are so powerful, that a pregnant woman may transmit to her infant what she attentively observed. Multiple forms and marks may be passed on, as small bumps, blemishes, spots, marks and warts that are not easy to wash off and remove.' Scevola de St. Marthe, administrator in Poitiers, published a three-volume poem *Paediotrophia* in 1584, with one verse on imagination [37]:

> 'Then (wonderful to tell) if you deny
> The strange request, nor with their wish comply,
> Avenging Nature, from unknown designs,
> With spots and marks the foetus' body signs,
> With stains indelible, that never can
> Wear out, thro' life, in woman, or in man.
> And! (stranger still) while in the mother's breast
> This passion sways, and rages o'er the rest,
> Whatever place she scratches, or besmears,
> A mark, in the same part, her infant bears.'

Beggars' and guardians' rules

Legislators aimed to protect pregnant women from the assumed harm of terror and unfulfilled desires. In 1298, the county of Rommersheim (Mosel) restricted fishing rights to the abbot and governor, with one exception [38]: 'Pregnant and confined women are allowed to fish with one foot inside the water, and the other on land.' In 1514, Regensburg's beggars' rule stated [39]: 'Who have such ailments as pregnant women may loathe or dread, should be separated from other people at cemeteries and churches, and must properly cover their gruesome disease or wound.' The Salzburg *Landtag* decreed in 1534: 'If a woman walks through a fruit orchard, and the trees bear fruit for which she feels particular desire, she or someone else may procure her a fruit that she may satisfy her wish' [40]. Vineyards were heavily guarded at vintage time by a *Saltner* (custodian) equipped with weapons, clappers, and a frightening outfit. The Reutlingen *Guardians' Rule* of 1578 cautioned [41]: 'If a woman, great with child, enters a vineyard to cut a vine, and the guardian recognizes her, he should approach her cautiously, making himself recognizable by slight coughing, and should not address her with rough or harsh words, and terrify her: but should warn her friendly, and, if she has not yet got a vine, should cut one for her himself.' The *Ratsprotokoll* of the imperial city of Hall ruled in 1622 [4]: 'The goitrous beggars' master shall be done away with because of his laziness, but in particular because of his abominable goiter, for the pregnant women's sake.' As late as 1783, Johann Wilhelm Casparson proposed a legislation for the beggars in Hessia-Cassel [42]: 'Because each frightening object may act awfully on pregnant women and hence on their enclosed fruit … mutilated, malformed, unnatural [beggars] and those afflicted with festering cancer sores in their face, must be entirely rejected from public places, especially from church portals, where they seek pity from the by-passers.'

Theories of imagination of the 17th century

In 1601, Scipione Mercurio believed that malformations and skin marks resulted from imagination, especially a naevus flammeus from watching fire [43]. He rejected the 'ridiculous' opinion that by touching her body the pregnant woman located the fetal birthmark, and reported a prospective trial on this topic with three pregnant women. Terror was considered the strongest teratogenic stimulus, as explained by Thomas Fienus in 1608 [44]. In 1614, Fabricius Hildanus, surgeon in Bern, related 'a red crescence on the nose of 3-year-old [son of prefect Nicolai Sinner], grown from lentil to cherry size … to the mother's unfulfilled longing for this fruit during pregnancy' [45]. The French philosopher René Descartes, banned by the church, proposed a theory of imagination in his *Treatise on Man*, composed in 1633 and published after his death [46]: maternal impressions are projected onto the pineal gland, principal seat of the soul (Fig. 5.5.3): 'Leaving the maternal pineal gland, the spirits transmit the ideas via the umbilical arteries to the pineal gland of the fetus, possibly modified by certain actions of the mother.' In 1672, Utrecht anatomist Isbrand van Diemerbroeck assumed that maternal imagination caused fetal marks and spots, but also 'replaced defects of the parents' body … so that the child is born with perfect limbs' [47]. In Brussels, Johannes Baptista van Helmont localized the 'power of imagination in the spleen … which is connected to the heart and uterus' [48]. He distinguished two ways of transmitting the impression: (1), for skin marks, 'by the mere thought a cherry is created from nothing at the very spot which the mother's hand touched, specifically the right, if she is right-handed, and the left if she is left-handed, as this hand is used to execute the orders of the soul … (2), in the cases of terror, which are much more powerful, the mother's hand is not required … but malformations result from viewing [horrible] things that are already created, and are reproduced by the soul.'

Johann Moritz Hofmann, professor and rector of the Altdorf school of medicine, described a girl with a sacral teratoma in 1689 [49]: 'A farmer's wife from Endenberg brought forth a girl with a large tumor hanging on sacrum and buttocks [Fig. 5.5.4] … [questioned about fantasies] she answered that, in the second month of gestation, at the farmer's next-door, she saw a large pig's stomach stuffed with clots and bacon, called *Säusack* [brawn] in this region … She lifted it with her hands, and then touched her own backside.'

Academic debates in the 18th century

When the unborn's assumed vulnerability was extended over the entire gestation, mainly maternal and no longer paternal imagination was blamed. A sharp shift cannot be identified. In 1720 [50], Amsterdam pathologist Frederik Ruysch, a founder of teratology, denied 'the false opinion that by imagination during intercourse, [the parents] might disfigure their own progeny'. In his treatise on

CHAPTER 5.5 Birthmark and blemish: the doctrine of maternal imagination

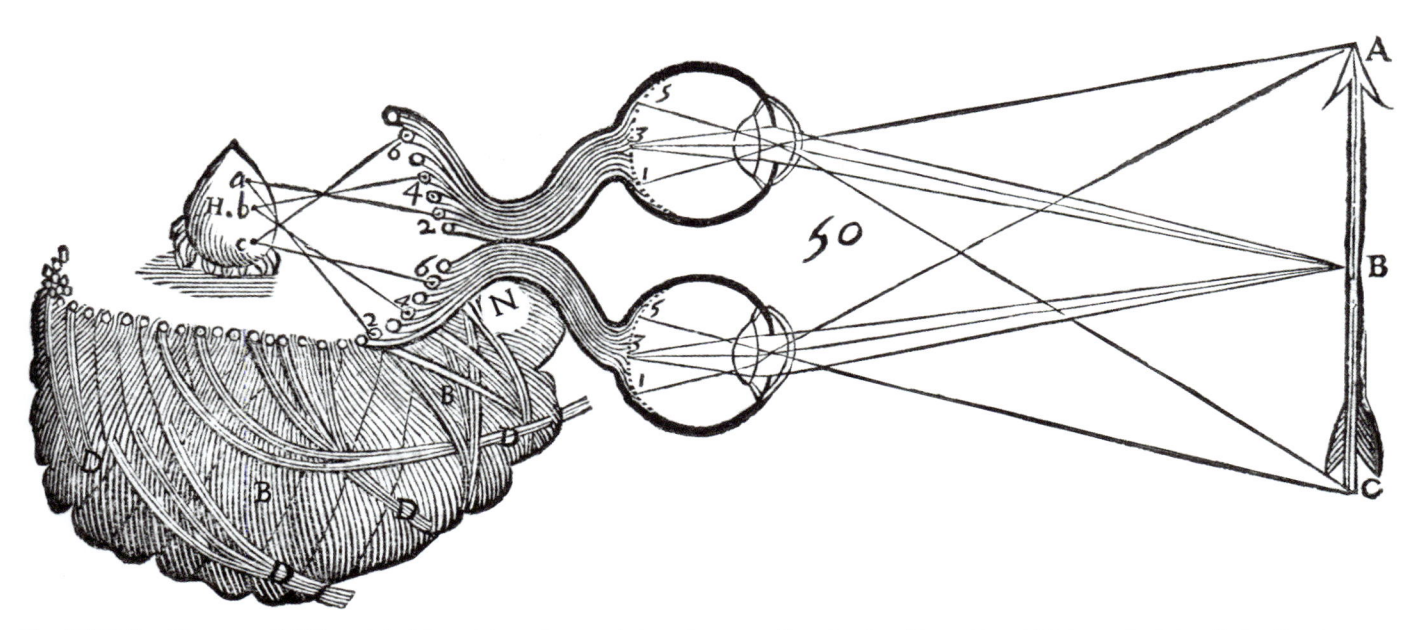

Fig. 5.5.3 René Descartes' 1633 model of the origin and transmission of maternal imagination. 'The spirits which leave the [pineal] gland having received the impression of a specific idea, pass through the tubules 2,4,6 and others into the pores or intervals which are between the small fibers of which this part of the brain (B) is composed' [46]. The transfer to the fetus was believed to occur via the bloodstream.

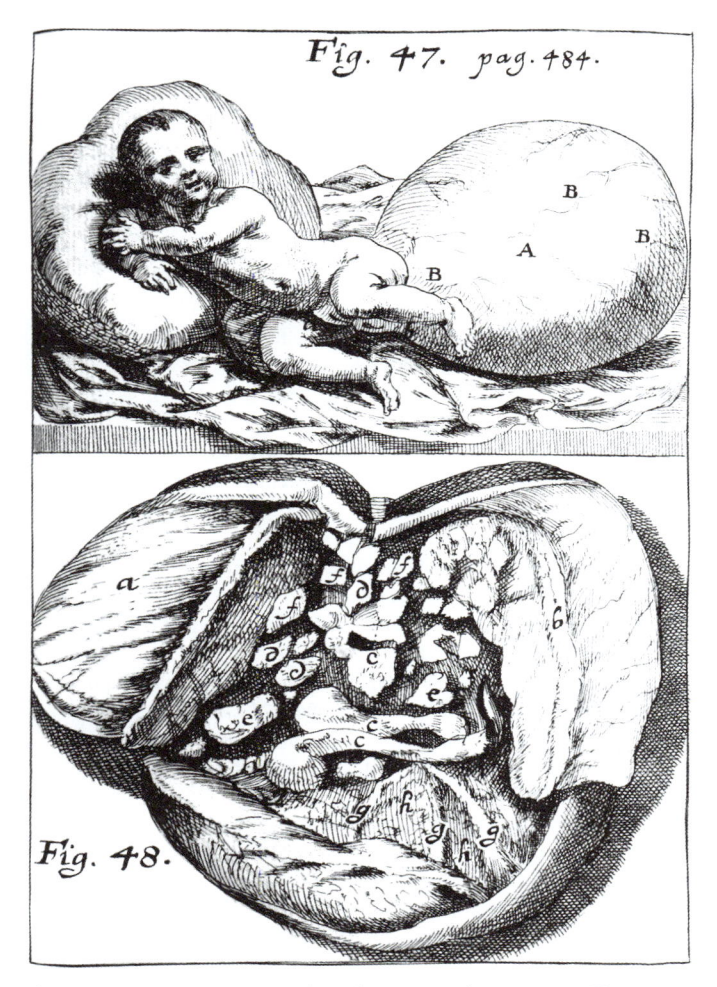

Fig. 5.5.4 Sacral teratoma attributed to maternal imagination. The tumour was described by Johann Moritz Hoffmann 1689 [49]. See text for details.

skin diseases of 1714, London surgeon Daniel Turner presented a chapter on 'the strange and almost incredible power of imagination in pregnant women' [51] in which he associated congenital marks with 'mother's fancy'. In 1727 he was contradicted by James Blondel, mainly with the argument that there were no nerve connections between mother and fetus [52]: 'The opinion that marks and deformities are from them, demonstrated to be a vulgar error.' A pamphlet war between Turner and Blondel, continued even beyond the latter's death in 1734, has been detailed by Wilson [53]. In Paris, exogenous (Lémery) and endogenous (Winslow) origin of malformations was debated, as detailed by Monti [54], but left the role of imagination unclear. In 1756 the Imperial Academy of St. Petersburg announced a prize for 'describing the direct cause afflicting the fetal, but not the mother's body in strong emotion … and affects especially that part of the infant's body the mother has touched on hers'. The prize was won by Carl Christian Krause of Leipzig, faithful promoter of the imagination theory, who claimed emotions 'transmitted by nerves penetrating the umbilical cord and branching in placenta and membranes' [55]. His opponent Georg Roederer denied the existence of imagination in the same booklet. The influential Padovan pathologist Giambattista Morgagni still defended imagination in 1761 [56]. Describing several severe malformation syndromes, he concluded: 'Even if they could be fairly deduc'd from external violence, a part is nevertheless assign'd to the imagination likewise.'

Replaced by teratology and genetics

Scientific teratology began with the anatomical collections of the families Geoffroy Saint Hilaire in Paris, Vrolik in Amsterdam, and Meckel in Halle. These enabled larger series of malformations to be observed, repeated patterns to be perceived, and different species to be compared. In his dissertation of 1759, Caspar Friedrich

Wolff demonstrated the embryo's stepwise development and growth and explained malformations as a natural consequence of disturbed development [57]. In 1791, Göttingen professor Johann Friedrich Blumenbach described the *nisus formativus* (formative drive) that regulates embryonic differentiation, and pointed out that 'even malformations, in which this drive is wrongly directed, reveal marvelous uniformity' [58].

Scientific progress barely affected the public memory, millennia-old convictions died slowly. In the 18th century, the direct gaze of women was considered immoral: cast-down eyes remained the epitome of female virtue [Sura 24:31] but also protected the pregnant woman from 'miswatching'. Many stayed at home while pregnant. The imagination doctrine was scientifically eradicated by the end of the 18th century. But throughout the 19th, the debate between defenders [59] and deriders [60] of maternal imagination persisted in medical textbooks. No prospective studies were conducted. As late as 1840, Berlin physiologist Johannes Müller assured that 'sudden, vehement states of the mother may retard or arrest stages of [fetal] metamorphosis' [61]. In the public mind, the time-honoured superstition remained alive. In 1981, one in four Cardiff women believed that portwine naevus resulted from unsatisfied cravings for strawberries or red cabbage [62].

Conclusion

The doctrine of imagination is of great antiquity, persisting as long as science failed to explain the origin of congenital abnormalities. It did not originate from public superstition, but was promulgated and interpreted by eminent scientists. Ascribed to sexual misconduct, malformations threatened mother and child up to the Middle Ages. By assigning diminished responsibility to the pregnant woman, she was no longer saddled with the burden of shame, and protected from the law's prosecution, the Church's penance, and society's disdain. Given the high frequency of malformations, the doctrine was urgently needed for the mother to survive; its price was assigning irrationality to women. It alluded to a specifically female lack of control or self-restraint, which led to the prejudice of women's spiritual or intellectual inferiority. Feelings of guilt and self-blame remained common among mothers who gave birth to a malformed infant.

REFERENCES

1. Källén B: Epidemiology of human congenital malformations. Cham, Switzerland: Springer, 2014.
2. Paré A: Of monsters and prodigies (1st French ed. 1573). London: Cotes and Du-gard, 1649: p. 648–9.
3. Preuss J: Vom Versehen der Schwangeren. Rudolstadt: Sammlung klinischer Vorträge, 1892: Vol. **5**.
4. Kahn F: Das Versehen der Schwangeren in Volksglaube und Dichtung. Frankfurt: Sauerländer, 1912: p. 33.
5. Ballantyne JW: Manual of antenatal pathology and hygiene. The embryo. Edinburgh: Green, 1904: p. 105–28, 252–7.
6. Harper DJ: MSV Taichan shu: book of the generation of the fetus. London: Routledge, 2009: p. 372–84.
7. Temkin O: Soranus' Gynecology. Baltimore, MD: The Johns Hopkins Press, 1956: p. 37, 176, 189.
8. Galen: On the usefulness of the parts of the body. Ithaca, NY: Cornell University Press, 1968: Vol. **2**, p. 637, 661, 712.
9. Claudii Galeni Pergameni: De theriaca, ad Pisonem commentariolius. Basileae: Cratandrus, 1531: Fol. 78v.
10. Aetii Medici Graeci: Contractae ex veteribus medicinae tetrabiblos. Basileae: Froben, 1549: p. 850.
11. Gruner OC: A treatise on the canon of medicine of Avicenna, incorporating a translation of the first book. London: Luzac & Co., 1930: p. 213.
12. The Trotula: An English translation of the Medieval compendium of women's medicine. Philadelphia, PA: University of Pennsylvania Press, 2002: p. 80.
13. Getty A: Ganesha. A monograph on the elephant-faced God. 2. ed. New Delhi: Munshiram, 1992: p. 8.
14. Titus Livius: History of Rome. Book 27: Scipio in Spain. London: Dent, 1905: p. 27.11.
15. Plinius the Elder: Natural history. London: Wernerian Club, 1847: Vol. **1**, Book 7, cap. 3: p. 187, 192–9.
16. Licetus F: De monstris (1st ed. Patavii 1616). Amstelodami: Frisius, 1665: p. 135, 185.
17. Bartholin T: Historiarum Anatomicarum Rariorum Centuria IV. Hagae-Comitis: Vlacq, 1657: p. 269.
18. Vrolik W: Tabulae, illustrating normal and abnormal development (lat ed. 1844). Amsterdam: Londonck, 1849: plate 53.8.
19. Kundrat H: Arhinencephalie als typische Art von Mißbildung. Graz: Leuschner & Lubensky, 1882.
20. Ahlfeld F: Die Missbildungen des Menschen. Leipzig: Grunow, 1880: Vol. **2** and Atlas in 2 parts, plate 46.18.
21. Batman S: The doome warning all men to the judgement. Translated from Conrad Lycosthenes. London: Nubery, 1581: p. 243.
22. Montaigne M: Essays (1st French ed. 1580). New York: Hill, 1910: Vol. **1**, p. 234.
23. Anonymus: Monstri in Neapolitano regno nati descriptio (1670). In: Holländer F: Wunder, Wundergeburt und Wundergestalt in Einblattdrucken. Stuttgart: Enke, 1921: p. 359.
24. Leeuwenhoek A: Concerning scales within the mouth, the scaly child .... Phil Trans 1684;**14**:586–92.
25. Heliodorus Emesenus: An Ethiopian romance (1587). London: Routledge, 1923: p. 118–9.
26. Cavazzi de Montecuculo GA: Historische Beschreibung der in dem untern Occidentalischen Mohrenland ligenden drey Königreichen Congo, Matamba, und Angola. München: Jäcklin, 1694: p. 104.
27. Parsons J: An account of the white negro shewn before the Royal Society. Phil Trans 1765;**55**:45–53.
28. McCrackin RH: Albinism and unialbinism in twin African negroes. Am J Dis Child 1937;**54**:786–94.
29. Hong ES, Zeeb H, Repacholi MH: Albinism in Africa as a public health issue. BMC Public Health 2006;**6:212**, 1–7.
30. Weisser U: Muhammad Al-Balawi: on the therapy of pregnant women, infants and children. Erlangen: Lüling, 1983: p. 313–8.
31. Megenberg Kv: Das Buch der Natur (1349). Edited by: Franz Pfeiffer. Stuttgart: Aue, 1861: p. 488.
32. Porta JB: Magiae naturalis sive de miraculis rerum naturalium. Antverpiae: Plantini, 1560: p. 76r.
33. Paré A: Concerning the generation of man (French ed. 1573). In: The workes of that famous chirurgion Ambrose Parey. London: Cotes, 1649: p. 605.

34. Barnes CM, Huang S, Kaipainen A, et al.: Evidence by molecular profiling for a placental origin of infantile hemangioma. PNAS 2005;**102**:19097–102.
35. Joubert L: Pourquoy conseilhe on a la fame grosse, de mettre la main a son derrière, si elle ne peut soudain estre satisfaite de son appetit. In: Erreurs populaires au fait de la medicine. Bourdeaux: Millanges, 1578: p. 310–6.
36. Irenaeus C: De monstris. Von seltzamen Wundergeburten. Ursel: Nicolaus Henrich, 1584: p. 302.
37. Scevole de St Marthe: Paedotrophia or the art of nursing and rearing children (1st Latin ed. 1584). London: Nichols, 1797: p. 36–7.
38. Markgraf LT: Mutter und Kind in den Weistümern des Mosellandes. Zeitschr Ver. Rhein. und westfäl. Volkskunde 1906;**2**:118–24.
39. Gemeiner CT: Stadt Regensburgische Jahrbücher vom Jahre 1497 bis zum Jahre 1525. Regensburg: Montag & Weiß, 1824: p. 249.
40. Grimm J: Deutsche Rechtsaltertümer. Göttingen: Dieterich 1828: p. 408–9.
41. Gayler R: Historische Denkwürdigkeiten der Freien Reichsstadt Reutlingen bis 1577. Reutlingen: Kurtz, 1840: p. 604.
42. Casparson WJCG: Abhandlung von Verhütung des Bettelns in einer Haupt- und Residenzstadt. Cassel: Cramer, 1783: p. 10–1.
43. Mercurio S: Kinder-Mutter oder Hebammen-Buch (Italian ed. 1601). Wittenberg: Mevius, 1671: p. 54, plate 3.
44. Fienus T: De viribus imaginationis tractatus (1st ed. 1608). London: Daniel, 1657: p. 282.
45. Fabricius Hildanus G: Observationum et curationum chirurgicarum centuria V. Francofurti: Merian, 1627: Vol. Obs. 3, 49, p. 18, 144.
46. Descartes R: L'homme et la formation du foetus. 2. ed. Paris: Bobin & le Gras, 1677: p. 67, 307–8.
47. Diemerbroeck I: Anatome corporis humani (1st ed. Ultrajecti 1672). Lugduni: Huguetan, 1679: p. 196–200.
48. Helmont JB: Aufgang der Artzney-Kunst (1st Latin ed. Venice 1651). Sultzbach: Endters, 1683: p. 867–9, 961.
49. Hoffmann JM: De foetu monstroso ex imaginatione matris. Miscellanea curiosa sive Ephemeridum Leopoldinae Naturae Curiosorum Decuriae II 1689;**8**:483–5.
50. Ruysch F: Adversariorum anatomico-medico-chirurgicorum decas secunda. Amstelodami: Janssonio-Waesbergios, 1720: p. 28.
51. Turner D: Of spots and marks of a diverse resemblance, imprest upon the skin of the foetus, by the force of the mother's fancy. In: De morbis cutaneis. London: Bonwicke et al., 1714: p. 102–28.
52. Blondel J: The strength of imagination in pregnant women examin'd. London: Pamphlet, 1727.
53. Wilson PK: 'Out of sight, out of mind?' The Daniel Turner–James Blondel dispute over the power of the maternal imagination. Ann Sci 1992;**49**:63–85.
54. Monti MT: Epigenesis of the monstrous form and preformistic 'Genetics' (Lémery–Winslow–Haller). Early Sci Med 2000;**5**: 3–32.
55. Krause CC: Abhandlung von den Muttermälern; nebst einer andern Abhandlung [Röderer]. Leipzig: Gollner, 1758: p. 7–8.
56. Morgagni GB: The seats and causes of diseases investigated by anatomy (1st Latin ed. Venice 1761). London: Millar, 1769: Vol. **2**, p. 758, 766.
57. Wolff CF: Theoria Generationis. Halle: Hendelianis, 1759.
58. Blumenbach JF: Über den Bildungstrieb. Göttingen: Dieterich, 1791: p. 111.
59. Welsenburg Gv: Das Versehen der Frauen in Vergangenheit und Gegenwart. Leipzig: Barsdorf, 1899.
60. Jacquemet E: Les Maladies de la premiere enfance. Paris: Baillière, 1892: p. 175.
61. Müller J: Mutter und Foetus. In: Handbuch der Physiologie des Menschen. Coblenz: Hölscher, 1840: Vol. **2**, p. 575.
62. Shaw WC: Folklore surrounding facial deformity and the origins of facial prejudice. Br J Plastic Surg 1981;**34**:237–46.
63. Dupré J: Le palais des nobles dames, auquel a treze parcelles ou chambres principales. Basiliae: Henricipetri, 1571: p. 182.
64. Lycosthenes C: Wunderwerck oder Gottes unergründliches Vorbilden. Basel: Henrichus Petri, 1557: p. 123, 201, 546.

5.6
Cast aside
Infants with Down's syndrome

Introduction

Trisomy 21 is the most frequent identifiable cause of mental retardation. Its terminology is flawed: terms connected with intelligence (idiot, imbecile, cretin, insane, foolish, lunatic, feeble-minded, and many more) changed their meaning, were perceived as insulting or offensive, and became politically incorrect. Moreover, their meaning changed. 'Cretinism' was used as a generic term for all forms of retarded development up to 1858; since then, it has been associated with hypothyreosis. Trisomy 21 also bore many names: Mongoloid idiocy, Mongolism, Kalmuc idiocy, Down's syndrome (frequently: Down-Syndrome), acromicria [1] and so on, after better understanding and an intervention by the People's Republic of Mongolia [2]. The terms 'Down's syndrome', 'trisomy 21', and 'mental retardation' are used in this chapter. For historical accuracy, original terms were not altered in the quotations.

Prevalence is difficult to determine because spontaneous miscarriage is frequent, pregnancies are selectively terminated, postnatal mortality is high, and many cases are not yet diagnosed at birth. In 1932, Bleyer estimated 'there are about 28,000 mongoloid idiots in the United States at this time ... 70% dying before the age of 20' [3]. The incidence in 1942–1952 in Birmingham, UK, was 1.1 per 1000 liveborn neonates [4]. The history of trisomy 21 has been described by Benda [5] and Berg [6]. Its perception grew with the recent rise in childbearing age.

Prehistory and archaeological findings

Trisomy 21 originated together with *Homo sapiens* 500,000 years ago, or even earlier, as other primates such as chimpanzees [7, 8] and orangutans [9] are also affected. The skull of a prehistoric native Californian from the 7200-year-old cemetery on Santa Rosa Island [10] and another skull from the late Saxon period [700–900 C.E.] excavated in Leicestershire [11] revealed features of Down's syndrome. However, Down's syndrome was rare in antiquity: among 7063 skeletons from European cemeteries used from 3200 B.C.E. until 800 C.E., only one skull with the specific features of trisomy 21 was found [12]. A child's skull from the 5th–6th century C.E. excavated in northeastern France [13], showed features of trisomy 21, but none were specific: a flattened back of the head could also result from head shaping, positional plagiocephaly, or rickets. The condition was rare because mothers were younger, their offspring had few chromosomal anomalies, affected individuals did not reach adulthood, and the infants' skeletons were undercounted as they often were not buried in regular cemeteries (see Chapter 8.7).

Depictions in premodern art

Trisomy 21 has been poorly documented in human history. A Neolithic clay figurine from West Thessalia (Greece, ca. 6500–3000 B.C.E.) [14] and a Toltec terracotta head from Mexico (500 C.E.) [15] seem to be the most probable early depictions. John Ruhräh called attention to Mantegna's 1506 altar painting 'Madonna with Child' [16], and many publications since then have claimed [17–19] or doubted [6, 20] the depiction of trisomy 21 in that and other paintings.

Confused with hypothyreosis

Alexander Haindorf studied at the Juliusspital Würzburg, one of Bavaria's oldest psychiatric asylums, and wrote in 1811 'cretinism and inborn feeblemindedness are the same' [21]. Children with trisomy 21 and those with hypothyreosis have been confused with one another for centuries. Indeed, there is a superficial likeness between the two conditions: both are mentally retarded, have short heads, large tongues, and low muscle tone. Shuttleworth in 1909 [22] published a table describing '16 leading diagnostic differences of the Cretinoid and the Mongolian type'.

Reports from asylums

In 1614, Felix Platter, city physician of Basel, described endemic cretinism [23]: 'In some regions they are frequent: in the Wallisian village Bremis I saw many sitting near the streets, and some were brought to me to Sedun ... with a misshapen head, a huge and swollen tongue, some mute, some deformed by goiter, gazing into the sun, twisting their body, and making bystanders laugh.' In Europe, there was no institution for the mentally retarded before 1800. Reluctantly, and after the French Revolution, the medical profession took responsibility for alleviating the suffering resulting from mental retardation. Early asylums were private institutions for well-to-do offspring. Public asylums resembled jails more than homes (German: '*Tollhaus*'). In Switzerland, clusters of 'cretins' were long known, and Napoleon ordered a census to be taken in 1811 of the endemic cases in the Wallis canton which revealed 3000 cases [24]. In 1841, Johann Jakob Guggenbühl established the *Abendberg* near Interlaken 4000 feet above sea level, devoted to the 'cure and prophylaxis of cretinism' [25].

It has been suggested [3, 6, 18] that Edouard Séguin, psychiatrist at the Paris Bicêtre hospital, described Down's syndrome in his 1846 book, but I was unable to find it therein [26]. After emigrating to New York, and already citing Down's paper, he clearly distinguished endemic from sporadic forms of cretinism, writing in 1866 [27]: 'So does [related to idiocy] the furfuraceous cretinism, with its milk-white, rosy, and peeling skin; with its shortcomings of all the integuments, which give an unfinished aspect to the truncated fingers and nose; with its cracked lips and tongue; with its red, ectropic conjunctiva, coming out to supply the curtailed skin at the margins of the lids.' In Scotland, Richard Poole, who directed the Royal Lunatic Asylum Montrose (near Edinburgh) from 1838, wrote in 1825 [28]: 'Would it be, ought it to be, enough for us, that these unfortunates were removed from our sight?'

John Langdon Down was appointed Medical Inspector of the newly built Royal Earlswood Asylum in Surrey in 1858, a castle for patients from wealthy families (Fig. 5.6.1). Here he wrote his famous 'Ethnic classification of idiots' in 1866 [29], with accurate description of the syndrome that was to bear his name: 'There can be no doubt that these ethnic features are the result of degeneration. The Mongolian type of idiocy occurs in more than ten percent of the cases presented to me [at Earlswood] … examples of retrogression, or at all events, of departure from one type [of human species] and the assumption of the characteristics of another.'

In 1877, John Fraser published clinical and postmortem findings in a woman with 'Kalmuc idiocy' [30]: 'Upper limbs short … lax finger joints … third and fourth toes half the length of the second … head small and round … plain face, plain back of the head, forming two parallel lines … face almost square … tongue long and round … skull: five wormian bones … the most important peculiarity is the absence of the nasal bones' (Fig. 5.6.2). To Fraser's case Arthur Mitchell, Commissioner of the Scottish Board of Lunacy, added notes on 62 cases of 'Kalmuc idiocy'. In the same year, 1877, William Ireland, at the Scottish National Institution at Larbert, described [31] 'genetous idiots. Many of them are dwarfish, and have broad faces offering some of the most striking features of the Tartar or Mongol'.

Within the same decade as Morel's *Degeneration*, Darwin's *Natural Selection*, Galton's *Eugenics*, and Haeckel's *Natural Creation*, Down, Mitchell, Fraser, and Ireland were influenced by the atmosphere of racism and social Darwinism of their time. Their racist language should not hide the fact that they were also pioneers of the empathic, individualized, and respectful education of mentally retarded children.

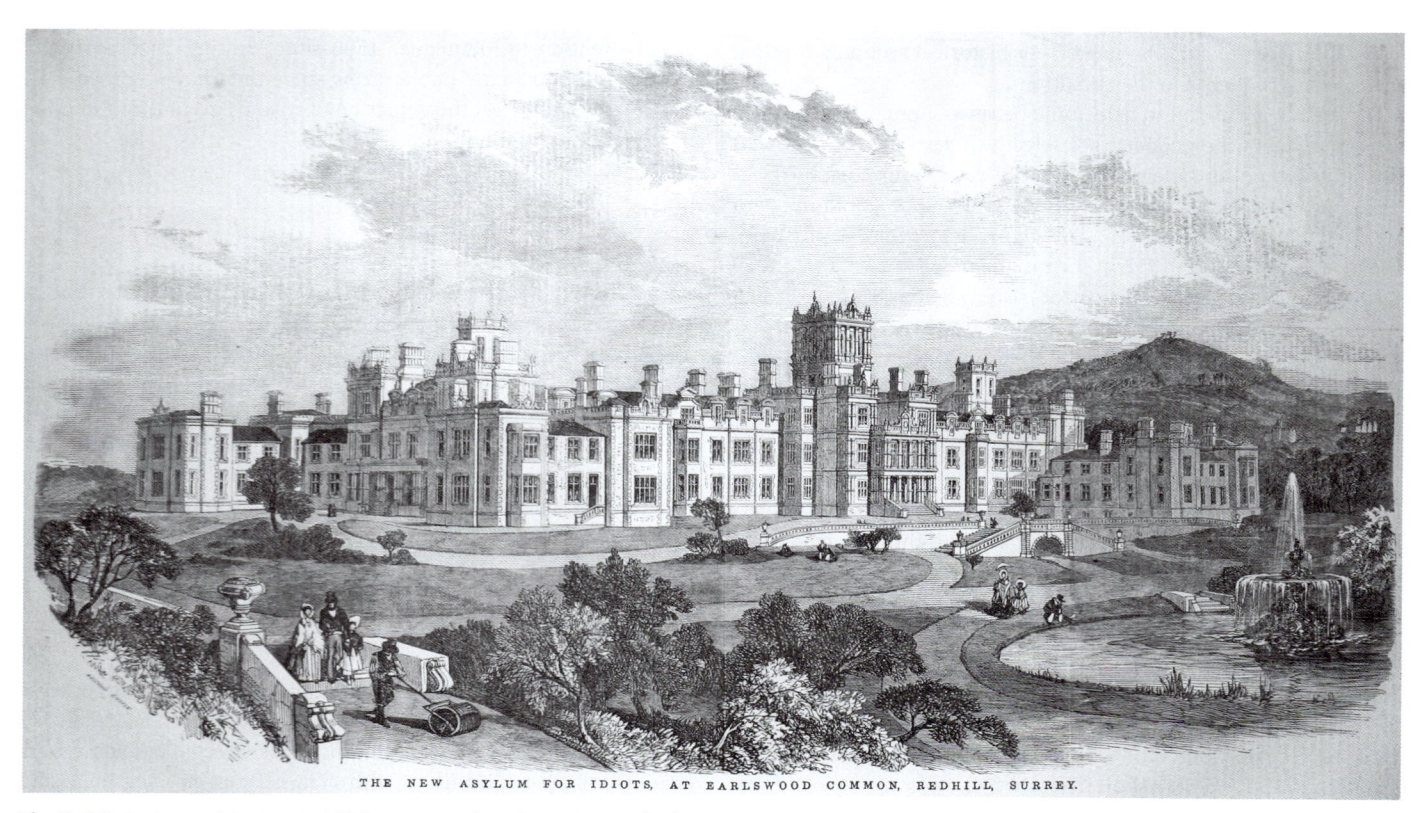

Fig. 5.6.1 Earlswood Asylum in 1854: engraving by Edmund Evans [59]. This institution was directed by John Langdon Down from 1858 to 1868.

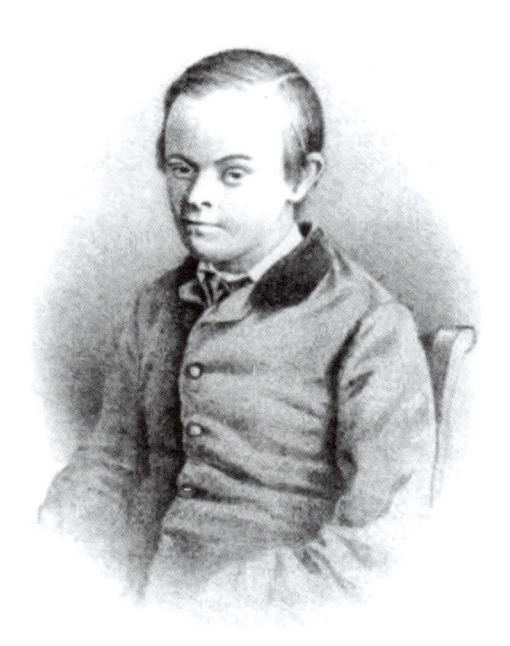

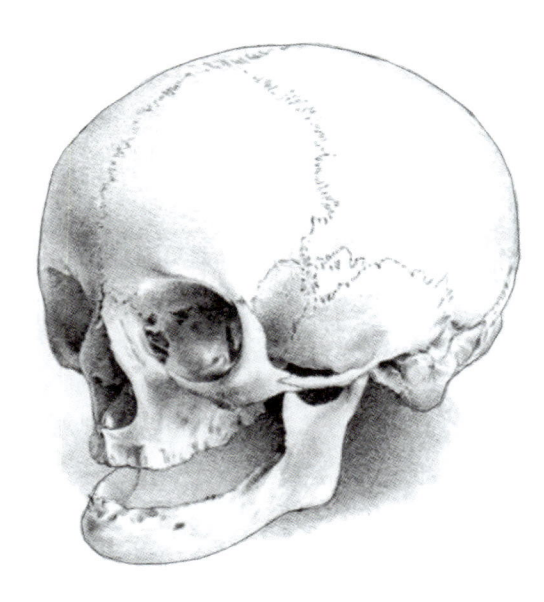

Fig. 5.6.2 Depiction of 'Kalmuc idiots' by Fraser and Mitchell 1876 [30]. Left: boy of Mitchell's collection showing 'obliquity of the eyes and palpebral slits'; right: skull of Elizabeth M. who died at 40 years of age, showing flat face, absence of nasal bone, and wormian bones.

Anthropology and racism: segregating the unfit

In Europe, most societies rejected obviously disabled babies and killed them at birth (see Chapter 8.1) or exposed them in the forest. Infants with heart defects died within a few weeks after birth. In September 1540, reformer Martin Luther described a 'changeling [*kielkropf*], eight years old, who did nothing but guzzle a lot and scream when touched ... If I were the ruler, I would drown the child in the river ... but the elector of Saxony objected to my suggestion' [32]. The spectrum of trisomy 21 was different in the 18th and 19th centuries from today: The obvious symptom was mental retardation, termed 'idiocy' when more, or 'imbecility' when less severe. Life expectancy of persons with trisomy 21 has risen from less than 30 to greater than 50 years from 1960 to 2000 [33]. Influenced by Galton and rising nationalism, a eugenics movement arose in many states. In Germany, crude theories on 'racial inferiority' or 'degeneration' evolved into Binding and Hoche's 1920 doctrine of 'useless eaters' who were 'unworthy of life' [34]. These ideas culminated in the murder of 'hereditarily diseased offspring' in Nazi Germany from 1939: 'idiocy and mongolism' were in first place on the report form from midwives and doctors (see Chapter 8.4). After World War II, infants with Down's syndrome were no longer killed, but still considered to be of little value, not only in Germany. In 1947, C. Anderson Aldrich at the Mayo Clinic wrote [35]: 'From the standpoint of the child ... they are happiest when allowed to grow up in situations where they can compete with their normal peers, in institutions ... The difficulties faced by the mothers ... as they become slaves to the child's dependency ... The father is placed in a very trying situation ... Many separations and divorces follow the birth of mongolian idiots ... The only adequate way to lessen all this grief ... is immediate commitment to an institution.'

Despite the fact that with appropriate support many people with Down's syndrome lead healthy and happy lives, and their malformations can be surgically corrected, most live in sheltered homes. A recent survey showed that in Italy and the US, 89 and 84% of adults with Down's syndrome lived in private homes, whereas in Canada 56% were in institutions and 44% in group homes [36].

Congenital malformations

About half the infants with Down's syndrome have major congenital malformations, which in the past caused their death and today means that the neonatologist encounters them. The prevalence of heart defects is 40%, mostly atrioventricular canal or ventricular septum defect leading rapidly to pulmonary hypertension [37]. The prevalence varies according to whether prenatal ultrasound, neonatal echocardiography, population-based screening, or autopsy have been carried out.

Down, Fraser, and Ireland did not mention heart defects, despite frequent post-mortem examinations. Archibald Garrod observed his first case at London's St Bartholomew Hospital in 1894 [38], and presented five cases to the London Clinical Society in 1898 [39], 'in which congenital cardiac lesions were associated with the Mongolian Type of Idiocy'. The combination had been overlooked in the asylums 'due to the failure of these children to survive to the age for admission to such institutions'.

Chromosomes, genes, and age

Chromosomal anomalies were suspected of causing Down's syndrome since 1923 [40]. However, the human chromosome number was incorrectly identified as 48 in 1923 [41]. In 1956, Tjio and Levan correctly determined the human chromosome set as 46 [42], and in 1959, Jérôme Lejeune and co-workers found an additional chromosome 21 in nine patients with Down's syndrome [43]. Chromosome 21 is the smallest human autosome, with 48 million base pairs and 225 genes, representing 1.5% of the genome. A highly conserved 'Down syndrome critical region' of human chromosome 21 band q22.3 was characterized [44]. This region causes Down's syndrome via the gene regulator 'nuclear factor of activated T cells' [45]. It is conserved on chromosome 22 of chimpanzees and orangutans. Humans have two chromosomes fewer than their cousins due to a fusion that occurred 5 million years ago that yielded the large human chromosome 2 [46]. In 1976, of 4760 patients with Down's syndrome, 93% had free (non-disjunction) trisomy, 4% had translocation (family-type), and 3% had mosaicism [47].

In 1846, among many causes of mental impairment, Edouard Séguin listed 'old age of the father and of the mother' [26]. In 1927, George Still studied 420 cases of Down's syndrome and concluded [48]: 'It is the age of the mother rather than the number of the particular pregnancy which determines the occurrence of Mongolism.' In 1933, Penrose studied 154 families of 'mongolian imbeciles' and confirmed [49] 'maternal age is of more etiological importance than the paternal age'. In statistics from the 1970s, the prevalence of trisomy 21 was 0.6 ‰ for mothers of age 20, 1.6‰ at age 30, and 10‰ at age 40 years [50]. For various reasons, maternal age has increased markedly in developed countries, as has the prevalence of trisomy 21. Since oral contraceptives became available in the 1960s, the mean mother's age at birth of her first child rose from 24 to 30 years, with some variation among European states.

Abrogating the trisomic fetus

In 1968, Carlo Valenti reported on a family with repeated, translocation type of Down's syndrome. From amniotic fluid cells, prenatal diagnosis of unbalanced trisomy 21 was made at 19 weeks of gestation, followed by a pregnancy interruption [51]. Since that time, eliminating fetuses with trisomy 21 has been a major motive for prenatal diagnostics [52]. This is not the place to discuss the well-documented history of prenatal diagnosis [53, 54]. Suffice it to say that prenatal diagnostic's aim was primarily to rule out Down's syndrome, and that most women did not want to give birth to a mentally retarded child. In the Zurich region from 1980 to 1996, '396 cases of trisomy 21 were detected prenatally, 92% of which were aborted' [55]. Nevertheless, the trisomy 21 livebirth rate remained constant, probably due to the trend towards higher maternal age at pregnancy. Society and the medical profession remained ambivalent: in the same hospital, in one operation theatre a pregnancy may be terminated because of fetal trisomy 21, whereas in another a ventricular septum defect is closed in a 2-month-old infant with trisomy 21. Few examples so drastically reveal the shift that occurs at birth (see Chapter 1.1), whom we consider a person.

The assessment of cell-free fetal DNA analysis and of prenatal screening in maternal blood changed this situation: non-invasive techniques allowed chromosomal anomalies to be diagnosed earlier, with less risk, and with great precision. The American College of Medical Genetics recommended that serum screening be offered to all pregnant women, regardless of their age [56]. With this option, each pregnant woman must weigh up two possibilities: the chromosomally normal fetus allowed to be born, and the chromosomally abnormal fetus, who is aborted. This dilemma will intensify when, which is only a matter of time and money, whole-genome sequencing from maternal blood becomes possible, revealing a host of congenital disorders. Many ethical issues arise, especially when, in addition to the parents' moral conflict, society's financial interests are involved [57]. It will be of utmost importance that parents understand the possible consequences of prenatal diagnostics. Physician providing this information may resemble 'the sorcerer's apprentice' in Goethe's famous poem [58]:

> 'Sir, my need is sore:
> Spirits that I've cited
> My commands ignore.'

Conclusion

The infant—and even more, the fetus—with Down's syndrome is the prototype of partial personhood, an individual to whom a restricted right to live is attributed. The historic evidence shows that mentally retarded children were never welcome: they were killed, abandoned, neglected, or hidden away in asylums. Prenatal diagnosis has led to their selective abortion. In many countries, ethical debates are intense and likely to continue, and a consensus across societies is unlikely. With today's prevailing views and values, Down's syndrome will probably become rare in developed countries. National legislation cannot halt global scientific progress. But legislation must ensure that opposing attitudes can coexist respectfully and respected within the same society: the right to know and the right not to know; the right to accept a disabled infant and the right not to accept it.

REFERENCES

1. Schüller A: Über Infantilismus. Wien Med Wochenschr 1907;**57**: 625–30.
2. Howard-Jones N: On the diagnostic term "Down's disease". Med Hist 1979;**23**:102–4.
3. Bleyer A: The frequency of mongoloid imbecility. Am J Dis Child 1932;**44**:503–8.
4. Record RG, Smith A: Incidence, mortality, and sex distribution of mongoloid defectives. Br J Prev Soc Med 1955;**9**:10–5.
5. Benda CE: Mongolism and cretinism. 2. ed. New York: Grune & Stratton, 1949.
6. Berg JM, Korossy M: Down syndrome before Down. Am J Med Genet 2001;**102**:205–11.
7. McClure HM, Belden KH, Pieper WA: Autosomal trisomy in a chimpanzee. Science 1969;**165**:1010–1.
8. Hirata S, Hirari H, Nogami E, Morimura N: Chimpanzee Down syndrome. Primates 2017;**58**:267–73.
9. Andrle M, Fiedler W, Rett A, et al.: A case of trisomy 22 in Pongo pygmaeus. Cytogenet Genome Res 1979;**24**:1–6.
10. Walker PL, Cook DC, Ward R, et al.: A Down syndrome-like congenital disorder in a prehistoric Californian Indian. Am J Physical Anthropol Suppl 1991;Suppl **12**:179.
11. Brothwell DR: A possible case of mongolism in a Saxon population. Ann Hum Genet 1959;**24**:141–50.
12. Czarnetzki A: Down's syndrome in ancient Europe. Lancet 2003;**362**:1000.
13. Rivollat M, Castex D, Hauret L, Tillier AM: Ancient Down syndrome: an osteological case from the 5–6th century. Int J Paleopathol 2014;**7**:8–14.

14. Diamandopoulos AA, Rakatsanis KG, Diamantopoulos N: A neolithic case of Down's syndrome. J. Hist Neurosci 1997;**61**:86–9.
15. Martinez-Frias ML: The real earliest historical evidence of Down syndrome. Am J Med Genet 2005;**132A**:231.
16. Ruhräh J: Paediatrics in art. Cretin or Mongol or both together? Am J Dis Child 1935;**49**:477–8.
17. Zellweger H: Mongolismus—Down's Syndrom. Ergeb Inn Med Kinderheilkd 1965;**22**:268–99.
18. Stratford B: In the beginning. In: Stratford B, Gunn P: New approaches to Down syndrome. London: Cassell, 1996: p. 3–11.
19. Levitas AS, Reid CS: An angel with Down syndrome in a sixteenth century Flemish nativity painting. Am J Med Genet 2003;**116A**:399–405.
20. Starbuck JM: On the antiquity of trisomy 21. J Contemp Anthropol 2011;**2**:18–44.
21. Haindorf A: Versuch einer Pathologie und Therapie der Geistes- und Gemüthskrankheiten. Heidelberg: Braun, 1811: p. 37–44.
22. Shuttleworth GE: Mongolian imbecility. BMJ 1909;**2**:661–5.
23. Platter F: Observationum in hominis affectibus plerisque libri tres. Basileae: König, 1614: Vol. **1**, p. 35.
24. Froriep R: Die Rettung der Cretinen. Bern: Wüterich-Gaudard, 1857.
25. Kanner L: Johann Jakob Guggenbühl and the Abendberg. Bull Hist Med 1959;**33**:489–502.
26. Séguin E: Le traitement moral, l'hygiène et l'éducation des idiots et des autres enfants arrières. Paris: Baillière, 1846: p. 181.
27. Seguin E: Idiocy: and its treatment by the physiological method. New York: Wood, 1866: p. 44, 381–2.
28. Poole R: An essay on education, applicable to children in general. Edinburgh: Waugh and Innes, 1825: p. 243.
29. Down JLH: Observations on an ethnic classification of idiots. Lond Hosp Rep 1866;**3**:259–62.
30. Fraser J, Mitchell A: Kalmuc idiocy: report of a case with autopsy. J Ment Sci 1876;**22**:169–79.
31. Ireland WW: On idiocy and imbecility. London: Churchill, 1877: p. 53–6.
32. Luther M: Tischreden 1540. Nr. 5297. Weimar: Böhlau, 1919: Vol. **5**, p. 9.
33. Mégarbané A, Ravel A, Mircher C, et al.: The 50th anniversary of the discovery of trisomy 21. Genet Med 2009;**11**:611–6.
34. Binding K, Hoche A: Die Vernichtung lebensunwerten Lebens. Leipzig: Meiner, 1920.
35. Aldrich CA: Preventive medicine and mongolism. Am J Ment Defic 1947;**52**:127–9.
36. Carfi A, Vetrano DL, Mascia D, et al.: Adults with Down syndrome. J Intellect Disab Res 2019;**63**:624–9.
37. Park SC, Mathews RA, Zuberbuhler JR, et al.: Down syndrome with congenital heart malformation. Am J Dis Child 1977;**131**:29–33.
38. Garrod AE: On the association of cardiac malformations with other congenital defects. St Bart Hosp Rep 1894;**30**:53.
39. Garrod A: Report at the London Clinical Society. Lancet 1898;**152**:1062.
40. Halbertsma T: Mongolism in one of twins and the etiology of mongolism. Am J Dis Child 1923;**25**:350–3.
41. Painter TS: Studies in mammalian spermatogenesis: II: The spermatogenesis of man. J Exp Zool 1923;**37**:291–336.
42. Tjio JH, Levan A: The chromosome number of man. Hereditas 1956;**42**:1–6.
43. Lejeune J, Gautier M, Turpin R: Étude des chromosomes somatiques de neuf enfants mongoliens. Compt Rend Acad Sci 1959;**248**:1721–2.
44. McCormick MK, Schinzel A, Petersen MB, et al.: Molecular genetic approach to the characterization of the "Down syndrome region" of chromosome 21. Genomics 1989;**5**:325–31.
45. Epstein CJ: Critical genes in a critical region. Nature 2006;**441**:582–3.
46. Kasai F, Takahashi E, Koyama K, et al.: Comparative FISH mapping of the ancestral fusion point of human chromosome 2. Chromosome Res 2000;**8**:727–35.
47. Giraud F, Mattei JF: Aspects epidémiologiques de la trisomie 21. J Genet Hum 1975;**23**:1–30.
48. Still GF: Place in family as a factor in disease. Lancet 1927;**210**:795–800, 853–8.
49. Penrose LS: The relative effects of paternal and maternal age in mongolism. J Genet 1933;**27**:219–24.
50. Pueschel SM, Rynders JE: Down syndrome. Cambridge, MA: Ware Press, 1982: p. 48, 167.
51. Valenti C, Schutta EJ, Kehaty T: Prenatal diagnosis of Down's syndrome. Lancet 1968;**292**:220.
52. Nicolaides KH: Turning the pyramid of prenatal care. Fetal Diagn Ther 2011;**29**:183–96.
53. Cuckle H, Maymon R: Development of prenatal screening—a historical overview. Semin Perinat 2016;**40**:12–22.
54. Hui L: Noninvasive approaches to prenatal diagnosis. In: Brynn L: Prenatal diagnosis. New York: Springer, 2019: p. 45–58.
55. Mutter M, Binkert F, Schinzel A: Down syndrome livebirth rate in the eastern part of Switzerland between 1980 and 1996. Prenat Diagn 2002;**22**:835–6.
56. Gregg AR, Skotko BG, Benkendorf JL, et al.: Noninvasive prenatal screening for fetal aneuploidy, 2016 update. Genet Med 2016;**18**:1056–65.
57. De Jong A, Dondorp WJ, de Die-Smulders C, Frints SGM, de Wert GMWR: Non-invasive prenatal testing: ethical issues explored. Eur J Hum Genet 2010;**18**:272–7.
58. Goethe JW: The sorcerer's apprentice. In: Zeydel EH: Goethe, the lyrist. 100 poems in new translation facing the originals. Chapel Hill, NC: University of North Carolina Press, 1955
59. Evans E. The new asylum for idiots at Earlswood Common, Redhill, Surrey [Engraving]. In: Illustrated London News, Is. 672, 1854; p. 213.

5.7
Crooked limbs
The thalidomide catastrophe

Introduction: crooked limbs

About 350 million years ago, fin-to-limb transition enabled marine vertebrates to conquer land and colonize various terrestrial habitats. The molecular mechanisms operating during embryonic development explain how their morphology diversified. As limbs developed, HoxD genes became sequentially activated in a progressive switch from proximal, Hox9, to distal, Hox13 [1]. The result was always a four-limb and usually five-digit pattern. Deviations from this deeply rooted image were perceived to be incompatible with human dignity, regarded with fascination, or loathed. Neolithic cave paintings of hands with extra digits document early interest in limb malformations [2].

Before prenatal diagnostics reduced the number of malformed infants, limb malformations had a prevalence of around 1 per 1000 newborns [3]. The defect was visible immediately at birth, and the infants did not die spontaneously shortly thereafter. Nevertheless, they were dreaded, because agrarian societies valued their offspring according to their bodily fitness. In the tense atmosphere of the delivery room, the limbs' integrity was the second concern after the baby's sex. The words 'monster', 'cripple', 'crook', and 'invalid' as insulting nicknames reveal the low esteem that limb malformations encountered. Using the thalidomide disaster as a prototype of disturbed development, this chapter aims to shed light on early views of limb teratogenesis and on legislators' efforts to prevent damage by drugs.

Antiquity and mythology

The omens' list on Chaldean clay tablets in Assurbanipal's Royal Library in Niniveh [4] contained a classification of limb malformations that included amelia and phocomelia: 'When a woman gives birth to an infant that has no feet, the canals of the country will be cut, and the house ruined … When … an infant whose hands and feet are like four fishes' tails [fins], the master [king] shall perish, and his country shall be consumed.'

Early reports

In the Middle Ages, sexual intercourse with animals or the devil were blamed for causing specific malformations, as mentioned in Luther's 'table talks' [5], and witchcraft was associated with children's diseases as late as 1751 [6]. Giving birth to a malformed infant could endanger the mother, as can be imagined from Conrad Lycosthenes' report from 1557 [7]: 'A child, marvellous and gruesome to look at … had neither arms nor feet, and the hips ended in a thick fish's tail … The mother was tortured to find out whether such monster had been conceived by infamy, but she was declared innocent and set free.' During the 17th century, the medical profession replaced the theory of cohabitation with animals by the more innocuous one of maternal imagination (see Chapter 5.5). In 1614, Basel anatomist Caspar Bauhin took great pains to define different levels of malformation and to compile previous theories on the origin of developmental anomalies in a table [8] (Figs. 5.7.1 and 5.7.2).

Phocomelia and amelia captured the imagination of medieval observers. Ambroise Paré wrote [9] (Fig. 5.7.3, left): 'In the year 1573, I saw at St. Andrew's Church in Paris, a boy nine years old, born in the village Parpavilla, six miles from Guise; his father's name was Peter Renard, and his mother, Marquete: He had but two fingers on his right hand, his arm was well proportioned from the top of his shoulder almost to his wrist, but from thence to his two finger's ends it was verie deformed, hee wanted his legs and thighs, although from the right buttock a certain unperfect figure, haveing only four toes, seemed to put it self forth; from the midst of the left buttock two toes sprung out.'

In his monumental *Observationes Medicarum*, Freiburg city physician Schenck von Grafenberg devoted no fewer than 24 folio pages [10] to cases of limb malformations published before 1596 and classified reduction defects in amelia (total absence of one or more limbs), phocomelia (shortened limb with lack of a proximal bone), defective forelimb/radius aplasia, finger or foot defects, and others. 'Dwarfs' with phocomelia were found among medieval court jesters and artists, or were put on show, displayed on markets. Some famous phocomeles who reached adulthood include Matthias Buchinger born 1674, Marco Catozze (le petit Pepin) born ca. 1750 (Fig. 5.7.4), Thomas Inglefield born 1769, Sarah Biffin born 1784, and Ruth Davis (the penguin girl) born ca. 1910.

Combined with the doctrine of maternal imagination, witnessing torture was believed to cause fetal injury and deformation, as Nicolas Malebranche reported in 1690 from the Paris Hospital of Incurables [11]: 'A young man who was born an Idiot, and whose Body was broken in the same places that Malefactors are broken on the Wheel … the cause of this Calamitous Accident was, That his

Tabula *** notata ad pag. 59

Sequitur Typus causas monstrosorum partuum exhibens.

Causæ monstrosorum partuum sunt vel.

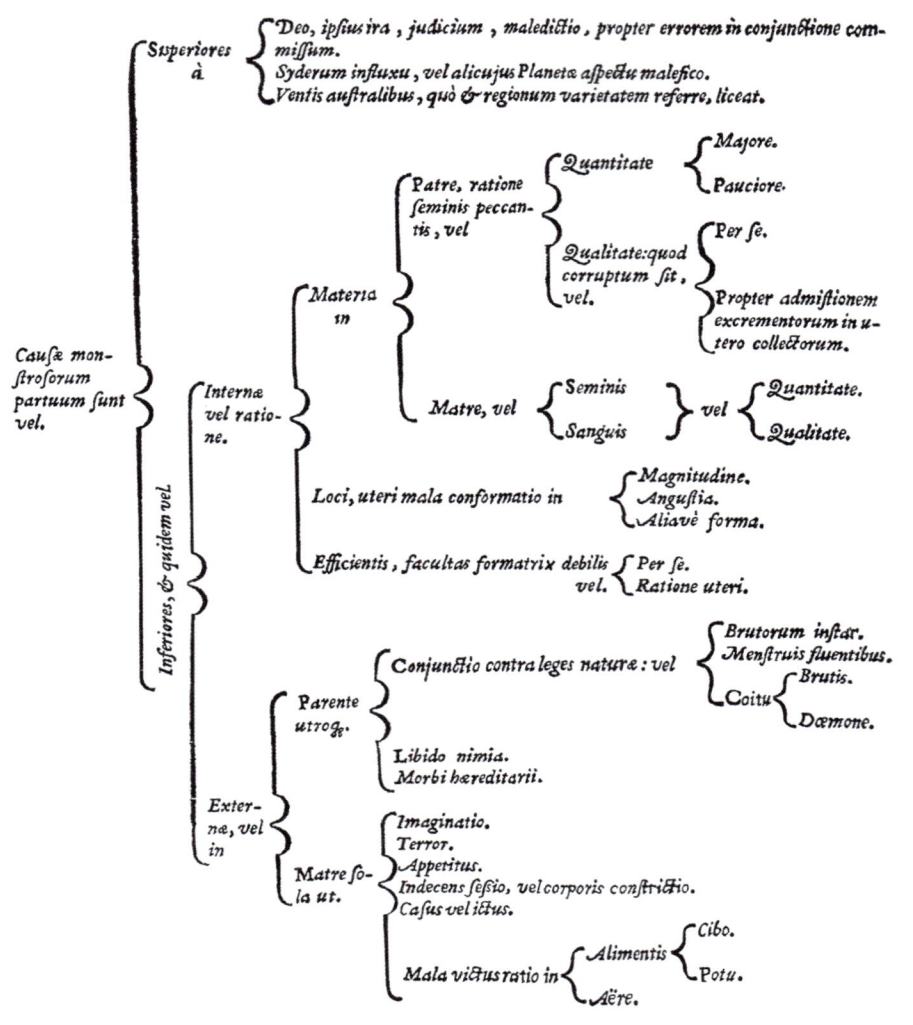

- Superiores à
  - Deo, ipsius ira, judicium, maledictio, propter errorem in conjunctione commissum.
  - Syderum influxu, vel alicujus Planetæ aspectu malefico.
  - Ventis australibus, quò & regionum varietatem referre, liceat.
- Inferiores, & quidem vel
  - Internæ vel ratione.
    - Materia in
      - Patre, ratione seminis peccantis, vel
        - Quantitate { Majore. Pauciore.
        - Qualitate: quod corruptum sit, vel. { Per se. Propter admistionem excrementorum in utero collectorum.
      - Matre, vel { Seminis / Sanguis } vel { Quantitate. Qualitate.
    - Loci, uteri mala conformatio in { Magnitudine. Angustia. Aliavê forma.
    - Efficientis, facultas formatrix debilis vel. { Per se. Ratione uteri.
  - Externæ, vel in
    - Parente utroq.
      - Conjunctio contra leges naturæ: vel { Brutorum instar. Menstruis fluentibus. Coitu { Brutis. Dæmone.
      - Libido nimia.
      - Morbi hæreditarii.
    - Matre sola ut.
      - Imaginatio.
      - Terror.
      - Apperitus.
      - Indecens sessio, vel corporis constrictio.
      - Casus vel ictus.
      - Mala victus ratio in { Alimentis { Cibo. Potu. Aëre.

Fig. 5.7.1 Caspar Bauhin's table of 1614 classifying higher (supranatural) and lower (biological) causes of malformations [8].

[pregnant] Mother hearing a Criminal was to be broken, went to see the Execution. All the blows which were given to the Condemned, struck violently the Imagination of the Mother; and by a kind of Repercussive blow, the tender and delicate Brain of her Infant … The violent course of the Animal Spirits of the Mother, made a forcible descent from her brain, towards all the Members of her Body, which were Analogous to those of the Criminal, and the same thing happened to the Infant. But because the Bones of the Mother were capable of withstanding the violent Impression of these Spirits, they receivd no dammage by them.'

Torture in public was a frequent execution method that included dismembering and stretching on the rack, and was done in many countries. It was forbidden in Scotland in 1708 and in most German states at the end of the 18th century [12]. Salomon Reisel, consultant to the Duke of Wuerttemberg, observed a case of total amelia [13] (**Fig. 5.7.3**, centre and right): 'In Wangen near Stuttgart a son was born to the farmer Hans Cunrad Hahn and his wife Ephrosine on May 10, 1689. He was living, with a vivid color, and was baptized on his father's name … He had the right [sic!] mouth corner longer than the left, a small naevus on his nose, and his anus was closed. The latter was dissected by the surgeon shortly after birth, so that he could suck, eat mash, and excrete stool. But his arms and legs were totally absent … His mother had been truly terrified at midgestation by a beggar with mutilated arms and legs, and transmitted her impression of his extremities to the embryo … I depicted him alive on the 14th, he died on the 17th day of life.'

Modern teratology

In 1759, Caspar Friedrich Wolff demonstrated stepwise embryonic development, coined the term 'germ layer', and explained

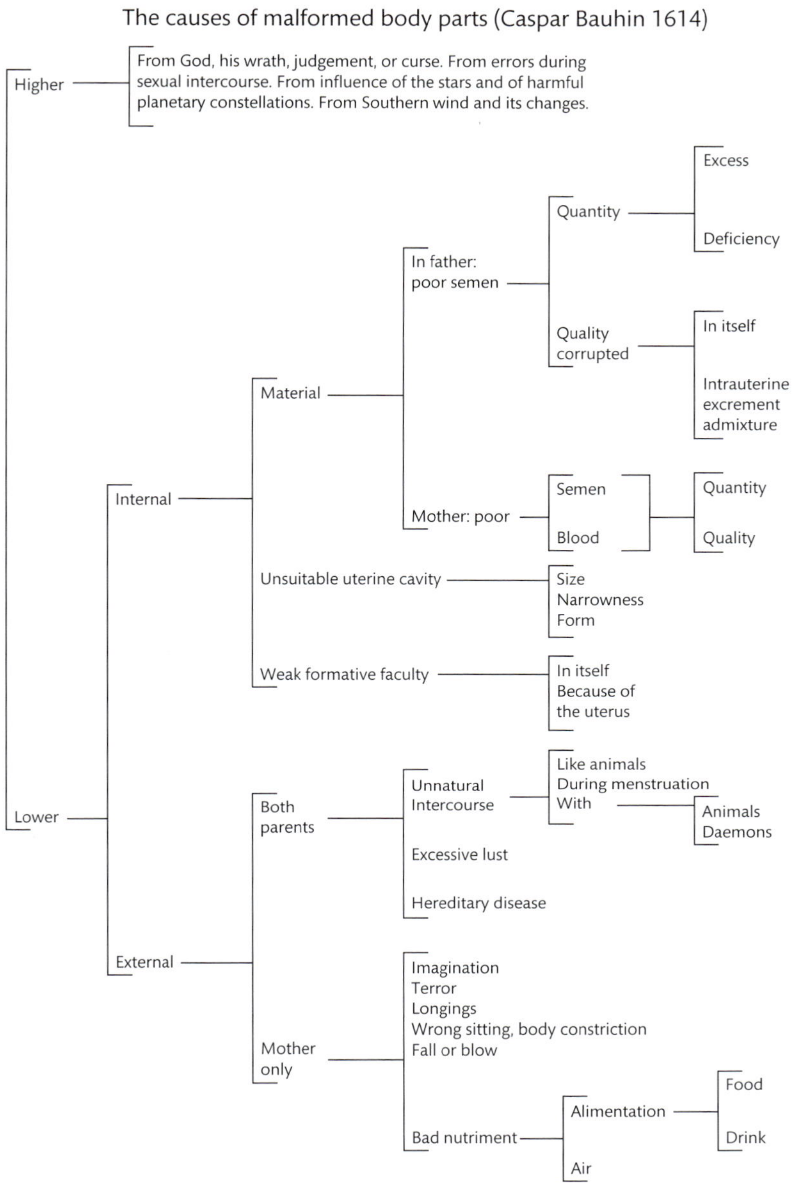

The causes of malformed body parts (Caspar Bauhin 1614)

- **Higher**: From God, his wrath, judgement, or curse. From errors during sexual intercourse. From influence of the stars and of harmful planetary constellations. From Southern wind and its changes.
- **Lower**
  - **Internal**
    - **Material**
      - In father: poor semen
        - Quantity: Excess / Deficiency
        - Quality corrupted: In itself / Intrauterine excrement admixture
      - Mother: poor
        - Semen: Quantity
        - Blood: Quality
    - Unsuitable uterine cavity: Size, Narrowness, Form
    - Weak formative faculty: In itself / Because of the uterus
  - **External**
    - Both parents
      - Unnatural Intercourse: Like animals, During menstruation, With Animals / Daemons
      - Excessive lust
      - Hereditary disease
    - Mother only
      - Imagination
      - Terror
      - Longings
      - Wrong sitting, body constriction
      - Fall or blow
      - Bad nutriment
        - Alimentation: Food / Drink
        - Air

Fig. 5.7.2 Caspar Bauhin's table, translated.

malformations as a natural consequence of disturbed differentiation [14]. In 1791, Johann Blumenbach described a formative drive that regulates embryonic differentiation, including malformations [15]. Albrecht von Haller described the development of the chicken heart from a loop in 1758 [16]. Teratology started as a descriptive science with collections of malformations in the anatomist families Geoffroy Saint Hilaire in Paris, Vrolik in Amsterdam, and Meckel in Halle (**Fig. 5.7.4**). Isidore Geoffroy Saint-Hilaire introduced the term 'teratology', studied dwarfs, distinguished rickets and diminished growth from malformations, and classified many congenital anomalies [17]. Camille Dareste induced 'monstrosities' by mechanical impulses while incubating hen eggs in 1877 [18]. In his scholarly *Manual of Antenatal Pathology and Hygiene*, Edinburgh obstetrician John Ballantyne devoted several chapters to limb malformations, and explained reduction anomalies as resulting from pressure, mechanical injury, or disturbed or arrested formation during embryonic life [19], and confessed: 'In all this, there is much that is uncertain, obscure, dark.'

Thalidomide embryopathy

Both the chronology and clinical manifestations of the thalidomide epidemic have been investigated [20, 21], therefore only its causes and consequences will be reported. The substance was produced by the German company Chemie Grünenthal from 1955 [22]. As usual at that time, no embryological testing had been done. Chemically similar to barbiturates but nontoxic in rodents, thalidomide was unsuitable as a suicide drug, and rapidly became a popular sleeping pill. It was advertised as 'non-toxic' and also used to alleviate morning

200 PART 5 Odd shape

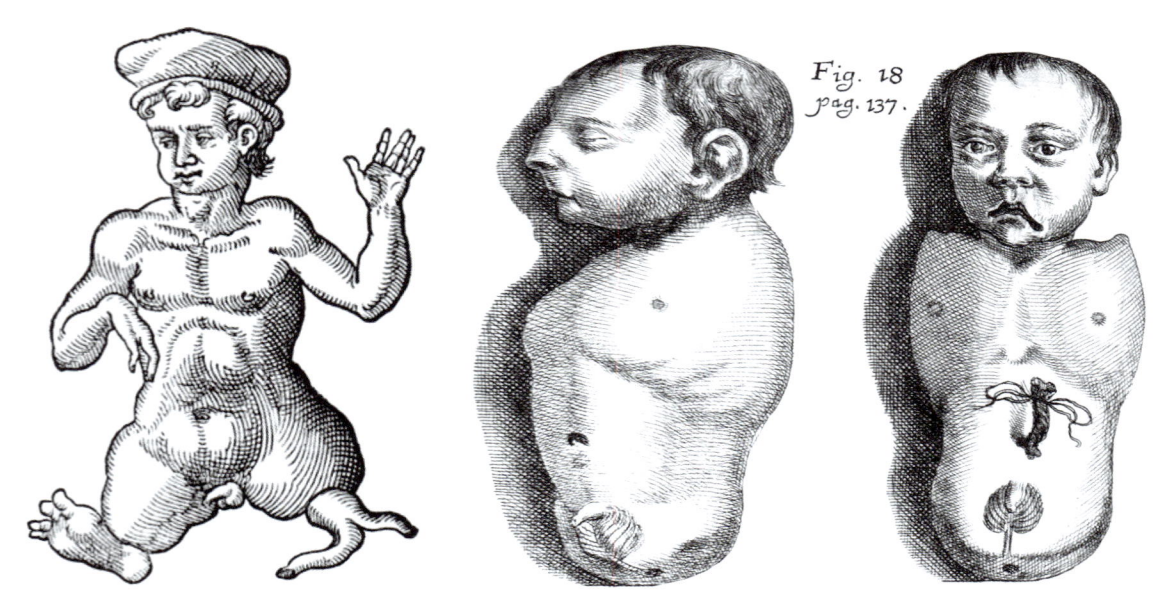

Fig. 5.7.3 Phocomelia and amelia observed during the 17th century. Left: phocomelia described by Ambroise Paré [9]; centre and right: amelia described by Salomon Reisel [13]. See text for details.

sickness of pregnancy. Following the then usual registration procedure lasting 4 weeks, the drug was licensed in July 1956 and marketed in Germany from October 1957, in Britain from April 1958, in Sweden from September 1958, in Canada from April 1961, and in 42 other countries as 'Contergan', 'Distaval', and under 40 other names, but not in the US, where Grünenthal had applied for approval in September 1960, but the Food and Drug Administration (FDA) posed questions the company could not answer [23].

Nine months later, the epidemic began.

In 1959, Munich gynaecologist Arnulf Weidenbach published 'a very unusual case of total phocomelia', born on 10 November 1958, and concluded 'it cannot be discerned if the phocomelia resulted from gene anomaly or a harmful environmental factor' [24]. Clusters of malformations were observed in Germany during 1961. At a scientific meeting on 18 November 1961, Hamburg geneticist Widukind Lenz suspected that 'Contergan' was responsible [25], and notified the producer, Grünenthal. In Sydney, William McBride had observed six cases of phocomelia, all exposed to 'Distaval', notified the producer Distillers Ltd. on 27 November, and published his results in a letter to *The Lancet* on 16 December [26]. On 27 November 1961, thalidomide was withdrawn from the market [27]. On 6 January 1962, Lenz published 52 cases from Germany, also in

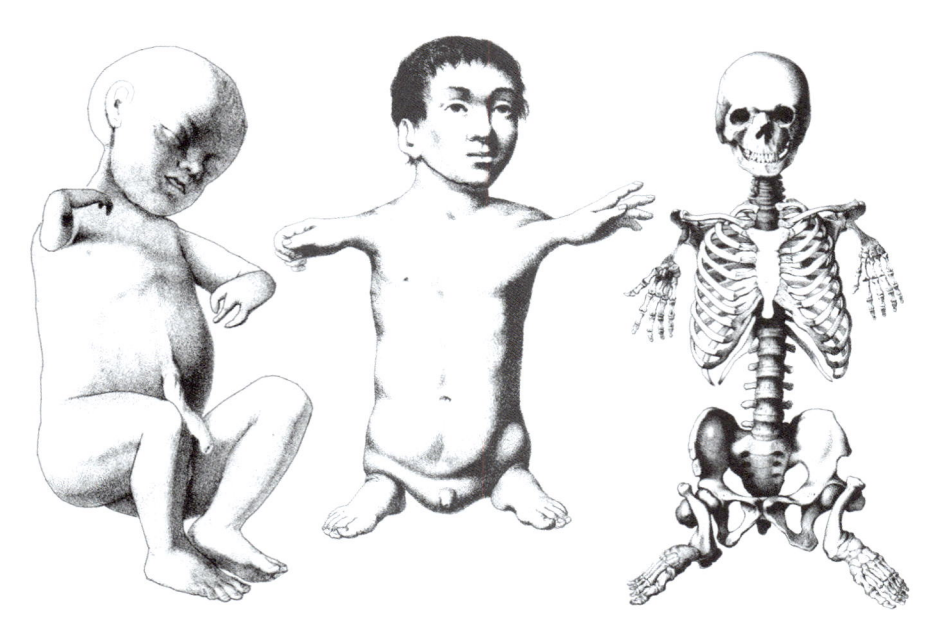

Fig. 5.7.4 Arm reductions depicted by Willem Vrolik in 1849 [43]. Left: newborn from Hovius' collection in Amsterdam, bilateral absence of forearm; centre and right: the famous dwarf Marco Catozze, named 'Petit Pepin', dissection performed by Auguste Dumeril. See text for details.

Table 5.7.1. Some types, frequencies, and chronology of malformation in thalidomide embryopathy. More severe cases involve arms and legs, some resemble Holt–Oram syndrome (phenocopy)

	Definition	Frequency	Time-sensitive window (postmenstrual)
Limb reduction			
Amelia	Absence of one or more limbs		d. 38–43 arms d. 41–45 legs
Micromelia	Abnormally small and imperfectly developed extremity		
Phocomelia	Shortened limbs, feet or hands arising close to the trunk ('seal extremities'), mostly bilateral	88% (all) 69% upper limb 40% lower limb	d. 38–47 arms d. 42–47 legs
Ectromelia	Hypoplasia or aplasia of one or more long bones		d. 39–45 arms d. 45–47 legs
Radius aplasa	Absent or defective radial bone		
Thumb hypoplasia/ triphalangea thumb	Small thumbs/thumb that has three phalanges instead of two	80%	d. 38–40 d. 46–50
Other malformation			
Hydrocephay	Accumulation of fluid within the brain		
Anophthalma	Absence of the eye(s)	10%	d. 40–48
Haemangioma	Capillary		
Coloboma	Defect of iris or lens		d. 38–46
Ear defects	Absence of the ears or inner ear defect	38%	d. 34–38
Heart malformation	Septum defects, Fallot tetralogy	8%	d. 46–50
Renal malformation	Multicystic kidney, ureter anomaly	8%	d. 42–52

d = days from last menstrual bleeding.
Source: Data from Lenz & Knapp 1962 [35]; Nowack 1965 [29], Leck 1962 [36]; Smithells and Newman 1992 [37]; Mansour 2018 [38].

The Lancet [28]. Symptoms and frequencies of thalidomide embryopathy are listed in Table 5.7.1. The reduction defects were usually more severe in the upper than in the lower extremities. Phocomelia, ectromelia, and amelia are not specific to thalidomide—they have been observed at all times (Figs. 5.7.3 and 5.7.4). In August 1962 the epidemic waned, but by then more than 3000 malformed infants had been born in Germany and about 10,000 worldwide within 4 years, the number of cases directly proportional to the thalidomide sales [20].

Sensitive windows and pathogenetic concepts

The thalidomide catastrophe was the greatest disaster in the history of pharmacology and soon researchers began to study how it came about. It became obvious that the drug's toxicity to the embryo is highly species specific, and acts in a short, time-sensitive developmental window [29] from 24 to 33 days after fertilization. This corresponded to 38–47 days after the start of the last menstruation (Table 5.7.1), maliciously a date when many women do not yet know they are pregnant.

From 1960 to 2000, more than 5000 papers were published on thalidomide, more than 2000 of them concerned with its teratogenic action [30]. Various and contradicting theories have been promulgated, but the mechanism by which the drug causes the malformations remained elusive. Trent Stephens classified several entirely different categories [30], affecting: (1) DNA replication or transcription; (2) synthesis or function of growth factors; (3) synthesis or function of integrins; (4) formation of blood vessels; (5) formation of cartilage; and (6) cell death or injury. In non-human primate embryos, Reinhard Neubert and colleagues detected a drastic down-regulation of surface adhesion receptors after exposure to thalidomide, acting on the trunk even before the limb bud exists [31]. Another injury attributed to the drug is the inhibition of small vessel formation, induced by basic fibroblast growth factors [32]. It has been shown in chick embryos that the drug causes a loss of immature blood vessels which may be the primary cause of the limb defects [33]. The drug has recently returned to medical use as an angiogenesis inhibitor in some malignancies. Thalidomide embryopathy—undoubtedly resulting from exogenous toxicity to the embryo—reveals striking similarities to Holt–Oram syndrome, an autosomal dominant inherited disorder caused by mutations in the TBX5 gene [34]. This 'phenocopy' may indicate a common terminal pathway for thalidomide embryopathy, Holt–Oram syndrome, and sporadic dysmelia, making these malformations resemble each other despite having completely different causes due to a similar biochemical reaction interfering with differentiation of the upper extremities and the heart.

Legislation for drug approval

Despite various efforts since 1876, there was no drug law in Federal Germany until February 1961. It was up to the manufacturers to determine which safety tests should be conducted. Even the law that was finally passed could not have prevented the thalidomide disaster, as it required neither the central registration of side effects nor the testing of new drugs on pregnant animals [39]. Surveillance of drug side effects was the responsibility of multiple provincial state offices, and a prescription requirement for new drugs was introduced as late as 1984. The Federal Ministry of Health was founded in 1962. The Contergan trial lasted 9 years, one of the longest court cases ever in Germany, but the absence of effective drug laws precluded a verdict. The trial revealed severe shortcomings in German drug legislation and ended in 1970 with a settlement: Grünenthal paid 110 million DM (30 million US$) to the victims, and the court admonished the legislators [40]: (1) to put new drugs under prescription requirement for 5 years; (2) to introduce federal oversight to ensure drug safety; and (3) to ensure patient protection priority over economic interests. Since 1978, the drug approval laws of Germany have been repeatedly tightened and today are so timid and restrictive that drugs to which fetuses and newborns may be exposed can no longer be developed in Germany [39, 41].

In the US, the Food, Drug, and Cosmetic Act was passed in 1938, and from 1950 the FDA was authorized to oversee the licensing of new drugs and to register side effects. The law required that before a new drug could be distributed, the manufacturer must submit extensive information on its safety to the FDA—a law that spared American babies the thalidomide catastrophe. In October 1961, shortly *before* the thalidomide–phocomelia relationship was published, the FDA pointed out that tests on mature animals and human adults or older children do not suffice to make recommendations concerning the fetus and newborn [23]. In January 1962, world-famous American cardiologist Helen Taussig travelled to Germany to study the phocomelia outbreak [42] which led to further tightening of the American drug laws. In 1962, John F. Kennedy awarded FDA physician Frances Kelsey the President's Medal of Honor for averting a thalidomide disaster in the US [21].

The European process of drug approval began with the European Economic Community directive in 1965. In 1995, the European Medicines Agency was founded, charged with harmonizing the process of drug approval and mutual recognition [41]. Today, European drug approval, tightened nearly every year, is very similar to the FDA process in the US.

Conclusion

What was disquieting about the thalidomide disaster was not the pharmaceutical manufacturer's delayed reaction: within a week of the first notification of its teratogenic potential, the drug was withdrawn. More worrying was the absence of effective control mechanisms during the registration process, which gave a highly toxic drug access to the market. But most appalling was the medical community's slow reaction and the late acknowledgement of its teratogenicity once the drug was distributed: the epidemic raged for 4 years and 'unusual' cases of malformation were observed for 3 years before McBride and Lenz independently linked them with thalidomide intake. Given the limited understanding of teratogenesis, the lack of a malformation registry, and the absence of laws protecting patients in the 1950s, the tragedy was not preventable. *First do no harm*: the Hippocratic principle demands we reflect on the risk–benefit trade-off. This is especially important when prescribing drugs for women of childbearing age: physicians must remember that the damage to the embryo typically occurs at or before the mother can know she is pregnant. *Big oaks from little acorns grow*: as in the cot death epidemic (see Chapter 8.5), it was not a 'life-saving' intervention that caused the catastrophe, but a 'simple and harmless sleeping pill' taken to relieve sleeplessness and morning sickness, conditions only recently promoted as diseases deserving treatment. *Blessing and curse*: in the aftermath of the 'Contergan' catastrophe, patient safety has greatly increased, but the price is that in some European countries, children cannot benefit from medical progress because new drugs for infants can in practice no longer be developed.

REFERENCES

1. Kherdjemil Y, Kmita M: Insights on the role of hox genes in the emergence of the pentadactyl ground state. Genesis 2017;**56**:e23046.
2. Lange A, Müller GB: Polydactyly in development, inheritance, and evolution. Q Rev Biol 2017;**92**:1–38.
3. Ermito S, Dinatale A, Carrara S, et al.: Prenatal diagnosis of limb anomalies: role of fetal ultrasonography. J Prenat Med 2009;**3**:18–22.
4. Ballantyne JW: The teratological records of Chaldea. Teratologia 1894;**1**:127–43.
5. Luther M: Tischreden (1556). Weimar: Böhlau, 1919: Vol. **5**, p. 613.
6. Storch J: Theoretische und practische Abhandlung von Kinder-Kranckheiten. Eisenach: Grießbach, 1751: Vol. **4**, p. 258.
7. Lycosthenes C: Wunderwerck oder Gottes unergründliches Vorbilden. Basel: Petri, 1557: p. 123, 201, 310, 546.
8. Bauhin C: De Hermaphroditorum monstrosorumque partuum natura. Oppenheim: Galler, 1614: p. 44–140 (Tabula *** notata ad pag. 59).
9. Paré A: Of monsters and prodigies (1st French ed. 1573). In: The workes of that famous Chirurgion Ambrose Parey. London: Cotes & Du-gard, 1649: p. 657.
10. Schenck von Grafenberg J: Observationes medicarum rararum, novarum, admirabilium, & monstrosarum (1st ed. 1596). Lugduni: Huguetan, 1644: p. 504, 628–52.
11. Malebranche N: Treatise concerning the search after truth (1st Latin ed. 1690). 2. ed. London: Bowyer, 1700: p. 55–6.
12. Melville RD: The use and forms of judicial torture in England and Scotland. Scot Hist Rev 1905;**2**:225–48.
13. Reisel S: Infans truncus sine artubus. Miscell Cursive Ephemeridum Decur II 1689;**8**:136–7.
14. Wolff CF: Theoria Generationis. Halle: Hendelianis, 1759.
15. Blumenbach JF: Über den Bildungstrieb. Göttingen: Dieterich, 1791: p. 111.
16. Haller Av: Sur la formation du coeur dans le poulet. Lausanne: Bousquet, 1758.
17. Geoffroy Saint-Hilaire I: Histoire générale et particulière des anomalies de l'organisation chez l'homme et les animaux. Paris: Baillière, 1832: Vol. **3**, p. 391.
18. Dareste C: Recherches sur la production artificielle des monstruosités. Paris: Reinwald, 1877.
19. Ballantyne JW: Manual of antenatal pathology and hygiene. The embryo. Edinburgh: Green, 1904: p. 105–28, 224.
20. Lenz W: A short history of thalidomide embryopathy. Teratology 1988;**38**:203–15.
21. Vargesson N: Thalidomide-induced teratogenesis: history and mechanisms. Birth Defects Res C 2015;**105**:140–56.
22. Franks ME, Macpherson GR, Figg WD: Thalidomide. Lancet 2004;**363**:1802–11.

23. Kelsey FO: Problems raised for the FDA by the occurrence of thalidomide embryopathy in Germany, 1960–1961. Am J Public Health 1965;**55**:703–7.
24. Weidenbach A: Totale Phokomelie. Zentralbl Gynäk 1959;**81**: 2048–52.
25. Pfeiffer RA, Kosenow W: Thalidomide and congenital abnormalities. Lancet 1962;**279**:45–6.
26. McBride WG: Thalidomide and congenital abnormalities. Lancet 1961;**278**:1358.
27. Hayman D: Distaval. Lancet 1961;**278**:1262.
28. Lenz W: Thalidomide and congenital abnormalities. Lancet 1962;**279**:45.
29. Nowack E: Die sensible Phase bei der Thalidomid-Embryopathie. Humangenetik 1965;**1**:516–36.
30. Stephens TD, Bunde CJW, Fillmore BJ: Mechanism of action in thalidomide teratogenesis. Biochem Pharmacol 2000;**59**:1489–99.
31. Neubert R, Hinz N, Thiel R, Neubert D: Down-regulation of adhesion receptors on cells of primate embryos as a probable mechanism of the teratogenic action of thalidomide. Life Sci 1996;**58**:295–316.
32. D'Amato RJ, Loughnan MS, Flynn E, Folkman J: Thalidomide is an inhibitor of angiogenesis. PNAS 1994;**91**:4082–5.
33. Therapontos C, Erskine L, Gardner ER, et al.: Thalidomide induces limb defects by preventing angiogenic outgrowth during early limb formation. PNAS 2009;**106**:8573–8.
34. Al-Qattan MM, Abou Al-Shaar H: Molecular basis of the clinical features of Holt-Oram syndrome resulting from missense and extended protein mutations of the TBX5 gene as well as TBX5 intragenic duplications. Gene 2015;**560**:129–36.
35. Lenz W, Knapp. K: Thalidomid-Embryopathie. Dtsch Med Wochenschr 1962;**87**:1232–42.
36. Leck IM, Millar ELM: Incidence of malformations since the introduction of thalidomide. BMJ 1962;**2**:16–20.
37. Smithells RW, Newman CGH: Recognition of thalidomide defects. J Med Genet 1992;**29**:716–23.
38. Mansour S, Baple E, Hall CM: A clinical review and introduction of the diagnostic algorithm for thalidomide embryopathy (DATE). J Hand Surg 2018;**44**:96–108.
39. Körner HH: Gesetz über den Verkehr mit Arzneimitteln (AMG). München: Beck, 2007.
40. Landgericht Aachen: Contergan-Einstellungsbeschluss vom 18.12.1970. Juristenzeitung 1971;**15/16**:507.
41. Van Norman GA: Drugs and devices. Comparison of European and U.S. approval processes. J Am Coll Cardiol Basic Trans Sci 2016;**1**:399–412.
42. Taussig HB: A study of the German outbreak of phocomelia. JAMA 1962;**180**:1106–14.
43. Vrolik W: Tabulae ad illustrandam embryogenesin hominis et mammalium. Amsterdam: Londonck, 1844–1849: p. plate 29, plate 76, fig 2; plate 77.

5.8

A wretched condition
Cleft urinary bladder

Introduction

The incidence of cleft bladder is 1:50,000 among male newborns, rarer than many other major malformations. But it was well known to the ancients because it was not (rapidly) lethal. The infants grew up with a continence problem for which therapeutic interventions were sought [1]: 'Of all instances in which an arrest of development of parts has taken part during human foetal life, none surpasses in interest or importance that which affects the genito-urinary organs … The sufferer from such structural defect may attain mature age—in the great majority of instances sexually incapacitated—a burden to himself and repulsive to those around.' The malformations of the exstrophy–epispadias complex have been classified early [2–5]. The following chapter delineates thoughts on the origin of this malformation and steps taken to lessen the children's suffering.

Perceived as hermaphrodites

Bladder malformation was usually accompanied with malformed genitalia, and the infants were confused with hermaphrodites, the most loathed of all congenital anomalies [6]. Etruscan diviners known as *haruspices* were given the task of averting or expiating the evil omen and of deciding on infants with ambiguous genitalia. Livius reported [7]: 'At Sinuessa [a child was born and] it was uncertain whether male or female. In fact the soothsayers summoned from Etruria said it was a terrible and loathsome portent; it must be removed from Roman territory, far from contact with earth, and drowned in the sea. They put it alive into a chest, carried it out to sea and threw it overboard'.

Forms and grades

A boy was examined in Freiburg by the surgeon Tobias Cneulin and reported by city physician Schenck von Grafenberg in 1596 [8]: 'A few days ago a deplorable infant was born here, in whom the abdominal wall had disappeared: the male member was wanting, in its place an opening was seen from which the urine poured. The scrotum with both testicles was normally formed. The parents asked for help from a surgeon, but I don't believe the baby survived.'

Descriptions from the 17th century were more precise (Fig. 5.8.1) [9–11] and discerned three grades: the mildest form, epispadias, where the urethra opens at the anterior side of the penis instead of its tip; more severe was bladder exstrophy, where the bladder's anterior wall is open; and most severe, cloacal exstrophy, entailing an open abdominal wall and common outlet for stool and urine. The affected children suffered most from painful inguinal eczema due to the urine continuously irritating the skin. Jacques Tenon reported three different types in 1761 [12]. In February 1782, a 6-week-old infant was referred to M. Castara, surgeon in Luneville, because the infant's sex could not be determined [13]. He described and depicted (Fig. 5.8.2) the infant, interpreting the protruding red swelling as the dorsal wall of the bladder, and the two continuously dripping openings as the ureters. Many other cases were reported in the 18th century, mostly males. Females with bladder exstrophy could become pregnant and give birth, albeit with difficulty, as surgeon John Bonnet of Fowye in Cornwall experienced on 18 July 18 1722 [14]: 'Agony had almost quite exhausted the poor Woman's spirits; but the Orifice of the Vagina was no way sensibly dilated. In vain were all Endeavours to relieve her … I told the Mother and the other Persons in the Room, that Death was inevitable without making the passage wider by Incision … I thrust my Scalpel into the inferior oblong orifice and cut into the orifice of the Vagina, so brought them into one: Then presently with my scissors, snipp'd the transverse membrane … drew forth a Female Infant, living and well form'd, to my own Surprize and Admiration of all … [Mother and child survived, but] ever since she was deliver'd, in the Manner recited, she hath suffer'd a *prolapsus uteri*, upon the least standing or walking.'

Thoughts on pathogenesis

As variable as this malformation's spectrum, so were the theories explaining its origin. The traditional view, blaming maternal imagination, was mentioned by Gottfried Herder as late as 1789 [15]: 'Nature seems to spare the female fetuses … The mother recounted that in the third month of pregnancy she was awakened by a fire alarm … she hurried to help extinguish the fire, but in the darkness and in the crowd bumped against a shaft, with severe and prolonged pain at her pubic region … Could it be that the violence the mother suffered caused a rupture of the embryo's pubic symphysis? … The shuttered

PART 5 Odd shape

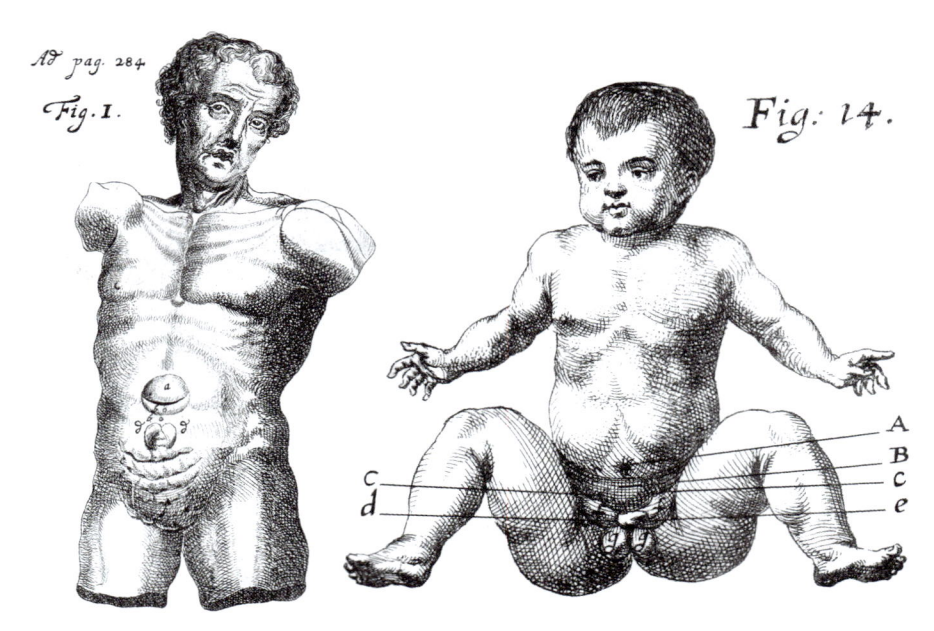

Fig. 5.8.1 Descriptions of cleft bladder from the 17th century. Left: male adult published by Ten Rhyne 1672 [9]; a, umbilical swelling with rudimentary penis; b, ureter orifices; g, rudimentary and split penis; f, skin eczema. Right: male newborn infant described by Gockel 1686 [11]. A, umbilicus; B, extroverted bladder; C, penis rudiments; F, ureter orifices; g, testicles.

and weakened parts could not subsequently develop properly … arrest of development … consent between body parts of the mother and those of the fetus.' Concerning the same case, the journal editor Johann Christian Stark commented [16]: 'Obviously a rupture of the integument occurred during development, whereby also the pubic bones were separated together with the peritoneum and the bladder. The latter then was inverted, so that the dorsal, normally concave, surface became convex.' Other mechanical theories included primary obstruction of the urethra with congested urine [2], short umbilical cord [17], or an atypically located yolk sac [18]. Several

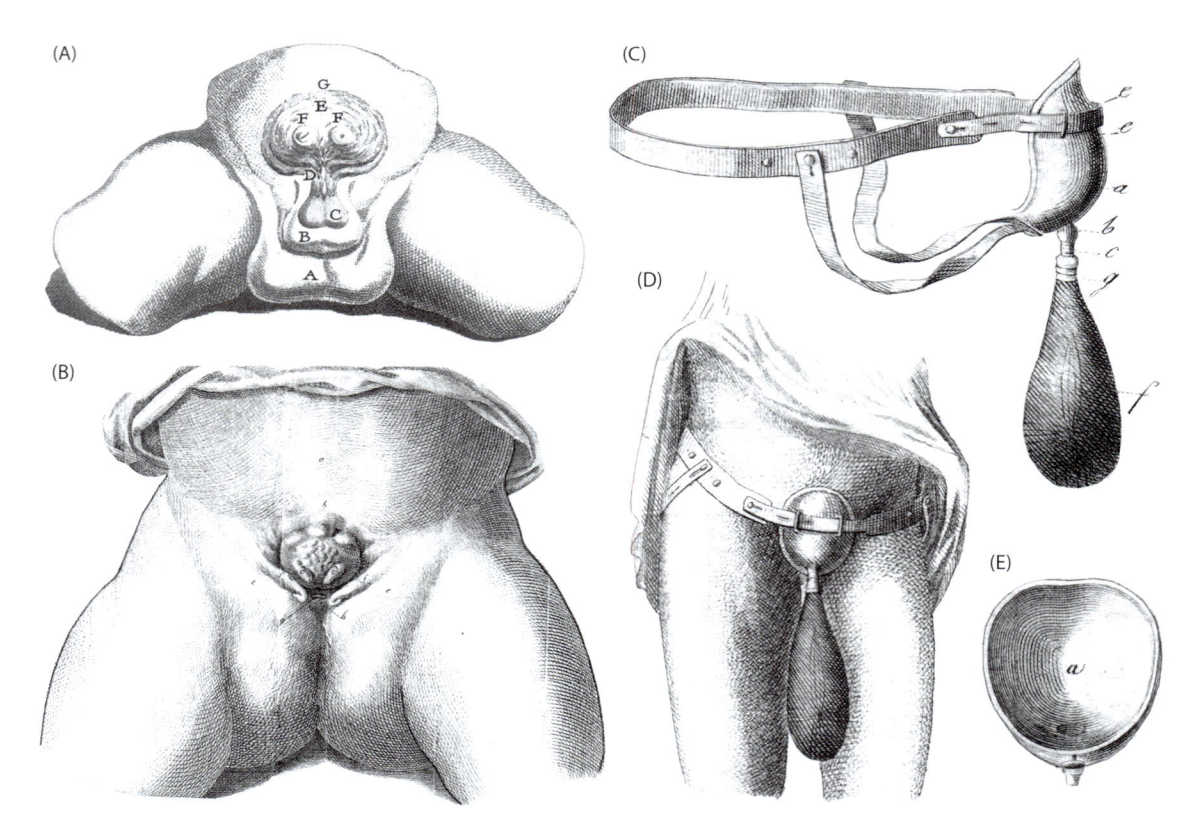

Fig. 5.8.2 Descriptions of cleft bladder from the 18th century: A, a 6-week-old male infant described by Castara in 1785 [13] (A, scrotum with testicles; B, transverse fold; F, ureter orifices; G, inflamed skin); B, female infant depicted by Herder in 1789 [15]; C–E, the same female as in B, with urine collecting device constructed by Stark in 1785 [16].

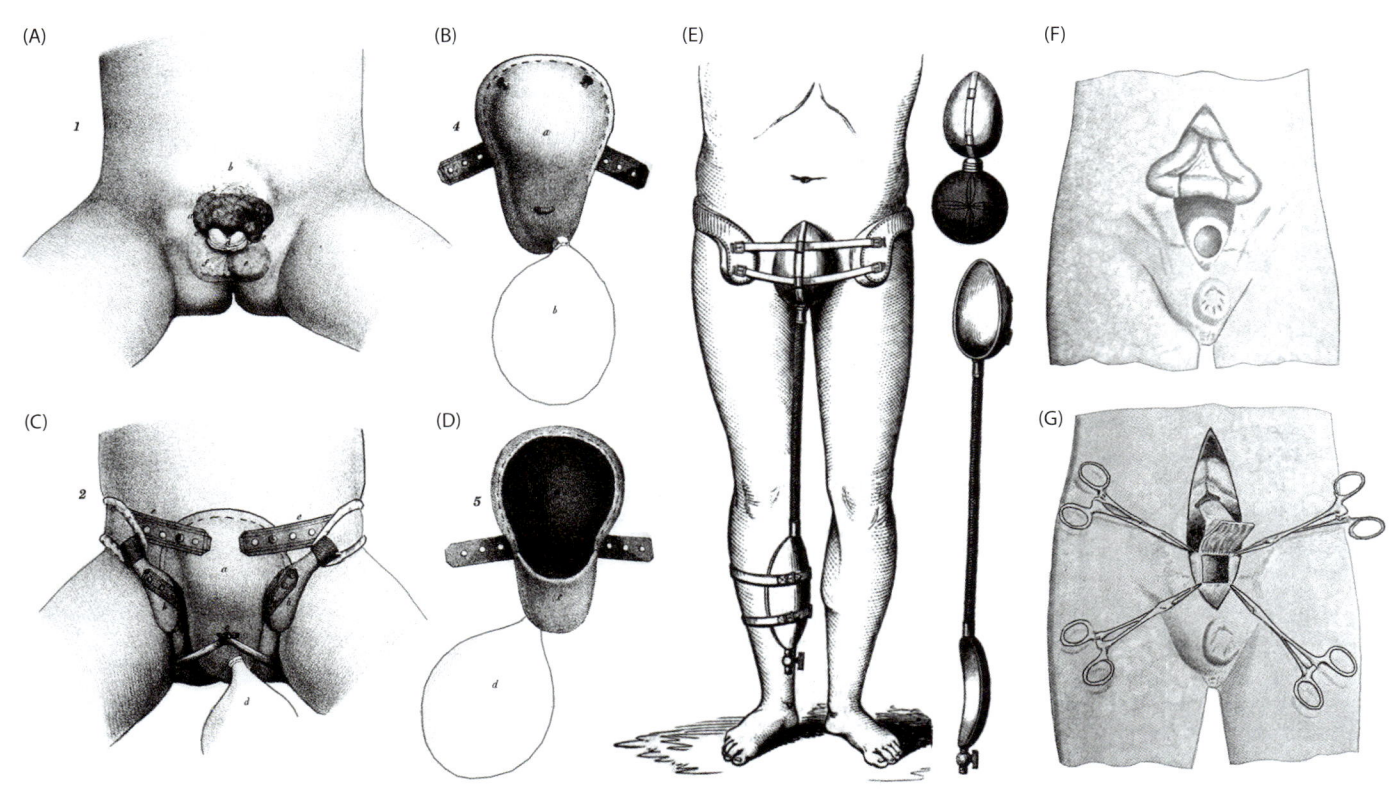

Fig. 5.8.3 Therapeutic approaches to cleft bladder in the 19th century: A–D, case description of Vrolik 1834, plate 29 [29], and collecting device from his instrument maker Smit. E, drainage system by McWhinnie 1850 [1]; F and G, operative formation of a bladder from an isolated gut loop described by Rutkowski in 1899 [36].

bursting theories were promulgated, with disruption of the allantois [3, 19], the bladder and ventral abdominal wall [20], or the cloacal membrane [18]. Other authors argued for arrested development [21] or disturbed migration of the infraumbilical mesenchyme [22]. Chromosomal aberrations have been reported, in particular duplications of 22q11.2, a region responsible for many anomalies [23]. The underlying pathogenesis of the bladder exstrophy–epispadias complex remained elusive. As the umbilical cord is always and the hindgut often involved, the lesion must occur before the 10th embryonal week, when part of the gut develops within the umbilical cord. Possibly, various pathogenetic ways or timing of the cloacal membrane's rupture may be responsible for different malformation grades within the exstrophy–epispadias spectrum [17].

Incontinence apparatuses

Dozens of urine collecting devices were constructed over the centuries to give relief to the tortured children, some of them depicted in Figs. 5.8.2 and 5.8.3. Around 1770, a centre of expertise evolved in Amsterdam [2, 24, 25], where receptacles were manufactured from sheet copper or pewter. Another centre for these devices was in Edinburgh in 1805 around Andrew Duncan [3, 26, 27]: 'This [tin] contrivance ... protects the bladder's sensitive surface from being irritated and inflamed by the clothes rubbing against it; and, by collecting the urine, it prevents the clothes from being spoiled, and becoming intolerably fetid. It is, in fact, an artificial bladder.'

Around 1740, natural rubber was imported from Meso-America, but it did not become medically useful until Charles Goodyear invented vulcanization in 1844 [28]. Rubber changed the world of infants by enabling teats to be sterilized (see Chapter 6.7). It changed the world for infants with cleft bladder even more, as elastic drainage systems became available. Fig. 5.8.2 C–E shows Stark's *Urinfänger* (urine catcher) constructed in 1798 [16]. In 1844, Willem Vrolik and his instrument maker Smit [29] 'imitated the device of Prof. Bonn' in constructing 'a copper receptacle placed against the pubic bones with three openings and a flask of elastic gum'. In 1850, Melville McWhinnie described the children's symptoms [1]: 'Besides the urinous smell which aggravates so much their wretched condition, there is frequently that peculiarity in the movements ... resulting from the soreness of the parts, and the consciousness that the tumor [bladder] will bleed from the slightest friction.' He described the device depicted in Fig. 5.8.3E: 'The urine here collected flowed through a funnel at its lower part into an India rubber bottle placed between the widely-separated thighs ... The urine passes down a vulcanized India rubber pipe into a metallic reservoir, adjusted to the inner side of the calf of the leg, and which can be evacuated at pleasure by means of a stop-cock.'

Corrective surgery

In France in 1839, Richard de Nancy proposed, in theory [30], 'a high grade extroversion can be operated by using the skin of the abdomen to close the anterior bladder wall … and it would be necessary to free the urethra-canal by a sonde to avoid accumulation of urine.' Paul Guersant, who had been surgeon at the Paris Hôpital des Enfants Malades for 20 years, described operations for many congenital malformations in 1864 [31], but gave up on cleft bladder: 'We confess that [this operation] never succeeded in our hands and that we do not dare to undertake it unless the parents urge us.' From 1852 to 1885 surgeons tried to transplant the ureters into the rectum [32], perineum [33], or to leave a catheter in the bladder [34], but without enduring success. Disappointed and honest, John Simon published a statement in 1852 not far from Guersant's opinion [32]: 'A train of thought will naturally arise in reviewing the nature of the malformation, the misery thereby entailed upon the patient, the persevering investigations of the surgeon, the attempt to remedy a distressing inconvenience … and the unfavourable termination … This novel operation testifies to the ardent wish of the surgeon to benefit his patient, but that the risks are perhaps disproportionate with the annoyance of a malformation which improved apparatuses may render bearable.'

An operation that enabled continence was developed in Prague by Karel Maydl in 1894 [35]. He excised the bladder triangle and transplanted it into an isolated loop of the sigmoid flexure (ureterosigmoidostomy). In 1899, Max Rutkowski in Krakau modified Maydl's operation, replacing the malformed bladder by an isolated ileum loop and closing the abdominal wall (Fig. 5.8.3F, G) [36]. Maydl's operation appeared to succeed technically, but half of the infants were dead by the age of 10 years [37]. Following many adaptations and modifications, the technique was widely used for around 100 years. But the concept ignored that evolution abandoned the cloaca in mammals and organized different outlets for urine and stool for good reasons: it took nearly a century to discover that, after decades, ureterosigmoidostomy was followed by colon cancer, usually at the site of the trigonum implantation [38, 39]. Bladder neck reconstruction was developed in 1942 to achieve continence [40] and from 1977 complete primary repair without urinary diversion became possible [41]. Today, diversion into the gut has been largely replaced by correcting operations in two or three steps, beginning with closure of the bony pelvis, the bladder, and anterior abdominal wall, followed later by epispadias repair and penis remodelling [42]. But even with bladder neck reconstruction, sustained continence could be achieved in only half of the children and chronic infection with urease-producing bacteria led to stone formation in every fourth child [43], although results were somewhat better in high-volume centres [44]. Despite the grim prognosis, no multicentre or randomized controlled trials have been done, and evidence for the best intervention is weak.

Conclusion

Thoughts on this malformation's origin evolved in the usual sequence: maternal imagination in the 17th, mechanical lesion in the 18th, developmental arrest in the 19th, and genetic misdirection in the 20th century. Urine collecting devices followed the use of rubber. The slow progress in surgical correction sheds light on the systemic problems of small-volume hospitals and the absence of regional or national study centres. Instead of multicentre protocols and long-term follow-up, hundreds of single-centre publications have recommended countless operations and techniques barely comparable with each other, without control groups. Cleft bladder is rare—and it will become even rarer due to prenatal diagnostics and abortion of malformed fetuses. Its long-term prognosis is all but satisfactory.

REFERENCES

1. McWhinnie AM: Account of the history and dissection of a case of malformation of the urinary bladder. Lond Med Gaz 1850;**45**:360–7.
2. Bonn A: Über eine seltene und widernatürliche Beschaffenheit der Harnblase und Geburtstheile eines zwölfjährigen Knabens. Strasburg und Kehl: [NN], 1782.
3. Duncan A: An attempt towards a systematic account of the appearances connected with that malconformation of the urinary organs, etc. Edinb Med Surg J 1805;**1**:43–60, 132–42.
4. Weidmann F: De nativo vesicae urinariae prolapsu. Gottingae: Dieterich, 1833.
5. Schmitt P: Ueber die Harnblasenspalte nebst Beschreibung und Abbildung. Würzburg: Zürn, 1836.
6. Martin E: Histoire des monstres (1st ed. 1880). Grenoble: Millon, 2002.
7. Titus Livius: History of Rome. Book 27: Scipio in Spain. London: Dent, 1905: p. 27.37, 6–7.
8. Schenck von Grafenberg J: Observationes medicarum rararum, novarum, admirabilium, & monstrosarum (1st ed. 1596). Lugduni: Huguetan, 1644: p. 504, 628–52.
9. Ten Rhyne W: Meditationes in magni Hippocratis textum XXIV. De veteri Medicina. Lugnuni Batavorum: Schuylenburgh, 1672: p. 284.
10. Stalpart van der Wiel C: Observationum rariorum medic. centuriae posterioris pars prior (1st ed. 1687). Leidae: Kerkhem, 1727: p. 327–33.
11. Gockel CL: Vesica spongiosa extra abdomen posita cum defectu penis. Ephem Miscell Nat Cur 1686;**6**:84–5.
12. Tenon J: Mémoire sur quelques vices des voies urinaires. Mém Acad Roy Sci 1761;115–24, 3 tables.
13. Castara M: Description d'un vice singulier de conformation. Paris: Histoire de la Société Royale de Médecine, 1780–1981: Vol. **4**, p. 323; plate p.354.
14. Bonnet J: A letter to Claudius Amyand, concerning the preternatural structure of the pudenda in a woman. Phil Trans Lond 1724;**33**: 142–6.
15. Herder G: Beschreibung eines angebohrnen Vorfalls einer umgestülpten Urinblase bei einem Mädchen. Neues Archiv für die Geburtshilfe, Frauenzimmer- und Kinderkrankheiten 1798;**1**:21–48.
16. Stark JC: Ein Urinfänger oder Halter für das Kind in den vorhergehenden Fall. Neues Archiv für die Geburtshilfe, Frauenzimmer- und Kinderkrankheiten 1798;**1**:49–57, 190–2.
17. Johnston TB: Extroversion of the bladder, complicated by the presence of intestinal openings on the surface of the extroverted area. J Anat Physiol 1913;**48**:89–106.
18. Patten BM, Barry A: The genesis of exstrophy of the bladder and epispadias. Am J Anat 1952;**90**:35–57.
19. Ahlfeld F: Die Entstehung des Nabelschnurbruches und der Blasenspalte. Arch Gynäk 1877;**11**:85–109.
20. Wood J: Fission and extroversion of the bladder and epispadias. Lancet 1869;**1**:259–60.

21. Meckel JF: Handbuch der pathologischen Anatomie. Leipzig: Reclam, 1812: Vol. **1**, p. 698–743.
22. Wyburn GM: The development of the infra-umbilical portion of the abdominal wall. J Anat 1937;**71**:201–31.
23. Beaman GM, Woolf AS, Cervellione RM, et al.: 22q11.2 duplications in a UK cohort with bladder exstrophy-epispadias complex. Am J Med Genet 2019;**179A**:404–9.
24. Veltkamp J: Beschryving der tegennatuurlijke teeldeelen van een manspersoon, en eenes werktuigs dienende etc. Zwolle: Verhand. der Hollandsche Maatsch. der Wetensch. 1770: Vol. **4**, p. 135.
25. Stolte JH: Beschryving der wanschapene Teeldeelen en Waterwegen van een Man, en eenes Werktuigs dienende om de Pis op te vangen. Zwolle: Hoffman, 1770: p. 29.
26. Coates WH: Case of a remarkable conformation of the urinary and genital organs in female child. Edinb Med Surg J 1805;**1**:39–43.
27. Cooper A: Case of malconformation of the urinary and genital organs in a female. Edinb Med Surg J 1805;**1**:129–32.
28. Goodyear C: Improvement in India-Rubber Fabrics. United States Patent Office 1844;Pat.-Nr. 3633.
29. Vrolik W: Tabulae ad illustrandam embryogenesin hominis et mammalium. Amsterdam: Londonck, 1844–1849: plates 29, 76, 77.
30. Richard (de Nancy) CJF: Traité pratique des maladies des enfants. Paris, Lyon, Montpellier: Baillière, 1839: p. 69.
31. Guersant MP: Notice sur la chirurgie des enfants. Paris: Asselin, 1864–1867: p. 252.
32. Simon J: Ectropia vesicae (absence of the anterior walls of the bladder and pubic abdominal parietes). Lancet 1852;**60**:568–70.
33. Holmes T: On congenital extroversion of the bladder; and on a method of alleviating some of its effects by a plastic operation. Lancet 1863;**81**:714–5.
34. Wyman HC: Operation for congenital extroversion of the bladder of an infant five days old. Med Rec 1885;**28**:646.
35. Maydl K: Über die Radikaltherapie der Blasenektopie. Wien Med Wochenschr 1894;**44**:1113–5, 1169–72, 1209–10, 1256–8, 1297–301.
36. Rutkowski M: Zur Methode der Harnblasenplastik. Zentralbl Chir 1899;**26**:473–8.
37. Mayo CH, Hendricks WA: Exstrophy of the bladder. Surg Gynecol Obstet 1926;**43**:129–34.
38. Husmann DA, Spence HM: Current status of tumor of the bowel following ureterosigmoideostomy. J Urol 1990;**144**:607–10.
39. Strachan JR, Woodhouse CRJ: Malignancy following ureterosigmoidostomy in patients with exstrophy. Br J Surg 1991;**78**:1216–8.
40. Young HH: Exstrophy of the bladder: the first case in which a normal bladder and urinary control have been obtained by plastic operation. Surg Gynecol Obstet 1942;**74**:729–37.
41. Jeffs RD: Functional closure of bladder exstrophy. Birth Defects Orig Artic Ser 1977;**13**:171–3.
42. Mitchell ME: Bladder exstrophy repair: complete primary repair of exstrophy. Urology 2005;**65**:5–8.
43. Mouriquand PD, Bubanj T, Feyaerts A, et al.: Long-term results of bladder neck reconstruction in children with classical bladder exstrophy. Br J Urol Int 2003;**92**:997–1002.
44. Woodhouse CRJ, North AC, Gearhart JP: Standing the test of time: long-term outcome of reconstruction of the exstrophy bladder. World J Urol 2006;**24**:244–9.

PART 6
Breast is best

6.1 Bad milk: medical doctrines that impeded breastfeeding *213*

6.2 Regulated wet nursing: managed care or organized crime? *221*

6.3 Guttus, tiralatte, and téterelle: breast pumps *227*

6.4 Pap, gruel, and panada: early approaches to artificial feeding *233*

6.5 Milk demystified by chemistry *241*

6.6 From swill milk to certified milk: progress in cow's milk quality *247*

6.7 Technical inventions that enabled artificial infant feeding *253*

6.8 Selling safety: commercial production of infant formula *259*

6.9 Feeding the feeble: steps towards nourishing preterm infants *265*

6.10 Much ado about nothing: controversies on tongue-tie *273*

6.11 Lethal lullabies: opium use in infants *279*

INTRODUCTION

Part 6 highlights infant nutrition. Deeply rooted prejudices against colostrum and the ban of sexual intercourse impeded breastfeeding. Commercial wet nursing was a dangerous and expensive alternative and relied on the exploitation of poor, unmarried mothers. Homemade substitutes were even more dangerous, especially in summer, due to bacterial contamination and poor milk quality. Women never had a real choice between breast and bottle. The 19th century de-emotionalized milk. With chemical analysis, evaporation, pasteurization, and cooling, safe but expensive artificial formula became available. The female breast became sexualized in the 20th century which threatened its nourishing function and caused a decline in breastfeeding. Breast pumps were used since antiquity for various reasons. Enteral nutrition of preterms became possible with gavage, pipettes, fortifiers, and probiotics. For millennia, infants were intoxicated with opium for excessive crying, suspected pain, teething, and diarrhoea.

6.1 Bad milk
Medical doctrines that impeded breastfeeding

Introduction: breastfeeding and survival

Even though philosophical and medical authorities explicitly promoted breastfeeding, a large proportion of infants were not breastfed by their mother and had diminished chances to survive. This was even more true longer ago [1], especially in summer, when bacterial growth was rapid in unrefrigerated milk. In Paris in 1899, Budin reported an infant mortality of 4.9% in breastfed and of 45.8% in bottlefed infants [2]. Compared to October through June, summer mortality in Berlin was 2.2 times higher in breastfed and 5.7 times higher in bottlefed infants in 1901 [3]. As late as 1977, in the absence of toilets and piped water, the risk to die postnatally was 5.2 times higher when Malaysian infants were bottlefed than when breastfed [4]. Recommendations were given as general, ritual endorsement with little impact. A remarkable degree of ambivalence is revealed by the host of qualifying phrases and conditions: 'If the mother's health permits ...', 'If she has enough milk ...', 'If her husband permits ...', and so on. Breastfeeding was never a matter of morals or fashion, as alluded to in medical texts, but social and economic pressure forced mothers to abandon the natural means of infant feeding. In addition, false medical doctrines had erected obstacles practically insurmountable by most women. The following chapter searches for explanations.

Classic theory of lactation

Being ignorant of hormones and blood circulation, Greek scholars imagined a physical connection to transfer *concocted* menstrual blood to the breasts. The raw material for milk originated in the uterus. Hippocratic writers stated (5th century B.C.E.) [5]: 'Milk is akin to the menses when the eighth month is gone and the nutriment passes over [to the breasts].' Also Aristotle (384–322 B.C.E.) equalled milk with retained menstrua [6]: 'In [thirty] days after conception the discharge [catamenia] no longer takes its usual course, but is turned towards the mammae, in which the milk begins to make its appearance.' Galen (129–210 C.E.) wrote [7] 'While in the uterus, we are wont to be nourished by blood, and the source of milk is from blood undergoing a slight change in the breasts' and believed a vessel existed to connect the uterus to the breasts [8]: 'It was my special aim to tell the usefulness of the close relation between the breasts and uteri ... Only to the testes [ovaries] and breasts did [nature] bring [blood] not from vessels nearby, but from those at a distance, not to be forgetful of her first aim, by Zeus, but choosing a better one; for both milk and semen are generated from perfectly concocted blood. It is the length of time which the blood spends in the vessel conducting it that permits the perfect concoction of these, and of necessity blood spends more time in longer vessels and the longer vessels are always those that come from a distance.' Galen's teachings were transmitted into medieval medicine by Avicenna (11th century C.E.) [9]: 'During pregnancy, the blood which is otherwise discharged from the female at the time of menstruation becomes nutriment [for the embryo].'

In the 13th century, the Franciscan scholar Bartholomäus Anglicus (1190–1250) wrote [10]: 'For aftir the burthe of a childe yif blood is not iwastid with fedinge, it cometh by a kynde wey into the pappis [breasts] and waxith whit by vertu of ham and taketh the qualite of melk ... The pappes ben isette to the brest to be near to the herte and turne into the kynde of melk. For blood cometh by an *holough veyne* to the hearte and thanne to the brest.' The widely distributed *Women's Secrets*, ascribed to Albertus magnus (1192–1260) [11] but compiled in the 14th century, specified: 'The first thing that develops is a certain vein or nerve which perforates the womb and proceeds from the womb up to the breasts. When the fetus is in the uterus of the mother her breasts are hardened, because the womb closes and the menstrual substance flows to the breast.'

Pre-Vesalian anatomy persisted

Mondino dei Luzzi, pathologist in Bologna, dissected two female corpses in 1315, and described 'from the side of the uterus originate two vessels. One penetrates the abdominal wall [diaphragm?] and ascends, the other ascends less hidden and close to the skin, until it

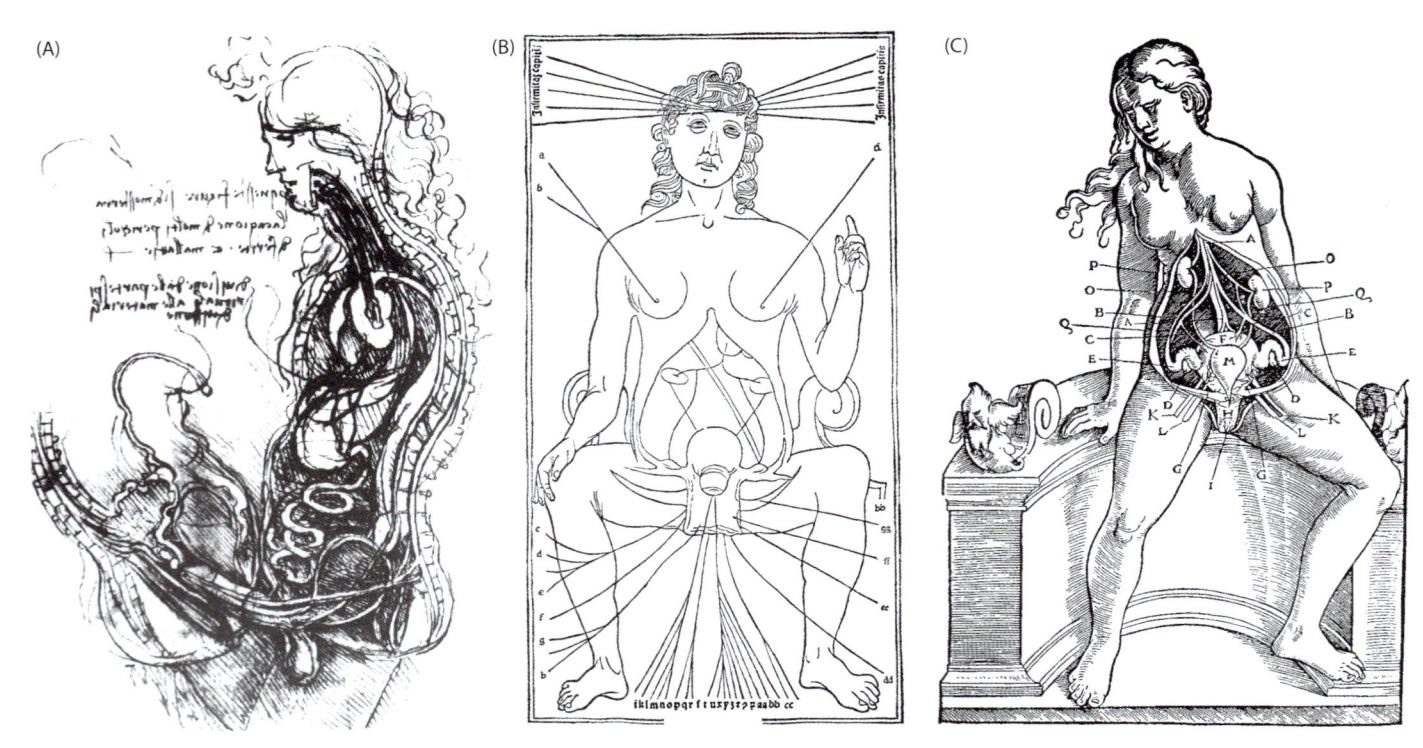

Fig. 6.1.1 Presumed vascular connections between uterus and breast as depicted by pre-Vesalian anatomists: A, *vasa menstrualia* of Leonardo da Vinci's *Anatomic Plates* ca. 1489 [13]; B, *vena lacteae* (ff) of Johannes de Ketham's *Fasciculus Medicinae* 1495 [14]; C, *venae seminales candidae* (B,B) of Walter Ryff's *Humani Corporis Descriptio* 1541, woodcut by Hans Baldung Grien [16].

reaches the breasts' [12]. Leonardo da Vinci, in his anatomical drawings, described 'two creatures cut through the middle' [13] and explained: 'We shall make 3 figures of the female to show the womb and menstrual veins which go to the breasts [Fig. 6.1.1A] … I display to men the origin of their second-first or perhaps second cause of existence.'

From Galen came the belief that the sperm is derived from the testes, the 'first cause', and from Hippocrates by way of Avicenna the idea that the soul, the 'second cause', is infused from the spinal cord. Therefore, Fig. 6.1.1A shows two tubes in the penis. When printing disseminated anatomical knowledge, the *vasa menstrualia* assumed different shapes, were confused with the ductus thoracicus or with epigastric vessels, and sometimes became a product of sheer fantasy. Ascribed to Johannes Ketham [14], the *Fasciculus Medicinae* depicted in 1491 (Fig. 6.1.1B): 'The female breasts are large in order to reduce the heat received from the heart … vessels ascend from the uterus to the breasts.' The field surgeon Hans von Gersdorf stated in 1528 [15]: 'Between [uterus] and the breasts are the milk-vessels and the menstrual vessels.' Walter Ryff's anatomy of 1541 depicted and named the *venae seminales candidae* (Fig. 6.1.1C) [16]. Padovan anatomist Andreas Vesalius dissected many human bodies and depicted the intra-abdominal vessels meticulously—his *Fabrica* (1st ed. 1543) did not mention any connection between uterus and breast [17]. However, Aristotle's and Galen's doctrine of lactation had made its way into the paediatric texts and remained highly influential well into the 19th century. Leuven anatomist Philipp Verheyen denied a vascular and proposed a nerve connection in 1726 [18]. Leiden professor Herman Boerhaave, usually not afraid to attack traditional doctrines, described a 'miraculous vascular connection' [19], whereas his pupil Albrecht von Haller referred to Vesalius, who could not find these vessels [20]: 'Moreover, there is a certain nervous sympathy between the breasts and the uterus.'

The condemnation of mothers who did not breastfeed started after the Reformation [21]. However, breastfeeding remained an exception among the wealthy. Defining the class *mammalia*, Linnaeus in 1758 abandoned Aristotle's classification *quadrupedia* [22]. In Germany, *Rabenmutter* became the favourite stereotype, unjustly attributed to the raven by Konrad von Megenberg in 1349: 'The ravens throw quite a few kids out of the nest when annoyed by the trouble to bring them enough food' [23]. In the US, the La Leche League referred to woman who chose not to breastfeed as *bad yuppie mothers* [24].

Modern theory of lactation

Astley Cooper characterized the anatomy and function of the mammary gland in his monumental *On the Anatomy of the Breast* in 1840 [25]: 'The secretion of milk proceeds best in a tranquil state of mind and with a cheerful temper; on the contrary, a fretful temper lessens the quantity of milk.' He correctly described the lobular structure of the gland (Fig. 6.1.2) and the letdown reflex. His description of dilated mammary ducts, however, was based on the injection technique of coloured wax: recent ultrasound studies revealed that there are no lactiferous sinuses [26].

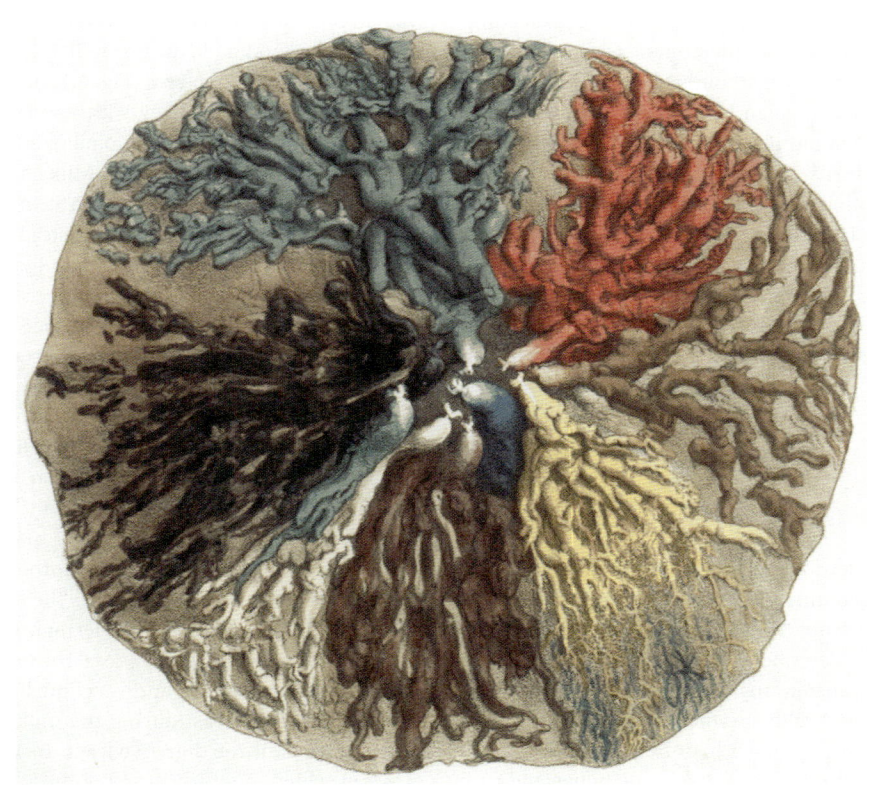

Fig. 6.1.2 Injection of the lactiferous ducts with coloured wax before dissection, from Cooper 1840 [25]. The preparation shows separated lobes of the lactating gland and the 'dilated' mammary sinuses.

Hormones entered the stage in 1905 with Ernest Starling. In 1928, Stricker and Grueter induced copious lactation in rabbits with extracts from the anterior pituitary [27], and in 1932 Riddle and colleagues isolated and named the proteohormone *prolactin* [28]. Its amino acid sequence was identified by Shome in 1977 [29]. Milk production is regulated by a supply and demand process in which the key factor is the infant's sucking. It causes prolactin to be released from the mother's anterior pituitary and oxytocin to be released from the posterior pituitary; the former triggers milk production in the mammary alveoli, the latter the milk ejection reflex. Any reduction of sucking frequency will reduce the amount of prolactin secreted and jeopardize breastfeeding success.

'Abstain completely from sexual relations'

Derived from the classical theory, scientists prohibited intercourse during lactation, usually with Galen's words [7]: 'I order all women who are nursing babies to abstain completely from sex relations. For menstruation is provoked by intercourse, and the milk no longer remains sweet. Moreover some women become pregnant, than which nothing could be worse for the suckling infant. For in this case the best of the blood goes to the foetus ... Meantime the blood of the pregnant naturally becomes less and of inferior quality, so that not only less, but inferior, milk collects in the breasts; so that if a nursing mother should become pregnant, I should strongly advise that another nurse should be procured, thinking and considering that her milk would be better in taste, appearance, and odor.'

In Roman Egypt, sexual restrictions were an obligatory part of wet-nursing service contract papyri [30]: 'So long as she is duly paid she shall take proper care both of herself and of the child, not injuring her milk nor sleeping with a man nor becoming pregnant.' Soranus explained [31]: 'For coitus cools the affection toward [the] nursling by the diversion of sexual pleasure and moreover spoils and diminishes the milk.' Avicenna transmitted the doctrine [9]: 'The wet-nurse should not allow coition, for this disturbs the menstrual blood and diminishes the quantity of milk and alters its composition, as shown by change of odor. Moreover, she might become pregnant, in which case there would be a dual unpropitious influence.'

Practically all authors from the 15th to the 18th century reiterated the intercourse ban during lactation, with varying reasons: Augsburg city physician Bartholomäus Metlinger 1473: 'very harmful' [32]; Frankfurt city physician Eucharius Roesslin 1513: 'bad taste' [33]; Simon de Vallambert, physician to the Duke of Orléans 1565: 'bad smell' [34]; Verona physician Omnibonus Ferrarius 1577: 'odor deteriorates' [35]; Royal midwife Louise Bourgeois 1609 [36]: 'Above all, [lactating women] should beware of the loving mood: this happens often in good-looking women returning to their husbands, their milk is a real venom for the infants.' Zurich city physician Johann Muralt 1697: 'disgusting impression' [37]; and the widely distributed *Nurse's Guide* from London 1729 [38]: 'If a Nurse, by Frequent Entercourse with her Husband, should give her Foster-Child an ill-flavour'd Milk, destitute of its fattest and richest Part, the purest Blood, of which it ought to be made, having been spent on the Parts serving to Generation.'

In the Scandinavian countries, the notion that breastfeeding women should abstain from sexual intercourse was introduced as late as the 17th century [39]. In his famous book on childhood diseases [40], Uppsala Royal Physician Nils Rosén von Rosenstein adopted the prejudice: 'She should not indulge in love, because the child suffers and the milk turns unhealthy and salty. If a married nurse desires intercourse with her husband, she is no longer capable to be a wet-nurse.' As late as 1917, Pierre Garnier claimed that 'copulation makes the milk serous, tasteless, and yellowish' [41]. Galen's ban on intercourse isolated the mother, provided an alibi for paternal infidelity, and made the infant its own father's rival. To comply to the doctrine, the rich hired wet-nurses and the poor took refuge in artificial feeding.

'Delay feeding as colostrum is poisonous to the infant'

Soran's highly influential obstetrics text impeded breastfeeding more than any other author. He recommended the infant be fed by a nurse from day 3 and by its own mother from 20 days of age [31]. Delayed feeding persisted, as Metlinger described in 1473 [32]: 'In the first fourteen days it is better that another woman suckles the infant than its mother, because her milk is not healthy for the child. During this time the mother should let herself suck by a whelp or by an [adult]. If, however, she suckles her infant from the beginning, some honey and rose honey should be applied [into the infant's mouth] before breastfeeding so that the milk injures it less.' Midwife Jane Sharp recommended in 1671 to postpone breastfeeding until the lochia cease [42]: 'It is not good for a woman presently to suckle her child because those unclean purgations cannot make good milk, the first milk is naught.' In the Netherlands, as shown by Brueghel's pictures (Fig. 6.1.3), breastfeeding was associated with wealth and handfeeding with poverty [43]. Delayed feeding deprived the neonate of immunoglobulins and exposed the mother to the risk of engorgement and mastitis. 'Milk fever' was considered a natural phase of lactation. Cassel obstetrician Stein's text of 1774 recommended removing colostrum using a pump instead of young dogs [44]: 'Several times a day to draw the unclean milk [colostrum, named 'the beestings'] until it loses the creamy characteristic and appears nicely white and all in one color. This usually lasts for 5–7 days … during which the child flourishes better with a drinkable gruel than with the first unclean mother's milk.'

Few mothers could maintain lactation by pumping for several weeks, and delayed breastfeeding usually meant no breastfeeding. In 1750, William Cadogan, physician to the London Foundling Hospital, did away with the ban [45]: 'I am confident that there would be no Fever at all, were things managed rightly: It should be just after the Birth applied to the Mother's Breasts … The Mother's first milk is purgative, and cleanses the child from its long hoarded Excrement' (see Chapter 7.4). Herman Boerhaave also considered colostrum beneficial in 1759 [46]: 'The first milk after delivery is not thick, but watery, subtle, and very much different to that which accumulates in the breast during the milk fever. It purges the infant gently and cleans the digestive tract.' In 1788, Jean Baptiste Baumes of Montpellier mocked 'the prejudice, tyrant of all states, which claims that the first milk rising to the breast after birth is murderous for the nursling' [47]. Prejudices against colostrum feeding persist in many regions up to the present day, including Guinea-Bissau [48],

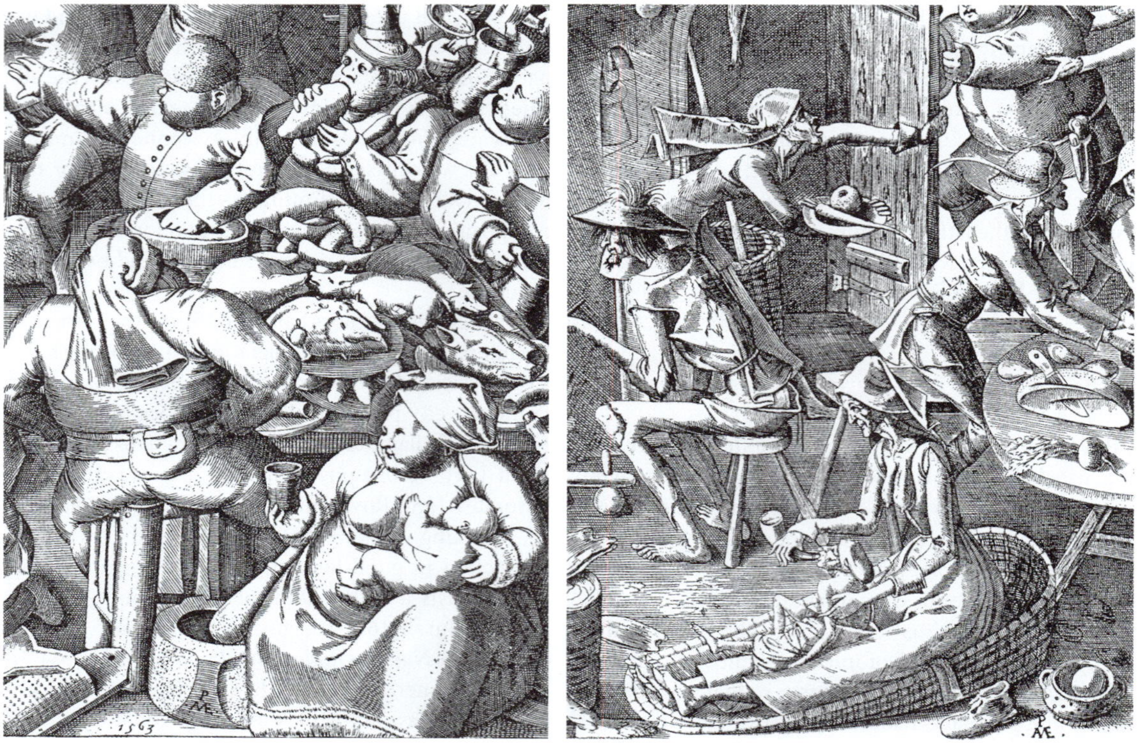

Fig. 6.1.3 The rich kitchen (left, detail) was associated with breastfeeding, the poor kitchen (right, detail) with handfeeding using a horn. Copper engravings by Pieter Brueghel the Elder, 1562 [43].

India, Pakistan, and several African states [21, 49]. A third of the mothers in modern Turkey still believe that colostrum should not be given to the newborn and that at least three calls to prayer should have occurred before the first postpartum breastfeeding [50].

'Bad milk causes neonatal convulsions'

The *Nurse's Guide* of 1729 [38] listed 'several disorders that happen to young Children, from their nurse's bad milk … he will be subject to the Epilepsy, or Falling-Sickness, which is a periodical Convulsion of the whole Body'. Schütte's midwives' book of 1773 advised against breastfeeding if 'the mother is sickly, afflicted with female or nervous disorders, or if irascible, impatient, or melancholic' [51]. All arguments against breastfeeding convene in Morton's monograph of 1831 [52]: 'Violent affections of the mind will cause the milk to become thin and yellowish, and to acquire noxious properties: … milk is liable to deterioration from another cause, namely, the recurrence of the usual periodical appearance—for should this take place in a nurse, it is agreed that her milk is liable to produce disorders in the child who imbibes it; … Diseases which frequently arise in children from lactation, especially when protracted: … the nurse's milk becoming either simply impoverished, or of a positively injurious quality … rickets, convulsions, epilepsy—and lastly meningitis, which gives rise to the effusion of serum, constituting the well known and very fatal disease termed Hydrocephalus.'

As late as 1879, London obstetrician Charles Routh, in a book meant to propagate breastfeeding [1], listed among the 'circumstances [when] a mother should not suckle her infant … Evidence that the mothers milk does not agree with the child: It may produce diarrhea, insomnia, it may be convulsions. This is more especially the case in very impressionable women'. And in 1896, Boston paediatrician Thomas Morgan Rotch [53] taught: 'The mothers who have uncontrollable temperaments, who are unhappy, who are unwilling to nurse their infants, who are hurried in the details of their life, are unfit to act as the source of food-supply for their infants. Even if their milk happens to be sufficient in quantity, it will be so changeable in quality as to be a source of discomfort and even danger for their offspring.'

'Frequent and prolonged feeding spoils the child'

Avicenna [9] recommended 'at first, the infant is allowed the breast three times only in the day', which was repeated by Rößlin in 1513 [33], Guillemeau in 1643 [54] and Muralt in 1697 [37]. Rotch [53] and Holt [55] advocated strongly regulated feeding. The 20th century added more medical advice which impeded breastfeeding: the scheduled feeding every 4 hours, addition of tea, water, or formula, and use of a pacifier led to decreased milk production and early cessation of breastfeeding. Berlin paediatrician Adalbert Czerny published *The Physician, The Child's Educator* in 1908 [56]: 'The first important educational measure is familiarizing with time regulation. For this aim, nutrition is well-suited … Scheduled feeding intervals are not only an important regulation for nutrition, but indeed the first to control the desires'. Most physicians and nurses received minimal training in nutrition, and little high-quality, prospective research was performed on this topic. False medical advice softened when professional lactation consulting became available. The La Leche League, founded in Chicago in 1957 [24], paved the way for the Babyfriendly Hospital Initiative of the World Health Organization. Paediatricians did not support this movement, and their knowledge about breastfeeding continued to be remarkably limited [57].

'Breastfeeding destroys maternal health and beauty'

It was again Soran who had erected another obstacle [31]: 'But if anything prevents it one must choose the best wet nurse, lest the mother grow prematurely old, having spent herself through the daily suckling. For just as [the earth] is exhausted by producing crops after sowing and therefore becomes barren of more, the same happens with the woman who nurses the infant; she either grows prematurely old having fed one child, or the expenditure for the nourishment of the offspring necessarily makes her own body quite emaciated. Consequently, the mother will fare better with a view to her own recovery and to further childbearing, if she is relieved of having her breasts distended too. For as vegetables are sown by gardeners into one soil to sprout and are transplanted into different soil for quick development, in the same way the newborn, too, is apt to become more vigorous if borne by one woman but fed by another.'

William Cadogan contradicted in 1750 [45]: 'Were it rightly managed, there would be much Pleasure in it, to every Woman that can prevail upon herself to give up a little of the Beauty of her Breast to feed her offspring; though this is a mistaken Notion, for the Breasts are not spoiled by giving suck but by growing fat.' Morton insisted in 1831 [52]: 'Disorders frequently produced in Women by that process: … lose their good looks, become gradually weaker, and as their strength declines, their milk is simultaneously lessened in quantity, and altered in its other properties … pain in the head … perspirations by night … pulmonary consumption.'

As late as 1957, paediatrician Benjamin Spock conceded a 'disadvantage' that breastfeeding alters the breasts in an undesirable way as sagging or dropping, and renders them 'unattractive' [58]. However, breastfeeding women tend to be slim, and sagging is not a consequence of breastfeeding, but of excessive weight gain during pregnancy [59]. In 1991, 55% of underprivileged Chicago women had negative attitudes toward breastfeeding [60], and in 1999, a large proportion of low-income men in Britain felt *uneasy* with breastfeeding [61].

Conclusion

From antiquity, medical doctrines impeded rather than promoted breastfeeding. They separated the infant from its mother and hampered lactation, whereas the authors ritually declared that the 'breast is best'. That medical authors were predominantly men may play a role in this misinformation and indoctrination, as breastfeeding is an exclusively female activity. The prerogative of interpretation was a matter of power, as pointed out in 1950 by Frank Richardson

[62]: 'Most formidable of all obstacles to breast feeding is the indifference, and at times the actual opposition, of a large segment of the medical profession.' The 20th century brought an erotization of the female breast to a degree that its nourishing function was seriously threatened by its sexual role. This process met little opposition from the medical profession. Maternal risk factors for early cessation of breast feeding include age under 25 years, smoking, full-time employment, and lower educational attainment [63]. Long-standing and deeply rooted prejudices extending into the motives of modern societies, including those of health professionals, may contribute to a hostile environment for breastfeeding.

REFERENCES

1. Routh CHF: Infant feeding and its influence on life. 3. ed. New York: Wood, 1879: p. 31–3, 50, 104, 150.
2. Budin P: Le Nourrisson. Paris: Doin, 1900: p. 23, 41, 99, 213.
3. Rietschel H: Die Sommersterblichkeit der Säuglinge. Erg Inn Med Kinderheilk 1910;**6**:369–490.
4. Habicht JP, DaVanzo J, Butz WP: Mother's milk and sewage: their interactive effects on infant mortality. Pediatrics 1988;**81**:456–61.
5. Littré E: Oevres complètes d'Hippocrate. 2e livre des epidemies. Amsterdam: Hakkert, 1962: Vol. **5**, p. 119.
6. Aristotle: History of animals. In ten books. London: Bell, 1883: p. 72, 192.
7. Green RM: A translation of Galen's Hygiene (de sanitate tuenda). Springfield, IL: Thomas, 1951: p. 24–9.
8. Galen: On the usefulness of the parts of the body. Ithaca, NY: Cornell University Press, 1968: Vol. **2**, p. 639, 712.
9. Gruner OC: A treatise on the canon of medicine of Avicenna, incorporating a translation of the first book. London: Luzac & Co., 1930: §126, §696–709.
10. Anglicus B: De Proprietatibus Rerum, 1601. Translated by: John Trevisa: On the properties of things. A critical text. Oxford: Clarendon Press, 1975: Lib. 5, p. 233–4.
11. Lemay HR: Women's secrets: A translation of Pseudo-Albertus Magnus's De secretis Mulierum with Commentaries. New York: State University of New York Press, 1992: p. 109.
12. Mondino dei Luzzi: Anatomia Mundini. Lugduni: Blanchard, 1531: Fol. 17.
13. Vangensten OCL, Fonahn AM, Hopstock H: Quaderni d'anatomia I–IV. Fogli della Royal Library of Windsor. Leonardo da Vinci. Christiania: J. Dybwad, 1914: Vol. **3**, Fol. 7r.
14. Ketham J: Fasciculus medicinae. Venetiis: per Johannem et Gregorium de Gregoriis, 1495.
15. Gersdorff Hv: Feldtbuch der Wundartzney, newlich getruckt vnd gebessert. Strassburg: Schott, 1528: p. Fol. 14.
16. Ryff W: Omnium humani corporis partium descriptio, seu vocant Anatomia. Strassbourg: Pistor, 1541.
17. Leveling HP: Anatomische Erklärung der Original-Figuren von Andreas Vesal. Ingolstadt: Industriecomptoir, 1800.
18. Verheyen P: Corporis humani anatomiae liber secundus. Accedit descriptio anatomica partium foetui et recenter nato propriarum. 2. ed. Bruxellis: Serstevens, 1726: p. 42.
19. Boerhaave H: Praelectiones academicae in proprias institutiones rei medicae. Venetiis: apud Simonem Occhi, 1745: Vol. **5**, p. 38, §666.
20. Haller A: Elementa physiologiae corporis humani. 2. ed. Lausannae: Sumptibus Societatis Typographicae, 1778: Vol. **7**, p. 20–4.
21. Fildes V: Breasts, bottles, and babies. Edinburgh: Edinburgh University Press, 1986: p. 98–121, 307.
22. Linnaeus C: Systema naturae per regna triae naturae. 10. ed. Holmiae: Laurentii Salvii, 1758: Vol. **1**, Animalia.
23. Megenberg Kv: Das Buch der Natur [1349]. Edited by: Franz Pfeiffer. Stuttgart: Aue, 1861: p. 176.
24. Blum LM: At the breast: ideologies of breastfeeding. Boston, MA: Beacon, 1999: p. 63.
25. Cooper AP: On the anatomy of the breast. London: Longman & Co, 1840: Vol. **2**, p. 129, plate VI.
26. Ramsay DT, Kent JC, Hartmann RA, Hartmann PE: Anatomy of the lactating human breast redefined with ultrasound imaging. J Anat 2005;**206**:525–34.
27. Stricker P, Gruter F: Action du lobe antérieur de l'hypophyse sur la montée laiteuse. Compt Rend Soc Biol 1928;**99**:1978–80.
28. Riddle O, Bates RW, Dykshorn SW: A new hormone of the anterior pituitary. Proc Soc Exp Biol 1932;**29**:1211–2.
29. Shome B, Parlow AF: Human pituitary prolactin (hPRL). J Clin Endocrinol Metab 1977;**45**:1112–5.
30. Bradley KR: Sexual regulations in wet-nursing contracts from Roman Egypt. Klio 1980;**62**:321–5.
31. Temkin O: Soranus' Gynecology. Baltimore, MD: The Johns Hopkins Press, 1956: p. 79–117.
32. Metlinger B: Ein vast nützlich Regiment der jungen Kinder. Augsburg: Zainer, 1473: p. 9–17, Fol. 17.
33. Rößlin E: Der Swangern Frauwen und hebammen Rosegarten. Facsimile Antiqua Verlag Wutöschingen 1993. Straßburg: Flach, 1513: p. 79.
34. Vallambert Sd: Cinq livres de la manière de nourrir et gouverner les enfants dès leur naissance. Reprint Droz, Geneve 2005. Poitiers: Manefz et Bouchetz, 1565: p. 89–101, 112, 207–8.
35. Ferrarius O: De arte medica infantium. Brescia: Marchetti, 1577: p. 11, 31.
36. Bourgeois L: Observations Diverses sur la Sterilité, Perte de Fruits, Foécondité, Accouchments, et Maladies de Femmes, et Enfants Nouveaux-naiz. Paris: Dehoury, 1609: p. 98–100, 155.
37. Muralt J: Kinder- und Hebammen-Büchlein. Basel: König, 1697: p. 206, 212.
38. Eminent Physician: The nurse's guide. London: Brotherton and Gilliver, 1729: p. 28–39.
39. Benedictow OJ: On the origin and spread of the notion that breastfeeding women should abstain from sexual intercourse. Scand J Hist 1992;**17**:65–76.
40. Rosenstein NRv: Anweisung zur Kenntnis und Chur der Kinderkrankheiten (1st Swedish ed. 1764). 4. ed. Göttingen: Dieterich, 1781: p. 1–29.
41. Garnier P: Le mariage, dans ses devoirs, ses rapports, et ses effets conjugaux. Paris: Garnier, 1917.
42. Sharp J: The midwives book. London: Miller, 1671: p. 351–71.
43. Bastelaer Rv: Les estampes de Pieter Bruegel l'Ancien. La cuisine maigre. La cuisine grasse. Bruxelles: van Oest & Co, 1908: p. 154, 159.
44. Stein GW: Beschreibung einer Brust- oder Milchpumpe. Kleine Werke zur praktischen Geburtshülfe. Marburg: Academische Buchhandlung, 1774: p. 49, 64–8.
45. Cadogan W: An essay upon nursing and the management of children. London: Roberts, 1750: p. 15, 18–27, 34.
46. Boerhaave H: Traité des maladies des enfans. Avignon: Saillant & Nyon, 1759: p. 38.
47. Baumes JBT: Mémoire sur l'ictère des nouveau-nés. Nismes: Castor Belle, 1788: p. 16.

48. Gunnlaugsson G, Einarsdottir J: Colostrum and ideas about bad milk. Soc Sci Med 1993;**36**:283–8.
49. Rangroo V: The evolution of paediatrics from archaeological times to the mid-nineteenth century. Acta Paediatr 2008;**97**:677–83.
50. Hizel S, Ceyhun G, Sanli C: Traditional beliefs as forgotten influencing factors on breast-feeding performance in Turkey. Saudi Med J 2006;**27**:511–8.
51. Schütte JH: Wohlunterwiesene Hebamme. 2. ed. Franckfurt am Mayn: Joh. G. Fleischer, 1773: p. 230–5.
52. Morton E: Remarks on the subject of lactation. London: Longman &Co, 1831: p. 3, 14, 24.
53. Rotch TM: Pediatrics. The hygienic and medical treatment of children. Edinburgh: Pentland, 1896: Vol. **I**, p. 159.
54. Guillemeau J: De la grossesse et accouchement des femmes. Paris: Jost, 1643: p. 551–87.
55. Holt LE: The diseases of infancy and childhood. New York: Appleton, 1898: p. 159, 184.
56. Czerny A: Der Arzt als Erzieher des Kindes. 11. ed. Wien: Deuticke, 1946: p. 25.
57. Schanler RJ, O'Connor KG, Lawrence RA: Pediatricians' practices and attitudes regarding breastfeeding promotion. Pediatrics 1999;**103**:e35.
58. Spock B: Dr. Spock's baby and child care. New York: Pocket Books, 1957.
59. Pisacane A, Continisio P: Breastfeeding and perceived changes in the appearance of the breasts. Acta Paediatr 2004;**93**:1346–8.
60. Dix DN: Why women decide not to breastfeed. Birth 1991;**18**:222–5.
61. Henderson L, McMillan B, Green JM, Renfrew MJ: Men and infant feeding. Birth 2011;**38**:61–70.
62. Richardson FH: Breast feeding comes of age. JAMA 1950;**142**:863–7.
63. Baxter J, Cooklin AR, Smith J: Which mothers wean their babies prematurely from full breastfeeding? Acta Paediatr 2009;**98**:1274–7.

6.2

Regulated wet nursing
Managed care or organized crime?

Introduction

Wet nursing was common in all cultures from prehistoric times; motives included: (1) to preserve the infant's life after maternal death, so frequent over centuries of pelvic constriction and puerperal sepsis; (2) to unburden the mother during illness or supposed weakness; (3) to exploit female slaves and restore their working ability after birth; (4) to maintain marital relations by bypassing the intercourse ban during lactation; and (5) to increase offspring by avoiding lactational amenorrhea. In the aristocracy, having an heir was a particular aim—understandable, given the high infant mortality rate.

In much of history the modern term *choice* was inappropriate to describe a mother's ability to breastfeed her infant. An ever-increasing demand for wet nurses, the variety of motives, the societal inequality between employer and wet nurse, the elevated infant mortality rate, and a combination of cultural, emotional, and economic pressures produced a need for rules. In many states the rights and duties of both the wet nurses and those who procured them were meticulously regulated.

Antique contracts

In Egypt, wet nursing was an organized profession: 'Pharaoh's daughter said unto her: Take this child away, and suckle it for me, and I will give [thee] thy wages' [Exodus 1:2]. In Babylonia, a wet nurse was paid about 3 shekels, and deceit was regulated in the Code of Hammurabi (ca. 1700 B.C.E.) [1]: 'If a man gives his child to a nurse and the child die in her hands, but the nurse unbeknown to the father and mother nurse another child, then they shall convict her of having nursed another child without the knowledge of the father and mother and her breasts shall be cut off.'

Greece—choosing a wet nurse

In the Homeric age, wet nurses were slaves [2]. In the 5th century B.C.E., Plato proposed a central nursery [3], where 'they will take mothers when their breasts are full, using every device so that none is aware of her own; and they will provide wet nurses if the mothers do not have enough milk, and supervise the mothers.' Aristotle believed ca. 450 B.C.E. [4] 'black women are better nurses than white women', and Soranus canonized the qualities to be fulfilled by a mercenary wet nurse [5]. The vote for brown hair, phlegmatic temper, and the nail milk test ('if a drop is made to fall on the finger nail or a leaf of sweet bay, it spreads gently and when rocked it retains the same form') illustrate how nonsense could persist in medicine for two millennia when concocted by an authority (Table 6.2.1).

In the 1st century C.E., Plutarch defavoured wet nursing [23]: 'But the good-will of foster-mothers and nursemaids is insincere and forced, since they love for pay … So mothers must endeavour, if possible, to nurse their children themselves; but if they are unable to do this, either because of bodily weakness (for such a thing can happen) or because they are in haste to bear more children, yet foster-mothers and nursemaids are not to be selected at random, but as good ones as possible must be chosen. And first of all, in character they must be Greek.'

Roman laws, Constantine's reform, and medieval Italy

Many wet nursing contracts endured from Roman Alexandria, one of which was translated by Schubart [24]: 'Theodote agrees to breastfeed the slavechild Tyche belonging to Marcus [Aemilius], which he entrusted to her, for the duration of 18 months, with her own clean and unspoiled milk … She has received 72 silver drachms from Marcus' own hand to cover the first nine months. Should anything human happen to the infant during these months, she will admit another infant and raise and suckle it for the duration of nine months without payment.' Before the delivery of a patrician, a slave was bought to act as a wet nurse [25]. The less rich hired one of the wet nurses who stayed around the *Columna lactaria* on the *forum olitorium*, the vegetable market, at least from the 1st century B.C.E. (Fig. 6.2.1) [26]. This was the same place where unwanted neonates

---

Reproduced with permission from Obladen, M. Regulated wet nursing: managed care or organized crime? *Neonatology*, 102(3):222–228. Copyright © 2012 S. Karger AG, Basel.

Table 6.2.1 Qualifications to be fulfilled by a hired wet nurse and to be examined by the recommending physician, as defined in some highly influential texts over 1800 years

Author	Publication date	Age (years), origin	Nurse's delivery	Health features	Mental features	Skin/hair colour	Body features	Breasts	Milk	Reference
Soranus	Ca. 150 C.E.	20–40 Greek	2–3 mo, 2–3 para	*, healthy	Sympathetic not angry	Good colour	Strong, of large frame	Medium size	White, no smell, #	[5]
Oribasius	Ca. 360 C.E.	25–35	As mother	No epilepsy or gastroenteritis	Prudent, pleasant	–	Broad shoulders	Medium size symmetrical	White, good smell, #	[6]
Avicenna	Ca. 1020	25–35	6–8 wks, term, male	*, no diarrhoea, no constipation	Phlegmatic, not stupid	Good colour Not pale	Strong neck	Firm nipples	White and sweet, #	[7]
B. Metlinger	1473	20–30	6–12 wks, full term	No disease	Not angry, not timid	Brown	Strong neck	Large and firm	White, sweet no smell, #	[8]
E. Rösslin	1513	–	>2 mo, best male	No diarrhoea	Quiet, not stupid	Good colour	Strong neck	Medium size	Not brown or red, #	[9]
S. Vallambert	1565	25–35	>6 wks, best male	Healthy	Prudent, gentle	–	Strong neck	Large and firm	White, sweet abundant, #	[10]
L. Bourgeois	1609	–	–	White teeth, no epilepsy or leprosy	Not choleric	Brunette, not red	Upright	Medium size	Abundant	[11]
J. Guillemeau	1643	25–35	1–2 mo	No disease in family	Prudent	Brunette, not red	Strong neck	Medium size	White, sweet no smell, #	[12]
J. Sharp	1671	18–40	Identical gender	No squinting, good teeth	Sanguine, prudent	Light brown	Medium stature	Well proportioned	Not too much	[13]
F. Mauriceau	1680	25–35	1–3 mo	No epilepsy, no venereal	Sanguine, friendly	Black/brown, not red	Medium stature	Large	White, sweet no smell, #	[14]
Nurse's Guide	1729	25–35	3–4 mo 2–3 para Term, male	No squinting, no ulcers white teeth	–	Brown, not red, no freckles	Medium stature	Large and firm	White, good smell, #	[15]
N. Rosenstein	1781	20–30	>6 wks	No infectious or unclean dis.	Quiet, friendly	–	Similar to mother	Well-shaped nipples	White-blue Sweet, #	[16]
A. Henke	1821	<30 Rural	<8 wks, 1 or 2 para	*, no venereal symptoms	Quiet, never violent	–	Strong	Not flat and not fat	No colour, no smell, #	[17]
C. West	1865	20–25	3–5 mo, multipara	*, no syphilis or phthisis	–	Brunette	Robust	Small but secreting	Spec. gravity 1032	[18]
L. E. Holt	1898	20–30	1–5 mo, primipara	*, no syphilis	Phlegmatic, good moral	No anaemia	–	Small but not flat	Abundant	[19]
H. Finkelstein	1921	–	>6 wks	*, no syphilis, tbc, or caries	–	–	–	Conical	Few colostrum Corpuscles	[20]
J. Hess	1923	18–35 Teutonic Slavic	>8 wks, multipara	*, no infection or skin disease	Phlegmatic, no insanity or epilepsy	Not black	–	Spherical	Enough volume	[21]
M. Pfaundler	1924	20–30 Slavic	>8 wks, pluripara	*, no lues/tbc in nurse's child	–	No anaemia	–	Medium size cylindrical	No colostrum corpuscles, #	[22]

*, health of the nurse's child should be considered; #, nail test of the milk, see text. mo, months; tbc, tuberculosis; wks, weeks.

could be officially abandoned. Analysing epitaph inscriptions from the city of Rome, Keith Bradley found that most wet nurses were slaves or ex-slaves, but many nurslings were also slaves: despite high infant mortality, it was more economical to breed *vernae* (house slaves) than to buy adults [27]. In addition to the wet nurses there were *assae nutrices* (dry nurses), specialized in hand feeding. Constantine's legislation (318–331 C.E.) suppressed infanticide and regularized abandonment, but did not reduce wet nursing. The belief in the transmission of character traits from the nurse persisted and, beginning with a Lateran Council decree of 1179, the Church reiterated that Christians must not wet nurse Jews or Muslims [28]. The search for a *balia*—the father's task—could be difficult, as reported by Ross for the Datini family in Florence in 1391 [29]: 'I have found one … whose milk is two months old; and she has vowed that if her babe, which is on the point of death, dies tonight, she will come as soon as it is buried.' Despite the rules in the contract, pregnancy of the *balia* more frequently terminated the infant's stay than the early death of the child.

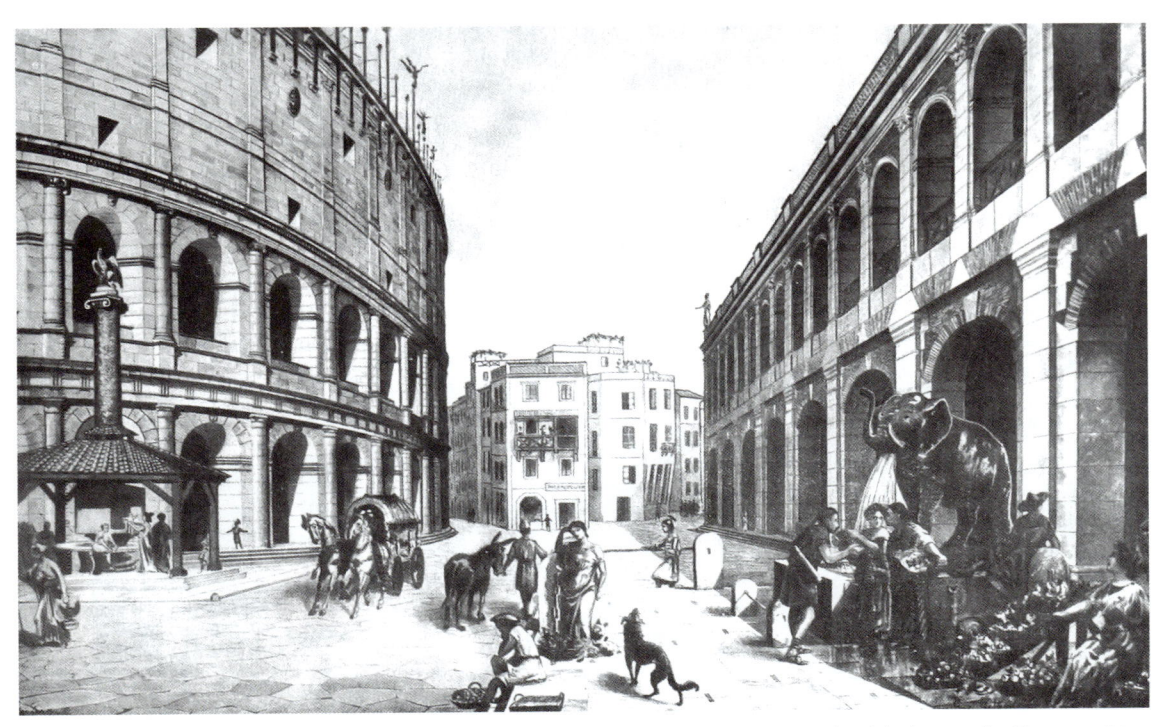

Fig. 6.2.1 The *Forum olitorium* (vegetable market) in Rome with the *Columna lactaria* (milk column, left side), close to the *Theatrum Marcellum*, which held 13,000 spectators. Reconstruction by Gatteschi [26]. Right side: fountain decorated with the elephant *Herbarius* and the *Minutia frumentaria* (granary, where the poor received wheat and cereal for free).

Britain—from Elizabethan times

From the Reformation, wet nursing was officially frowned upon, but persisted privately. 'Until the late 18th century it was a social norm for [British] upper- and middle-class mothers to employ wet nurses rather than feed their own children' [30]. In certain parishes in Buckinghamshire and Herefordshire, wet nursing was a major source of income, as studies of burial registries by Dorothy McLaren [31] and Valerie Fildes [32] revealed. The mortality of these infants sent out from London was high, as Walter Harris [33] reported in 1689: 'To the same Causes was owing an Observation, which was made not long ago by a worthy Divine, Rector of a Parish 12 miles from London, who with great Grief in Mind told me seriously, that his Parish was, when he first came to it, filled with sucking infants, and yet in the Space of one Year, that he had buried them all except two, and that the same Number of small Infants being soon twice supplied, according to the usual Custom of hireling Nurses, from the very great and almost inexhaustible City, he had committed them all to their Parent Earth, in the very same Year.'

As described by Alexander Hamilton [34] 'in the year 1767, in consequence of the humane suggestion of Mr. Jonas Hanway, an act of parliament was passed, obliging the parish-officers of London and Westminster to send their infant poor to be nursed in the country, at proper distances from the town'. These infants had a high mortality, whitewashed by incomplete reporting, as pointed out by Baines in 1861 [35]: 'Amongst its most disastrous results may be regarded the fate of the wet nurse's child, which is in most cases put out to *dry-nurse*, falls into ignorant or unprincipled hands, and, as a consequence, too often meets with premature death … I refer to … the system carried on with regard to children whose names are entered on the books of burial clubs … Some restrictive clauses are urgently needed in the Burial Act with reference to the disposal of infants said to be "still-born", such subjects having been hitherto enclosed in the coffins of adults without the payment of regular fees, and without requiring the production of a medical certificate … I suggest that it would be interesting and instructive to know how many of the mothers of "still-born" children had, previously to the birth, decided upon taking up the vocation of wet nurse.'

Under the heading 'Child murder and wet-nursing' a campaign against infanticide and 'baby farming' was led by the *British Medical Journal* from 1860 [36, 37]. The trials against baby farmers Charlotte Winsor in 1865 and Margaret Waters in 1870 met widespread public interest, even more when Waters was found guilty of murder and hanged in October 1870. Following the execution, the *Infant Life Protection Act* was passed, declaring it unlawful to take in infants to nurse, except in a house duly registered and frequently inspected for this purpose [38]. A *Lancet* editorial of 1872 hoped the law 'stops the system of child-murder which baby-farming is believed to have so largely induced' [39].

France—before and after the Revolution

For the urban French, wet nursing in the countryside was the normal way of baby feeding, legislated by King John the Good in 1350: 'Wet nurses sucking out of the infant's house will earn hundred sols per year and not more … *recommandaresses* [brokers] two sols from each party.' In 1611, a law was needed for the *meneurs* (nurse procurers): 'By 50 francs fine and prison for the first time it is forbidden to lead the nurses anywhere but to the broker's office' [40]. A law of

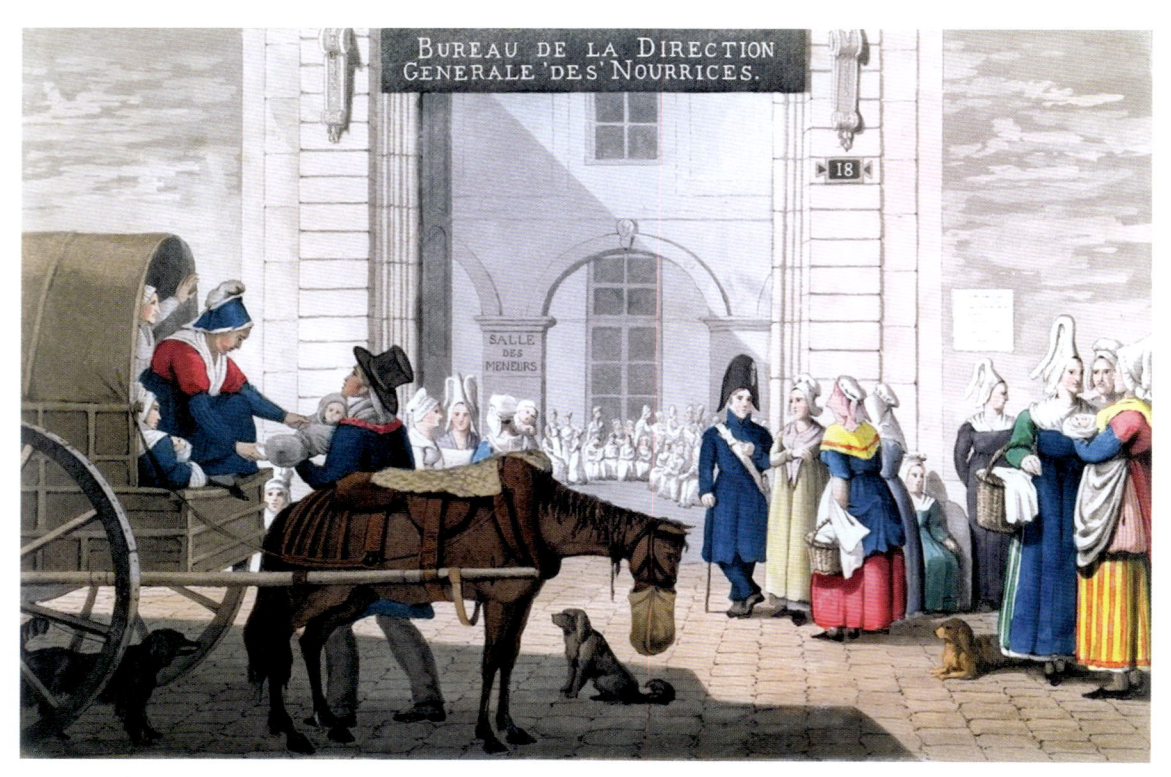

Fig. 6.2.2 The nurses' office in Paris, lithography by Jean Henri Marlet 1820. Located at 18, rue Sainte-Apolline, the office supplied wet nurses from the countryside to Parisian families. The nurses' headdresses indicate various provenance. To the left, a wet nurse sitting in the cart receives the nursling from the *meneur*.
Collection d'histoire de la pharmacie, Ordre National des Pharmaciens, Paris, with permission.

Louis XIV of 1715 granted four brokers the sole right to place wet nurses, established the central wet nurses' office in the Rue d'Apolline (Fig. 6.2.2), and regulated: 'We interdict the nurses to accept at the same time two nurslings, by punishment of whipping against the wet nurse and a fine of fifty livres against her husband.' The revolution reduced the brokers' privileges. Between necklace and high treason trials, Marie-Antoinette founded the Société de Charité Maternelle in 1787 [41]. In 1790, the police lieutenant Jean LeNoir reported that of 21,000 infants born in Paris, fewer than 1000 were nursed by their own mothers: 'The *meneurs* are the persons … who recruit all the women of their neighbourhood disposed to nurse, and conduct them to a bureau known as the *Bureau de Recomanderesses*' [42]. In 1816, the bureau in the rue Apolline admitted 6292 wet nurses, 5081 of whom were provided with an infant [43]. Following a decree of 1842, the nurse had to obtain a mayor's certificate assuring 'that she has sufficient means for existence, is of good lifestyle and morals, has no other nursling, and the age of her last infant allows her to accept one; it should indicate the date of birth of her infant, if it is alive or dead, and that she is equipped with a fireguard and a cradle for the infant entrusted to her.'

In 1867, Charles Monot, mayor of Montsauche, Nièvre, published a series of letters [44] revealing continued abuse of the wet nursing business: 'To withdraw from the hands of Mrs. Jeantin the babywear which belongs to me … This woman had the infant from December 29 to February 26, the time he died … She demands 10 francs and 50 centimes for the costs she had, but because she had him for two months only and cashed 16 francs for three, 5 fr. 50 must return to me plus the babywear.' In many cases, wet nursing was unsuccessful, as Charles Routh reported [45]: 'In one [Gironde community] the mothers suckle their own children; in the other a number of mercenary wet nurses take in children from Bordeaux in large numbers to nurse. In the first commune the mortality is 13 per cent. In the second 87 per cent.'

In December 1874, following an initiative of Théophile Roussel, a law was voted 'for the protection of infants sent out to nurse', which more or less ended the wet nursing business in France [46]: '§1, every infant under two years of age who is placed for paid wet-nursing outside its parents' home, must be under surveillance by the public authority [Prefecture] … §3, the superior committee on infant protection must report the infants' mortality to the minister of the interior each year … §4, the minister of the interior must publish detailed statistics on infant mortality each year and report to the president of the Republique on carrying out the present law … §7, Each person who wishes to nurse an infant must obtain a certificate by the mayor indicating if her last infant is alive and at least 7 months old.' During the 25 years following the *Loi Roussel*, the infant mortality in France fell from 39% to 8% [47].

US—milk depots and public health

In colonial America, wet nursing began late because of the relative paucity of women [48], but by 1706, breast milk was the most common commodity advertised by colonial newspapers [28]. Wet nurses became standard, especially in the south, and were recently immigrated, poor, of colour, or all three [32]. 'No more wet nurses!'

was the advertisement for Liebig's food in 1869 [49], even though Luther Emmett Holt warned in 1898 [19]: 'It is no small thing to deprive an infant of its mother's breast when, as statistics show to be true of the children of wet nurses, this fact reduces its chance of survival to one in ten.' Isaac Abt complained in 1917 [50]: 'In Chicago at present no directory for wet nurses exists such as those in New York and in Boston … It has been our experience that wet nurses have practiced deceit, either by diluting the milk or by substituting cow's milk for their own product.' The Boston wet nurse directory became a donor bank in 1919 [51]. At the Floating Hospital, a technique was developed to dry breast milk [52], but was never commercialized. In 1912, the US Children's Bureau was founded, devoted to the welfare of mothers and children and vigorously supporting breastfeeding. Its first investigation revealed that the US ranked 11th in infant mortality, and found a correlation between poverty and the infant mortality rate. The activities culminated in the *Sheppard Towner Maternity and Infancy Protection Act* of 1921, which provided for instruction in hygiene through public health nurses, visiting nurses, and consultation centres, but met much opposition from conservative forces ('feminist-socialist-communist plot') and was repealed in 1927 [53]. In 2008, the US infant mortality rate ranked 31 of 34 countries in the Organisation for Economic Co-operation and Development.

Present situation and conclusions

Rarely expressed outright, wet nursing depended on the diminished survival of the nurse's child: it had either died during or after birth, or was given to a foundling asylum, farmed out to an even poorer woman, or exposed to risky artificial feeding (dry nursing). With improved sanitation, plumbing, refrigerators, and canned sterile formula, artificial feeding became safer, and wet nursing gradually declined during the second half of the 19th century. A series of international congresses (Gouttes de Lait congresses of Paris 1905, Brussels 1907, and Berlin 1911) followed the successes of the British and French infant protection laws, and led to legislation to protect mother and infant in most countries. The last relics of wet nursing were donor milk banks for sick or very immature infants, with considerable laboratory expenses to make this nutrient safe [51]. In the historiography of wet nursing, a female topic insufficiently appreciated by male authors, emotional factors may have been over-emphasized and economic needs were barely considered. Wet nursing regulations became the foundation of legislation concerning infant protection and public health.

REFERENCES

1. Harper RF: The code of Hammurabi, King of Babylon. Chicago, IL: University of Chicago Press, 1904: §194.
2. Rosaria SM: The nurse and the child in Greek life. J Pediatr 1947;**30**:205–13.
3. Plato: The republic. New Haven, CT: Yale University Press, 2006: p. 162.
4. Aristotle: History of animals. In ten books. London: Bell, 1883: p. 72, 192.
5. Temkin O: Soranus' Gynecology. Baltimore, MD: The Johns Hopkins Press, 1956: p. 79–117.
6. Lascaratos J, Poulakou-Rebelakou: Oribasius (fourth century) and early Byzantine perinatal nutrition. J Pediat Gastroent Nutr 2003;**36**:186–9.
7. Gruner OC: A treatise on the canon of medicine of Avicenna, incorporating a translation of the first book. London: Luzac & Co, 1930: p. §126, §696–709.
8. Metlinger B: Ein vast nützlich Regiment der jungen Kinder. Augsburg: Zainer, 1473: p. 9–17, Fol. 17.
9. Rößlin E: Der Swangern Frauwen und hebammen Rosegarten. Facsimile Antiqua Verlag Wutöschingen 1993: Straßburg: Flach, 1513: p. 79.
10. Vallambert Sd: Cinq livres de la manière de nourrir et gouverner les enfants dès leur naissance. Reprint Droz, Genève 2005. Poitiers: Manefz et Bouchetz, 1565: p. 89–101, 112, 207–8.
11. Bourgeois L: Observations Diverses sur la Sterilité, Perte de Fruits, Foecondité, Accouchements, et Maladies de Femmes, et Enfants Nouveaux-naiz. Paris: Dehoury, 1609: p. 98–100, 155.
12. Guillemeau J: De la grossesse et accouchement des femmes. Paris: Jost, 1643: p. 551–87.
13. Sharp J: The midwives book. London: Miller, 1671: p. 351–71.
14. Mauriceau F: Tractat von Kranckheiten schwangerer und gebärender Weibspersonen. Basel: Bertsche, 1680: p. 332–47, 393.
15. Eminent Physician: The nurse's guide. London: Brotherton and Gilliver, 1729: p. 28–39.
16. Rosenstein NRv: Anweisung zur Kenntnis und Chur der Kinderkrankheiten (1st Swedish ed. 1764). 4. ed. Göttingen: Dieterich, 1781: p. 1–29.
17. Henke A: Handbuch zur Erkenntniß und Heilung der Kinderkrankheiten. 3. ed. Frankfurt: Wilmans, 1821: Vol. **1**, p. 89–106.
18. West C: Lectures on the diseases of infancy and childhood. 5. ed. London: Longman & Co, 1865: p. 538–40.
19. Holt LE: The diseases of infancy and childhood. New York: Appleton, 1898: p. 159, 184.
20. Finkelstein H: Lehrbuch der Säuglingskrankheiten. 2. ed. Berlin: Springer, 1921: p. 149, 355, 542.
21. Hess JH: Premature and congenitally disabled infants. London: Churchill, 1923: p. 114–30, 171–204.
22. Pfaundler Mv: Physiologie, Ernährung und Pflege der Neugeborenen. Döderlein: Handbuch der Geburtshilfe, Band 1. 2. ed. München: Bergmann, 1924: p. 146–65.
23. Pseudo-Plutarch: Moralia: De liberis educandis. Loeb Classical Library. London: Heinemann, 1927: Vol. **1**, p. 15.
24. Schubart W: Die Amme im alten Alexandrien. Jahrb Kinderheilk Phys Erziehung 1909;**70**:82–95.
25. Joshel SR: Nurturing the master's child: Slavery and the Roman child-nurse. Signs 1986;**12**:3–22.
26. Gatteschi G, Trabacchi A: Teatro di Marcello—Foro Olitorio—Elefante Erbario. In: Restauri della Roma imperiale. Roma: Bretschneider, 1924: p. 63.
27. Bradley KR: Wet nursing at Rome: a study in social relations. In: Rawson B: The family in ancient Rome. Ithaca, NY: Cornell University Press, 1986: p. 201–29.
28. Fildes VA: Wet nursing: a history from antiquity to the present. Oxford: Blackwell, 1988: p. 127–30.
29. Ross JB: The middle-class child in urban Italy, fourteenth to early sixteenth Century. In: deMause L: The history of childhood. New York: The Psychohistory Press, 1974: p. 183–228.
30. Fildes V: Breasts, bottles, and babies. Edinburgh: Edinburgh University Press, 1986: p. 98–121, 307.
31. McLaren D: Nature's contraceptive. Wet-nursing and prolonged lactation. Med Hist 1979;**23**:426–41.

32. Fildes V: The English wet-nurse and her role in infant care 1538–1800. Med Hist 1988;**32**:142–73.
33. Harris W: A treatise of the acute diseases of infants (1st ed. 1689). London: Astley, 1742: p. 17–8, 36.
34. Flügge C: Die Aufgaben und Leistungen der Milchsterilisierung gegenüber den Darmkrankheiten der Säuglinge. Zeitschr Hyg 1894;**17**:272–342.
35. Baines MA: Infant alimentation; or artificial feeding. Lancet 1869;**77**:33–4.
36. Davis JH: Child-murder and wet-nursing. BMJ 1861;**1**:183.
37. Acton W: Child-murder and wet-nursing. BMJ 1861;**1**:183–4.
38. Homrighaus RE: Wolves in women's clothing: baby-farming and the British Medical Journal. J Fam Hist 2001;**26**:350–72.
39. Editorial: The Infant Life Protection Act. Lancet 1872;**100**:612.
40. DuMesnil O: L'industrie des nourrices et la mortalité des nourrissons. Paris: Baillière, 1867: p. 7–22.
41. Lecomte J: La Charité de Paris. Paris: Dent, 1862: p. 2–6.
42. LeNoir JCP: Détail sur quelques établissements de la ville de Paris demandé par sa Majesté impérial, la Reine de Hongrie. Paris: Le Noir, 1780: p. 28–9.
43. Horn W: Reise durch Deutschland, Ungarn, Holland, Italien, Frankreich, Großbritannien und Irland. Berlin: Enslin, 1831: Vol. **2**, p. 695.
44. Monot C: De l'industrie des nourrices et de la mortalité des petits enfants. Paris: Baillière, 1867: p. 118.
45. Routh CHF: Infant feeding and its influence on life. 3. ed. New York: Wood, 1879: p. 31–3, 50, 104, 150.
46. Martin-Fougier A: La fin des nourrices. In: Le mouvement social, No. 105: Traveaux des femmes dans la France du XIXe siècle. 1978: p. 11–32.
47. Paterne: Critique de la loi Roussel. In: Keller A: Bericht über den III. internationalen Kongress für Säuglingsschutz (Gouttes de lait). Berlin: Stilke, 1912: p. 1058–91.
48. Treckel PA: Breastfeeding and maternal sexuality in Colonial America. J Interdiscip Hist 1989;**20**:25–51.
49. Apple RD: "Advertised by our loving friends": the infant formula industry and the creation of new pharmaceutical markets, 1870–1910. J Hist Med All Sci 1986;**41**:3–23.
50. Abt I: The technic of wetnurse management in institutions. JAMA 1917;**69**:418–20.
51. Jones F: History of North American donor milk banking: one hundred years of progress. J Hum Lact 2003;**19**:313–8.
52. Smith LW, Emerson PW: Notes on the experimental production of dried breast milk. Boston Med Surg J 1924;**191**:938–40.
53. Lemons JS: The Sheppard-Towner Act: progressivism in the 1920s. J Am Hist 1969;**55**:776–86.

6.3

Guttus, tiralatte, and téterelle
Breast pumps

Introduction: why breast pumps?

Before commercially produced, sterile formula became available (ca. 1870), the failure of breastfeeding was life-threatening for the infant, and it was frequent, as traditional medical recommendations impeded rather than promoted successful breastfeeding (see Chapter 6.1). Like other household items, breast pumps go back to antiquity, were used for a variety of reasons, and manufactured in various forms. Small volume devices with continuous suction or sucking glasses were used to elevate or elongate small, flat, or retracted nipples; to prevent or treat cracked or sore nipples; to prevent or treat retention or 'milk fever'; and to give relief from engorgement. Larger volume devices, self-sucked or with mechanically produced negative pressure, were used to remove and discard milk regarded as 'unhealthy' (e.g. colostrum) and to maintain lactation, while the infant was being wet nursed (at the breast of a mercenary nurse) or dry nursed (hand-fed), to extract, store, or sell human milk as a remedy [1], and to allow the breastfeeding mother to temporarily leave her baby, usually for work. Large volume, electrical pumps with intermittent suction, usually bilateral, were widely used in hospitals to augment the milk production by thoroughly emptying the breast, to feed preterm, sick, multiple or malformed infants, or those whose suck was weak due to neurological impairment, and to protect the breastfeeding mother after discharge from the hospital from embarrassment, prejudices against breastfeeding in public, and to maintain lactation while returning to work outside the home.

Antique milk pumps

A large number of ceramic vessels from the 6th to the 5th century B.C.E. were found in infant graves and votive deposits in Boeotia, Attica, Cyprus, and the Greek colonies in southern Italy. Many of them belong to the *guttus* type with a narrow mouth or neck, as described by M. Terentius Varro [2], 'which release the wine in small sips, and from the drops are called guttus'. They frequently were varnished black and had the shape of a female breast, some with a nipple on top, and a complex internal construction (Fig. 6.3.1D). Archaeologists believed them to be oil distributors for lamps, or Boeotian trick vases [3]. Roman collector Luigi Sambon interpreted them as feeding bottles in 1895 [4]: 'Among the pottery I have found invalid medicine cups and feeding bottles for infants (gutti). Many of these are ingeniously fashioned in the shape of the female breast, some offer curious shapes of animals. I have found some which have a woman suckling her infant worked in relief on their surface evidently indicating their use, but what positively confirms these *gutti* to be feeding bottles is that they have been found in the tombs of children who died during the period of lactation … These old feeding bottles are so constructed that no flies or dust can reach their contents.'

In 1933, Geert Snijder, director of the Amsterdam Allard Pierson Museum, identified [5] their dual purpose, breast pump and feeding bottle: 'Remarkable that in some specimens the basal opening is quite large, and little suitable for vase tricks … I am convinced that this *guttus* subtype is an apparatus to withdraw milk from the maternal breast … My colleague, Prof. van Rooy, has used it upon my suggestion with optimal success in his [Amsterdam] obstetrics hospital, and his results are in this paper's appendix.' Van Rooy's report specified: 'The vessel was filled with water and applied with its lower opening upon the nipple. By opening and closing the spout with the finger, small volumes of water drained, an intermittent vacuum resulted in the vessel, which enlarged the nipple and allowed the milk to flow … When the sucking force of the draining water was replaced by that of the mouth, the milk flow was abundant and accumulated inside the vessel.'

Specific glass vessels have been excavated around the Mediterranean, and shown to originate from Roman glass factories [6]. These milk drawers were made of glass, and their shape allowed few intact devices to survive. A sucking glass dating from the 2nd century C.E. was unearthed in Zadar, Croatia, and is depicted in Fig. 6.3.1E [7].

Middle Ages

Medical progress was slow in medieval times, and next to nothing was published. From 712 C.E. to 1260 C.E., the greater part of the

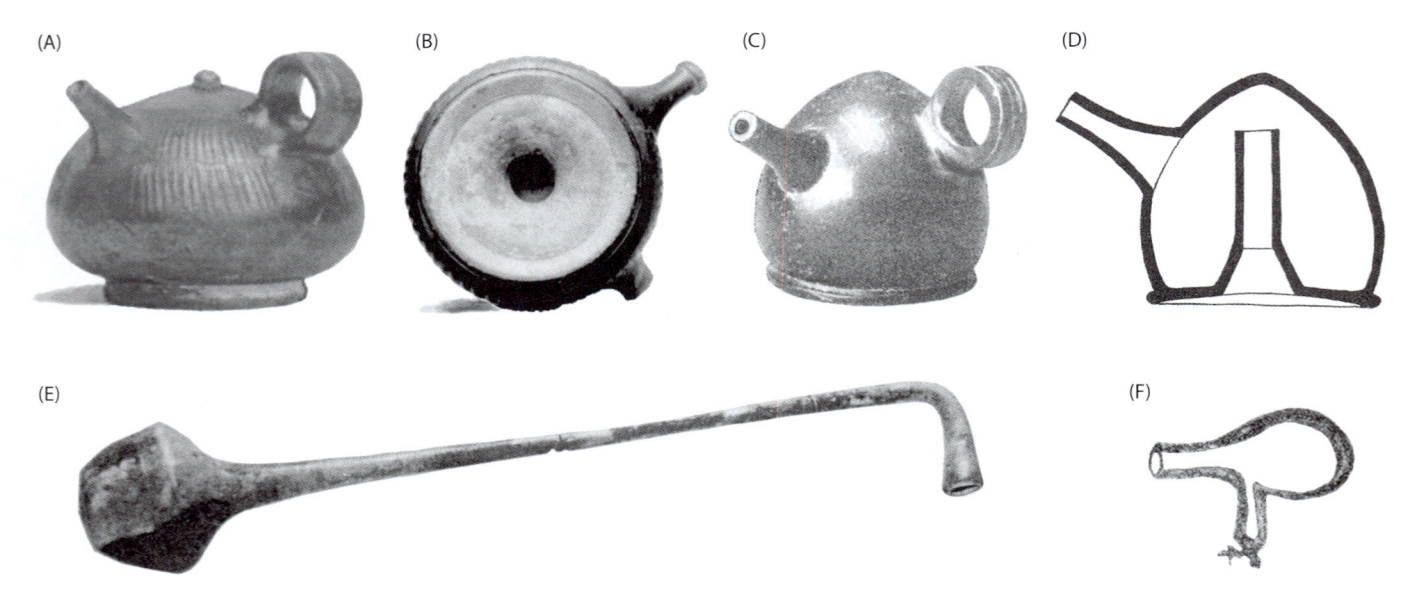

Fig. 6.3.1 Antique breast pumps: A–D, *guttus*-type ceramic breast pumps from Greece, 5th century B.C.E.; A, Allard Pierson Museum Amsterdam, typical form; B, British Museum London, both pumps described by Snijder 1933 [5]; C, specimen in the Geneva Museum, described by Noll 1936 [37]; D, internal structure of the Geneva *guttus*, described by Sambon 1895 [4]; E, Roman glass *tiralatte* from Zadar, Croatia, 31 cm long, 2nd century C.E., described by Sudhoff 1918 [7]; F, medieval glass vessel from the Roger Frugardi codex, 10th century C.E. [7].

Iberian Peninsula belonged to various Islamic caliphates, and became the centre of intellectual activity in Europe. Famous Muslim medical faculties were founded in Cordova, Granada, Sevilla, and Toledo, whereas the rest of Europe had but the universities of Bologna, Salerno, and Oxford. The Golden Age of Umayyad rule in Andalusia, in which the majority of the population was able to read and write, brought forth Albucasis (936–1013 C.E.), scholar of the University of Cordova. Around 1170, part of his important treatise *On Surgery* made its way into the *Codex Latinus* 161 by Roger Frugardi of Salerno [7], showing a small figure (Fig. 6.3.1F) and the text: 'After birth the tip of the breast is often retracted inwards, so that the child cannot attach to it. Here a vessel [*cuffa*] can be applied to the nipple, the head of which [*capitellum*] is sucked to draw the nipple out.'

The 16th and 17th centuries

Colostrum was regarded as unwholesome in many cultures as Metlinger explained in 1473 [8]: 'During the first fourteen days another woman should suckle the infant, because the mother's milk is not healthy ... Meanwhile the mother should be sucked by a whelp.' Delayed emptying of the breast invariably led to engorgement, and *milk fever* was regarded a normal postpartum state. For those without access to young dogs, Verona physician Omnibonus Ferrarius published a sucking glass called *tiralatte* in 1577 [9]: 'To prevent the milk from deteriorating, it should be sucked out with the small instrument [Fig. 6.3.2A, B] produced for this purpose in Italy; its large opening is placed over the nipple, the long tube is sucked with the mother's own mouth, so that the breast is emptied twice daily, as long as the milk flows.' The surgeon Johannes Scultetus described many instruments in 1665 [10] and 1666 [11]: 'In some lactating women the nipples are so deeply hidden, that it is impossible for the neonate to grasp them ... In such case, she should apply the base of the sucking glass [Fig. 6.3.2D] to the nipple and fix it with a band [Fig. 6.3.2E], then take the long tube into her mouth and elevate the nipple by suction. Or, a fairly robust girl [1655 edition: 'one who is of years'] can be ordered to bring forth the hidden nipple by strong sucking [Fig. 6.3.2C, K]. Another technique ... is to fill a small drinking glass [Fig. 6.3.2L] with hot water, pour it out, and turn the glass over the nipple, on which it attaches so firmly, that afterwards the infant can easily grasp it with its mouth. With all three techniques not only the nipple is elongated, but also the milk drawn into the breasts.' Royal *accoucheur* François Mauriceau depicted a similar pump to treat sore nipples in 1680 [12]: 'Avoid suckling the infant until [the nipples] are completely healed; hence for some time the milk must be milked out ... One can also use the small instrument depicted at the beginning of this chapter [Fig. 6.3.2F].'

From the 16th to the 18th century, corsets were worn in most of Europe by well-to-do women from school age for most of the day. They flattened the breast and were responsible for a high incidence of inverted nipples among the wealthy. Manchester man-midwife Charles White complained in 1791 [13]: 'The small flat nipple which lies buried in the breast is generally occasioned by the tight dress, which has for some centuries been so constantly worn in this island by the female sex of all ages, and of almost all ranks. This dress, by constantly pressing upon the breast and nipple, reduces it to a flat form, instead of a conical one, with the nipple in its apex, which it ought to preserve.' In 1800, William Roscoe, in the notes of his translation of Tansillo's *Balia* of 1534: [14]: 'By a certain absurd custom, which has often prevailed, and may soon prevail again in this island, the nipple of the female breast is frequently so depressed, as to render it, throughout life, totally unfit for the purpose for which it was by nature intended.' Similar reports came from other countries [15].

A *tétine* (milk drawer) very similar to Ferrario's and Mauriceau's devices was depicted by the Paris Royal surgeon Pierre Dionis

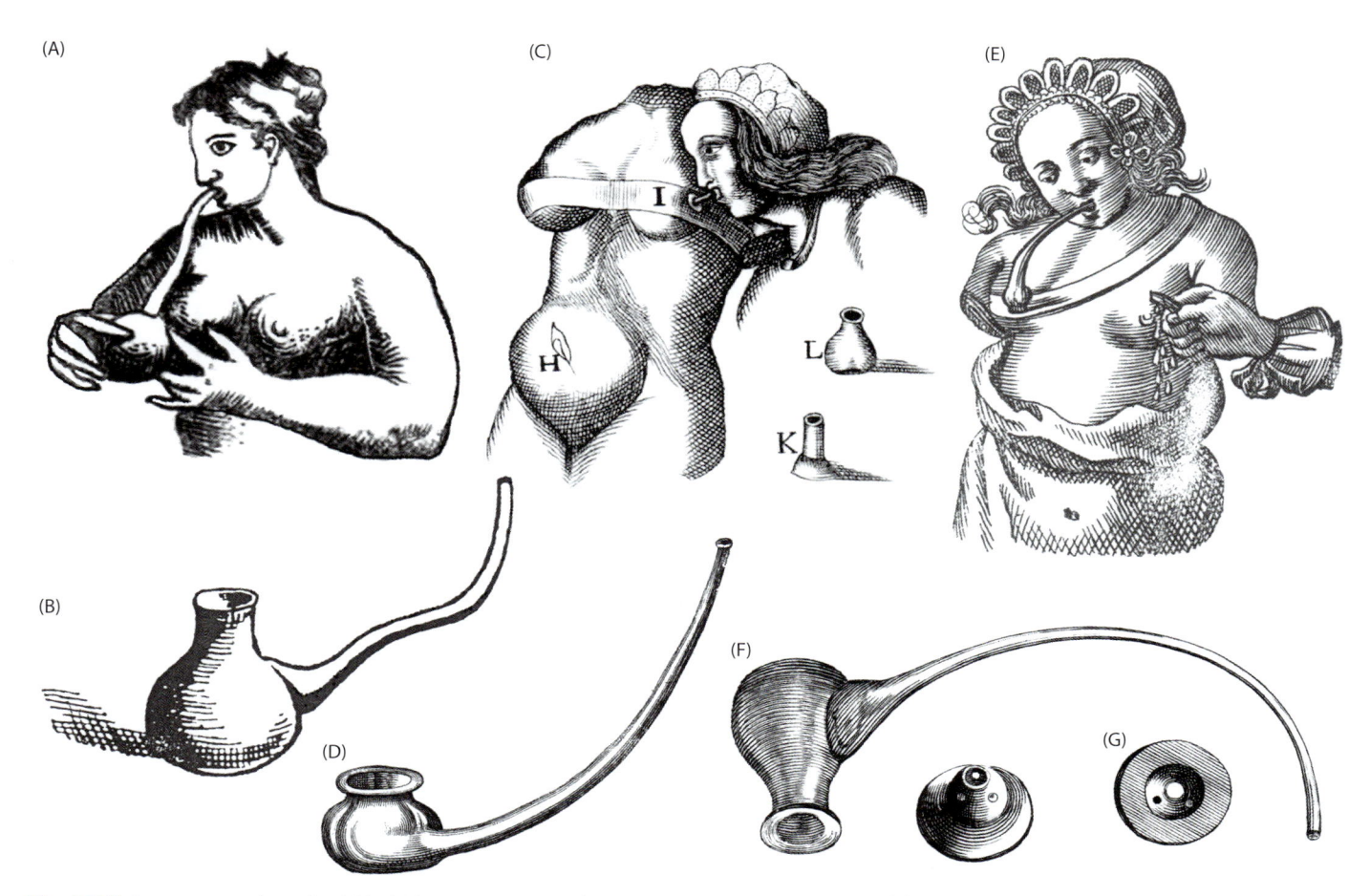

CHAPTER 6.3 Guttus, tiralatte and téterelle: breast pumps   229

Fig. 6.3.2 Breast pumps from the 16th–17th century: A, B, *tiralatte* as described by Ferrario 1577 [9]; C, sucking tube to empty the breast with the help of another woman, and K, L, sucking glass described by Scultetus 1665 [10]; D, E, sucking glass and its use for self-sucking, described by Scultetus 1666 [11]; F, sucking apple and G, two nipple shields described by Mauriceau 1680 [12].

in 1718 [16]. Jacques Mesnard, *accoucheur* in Rouen, published a book on midwifery in question–answer form in 1753 [17]: 'Question: If, by its suction, an infant has excoriated the nipple of its nurse … Answer: One should forbid the nurse to breastfeed the infant, and order to draw her milk using an ivory tube with small head end, or a similar device, or a new smoking pipe: It is used by applying the head end over the nipple and sucking strongly through the tube. In this manner the breasts must be relieved until the fissures are healed' (Fig. 6.3.3A, B).

Georg Wilhelm Stein, director of the Foundling Hospital in Kassel, described a piston breast pump in 1774 which was not easily cleaned (Fig. 6.3.3C–F), given the fact that it also was used as clyster syringe and cupping glass [18]: 'Now we can do without the young dogs and the old matrons, whom the noble ladies made good use of … My first concern is the frequently necessary elongation of the nipples, and the opening of the milk ducts. For this purpose I apply the tool already eight days before the expected delivery, twice or thrice daily … When the nipples withdrew too deeply into the breasts, I apply the small and flat recipient with the stopcock, pull out the nipple with the pump, close the syringe and leave the glass sitting on the breast from morning to evening.'

Rubber, obtained from trees, had long been used by Mayas and Incas for ball games, and was brought to Europe and presented to the Paris Academie des Sciences by the geographer Charles Marie de la Condamine in 1745 [19]. Brittle in winter and sticky in summer, it remained a museum curiosity and found limited use for boots and garments. In 1839, Massachusetts inventor Charles Goodyear heated India rubber with sulphur and lead oxide—vulcanization—which greatly improved its elasticity. Half a century earlier, Prussian field surgeon Johann Theden described the use of unvulcanized rubber, obviously imported from American natives, in a breast pump in 1782 [20]: 'For a woman desiring to breastfeed it is most beneficial if already during the last months of pregnancy the nipples are elevated by a female, by young dogs, or by a machine, and the milk flow is started early; she will be able to feed her infant properly, and will be less affected by milk fever … The best machines to extract the nipples from the breast and to start the milk flow are the milk pumps made of elastic resin [Fig. 6.3.3G]. I take such a resin bag in the shape of a hollow sphere, an animal head, or however else the Indians produce it, and fix it to a broad, funnel-shaped sucking glass with a button on its back. The button is fixed in the bag with a tightly bound ligature. To attach the milk pump, the glass is humidified slightly and the funnel attached over the nipple. When releasing the compression of the hand onto the bag, the glass adheres like a cupping glass, and extracts both nipple and milk, without any inconvenience … Compared to Stein's milk pump, the device has the

230 PART 6 Breast is best

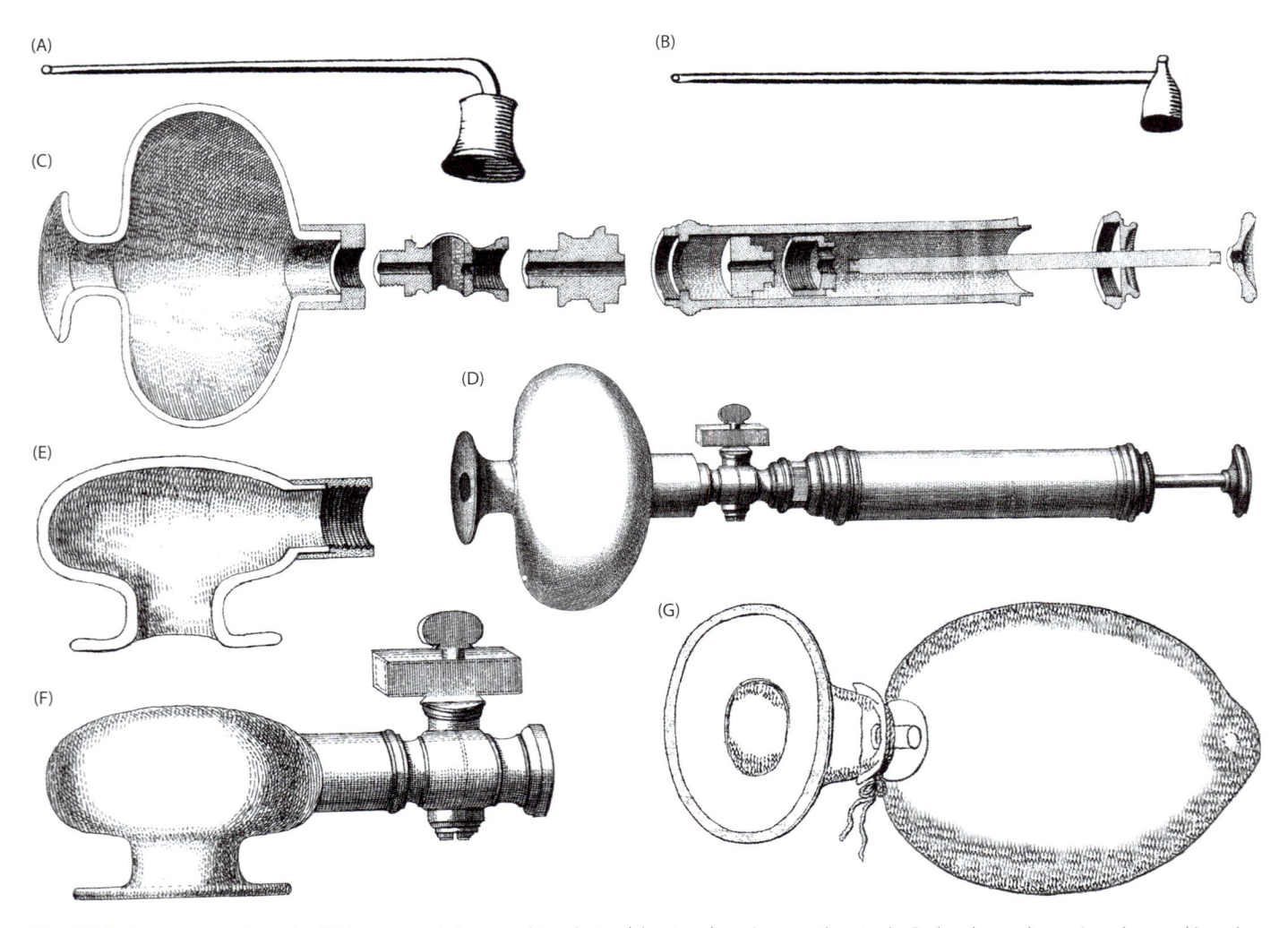

Fig. 6.3.3 Breast pumps from the 18th century: A, ivory sucking device (*chapiteau*) to elongate the nipple; B, the cheap alternative, clay smoking pipe, both described by Mesnard 1753 [17]; C–F, piston-driven breast pump described by Stein 1774 [18]; C, disassembled; D, assembled; E, F, cupping glass to form the nipples; G, breast pump with bag of unvulcanized India rubber, described by Theden 1782 [20].

advantages of being less complex, less expensive, and less breakable.' Given the fact that babies latch on the areola rather than the nipple, the emphasis of many authors on nipple forming is astonishing.

The 19th century

In the 19th century, techniques advanced which gave the sick, the premature, and the malformed infant a chance to survive. As early as 1839, Charles Richard de Nancy succeeded to bring up a 6-month preterm infant up to the end of the first year in a heated bed with feedings by a *téterelle à pompe* [21]. A nasal spoon and gavage were used in French hospitals from 1851 and required previous milk expression or pumping [22]. In 1892, Lyon paediatrician Edouard Jacquemet described a double-suction breast pump to facilitate the sucking effort for the preterm infant [23] (**Fig. 6.3.4A**). The *téterelle biaspiratrice* by Paris obstetrician Alfred Auvard was used to treat cracked nipples, but also to feed preterm or weak infants. The milk accumulated in the lower part of the glass vessel. A valve in the infantile outlet allowed the mother to create negative pressure while the infant breas feeding [24]. When bacteria became known around 1860, breast pumps were designed which were easy to clean and whose glass parts could be sterilized.

The 20th century: modern devices

Manual expression had been long used to enhance lactation, especially for preterm infants [25]. The US, where Thomas Edison opened the first electric power plant in New York in 1882, were also the cradle of the electric breast pump. Abt's electrical breast pump [26] remained a hospital-based technology for decades. The *téterelle biaspiratrice* was reinvented by Fred Caldwell in 1915 [27]. The 20th century saw the erotization of the female breast, especially in the US [28] to a degree that its nourishing function was seriously threatened by its sexual role. As early as 1910, a device was patented 'to avoid unpleasant and embarrassing situations by the necessary exposure of the breast in suckling the child' [29] (**Fig. 6.3.5A**). It remains difficult to imagine how the nursing attachment was kept clean. Mothers breastfeeding in public were arrested for indecent exposure [30], breastfeeding beyond the first year of life was judged as sexual abuse with the consequence of loss of custody [31]. And it required legislation in most states to clarify that breastfeeding in

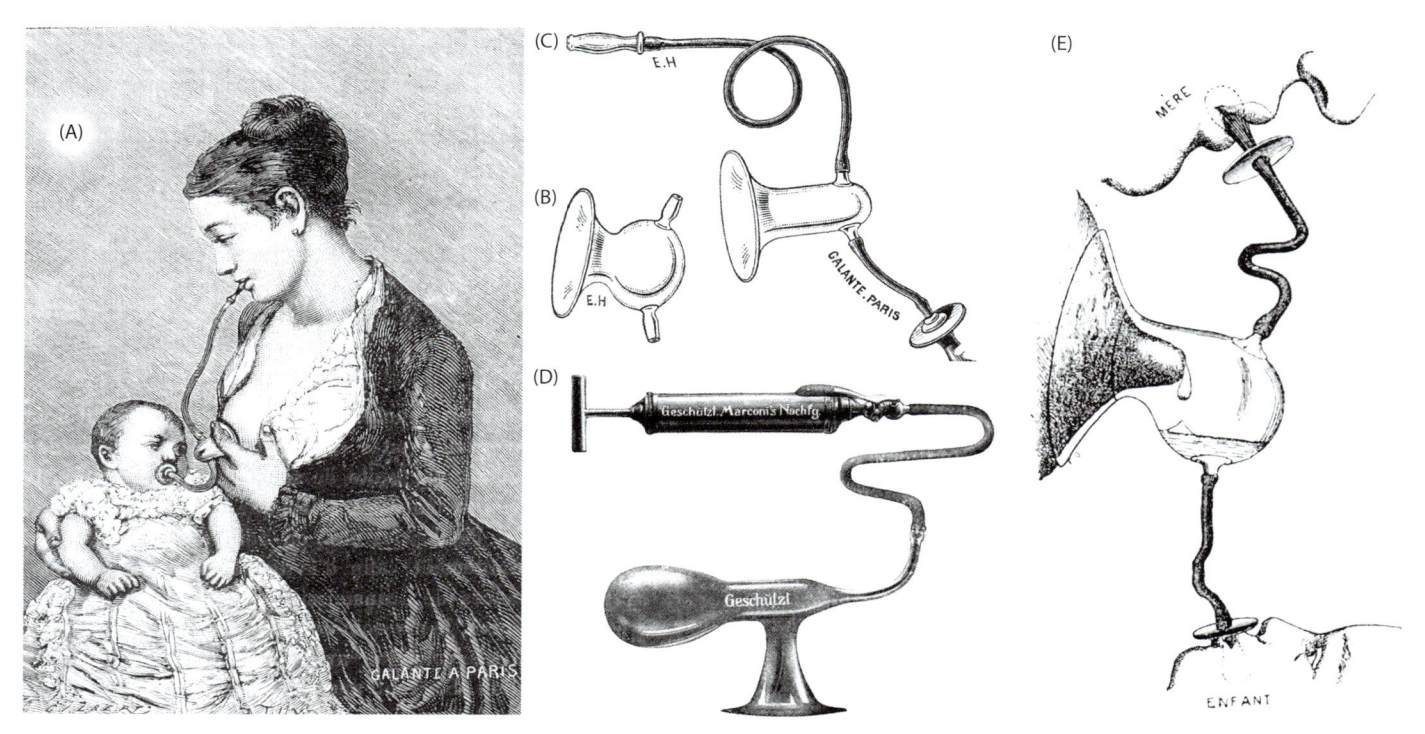

Fig. 6.3.4 Breast pumps from the 19th century: A, *téterelle biaspiratrice* to feed weak infants, depicted by Jacquemet 1882 [23]; B and C, alternatively shaped glass parts of A; D, piston-driven milk pump described by Jaschke 1909 [38]; E, téterelle with valve in the lower tube, described by Auvard 1889 [24].

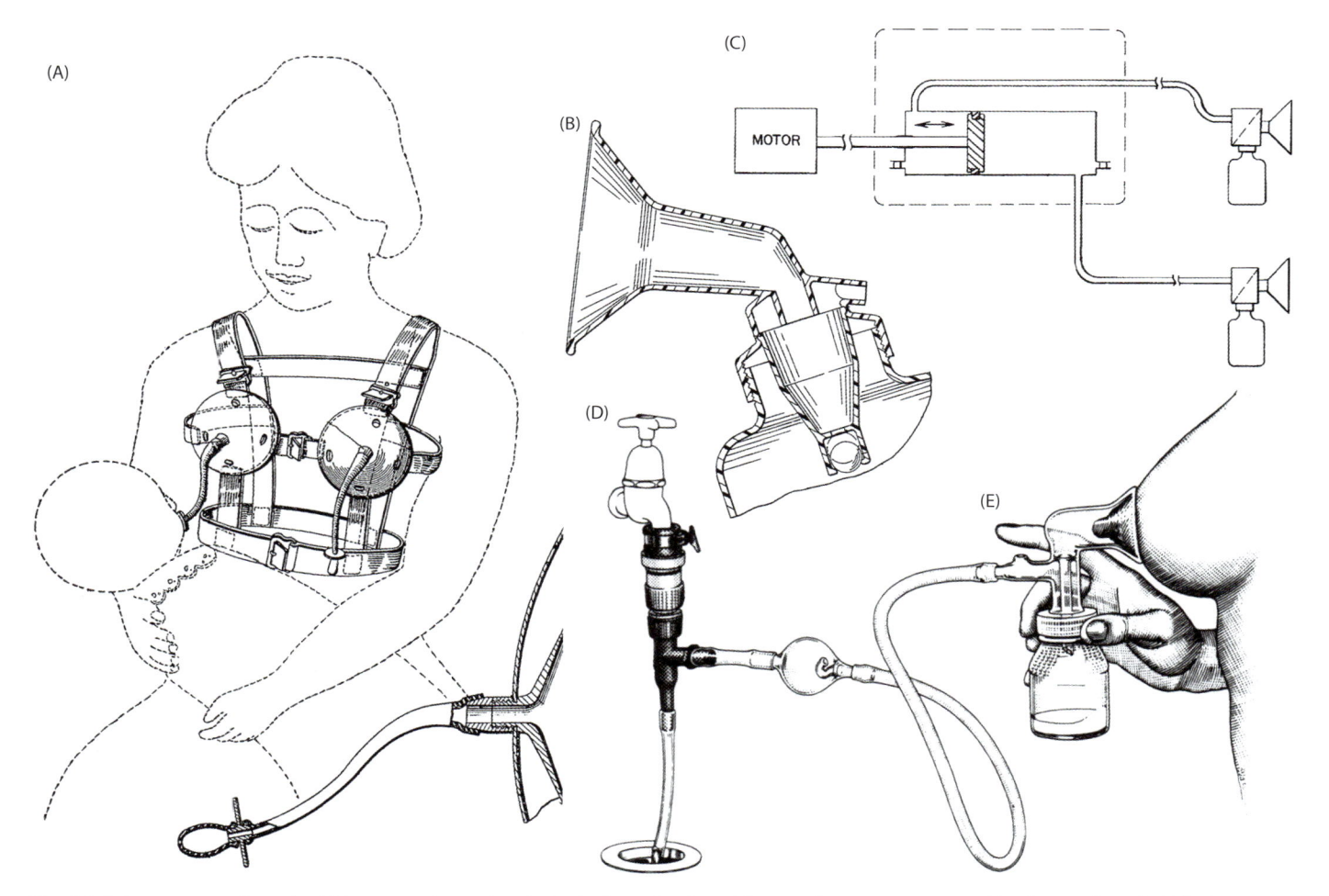

Fig. 6.3.5 Breast pumps from the 20th century: A, nursing device for breastfeeding without *embarrassment*, patented by Cunningham 1910 [29]; B, cup with ball valve, patented by Larsson 1989 [39]; C, bilateral pump patented by Larsson 1999 [40]. D, E: Water-jet pump described by Sponsel in 1983 [41].
D, E: Reproduced with permission from Sponsel, W.E., Simple and effective breast pump for nursing mothers. *BMJ*, 286:1180–1181. Copyright © 1983 BMJ Publishing Group Ltd.

public was *not* illegal [32]. Realizing that women were embarrassed and men felt uneasy by breastfeeding [33, 34], the industry reacted promptly: electric pumps were developed for bilateral application (Fig. 6.3.5B, C) which were small and portable and had disposable parts. The long-known water-jet pump was proposed as a cheap alternative (Fig. 6.3.5D, E). Randomized trials did not establish differences between various breast pumps regarding expressed volume, bacterial contamination, and transfer to feeding at the breast [35]. In the US, 85% of breastfeeding women are presently using breast pumps [36] and workplace pumping has become a major issue. However, workplace lactation requires time, space, and cooling facilities, all of which not every employer is willing to provide.

Conclusion

For two-and-a-half millennia, breast pumps have been used and their form changed with the material available. Despite their longstanding and extensive use, the scientific literature on breast pumps is limited. More than paediatricians' appeals (which focused on the benefit for infants and were often based on incomplete understanding of lactation physiology), breast pump manufacturers effectively promoted breastfeeding and are nowadays in keen competition with the formula industry. During the last century, rapid technical development occurred associated with widespread use of breast pumps in some countries. This change is both an indicator of technical progress and reflects women's changing position in society.

REFERENCES

1. Gourevitch D: Les tire-lait antiques et la consommation médicale de lait humain. Hist Sci Med 1990;**24**:93–8.
2. Varro MT: On the Latin language. Loeb Classical Library 333. London and Cambridge, MA: Harvard University Press, 2006: p. V, 124.
3. Kilinski K: Boeotian trick vases. Am J Archaeol 1986;**90**:153–8.
4. Sambon L: Donaria of medical interest in the Oppenheimer Collection of Etruscan and Roman Antiquities. BMJ 1895;**2**: 146–50.
5. Snijder GAS: Guttus und Verwandtes. Mnemosyne 1933–1934;**1**: 34–60.
6. Tantrakarn K, Kato N, Hokura A, et al.: Archeological analysis of Roman glass excavated from Zadar, Croatia. X-Ray Spectrom 2009;**38**:121–7.
7. Sudhoff K: Beiträge zur Geschichte der Chirurgie im Mittelalter. 2. Abbildungen in einer Rogerhandschrift des 13. Jahrhunderts. Stud Gesch Med 1918;11–12:13–4, plate I.
8. Metlinger B: Ein vast nützlich Regiment der jungen Kinder. Augsburg: Zainer, 1473: p. 9–17, Fol. 17.
9. Ferrarius O: De arte medica infantium. Brescia: Marchetti, 1577: p. 11, 31.
10. Scultetus J: Armamentum chirurgicum. 5. ed. Venetiis: Combi, & LaNou, 1665: p. 37, 137, Tab. 16, 37.
11. Scultetus J: Wund-Artzneyisches Zeug-Hauß. Franckfurt: Gerlin, 1666: p. 27, 124.
12. Mauriceau F: Tractat von Kranckheiten schwangerer und gebärender Weibspersonen. Basel: Bertsche, 1680: p. 332–47, 393.
13. White C: A treatise on the management of pregnant and lying-in women. London: Dilly, 1791: p. 57.
14. Tansillo L: The nurse. A poem 1534. Translated from the Italian by: William Roscoe. 2. ed. Liverpool: Cadell & Davies, 1800: p. 8.
15. Fildes V: Breasts, bottles, and babies. Edinburgh: Edinburgh University Press, 1986: p. 98–121, 307.
16. Dionis P: Traité général des accouchements. Paris: Dehoury, 1758: p. 358.
17. Mesnard J: Le guide des accoucheurs ou le maistre dans l'art d'accoucher les femmes et de les soulager. Paris: De Bure & Co. 1753: p. 360.
18. Stein GW: Beschreibung einer Brust- oder Milchpumpe. Kleine Werke zur praktischen Geburtshülfe. Marburg: Academische Buchhandlung, 1774: p. 49, 64–8.
19. Labey R: Christophe Colomb, le caoutchouc et les tétines. Rev Hist Pharm 1994;**82**:55–64.
20. Theden JCA: Neue Bemerkungen und Erfahrungen zur Bereicherung der Wundarzneykunst und Arzneygelahrheit. Berlin und Stettin: Nicolai, 1782: Vol. **2**, p. 257–60, Tab. 3.
21. Richard (de Nancy) CJF: Traité pratique des maladies des enfants. Paris: Baillière, 1839: p. 128.
22. Budin P: Le Nourrisson. Paris: Doin, 1900: p. 23, 41, 99, 213.
23. Jacquemet E: Les Maladies de la première enfance. Paris: Baillière, 1892: p. 15–6.
24. Auvard A: Travaux d'obstetrique. Paris: Lecrosnier et Babé, 1889: Vol. **I**, p. 353.
25. Sedgwick JP: Establishment, maintenance, and reinstitution of breast feeding. J Am Med Assoc 1917;**69**:417–8.
26. Tarr EM: Development and re-establishment of breast milk by use of Dr. Abt's electric breast pump. Cal West Med 1925;**23**:728–32.
27. Caldwell FC: An effective breast pump. Am J Dis Child 1915;**9**:381–6.
28. Saha P: Breastfeeding and sexuality: professional advice literature from the 1970s to the present. Health Educ Behav 2002;**29**:61–72.
29. Cunningham HB: Nursing attachment. United States Patent Office 1910; Pat.-Nr. 949414.
30. Jelliffe DB, Jelliffe EFP: Human milk in the modern world. Oxford: Oxford University Press, 1978: p. 302–7.
31. Umansky L: The Karen Carter case and the politics of maternal sexuality. In: Ladd-Taylor M, Umansky L: Bad mothers: the politics of blame in twentieth century America. New York: New York University Press, 1998, p. 209–309.
32. Vance MR: Breastfeeding legislation in the United States. Leaven 2005;**41**:51–4.
33. Dix DN: Why women decide not to breastfeed. Birth 1991;**18**:222–5.
34. Henderson L, McMillan B, Green JM, Renfrew MJ: Men and infant feeding. Birth 2011;**38**:61–70.
35. Becker GE, Cooney F, Smith HA: Methods of milk expression for lactating women. Cochrane Database Syst Rev 2011;**12**:CD006170.
36. Labiner-Wolfe J, Fein SB, Shealy KR, Wang C: Prevalence of breast milk expression and associated factors. Pediatrics 2008;Supp. **2**:S63–8.
37. Noll R: Ein griechischer Milchsaugapparat. Ciba Zschr 1936;**3**:1213.
38. Jaschke RTh: Eine neue Milchpumpe. Zentralbl Gynäk 1909;**33**: 556–9.
39. Larsson KO: Breastpump. United States Patent 1989; Pat.-Nr. 4857051.
40. Larsson MN: Alternating suction breastpump assembly and method. United States Patent 1999; Pat.-Nr. 5945690.
41. Sponsel WE: Simple and effective breast pump for nursing mothers. BMJ 1983;**286**:1180–1.

6.4

Pap, gruel, and panada
Early approaches to artificial feeding

Introduction

Contemporary publications on infant feeding claim that 'up to the nineteenth century, the overwhelming majority of infants received their nourishment at the breast' [1, 2]. But is this statement true? The 'scientific' development of infant nutrients from 1870 to 1910 was described in excellent reviews by Apple [1], Mepham [3], and Weaver [4]. But relatively little is known about infant feeding in the 'prescientific' era before 1860. The aim of this chapter therefore is to track down even earlier approaches to artificial feeding, to characterize feeding in different epochs, and to compare their recipes. Special attention was paid to artificial feeding as an exclusive substitute for breastfeeding or wet nursing (see Chapter 6.2) in very young infants. The following foods were analysed: (1), *pap* (Pappe, Brei, bouillie), a semi-solid food made from flour or bread, cooked in water with or without milk; (2), *gruel* (Schleimsuppe, decoction), a thin porridge resulting from boiling cereal (oat, wheat, rye) in water or milk; and (3), *panada* (Brotsuppe, panade), a preparation of flours, cereals, or bread cooked in broth. These mixtures were usually cooked and kept warm for some time. Some authors used various terms synonymously. In German, the verbs *päppeln* (to nourish) and *pappen* (to stick) originated from *pap* in the 15th century.

Antiquity

The domestication of large mammals began with sheep and goats in Mesopotamia around 8000 B.C.E. and proceeded to cows in India and Southwest Asia around 6000 B.C.E. [5]. A 5000-year-old stone frieze in the Ninhursag temple in the Sumerian City Tell al-'Ubaid in the Euphrates delta depicts the milking of cows and preparation of dairy products [6]. Aristotle [7] and Galen [8] described animal milk as a nutrient for infants. In the 2nd century C.E. Soranus, who disliked early breastfeeding, did not object to breast milk substitutes: 'If, however, a woman able to provide milk is not at hand, during the first three days one must use honey alone, or mix goat's milk with it.' Moreover, he described nutrition with 'artificial nipples' [9].

Evidence from artefacts

Feeding vessels for infants date from about 4000 B.C.E., and have been unearthed in large numbers from infant graves throughout the Roman empire including Britain [10], Hungary [11], and Germany [12]. They have been described extensively [13–17] and were sometimes misunderstood as lampfillers [18], until gas chromatography and mass spectroscopy proved they had been used for milk [12, 19]. There are famous collections in Paris, Fécamp, Geneva, Cologne, the Wellcome Museum in London, Drake Collection in Toronto, and Eisenberg Collection in New Mexico [19, 20]. In Colonial America, infant feeders made of pewter were produced and sold from 1666 [21]. The history of artificial infant feeding in the US has been described by Thomas Cone [22]. Fig. 6.4.1 illustrates feeding vessels from various cultures.

Early printed books

The artificial feeding of infants figured prominently in scientific texts soon after the printing press became available (Table 6.4.1). In 1473, Bartholomäus Metlinger stated [23]: 'One should also know about the gruel that is given to it after it has nursed; when the milk of the nurse is good and she has enough, the child needs less gruel especially when the nursing agrees with it; when the milk is not good or when the wet-nurse is sick or has little milk or the baby does not thrive on the nursing one should give more gruel. One should be careful not to burn the child by giving it gruel that is too hot as it is an old wife's opinion that if the gruel will not burn a coarse finger it will not burn the tender child.'

Cornelius Roelans used goat's milk as a remedy for diarrhoea in 1485. Eucharius Roesslin did not mention artificial feeding in 1513, but did list several recipes to augment lactation [24]. For infantile diarrhoea, he recommended 'white bread … or a thin mush made from bread roll cooked in water'. Thomas Phaire (first ed. 1544) mentioned 'playsters for the encrease of mylke' rather than recipes for pap [25]. Artificial feeding was accepted earlier in France; Simon Vallambert

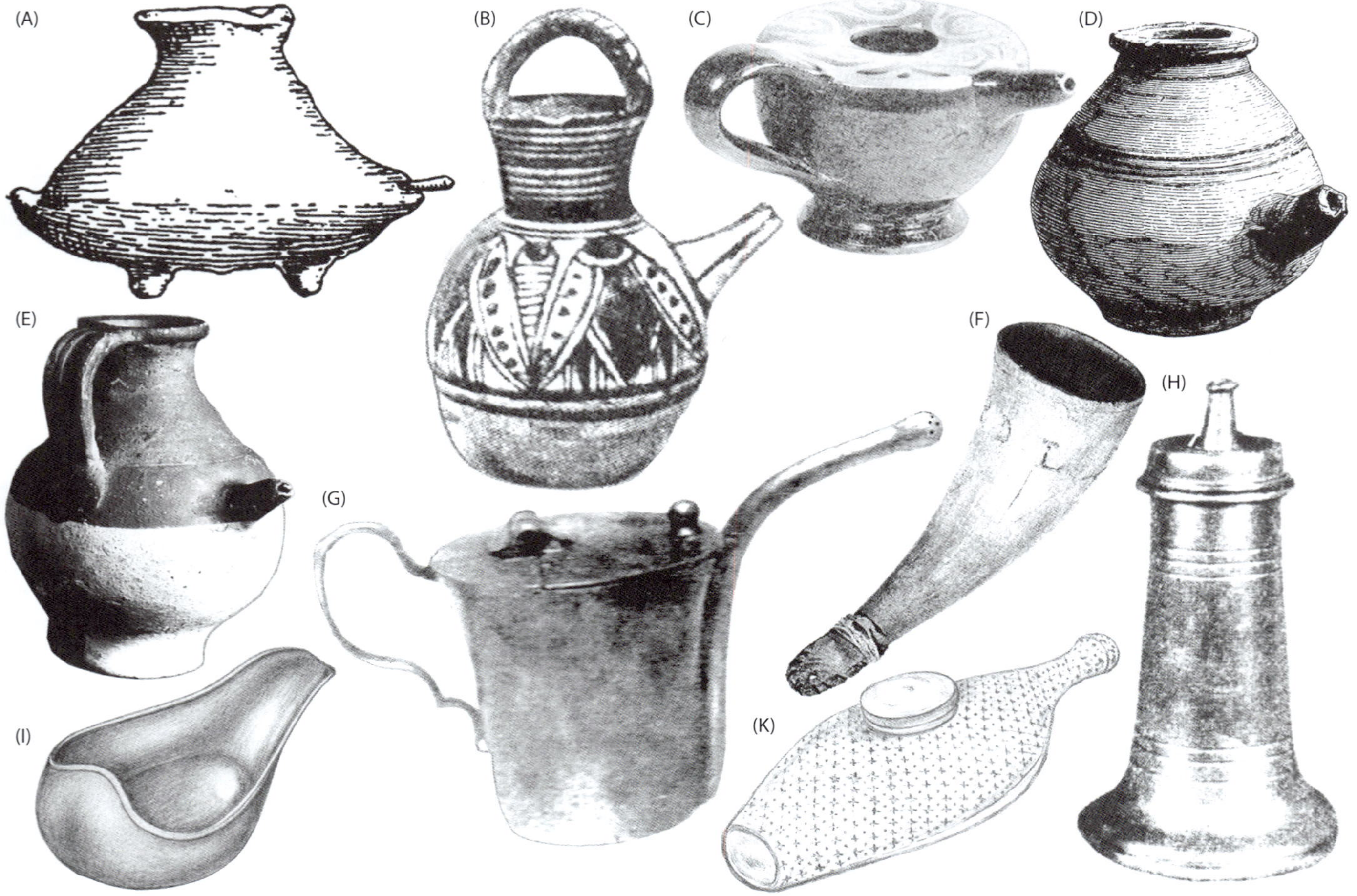

Fig. 6.4.1 Infant feeders from different cultures used before 1860: A, four-footed terracotta jug, Nierstein, late Bronze Age, ca. 1400 B.C.E. (Roman Museum Cologne); B, Mycenic-style painted earthenware, Cyprus, 10th century B.C.E. (Metropolitan Museum New York); C, varnished clay guttus, Greek, 5th century B.C.E.; D, clay, Gallo-Roman, ca. 100 C.E. (Roman Museum Cologne); E, clay, Germanic-Roman, ca. 300 C.E. (Roman Museum Cologne); F, cow's horn with parchment tip, Sweden ca. 1740 (Nordisk Museum Stockholm); G, spouted tin feeder ('bubby pot') from Britain, ca. 1780 (Wellcome Museum London); H, screw capped pewter bottle, Germany, ca. 1780 (Drake Collection, Toronto); I, open silver pap-boat, France ca. 1820 (Dufour collection, Fécamp Museum); K, capped china pap-boat, Britain, ca. 1830 (Drake Collection, Toronto).

discerned three types in 1565 [26]: '(1), *Souppe de pain*: cut little pieces of bread and, having removed the crust, soak them in one of the following liquids, and when they are dissolved, knead them with the fingers ... (2), *panade*: the soft part of the bread is grated or kneaded, put with a broth of good meat into a small covered pot, and is cooked on small coal fire while being continuously stirred with a silver or wooden spoon ... It may be cooked with vegetable broth or, more often, with milk from a goat or a cow ... (3), *bouillie*: is made from cow's milk and rice or wheat flour, or the soft part of white bread, cooked together until it thickens, sometimes yolk or eggwhite is added, and it is applied with a horn perforated at both sides, one end adapted similar to a teat.' Fig. 6.4.2 shows an example of pap used for a neonate in 1470, and Fig. 6.4.3 shown that even under difficult perinatal conditions breastfeeding was avoided in favour of pap.

The 17th and 18th centuries

In 1643, Jacques Guillemeau [27] recommended recipes similar to Vallambert's: ' In the beginning, one should give *pannade*, or infants soup ... The white part of dry bread should be grated to make it soft and soluble. Then it should be placed into a small varnished vessel with well seasoned broth of calf, fowl, or sheep ... For *bouillie*, we take cow's milk ... it should be neither too thick nor too liquid ... The flour is cooked carefully and dissolves, the milk should not lose its watery substance.' Ambroise Paré specified in 1573 [28]: 'Pap ... must be answerable [similar] in thickness to the milk, so that it may not be difficult to be concocted or digested. For pap hath these three conditions, so that it bee made with wheaten flower, and that not crude, but boiled: let it bee put into a new earthen pot or pipkin, and so set into an oven at the time when bread is set thereinto to bee baked.' This does not mean that artificial feeding was ever safe. Men entered midwifery and became aware of infants' needs, and authors began to shake their heads when mothers could not or would not breastfeed, as Walter Harris in 1742 [29]: 'But let us take a survey of the Advantages that prompt Mothers so commonly to sacrifice their beloved Offspring. They are the more free Enjoyment of Diversions; the greater Niceness of adorning their Persons; the Opportunity of receiving impertinent Visits, and returning those insipid Favours; the more frequent

Table 6.4.1 Recipes for homemade pap, panada, or gruel 1473–1851

Author, reference	Year, place	Pap	Panada	Gruel and others
Metlinger [23] A, S, W	1473 Augsburg	One-fourth goat's milk	White bread, sugar, milk	–
Vallambert [26] A, W	1565 Orleans	Sieved flour, goat's milk, egg yolk, honey	Breadcrumbs, legume or meat broth, egg yolk	Souppe de pain: breadcrumbs, water
Paré [28] A, W	1573 Paris	Wheat flour, milk	–	–
Van Helmont cited from [16]	1612 Brussels	Barley bread in water, milk	–	–
Guillemeau [27] A, W	1643 Paris	Cow's or goat's milk, flour, sugar, butter	Breadcrumbs, calf or chicken broth	–
Mauriceau [40] A, S, W	1673 Paris	Baked wheat flour, cow's milk, water	–	–
Culpeper cited from [16]	1676 London	Barley bread in water, milk	–	–
Ettmüller [41] A, W	1699 Leipzig	Flour, milk	White bread, milk, egg yolk, aniseed	–
The Nurse's Guide [42] S, W	1729 London	Fine baked flour, cooked in milk, salt	–	–
Cadogan [30] A, S, W	1748 Bristol	Bread, water, unboiled milk	Bread, meat broth	Rice, water
Smellie [43] S	1752 Edinburgh	Loaf bread, water, cow's milk	Loaf bread, broth of fowl or mutton	Oatmeal, water
Ballexserd [32] A, W	1762 Paris	Bread crust or baked flour, milk, butter	Baked flour, beef broth	Rice water
Raulin [33] S, W	1769 Paris	Cow's or goat's milk, honey, water, egg	Dry bread or biscuit, water, oil/butter, honey	Rye or oatmeal, water, aniseed
Armstrong [35] A, S, W	1771 London	Dry roll/biscuit, water, cow's milk, sugar	Breadcrumbs, water	–
Baudelocque [44] A, S, W	1781 Paris	Diluted cow's or goat's milk, flour, water, sugar	–	Barley, water
Moss [45] A, S	1781 Liverpool	Dry bread, water; milk, sugar	Bread, water, sugar	Oatmeal, sugar, water
Underwood [46] S, W	1784 London	Bread roll, water, cow's milk, sugar	Bread, meat broth	Barley, water
Smith [37] S, W	1792 London	Cow's milk, water, brown sugar	Mixture of milk and broth	Rice, cinnamon, water
Hamilton [47] A, S, W	1813 Edinburgh	Cow's milk, bread, water	Spoon meat, milk, broth	Arrowroot, water, milk
Henke [48] S, W	1821 Erlangen	Rusk cooked in 2 parts water, 1 part cow's milk, sugar	Rusk cooked in calf broth or thin beer	Rice or barley in water
Meissner [49] S, W	1844 Leipzig	Rusk, milk, water, later egg yolk	Rusk in fennel tea or pigeon broth	Fennel tea
Barrett [50] A, S, W	1851 Bath	Rusk in warm water, milk, sugar	Crust of bread, sugar, milk/broth	Oatmeal, prepared barley, water

First column identifies the available (not necessarily the first) edition, and the type of artificial feeding: A, additive to breastfeeding; S, substitute for breastfeeding; W, use after weaning. Van Helmont and Culpeper cited from Fildes [16]. Proportions were usually not provided, the mixtures cooked for 10–30 min.

Attendance on the Theatre, or the spending the greatest Part of the Night on their beloved Cards.'

Handfeeding was near generally practised in most foundling hospitals, but not in Bristol, where director William Cadogan wrote in 1750 [30]: 'If I could prevail, no Child should ever be cramm'd with any unnatural Mixture ... nor afterwards fed with any ungenial alien Diet whatever, the first three Months ... most mother cannot, or will not undertake the troublesome Task of suckling their own Children ... I am very glad, that [artificial feeding] is not the method of the hospital.' In 1753, the London apothecary James Nelson described the dilemma: 'Where [breastmilk] cannot be obtain'd, then Cows-milk, made thinner and lighter by the addition of water, is to supply its place ... I have often seen Children wash'd away with the watery Gripes, when it appeared they had no other Food but Water-Pap' [31]. Despite the head-shaking, most authors provided recipes for farinaceous pap and gruel made from sheep's milk and barley

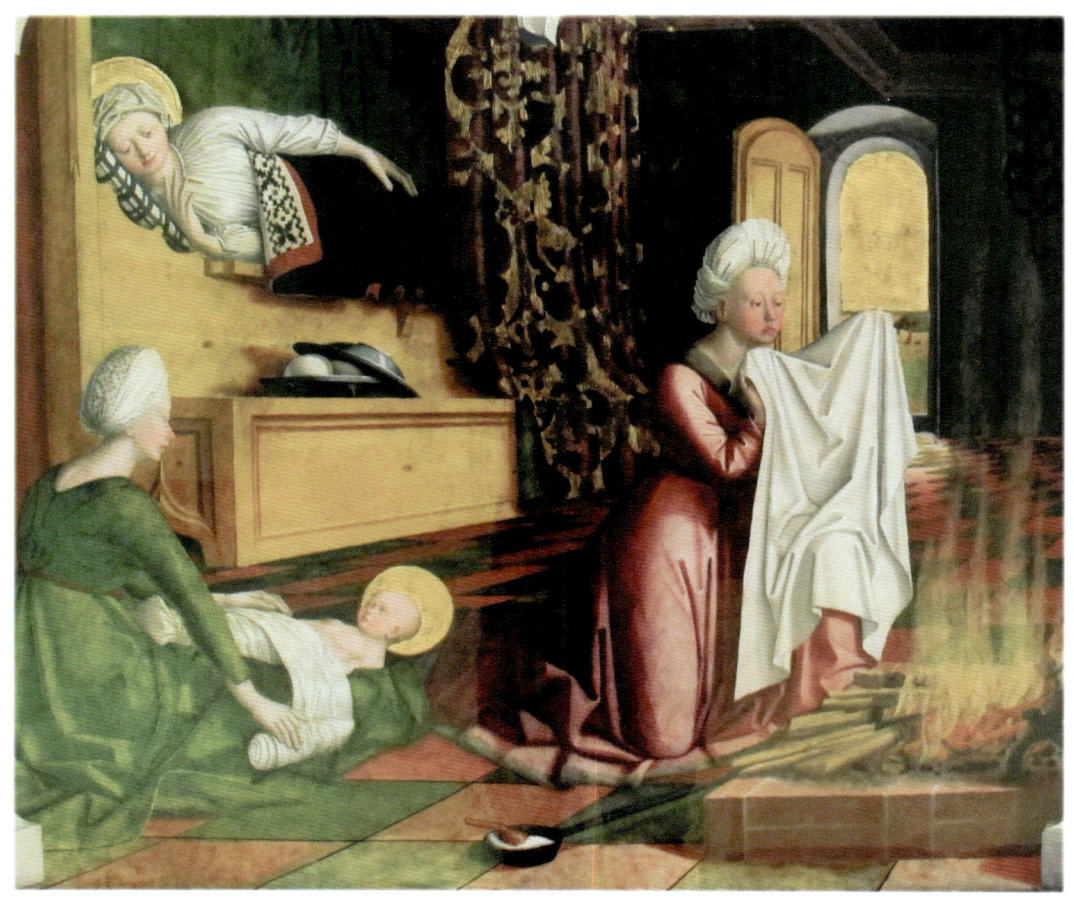

Fig. 6.4.2 Altarpiece showing the birth of Virgin Mary, mother's postpartum meal is waiting on a sideboard, infant's first food in a pap-pan on the floor.
Master of Uttenheim, ca. 1470, Germanisches Nationalmuseum Nürnberg, Gm 1180, with permission.

flour (Table 6.4.1). Several of them knew that pap made from baked flour, breadcrumbs, rusk, or biscuit was better tolerated than pap made of fresh flour. Jacques Ballexserd described roasting in 1762 [32]: 'Unfermented flour sours in the stomach … therefore it must be baked first; for this effect, it is put into the oven in a large pan, and stirred from time to time. The pap made from this baked flour is less noxious than the ordinary pap.' Joseph Raulin confessed in 1770 [33]: 'In all parts of the world there are cities and many families who raise their infants with cow's or goat's milk … In Montreuil-sur-Mer it's the exclusive way of infant feeding.'

Alexander Hamilton was not in favour of hand-feeding in 1781 [34]: 'Nothing can be more ridiculous than an opinion some have entertained, that milk of other animals is preferable to that of the child's mother or that an infant can be reared by any other food better than by that provided by nature.' His advice for weaning was less natural: 'There can be no harm in giving the child a little weak white-wine whey, diluted brandy punch, or even a tea-spoonful or two of syrup of poppy, for a few nights after weaning, to prevent restlessness and fits of crying, till the breast is forgotten.' Eighteenth-century authors deplored and discouraged the use of breast milk substitutes and gave advice while blushing, such as Armstrong in 1771 [35]: 'Though I am no advocate for bringing up children by hand, as it is called, … I thought it might not be impertinent to offer a few directions about dry-nursing.' Dutch professor of surgery Peter Camper wrote in 1777 [36]: 'Usually infants suck milk or whey from a tinpot whose spout is covered with soft leather. But simultaneously they suck much air with it. To alleviate this fault, the spout canal was extended to the pot's bottom; but then much force was needed to suck up the liquid.' Hugh Smith described a similar vessel in 1792 which combined the advantages of a sauce-boat with the convenience of a sucking-teat and was called 'bubby-pot' [37]: 'An infant in the first month will receive from one pint of milk more real and good nourishment, than from ten quarts of pap … I frequently order milk and broth to be mixed together, and think it proper food … This pot is somewhat in form like an urn; it contains a little more than a quarter of a pint … The neck of the spout is a little raised, and forms a roundish knob, somewhat in appearance like a small heart; this is perforated by three or four small holes: a piece of fine rag is tied loosely over it, which serves the child to play with instead of the nipple.' Cookbooks and housefather literature addressing the laity of the 18th century often contained recipes for pap, gruel, or panada [38, 39].

The 19th century

With industrialization, mothers went out to work, and the 7th edition of Hamilton's book noted in 1813 [47]: 'Pap and panada

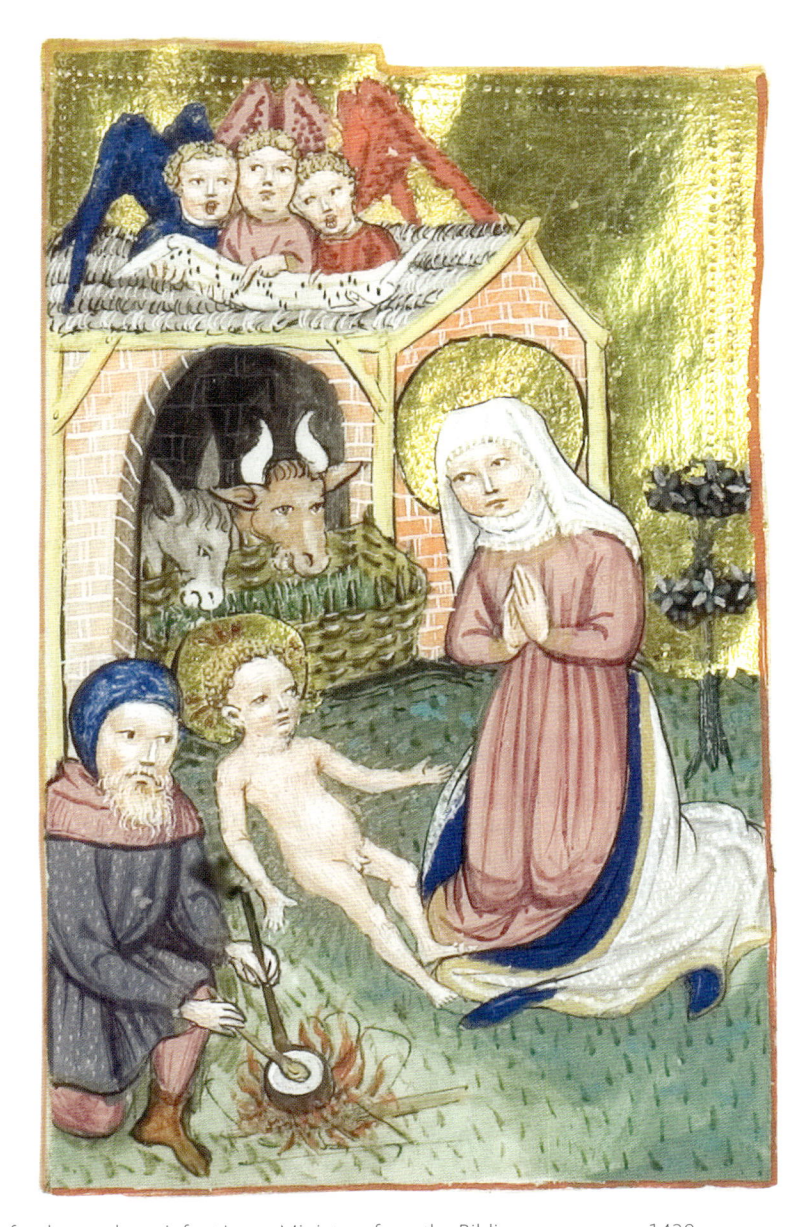

Fig. 6.4.3 Joseph cooking pap for the newborn infant Jesus. Miniature from the Biblia pauperum ca. 1430. Heidelberg University Library, Cod. Pal. Germ 148, with permission.

be now almost universally used for the first food of infants, as a substitute for mother's milk.' Another piece of evidence specific for this era is the abundance of patents concerning infant bottles and mouthpieces: Theodore Drake collected 232 US patents from 1841 [51]. Munich hospital founder Hauner complained in 1853 [52]: 'The only beneficial nutrition [breastfeeding] has become rarer and rarer, especially in the large cities, where the rich from idleness, the employed from work burden, and the unmarried from the need to resume service, all fail to nurse their offspring themselves.' A *Lancet* editorial of 1858 [53] referred to Schöpf-Merei's statistics from Manchester, where 'the majority of mothers in the operative ranks are unable to discharge satisfactorily the duties of mothers and the mortality amongst young children during one year amounted to 55.4 per cent'. In Derby, 20% of the infants born in 1900–1903 were never breastfed, and 17% only briefly [54].

Gastroenteritis/cholera infantum

Hand-feeding was associated with diarrhoea in the earliest books. Paul Bagellardo held *fluxus ventris* (diarrhoea) to be caused by a corruption or excess of milk in 1472 [55] and Walter Harris wrote in 1742 [29]: 'From the middle of July to about the middle of September, the Epidemical Gripes of Children are so rife every Year, that more of them usually die in one Month, than in three or four at any other Time: For the Heat of that Season commonly weakens them at least, if it does not entirely exhaust their Strength.' Hugh Smith analysed

London child burials from 1762 to 1771, and concluded [37]: 'The thrush and watery gripes are, in the author's opinion, artificial diseases, and both of them totally occasioned by improper food, such as all kinds of pap, whether made from flour, bread, or biscuit; they all cause too much fermentation in an infant's stomach, and irritate their tender bowels beyond what Nature can support.'

'Summer diarrhoea' accounted for two-thirds of the deaths of all infants [56], and even more in large towns as New York [57, 58]. Infection was suspected for centuries but not associated with living microorganisms invading the body. Persisting miasmatic doctrines (see Chapter 7.9) held bad air and weather changes responsible and neglected both milk-borne disease and infection transmitted by contaminated water. As late as 1900, McCook Weir believed that 'the cause is … fermentation in the alimentary canal. Heat is the leading factor, and direct solar heat will suffice without a higher ground temperature … a form of heat stroke with high temperature is present in almost all of these cases' [59]. Controlled trials and long-term studies were few and population or birth-based statistics rare. Louis Jurine of Geneva studied 52 artificially fed infants longitudinally in 1807 [60], some with bold diets: 'Observation 52: During the first ten days of life chicken broth was given, then panada of the same broth hoping to moderate abundant diarrhea. Soon this panada was followed by others prepared from butter and sugar and by veal broth … none of which ameliorated diarrhea. As the infant made no progress, chicken broth was resumed with the addition of Malaga wine, later substituted by a pap of flour, water, sugar, and egg yolk, which moderated diarrhea but provoked vomiting.' Remarkably, of 24 boys only three and of 28 girls only two died up to the age of 8 years. Despite the paucity of data, many authors held strong opinions, a phenomenon which accompanied the literature on artificial infant feeding up to the present day. Simard claimed in 1895 [61]: 'Wrongly directed artificial feeding is the main and almost sole cause of the very frequently fatal diseases of the digestive organs.'

In 1898, Holt stated [62]: 'The number of cases which cannot be managed by simply varying the different elements of cow's milk, is small …, the exceptions being premature and delicate infants.' The bacteriology of infantile diarrhoea was clarified by Theodor Escherich in 1885 [63], even though he initially held streptococci and not *Escherichia coli* for the pathogen. But the composition of breast-milk substitutes would remain overestimated and the hygiene of their preparation underestimated for decades.

Conclusion

The failure to breastfeed is no recent phenomenon. Literature and artefactual evidence reveal that it was widespread throughout history. It is unlikely that it originated from the availability of commercial formula. More probable reasons, each valid for significant parts of the population, included: (1) maternal death; (2) infant abandonment or admission to a foundling hospital; (3) lack of maternal milk, for whatever reason; (4) wet-nurses' own infants usually were deprived of their natural food; (5) decline of the wet-nursing business because of fear of milk-borne infection; (6) need for unmarried women to work; and (7) urbanization and industrialization urging women into paid outside work. The moralistic assumption that not need, but choice was a major motive for bottle-feeding originated in the 18th century. In the reality of urban life, however, it was often the only way to save the infant's life.

REFERENCES

1. Apple RD: Mothers and medicine. Madison, WI: University of Wisconsin Press, 1987: p. 4, 66.
2. Schwab MG: Mechanical milk. An essay on the social history of infant formula. Childhood 1996;**3**:479–97.
3. Mepham TB: "Humanizing" milk: the formulation of artificial feeds for infants (1850–1910). Med Hist 1993;**37**:225–49.
4. Weaver LT: "Growing babies": defining the milk requirements in infants 1890–1910. Soc Hist Med 2009;**23**:320–37.
5. Diamond J: Guns, germs, and steel. The fates of human societies. New York: Norton, 1999: p. 167.
6. Hall HR, Woolley CL: Ur Excavations. Volume 1: Al-'Ubaid. Oxford: Oxford University Press, 1927.
7. Aristotle: History of animals. London: Bell, 1883: Vol. **3**, chapter 20, p. 71.
8. Galen: De alimentorum facultatibus. Cambridge: Cambridge University Press, 2003: p. 123–5.
9. Temkin O: Soranus' Gynecology. Baltimore, MD: The Johns Hopkins Press, 1956: p. 79–117.
10. Eckardt H: The Colchester 'Child's Grave'. Britannia 1999;**30**:57–89.
11. Bókay Jv: Tönerne Sauggefäße aus dem Bronzezeitalter auf dem Gebiete Ungarns. Jahrb Kinderheilk 1937;**148**:226–8.
12. Huttmann A, Greiling H, Tillmanns U, Riedel M: Inhaltsanalysen römischer Säuglingstrinkgefässe. Kölner Jahrbuch für Vor- und Frühgeschichte 1989;**22**:365–72.
13. Brüning H: Geschichte der Methodik der künstlichen Säuglingsernährung. Stuttgart: Enke, 1908: p. 45–123.
14. Drake TGH: Infant feeding in England and in France from 1750 to 1800. Am J Dis Child 1930;**34**:1049–61.
15. Lacaille AD: Infant feeding bottles in prehistoric times. Proc R Soc Med 1950;**43**:565–8.
16. Fildes V: Breasts, bottles, and babies. Edinburgh: Edinburgh University Press, 1986: p. 98–121, 307.
17. Spaulding M, Welch P: Nurturing yesterday's child. Toronto: Natural Heritage/Natural History, 1994: p. 69–109.
18. Schäfer S, Marczoch L: Lampen der Antikensammlung. In: Archäologische Reihe. Frankfurt: Museum für Vor- und Frühgeschichte, 1990: Vol. **13**, p. 68.
19. Weinberg F: Infant feeding through the ages. Can Fam Physician. 1993;**39**:2016–20.
20. Nowell-Smith F: Feeding the nineteenth-century baby. Mater Hist Bull 1985;**21**:15–23.
21. Caulfield E: Infant feeding in Colonial America. J Pediatr 1952;**41**:673–87.
22. Cone TE: 200 years of feeding infants in America. Columbus, OH: Ross Laboratories, 1976: p. 17–92.
23. Metlinger B: Ein vast nützlich Regiment der jungen Kinder. Augsburg: Zainer, 1473: p. 9–17, Fol. 17.
24. Roelans von Mecheln C: Das Buch der Kinderkrankheiten. Übersetzt von: Hermann Brüning. Rostock, 1485: Vol. **3**, p. 17–107.
25. Phaire T: The boke of children. Edinburgh: Livingstone, 1955: p. 19–22.
26. Vallambert Sd: Cinq livres de la manière de nourrir et gouverner les enfants dès leur naissance. Reprint Droz, Geneve 2005. ed. Poitiers: Manefz et Bouchetz, 1565: p. 89–101, 112, 207–8.

27. Guillemeau J: De la grossesse et accouchement des femmes. Paris: Jost, 1643: p. 551–87.
28. Paré A: The workes of that famous chirurgion Ambrose Parey. Lib 24, chap. 23: How to make pap for children. London: Cotes and Du-gard, 1649: p. 610.
29. Harris W: A treatise of the acute diseases of infants. London: Astley, 1742: p. 17–8, 36.
30. Cadogan W: An essay upon nursing and the management of children. London: Roberts, 1750: p. 15, 18–27, 34.
31. Nelson J: An essay on the government of children. 2. ed. London: Dodsley, 1753: p. 66–71.
32. Ballexserd J: Dissertation sur l'éducation physique des enfans, depuis leur naissance jusqu'a l'âge de puberté. Paris: Vallat-la-Chapelle, 1762: p. 111.
33. Raulin J: Von Erhaltung der Kinder. Leipzig: Crusius, 1770: Vol. **2**, p. 182.
34. Hamilton A: A treatise of midwifery. Edinburgh: Dickson & Co, 1781: p. 384–5.
35. Armstrong G: An account of the diseases most incident to children. 2. ed. London: Cadell, 1783: p. 157–68.
36. Camper P: Betrachtungen über einige Gegenstände aus der Geburtshülfe und über die Erziehung der Kinder. Leipzig: Schneider, 1777: Vol. **2**, p. 33.
37. Smith H: Letters to married women on nursing. 6. ed. London: Kearsley, 1792: p. VII, 125–32, 189.
38. Liger L: Dictionaire pratique du bon menager de campagne et de ville. Paris: Ribou, 1715: p. 189.
39. Glasse M: The art of cookery, made plain and easy. London: Strahan, 1784: p. 243.
40. Mauriceau F: Tractat von Kranckheiten schwangerer und gebärender Weibspersonen. Basel: Bertsche, 1680: p. 332–47, 393.
41. Etmuller M: Etmullerus abridg'd; or, a compleat system of the theory and practice of physic. 2. ed. London: Bell and Wellington, 1703: p. 620–32.
42. Eminent Physician: The nurse's guide. London: Brotherton and Gilliver, 1729: p. 28–39.
43. Smellie W: A treatise on the theory and practise of midwifery. London: Sydenham Society, 1878: Vol. **1**, p. 425.
44. Baudelocque JL: De l'allaitement au biberon. In: Principes sur l'art des accouchemens. Paris: Méquignon, 1787: p. 313–9.
45. Moss W: An essay on the management and nursing of children. London: Johnson, 1781: p. 56.
46. Underwood M: A treatise on the disorders of childhood. 2. ed. London: Matthews, 1801: Vol. **3**, p. 157–78.
47. Hamilton A: A treatise on the management of female complaints. 7. ed. Edinburgh: Ramsay, 1813: p. 253–5.
48. Henke A: Handbuch zur Erkenntniß und Heilung der Kinderkrankheiten. 3. ed. Frankfurt: Wilmans, 1821: Vol. **1**, p. 89–106.
49. Meissner FL: Die Kinderkrankheiten nach den neusten Ansichten und Erfahrungen. 3. ed. Leipzig: Fest, 1844: Vol. **1**, p. 36–49.
50. Barrett T: Advice on the management of children in early infancy. Bath: Binns and Goodwin, 1851: p. 48.
51. Drake TGH: American infant feeding bottles, 1841 to 1946, as disclosed by United States Patent specifications. J Hist Med Allied Sci 1948;**3**:507–24.
52. Hauner A: Über Pflege und Wartung der Kinder in den ersten Lebensjahren. J Kinderkrankheit 1853;**21**:209–30.
53. Editorial: The murder of the innocents. Lancet 1858;**71**:345–6.
54. Howarth WJ: The influence of feeding on the mortality of infants. Lancet 1905;**166**:210–3.
55. Bagellardo P: Opusculum recens natum de morbis puerorum. Lyon: Barbou, 1538: Vol. **1**, p. 60.
56. Rietschel H: Die Sommersterblichkeit der Säuglinge. Erg Inn Med Kinderheilk 1910;**6**:369–490.
57. Straus LG: Disease in milk—the remedy: pasteurization. New York: Dutton, 1913: p. 47, 161.
58. LaFétra LE: The development of pediatrics in New York City. Arch Pediat 1932;**49**:36–60.
59. McCook Weir A: "Summer diarrhoea". BMJ 1900;**2**:459.
60. Jurine L: Abrégé d'un mémoire sur l'allaitement artificiel. Bibliothèque Universelle des Sciences (Genève) 1830;**43**:439–51.
61. Simard A, Fortier R: Notes concerning the nourishment of children in their earliest infancy. J Am Public Health Assoc 1895;**20**:367–79.
62. Holt LE: The diseases of infancy and childhood. New York: Appleton, 1898: p. 159, 184.
63. Escherich T: Die Darmbakterien des Neugeborenen und Säuglings. Fortschr Med 1885;**3**:512–22; 547–55.

6.5 Milk demystified by chemistry

Introduction

Early cultures regarded milk not as a simple nutrient, but a living fluid, the elixir of life. Several mythologies maintained that clustered stars in the universe originated from milk. The term galaxy (via lactis, Milky Way, Milchstrasse) is derived from a Greek myth. The newborn Heracles, the story goes, was removed from his mother Alcmene and carried to the breast of the sleeping Hera. Awaking, she indignantly pushed the child (fruit of her husband's unfaithfulness) away, spilling her milk over heaven. Hindu mythology connected the origin of the galaxy to the celestial bitch Sarama crossing the sky and scattering her milk [1]. The following chapter traces the deep fall of milk from a heavenly elixir to a tradeable nutrient.

Milk myths

In India, veneration of the cow originated in the Vedic Period and was based on a mystical relationship between the cow and the universe. The Rig-Veda (1500 B.C.E.) described sacrificing butter to have sins forgiven [2]. From Abraham's time (2000 B.C.E.), ancient Hebrews likewise used milk and butter as a sacrifice [Genesis 18:8]. For Moses, milk symbolized wealth and peace with the promise 'to bring them … unto a land flowing with milk and honey' [Exodus 3:8]. At Salomo's time (970–930 B.C.E.), Hebrews regarded milk a nutrient: 'And thou shalt have goats' milk enough for thy food' [Proverbs 27:27]. In Egypt, cows were consecrated to Isis. The cow-headed goddess Hathor personified motherhood and was believed to help women in childbirth. Greek mythology held that Zeus had been hidden from his father's wrath in a cavern in Crete, where he was nourished by the goat-nymph Amalthea (Fig. 6.5.1) [3]. As it decayed so rapidly, animal milk was generally not available in antiquity except in the form of cheese. But Athen's nobility used it as a remedy in 367 B.C.E. [4]: 'Timagoras … wanted cow's milk for some ailment.' Romans ascribed their strength to the belief that the city founders Romulus and Remus had been nourished by a she-wolf. Roman Emperor Caesar (ca. 50 B.C.E.) was astonished that the Germanic peoples 'have no zeal for agriculture, and the greater part of their food consists of milk, cheese, and flesh' [5]. And Tacitus wrote in Germania (100 C.E.) [6]: 'Their foods are simple, wild fruits, fresh game, or curdled milk.'

The Christian attitude towards milk was not rational: St Peter attributed spiritual power to it [1. Peter 2:2]: 'As newborn babes, desire the sincere milk of the word, that ye may grow thereby.' The *milk of salvation* became a symbol for piety and eternal peace, and Augustinus wrote in the *Confessions* (398 C.E.) [7]: 'The name of my Saviour had my tender heart even together with my mother's milk devoutly drunken in.' Character traits and emotions were believed to be transmitted by milk, infantile diseases were attributed to 'bad milk' (see Chapter 6.1); while 'good milk' (also of human origin) was used as a remedy for a host of diseases [8, 9]. Some cultures regarded infants breastfed by the same woman as milk siblings. Islamic law codified the relationship between such individuals, the Koran forbade them to marry each other [10]. A book entirely devoted to milk was published by Conrad Gesner in 1541 [11].

Milk of different mammals

In the 4th century B.C.E., Aristotle knew that milk of different species varied in composition, and discerned watery, cheesy, and oily compounds [12]: 'There is more cheese in cow's milk than in goat's milk.' Galen also wrote about differences in milk [13]: 'Cow's milk is very thick and fatty, while milk from the camel is very liquid and much less fatty; and next to the latter animal is that from mares, and following this, ass's milk. Goat's milk is well proportioned in its composition, but ewe's milk is thicker.' In the 10th edition of *Systema Naturae* published in 1758, Carl Linné replaced Aristotle's taxonomic term *quadrupedia* by *mammalia*, characterizing the entire class by its ability to suckle milk [14].

More detailed analyses of different animals' milk were published in the middle of the 18th century (Table 6.5.1). Usually they underestimated the carbohydrate content (by analysing ethanolic extracts), and overestimated the amount of protein (by weighing the coagulum). Measurements taken by Boyssou and of Van Stipriaan and colleagues became widely known when Michael Underwood reproduced them in his *Treatise on the Diseases of Children* [15], which went through more than ten editions from 1784 to 1848. Some mystery remained, as the methods were not precise. But all authors understood that human milk was higher in sugar and lower in protein than cow's milk. Hugh Smith pointed out in 1792 [16]: 'Asses'

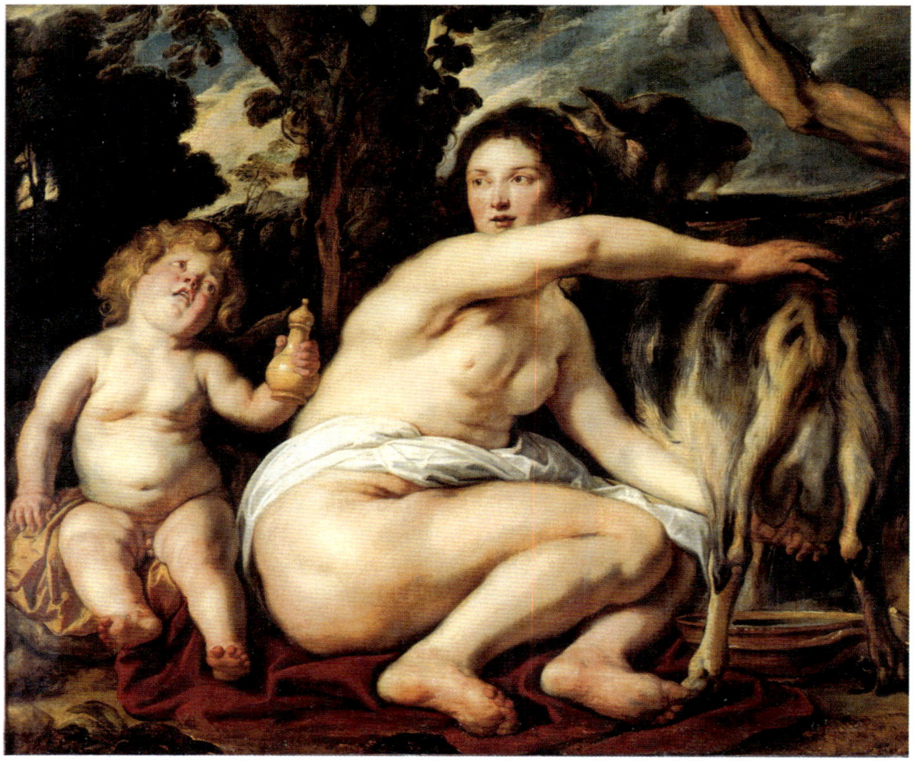

Fig. 6.5.1 Heroes and gods were believed to be nurtured by animals after being abandoned. Zeus nourished by the she-goat Amalthea assisted by a nymph and a wooden bottle. Detail of a painting by Jacob Jordaens, 1640.
Grand Palais, Musé du Louvre, Paris. Photo RMN, Jean-Gilles Berizzi, with permission.

milk is generally allowed to be the nearest to the human, and according to the above experiments we find it so, abounding mostly with whey, and having little of the cream or curd in it.' Once the dissimilarities in milk composition were understood, it was a logical step to alter animal milk to make it 'resemble' human milk.

In 1838, Berlin chemist Franz Simon analysed and compared the constituents of human, cow, and dog milk [22], finding casein contents of 3.4–4.0%, 6.8–7.2%, and 14.6–17.4%, lactose contents of 4.3–7.0%, 2.8–3.0%, and 2.9–3.0%, and fat contents of 0.8–5.4%, 3.8–4.0%, and 13.3–16.2%, respectively. His figures were still too high for protein and too low for sugar, but his analysis was widely cited and translated into German and English. As late as 1853, Vernois and Becquerel published a mean percentage of 4.3% sugar, 3.9% casein, and 2.7% fat for human milk [23]. It was Arthur Vincent Meigs of Philadelphia who in 1884 reported that human milk contained 1.05% protein and 7.4% sugar [24], measurements very similar to present day analyses. Milk analyses had little impact as long as no infant food was produced commercially. In 1853, Ploss compiled 67 remarkably different proposals for breast milk substitutes published within 50 years [25], and concluded: 'It is high time to follow different paths

Table 6.5.1 Eighteenth-century milk analyses of various mammal species, compared with 1925 measurements

Weight (%)	Rang, Spielmann 1753 [17] Strasbourg			Young 1776 [18] Edinburgh		Boyssou 1790 [19] Aurillac, Auvergne			Van Stipriaan Luiscio, Bondt 1790 [20] Delft/Amsterdam				Powers 1925 [21] New Haven, CT		
Species	Cream	Butter	Cheese	Sach.salt	Res.	Sach.salt	Butter	Cheese	Sugar	Cream	Butter	Cheese	Carb.	Fat	Protein
Women	4.69	2.34	1.56	3.18	1.11	4.43	3.65	1.30	7.31	8.69	3.00	2.69	7.3	4.0	1.5
Cows	7.81	2.34	9.37	2.78	1.10	3.56	2.83	4.46	3.06	4.06	2.69	8.94	4.7	3.5	3.5
Goats	3.12	1.17	10.5	2.51	1.35	2.34	3.39	5.99	4.37	7.94	4.56	9.12	4.3	4.0	4.6
Asses	1.17	–	1.17	4.22	1.03	4.86	0.11	2.22	4.50	2.94	–	3.31	6.1	1.3	1.8
Sheep	6.24	5.47	12.5	1.77	–	2.34	4.34	5.79	4.19	11.6	5.81	15.7	5.0	7.0	5.6
Mares	1.17	–	6.63	3.62	0.98	3.65	0.07	2.08	9.06	0.81	–	1.62	5.8	1.1	2.5

Original measurements were converted into weight percentages (Ancien Régime measures: livre = librum, 490 g; once = uncia, 30.6 g; gros = drachma, 3.82 g; grain = granum, 53 mg. Young study based on apothecary measures: Troy pound = librum, 373 g; ounce = uncia, 31.1 g; drachm, 3.89 g; grain, 65 mg) (Alberti, 1957; Zupko, 1990). Largely, *butter* corresponds to fat and *cheese* to protein. In the study of Rang and Spielmann, *cream* corresponds to phlegm and includes carbohydrates. In the studies of Young and Boyssou, *sach. salt*, saccharine salt, corresponds to sugar. In the study of Young, *Res.*, residue, corresponds to protein and fat insoluble in water. The two 1790 studies were submitted simultaneously for a prize sponsored by the Paris Royal Society of Medicine.

than heretofore and to develop generally valid rules.' However, it was not the scientists who followed new paths, but the manufacturers of proprietary infant food. Paediatricians had nothing to counter these developments: in 1925, Grover Powers of Yale studied no fewer than 27 milk mixtures available on the US market [21].

The body, a chemical factory

In 1553, Servetus had paid with his life for replacing the holy spirit by pulmonary gas exchange. Scheele und Priestley had isolated oxygen in 1772, but it was Antoine Lavoisier who drew the far-reaching conclusions and envisioned the living body as a biochemical factory in 1785. The French Revolution shattered nutritional myths and opened the door for the secularization of science. Rational doctrines, however, disregarded the highly emotional aspect of breastfeeding. Lavoisier's ideas were corroborated by the experimental physiologist Claude Bernard, and applied to infant feeding by Justus von Liebig. It was no coincidence that Liebig had trained in Paris from 1822 with Joseph Gay-Lyssac, who was a student of Lavoisier.

Scientific feeding: the percentage method

Observing the striking association between infant mortality and hand-feeding, and underestimating the importance of bacterial infection, the pioneers of paediatrics sought the cause in unwholesome composition of the nutrients. From 1880 to 1920, the printing press was extensively used in the quest for the philosopher's stone—the appropriate formula composition. The most influential person in this endeavour was Thomas Morgan Rotch, from 1893 head of Boston Children's Hospital. It was his theory that slight changes (even fractions of a per cent) in the proportions of sugar, fat, and protein could seriously affect an infant's health, growth, and development [26]. He established the Walker-Gordon Laboratory in Boston and by 1907, in 20 other US cities [27]. Ironically and tragically, although Rotch intended to promote breastfeeding, he became America's promoter of hand-feeding: formulas became so complex that they had to be prepared in commercial laboratories. By complicating the percentage method even further, Rotch wanted to consolidate the young specialty of paediatrics. However, paediatricians complained about the mathematics required for the prescription and there were no genuinely scientific methods to study the pros and cons of artificial feeding. All this activity ultimately paved the way for industrially produced formula, which was easy to prepare. Grover Powers noticed in 1925 [21] that 'the multitude of milk mixtures are essentially alike or identical except in concentration' and proposed 'to express their constitution in terms of their actual nutrients independent of the medium, water, in which they are carried'. This proposal modified percentage feeding and remained the preferred method to characterize infant foods in America.

Calorimetry

On the other side of the Atlantic, infant feeding became complicated in a different manner. In 1777, Laplace and Lavoisier used an ice calorimeter (Fig. 6.5.2A) to measure heat production and oxygen consumption in guinea pigs [28]: 'Respiration is therefore a combustion, much slower, but perfectly similar to that of carbon.' In 1848, Claude Bernard demonstrated that the liver metabolizes all kinds of food into sugar, thereby fuelling tissue respiration [29]. More sophisticated and reliable calorimeters were developed by Regnault and Reiset in Paris in 1849 [30] and by Pettenkofer and Voit in Munich in 1866 [31], and were soon applied to study neonatal nutrition: in Munich in 1877, Josef Forster used the Pettenkofer calorimeter with an open circuit to study infants aged 2 and 7 weeks. He found that even hungry infants produced twice as much carbon dioxide and metabolized twice the amount of fat as adults [32]. At the Prague Foundling Hospital in 1895, Franz Scherer modified Regnault's calorimeter with a closed respiratory chamber (Fig. 6.5.2C,D) to study the influence of ambient temperature on the metabolism of 85 breastfed infants [33]: in winter at a mean temperature of 13.6°C, their oxygen consumption during the first week was 685 mL/kg/h as compared to 529 mL/kg/h in summer at a mean temperature of 20.1°C.

Max Rubner had modified the Pettenkofer apparatus and performed metabolic studies for years in Munich and Marburg, proving that the thermodynamic laws are valid in the living mammal. After being called to Berlin, with Otto Heubner he studied a breastfed boy aged 5 weeks for 9 days in 1897 [34]. The boy produced 0.94 g CO_2 and 1.6 g H_2O per kg and hour, his nitrogen uptake was 0.99 g per day, whereof the accretion was 0.26 g per day. The energy content of the breastmilk was 61–72 Cal/100 mL, and the infant's energy consumption was 2.93 Cal per kg and hour. A year later, Rubner and Heubner repeated the study with an artificially fed infant [35]. Their data enabled another form of 'scientific' feeding guided by the energy quotient in Cal/kg/day.

Regulated feeding

In 1906, Adalbert Czerny and Arthur Keller of Breslau published a voluminous book on child nutrition [36] which established the idea that infants should be fed at fixed times, five meals per day, and which impeded breastfeeding for decades. Social-Darwinistic theories basing education on uniformity and care on obedience shaped German paediatrics for half a century. Diarrhoeal diseases, the authors believed, were caused from 'too much' of certain nutrients, especially flour ('Mehlnährschaden') or cooked milk ('Milchnährschaden'). In France, where many infants were hand-fed in the 19th century, Pierre Budin studied the growth of numerous artificially fed infants and recommended not exceeding a cow's milk volume equivalent to 10% bodyweight to avoid overfeeding [37]. In 1898, Abraham Jacobi mocked the paediatricians' recommendations [38]: 'No subject has been treated more extensively, more eagerly, sometimes even more spitefully, than that of infant feeding. The philosopher's stone has not been so anxiously sought for nor so often found in medical journals, books, and societies as the correct infant food and the appropriate treatment of cow's milk.' Jacobi alluded to the enrichment with fat by Gaertner [39], with 'second carbohydrate' by Czerny and Keller [36], and with protein by Finkelstein [40]. Despite hundreds of ever-more accurate analyses of human milk, the medical

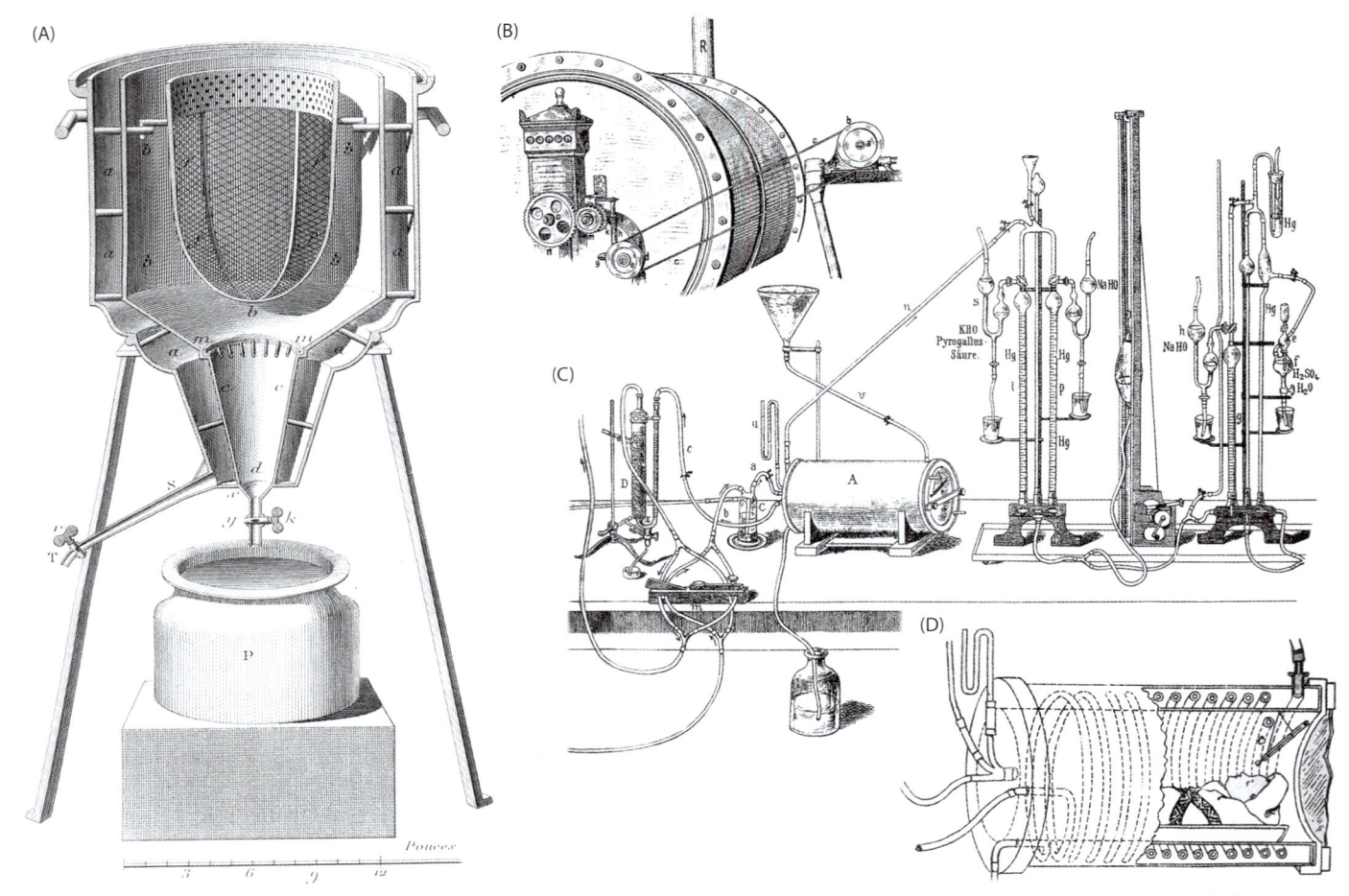

Fig. 6.5.2 Calorimeters used to measure respiration and energy metabolism. A, ice calorimeter used by Lavoisier and Laplace in 1777 [28]; B, Rubner's respiration apparatus of 1889 used in conjunction with a Pettenkofer calorimeter to measure energy uptake in neonates [34]; C, Scherer's modification of Regnault's calorimeter used to measure neonatal oxygen consumption in summer and winter of 1895 [33]; D, infant respiration chamber of Scherer's calorimeter.

profession remained quite uncertain as to the appropriate composition of nutritional substitutes.

Decline of breastfeeding

In 1906 Emil von Behring asserted prosaically 'In a town like Berlin more than two-thirds of the babies must be bottle-fed' [41]. David Forsyth stated for Britain in 1911 [42]: 'The period of sucking has been steadily growing shorter from the middle ages until now.' Twenty per cent of the infants born in Derby from 1900 to 1903 were never breastfed, and 17% only briefly [43]. In eight US cities surveyed from 1911 to 1915, at 12 months of age 13% of infants had been exclusively breastfed and 45% partially breastfed [44]. The American decline of breastfeeding rates began in the 19th century and was most pronounced between the two world wars [45]. It reached its all-time low in 1971, when less than 25% of infants in the US were initially breastfed and only 14% between 2 and 3 months of age. Then began a slow resurgence of breastfeeding, and by 1998, two-thirds of infants were breastfed initially and 50% at 3 months of age [46].

The present research focuses are the immune function and the neuroprotection of breastmilk and its supplementation for the needs of immature infants.

Conclusion

Secularization during the French Revolution de-emotionalized infant nutrition. Chemical methods and calorimetric studies promoted understanding of milk's composition and energy metabolism. At the end of the 19th century, microbiology transformed artificial nutrition from a risky custom to a rational system. Experts' opinions on nutrition were highly discrepant and their recommendations largely unsuccessful, and over the long term had no chance against the corroborating basics of food chemistry. The attempt of physicians to claim infant nutrition as their responsibility failed because it was contaminated by empiricism, tradition, moral prejudices, and selfishness—and because it neglected the emotional aspect of infant feeding. Demystification made artificial nutrition safer for infants, but it also paved the way for commercially produced proprietary formulas. This approach ignored the anti-infective properties of human milk which contains antibodies, complement, lysozyme, lactoperoxidase, lactoferrin, and cellular components. Establishment of rules for artificial feeding did not encourage breastfeeding but paid lip service to 'breast is best', more often based on persistent mystical beliefs in 'living milk' than on scientifically sound information on its properties.

REFERENCES

1. Kramrisch S: The Indian Great Goddess. Hist Religions 1975;**14**:235–65.
2. Siqueira TN: Sin and salvation in the early Rig-Veda. Anthropos 1933;**28**:179–88.
3. Ovidii Nasonis P: Fastorum libri sex. Fast. 5, chapter 115. London: Macmillan, 1929: p. 255.
4. Plutarch: Lives of illustrious men. Volume 5: Pelopidas. Book 30. Loeb Classical Library 87. London: Heinemann, 1968: p. 419.
5. Caesar GJ: The Gallic war. Book 6, chapter 22. Loeb Classical Library 72. Cambridge, MA: Harvard University Press, 1970: p. 347.
6. Tacitus: Germany. Cap. 23. Warminster, England: Aris & Phillips, 1999: p. 37.
7. Augustine: Confessions. Book 3, chapter 4. Loeb's classical library 26. London: Heinemann, 1977: p. 112.
8. Hentschel G: De seri lactis virtute longe saluberrima. Halae Magdeburgicae: Hilligei, 1725.
9. Petit-Radel P: Essai sur le lait, considéré médicinalement sous ses differens aspects. Paris: Boudet, 1786.
10. The Koran. Sura 4, 23. Translated from the Arabic by: John M. Rodwell. London: Dent, 1963: p. 413.
11. Gesner C: Libellus de lacte et operibus lactariis philologus pariter ac medicus. Tiguri: Froschauer, 1541.
12. Aristotle: History of animals. London: Bell, 1883: Vol. **3**, chapter 20, p. 71.
13. Galen: De alimentorum facultatibus. Cambridge: Cambridge University Press, 2003: p. 123–5.
14. Linnaeus C: Systema naturae per regna triae naturae. 10. ed. Holmiae: Salvius, 1758: Vol. **1**, Animalia.
15. Underwood M: A treatise on the disorders of childhood. 2. ed. London: Matthews, 1801: Vol. **3**, p. 157–78.
16. Smith H: Letters to married women on nursing. 6. ed. London: Kearsley, 1792: p. VII, 125–32, 189.
17. Rang BH: De optimo infantis recens nati alimento. Diss. sub praeside de Jac. Reinboldus Spielmann. Reprinted in: Delectus dissertationum medicarum Argentoratensium, Nuremberg 1777, pp. 49–91: Strasbourg: Heitz, 1753.
18. Young T: Dessertatio medica de natura et usu lactis in diversis animalibus. Edinburgi: Drummond, 1776.
19. Boyssou L: Recherches sur la nature et les propriétés physiques et chymiques des differens laits de femme, de vache, de chèvre, d'anesse, de brebis et de jument. Hist Mém Soc Roy Méd 1790;**9**:615–27.
20. Van-Stipriaan Luiscio A, Bondt N: Dissertatio in qua determinetur, per examen comparatum proprietatum physicarum et chemicarum, natura lactis muliebris, vaccini, caprilli, asinini, ovilli et equini. Hist Mém Soc Roy Méd 1790;**9**:525–40.
21. Powers GF: Comparison and interpretation on a caloric basis of the milk mixtures used in infant feeding. Am J Dis Child 1925;**30**:453–75.
22. Simon JF: De lacte muliebris ratione chemica et physiologica. Berolini: Inaug.-Diss, 1838.
23. Vernois AGM, Becquerel A: Recherches sur le lait. Deuxieme partie. Ann Hyg Publ Med Leg 1853;**50**:43–147.
24. Meigs AV: Proof that human milk contains only about one percent casein: with remarks on infant feeding. Arch Pediatr 1884;**1**:216–41.
25. Ploss HH: Ueber das Aufziehen der Kinder ohne Brust. J Kinderkrankh 1853;**20**:217–225, Tab.
26. Rotch TM: Some important aspects connected with the scientific feeding of infants. In: 'Festschrift' in honor of Abraham Jacobi, to commemorate the seventieth anniversary of his birth. New York: Knickerbocker, 1900: p. 318–26.
27. Apple RD: Mothers and medicine. Madison, WI: University of Wisconsin Press, 1987: p. 4, 66.
28. Lavoisier A-L, Laplace P-S: Mémoire sur la chaleur. Mémoires de l'Académie des Sciences (Paris) 1780;355–408.
29. Bernard C: De l'origine du sucre dans l'économie animale. Arch Gén Méd 1848;**18**:303–19.
30. Regnault HV, Reiset J: Recherches chimiques sur la respiration des animaux des diverses classes. Ann Chim Phys 1849;**26**:299–519.
31. Pettenkofer Mv, Voit C: Untersuchungen über den Stoffverbrauch des normalen Menschen. Zeitschr Biol 1866;**2**:459–573.
32. Forster J: Amtlicher Bericht der 50. In: Versammlung Deutscher Naturforscher und Ärzte. München: 1877: p. 355.
33. Scherer F: Die Respiration des Neugeborenen und Säuglings. Jahrb Kinderheilk 1896;**43**:471–96.
34. Rubner M, Heubner O: Die natürliche Ernährung eines Säuglings. Zeitschr Biol 1898;**36**:1–55.
35. Rubner M, Heubner O: Die künstliche Ernährung eines normalen und eines atrophischen Säuglings. Zeitschr Biol 1899;**38**: 315–98.
36. Czerny A, Keller A: Des Kindes Ernährung. Leipzig: Deuticke, 1906: Vol. **1**.
37. Budin P: Le Nourrisson. Paris: Doin, 1900: p. 23, 41, 99, 213.
38. Jacobi A: Therapeutics of infancy and childhood. 2. ed. Philadelphia, PA: Lippincott, 1898: p. 27–9.
39. Gaertner G: Ueber die Herstellung der Fettmilch. Wiener Med Wochenschr 1894:1870.
40. Ylppö A: Premature children: should they fast or be fed in the first days of life? Ann Paediatr Fenn 1954;**1**:99–104.
41. Straus LG: Disease in milk—the remedy: pasteurization. New York: Dutton, 1913: p. 47, 161.
42. Forsyth D: The history of Infant-feeding from Elizabethan times. Proc R Soc Med 1911;**4**:110–41.
43. Howarth WJ: The influence of feeding on the mortality of infants. Lancet 1905;**166**:210–3.
44. Woodbury RM: Infant mortality and its causes. Baltimore, MD: Williams & Wilkins, 1926.
45. Hirschman C, Butler M: Trends and differentials in breast feeding. Demography 1981;**18**:39–54.
46. Fomon S: Infant feeding in the 20th century. J Nutr 2001;**131**: 409S–20S.

6.6

From swill milk to certified milk
Progress in cow's milk quality

Introduction

During the industrial revolution in the first half of the 19th century, the European population doubled, and the proportion of city dwellers rose to 50%. Urbanization jeopardized infant nutrition in at least three ways: (1) mothers accepted paid work far from their homes, undermining breastfeeding; (2) cow's milk was either produced in the cities under questionable circumstances, or was transported long distances and sold under likewise suspect conditions; and (3) working class neighbourhoods usually lacked sanitation and rarely had access to clean water. The following chapter identifies actions taken during the second half of the 19th century to improve the quality of cow's milk in the metropoles.

Contaminated and adulterated milk

Although there was no knowledge of pathogenic microbes until 1841, Naples professor Filippo Baldini, a protagonist of artificial infant feeding, worried about dirty stables in 1786: 'One must take care that the goats do not lay down in their excrements or in humid places, and should be afraid if they absorb the volatile matter through the pores of their skin.' In London, the *Commission on Adulterations* painted a gloomy picture in 1855 [1]: 'He [Dr. Normandy] saw from thirty to forty cows in a most disgusting condition, full of ulcers, their teats diseased and their legs full of tumours and abscesses—in fact, quite horrible to look at; and a fellow was milking them in the midst of all this abomination. This was by no means an exceptional case, a great many dairies being in the same condition. The milk, in consequence, is really diseased milk.'

John Mitchell published an entire book on 'the falsification of food' in 1848 [2] and the 'cow with the iron tail' became subject of a satirical poem in 1867 [3]: 'For he won't want milk, if the truth they talk, while he has his pump, and his lump of chalk.' Vernois and Becquerel described milk manipulation in France in 1853 [4]: 'Milk is alterated in Paris by the following substances, listed in the order of frequency: water, glucose, flour, starch, dextrine, infusion of amylaceous matter (rice, barley, bran), yolk of egg and white of egg, sugar, caramel, cassonade; gelatine, liquorice, boiled carrots, broken-down calves brains, serum of blood, several salts, bicarbonate of soda.'

The situation was no better in Germany and Carl Hennig, director of the Leipzig Childrens Hospital, stated in 1874 [5]: 'Often the milk is diluted with water to raise profits. The conscientious landowners know that this occurs most frequently during transport and therefore send their products in sealed vessels.' All over Europe, a plethora of *lactometers* was developed to detect falsifications. Martiny's monograph on milk of 1871 devoted 51 pages to these devices [6], some of which are depicted in Fig. 6.6.1. Fig. 6.6.1A–D and I show hydrometers that measured specific density at defined temperature. The deeper the metered bulbs sink, the lower the specific gravity, which may reveal dilution. Fig. 6.6.1B, G, and H measured the percentage cream layer that ascended after a defined time. Fig. 6.6.1F is an optical instrument that assessed the translucency of candlelight through a thin layer of milk, believed to indicate its fat content.

Swill milk and milk transport

With the invention of the column distillery, mass production of cheap spirits became possible in the early 19th century, and hard liquors abounded in the growing suburbs. The distillery waste *slop* was fed to cows who became sick and produced thin and contaminated *swill milk*. Robert Hartley, secretary of the New York Association for Improving the Conditions of the Poor, described the situation in his city in 1842 [7]: 'During the winter season, about two thousand cows are said to be kept on the premises ... All the cows are most inhumanly condemned to subsist on this most unnatural aliment ... At the distilleries, the slop is drawn off hot into tanks, at short intervals through the day, and in this state is distributed and eaten by the cows on the premises, and also by those in the adjacent parts, as before it cools it may be transported to a considerable distance ... cases have occurred where, owing to lameness from debility or disease, and sometimes by a paralysis of the limbs, the cattle, unable to stand, have been supported

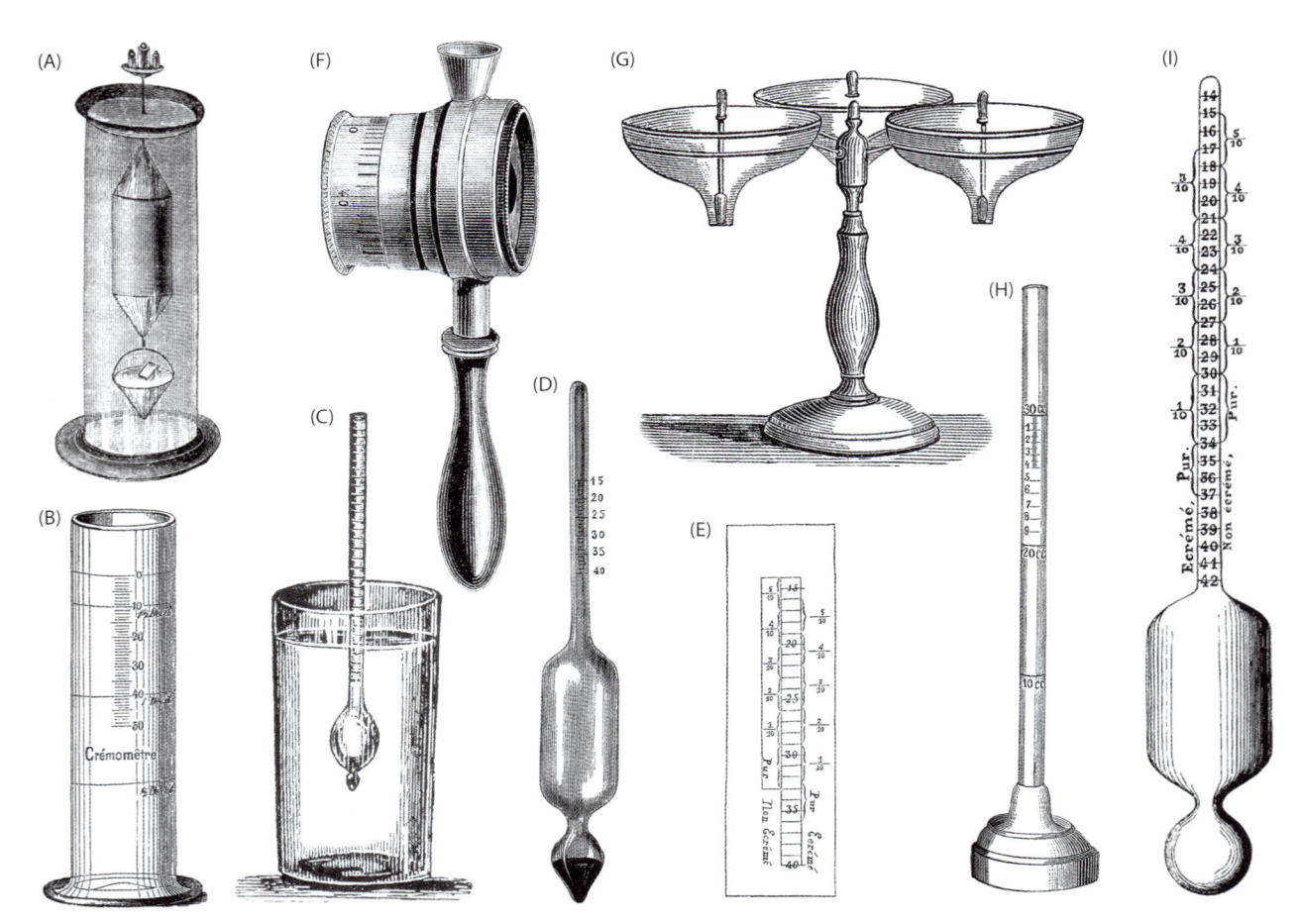

Fig. 6.6.1 Instruments used in the 19th century to prove milk falsification: A, hydrometer of Nicholson 1790; B, cremometer of Schübler 1817; C, lactometer of Hartley 1842; D, lactodensimeter of Quevenne 1842; E, Quevenne's scales for full-cream and skim milk; F, lactoscope of Donné 1843; G, butyrometer of Krocker 1856; H, lactobutyrometer of Marchand 1854; I, galactometer of Bouchardat 1857.
Figures modified from Martiny 1871 [6] and Krafft 1885 [46].

by straps passed under the body, and yet have been retained as milkers … Slop milk is naturally very thin, and of a pale bluish color. In order to disguise its bad qualities and render it saleable, it is necessary to give it color and consistence … Starch, sugar, flour, plaster of Paris, chalk, eggs, anatto, etc. are used for this purpose … more than three-fourths of the infants born in our cities, are sustained in whole or in part on artificial diet.' New York City Inspector David Reese agreed in 1857 [8]: 'Distilleries in or near large cities … an intolerable nuisance and curse … wherever they exist, their slops will furnish the cheapest food for cows, the milk from which is more pernicious and fatal to infant health and life than alcohol itself to adults … So long as distilleries are tolerated in cities, cow stables will be their appendages, and the milk, fraught with sickness and death, will still perpetuate mortality.' From May 1858, a series of eight articles with a total of 36 drastic pictures (Fig. 6.6.2) appeared in *Frank Leslie's Illustrated Newspaper*, 'exposing the milk trade of New York and Brooklyn' [9]. The pictorial campaign prompted a law prohibiting the sale of swill milk in April 1861, and Leslie triumphed 'a great victory won' [10].

Cows fed on slop were not a specific US problem: city distilleries were described and opposed by authors in England, Germany, France, and other countries. For Germany, Hennig complained in 1874 [5]: 'In the large cities dairies and cowstables make room for distilleries, dyeing works, steam laundries, and cigar factories … Milk of cows fed spent corn, rape, distillery slop and the like is noxious for newborn infants.' Milk transport from the allegedly healthier countryside was no real alternative. In Detroit, Sutherland had patented a refrigerator-railway car in 1867 [11], nevertheless in 1905 Fabian Society member Lawson Dodd observed [12]: 'The railway companies have no financial or other interest in the delivery of clean milk, and therefore very seldom provide proper vans for its conveyance. Fish, paint, petroleum, or other unsuitable goods are packed along with the milk. The churns from the farms are allowed to stand for hours on platforms of rural stations to be dealt with as ordinary goods, or to await the slow milk train. While thus waiting, the milk is often exposed to the hot rays of the sun and the dust of passing traffic, which both make for increased bacterial contamination.'

Milk-borne disease

The triumph of bacteriology contributed to improving the quality of milk. In 1881, Henri Fauvel, chemist in the Paris police headquarters, detected vast numbers of bacteria and cryptogams in 28 of 31 milk bottles used in ten different nurseries [13]. At the turn

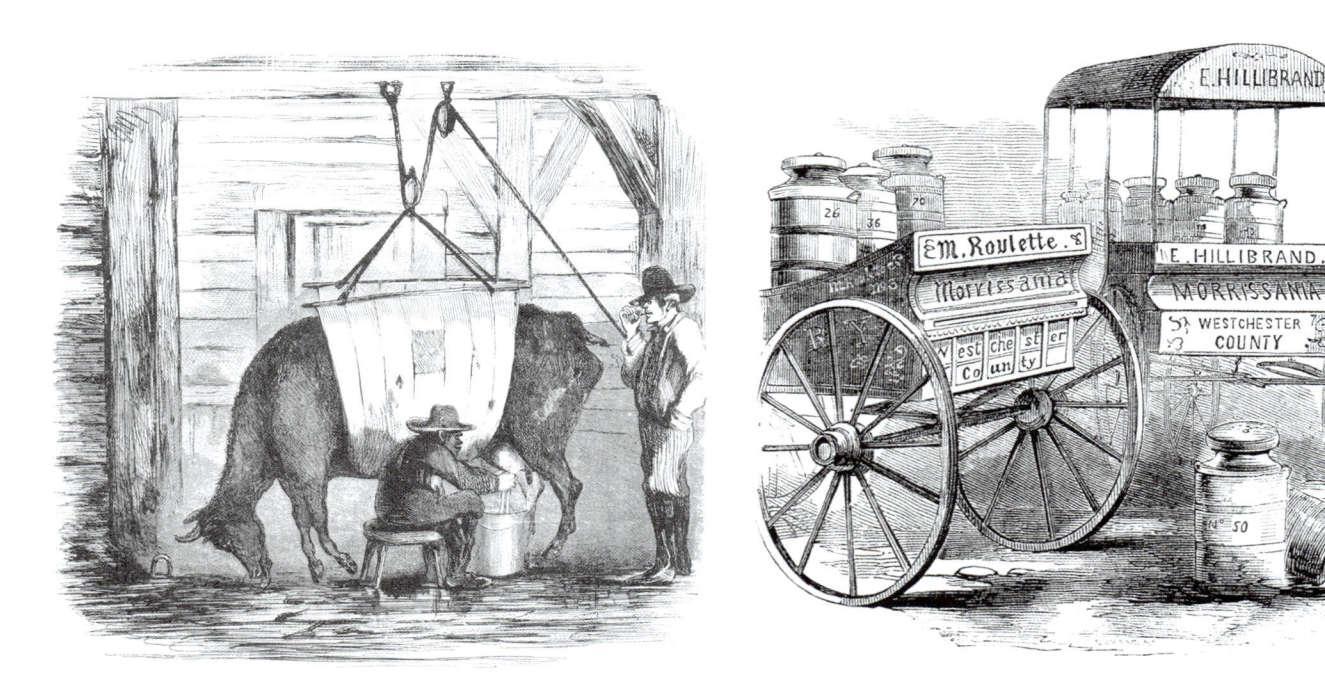

Fig. 6.6.2 Left: sick cow being hoisted for milking; right: milk wagons for the transport of swill milk. Both figures from *Leslie's Illustrated Newspaper*, 1858 [9].

of the century, cow's milk was known to be highly contaminated, and Dodd stated ironically [12]: 'If the almighty had intended that there should be no manure in the milk, he would have placed the udder at the other end of the cow.' For his review 'White Poison' Peter Atkins carefully collected data on milk microbiology from Britain: in 1901, 10% of London samples were classified as *dirty* and Liverpool samples contained *Escherichia coli* in 72% when transported by rail, and in 44% when produced in the town; 10% of milk samples contained tubercle bacilli [14]. Concerning *Mycobacterium bovis*, Robert Koch stated in 1901 [15]: 'It is not decided whether man is susceptible to bovine tuberculosis… If such a susceptibility really exists, the infection of human beings is but a very rare occurrence… I therefore do not deem it advisable to take any measures against it.' British scientists, especially Sir John McFadyean, contradicted Koch's view, which led to appoint the Royal Commission on Tuberculosis, ruling in 1907 [16]: 'A very considerable amount of disease and loss of life, especially among infants and children, must be contributed to the consumption of cow's milk containing tubercle bacilli.' The ensuing acrimonious controversy on *M. bovis* ('Milk War') persisted for half a century and has been described by Barbara Orland [17]. Governments ordered tuberculin testing—or slaughtering—and certified 'tuberculosis-free herds'. Less belligerent but also long standing was the debate on group B streptococci. Recognized as causing bovine mastitis (*gelber galti*, *garget*) by Nocard in 1887 [18], the germ was initially termed *Streptococcus agalactiae*. Rebecca Lancefield identified type B serologically in 1933 [19] and described sporadic infections in humans. But as late as 1966 it was recognized that group B streptococci had become the most frequent single cause of neonatal sepsis in Boston (see Chapter 7.9) [20]. As with *M. tuberculosis*, there was extensive debate whether human and bovine strains are identical. Today group B streptococci are frequent contaminants in the female genital tract and there is no evidence that cattle are a significant resource for transmission.

Fresh water, sewage, and drainage

An uninterrupted supply of fresh water is a precondition of urbanization. Early human cultures exerted great effort to construct and operate aqueducts, cisterns, wells, and highly sophisticated distribution systems. Breakdowns of their water supply probably contributed to the collapse of the Indus valley civilization, the Akkadian Empire in Mesopotamia, and the Nabatean civilization in Petra, Jordan. In addition to freshwater distribution and public baths, the Romans built a sewer system connected to the *cloaca maxima*, described by Plinius in the 1st century C.E. [21]. Much of that ancient knowledge seems to have been lost during the Middle Ages. The large metropoles lacked sewage systems that separated the supply of freshwater and drainage of wastewater. Between 1831 and 1866, four pandemics of Asiatic cholera ravaged Europe, taking millions of lives in the ever-growing cities, firstly and mainly infants. It was not until such catastrophes that the European capitals finally built efficient sewage systems and freshwater supplies.

François I ordered French houses to be equipped with cesspits in 1530. The cities were ill-smelling agglomerations of houses with sinks and cowstables nearby. Freshwater of doubtful quality was supplied to the houses by water carriers as Sebastien Mercier reported in 1802 [22]: 'The night-men, to spare themselves the trouble of conveying the filth to a sufficient distance from the town, empty their carts at break of the day into the common sewers and rivulets, these filthy drags are slowly floated down the streets towards the river Seine, and infect those parts of the shore, where the men who carry water about, go on a morning to fill their buckets.' The Paris

Cemetery of the Innocents, adjoining the main market, was removed in 1780 because of its evil smell. Within Haussmann's newly constructed city, the engineer Eugène Belgrand began building a 600 km sewage system in 1853. The central freshwater reservoir Montsouris was finished in 1874. In 1906 the river Bièvre, filthy since 1577, was transferred underground to become the main collecting canal [23].

The situation was no better in Tudor England, as pointed out by David Forsyth [24]: 'There were latrines, but no drains. At the back of every house stood a cesspool.' Erasmus of Rotterdam, who lived in England between 1499 and 1506, described English houses in which 'the floors are commonly of clay, strewn with rushes, under which lies an ancient collection of spittle, vomit, urine of dogs and men, spilled beer, relics of fishes, and other unnamable filth' [25]. In such surrounding, artificial feeding of infants had little chance of success. In 1613, the 'New River' was finished, transporting fresh water to London over a distance of 67 km [26]. Its population, 250,000 at that time, quadrupled up to 1800 and additional water supplies had to be procured. Disposing of the waste water of 3.2 million inhabitants and a quarter of a million tons of manure produced by London's cows each year in the early 1860s was a logistic challenge and environmentally hazardous [14]. Following the Metropolitan Water Act of 1852 and a final cholera epidemic, the London sewage system was built by Joseph Bazalgette, transforming the former Fleet River into a main sewer [27].

The freshwater supply of New York City was ensured by the Croton aqueduct. But the few existing drains were frequently clogged up by dead animals, garbage, and refuse, and were cleansed by prisoners [28]. Construction of a modern sewage system began in 1871. In Berlin, most backyards hosted a latrine right next to the well pump. From 1872, after repeated urging by Rudolf Virchow, a radial sewerage and drainage system was constructed by James Hobrecht [29].

Certified milk

The first milk depot in America was established by Henry Koplik in the Eastern Dispensary in New York in 1889 [30]. It distributed sterilized milk mixtures according to physician's prescription for sick infants. Henry Coit of New Jersey was another pioneer of clean and safe milk for infants. He was motivated by the death of his own son in 1887 [31]: 'I was driven from one source of impoverished and contaminated milk to another, until, in desperation, I sought a small suburban dairyman … Honest and industrious, but without a knowledge of hygiene, he became a dangerous element in my family life.' In 1893, Coit founded the 'Medical Milk Commission' which gave a certificate to milk sealed in separate quart containers that fulfilled three criteria: 'Uniform nutritive value; reliable keeping qualities; and freedom from pathogens' [32]. The Fairfield Dairy sold it for 12 cents a quart, 6 cents more than ordinary milk. Coit wrote 'the poorest baby in Coomes Alley will now fare equally well with Thomas Edison's baby in Lewellen Park' [31]. In 1896 the New York Medical Society likewise formed a milk commission, and by 1906 there were 36 commissions throughout the US requiring the formation of an 'Association of Medical Milk Commissions' to ensure bacteriological and chemical standards for certification, and Henry Coit was elected its president. Mostly maintained by private charity, the milk depots supplied 'best', 'proper', 'clean', or 'certified' milk to 'needy persons' or 'the worthy poor' and provided visits 'to educate mothers in the care of infants' [33].

Certified milk was not sterile, but it did contain under 10,000 bacteria per millilitre. In the worldwide raw-versus-pasteurized milk debate, Coit held the opinion that boiling destroys important properties and encourages the careless handling of milk. Over the long term, however, certified milk could not compete with the trend towards pasteurization. Atkins described how from 1922, British legislation ensured bacteriological quality grading of milk and its protection from contamination in transit [34].

Pasteurization plants, depots, and dispensaries

The impact of pasteurization has been described previously. French physicians (Budin, Auvard, Dufour) were in favour of boiling, whereas Germans (Heubner, Finkelstein) preferred raw milk. In the US, Abraham Jacobi advised the boiling of all milk for children feeding as early as 1873, whereas Coit, Henry Arthur Meigs, and Alfred Hess opposed boiling. In 1891, Thomas Morgan Rotch together with Gustavus Gordon and George Walker established the Walker–Gordon Laboratory (from 1897 *farm*) for the production of clean *guaranteed* milk [35].

The New York philanthropist Nathan Straus, co-owner of Macy's storehouse, became convinced that impure milk was responsible for the deaths of many babies [36]: 'Here in New York the lives of thousands of children are sacrificed every summer, simply and solely because they are fed impure milk.' From 1893 he organized large pasteurization plants and used cooled cars to distribute 34,400 bottles per year: 'Only *Certified Milk* is used, containing not more than 10,000 bacteria per cubic centimeter. This purest milk obtainable is modified and pasteurized in the laboratory at 348 East 32d Street.' Pasteurization meant heating the milk to a temperature of from 140°F to 157°F and holding it at this temperature for 20 min and then rapidly cooling it. Milk for the 1st to 3rd month of life followed the recipes of Drs. Green and Freeman (1.5 oz of 16% cream; 3 oz full milk; 13 oz. water; 0.5 oz lime water; 1 oz milk sugar, fills 6 bottles à 3 oz); for the 3rd to 7th month of Dr Jacobi (18 oz full milk; 18 oz barley water; 1 oz cane sugar; 20 grains table salt; fills 6 bottles à 6 oz.). 'Coupons were placed without cost, and without restriction as to quantity, at the disposal of any physician giving his services freely to the poor.' In 1895, Straus wrote to the mayors of every city in the US [36]: 'I have long held that the day is not far distant when it will be regarded as a piece of criminal neglect to feed young children on milk that has not been sterilized.' In 1908, Chicago mandated milk pasteurization, followed by many cities throughout the United States. In 1911, 43 milk depots were in operation in 30 US cities [33].

In Britain, the pioneer Infant Milk Depot opened in St Helens in 1899, equipped with automated sterilizers and bottle washing machines. It was followed by Liverpool, Battersea, York, and Glasgow up to 1904 [37, 38], predominantly supplying milk for the poor. The technical standard in the Glasgow depot was described by Bailie Anderson in 1905 [39]: 'Each trolley is capable of holding 540 bottles, or 60 baskets. The milk sterilizer has a capacity of 1,080 bottles, or one day's supply for 120 children … The cold chamber had a total capacity of 2,000 bottles ... bottle washing machine had an output of 20 bottles per minute ..., each bottle is washed three times.' The National Clean Milk Society was founded by Wilfried Buckley in 1916 [14].

A debate on pasteurization ('killing the milk') continued even after an editorial of the *Boston Medical & Surgical Journal* stated in 1923 [40]: 'Boiled fresh milk is the only entirely safe milk that can be fed to infants.' The terms pasteurization and sterilization were used somewhat interchangeably until being defined in 1927. Milk pasteurization became mandatory by law in the UK in 1985 [41] and in Australia in 1994. For the European Union, council directive 92/46 regulated the sale of raw and heated milk in 1992. Selling raw milk is illegal in 25 of the US [42]. In Germany at the begin of the 20th century, the infant hospitals in Dresden and Berlin had model cowstables providing showers for the cows.

In the Maternité of Nancy, Adolphe Herrgott founded the consultation and follow-up service *oeuvre de la maternité* for neonates in 1890. The infants were brought by their mothers for medical examination 1 month after birth and when the child's progress was satisfactory, the mother received a gift of money. In 1892, Gaston Variot founded the consultation service in Belleville, Paris (**Fig. 6.6.3**), and Pierre Budin that in the Paris Charité, named *goutte de lait*. They encouraged breastfeeding and distributed undiluted cow's milk sterilized in small bottles. The goutte de lait in Fécamp, France, founded by Léon Dufour in 1894, was associated with a dramatic fall in infant mortality and became a model for milk dispensaries throughout Europe. As pointed out by Deborah Dwork [43], the clean milk movement did not directly lower infant mortality, but it did become the root of infant welfare. In 1912, 200 *gouttes* took part in a national conference, their successor organization *école maternelle* is still found in every French town.

International congresses

The International Congresses for the Study and Prevention of Infantile Mortality (Paris 1905, Brussels 1907, Berlin 1911) carried the subtitle *goutte de lait*. Their history and impact on infant welfare has been described by Catherine Rollet [44]. Nathan Straus lectured in Brussels: 'However, as the infantile death rate in New York went steadily down ... coincident with the increased use of pasteurized milk, the significance of my work became apparent ... 3.14 million bottles in 1906.' In Berlin in September 1911, Straus was the official delegate of the US, and announced proudly 'to save 125,000 babies a year ... infant death rate cut in half' and reported to President Taft the 'necessity for accurate and uniform vital statistics' [36]. With delegates from 28 countries, the trilingual proceedings of the Berlin *goutte de lait* has 1256 pages. It appeared 2 years before World War I terminated the plans for a congress in London in 1915—and global scientific efforts for infant welfare. Carlo Agostoni and Dominique Turck have shown how concerns that cow's milk may harm a child's health repeatedly became fashionable up to the present day [45].

Conclusion

Progress in bacteriology and hygiene lowered the risk of cow's milk as a human nutrient. This was especially helpful for artificially fed infants and even more so during the summer months. From 1882, the clean milk movement paralleled the efforts pioneered by Philipp Biedert in Alsatia and Arthur Vincent Meigs in Philadelphia to modify the protein, fat, and mineral concentration of cow's milk which in the future was to improve the outcome of infants with gastroenteritis [35]. For city dwellers it remained

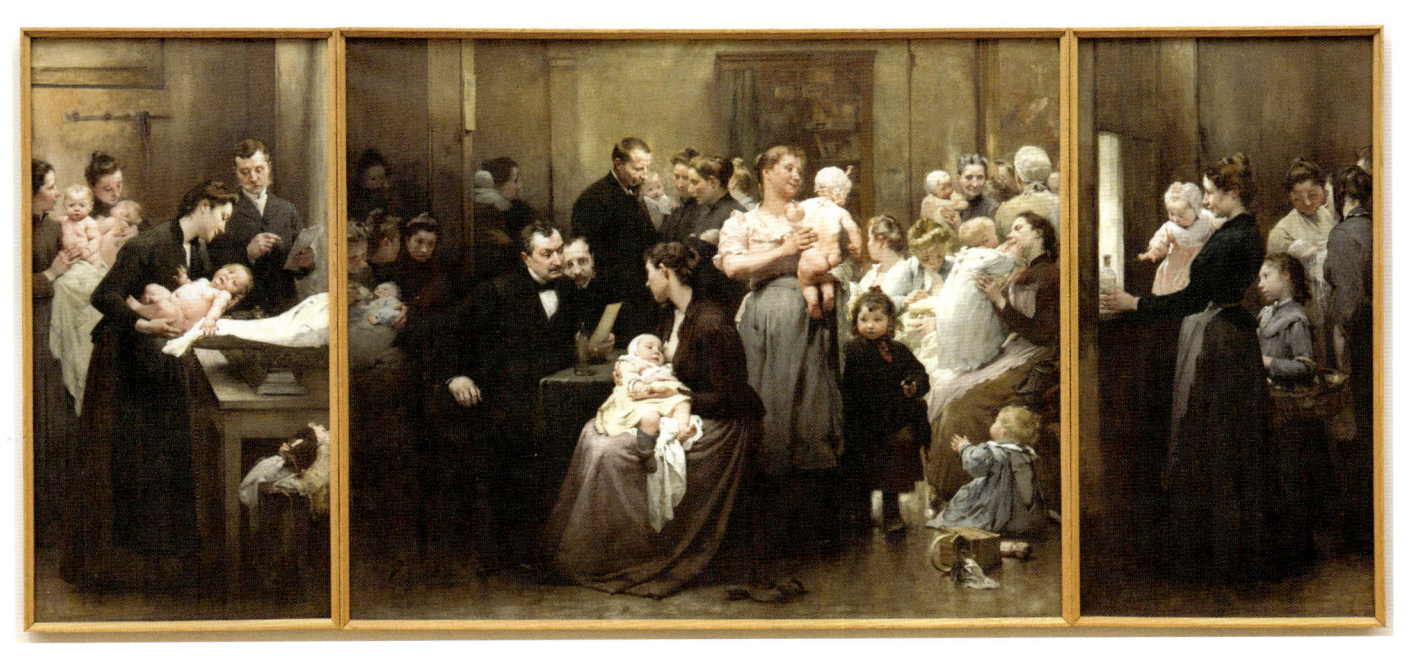

Fig. 6.6.3 The *Goutte de Lait* at Belleville Dispensary, Paris, opened in 1892. Painting by Jean Geoffroy 1901. Left: weighing; centre: consultation; right: milk distribution. Musée du Petit Palais, IMG 3839.
Parisienne de Photographie, with permission.

hazardous to consume raw milk until after World War I. The physician-initiated clean milk movement of Koplik and Coit in the US and of Budin and Dufour in France improved the quality of cow's milk used for infant feeding, but, against their will, did not promote breastfeeding. Pasteurization plants and infant milk depots provided clean milk at affordable prices. Born of humanitarian motives, neither approach could withstand the power of global marketing. Moreover, they were internally inconsistent and physicians were not unanimous. Decades of debate on milk-borne disease, pasteurization, and the optimal composition of infant food delayed governmental legislation. Moreover, the debates paved the way for industrially produced formula for which neither physician nor parents had to worry about quality. Within the broader context of protecting nurslings, efforts to improve the quality of cow's milk were key. Although a direct connection between the clean milk movement and declining infant mortality rate cannot be proven, the former doubtless encouraged international cooperation supporting infant welfare and public health.

REFERENCES

1. Commission on adulteration: London milk and London cows. Lancet 1855;**66**:551.
2. Mitchell J: Treatise on the falsifications of food. London: Baillière, 1848: p. 74–81.
3. Griset E, Hood T: The cow with the iron tail. In: Griset's Grotesques. London: Routledge, 1867: p. 80.
4. Vernois AGM, Becquerel A: Recherches sur le lait. Deuxième partie. Ann Hyg Publ Méd Légale 1853;**50**:43–147.
5. Hennig C: Neuere Erfahrungen über Ersatzmittel der Muttermilch. Jahrb Kinderheilk 1874;**7**:41–60.
6. Martiny B: Die Milch, ihr Wesen und ihre Verwerthung. Danzig: Kafemann, 1871: Vol. **1**, p. 126–69.
7. Hartley RM: An historical, scientific, and practical essay on milk as an article of human sustenance. New York: Leavitt, 1842: p. 132–46, 198.
8. Reese DM: Report in infant mortality in large cities. Philadelphia, PA: Collins, 1857.
9. Berghaus A, Nast T: Exposure of the milk trade of New York and Brooklyn/the swill milk trade. Frank Leslie's Illustrated Newspaper 1858;**5**:358–410.
10. Leslie F: A great victory won! Swill milk abolished by law. Frank Leslie's Illustrated Newspaper 1861;**11**:305.
11. Sutherland JB: Improved refrigerator-car. United States Patent Office 1867; Pat.-Nr. 71423.
12. Dodd FL: Municipal milk and public health. Fabian Tracts 1905;**3**:1–19. Reprint London 1969.
13. Fauvel H: Note sur les altérations du lait dans les biberons. Bull Acad Méd 1881;**10**:614–7.
14. Atkins PJ: White poison? The social consequences of milk consumption, 1850–1930. Soc Hist Med 1992;**5**:207–27.
15. Koch R: The combating of tuberculosis in the light of the experience that has been gained in the successful combating of other infectious diseases. Lancet 1901;**158**:187–91.
16. Francis J: The work of the British Royal Commission on Tuberculosis, 1901–1911. Tubercle (London) 1959;**40**:124–32.
17. Orland B: Cow's milk and human disease. Food Hist 2003;**1**:179–202.
18. Nocard M: Mammite contagieuse. Bull Mém Soc Centrale Méd Vét 1885;**39**:296–302.
19. Lancefield RC: A serological differentiation of human and other groups of hemolytic streptococci. J Exp Med 1933;**57**:571–95.
20. Eickhoff TC, Klein JO, Daly K, et al.: Neonatal sepsis and other infections due to group B beta-hemolytic streptococci. N Engl J Med 1964;**271**:1221–8.
21. Plinius the Elder: Naturalis historia. Darmstadt: Wissenschaftliche Buchgesellschaft, 1992: p. 75.
22. Mercier LS: Paris delineated. London: Symonds, 1802: Vol. **1**, p. 21–5.
23. Brunfaut J: Hygiène Publique. Les Odeurs de Paris. 2. ed. Paris: Lefèvre, 1882.
24. Forsyth D: The history of infant-feeding from Elizabethan times. Proc R Soc Med 1911;**4**:110–41.
25. Furnivall FJ: Early English meals and manners. London: Trübner, 1868: p. LXVI.
26. Ward R: London's new river. London: Historical Publications Ltd, 2003.
27. Halliday S: Great stink of London. Stroud: Sutton, 1999.
28. Duffy J: A history of public health in New York City 1625–1866. New York: Russell Sage, 1968.
29. Hobrecht J: Die Canalisation von Berlin. Berlin: Ernst & Korn, 1884.
30. Koplik H: The history of the first milk depot or Gouttes de Lait with consultants in America. JAMA 1914;**63**:1574–5.
31. Waserman M: Henry L. Coit and the certified milk movement in the development of modern pediatrics. Bull Hist Med 1946;**46**:359–90.
32. Coit HL: Certified milk. Arch Pediatr 1897;**14**:824–6.
33. Kerr JW: Data regarding operations of infants' milk depots in the United States in 1910. Public Health Rep 1911;**26**:1227–45.
34. Atkins P: Liquid materialities. A history of milk, science and the law. Farnham: Ashgate, 2010.
35. Morse JL: Recollections and reflections on forty-five years of artificial infant feeding. Pediatrics 1935;**7**:303–24.
36. Straus LG: Disease in milk—the remedy: pasteurization. New York: Dutton, 1913: p. 47, 161.
37. Harris FD: The supply of sterilised humanised milk for the use of infants in St Helens. BMJ 1900;**2**:427–31.
38. McCleary GF: The infants' milk depot: its history and functions. J Hyg (Lond) 1904;**4**:329–68.
39. Anderson BWF, Straus N, Lister TD, et al.: A discussion on infant milk depots. BMJ 1905;**2**:643–7.
40. Editorial: Milk: Safe or unsafe? Boston Med Surg J 1923; **188**:177.
41. Sharp JCM, Paterson GM, Barrett NJ: Pasteurisation and the control of milkborne infection in Britain. BMJ 1985;**291**:463–4.
42. Weisbecker A: A legal history of raw milk in the United States. J Environ Health 2007;**69**:62–3.
43. Dwork D: The milk option. Med Hist 1987;**31**:51–69.
44. Rollet C: La santé et la protection de l'enfant vues a travers les congrès internationaux (1880–1920). Ann Dém Hist 2001;**1**:97–116.
45. Agostoni C, Turck D: Is cow's milk harmful to a child's health? J Pediatr Gastroenterol Nutr 2011;**53**:594–600.
46. Krafft G: Lehrbuch der Landwirtschaft. 4. ed. Berlin: Parey, 1885: Vol. **3**: Tierzucht, p. 124–31.

6.7 Technical inventions that enabled artificial infant feeding

Introduction

Coal, steam, and steel fuelled the industrial revolution during the first half of the 19th century, and growing metropoles changed human life radically. The European population doubled, and the proportion of city inhabitants rose to 50%. Urbanization jeopardized infant nutrition in at least three ways: (1) mothers had to accept paid work far from their homes, which undermined breastfeeding; (2) cow's milk was either produced in the cities under questionable circumstances, or was transported long distance and sold under even more suspect conditions; and (3) pathogenic bacteria and hygienic precautions were unknown—the equipment for 'hand-feeding' was often a microbiological paradise. This chapter identifies technical innovations which made artificial feeding safer and paved the way for the industrial production of baby food.

Traditional teats

The developments of the baby bottle and pacifier have been described [1–5]. These reports often did not specify the feeding mouthpiece, the *teat*. Various materials and forms, resembling more or less a female nipple, were used over centuries, and as long as microbes were unknown, they remained the weak link in artificial feeding. Sponges, cloth, chamois leather, parchment, tanned heifer's teats (preserved in alcohol or soaked in water before use), cork, and softened ivory were used as nipples—and as ideal culture media for bacterial growth. Easily available sponges were among the earliest nipple substitutes. In 1787, Paris obstetrician Jean-Louis Baudelocque [6] described 'an infant bottle of glass … One adjusts a fine sponge in the form of a plug, protruding half an inch, which can be recovered by a thin line attached to the bottleneck. Each time the infant has been fed, the little sponge and the catchline are put in water and washed, also the bottle is cleaned, and it will never acquire that harsh smell which the other bottles take on after some days.' Adolf Henke of Erlangen recommended similar devices in 1821 [7]: 'A small thoroughly cleaned and suitably cut sponge is plugged into the bottleneck, covered with a fine linen cloth which is tightly fastened.' In Leipzig, the obstetrician Friedrich Meissner modified in 1844 [8] 'a sucking bottle to which an artificial nipple is attached, prepared from a wash-sponge that is covered by a bladder whose tip is perforated by several needle stitches. From this the infant sucks until satiated. Utmost cleanliness is necessary, the artificial teat must be rinsed after each use, because the humidity therein sours easily and spoils the infant's nutrition and digestion.'

Cow horns were used in many countries. George Armstrong, founder of the London Dispensary for the Infant Poor, discerned in 1777 [9]: 'Two ways of feeding children who are bred up by the hand; the one is by means of a horn, and the other is with a boat or spoon … The small end of [the polished horn] is perforated, and has a notch round it to which are fastened two small bits of parchment, shaped like the tip of the finger of a glove, and sewed together in such a manner, as that the food poured into the horn can be sucked through between the stitches.' And Hugh Smith observed in 1792 [10]: 'Some inventions of this kind, by means of parchment or leather sewed to the pointed end of a horn, which is no bad thought, and capable of great improvement … a piece of sponge covered with a linen cloth is tied over the smaller end. This serves the children very well as an artificial nipple.'

Cloth-covered teats were used in Munich's only children's hospital, as Hauner criticized in 1853 [11]: 'Usually flour and milk is cooked and this mash is smeared into the child's mouth with a cloth-sucker [*Sauglappen*], a spoon made of bone, or with the finger … The infant may hold the sucker in its mouth all night long.' Animal teats for attachment to feeding vessels were sold by tripe butchers for centuries. In 1826, the Paris midwife Madame Breton began to commercialize preserved (tanned) heifer's teats [12]: 'The nipples are furnished dry. They must be placed in fresh water four to five hours until they have regained their suppleness … When the infant has finished nursing they should be carefully washed and placed under an inverted glass to prevent drying out.' In 1839, the product received a medal of honour [13]: 'Madame Breton has developed a simple and economic procedure to prepare calves' teats … which can be used for a month or six weeks … and are delivered for one franc a piece … The jury accords her a bronze medal.'

Reproduced with permission from Obladen, M. Technical inventions that enabled artificial infant feeding. *Neonatology*, 106(1):62–68. Copyright © 2014 S. Karger AG, Basel.

When gutta-percha became available in 1848, Breton's competitor Swygenhofen attacked the versatile midwife [14]: 'Let me assert that my teats, made of best *goutta*, offer advantages which yours don't have: They are thinner and less subject to break, to disintegrate, or to crack.' Despite the competition, tanned heifer's teats remained in surgical instrument catalogues in 1860 [15]. In 1853, London obstetrician Thomas Bull identified teat materials as the weak link in artificial feeding [16]: 'The bottle must always be scalded out after use ... Various kinds [of artificial teats] are used: a prepared cow's teat, a piece of washed chamois leather, or a few folds of fine soft linen; whichever is preferred, it must be secured firmly to the bottle with thread, and care must be taken that its extremity does not extend more than half of an inch ... lest for the child will get the sides of the artificial teat so firmly pressed together between its gums, that there will be no channel for the milk to pass. It must be pierced with two or three very fine openings, and, lest the milk should flow through too rapidly, a small conical piece of sponge must be placed in the teat.' Bull claimed: 'Most cleanly and convenient apparatus of all is a cork nipple fixed in the sucking bottle, upon the plan of M. Darbo of Paris. The cork, being of a particularly fine texture, is supple and elastic, yielding to the infant's lips while sucking, and is much more durable than the teats ordinarily used.'

Vulcanization and rubber teats

Natural rubber is sticky in summer and brittle in winter. Caoutchouc (standard rubber) came from South America, 'gutta-percha' (tropical rubber) from Asia at the end of the 18th century. After years of experimenting, Charles Goodyear of New York patented vulcanization in 1844 [17]: 'My principal improvement consists in the combining of sulphur and white lead with the India-rubber, and in the submitting of the compound thus formed to the action of heat at a regulated temperature, by which combination and exposure to heat it will be so far altered in its qualities as not to become softened by the action of the solar ray ... nor will it be injuriously affected by exposure to cold.' Tyres were not the main business yet, and Goodyear earned his money with medical supplies needed in the Civil War. Rubber teats were patented by New York inventor Elijah Pratt in 1845 [18]: 'I introduce two small tubes, of glass, silver, wood, or ivory through the cork ... through one the child imbibes the liquid contents, while at the same time air enters through the other and replaces the liquid drawn out ... I adapt a contractile valve to the exterior orifice of the sucking-tube and another to the interior orifice of the air tube ... I also place an artificial nipple or sheath of India-rubber over the sucking tube.'

Thomas Barret did not welcome the innovation in 1851 [19]: 'The nipple for the bottle may be made of chamois leather, or a piece of sponge covered with washed leather; or, what has been recently invented, a teat of India-rubber; but, in my judgement, the best nipple is a calf's teat: whenever so used care must be taken that it is well secured to the bottle, or the child may swallow it. The bottle should be carefully and thoroughly washed after each use; the nipple should be always cleaned and changed frequently, or of course it soon becomes acid; and when a calf's teat is used it may be kept in spirit and water.' Traditional teats persisted besides rubber teats for three more decades, until the detection of bacteria showed that rubber teats, sterilizable, allowed more hygienic bottle feeding. Fig. 6.7.1 illustrates teat development during the 18th and 19th centuries.

The glass bottle

In 1784, Filippo Baldini of Naples invented a feeding vessel with a screwcap (Fig. 6.7.1A, B) [20]: 'It is a kind of glass bladder the mouthpiece of which is a spherical metal capsule, gilded to prevent the formation of rust or verdigris ... One inserts a sponge which fills the capsule's capacity and emerges from its other end ... The sponge replaces the nipple ... The vessel and especially the sponge must be cleaned carefully, even several times per day, with lukewarm water.'

Glass bottles in all forms began to replace pottery and pewter vessels: they were not necessarily easier to clean, but dirt and food remnants became visible, which augmented the chance of providing clean milk to infants. Charles Windship of Norfolk, Massachusetts, patented a glass bottle named 'lacteal, or artificial breast' in 1841 [21], with a broad teat covered with deerskin chamois leather 'to induce the child to think that it derives its nourishment directly from the mother, as it feeds in the natural position'. A very similar device named 'mamma feeding bottle' was recommended by Charles Routh in 1879 [22]: 'This [glass bottle] is so constructed as to prevent the child from taking down air with its food ... shaped like a female breast ... nipple of India-rubber ... stop-cock ... may be worn by the female in the position of the breast.'

Most popular was the 'Biberon Robert' sold from 1873; a rubber tube from its base supplied milk at the slightest suction (Fig. 6.7.1K). However, it had drawbacks: an inspection of 31 bottles from ten nurseries by Henri Fauvel in 1881 [23] showed 'in 28 cases ovoid cells and mycelia [thrush] in large number in teats, rubber tubes, and bottles'. The tube was also a bacterial paradise, 'tolerating it means promoting infanticide' wrote Léon Dufour in 1894 [24]. Acrimonious scientific debates for and against tube bottles continued for decades. From 1910, French law interdicted their import but not their production and the 'Biberon Robert' was produced until 1928 [25]. A hygienic dilemma characteristic of all bottles was recognized: open systems made the infant swallow air; closed systems impeded sucking by negative pressure. Valves or pipes designed to overcome these problems made the systems difficult to clean. Seamless rubber nipples fitted over the neck of the bottle were available in 1912 [26], but were not widely used.

Refrigeration

Until 1850, the only means to delay food spoilage was the icebox. Natural ice, harvested in winter and stored in specially constructed cellars, ran notoriously low in summer, the time when cooling foods was most necessary. Transporting ice from the lakeside stores in the north to the large cities in the south was complicated and expensive. Artificial refrigeration was demonstrated in Glasgow by William Cullen in 1748, for very small samples [27]. A continuous ammonia absorption machine for the production of large amounts of ice was invented by Ferdinand Carré in 1860 [28]. The machine produced 5 kg ice per kilogram of burned coal and was built on a large scale (Fig. 6.7.2). Big ice blocks were used to cool the milk chamber in the 'weaklings' pavillon' in Paris, the institution in which incubator

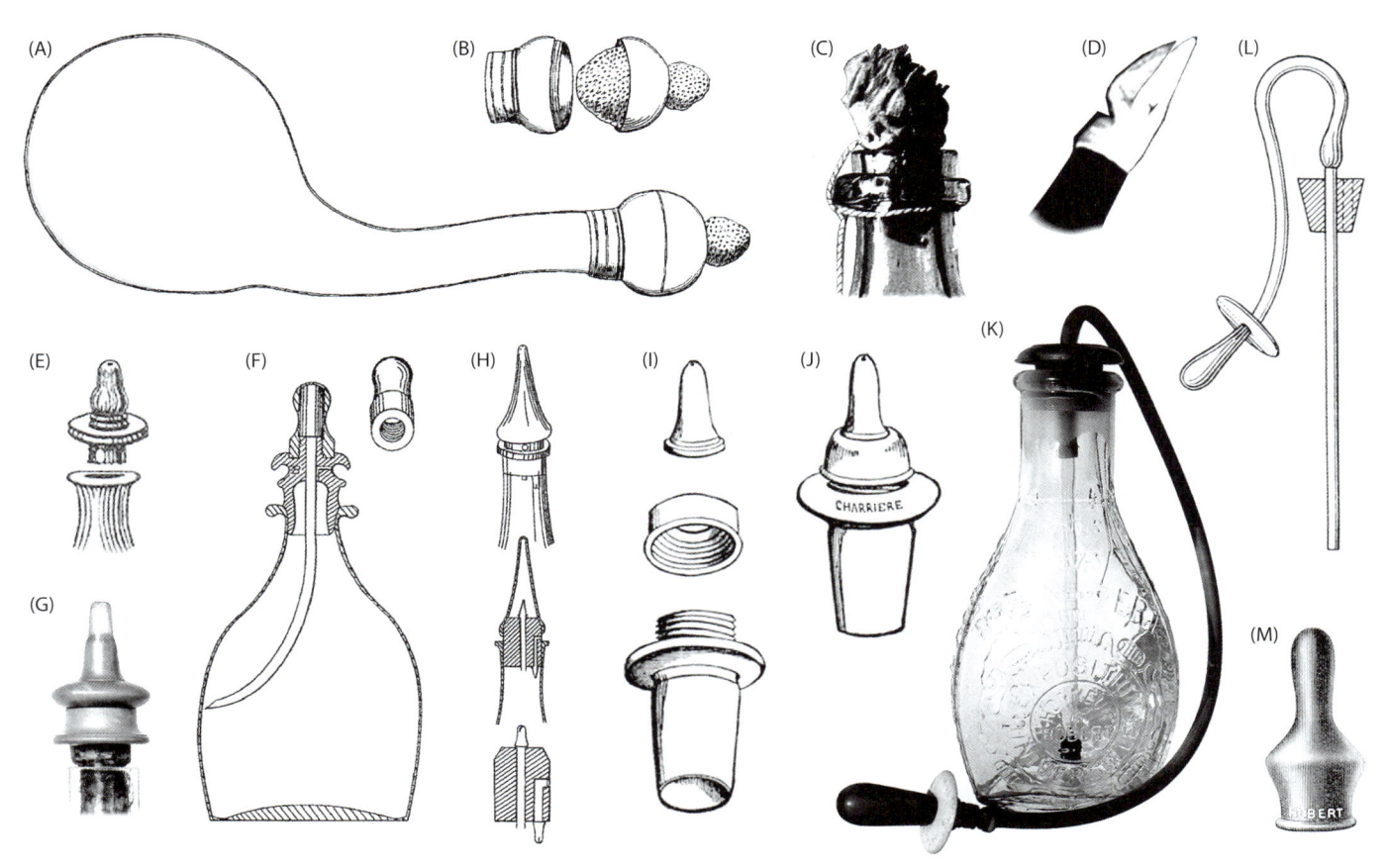

Fig. 6.7.1 Teat materials used during the 18th and 19th centuries: A, Baldini glass bottle of 1784 with spherical sponge capsule; B, Baldini's guilded sponge capsule, opened; C, Baudelocque sponge of 1787 with recovery thread; D, slitted parchment attached to a cow horn, ca. 1750; E, Madame Breton's tanned heifer's teat of 1826; F, Dupuy patented baby bottle of 1844 with softened ivory teat; G, Darbo cork teat of 1850; H, Pratt's patented teat of 1845, corkpiece with air inlet and outlet valves, cover of India-rubber; I, Charrière teat of 1862 from softened ivory, disassembled; J, Charrière teat, assembled; K, Robert *biberon* of 1873 with glass pipe, teat, and tube of rubber; L, Auvard rubber teat of 1889, glass pipe, rubber tube, and cork with air inlet; M, Robert rubber teat directly adaptable ('sens tube') to the bottleneck, 1895.

care was developed (see Appendix 3). Driven by competition among beer brewers, highly varied systems for producing ice were developed from 1860 to 1890 in Europe and the US by Gorrie, Harrison, Kirk, Toselli, Windhausen, Linde, and many others [29]. Priority fights, patent lawsuits, and national historiographies illustrate how capitalism and nationalism exploited scientific progress towards the end of the 19th century. Darcel reported on the difficulties which Carré's apparatus encountered in 1863 [30]: 'Businessmen came, ingenious in another way, who accused Monsieur Carré of imitation; but the Paris Imperial Court ruled that they had themselves counterfeited the apparatus of Monsieur Carré, who merits having first industrialized and published these principles.' The availability of efficient and economic refrigeration enabled new food technologies such as the transport of frozen meat and storage of milk products. Ice boxes were introduced to nurseries before 1880 and to private households from 1900; they were replaced by electric refrigerators in North America from 1930, in Europe after World War II.

Microbiology and pasteurization

A pioneer in the understanding of microbiology, Louis Pasteur discovered pasteurization (of wine) in 1860 [31]. It was not advocated for milk until 1886, when Munich chemist Franz Soxhlet described 'partial sterilization' of milk to prevent diarrhoeal disease in infants [32]: 'In the standard dairy, milk is contaminated with fodder and manure carrying fermenting agents ... Sterilization occurs within 35–40 minutes when the milk is heated in closed bottles to the temperature of boiling water ... I have elaborated such a system and realized in my own family that it is not difficult to apply ... The boy was nourished with milk that originated from an unclean city cowstable in which besides hay, distillery slop was fed, and he never suffered the slightest indigestion.' Soxhlet's apparatus (Fig. 6.7.3), soon found in many households, was adapted for Britain [33] and France [34]. In the US, Atwood patented an apparatus allowing large-scale pasteurization of milk in 1897 [35]. Abraham Jacobi wrote in 1898 [36]: 'Nothing has been more successful in that direction [to remove the dangers of intestinal disorders and the sources of excessive mortality] than the wide-spread practice of sterilization and pasteurization of cow's milk.' Pathogenic bacteria were detected in rapid sequence: *Mycobacterium tuberculosis* by Koch in 1882 [37], *Escherichia coli* by Escherich in 1885 [38], and group B streptococci by Nocard in 1887 [39]. Understanding their culturing conditions advanced the pasteurization technique. In Boston in 1908, Milton Rosenau described the thermal death of bacteria opening the door for high-temperature short-time ('flash') pasteurization [40]. Today

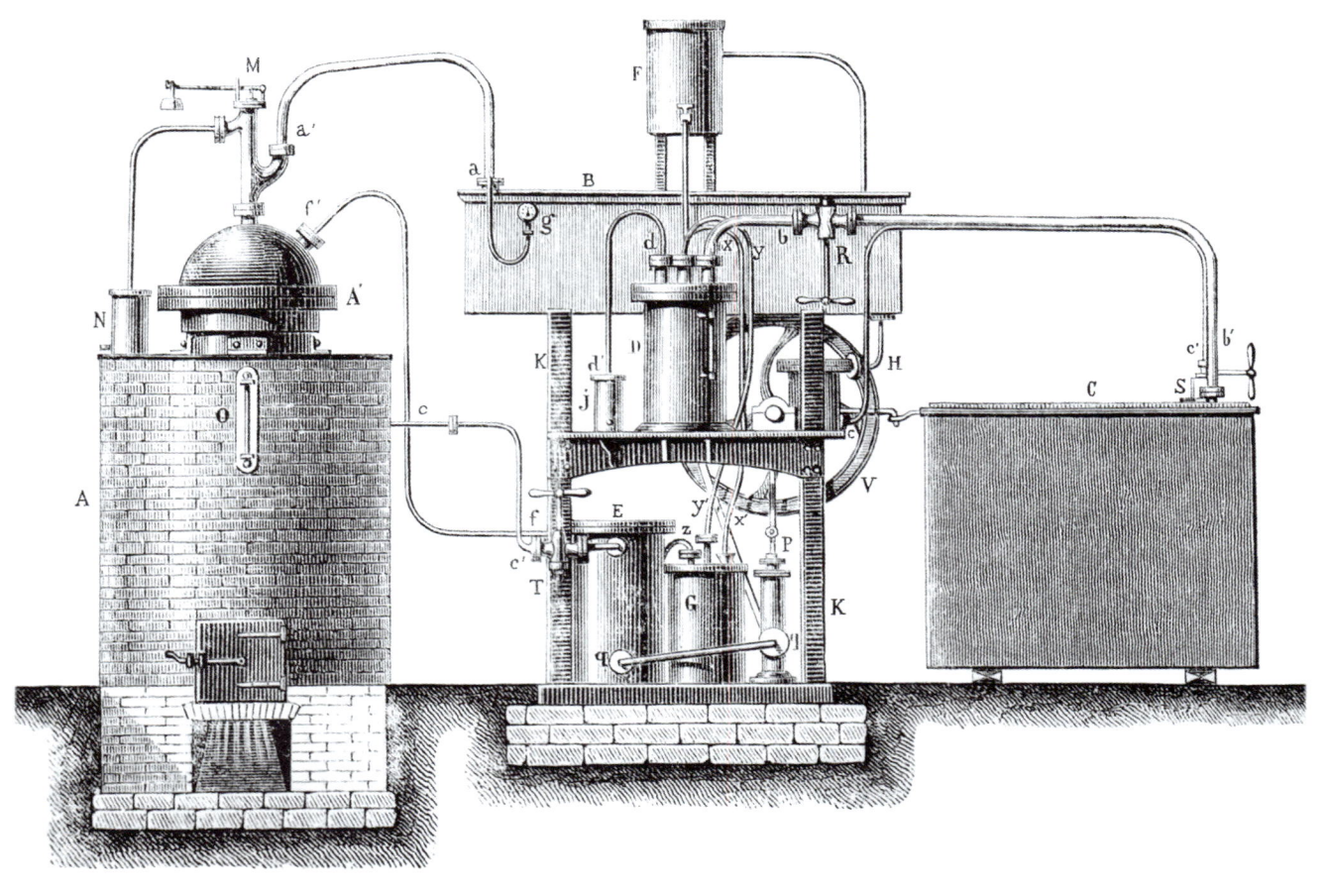

Fig. 6.7.2 Ammonia absorption cooling machine developed by Ferdinand Carré 1860 that could produce up to 250 kg ice per hour [28, 30].

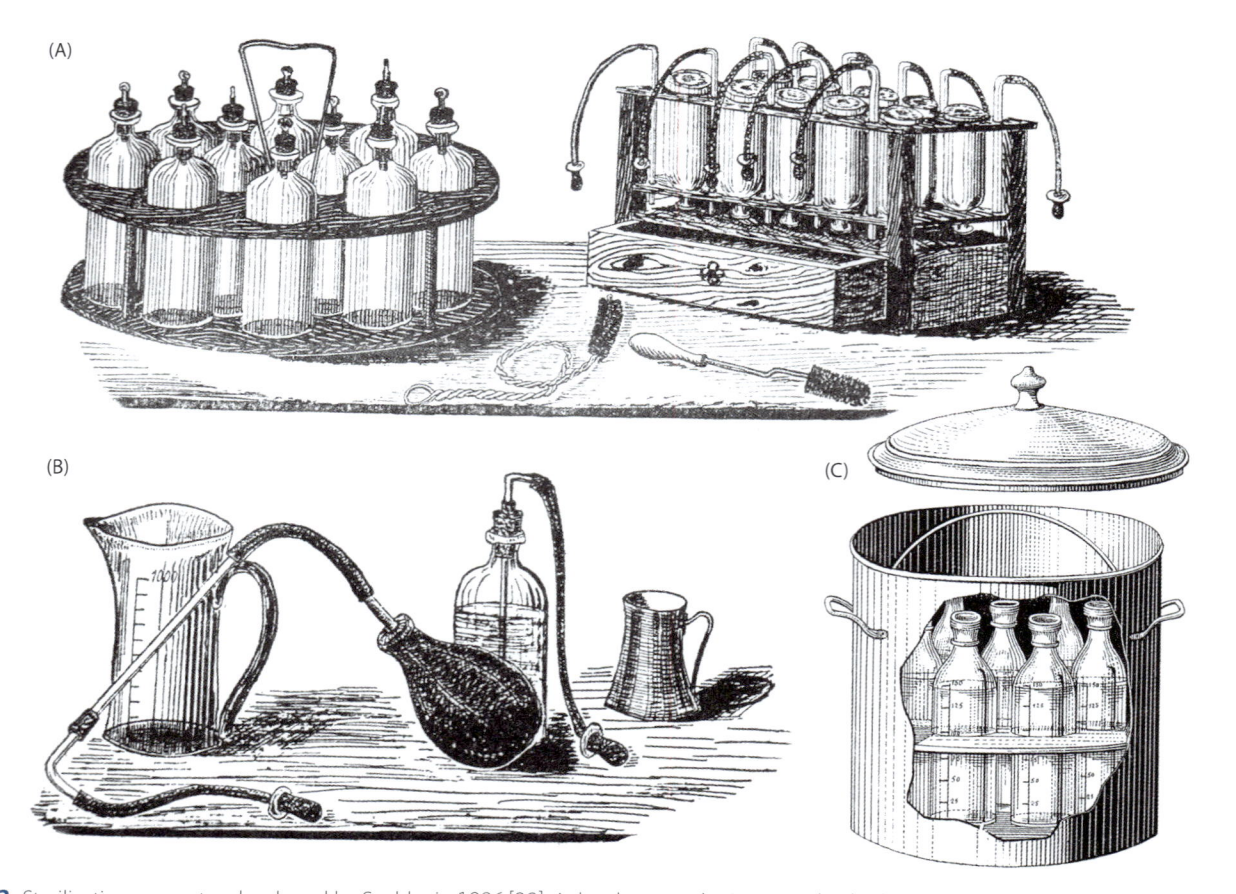

Fig. 6.7.3 Sterilization apparatus developed by Soxhlet in 1886 [32]. A, bottle tray to be immersed in boiling water; B, cleaning utensils for bottles and tubes; C, Budin's modification of the Soxhlet apparatus for rubber-capped bottles [34].

the pasteurization of cow's milk is compulsory in most countries. For very low birthweight infants, donated human milk is usually pasteurized, but the procedure brings no advantage for a mother's own milk [41].

Fuelled by the discovery that scurvy occurred when milk was boiled, reservations about and prejudice against pasteurization persisted for decades. As late as 1943, G.S. Wilson from the London School of Hygiene fought for the compulsory pasteurization of milk [42] and deplored that '5 to 10% of farms in this country are sending out milk containing tubercle bacilli; and a much higher proportion containing mastitis [i.e. group B] streptococci'.

Storing, preserving, and transport

Peter Durand of Middlesex patented the sealed metal container in 1810 [43]. In 1856, Gail Borden of Texas patented an evaporizer with which he could produce condensed milk [44]. Evaporation and tin-plate cans were used by Nestlé in Switzerland from 1875 [45], allowing transport and storage without microbial contamination. Tinned condensed milk was marketed on a commercial scale from 1870 and by 1892 accounted for 12% of all London's milk consumption [46]. In 1867, J.B. Sutherland of Detroit patented a refrigerated railroad car [47]. But in Britain most railroad cars remained unrefrigerated in 1904, even when travelling for several days, as described by Lawson Dodd [48]: 'The railway companies have no financial or other interest in the delivery of clean milk … The churns from the farms are allowed to stand for hours on platforms of rural stations … the milk is often exposed to the hot rays of the sun and the dust of passing traffic.' In the 20th century, the advent of the motor car drove horses, their stables, and their manure out of the cities, reducing the number of flies and their transport of bacteria into baby food.

Conclusion

In the middle of the 19th century, technical progress reduced the risk of milk-borne bacterial infection. Of vital importance were sterilizable glass bottles and rubber teats. With the advent of technical equipment for cooling, pasteurization, and evaporation, large-scale production of safe infant food became possible. The developing formula industry utilized these inventions more rapidly than private households, but left important issues unresolved, such as protection against necrotizing enterocolitis, the need for clean water, and high costs.

REFERENCES

1. Brüning H: Geschichte der Methodik der künstlichen Säuglingsernährung. Stuttgart: Enke, 1908: p. 45–123.
2. Forsyth D: The history of infant-feeding from Elizabethan times. Proc R Soc Med 1911;**4**:110–41.
3. Drake TGH: Infant feeding in England and in France from 1750 to 1800. Am J Dis Child 1930;**34**:1049–61.
4. Wickes IG: A history of infant feeding. I. Primitive peoples. Arch Dis Child 1953;**28**:151–8.
5. Fildes V: Breasts, bottles, and babies. Edinburgh: Edinburgh University Press, 1986: p. 98–121, 307.
6. Baudelocque JL: De l'allaitement au biberon. In: Principes sur l'art des accouchemens. Paris: Méquignon, 1787: p. 313–9.
7. Henke A: Handbuch zur Erkenntniß und Heilung der Kinderkrankheiten. 3. ed. Frankfurt: Wilmans, 1821: Vol. **1**, p. 89–106.
8. Meissner FL: Die Kinderkrankheiten nach den neusten Ansichten und Erfahrungen. 3. ed. Leipzig: Fest, 1844: Vol. **1**, p. 36–49.
9. Armstrong G: An account of the diseases most incident to children. 2. ed. London: Cadell, 1783: p. 157–68.
10. Smith H: Letters to married women on nursing. 6. ed. London: Kearsley, 1792: p. VII, 125–32, 189.
11. Hauner A: Über Pflege und Wartung der Kinder in den ersten Lebensjahren. J Kinderkrankh 1853;**21**:209–30.
12. Breton MV: Avis aux mères qui ne peuvent pas nourrir. Paris: Baillière, 1826: p. 4–6.
13. Jury central sur les produits de l'Industrie Française: Rapport. Paris: Bouchard-Huzard, 1839: Vol. **3**, p. 465.
14. Swygenhofen Chv: La Gutta-Percha, ou application de cette substance à la médecine. Bruxelles: Parent, 1848: p. 15–6.
15. Landrin H-C: Nouveau manuel complet du fabricant d'instruments de chirurgie. Paris: Roret, 1860: p. 83.
16. Bull T: The maternal management of children, in health and disease. 2. ed. Philadelphia, PA: Lindsay and Blakiston, 1853: p. 80–2.
17. Goodyear C: Improvement in India-Rubber fabrics. United States Patent Office 1844; Pat.-Nr. 3633.
18. Pratt E: Improvement in nursing bottles. US Patent Office 1845; Pat.-Nr. 4138.
19. Barrett T: Advice on the management of children in early infancy. Bath: Binns and Goodwin, 1851: p. 48.
20. Baldini F: Manière d'allaiter les enfants a la main au defaut de nourrices. Paris: Buisson, 1786: p. 66–75.
21. Windship C: Method of constructing Lacteal or artificial breasts. US Patent Office 1841; Pat.-Nr. 1985.
22. Routh CHF: Infant feeding and its influence on life. 3. ed. New York: Wood, 1879: p. 31–3, 50, 104, 150.
23. Fauvel H: Note sur les altérations du lait dans les biberons. Bull Acad Méd 1881;**10**:614–7.
24. Sautereau M: Le docteur Léon Dufour et l'oeuvre de la "Goutte de lait" (1894–1928). Ann Normandie 1991;**41**:217–33.
25. Julien P: Nouveaux documents sur le biberon Robert. Rev Hist Pharm 1996;**43**:25–37.
26. Fomon S: Infant feeding in the 20th century. J Nutr 2001;**131**: 409S–20S.
27. Cullen W: On the cold produced by evaporating fluids and of some other means of producing cold. Edinburgh: Hamilton, 1756: Vol. **2**, p. 145–56.
28. Carré FPE: Note sur un appareil propre à produire du froid. Compt Rend Acad Sci 1860;**51**:1023–7.
29. Reif-Acherman S: The early ice making systems in the nineteenth century. Int J Refrigeration 2012;**35**:1224–52.
30. Darcel A: Production économique du froid et de la glace. L'Illustration, J Univ 1863;**41**:303–4.
31. Pasteur L: Mémoire sur la fermentation alcoolique. Ann Chim Phys 1860;**58**:323–426.
32. Soxhlet F: Über Kindermilch und Säuglings-Ernährung. Münch Med Wochenschr 1886;**33**:253–6, 276–8.
33. Stewart CH: The sterilization of milk. BMJ 1896;**2**:626–8.

34. Budin P: Le Nourrisson. Paris: Doin, 1900: p. 23, 41, 99, 213.
35. Atwood H: Apparatus for pasteurizing milk. US Patent Office 1897; Pat. Nr. 586831.
36. Jacobi A: Therapeutics of infancy and childhood. 2. ed. Philadelphia, PA: Lippincott, 1898: p. 27–9.
37. Koch R: Die Ätiologie der Tuberkulose. Berlin Klin Wochenschr 1882;**19**:221–30.
38. Escherich T: Die Darmbakterien des Neugeborenen und Säuglings. Fortschr Med 1885;**3**:512–22; 547–55.
39. Nocard M: Mammite contagieuse. Bull Mém Soc Centr Méd Vét 1885;**39**:296–302.
40. Rosenau MT: The thermal death points of pathogenic microorganisms in milk. Hyg Lab Bull No. 42. Washington, DC: US Public Health and Marine Hospital Service, 1908.
41. Cossey V, Vanhole C, Eerdekens A, et al.: Pasteurization of mother's own milk for preterm infants does not reduce the incidence of late-onset sepsis. Neonatology 2013;**103**:170–6.
42. Wilson GS: The pasteurization of milk. BMJ 1943;**1**:261–2.
43. Durand P: A method of preserving animal food, vegetable food, and other perishable articles. Rep Art Manufact Agric 1811;**19**:193–6.
44. Borden G: Concentration of sweet milk and extracts. US Patent Office 1856; Pat.-Nr. 15553.
45. Pfiffner A: Henri Nestlé (1814–1890). Vom Frankfurter Apothekergehilfen zum Schweizer Pionierunternehmer. Zürich: Chronos, 1993: p. 150, 174.
46. Atkins PJ: White poison? The social consequences of milk consumption, 1850–1930. Soc Hist Med 1992;**5**: 207–27.
47. Sutherland JB: Improved refrigerator-car. United States Patent Office 1867; Pat.-Nr. 71423.
48. Dodd FL: Municipal milk and public health. Fabian Tracts 1905;**3**:1–19. Reprint London 1969.

6.8

Selling safety
Commercial production of infant formula

Introduction

Breastfeeding by the own mother is the best way to feed an infant. However, there have always been mothers who could not or would not breastfeed their own infant and who preferred artificial nutrition ('hand-feeding'). With industrialization, the breastfeeding rate and duration began to decline during the 19th century (see Chapter 6.4). Physicians and politicians criticized the practice because it was associated with gastroenteritis (cholera infantum) and elevated infant mortality. Up to the middle of the 19th century, substitutes were hand-made with whatever nutrients were available, often with dirty cow's milk or contaminated water. Weaver has delineated how our modern understanding of infant nutrition emerged [1]. The situation changed gradually when industrially processed infant foods came onto the market. The following chapter traces this development.

Gail Borden's *Condensed Milk*, 1856

In 1856, after years refining his apparatus (Fig. 6.8.1), the Texan inventor Gail Borden patented a 'milk concentrating process to be performed in a vacuum pan' [2]. He had already published a newspaper and produced the meat biscuit 'pemmican' with little success. He and his partner Jeremiah Milbank opened a factory in Burrville, Connecticut, in 1857. Renamed 'New York Condensed Milk Company', they sold evaporated milk to the Unionist army during the Civil War. Their evaporation technique was exported to Europe by George and Charles Page, who founded the 'Anglo-Swiss Condensed Milk Company' in Cham, Switzerland, in 1866 [3]. Borden pioneered the use of glass milk bottles in 1885 [4]. In addition to Eagle brand condensed milk, the company produced malted milk for infants.

Justus von Liebig's *Soup for Infants*, 1865

The Munich chemist Justus von Liebig was already famous for his 'meat extract' when in 1865 he invented 'a soup representing the most complete replacement of mother's milk' [5]. The product had to be heated for 1 h at 66°C to transform starch and malt to sugar (Table 6.8.1). Liebig initially denied having commercial interests and pretended to have philanthropic motives by feeding the 'soup' to his grandchildren, the sick son of the Munich obstetrician Carl Hecker [6], and to his biographer Volhard's children [7]. He published the recipe in 1865 [5], and several entrepreneurs immediately began producing and marketing it; the Munich pharmacy Pachmayr sold 30,000 packs within 11 months. Follow-up brands were produced by E. Löflund, J.P. Liebe, and J.R. Nichols, and soon many others were on sale in Stuttgart, London, Boston, France, and Switzerland from 1866 [3]. Liebig's infant food was sold in the US in 1869 for $1.00 a bottle.

Henri Nestlé's *Farine Lactée*, 1867

The tradesman and pharmacist Henri Nestlé invented an infant food in 1867 which became a worldwide success. He had previously manufactured bone meal fertilizer, lamp oil, and liquid gas in Vevey, Switzerland. Like Liebig, he claimed philanthropic motives by feeding a preterm infant (*le petit Wanner*), whom his biographer Pfiffner could not track down [8]. *Farine lactée* (Kindermehl) consisted of ground rusk-like wheaten bread, condensed milk, and potassium carbonate and was diluted with water. One box lasted for 5 days and was sold for 1.25 Swiss francs, 1.80 French francs, 50 German Kreuzer, and 50 cents in the US. Nestlé wrote in 1868: 'Liebig's children's soup is excellent, but laborious to prepare, to which adds the trouble of procuring flour, malt, milk and potash of high quality, which is no small thing.' An immigrant with limited rights in Switzerland, Nestlé aimed at large-scale industrial production and international marketing right from the start. His product met a need in the small town of Vevey [8]: 'I sell a dozen tins a day, a success exceeding all my expectations … When just as much were sold in the large cities, I must set up a colossal factory and will soon be a millionaire.' Both forecasts came true. Within 7 years the sales of *Farine lactée* rose to 3000 tins per day and Nestlé had to enlarge his factory several times. In 1875, he sold his company including his name for a million Swiss francs

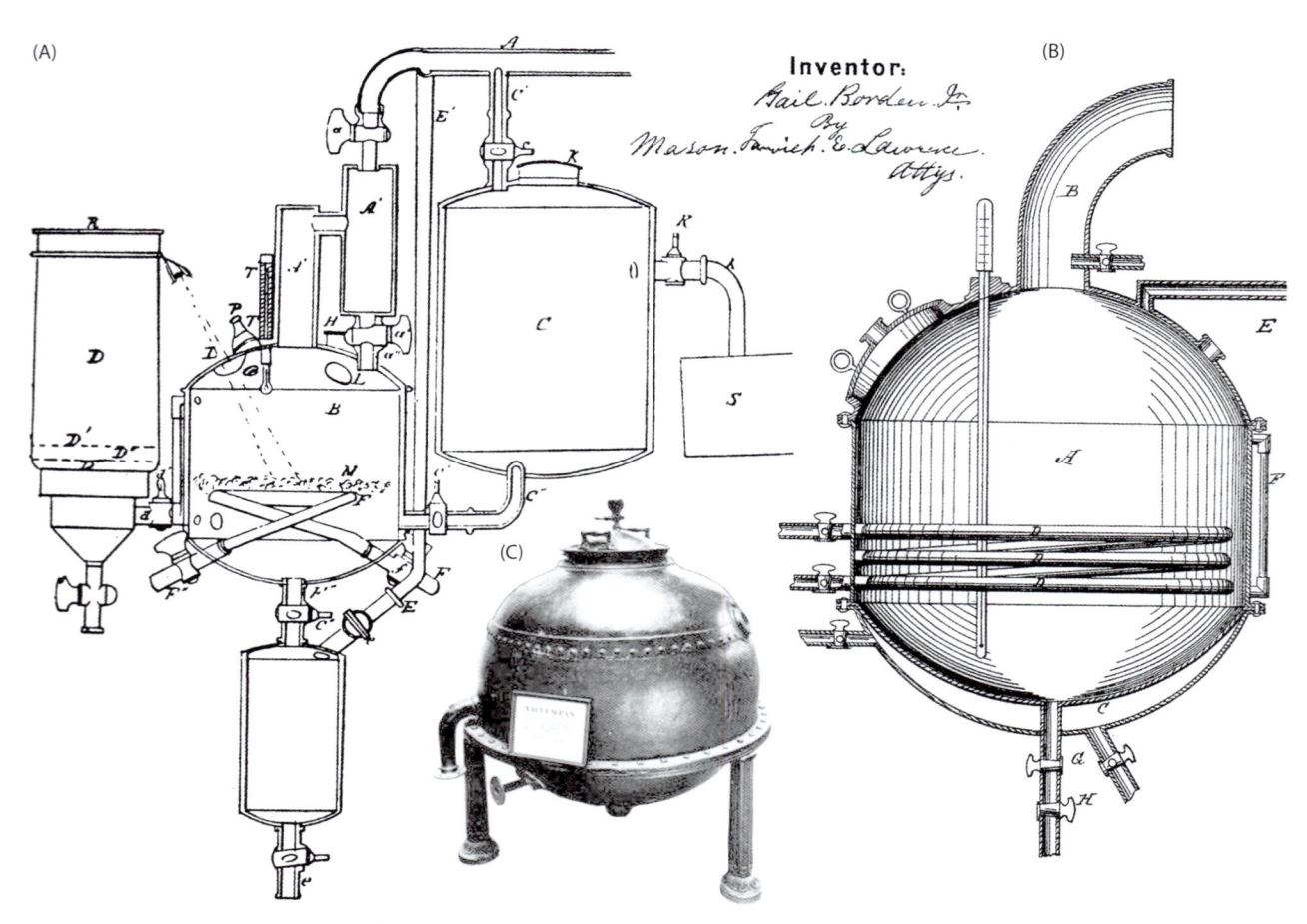

Fig. 6.8.1 A, evaporizer equipment for condensing milk, from Borden's 1856 patent [2]; B, improved vacuum pan from Borden's 1865 patent [61] (with B, pipe leading to the condenser and air pumps; C, steam jacket; D, coil pipe for steam; E, induction pipe for fresh milk); C, Borden's vacuum pan.

plus a carriage. In 1905, Nestlé and Anglo-Swiss merged, and today Nestlé S.A. is the world's largest food company with nearly 500 factories and annual sales exceeding US$1 billion.

Composition, competition, commerce, and cost

The early commercial formulas had remarkably different compositions, as summarized in Table 6.8.1. In most of them, the starch was converted into soluble maltose and dextrin, as proposed by Liebig. The London pharmacist Gustav Mellin invented a milk modifier in 1866, which was exported to the US from 1874 and became very successful when adapted to Rotch's percentage feeding. Also in the US, Mellin's former co-worker James Horlick produced malted milk, which combined dry milk and a milk modifier. To evaporation and maltose enrichment, Philipp Biedert of Alsace and Arthur Victor Meigs of Philadelphia added modification of the cream compound (Table 6.8.1). Physicians praised one or the other product without sound scientific evidence, and without consensus, 'a humiliating role', as Rotch complained in 1893 [9]. As outlined by Weaver [10], the control of nutritional intake differed among countries: the French favoured weight control, the Americans volumetry or percentage feeding, and the Germans calculated caloric intake. Within a few years, several companies grew from zero to large-scale industries. Competition persisted for some time between physician-prescribed and pharmacist-distributed products; those manufactured in pasteurization plants, especially the Walker–Gorden Laboratories; and proprietary formula. Formula feeding was expensive in relation to the family income: feeding an infant with Nestlé's food absorbed a quarter of a factory maid's or 10% of an average employee's income in 1875. A hundred years later in Costa Rica, feeding formula during the first 3 months was equivalent to 18% of the minimum wage [11]. It was no help for the poor, who needed safe nutrients most urgently.

The formulation of artificial feeds up to 1910 was reported by Mepham [12]. In 1925, Grover Powers from Yale characterized 27 widely used milk mixtures, classified them into seven groups, and stated [13]: 'The majority show higher values for total calories in protein and carbohydrate and a lower value for fat. Indeed, the popular mixtures are as unlike human milk as they are unlike unmodified cow's milk.'

Safety and health

Proprietary infant formulas put an end to the age-old threat of cholera infantum. But was it a causal relationship or a coincidence? Homemade infant food also profited from rubber teats, pasteurization, refrigeration, and sewerage (see Chapter 6.7). Formulas also introduced a new trouble: scurvy, which spread within the institutions housing artificially fed infants. Philipp Doepp, physician at the St.

Table 6.8.1 Nineteenth-century proprietary infant formulas

Author/company, year	Name of product	Weight percentages of carbohydrate (C), protein (P), and fat (F).	Preparation by mother	Reference
Borden 1856 US	Eagle brand condensed milk	Concentrated and sweetened cow's milk. C 71.9; P 13.4; F 6.1. Malted milk for infants from 1890	Reconstituted with 6 parts water	[17] [18]
Liebig 1865 UK 1868 US 1869	Suppe für Säuglinge	(Skim) milk, wheaten flour, malt, bicarbonate of potash. C 72.0; P 16.2; F 10.2	See text; usually prepared by pharmacy	[12]
Anglo-Swiss Co. 1866, Cham, Switzerland	Milkmaid	C 68.7; P 14.6; F 13.1	Concentrate of honey consistency, to be diluted with 1:6 warm water	[3]
Gustav Mellin, Britain 1866, US from 1874	Mellin's infant food	Milk modifier: malted carbohydrate Desiccated malt extract; maltose; dextrin C 80.3; P 11.4; F 0.5	Dissolved in hot water, then cold milk added	[19] [20]
Nestlé 1867, Vevey, Switzerland; US 1890	Farine lactée/malted milk	Dextrin and wheat starch C 79.0; P 11.1; F 5.1 1932: C 69.5; P 15.0; F 9.8	Boiled with water for a few minutes	[3] [21]
Horlick 1875, Racine, WI	Malted milk	Made from malted barley, wheat flour; starch converted to maltose + dextrin C 76.8; P 13.7; F 5.8	Water added	[22]
Biedert 1878, Hagenau/Alsace	Ramogen	Desiccated paste C 65.8; P 10.1; F 21.9	Pharmacy; marketed until 1935	[23] [24]
Maltine Manufacture Co. 1885, Bloomsbury, London	Carnrick's soluble food	Desiccated milk, malted wheat flour, lactose. C 80.6; P 14.4; F 2.6	1 part is mixed with 9 parts of water and boiled for a few minutes	[14]
AV Meigs 1885, Philadelphia	Meigs' mixture	Not sterilized C 50.8; P 9.0; F 38.5	5 mL milk, 10 mL cream, 10 mL lime water, 15 mL water, 2.2 g milk sugar	[12] [25] [26]
Allen & Hanbury 1892, Ware, Hertfordshire	Allenbury No. 1	Desiccated cow's milk, excess of casein removed, vegetable albumin and lactose added. C 70.9; P 10.3; F 14.8	Reconstituted with 6 parts of water	[14]
Frank Baum 1895, Smith & Kline	Eskay's albumenized food	Arrowroot, starch, lactose C 87.8; P 6.6; F 1.2	Pure cereal to be used with fresh cow's milk	[27]

Contents are given as weight percentages in the dry substance as analysed by Hutchison 1901 [14], Congdon in 1918 [15], and Hess in 1921 [16]. Protein determination is usually too high, differences to 100 are due to water, mineral matter, or ash. Comparative percentages for human milk were C 49.3; P 18.2; F 30.0; and for cow's milk C 38.0; P 27.9; F 28.6.

Petersburg foundling hospital, described a scurvy epidemic claiming 26 children in the spring of 1831 [28]. In Berlin in 1902, Neumann reported 27 cases of Barlow's disease occurring after 7 months of artificial feeding. He assumed that the 'antiscorbutic principle' was destroyed by extensive cooking or repeated heating in the Soxhlet apparatus [29]. In 1904, Lecornu described six cases of scurvy following feeding with industrial milk for several months in Paris [30]. In Zürich, Jacob Bernheim observed nine cases 'between September 1906 and May 1907, who had all received *Berner Alpenmilch*' and believed the disease resulted from homogenization [31]. In 1921, Finkelstein observed numerous scorbutic infants in Berlin—'exclusively a disease of bottle-fed infants' [32]. Vitamin C was detected by Holst and Frölich in 1912 and orange juice was given to infants [33]. The debate on pasteurization and vitamin loss continued until 1923 [34], when an editorial clarified that 'boiled fresh milk is the only entirely safe milk that can be fed to infants … Its loss of vitamin content is easily remediable by the addition of orange juice to the diet'.

'Humanization' during the 20th century

With advancing analyses of breast milk, formula composition was altered, a process euphemistically called 'humanization'. Hutchison classified the proliferating proprietary foods as: (1) dried cow's milk with some cereal, to be reconstituted with water; (2) farinaceous food, usually malted, requiring the addition of milk; and (3) farinaceous food with undigested starch [14]. Barness tabulated milestones in commercial formula development up to 1930 [35]. Fomon described formula enrichment with vitamins and iron [36]. Highlights are listed from these papers: 'dextri-maltose' introduced by Mead Johnson in 1911 to enrich energy; 'synthetic milk adapted' and vegetable fat by Gerstenberger in 1915; and cod liver oil, later synthetic vitamin D, in 1920. The antirachitic potency of cow's milk was increased by feeding the animals cod liver oil [37] or irradiated yeast [38]. In 1926, 'Similac' was marketed by Ross Laboratories; in 1929, a soybean-based formula for milk allergy; in 1931, 'Pablum', a mineral- and vitamin-fortified cereal; in 1942, 'Nutramigen', a hydrolysate; in 1951, iron fortification (Ross); and in 1959, 'Enfamil', fortification with choline and inositol. Weaver emphasized the importance of oligosaccharides [39]. However effectively the formula may have been improved, Abraham Jacobi's statement of 1898 remained true [40]: 'Ergo, cow's milk is not woman's milk.'

Subtle and aggressive marketing

The young field of paediatrics derived much of its identity from real or supposed difficulty to feed infants. Soon the industry realized that paediatric nutritional advice was rooted in neither scientific evidence nor personal experience but encouraged repeated consultations at the doctor's office. In 1932, the American Medical Association Committee on Foods ruled that 'the promulgation of feeding formulas in advertising to the laity is considered to be in conflict with the best experience, authoritative judgement, and basic principles in infant feeding and is not permissible' [41]. The industry joined forces with the paediatricians, ceased advertising to the laity and began supporting paediatric research and congresses. This allowed both sides to save face, to pay lip service to 'breast is best', and to use science in advertising. The products became 'to be used under the direction of a physician' [22]; the resulting conflict of interest has been described by Rima Apple [27] and Jacqueline Wolf [42]. There were and remain close connections between formula companies and paediatricians, but they developed after the market for formula rather than being a causal factor, and the marketing methods did not differ in Europe.

A modern war of faith

As early as 1939, Cicely Williams in Singapore gave a lecture entitled 'Milk and Murder' in which she emphasized the dangers of disrupting breastfeeding [43]. The conflict between the Swiss 'Third World Working Group' and the formula industry began in 1970 and illustrates how simplification and fixed opinions influence the interpretation of published data. Dobbing [44] and Newton [45] have reported on this long-standing controversy which had features of a crusade and class struggle. Nestlé S.A. was singled out as *pars pro toto* for a series of accusations: (1) steering mothers away from successful breastfeeding; (2) promoting baby food into developing countries without clean water; and (3) saleswomen masquerading as 'milk-nurses' who advertised formula in the Third World. In 1971, Derrick Jelliffe, director of the Caribbean Food and Nutrition Institute, linked advertising for industrial baby foods with less breastfeeding and elevated infant mortality: 'commerciogenic malnutrition', 'thoughtless promotion' [46]. 'There is alarming evidence that the sale of infant formula is leading directly to infant deaths' [45]. Mike Müller published a pamphlet in 1974: 'The baby killer: War on Want' [47]. His title was translated into 'Nestlé kills babies' and the company sued and won after a 2-year trial in Bern. A Pyrrhic victory, as its reputation had been severely damaged by the long and acrimonious public debate and by the judge's admonition: 'Nestlé must fundamentally rethink its methods of promotion for infant milks in developing countries ... to avoid the charge of immoral and unethical behavior' [44]. In July 1977, the US 'Infant Formula Action Coalition', endorsed by the National Council of Churches, started a boycott against all Nestlé products lasting 7 years. In May 1978, Senator Edward Kennedy held a public Senate hearing in which Jelliffe testified: 'We have calculated that if breast-feeding could be reinstituted in developing countries—and this is partly a guesstimate—some 10 million babies would be saved from diarrhea and marasmus each year.' Senator Kennedy asked: 'Can a product which requires clean water, good sanitation, adequate family income, and a literate parent to follow printed indications be properly and safely used in areas where water is contaminated, sewage runs in the streets, poverty is severe and illiteracy is high?' [44]. In 1981, Charles May, editor of *Pediatrics*, stated: 'No substantial, sound, scientific data were ever set forth by the critics of industry or officials of the WHO [World Health Organization] to support the claim that marketing practices for infant formulas have actually been a significant factor in decline in prevalence of breastfeeding' [48].

The WHO Code

After the hearings, the WHO issued recommendations for marketing infant formula in 1981 [49]. The 'International Code of Marketing Breast-Milk Substitutes' regulated advertising and sales promotion to the public and distributed to mothers free formula, feeding bottles, nipples, and pamphlets [44, 45]. Nestlé complied, and the boycott ended in October 1984. Violations of the Code were frequent, and complaints were listed each year [50, 51]. As late as 1996 in Thailand, where compliance with the WHO Code was voluntary, 26% of mothers received free samples of infant formula and/or feeding bottles or teats and 50% of the health workers received gifts donated by the companies [52]. National infant-formula legislation regulated the composition, labelling, and quality control of commercial formulas in most countries. The marketing code was one of several public health statements that contributed to the resurgence of breastfeeding at the end of the second millennium [53].

Artificial feeding and infant mortality

As early as 1860, London obstetrician Charles Routh published a book devoted to infant feeding and mortality [54]. The infant mortality rate remained around 150 per 1000 live births in England and Wales for half a century. Fig. 6.8.2 illustrates some of the multiple and interconnected factors that accompanied the decrease in the infant mortality rate during the 20th century. In the Third World, infant mortality remained elevated longer—but it decreased. Cessation of breastfeeding did not necessarily mean feeding commercial formula, which especially the poor could barely afford. In 1996, a large randomized trial in Belarus (PROBIT) investigated the effects of breastfeeding promotion based on the WHO recommendation. It proved that this intervention increased the duration and exclusivity of breastfeeding. The infants in the intervention group had significantly less gastroenteritis, but no significant difference in mortality, respiratory infection, asthma, and intelligence [55, 56]. Neither the WHO inquiry in developing countries [57] nor studies in the US and other industrialized countries [58] found the introduction of formula associated with increasing mortality. From 1977 to 1985, the Nicaraguan infant mortality rate declined from 122 to 65 per 1000 despite the fact that during that time breastfeeding rates (at 6 months) declined from 58% to 33% [59]. Nevertheless, *Lancet* editor Anna Coutsoudis insisted in 2009 [60]: 'Voracious global marketing by the formula-milk industry over the past 60 years has ... dislodged breastfeeding as a viable and desirable strategy for infant feeding.' However, it is even possible that an important part of the decrease in the infant mortality rate, in all countries, was due to safer artificial feeding; there is no proof that it occurred because of, or despite, the availability of commercial infant formula. The WHO emphasized that infants breastfed into their second year have significantly better survival than those who ceased breastfeeding

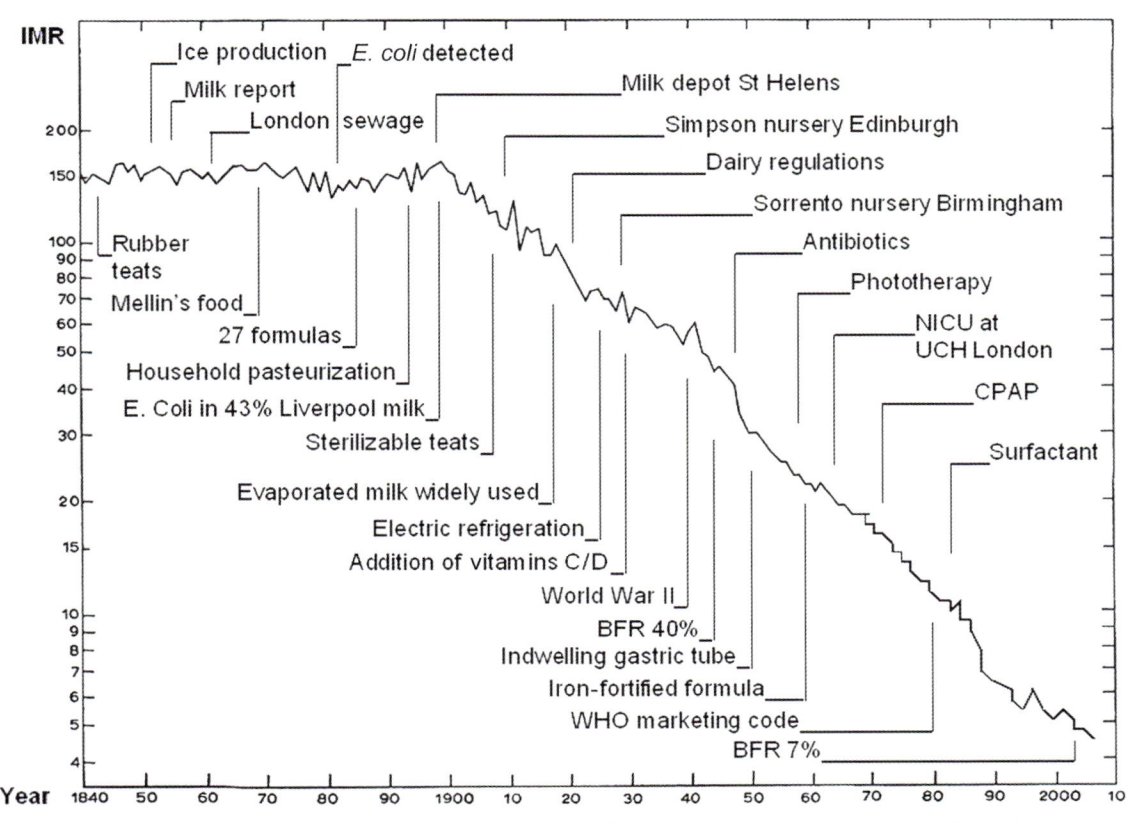

Fig. 6.8.2 Infant mortality rate per 1000 liveborn infants (IMR, logarithmic scale) of England and Wales 1840–2010. Above the curve: milestones in medicine and public health. Below the curve: milestones in infant nutrition. If not specified otherwise, lines indicate widespread use rather than first description. BFR, breastfeeding rate at 4 months; CPAP, continuous positive airway pressure; NICU, neonatal intensive care unit.
Source: Data from Beaver, M.W. Population, infant mortality and milk. *Population Studies*, 1973;27:243–254.

Conclusion

Preconditions for the production of safe and storable infant food were evaporation, pasteurization, and cooling. Once these requirements were fulfilled, a powerful market developed. Gross differences in the composition of proprietary formula did not affect their success. Industrially produced formula was expensive and of little benefit to those who needed it most. The decline in breastfeeding began early in the 19th century with paid female work. Women never had the choice of 'breast versus bottle', and poor women had no choice between safe and unsafe substitutes. The decision not to breastfeed is complex, influenced by cultural habits, cost considerations, and psychological and social factors. One remarkable aspect of the formula controversy is that neither the industry nor independent research had presented scientific proof for either of these two opinions: alleged increase or decrease in infant mortality due to feeding commercial formula.

REFERENCES

1. Weaver LT: The emergence of our modern understanding of infant nutrition and feeding 1750–1900. Curr Pediatr 2006;**16**:342–7.
2. Borden G: Concentration of sweet milk and extracts. US Patent Office 1856; Pat.-Nr. 15553.
3. Fürst L: Die künstliche Ernährung des Kindes im ersten Lebensjahre. Leipzig: Weber, 1870.
4. Frantz JB: Gail Borden: dairyman to a nation. Norman, OK: University of Oklahoma Press, 1951.
5. Liebig Jv: Suppe für Säuglinge. Ann Chem Pharm 1865;**133**: 374–83.
6. Hecker C: Eine Erfahrung über die Liebig'sche Suppe für Säuglinge. Ann Chem 1866;**138**:83–94.
7. Volhard J: Justus von Liebig. Leipzig: Barth, 1909: Vol. **2**, p. 304–8.
8. Pfiffner A: Henri Nestlé (1814–1890). Vom Frankfurter Apothekergehilfen zum Schweizer Pionierunternehmer. Zürich: Chronos, 1993: p. 116, 123, 210, 278.
9. Rotch TM: The general principles underlying all good methods of infant feeding. Boston Med Surg J 1893;**129**:505–6.
10. Weaver LT: "Growing babies": defining the milk requirements in infants 1890–1910. Soc Hist Med 2009;**23**:320–37.
11. Mata L: Breast-feeding: main promoter of infant health. Am J Clin Nutr 1978;**31**:2058–65.
12. Mepham TB: "Humanizing" milk: the formulation of artificial feeds for infants (1850–1910). Med Hist 1993;**37**:225–49.
13. Powers GF: Comparison and interpretation on a caloric basis of the milk mixtures used in infant feeding. Am J Dis Child 1925;**30**:453–75.
14. Hutchison R: Food and the principles of dietetics. 3. ed. London: Arnold, 1901: p. 445–7.
15. Congdon LA: A study of foods for infants. Trans Kansas Acad Sci 1918;**29**:209–16.

16. Hess JH: Principles and practice of infant feeding. 2. ed. Philadelphia, PA: Davis, 1921: p. 275.
17. Frantz AG: Prolactin. N Engl J Med 1978;**298**:201–7.
18. Cone TE: 200 years of feeding infants in America. Columbus, OH: Ross Laboratories, 1976: p. 17–92.
19. Cone TE: History of American pediatrics. Boston, MA: Little, Brown & Co., 1979: p. 146.
20. Apple RD: "Advertised by our loving friends": the infant formula industry and the creation of new pharmaceutical markets, 1870–1910. J Hist Med All Sci 1986;**41**:3–23.
21. Pfiffner A: Henri Nestlé (1814–1890). Vom Frankfurter Apothekergehilfen zum Schweizer Pionierunternehmer. Zürich: Chronos, 1993: p. 150, 174.
22. Apple RD: "To be used only under the direction of a physician": commercial infant feeding and medical practice, 1870–1940. Bull Hist Med 1980;**54**:402–17.
23. Biedert Ph: Das künstliche Rahmgemenge. Jahrb Kinderheilk N.F. 1878;**12**:366–75.
24. Powers GF: Infant feeding. JAMA 1935;**105**:753–61.
25. Bracken FJ: The history of artificial feeding of infants. Maryland State Med J 1956;**5**:40–54.
26. Meigs AV: Milk analysis and infant feeding. Philadelphia, PA: Blakiston, 1885: p. 49–60.
27. Apple RD: Mothers and medicine. Madison, WI: University of Wisconsin Press, 1987: p. 4, 66.
28. Doepp P: Notizen über das kaiserliche Erziehungshaus (Findlingshaus) zu St. Petersburg. Hamburg: Hoffmann & Campe, 1835: Vol. **5**, p. 306–50.
29. Paladin A, Wahl J, Zink A: Evidence of probable subadult scurvy in the Early Medieval cemetery of Castel Tirolo, South Tyrol, Italy. Int J Osteoarchaeol 2018;**28**:714–26.
30. Lecornu P: Les laits industriels, leur valeur dans l'allaitement artificiel. Paris: Rousset, 1904.
31. Bernheim-Karrer J: Säuglings-Scorbut bei Ernährung mit homogenisierter Berner Alpenmilch. Correspondenz-Blatt für Schweizer Ärzte 1907;**37**:593–8.
32. Finkelstein H: Lehrbuch der Säuglingskrankheiten. 2. ed. Berlin: Springer, 1921: p. 149, 355, 542.
33. Kreiter SR, Schwartz RP, Kirkman HN, et al.: Nutritional rickets in African American breast-fed infants. J Pediat 2000;**137**:153–7.
34. Editorial: Milk: safe or unsafe? Boston Med Surg J 1923;**188**:177.
35. Barness LA: History of infant feeding practices. Am J Clin Nutr 1987;**46**:168–70.
36. Fomon S: Infant feeding in the 20th century. J Nutr 2001;**131**:409S–20S.
37. Lesné E, Vagliano M: Production d'un lait de vache donné de propriétés antirachitiques. Compt Rend Acad Sci 1924;**179**:539–44.
38. Lomax E: Difficulties in diagnosing infantile scurvy before 1878. Med Hist 1986;**30**:70–80.
39. Weaver LT: Improving infant milk formulas. J Pediatr Gastroenterol Nutr 2003;**36**:307–10.
40. Jacobi A: Therapeutics of infancy and childhood. 2. ed. Philadelphia, PA: Lippincott, 1898: p. 27–9.
41. AMA Committee on Foods: Feeding formulas for infants in lay advertising. JAMA 1932;**99**:391.
42. Wolf JH: The first generation of American pediatricians and their inadvertent legacy to breastfeeding. Breastfeed Med 2006;**1**:172–7.
43. Baumslag N: Cicely Delphine Williams, 1893–1992. Am J Public Health 1993;**83**:1500–1.
44. Dobbing J: Infant feeding. Anatomy of a controversy 1973–1984. London: Springer, 1988: p. 4, 55, 85.
45. Newton LH: Truth is the daughter of time: the real story of the Nestlé case. Bus Soc Rev 1999;**104**:367–95.
46. Jelliffe DB: Commerciogenic malnutrition? Time for a dialogue. Food Technol 1971;**15**:55–6.
47. Müller M: The baby killer. War on Want. London: Oxfam, 1974.
48. May CD: The "infant formula controversy": a notorious threat to reason in matters of health. Pediatrics 1981;**68**:428–30.
49. WHO/UNICEF: International code of marketing breast milk substitutes. WHO Chron 1981;**35**:112–7.
50. Koletzko B: Marketing of dietetic products for infants and young children in Europe. Ann Nutr Metab 2011;**59**:70–2.
51. Brady JP: Marketing breast milk substitutes. Arch Dis Child 2012;**97**:529–32.
52. Taylor A: Violations of the international code of marketing of breast milk substitutes: prevalence in four countries. BMJ 1998;**316**:1117–22.
53. Wright AL, Schanler RJ: The resurgence of breastfeeding at the end of the second millennium. J Nutr 2001;**131**:421S–5S.
54. Routh CHF: Infant feeding and its influence on life. 3. ed. New York: Wood, 1879: p. 31–3, 50, 104, 150.
55. Kramer MS, Matush L, Vanilovich I, et al.: Effect of prolonged and exclusive breast feeding on risk of allergy and asthma: cluster randomised trial. BMJ 2007;**335**:815.
56. Kramer MS, Matush L, Bogdanovich N, et al.: Health and development outcomes in 6.5-y-old children breastfed exclusively for 3 or 6 mo. Am J Clin Nutr 2009;**90**:1070–4.
57. Raphael D, Davis F: Only mothers know: patterns of infant feeding in traditional cultures. Westport, CT: Greenwood, 1985.
58. Kovar MG, Serdula MK, Marks JS, Fraser DW: Review of the epidemiologic evidence for an association between infant feeding and infant health. Pediatrics 1984;**74**:615–38.
59. Sandifort P, Morales P, Gorter A, et al.: Why do child mortality rates fall? Am J Public Health 1991;**81**:30–7.
60. Coutsoudis A, Coovadia HM, King J: The breastmilk brand: promotion of child survival in the face of formula-milk marketing. Lancet 2009;**374**:423–5.
61. Borden G: Improvement in condensing milk. US Patent Office 1865; Pat.-Nr. 2103.

6.9

Feeding the feeble
Steps towards nourishing preterm infants

Introduction

Before specialized institutions allowed prematures to survive, there was little knowledge on how to feed them. The infant's weak suck usually led to the mother producing less milk, a vicious circle. Hospitalized preterm infants had next to no chance, as Charles Billard described [1]: 'Marie Loisel was brought to the [Paris] Foundling Hospital shortly after birth on August 4, 1826. She was 37 cm in length, her legs extremely small, face congested and very red, skin discolored, few movements. Her cry, albeit complete, was barely audible. She swallowed without vomiting, but refused the breast … During the following days she remained in the same condition and finally died on the morning of the 10th without any other symptom but extreme weakness.' In private households, favourable circumstances could improve the child's chances. In 1839, Charles Richard (de Nancy) described a boy born 12 weeks before term in Lyon [2]: 'The infant was extremely small, the skin red, nails incomplete … His room was well heated and his cradle flanked by stoneware jugs filled with warm water … His weakness was so great that he could not suck the breast, so he was spoonfed. The mother placed her milk drop by drop on his lips and into his mouth. For two weeks, he was nourished via a *téterelle à pompe*. During this time the mother first used puppies, then a stronger infant to empty her breast … [The premature boy] eventually learned to suck and developed from day to day.' Focusing particularly on the US, Thomas Cone described pioneers in the care and feeding of the preterm infant [3]. The aim of this chapter is to describe the development of feeding techniques for and the increase in knowledge on the nutritional needs of premature infants.

Weak sucking and swallowing

In 1851, not long after vulcanized rubber was invented, the Charenton obstetrician Marchant [4] described feeding by intermittent gavage: 'With such weakness, respiration is impaired and the swallowing of nutrients impossible, so infants perish within several hours and two days … In such cases, I propose artificial nutrition via an elastic rubber tube size 14 Charrière. Its introduction into the esophagus is neither dangerous nor difficult. With this method, the infant's weakness can be overcome and it can benefit from nourishment to save its life.' The thick rubber tube had to be inserted for each meal, possibly impairing respiration (Fig. 6.9.1A). Russian foundling hospitals harboured large premature special care units (see Appendix 2). From St. Petersburg, where 4416 wet nurses were employed in 1831, Philipp Doepp reported [5]: 'We keep premature and atrophic infants alive by carefully injecting good wet-nurses' milk into the mouth and by the perpetual concern for maintaining ambient warmth.' In Moscow, where 40 incubators were in operation, Nikolaus Miller treated 6036 preterm infants from 1869 to 1880 and reported on their nutrition [6]: 'We use an elastic tube to feed those infants who cannot swallow due to weakness or thrush, or we dribble milk through a funnel into the nose, which enhances reflex movements and induces them to swallow.'

Exhibitions of the Lion incubator—with living babies—preceded the establishment of premature infant wards in several cities. During the 1898 exhibition in Dr Frühwald's Poliklinik in Vienna, Fritz Passini [7] recorded the weight gain of 14 infants weighing less than 1800 g (Fig. 6.9.2): 'Wet-nurses' milk was expressed and administered with a beaked nasal spoon … a quantity corresponding to 16% of the body weight … each hour 3 spoons at 15g.' Ten infants were discharged alive. In Chicago's Michael Reese Hospital, Julius Hess did not place the catheter in the stomach 'to avoid irritating the gastric mucosa and stimulation of the reflexes of the cardia' … 'The distance to which the catheter is to be passed is of great importance, when we consider that this procedure must be repeated at least six to eight times daily over a considerable period of time. It has been our rule to measure the distance from the bridge of the nose to the tip of the ensiform cartilage … The catheter is marked at this point with indelible ink and is passed to this point or about 1 cm further than this distance which allows it to reach the lower end of the esophagus just above the cardia, from which point the food will flow through the patent cardia' [8]. Medicine droppers (pipettes) with rubber tips were in use since Goodyear's invention. The Boston Floating Hospital, located on a ship since 1894, held a special care

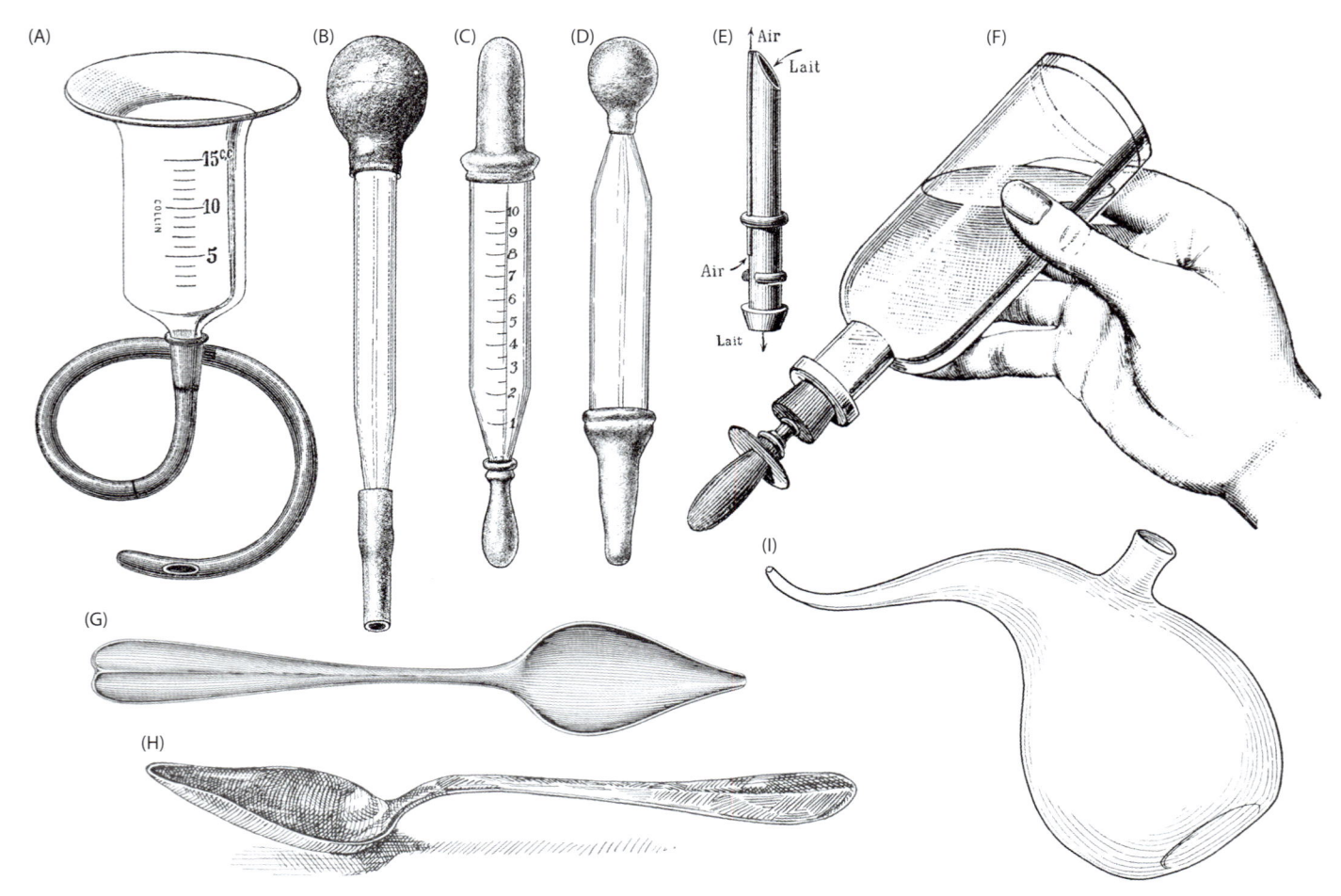

Fig. 6.9.1 Devices used 1890–1920 to nurture premature infants: A, gavage from Budin 1886 [13]; B, medicine dropper with soft rubber tubing over lower end; C, Breck feeder, original version [8]; D, modified Breck feeder with dropper bulb at the upper end (regarded unsafe by Hess) [8]; E, air inlet piece of Budin's galactophore 1892 [12]; F, use of Budin's galactophore; G, Kermauner's spoon for nasal feeding [59]; H, fruit spoon for nasal or oral feeding [8]; I, ondine used for nasal feeding by Engel [16].

unit for sick infants and a school of nursing in which Samuel Breck developed a device for feeding prematures [9]: 'The apparatus, first introduced by Dr. Breck, consists of a small glass tube holding about 1 oz.' It was also used by Blacker at the University College Hospital in 1898 [10]: 'One end is so shaped that a teat can be placed upon it, and to the other end is attached a rubber cot. The dropper being full of milk, and by squeezing the cot it is easy to fill the back of the child's throat with small quantities of milk at a time, which are then readily swallowed.'

In the Paris Hôpital St. Louis, Alfred Auvard used the *téterelle* in 1905 [11], an apparatus allowing the mother to support her infant's weak suck with a valved tube in her own mouth (see Chapter 6.3). Pierre Budin directed the Paris Maternité weaklings' pavillon from 1895 and described the mode of feeding in 'a puny infant who [initially] received milk from the wet-nurse until a stronger infant had induced the mother to lactate and the weak infant could suck'. Meticulous records were kept (**Fig. 6.9.3**); premature infants were fed maternal or wet-nurses' milk exclusively, applied by gavage or *galactophore* [12]. The latter was a feeding bottle with an air inlet tube to facilitate sucking (**Fig. 6.9.1E, F**). In even weaker infants, Budin highlighted [13]: 'When the infants are weak, they sometimes refuse to suck; one then pours the milk into their mouth either directly by applying pressure onto the nipple, or by using a little spoon until they are strong enough to take the breast. However, if they don't swallow or drool and spit out the offered milk, one must think about feeding by tube.'

Among German physicians, gavage feeding was less popular than nasal feeding. Ernst Oberwarth reported in 1911 [14]: 'Extremely weak infants cannot swallow milk, it flows back from the mouth. This can be remedied by dribbling milk into the nose with a bended nasal spoon, or better with a pipette, whereby pharyngeal irritation triggers swallowing.' Heinrich Finkelstein also preferred nasal feeding [15]: 'If the infant also rejects the rubber teat, milk must be poured in. This is achieved with spoons, small boat-like vessels, funnels, or ondines [**Fig. 6.9.1G–I**], syringes may also be used. Via oral application, milk spills out due to tongue movements. Better and safer is pouring through the nose, which provokes swallowing. This must be done slowly and cautiously to avoid overfilling the pharyngeal space with the danger of suffocation or aspiration.' Derived from an ophthalmological instrument, the *ondine* (**Fig. 6.9.1I**) was proposed by Stefan Engel to dribble human milk through the nose into the pharynx of prematures [16].

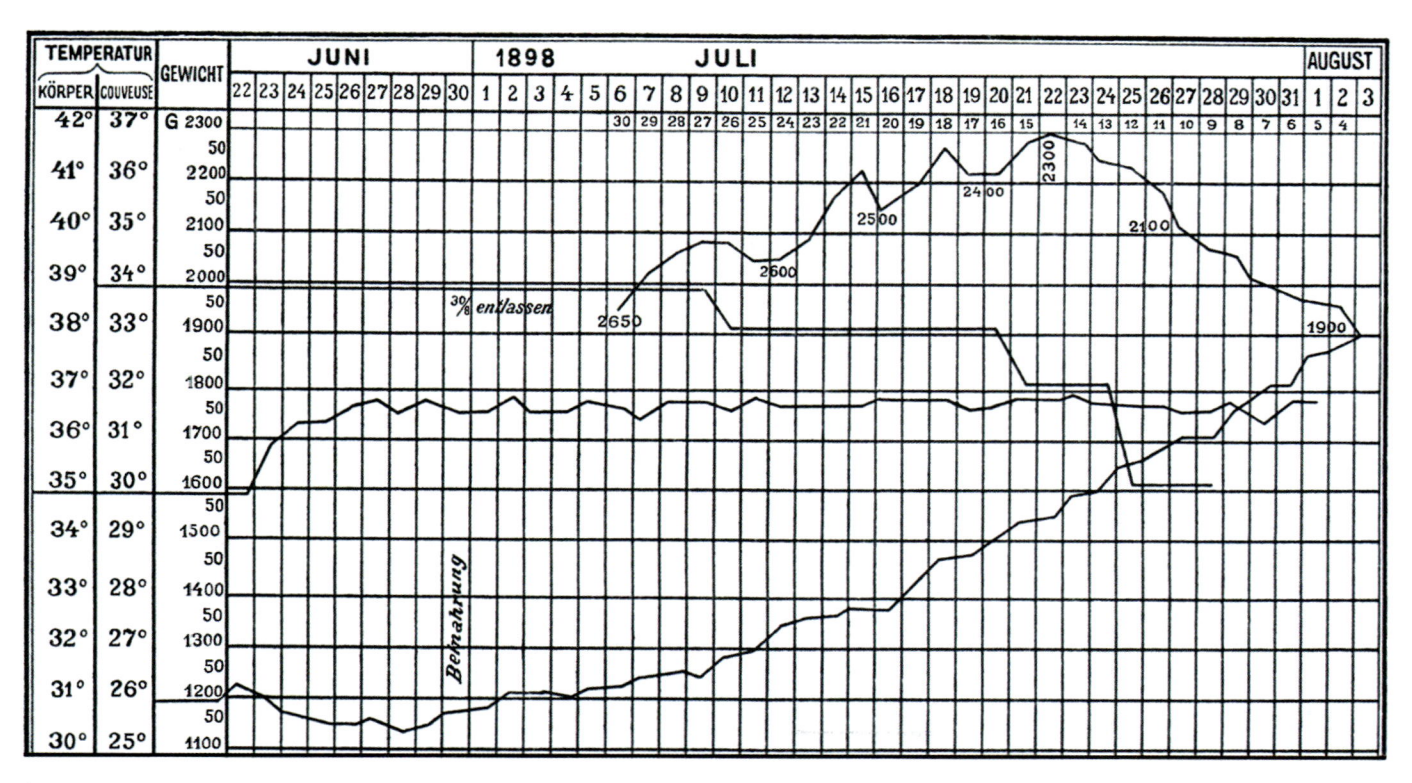

Fig. 6.9.2 Weight and temperature chart of baby girl Antonie, born 15 June 1898 and admitted to the Lion incubator exhibition at the *Vienna Policlinic of Prof. Frühwald* or 22 June with hypothermia and 1220 g body weight. She received 160 mL/kg expressed wet nurses' milk in 18 nasal spoon feedings daily, but did not thrive until Liebig's soup was added from 30 June. Thereafter her mean weight gain was 15 g/kg/d. Weight curve turns at chart edges on 3 and 15 August [7].

Indwelling nasogastric tube

Indwelling polyethylene tubes were used in 30 infants less than 1800 g by Stephen Royce and colleagues at New York Babies Hospital in 1951 for a total of 540 tube days [17]: 'With the bell of the stethoscope over the stomach area, air injected with a syringe can be heard to bubble into the stomach.' In Düsseldorf in 1955, Jörn Gleiss used indwelling polyvinylchloride tubes in 389 infants less than 2250 g for a mean duration of 27 days in survivors [18]: 'In the beginning, the tube sometimes glided into the duodenum, recognizable from yellowish discoloration and hardening of its distal part ... duodenal secretions seem to extract the softener from the polyvinylchloride.'

When to start enteral feeding

In 1913, James Goodhart of London's Evelina Hospital stated [19]: 'These feeble infants must not be allowed to wait 2 or 3 days for regular feeding with the mother's milk.' Gavage feeding from the second day on was the predominant technique in the premature infant ward at Kaiserin Auguste Victoria Haus in Berlin (Fig. 6.9.4): Fritz Rott published the nutritional protocols of 49 infants thus nourished in 1912 whose admission weights were 950–2270 g [20]. Delayed feeding seems to have originated from safety concerns. Julius Hess wrote in 1923 [8]: 'During the first day it is our custom to withhold milk for twelve hours until the respiratory and circulatory functions are well established.' This interval unfortunately became longer and longer until infants were starved for days. Clement Smith stated in 1949 [21]: 'Premature infants at the Boston Lying-in and Children's Hospital are given no food or water for two or three days after birth.' In the Birmingham Sorrento Hospital preterm infants had to survive a week of starvation in 1952 [22]: 'The caloric allowance of 28 calories per pound daily, which is required for the maintenance of a full-term infant, can be reduced to approximately 20–25 calories per pound daily for the less active premature infant and it is not necessary to reach even this maintenance requirement until the 7th to 10th day ... In recent years the survival rate has been improved by giving nothing by mouth for several days.' In Helsinki, Arvo Ylppö opposed this view in 1954 and recommended starting glucose by mouth or gavage on the first, and human milk on the second day [23]. In 1950–1952, Gleiss performed a controlled trial in 194 preterm infants weighing 500–2750 g in Düsseldorf [24]: mortality was 28% when feeding began at 12–24 hours, and 41% when begun at 36 hours of age. But starvation diets persisted until 1964, when three British women set the signal to modify neonatal treatment according to long-term outcome: from Edinburgh, Cecil Drillien reported alarmingly high rates of neurological handicaps in very low birthweight infants [25], associated with a delay in regaining birth weight. From Oxford, Victoria Smallpeice and Pamela Davies published an interhospital comparison of 164 infants of 1–2 kg birthweight. Those fed from birth had lower mortality, less jaundice, and shorter time to regain birthweight than those whose

PART 6 Breast is best

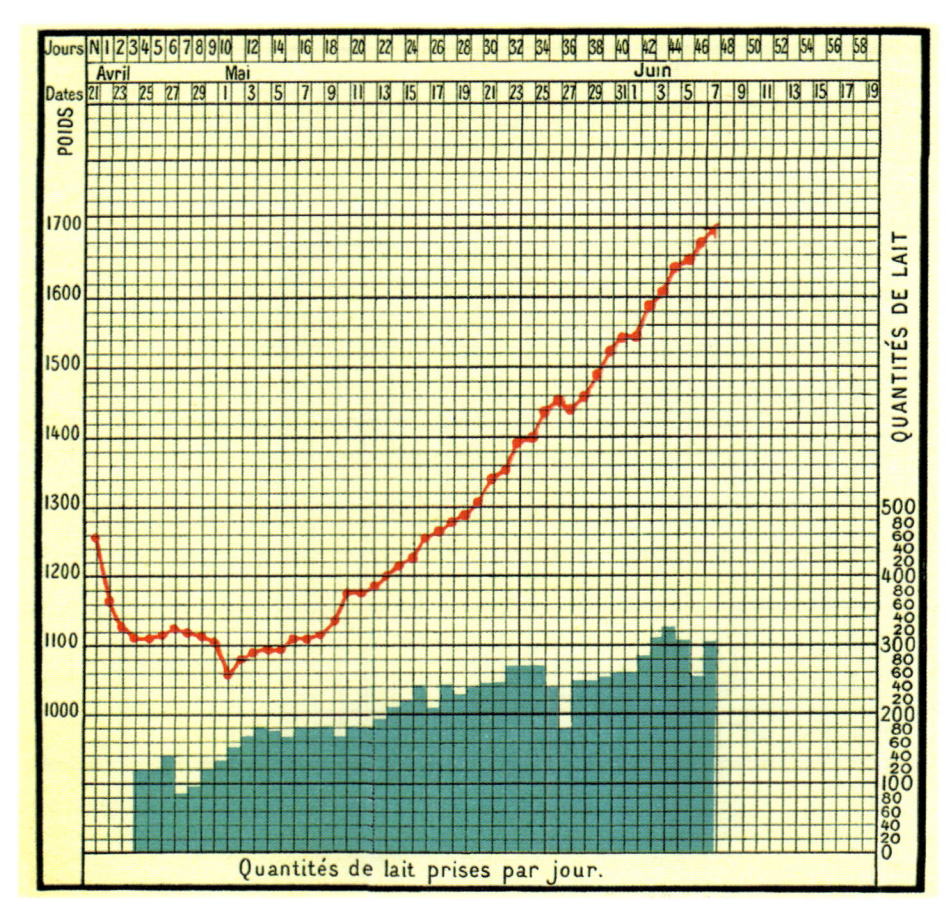

Fig. 6.9.3 Weight and nutrition chart of a boy of 1270 g body weight, about 29 weeks' gestation, born 21 April 1898 and admitted to the *Pavillon des Débiles* of the Paris Maternité. He was placed in a closed wood and glass incubator and received wet nurses' milk by *gavage* from day 5. Solid columns depict daily milk intake. His weight fell to 1070 g on day 10; thereafter, with a mean intake of 173 mL/kg (116 kcal/kg/d) his weight gain was 12.5 g/kg/d [13].

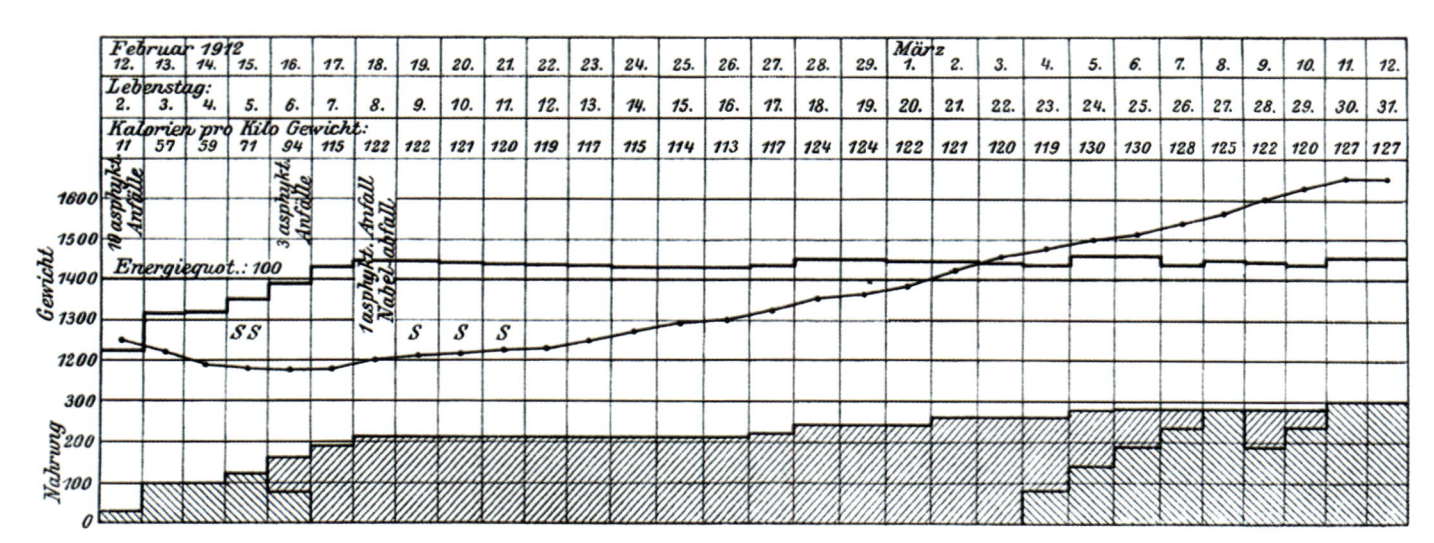

Fig. 6.9.4 Weight and nutrition chart of baby girl Katharina B, born 11 February 1912 and admitted to the prematures' ward of the Berlin *Kaiserin Auguste Victoria Haus* with a body weight of 1250 g. She was placed in a heated double-wall open bed and received wet nurses' milk, initially by bottle, from day 6 by *gavage* because of weak suck and repeated apnoeic spells (daily gavage volume depicted by ascendingly hatched columns). From day 23 she learned to bottle-feed. Her mean intake was 182 mL/kg/d (122 kcal/kd/d), her weight gain after the first week 15 g/kg/d [20].

nourishment was delayed 4–32 hours. They concluded [26]: 'This was not a controlled trial, but the alleged dangers and difficulties of early feeding have been overstressed ... We do not favor intravenous feeding because we think the infant's greatest need is milk.'

Energy and protein requirements

The quest for safe and effective energy and protein administration lasted over a century. In 1904, John Lovett Morse at Harvard applied the calorimetric method to the feeding of six premature infants, concluding 'that the caloric need of premature infants is relatively greater than that of full-term infants' [27]. Ylppö described shortcomings of human milk for preterm infants in 1919 [28]: 'It has not been proven that human milk is the ideal nutrient for prematures. On the contrary, we must imagine that its low mineral and protein content does not fulfil the requirements of their extraordinary growth, especially not that of their bones.' Hans Langer, also at the Berlin Kaiserin Auguste Victoria Haus, performed a controlled study in 115 preterm infants weighing under 2 kg in 1926: infants fed human milk enriched with 2% *Plasmon* but only 75 kcal/kg/d gained more weight than those fed 110 kcal/kg/d without protein supplement [29]: 'When nourishing preterm infants, meeting their protein need is the first priority.' In 1947, Harry Gordon of Denver and his colleagues in New York published a controlled study of 122 premature infants weighing 1–2 kg fed isocaloric amounts of human milk, evaporated milk, or a mixture of skimmed cow's milk. They found that 'mixtures of cow's milk in amounts designed to provide approximately 120 kcal/kg/d produced larger weight gains in premature infants than human milk' and assumed 'this superiority is due to the increased protein content of cow's milk' [30]. In 1951, Janet Hardy and colleagues performed a controlled trial in Baltimore proving that semi-demand feeding of a higher caloric supply shortened hospitalization as compared to the usual 120–130 kcal/kg/d [31]. In 1955 at Chicago's Michael Reese Hospital, B.M. Kagan and co-workers compared the growth of 1–2 kg infants fed isocaloric (82 kcal/kg/d) milks of human and cow's origin. Instead of relating the growth differences to protein, they concluded [32]: 'The increased weight gain over that provided by isocaloric amounts of human milk appears to be directly related to the increase in ash intake rather than to the percentage of protein, carbohydrate or fat.'

In 1967. M. Davidson studied eight different formulas in a randomized trial in 442 low birthweight infants in New York and found 'the minimal intake of protein associated with consistently high weight gain was 4 g/kg/d' [33]. In 1976, Niels Räihä of Helsinki and his colleagues in New York compared the quantity and quality of protein intake in infants under 2100 g in a randomized trial [34]. They varied protein content and whey-to-casein ratio in isocaloric human milk and formulas and detected no difference in growth, but metabolic acidosis in the group fed casein-predominant formula. In a lecture in 1957, Lewis Barness mentioned increased morbidity and mortality in premature infants fed a 4.1% protein diet [35]. This triggered much discussion and may have prevented sufficient recommendations by nutrition committees. In 1977, the American Academy of Pediatrics Committee on Nutrition suspected [36]: 'Appropriate requirement for the low-birthweight infant would appear to fall in the range of 2.5 to 5.0 g/kg/day'. In 1995, the Nutrition Committee of the Canadian Paediatric Society recommended protein intakes of 3.0–3.6 g/kg/day for infants above, and 3.5–4.0 g/kg/d for infants below 1000 g birthweight [37]. It was not until 2010 that the European Society of Paediatric Gastroenterology, Hepatology and Nutrition Committee on Nutrition recommended 3.5–4.0 g/kg/d for infants above, and 4.0–4.5 g/kg/d for infants below 1 kg [38].

Parenteral supplements—way out of the dilemma

To stabilize serum potassium in premature infants with respiratory distress, Robert Usher in Montreal administered intravenous glucose, insulin, and bicarbonate in 1959 'until adequate oral intake had been established' [39]. In Chicago, Marvin Cornblath and co-workers published a randomized trial in infants under 1500 g birthweight in 1966 showing 'a mortality of 30% in infants given intravenous glucose as compared to 50% in those given nasogastric fluids or who were starved' [40]. Casein hydrolysate, glucose, 1% ethanol but no fat was intravenously infused by Gerda Benda in 1971 [41]: 'We have trained our nurses in the technique of needle placement.' At Columbia University in 1972, John Driscoll and colleagues applied beef fibrin hydrolysate and glucose, but no fat to infants less than 1200 g via an indwelling central venous catheter [42]. Rosita Pildes and co-workers in Chicago randomized 54 infants less than 1500 g to receive glucose only, or glucose and crystalline amino acids via peripheral vein [43], and observed more rapid weight gain in the glucose-amino acid group.

Deficiencies and fortifiers

In his 1919 work, Ylppö described 'rickets in all prematures without exception, affecting not only the skull, but all bones, already in the second or third month of life' [44]. In 1936, Davidson and co-workers reported that premature infants developed clinical and radiological signs of rickets despite feeding 'vitamin D milk' from cows fed irradiated yeast [45]. In 1939, Genevieve Stearns of Iowa knew that two-thirds of the mineral content of term infants was deposited during the last trimester of pregnancy [46]: 'It is not surprising that prematurely born infants fed only human milk almost invariably develop rickets.' Helen Benjamin and co-workers in New York performed a balance study in five premature infants in 1943 and concluded [47]: 'Mineral retention with a diet of human milk supplemented with vitamin D was inadequate to meet even the lowest calculated requirement.' In 1949, Hess and Lundeen stated 'two to four times as much vitamin D as is given to the full-term infant, proportionate to its weight, is given to the premature infant' [48]. In 1964, Boissière and Cagnat described *dystrophie ostéomalacique* in preterm infants [49]. In 1971, radiologist Nathan Griscom and colleagues of the Boston Lying-In Hospital described 'fractures, generalized porosis, poorly mineralized subperiosteal new bone, epiphyseal separations, enlargement of costochondral junctions, and metaphyseal cupping' in three infants less than 950 g and concluded [50]: 'The illness from which these infants suffered was apparently metabolic and probably nutritional.' This was in line with bone densitometry measurements of Jean Steichen and co-workers of Cincinnati in 1980 [51]: 'The commonly seen osteopenia of prematurity results primarily from a mineral deficiency, rather than vitamin D deficiency' and recommended to 'increase the calcium and phosphorus content in formulas for low birthweight infants.' Feeding human milk to premature infants was not the top priority of the formula industry. Commercial fortifiers with protein, calcium and phosphorus were available from 1977 [52], more elaborate products that also contained sodium, iron, zinc, and vitamins from 1995 [53]. In a randomized trial published in 1996, Alan Lucas and co-workers reported improved short-term growth in infants less than 1850 g with a multi-nutrient fortifier, but no long-term benefit [54]. No randomized trials have been performed investigating calcium and phosphorus supplementation to prevent osteopenia in preterm infants [55].

Formula for prematures

Anaemia of prematurity was ubiquitous. In 1928, Helen Mackay of Queen's Hospital demonstrated that with 'iron and ammonia citrate in a daily dose between 4.5 and 9 grains' haemoglobin rose from 58% to 80% within 6 months. When Cow & Gate Co. supplied dried milk with the iron salt 'there was little likelihood of the food being thrown down the sink, in contradistinction to the possible fate of medicine' [56]. Many reinforced proprietary formulas for preterm infants came on the market during the 1950s (Similac, Alacta, Enfamil, etc.). When compared to human milk, they were associated with much higher incidence of necrotizing enterocolitis [57], therefore human milk remained the preferred nutrient for preterm infants, despite the need of fortification.

A recent advance in the nutrition of preterm infants was probiotics. Infants living in a special care unit from birth are inevitably colonized by pathogenic bacteria, paving the way for enteral infection. A Cochrane meta-analysis of 16 randomized trials performed from 1993 to 2010 revealed an incidence reduction of severe necrotizing enterocolitis to a third in preterm infants given enteral lactobacilli or bifidobacteria [58].

Conclusion

Whereas devices to overcome the preterm infant's weak sucking and swallowing were developed within three decades, its nutritional needs remained unfulfilled after more than a century of intense research. Many studies equated optimal development with maximum weight gain. Nutritional theory followed two principles that contradicted each other for decades: (1) breast is best, also for the preterm infant, (2) postnatal growth should approach fetal growth, say, 14 g/kg/d. Nutritional practice lagged behind the knowledge about metabolic need, and many infants received less protein and minerals than necessary for their growth. Less (and later than respiratory procedures proposed for preterm infants), nutritional protocols were subjected to rigorously controlled trials of sufficient size and entailing long-term follow-up. Consensus-based recommendations ignored the few existing randomized trials and attempted to meet the infant's needs without assessing the success. The evidence for nutritional interventions in the preterm infant remained poor.

REFERENCES

1. Billard CM: Die Krankheiten der Neugeborenen und Säuglinge (1st French ed. 1828). Weimar: Industrie-Comptoir, 1829: p. 65, 228.
2. Richard (de Nancy) CJF: Traité pratique des maladies des enfants. Paris: Baillière, 1839: p. 128.
3. Cone TE: History of the care and feeding of the premature infant. Boston, MA: Little & Co., 1985: p. 72–73, 92–105.
4. Marchant [de Charenton]: Soins à donner aux nouveau-nés. Gaz Méd Paris 1851;**21**:824.
5. Doepp P: Notizen über das kaiserliche Erziehungshaus (Findlingshaus) zu St. Petersburg. Hamburg: Hoffmann & Campe, 1835: Vol. **5**, p. 306–50.
6. Miller NT: Die Frühgeborenen und die Eigenthümlichkeiten ihrer Krankheiten. Jahrb Kinderheilk 1886;**25**:179–94.
7. Passini F: Beitrag zur Ernährung frühgeborener Kinder. Jahrb Kinderh 1899;**49**:411–24.
8. Hess JH: Premature and congenitally disabled infants. London: Churchill, 1923: p. 114–30, 171–204.
9. Morse JL: The care and feeding of premature infants. Am J Obstet Dis Women Child 1905;**4**:589–99.
10. Blacker GF: The care and feeding of premature infants. Practitioner 1898;**61**:28–37.
11. Auvard PVA: Le nouveau-né. Physiologie—Hygiène—Allaitement. 5. ed. Paris: Doin, 1905: p. 204.
12. Budin P: Femmes en couches et Nouveau-Nés. Paris: Doin, 1897: p. 266.
13. Budin P: Le Nourrisson. Paris: Doin, 1900: p. 23, 41, 99, 213.
14. Oberwarth E: Pflege und Ernährung der Frühgeburten. Ergeb Inn Med Kinderheilk 1911;**7**:191–223.
15. Finkelstein H: Lehrbuch der Säuglingskrankheiten. 2. ed. Berlin: Springer, 1921: p. 149, 355, 542.
16. Engel S, Baum M: Grundriss der Säuglings- und Kleinkinderkunde. 11. and 12. ed. München: J Bergmann, 1922: p. 164.
17. Royce S, Tepper C, Watson W, Day R: Indwelling polyethylene nasogastric tube for feeding premature infants. Pediatrics 1951;**8**:79–81.
18. Gleiss J: Zum Frühgeborenenproblem der Gegenwart. 10. Mitteilung Zeitschr Kinderheilk 1955;**76**:269–80.
19. Goodhart JF: The diseases of children. 10. ed. London: Still, 1913: p. 36.
20. Rott F: Zur Ernährungstechnik frühgeborener Säuglinge. Zeitschr Kinderheilk 1913;**5**:134–74.
21. Smith CA, Yudkin S, Young W, et al.: Adjustment of electrolytes and water following premature birth. Pediatrics 1949;**3**:34–48.
22. Crosse VM: The premature baby. 3. ed. London: Churchill, 1952: p. 49–81.
23. Ylppö A: Premature children: should they fast or be fed in the first days of life? Ann Paediatr Fenn 1954;**1**:99–104.
24. Gleiss J: Zum Frühgeborenenproblem der Gegenwart. 9. Mitteilung Zeitschr Kinderheilk 1955;**76**:261–8.
25. Drillien CM: The growth and development of the prematurely born infant. Edinburgh: Livingstone, 1964: p. 306.
26. Smallpeice V, Davies PA: Immediate feeding of premature infants with undiluted breast milk. Lancet 1964;**2**:1349–52.
27. Morse JL: A study of the caloric needs of premature infants. Am J Med Sci 1904;**127**:463–77.
28. Ylppö A: Das Wachstum der Frühgeborenen von der Geburt bis zm Schulalter. Zeitschr Kinderheilk 1919;**24**:111–78.

29. Langer H: Über die Ernährung frühgeborener Kinder in den ersten Lebenswochen. Zeitschrift Kinderheilk 1926;**41**:598–611.
30. Gordon HH, Levine SZ, McNamara H: Feeding of premature infants—a comparison of human and cow's milk. Am J Dis Child 1947;**73**:442–52.
31. Hardy JB, Goldstein EO: The feeding of premature infants. J Pediatr 1951;**38**:154–7.
32. Kagan BM, Hess JH, Lundeen E, et al.: Feeding premature infants—a comparison of various milks. Pediatrics 1955;**15**:373–82.
33. Davidson M, Levine SZ, Bauer CH, Dann M: Feeding studies in low-birth-weight infants. J Pediatr 1967;**70**:695–713.
34. Raiha NC, Heinonen K, Rassin DK, Gaull GE: Milk protein quantity and quality in low-birthweight infants: I. Metabolic responses and effects on growth. Pediatrics 1976;**57**:659–74.
35. Barness LA, Cornely DA, Valyasevi A, György P: Comparison of prematures fed high and low protein diets. Am J Dis Child 1957;**94**:480–2.
36. American Academy of Pediatrics Committee on Nutrition: Nutritional needs of low-birth-weight infants. Pediatrics 1977;**60**:519–30.
37. Nutrition Committee Canadian Paediatric Society: Nutrient needs and feeding of premature infants. Can Med Assoc J 1995;**152**:1765–85.
38. Agostoni C, Buonocore G, Carnielli VP, et al.: Enteral nutrient supply for preterm infants. J Pediatr Gastroenterol Nutr 2010;**50**:85–91.
39. Usher R: The respiratory distress syndrome of prematurity. I. Changes in potassium in the serum and the electrocardiogram and effects of therapy. Pediatrics 1959;**24**:562–76.
40. Cornblath M, Forbes AE, Pildes RS, et al.: A controlled study of early fluid administration on survival of low birth weight infants. Pediatrics 1966;**38**:547–54.
41. Benda GI, Babson SG: Peripheral intravenous alimentation of the small premature infant. J Pediatr 1971;**79**:494–8.
42. Driscoll JM Jr, Heird WC, Schullinger JN, et al.: Total intravenous alimentation in low-birth-weight infants. J Pediatr 1972;**81**:145–53.
43. Pildes RS, Ramamurthy RS, Cordero GV, Wong PW: Intravenous supplementation of L-amino acids and dextrose in low-birth-weight infants. J Pediatr 1973;**82**:945–50.
44. Ylppö A: Zur Physiologie, Klinik und zum Schicksal der Frühgeborenen. Zeitschr Kinderheilk 1919;**24**:1–110.
45. Davidson LT, Merritt KK, Chipman SS: Prophylaxis of rickets in premature infants with vitamin D milk. Am J Dis Child 1936;**51**:1–16.
46. Stearns G: The mineral metabolism of normal infants. Physiol Rev 1939;**19**:415–38.
47. Benjamin HR, Gordon HH, Marples E: Calcium and phosphorus requirements of premature infants. Am J Dis Child 1943;**65**:412–25.
48. Hess J, Lundeen E: The premature infant. Medical and nursing care. 2. ed. Philadelphia: Lippincott, 1949: p. 288.
49. Boissière H, Cagnat R, Poissonier M, D'Angely S: Dystrophie ostéomalacique du prématuré. Ann Pediatr (Paris) 1964;**11**:367–83.
50. Griscom NT, Craig JN, Neuhauser EB: Systemic bone disease developing in small premature infants. Pediatrics 1971;**48**:883–95.
51. Steichen JJ, Gratton TL, Tsang RC: Osteopenia of prematurity. J Pediatr 1980;**96**:528–34.
52. Fomon SJ, Ziegler EE, Vázquez HD: Human milk and the small premature infant. Am J Dis Child 1977;**131**:463–67.
53. Moro GE, Minoli I, Ostrom M, et al.: Fortification of human milk. J Pediatr Gastroenterol Nutr 1995;**20**:162–72.
54. Lucas A, Fewtrell MS, Morley R, et al.: Randomized outcome trial of human milk fortification and developmental outcome in preterm infants. Am J Clin Nutr 1996;**64**:142–51.
55. Kuschel CA, Harding JE: Calcium and phosphorus supplementation of human milk for preterm infants. Cochrane Database Syst Rev 2001;**4**:CD003310.
56. Mackay HMM: Anaemia in infancy: its prevalence and prevention. Arch Dis Child 1828;**3**:117–47.
57. Quigley MA, Henderson G, Anthony MY, McGuire W: Formula milk versus donor breast milk for feeding preterm or low birth weight infants. Cochrane Database Syst Rev 2007;**4**:CD002971.
58. Alfaleh K, Anabrees J, Bassler D, Al-Kharfi T: Probiotics for prevention of necrotizing enterocolitis in preterm infants. Cochrane Database Syst Rev 2011;**3**:CD005496.
59. Reuss ARv: Die Krankheiten des Neugeborenen. Berlin: Springer, 1914: p. 136.

6.10

Much ado about nothing
Controversies on tongue-tie

Introduction

Since Biblical times, the word 'tongue' besides naming an organ denominated the ability to speak: 'And Moses saith to the Lord, O my Lord, I am not eloquent, neither heretofore, nor since thou hast spoken unto thy servant: but I am slow of speech, and of a slow tongue' [Exodus 4:10]. Tongue-tied was synonymous with speechless: 'And looking up to heaven, he sighed, and saith unto him, Ephphatha, that is, Be opened. And straightway his ears were opened and the string of his tongue was loosened, and he spoke plain' [Mark 7:34–35].

Greek medicine

That something can or must be done with the neonate's tongue was rooted in Greek medicine. In the 3rd century B.C.E., Aristotle stated [1]: 'The human tongue is the freest, the broadest, and the softest of all: this is to enable it to fulfill both its functions … It has, also, to articulate the various sounds and to produce speech, and for this a tongue which is soft and broad is admirably suited, because it can roll back and dart forward in all directions; and herein too its freedom and looseness assists it. This is shown by the case of those whose tongues are slightly tied: their speech is indistinct and lisping, which is due to the fact that they cannot produce all the sounds.' Celsus, 1st century C.E., realized the uncertain benefit of frenotomy [2]: 'In some the tongue is really attached to its base from the first day of life onwards, who therefore cannot speak. In them, the tongue's tip should be seized with a small forceps and the membrane thereunder incised, with great care not to violate the veins which are close and may harm by profuse bleeding … Who is thereby healed, mostly can speak. But I have seen one who after cutting could protrude the tongue beyond the teeth, but still did not gain the ability to speak. In medicine it may be universally valid what should be done, but not universally valid what results and whom it helps.'

Galen of Pergamon believed in the 2nd century C.E. [3]: 'The tongue allows to speak in a distinguishable articulated voice; to which also contribute the teeth, lips, nostrils, palate, windpipe, and the tongue's median band. Therefore, in stutterers, lispers and others disabled in speech, one of these speaking instruments must be defect, either by malformation or acquired, like polyps, nostril obstruction, loss of incisor teeth, and lip mutilation.' But he did not advocate frenotomy [4]: 'Everything having to do with the tongue has been prepared most fully and perfectly by nature, and both the other arrangements and also the ligament (frenulum linguae) below the tongue display no little foresight of hers … To meet all these needs nature has marvellously prepared a ligament of the size that would be most suitable. It was made neither simply nor at haphazard, but with a marvellous, due proportion; if it ended farther out along the tongue or came to an end sooner than it should, it would certainly not be as good for the articulation of the voice and it would also be a hindrance to the motion in chewing.'

The Byzantine surgeon Paul of Aegina distinguished congenital and acquired forms of tongue-tie and specified the operative technique in the 7th century C.E. [5]: 'The fault of adhering tongue develops spontaneously when tight and short membranes fix the tongue, sometimes by hard scarring following a wound. Those who have the fault congenitally begin to speak late and have a tight band under the tongue.'

Competition of midwives and surgeons

Surgeons originated from barbers and village quacks and left few traces in the literature. Neonates were treated by midwives and, more than its need, the competence for frenotomy was widely disputed among midwives and surgeons. The decrees, by which the midwives had to swear, either obliged or prohibited them to separate the frenulum. In 1473, Bartholomaeus Metlinger recommended [6]: 'After the fruit has been born into the world, the midwife should grip into the infant's mouth with rose-honey or other honey spread unto her finger and should touch the infant's gums, palate, and tongue; and if something must be loosened, she should loosen it.' The Heilbronn 'midwives and sworn women's rule' interdicted frenotomy around 1480 [7]: 'She should not dare to loosen the tongue without medical advice, by which and because of incompetence many severe mistakes are made.' In contrast, the Passau midwives rule of 1595

Reproduced with permission from Obladen, M. Much ado about nothing: two millenia of controversy on tongue-tie. *Neonatology*, 97(2):83–89. Copyright © 2010 S. Karger AG, Basel.

demanded: 'When the infant's navel (string) is neatly removed, the midwife should reach under the infants tongue and detect, if it adheres; if this is the case, she must soon squeeze the vessel as long as it is tender.' To avoid profuse haemorrhage from sublingual vessels, Hieronymus Mercurialis admonished in 1584 [8]: 'Avicenna [1, 3. tract., 4.cap, 18] cautions very prudently, not to tear off the membrane itself, but to perforate it near its root with a needle, and with this needle to pull through a thread, and to ligate it. This thread, tightened daily, will soon and gently detach the membrane.'

In France, frenotomy and its complications were widely known, as indicated in the 1609 obstetric textbook of Louise Bourgeois [9]: 'One should also gently pass the finger under the tongue to find if they have the band (le filet), and if they do, one should not try to break it, because the fingernail which is poisonous will cause them chancre or ulcer; but the surgeon consulted to this business will remove it with a scissors tip without risk.' Bourgeois delivered Louis XIII who on 28 September 1610 was not spared the drastic procedure, as reported by Hérouard [10]: 'Seeing that he had trouble nursing we looked into his mouth. It was seen that the tongue-string was the cause. At five in the evening it was cut in three places by M. Guillemeau, the king's surgeon.'

The 1620 text of the Padovan surgeon Fabricius ab Aquapendente [11] was cited by his pupil Scultetus: 'Before I continue to describe this operation, I must emphasize the great presumptuousness the midwives exert everywhere; when they without exception, disrupt the band under each newborn infant's tongue using their forefinger's nail, which they maintain sharp and pointed for this purpose; under the pretext that, if they wouldn't do it, the infant never would learn to speak understandably; as if the ability of speech, which is peculiar to humans, would not be nature's gift but would be endowed by a silly woman's mediation … I wonder why the authorities do not pass a specific law forbidding in full seriousness this multiple child-murder committed by the midwives. Thereupon I warn you never to allow the midwife to even touch the tongue of your or other people's infants with their nails … But when in one in hundred thousand infants the tongue would be attached too much, the operation should be performed cautiously by an experienced surgeon … I make the infant cry, then I take a thin but rough cloth between my left hand's indexfinger and thumb; with which I grasp the tongue and pull it forward and upward, till the band below the tongue becomes visible; then I cut it with my right hand using a small curved knife. Fastidiously I take care not to violate the blood-vessels lying thereunder' (Fig. 6.10.1).

The borderline between midwives and surgeons was the use of instruments, which explains why midwives continued to detach the frenulum with their nails, and surgeons proceeded to invent instruments for the intervention, some of which are shown in Fig. 6.10.2. In 1666, the arsenal of operations and instruments known to the Ulm surgeon Scultetus included [12]: 'A silver instrument with which the surgeon lifts the newborns tongue and keeps it lifted until he has cut the band with a good scissors.' The Paris royal accoucheur François Mauriceau [13] used a fork-like instrument: 'It is not beneficial, as some women do, to disrupt the string with the nails, because an ulcer may result which is difficult to heal, but the infant should be brought to a surgeon who will cut the string with a pointed sharp scissors … But because the neonate's mouth is so small that it is difficult to insert two fingers in order to lift the tongue; and they would prevent the eyes to see properly what has to be done; therefore the surgeon may use a small fork, as depicted at the begin of this chapter, whose little arms (the tips of which should be blunt) he inserts to both sides of the band, thereafter he can lift and fix the tongue to perform the operation in comfort and safety.' In 1752, the Brandenburg court midwife Justine Siegmundin defined an indication [14]: 'For the need to loosen the tongue-band or membrane, these are the signs: That it cannot protrude the tongue or cannot move and wind it around the nipple. Among thousand infants there is barely one suffering from this defect.'

Uppsala pioneer of paediatrics Rosenstein emphasized in 1776 that he never saw any child's tongue tied (tunghäftan) [15] and the Berlin obstetrician Hagen's midwife catechism specified in 1791 [16]: 'Among ten infants, in whom the midwife or the nurse seek the reason for poor

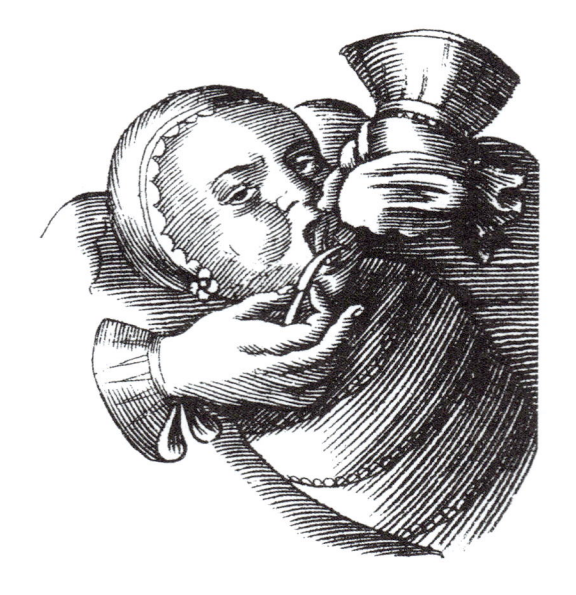

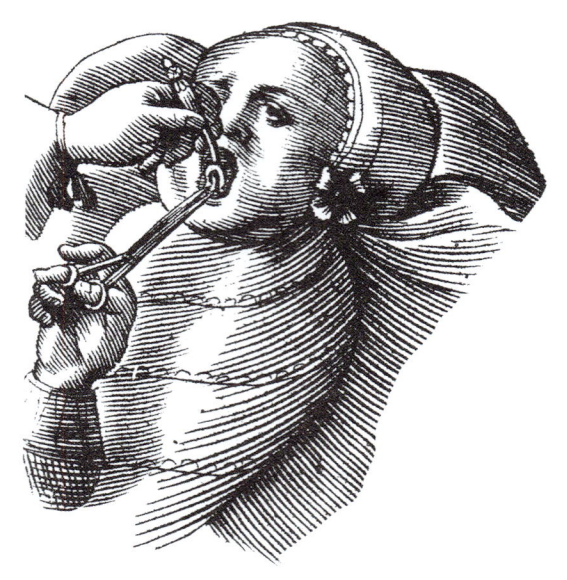

Fig. 6.10.1 Woodcuts showing the operative techniques of Fabricius 1620 [11] (left) 'the tongue is held with a handkerchief and the band loosened with a falciform knifelet' and Scultetus 1666 [12] (right) 'how the surgeon lifts the tongue with a silver instrument and dissects the attached band with a small sharp scissors'.

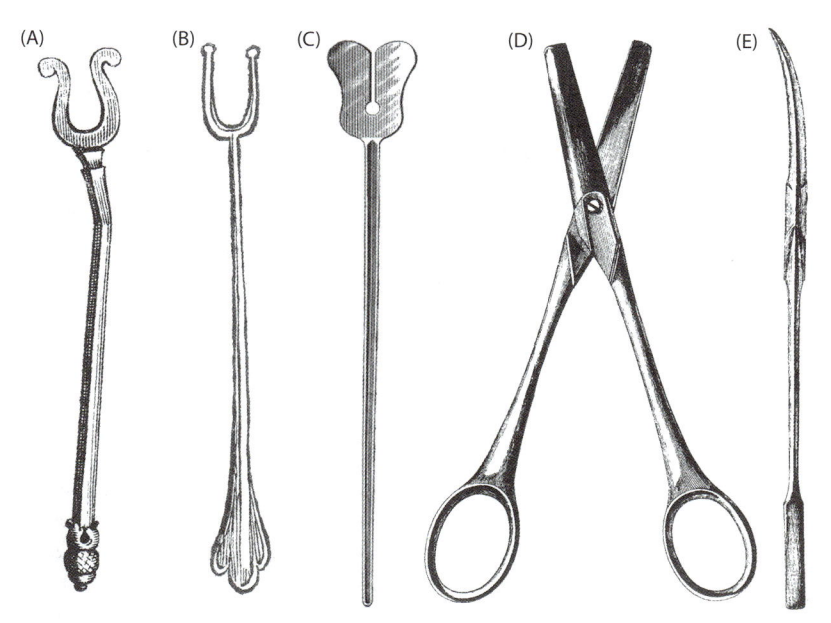

Fig. 6.10.2 Surgical instruments for frenotomy: A, tongue-lifter of Scultetus 1666 [12]; B, tongue fork of Mauriceau 1680 [13]; C, sonde cannelée of Petit 1774 [17]; D, blunt curved scissors proposed by Schmitt 1804; E, lateral view of scissors [46].

sucking in a short frenulum, barely one has this cause … Frequently the parents are deceived, for profit, greed and ignorance this aid is abused, and one unties where nothing is tied.' In 1774, the Paris surgeon Jean Louis Petit proposed the myrtle leaf-shaped handle, which had an incision meant to upload the frenulum (**Fig. 6.10.3**). It can still can be found in some modern instruments [17]. The instrument was propagated by Desormeaux in 1836 [18]: 'The midwives in Italy and Germany grow a nail of their little finger to use it for separation. The cutting edge of a coin was also used for this purpose. Now it is generally accepted that the little operation is rarely indicated and is performed as follows: The infant is positioned on its back or horizontally so that the light easily falls into its mouth; the tongue is lifted with a spatula or with the cleft handle, which J.L. Petit attached to the grooved probes for that purpose. Then the band, which lies in the handle's cleft is cut with a single stroke.'

The professional controversy over whose responsibility it was to perform frenotomy and when and how it should be performed, continued throughout the 19th century and is mentioned in the books of Rau 1807 [19], Jörg 1814 [20], Capuron 1820 [21], Wendt 1826 [22], Marjolin 1836 [23], Meissner 1844 [24], Guersant 1869 [25], and so on. In Paris, Eugène Bouchut moaned in 1867 [26]: 'Il y a beaucoup d'enfants qu'on dit avoir le filet et qui ne l'ont pas'.

Haemorrhage

In observation 301, Mauriceau reported [27]: 'April 12, 1682, an uncommon accident happened to a woman who had happily given birth to a nice male infant … Her surgeon, who had wanted to cut the tongue-band, which he pretended this child had, inadvertently opened a vessel under the tongue, of which such a great abundance of blood effused, that the infant died the same day … it seems to me that the second mistake of this surgeon, not to have the cleverness to stop this hemorrhage, was even greater than his first; because he could easily have repaired the open vessel by cauterizing with the heated tip of a simple probe.'

Severe haemorrhage following frenotomy was a tragedy which can be felt from the votive tablet in **Fig. 6.10.4**: 'In the year of 1731, the 8. April, it happened in Landtsperg that a small child who was only one day old, by loosening the tongue bled for 6 hours to such

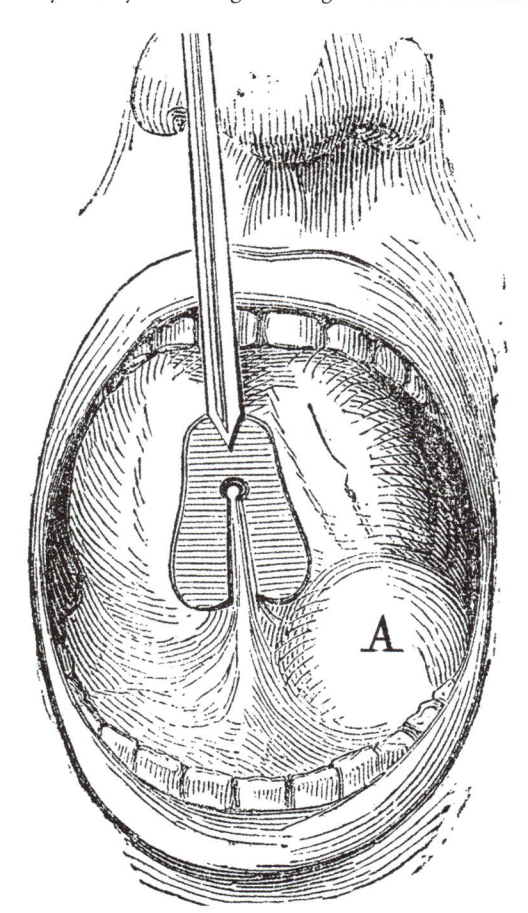

Fig. 6.10.3 Ranula (grenouillette, the froggy) with Petit's spatula on frenulum, 1867 [26].

a degree, that the barber and all others present ruled that it was impossible to staunch the bleeding and therefore the innocent child would give up its soul within half an hour. By vowing a holy mass and a votive table to the miraculous place of mercy, our dear Lord's rest, also by intercession of the Holy John of Nepomuk, the matter turned immediately and the child lives healthy up to the present day.' St John of Nepomuk was regarded patron of the tongue-sick, because under torture he refused to break the seal of confession. Lethal haemorrhage after frenotomy was described in each obstetric textbook published within the next 50 years [28–30] and Michael Underwood, a pioneer in perinatal medicine in London, wrote in 1801 [31]: ' I shall therefore only observe, that some little care and steadiness are required, or the veins under the tongue may be wounded, and in consequence an infant may lose its life. To avoid this danger, instead of making use of scissars, the bridle may be divided by a small curved bistoury; the back part of which will sufficiently press down the veins, so as to be entirely out of the way of being injured. These cautions have been judged by some people to be very trifling; but besides that infants have actually bled to death, the following equally fatal accident has arisen from cutting too deep, which I shall therefore notice in this place, as well as describe an instrument contrived to suppress the bleeding.' As late as 1931 Fischl wrote [32]: 'Given the futility of the procedure one should strongly object against it. I saw a case in whom the frenulum was cut despite my opposition and the child, who was hemophilic, bled to death from the wound.'

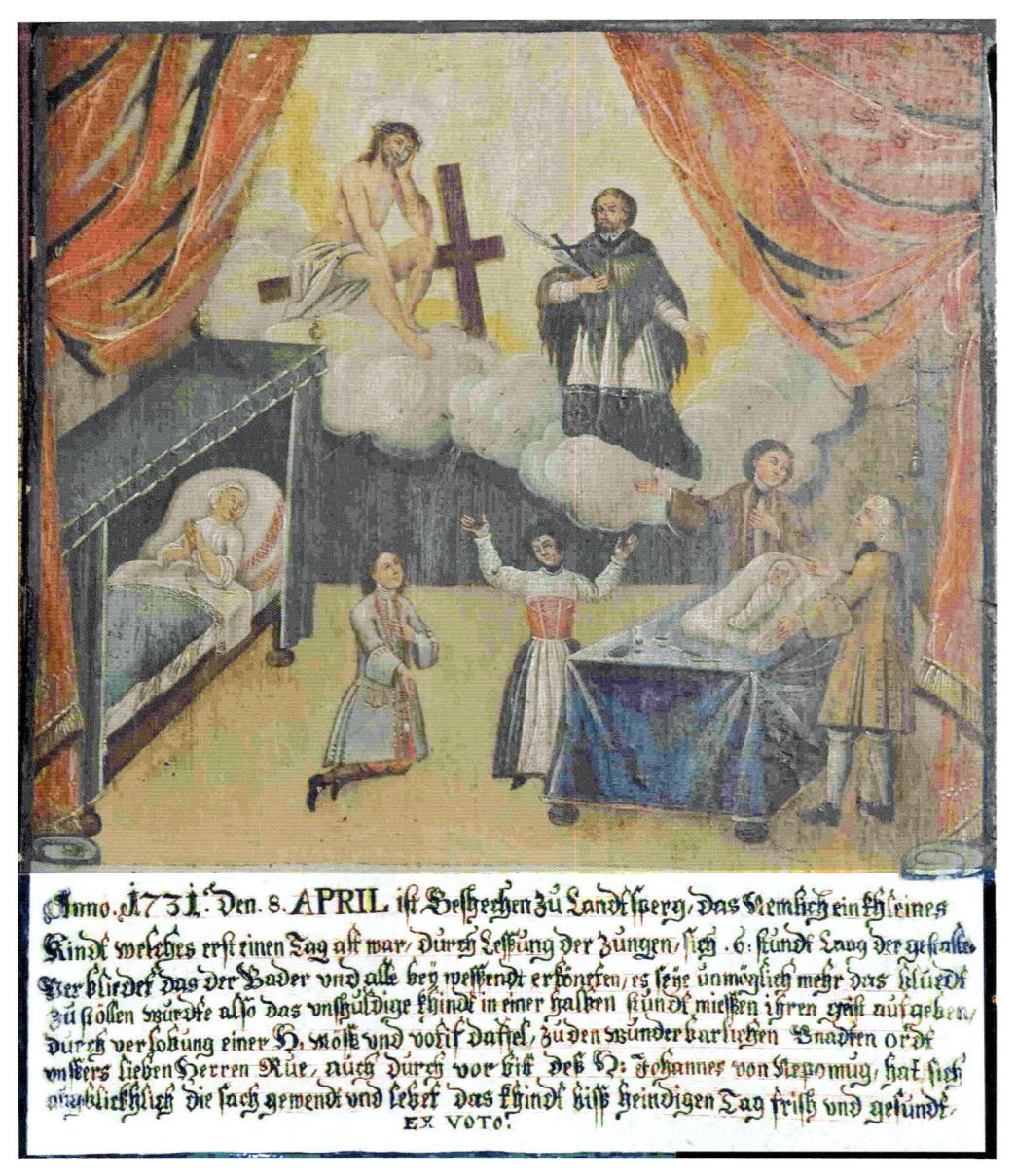

Fig. 6.10.4 Votive tablet of 1731 in the pilgrimage church of Herrgottsruh, Friedberg, Bavaria, thanking for salvation from severe haemorrhage following frenotomy (see text). The tablet shows the mother in childbed, the kneeing father, the injured neonate on the table, surrounded by the desperate midwive and two surgeons with their instruments, as well as Jesus Christ and St. John of Nepomuk in the clouds.
Votive tablet of 1731 in the pilgrimage church of Herrgottsruh, Friedberg, Bavaria, with permission.

Other complications

Ranula, a rare retention cyst of the sublingual duct, was among the most frequent diseases of the neonate in the 18th century. Stark characterized it in 1791 [33]: 'The so called froggy (ranula) is normally regarded as an infantile disease, because it usually develops within the first days after birth. Who knows, if intrauterine conditions add to its occurrence, as well as a broad and proliferated tongue-band.' The Göttingen physician Girtanner wrote in 1794 [34]: 'The most frequent diseases in the first days of life are apparent death, tongue-tie, ranula, tetanus, rose-rash, hydrocephalus.' He deplored the inability to treat ranula: 'It is sad for the philanthropist that hitherto no means could be detected to treat this disorder and without exception all affected infants become a victim of it and must die without rescue.'

In the Triest foundling hospital, Verson linked the froggy formation to previous frenotomy in 1838 [35]: 'The cause of the froggy is swelling and desorganisation of the Whartonian and sublingual ducts following occlusion of their orifice due to chronic inflammation, compression, or violation when cutting the tongue-band.' When routine frenotomy disappeared, ranula became so rare that some modern textbooks ignore this disorder altogether.

Modern indications

The diagnosis 'ankyloglosson' used since Galen, was coded Q38.1 in the International Classification of Diseases, Tenth Revision, but remained undefined and frenotomy (operations class 5-279.1) persisted. With controversial diagnostic criteria incidence statistics had little meaning. Motivated by midwives, the parents urged operations, as the Heidelberg paediatrician Ernst Moro stated in 1906 [36]: 'The anomaly rarely causes symptoms, but one can, to comply with the urgent wishes of mothers and midwives, cut the tongue-band with a scissors kick in order to calm them.' In 1941, McEnery pointed out that the neonatal frenulum is always short and should never be considered causally related to speech difficulties of any type [37]. In 1995, Peter Dunn realized [38] that 'tongue-tie has become a medical non-event' and contradicted: 'I became convinced that this condition was a very real one … We see a quite extraordinary difference in professional attitude … from earliest times up to the present century.' A 2007 methodological review of Segal and colleagues [39] concluded: 'There is no well-validated clinical method for establishing a diagnosis of ankyloglossia. Diagnostic criteria are needed to allow comparative studies of treatment.'

With the renaissance of breastfeeding, justification for frenotomy shifted from improved speech to supported feeding. Lactation consultants assumed the position traditionally held by midwives. The continuing diversity of opinion is illustrated by a modern survey of hundreds of otolaryngologists, paediatricians, lactation consultants and speech pathologists [40]: 'The majority of practising lactation consultants believe that tongue-tie frequently causes feeding difficulties, and that neonatal frenotomy is quite helpful. In marked contrast, 90% of pediatricians and 70% of otolaryngologists believe ankyloglossia never or rarely causes a feeding problem.' Hedonistic views enlarged the indication by nipple comfort and facilitated kissing, scientific medicine added randomized trials [41–43] and ultrasound diagnosis [44]. Wallace stated in 1963, that 'much entertaining nonsense has been written about tongue-tie' [45] and myriads of remarks on the topic are flooding internet blogs and websites. Like salting the infant's lips, piercing the ears, forming and deforming the skull, tight swaddling or bandaging, circumcision and genital mutilation, ritual bath and baptism, and other neonatal blessing or welcome rites, tongue manipulation originated in different cultures, was believed to be healthy for the infant, and persisted for thousands of years.

REFERENCES

1. Aristotle: Parts of animals. Loeb Classical Library. Edited by: G. P. Goold. Cambridge, MA: Harvard University Press, 1937: Vol. XII, p. II, XLV, 660 a, 17–27.
2. Celsus AC: De re medica libri octo. Lugduni Batavorum: Raphelengius, 1592: Vol. VII, p. 646.
3. Galenus C: De locis affectis. Edited by: Carolus Kühn: Leipzig: Cnobloch, 1825: Vol. **VIII**, p. 272.
4. Galenus C: De usu partium corporis. Ithaca, NY: Cornell University Press, 1968: p. 883.
5. Paulos von Aegina: Des besten Arztes sieben Bücher. Leiden: Brill, 1914: Vol. lib. 6, p. 492.
6. Metlinger B: Ein Regiment der jungen Kinder. Augsburg 1473. In: Sudhoff K: Erstlinge der Pädiatrischen Literatur; München 1925: p. cap. 1.
7. Burckhard G: Die deutschen Hebammenordnungen. Leipzig: Engelmann, 1912: Vol. **1**, p. 122, 247.
8. Mercurialis H: De puerorum morbis tractatus locupletissimi. Frankfurt: Wechelius, 1584: p. 261.
9. Bourgeois L: Observations diverses sur la sterilité, perte de fruits, foecondité, accouchments, et maladies de femmes, et enfants nouveaux-naiz. Paris: Dehoury, 1609: Reprint Paris, p. 96.
10. Hérouard J: Journal sur l'enfance et la jeunesse de Louis XIII. Paris: Soulié & Barthélemy, 1868: Vol. **I**, p. 7.
11. Fabricius Hieronimus ab Aquapendente: Opera chirurgica, in duas partes divisa. Francofurti: Hoffmannus, 1620: p. 105.
12. Scultetus J: Wund-Artzneyisches Zeug-Hauß. Franckfurt: Gerlin, 1666: p. 104–7.
13. Mauriceau F: Tractat von Kranckheiten schwangerer und gebärender Weibspersonen (1st French ed. 1668). Basel: Bertsche, 1680: p. 330, 358.
14. Siegemundin J: Königl.-Preußische und Chur-Brandenburgische Hof-Wehe-Mutter. Berlin: Voß, 1752: p. 248.
15. Rosenstein NRv: Anweisung zur Kenntnis und Chur der Kinderkrankheiten. (Swedish ed. 1764, English transl. 1766). 4. ed. Göttingen: Dieterich, 1781: p. 21.
16. Hagen JP: Hebammen-Catechismus. 4. ed. Berlin: Maurer, 1791: p. 376.
17. Petit JL: Traité des maladies chirurgicales et des opérations qui leur conviennent. Paris: Didot Jeune, 1774: Vol. **3**, p. 260.
18. Desormeaux M: Das Ancyloglossum oder die Verwachsung der Zunge. Analekten über Kinderkrankheiten 1836;**3**:115–23.
19. Rau G: Handbuch für Hebammen. Gießen: Heyer, 1807: p. 167.
20. Jörg JCG: Lehrbuch der Hebammenkunst. Leipzig: Industrie-Comptoir, 1814: §337.
21. Capuron J: Traité des maladies des enfans, jusqu' a la puberté. 2. ed. Paris: Croullebois, 1820: p. 59.
22. Wendt J: Die Kinderkrankheiten systematisch dargestellt. 2. ed. Breslau: Korn, 1826: p. 49.

23. Marjolin JN: Die Fröschleingeschwulst (Ranula). Analekten über Kinderkrankheiten 1836;**3**:124–9.
24. Meissner FL: Die Kinderkrankheiten nach den neusten Ansichten und Erfahrungen. 3. ed. Leipzig: Fest', 1844: Vol. **1**, p. 274.
25. Guersant PM: Notizen über chirurgische Pädiatrik. Erlangen: Enke, 1869: p. 256.
26. Bouchut E: Traité pratique des maladies des nouveau-nés. 5. ed. Paris: Baillière, 1867: p. 444, fig. 119.
27. Mauriceau F: Observations sur la grossesse et l'accouchement des femmes. Paris: Compagnie des Libraires, 1738: Vol. **2**, p. 249.
28. Levret A: L'art des accouchemens. 3. ed. Paris: Didot Jeune, 1766: p. 248.
29. Raulin J: Von Erhaltung der Kinder. Leipzig: Crusius, 1769: Vol. **2**, p. 68.
30. Deleurye F: Die Mutter nach der Anweisung der Natur. Frankfurt: NN, 1774: p. 60.
31. Underwood M: A treatise on the disorders of childhood (1st French ed. 1786). 2. ed. London: Matthews, 1801: Vol. 2: Every complaint of importance, falling under the more immediate Province of the Surgeon, p. 122.
32. Fischl R: Die Krankheiten der Mundhöhle im Kindesalter. In: Handbuch der Kinderheilkunde: 4. ed. Berlin: Vogel, 1931: Vol. **3**, p. 9.
33. Stark JC: Das Fröschlein. Archiv für die Geburtshülfe, Frauenzimmer- und neugebohrner Kinder-Krankheiten 1791;**3**:309–17.
34. Girtanner C: Abhandlung über die Krankheiten der Kinder. Berlin: Rottmann, 1794: p. 17, 25.
35. Verson FX: Der Arzt am Krankenbette der Kinder und an der Wiege der Säuglinge. Wien: Heubner, 1838: Vol. **1**, p. 114.
36. Moro E: Erkrankungen der Mundhöhle. In: Handbuch der Kinderheilkunde: 4. ed. Leipzig: Vogel, 1906: Vol. **2**, p. 35.
37. McEnery ET, Gaines FP: Tongue-tie in infants and children. J Pediatr 1941;**18**:252–5.
38. Dunn PM: Bridled babies: a history of tongue-tie. Proc Bristol Med Hist Soc 1995;**3**:15–23.
39. Segal LM, Stephenson R, Dawes M, Feldman P: Prevalence, diagnosis, and treatment of ankyloglossia. Can Fam Physician 2007;**53**:1027–33.
40. Messner AH, Lalakea ML: Ankyloglossia: controversies in management. Int J Pediatr Otorhinolaryngol 2000;**54**:123–31.
41. Ketty N, Sciullo PA: Ankyloglossia with psychological implications. J Dent Child 1974;**41**:43–6.
42. Lalakea ML, Messner AH: Ankyloglossia: does it matter? Pediatr Clin N Am 2003;**50**:381–97.
43. Dollberg S: Immediate nipple pain relief after frenotomy in breast-fed infants with ankyloglossia: a randomized, prospective study. J Pediatr Surg 2006;**41**:1598–600.
44. Geddes DT, Langton DB, Gollow I, et al.: Frenulotomy for breastfeeding infants with ankyloglossia. Pediatrics 2008;**122**:e188–94.
45. Wallace AF: Tongue-tie. Lancet 1963;**2**:377–8.
46. Schmitt WJ: Beschreibung und Abbildung einer neuen Zungenbandschere. In: Geburtshülfliche Fragmente. Wien: Lodersches Journal, 1804: p. 137–49.

6.11

Lethal lullabies
Opium use in infants

Introduction: opium, an ancient drug

The poppy plant has been cultivated since prehistoric times. Sumerian cuneiform tablets (3000 B.C.E.) describe narcotic drugs from the plant *gil* [1], but it has been doubted that these plants were *Papaver somniferum* due to ambiguous botanic nomenclature [2]. The term *opium* derives from the Greek word *opos* (juice). Whereas the historiography of opium [3–6] and its abuse [7, 8] is extensive, little attention has been paid to its widespread use in infants. The following chapter focuses on this aspect.

The crying infant

Announcing that the baby is alive, the birth cry is most welcome. This is less so for other kinds of infant crying and least so at night. In our evolutionary past, infants were constantly carried, their cry originated from isolation, as demonstrated by John Newman [9]: 'There is one situation that reliably evokes crying in most primate species: That is the physical separation of a baby from its mother … primates share the basic pattern of a gradually frequency-modulated tonality. This widespread similarity suggests that the mechanisms controlling infant cry patterns have had a conservative evolutionary history.' Charles Darwin stated in 1872 [10]: 'The chief expressive actions, exhibited by man and by the lower animals, are now innate or inherited—that is, have not been learnt by the individual … Infants scream from pain directly after birth, and all their features assume the same form as during subsequent years.' London psychologist John Bowlby hypothesized in 1957 that crying contributes to maternal–infant bonding [11]: 'There is plentiful evidence from the animal world … probably in all cases the mother responds promptly and unfailingly to her infant's bleat, call, or cry.' Selection pressure forced primates to live in groups. Crying infants attracted predators. Whoever did not react promptly, disappeared from the gene pool. Maternal attachment promoted both emotions and survival. Still today, infants cry less in gatherer-hunter societies [12]. Excessive infant crying has been associated with infant abuse in rhesus monkeys [13] and humans [14].

Infant sedation in antiquity

Putting babies to sleep with poppy derivatives was mentioned in the Egyptian papyrus *Ebers* (16th century B.C.E.): 'Capsules of the poppy plant and wasp droppings from the wall shall be mixed and sieved, and given on four days. The infant's crying ceases immediately.' [15] The third aphorism in the *Corpus Hippocraticum* (5th century B.C.E.) declared neonatal sleeplessness and dentition as diseases [16] and Galen (129–210 C.E.) recommended [17] 'to guess accurately what is moderate and comfortable [for the individual infant] and provide this before increasing distress throws its body and mind into excess of activity'. In the 10th century C.E., Baghdad author Rhazes recommended sedation in his booklet on the ailments of children [18]: 'Sleeplessness occurs in the first period of life from unwholesome milk … And give the child to suck syrup of poppy and smear the temples and forehead with oil of opium and saffron.' Avicenna (11th century C.E.) specified this treatment [19]: 'For [incessant crying] it is necessary to make [the baby] sleep if possible, by giving [a potion of] white poppy, yellow poppy, fennel seed, aniseed … If it is desired to make it still stronger, one should add an amount of opium equal to a third part of it or less.'

Praised and condemned by physicians

Once excessive infant crying had been defined a disease (*vigilia*) and opiates had Rhazes' and Avicenna's blessing, infant doping made its way into early medical treatises (Table 6.11.1) and from there into most paediatric texts. Opium often sailed through the literature under the flag of ancient recipes designed to conceal its bitter taste: *Mithridate* (Serapion, ca. 280 B.C.E.): poppy juice and lizard plus 40 herbs; *Theriac* (Andromachus 65 C.E.), also named *Galene* or *Venetian Treacle*: poppy juice, honey, and viper flesh plus 55 herbs; *Requies Nicolai* (Nicolaus Propositus, 1110 C.E.), also called *electuarium pro infantibus*: opium, nutmeg, and mandrakes; *Laudanum* (Paracelsus 1534): opium dissolved in alcohol and flavoured with saffron, cinnamon, or nutmeg; *Diascordium* (Fracastorius 1546), also misspelled *Diacodium*: poppy syrup, rose

---

Reproduced with permission from Obladen, M. Lethal lullabies: a history of opium use in infants. *Journal of Human Lactation*, 32(1):75–85. Copyright © 2016, SAGE Publications.

Table 6.11.1 Opiates and other treatments recommended for sleepless and teething infants in early printed medical textbooks

Author, year, reference	Sleeplessness	Teething	Other indication
Paolo Bagellardo 1472 [20]	Opium orally and as external ointment	Rubbing gums with hare's brain; lancing	Opium and aniseed in wine for loose stools
Bartholomäus Metlinger 1473 [21]	White P. extract to anoint temples	Hare's brain, violet oil	–
Cornelius Roelans 1485 [22]	External or oral white P. syrup or capsules, or opium	Hare's brain and chicken fat	Opium for diarrhoea and colic
Eucharius Roesslin 1513 [23]	External ointment of seed, capsule extract	–	–
Sebastianus Austrius (Roelans) 1540 [24]	White P. syrup and rose water	'Narcotics' and rose oil	P. and myrtle seed for diarrhoea
Thomas Phaire 1553 [25]	P. syrup on lips, or P. juice plaster	Hare's brain and chicken fat	Sorrel and P. seed, raisin, acorn apples for 'belly fluxe'
Simon Vallambert 1565 [26]	Mithridate or theriac at birth (!) and for excessive cry	'Quelque chose anodyne'	P. syrup for seizures, short breath, diarrhoea
Girolamo Mercuriale 1584 [27]	P. juice, 'Requies Nicolai'	Hare's brain	–
Jacques Guillemeau 1643 [28]	Diacodium and rose syrup for sleep	Hare's brain, chicken fat, lancing and diacodium	Opium syrup or theriac for seizures
Franciscus Sylvius 1674 [29]	Laudanum, anodyna, narcotica	Hare's brain, butter, and honey	Diascordium for belches, hicket, jaundice and 'curdled milk'
Walter Harris 1689 [30]	'Cordial', 'anodyne', 'narcoticks'	Incision of gums, diascordium	Theriac, anodynes for 'the gripes'
Michael Ettmüller 1688 [31]	P. syrup or laudanum opiatum	–	Anodynes for cough, Venetian treacle or mithridate for weaning, P. heads for seizures
Valentin Kräutermann 1740 [32]	P. emulsion or theriac Andromachi	Hare's brain, P. ointment, laudanum	Theriac for seizures, diacodium for colic

P., poppy. Application was oral if not otherwise specified.

honey, cinnamon, water germander (*teucrium scordium*) plus 14 other herbs.

Leipzig surgeon Michael Ettmüller considered opiates a cure-all in 1688 [31]: 'Forasmuch as all these Diseases of Children are deriv'd from one Cause [unwholesome milk], and consequently demand the same Method of Cure, 'twill be needless to trace every distinct Symptom apart … Tincture of Tartar …, and Venice Triacle or Mithridate given two grains … Syrup of Poppies, two drams.' George Armstrong, who founded the London Dispensary in 1769, was more cautious [33]: 'Some infants are more wakeful in the night than in the day, which is hurtful to themselves, and irksome to those about them; and therefore they ought to be broke of it as soon as possible … As to opiates, in this case, I reckon them very pernicious; though I am afraid some careless nurses use too much freedom with them, by giving them to children in the day as well as the night, in order to keep them quiet, and prevent their disturbing them in their business.' Swiss physician and chemist Christoph Girtanner stated in 1794 [34]: 'Sleeplessness is not a disease, but the symptom of a disease. One should therefore refrain from giving opiates to infants, to make them sleep.' Nevertheless, and in the same book, Girtanner listed a series of opiate recipes for infants, for example, to facilitate teething. Infant *soothers* were among the first proprietary drugs ever produced, and Michael Underwood disapproved of them in 1784 [35]: 'However wakeful a child may be in the night, it cannot receive a greater unkindness than from the exhibition of Godfrey's cordial, syrup of poppies, or any other opiate, to induce it to sleep better.' However, as they were about artificial feeding, physicians were remarkably ambivalent about opiates for infants: having once disapproved of them emphatically, they listed indications and concocted recipes. When the disaster became obvious in the 19th century, mothers, nurses, and quacks were blamed.

Breastfeeding and weaning

From antiquity, infants were often weaned abruptly from the breast which often involved the use of drugs. Soran warned in the 2nd century C.E. [36]: 'It is harmful to anoint the nipple with some bitter and ill-smelling things and thus wean the infant suddenly, the sudden change is injurious.' Avicenna recommended [19]: 'The best way is to apply a paste to the breast, made of myrrh and pennyroyal.' Guillemeau insisted in 1612 [28]: 'You must make him loathe the breast … rubbing the top of the nipple with mustard or aloe.' Ambroise Paré in 1649 [37]: 'Let the teat be annointed or rubbed with bitter things, as with Aloes, infusion of Colocynthus, or Wormwood, or with Mustard, or Soot stipped in water.' *The Nurse's Guide* in 1729 [38]: 'Rub her Nipples with Aloes, Wormwood, or Soot mixed with Water, to give him an adversion to it.' Fussy from sudden weaning, the baby was quieted with opium as Alexander Hamilton recommended in 1781 [39]: 'There can be no harm in giving the child a little weak white-wine whey, diluted brandy punch, or even a tea-spoonful or two of syrup of poppy, for a few nights after weaning, to prevent restlessness and fits of crying, till the breast is forgotten.'

With the onset of industrialization, mothers working in factories left their infants at home, often in custody of an older child. When poor, they could not afford a wet nurse and prolonged breastfeeding intervals, again with the help of opium, with disastrous consequences, as New York City superintendent David Meredith Reese described in 1857 [40]: 'Thousands thus perish in early infancy, their deaths being ascribed to colic, cholera, diarrhoea … though oftener produced by drugging for the relief of symptoms which the mother's milk would have prevented or cured, life being sacrificed by soothing syrup, Godfrey's cordial, Jayne's carminative.' In London, obstetrician Charles Routh reported similar experiences in 1879 [41]: 'To keep the child easy it was regularly drugged with some opiate after the breast had been given.'

Dentitio difficilis—cutting the teeth

The gums of teething infants had been rubbed with hare's brain since Soran and Galen (2nd century C.E.), with great faith and little harm. In the 18th century, this disgusting rite slowly fell from grace. Pliny the Elder (1st century C.E.) had recommended scarifying the gums for toothache [42]. With the development of surgery emerged the idea that teeth must be liberated from their prison, which lingered in textbooks for three centuries. In France, Ambroise Paré recommended lancing the gums in 1649 [37]: 'In such a caus, before the fore-named mortal accidents com, I would perswade the Chirurgian to open the gums in such places as the teeth bunch out, with a knife or lancet, so opening a waie for them.' Gum lancing and oral opiates became fashionable and teething became dangerous. The more threatening teething was considered, the riskier the treatments performed. Walter Harris lamented in 1689 [30]: 'Of all the disorders which threaten the lives of Infants, there is none that is wont to produce so many grievous Symptoms as a difficult and laborious Breeding of Teeth … The physician therefore ought to take care, that the Incision be always made with a proper instrument, whether it be a Penknife, or any other knife that has a thick Back … in slighter Cases of this Sort, the Use of *Diascordium*, and such like Medicines, has been found to do no harm.' Hugh Smith wrote in his letters to married women in 1792 [43]: 'A great assistance may be obtained by lancing of the gums … Let not a false tenderness prevent fond mothers from allowing such relief to their little babes, in the excruciating tortures they suffer by cutting of teeth … Let me advise you not to depend upon old women, to do it with crooked sixpences, and such like ineffectual means.' Nils Rosenstein's book appeared from 1764 to 1851 in 25 editions and eight translations, devoted ten pages to difficult teething, still recommended hare's brain, and sheds light on how opium was dosed [44]: 'The child is given as much poppy sirup (*syrupus e meconio*) as required to allow him a little rest. From repeated small doses the effective amount required to calm the infant can be assessed … If *syrupus e meconio* is not strong enough … one or several drops of *laudanum* may be given.' London obstetrician John Clarke affirmed in 1815 [45]: 'If the division of the gums should be unnecessarily performed, no inconvenience can result from it, but great mischief may arise from omitting it … It has been proposed, and often practised under these circumstances, to give opium in various forms to children, especially when the inflammation of the gums is attended with much pain; but this practice should be pursued with great caution.'

In retrospect, most infants with 'difficult teething' probably suffered from scurvy (see Chapter 7.6). Leonard Guthrie referred to the annual reports of the Registrar General [46]: 'For 1839 in London 709 deaths and in England 5,016 deaths were attributed to teething.' Although many of these deaths probably had other causes, it seems likely that treatment for 'difficult teething' was an early iatrogenic catastrophe for infants. As late as 1856, Charles West stated [47]: 'A great remedy in the diseases of early life is opium in its various preparations … perhaps no remedies are so often needed in the diseases of early life as sedatives, for at no other age is the nervous system so easily disturbed' and admitted 'the circumstances in which the gum-lancet is really indicated are comparably few'.

Use in institutions and by wet nurses

Opiates were an integral part of commercial wet nursing: William Buchan of Edinburgh complained in 1788 [48]: 'An indolent nurse, who does not give a child sufficient exercise in the open air to make it sleep … will seldom fail to procure for it a dose of laudanum, diacodium, saffron, or, what answers the same purpose, a dram of spirits or other strong liquors … I never knew a good nurse who had her Godfrey's cordials, Daffy's elixirs, &c. at hand.' Same city, same habit, different brands a century later, as Charles Routh reported [41]: 'There are some faults which [hired wet nurses] are especially liable to commit. One is drugging … The chemist's shop [is much frequented], especially on a saturday night … Gallons of laudanum, soothing syrups, Dalby's carminative, paregoric, disappear.' Although not mentioned in the official histories [49–51], opium was used extensively in the foundling asylums. Ludwig Ruland reported that in Paris already in the *Maison de la Couche* (founded 1326) 'the nurses gave a sleeping draught to the infants, probably a tea of *Papaver somniferum*, after which many never woke up' [52]. From the Dublin Foundling Hospital Thomas Jordan reported [53]: 'A sinister practice was use of Winslow's Soothing Syrup and Daffy's elixir; still more alarming was recourse to a draught composed of water and tincture of opium which left the infant *easy for an hour or two*.' In France, Napoleon's 1811 decree multiplied the foundling hospitals which were soon admitting more than 30,000 infants per year. A public scandal ('slaughter of the innocents') was elicited by *The New York Times* [54] and *Harper's Weekly* [55] headlines when it became known that several infants had died from opium intoxication and starvation in the hands of Mary Cullough, a baby farmer working for the New York Almshouse (Fig. 6.11.1).

Private use from the 16th to the 19th century

Soothers had been a part of the European habit of self-medication since the Middle Ages. In the German-speaking countries, poppy syrup was put into soups and pacifiers (Fig. 6.11.2) well into the 20th century. Besides *mohnschlotzer*, there were many names for them in different regions. From Görlitz (Saxony), Christian Struve reported in 1803 [56]: 'In the big immoral cities … they give infants mithridate or poppy soup, from which they become dazed or fall into convulsions … decoctions of poppy heads, mithridate, theriac, Philonium Romanum, and soothing powders don't provide natural sleep, they

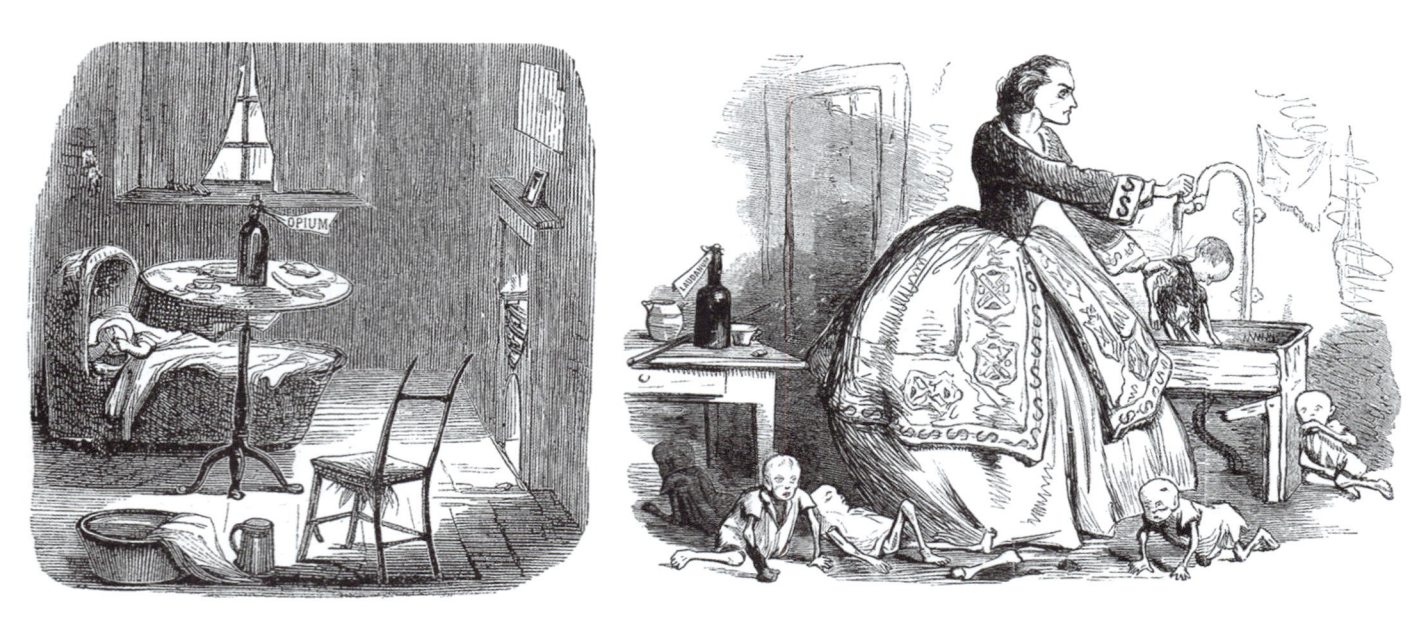

Fig. 6.11.1 *Harper's Weekly's* 1859 campaign against opium use in New York foundling asylums. Left: opium—the poor child's nurse [92]. Right: New York as nursing mother to her foundlings, depicting baby-farmer Mary Cullough, starving infants, and laudanum bottle on the table [55].

knock out the head.' In Cöthen (Anhalt), Arthur Lutze observed in 1862 'infants who suffocated from rag-bags' and stated 'it is a crime to administer poppy decocts and such like against crying, they make the infant stupid and dull'. In the English-speaking countries, numerous proprietary soothing syrups and teething powders for infants were on the market, some of which are listed in Table 6.11.2. In Quebec, Mrs Winslow's Soothing Syrup (Fig. 6.11.3), Children's Comfort, Dr. Groves Anodyne, and Dr. Moffetts Compound were so widely used that L.F. Dubé complained in 1915 [57]: 'Soothing syrups are a scandal and a disgrace to human intellect, maternal love, and civilization. They have killed more infants than a hundred Herodes.'

When legislation became effective (US 1915, UK 1920), several successful brands persisted without opiates.

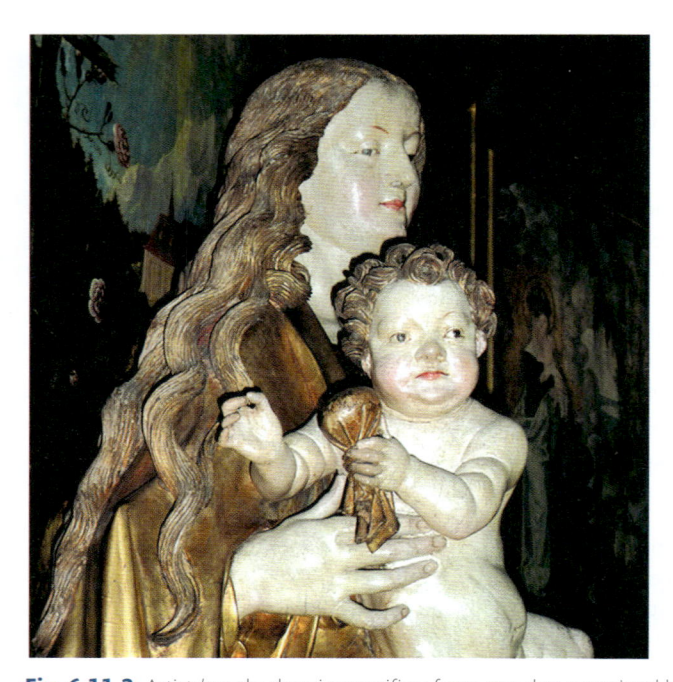

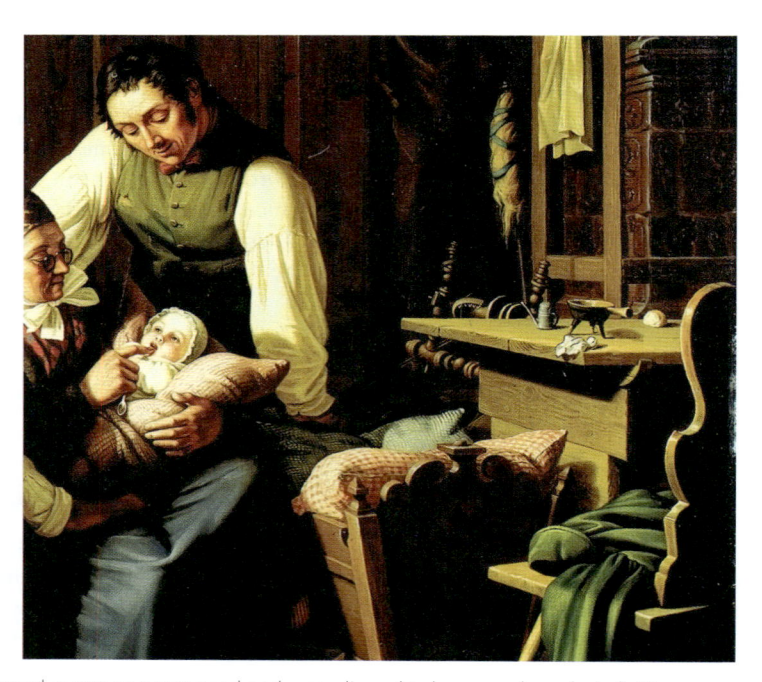

Fig. 6.11.2 Artists' works showing pacifiers from rags that contained bread, sugar, or poppyseed and were dipped in honey or brandy. Left, Hans Wydyz, detail of 'Rest during the flight', wood carving ca. 1514. Right, Johann Gottlieb Hantzsch, 'The first tooth', detail of an 1834 painting showing the poppy-rag side by side to pap-pan and pewter bottle.
Schnewlinaltar, Freiburg Cathedral, with permission. Right, Leipzig, Museum der bildenden Künste, Inv.-Nr. G 536, with permission.

CHAPTER 6.11 Lethal lullabies: opium use in infants

Table 6.11.2 Some 18th- and 19th-century proprietary soothing drugs widely used for infants

Drug, years sold	Producer, location	Typical ingredients	Opium content	Reference
Laudanum Sydenham, 1660–present	Pharmacies, local stores	Tincture of opium, wine, saffron, cinnamon, clover	3–10% powdered opium	[58]
Paregoric elixir, 1721–present	Bateman's drops, Benjamin Okell, New York	Tincture of opium, alcohol, camphor, aniseed oil	0.4–0.5%	[4]
Godfrey's Cordial, generic from 1750 to 1921	Thomas Godfrey, Hertfordshire; local stores had various recipes	Morphine (laudanum based), molasse, sassafras oil	1–3%	[6] [40]
Dover's Powder, 1762–1960	Thomas Dover, US	Ipecac powder, opium, saltpeter, tartar vitriolated	10%	[4]
James Dalby's Carminative, 1780–1920	London; from 1904 Fougerac Co. NY	Opium tincture, magnesium carbonate, nutmeg, aniseed	0.5–2%	[6]
Elixir of opium, 1837–1905	Dr John McMunn/AB Sands Co.	Ether-deodorized opium with alcohol		[59]
Mrs Winslow's Soothing Syrup, ca. 1849–1930	Charlotte Winslow/Curtis & Perkins, Anglo-American Drug Co.	Morphine sulphate, sodium carbonate, aqua ammonia, fennel spirit	2–3%	[6] [57]
Royal Infant's Preservative, 1853–1911	Atkinson & Barker, Manchester	Laudanum, magnesia carbonate, sugar, aniseed oil, saffron	0.7%	[6]
Children's Comfort, ca. 1850–1911	Gigault & Fairbanks, Worcester, MA	Morphine sulphate, until 1915	?	[57]
Dr. Groves' Anodyne for Infants, 1858–1919	Smith, Kline & French, Philadelphia	Morphine sulphate, chloral, sugar, spearmint oil	0.25%	[57]
Dr. Moffett's Teething Powder, ca. 1850–1915	C.J. Moffett Co., St. Louis, MO	Opium powder, calomel, bismuth	?	[57]
Street's Infants' Quietness, 1844	UK and US	Laudanum	1%	[6]

Opium content has been estimated according to the analyses of Paris [60], Taylor [61], and the Analytical Sanitary Commission 1853 [62]. For conversion to percentages, the following imperial/apothecary units were used: Weight: pound, 373 g; ounce, 31.1 g; drachm, 3.89 g; scruple, 1.3 g; grain, 64.8 mg. Volume: pint, 568 mL; fl. oz, 28.4 mL; fl. dram, 3.55 mL; fl. scruple, 1.18 mL; minim, 59 µL.

Dosage, withdrawal, and toxicity

A notorious problem of opiates was their inconsistent alkaloid content, due to biologic variability and adulteration. The composition and strength of *anodynes*, *nostrums*, and *specifics* was kept secret; chronic use led to tolerance, incomplete shaking to sedimentation in the bottle. The literature of all epochs abounds with reports on infant intoxication, a small selection of which follows. Galen warned [63]: 'In children one must avoid [theriac] entirely. For it is too strong for their inherent power and easily destroys their body and

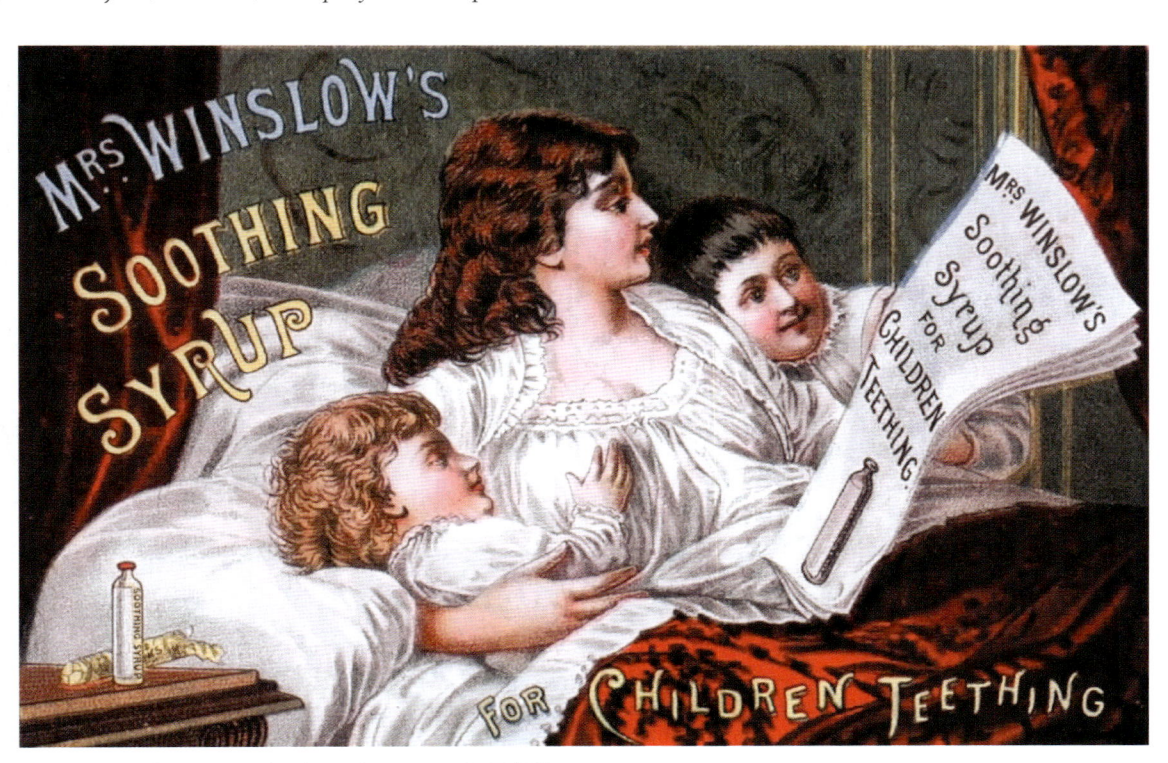

Fig. 6.11.3 Advertisement for Mrs Winslow's soothing syrup 1885 [93].

extinguishes breathing... I saw a child dying of the untimely use of the antidote.' The sarcophagus cover in Fig. 6.11.4, top left, illustrates that Galen's observation was not unique in ancient Rome. John Cook of Leigh/Essex, reported a personal tragedy in 1769 [64]: 'Opiates with infants ought to be used with the utmost caution. I lost a son above a year old, who was killed instantly, only with eight drops of liquid laudanum, when two drops are sufficient for a babe.' But this failed to change his opinion on teething: 'Should the pain become intolerable, *opium benignum* should be used.' John Clarke also encountered lethal opium intoxication in 1815 [45]: 'This last class of medicines has generally been exhibited in the forms of laudanum, syrup of white poppy, or under some empirical title, as Godfrey's Cordial, or Dalby's Carminative... Nothing is more uncertain than the effects of opium on young subjects... and has proved deleterious even in very small doses. Half a drachm [1.6 g] of genuine syrup of white poppy, and, in some instances, a few drops of Dalby's Carminative, have proved fatal in the course of a few hours to very young infants (since this paragraph was written the writer has seen another case in which forty drops of Dalby's Carminative destroyed an infant).'

Marshal Hall observed withdrawal symptoms in a 6-month-old boy at the Edinburgh Royal Infirmary on 10 February 1816 [65]: 'Being deprived of the breast at one month, its mother began the pernicious practice of giving it an *anodyne* every night; a practice which has been continued to the present day... The infant is thin, emaciated, sickly, and puny, and is said to be less in bulk than on the day of its birth... He is apt to be very restless and cross, frequently cries for a long time together unappeased, and sometimes appears to be affected with griping.' With or without physicians' prescription, myriads of *soothers* were given to infants during the 19th century, and *The Lancet* published reports of lethal intoxication annually [66–72]. In 1853, Thomas Bull compiled reports on 12 infants killed within 2 years from Godfrey's cordial alone [73]. In the same year, the London Sanitary Commission analysed laudanum samples prepared by 21 pharmacies [58]: their opium content ranged from 3% to 21%, and the alkaloid content of opium from 2.7% to 14%, which resulted in a 36-fold difference in morphine concentration. By 1863, infant deaths from opiates had become so frequent that the Registrar General Reports introduced the category 'narcotic deaths by age' which, for the years 1863–1867 disclosed 236 infant deaths under 1 year [6]. At the beginning of the 20th century, an Australian Royal Commission estimated that 15,000 infants a year were killed by proprietary medicines [74].

Not all poisoning was lethal: Hufeland's 1800 use of emetics [75], and the reports of Herapath in 1852 [76] and Kirk in 1853 [77], who used galvanism during many hours of laudanum-induced apnoea, are early descriptions of successful neonatal intensive care. Disastrous effects on mental development were known in 1866, when John Langdon-Down described 'the Mongolian type of idiocy' (see Chapter 5.6) and his very first idea was 'Has the nurse dosed the child with opium?' [78].

The opium trade

With the 12th-century crusades, the Serenissima Republic of Venice gained control of the trade between Europe and the Levant and became the central marketplace for silk, sugar, spices, and opium. Before export, the latter often was publicly refined to *Venetian Treacle*, as shown in Fig. 6.11.4, bottom left. The East India Company,

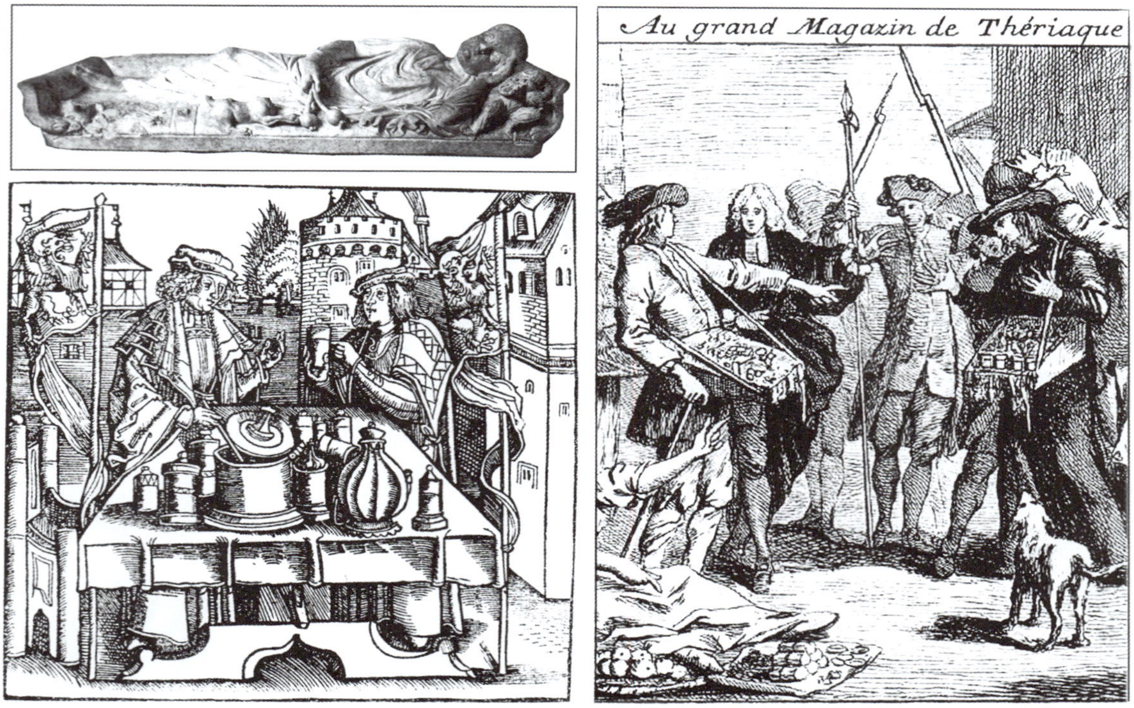

Fig. 6.11.4 Opium in everyday life. Top left, Prometheus sarcophagus cover with an infant holding two poppyheads. Rome, 3rd century C.E. [94]. Bottom left, public mixing of theriac in Venice, from Hieronymus Brunschweig, 1512 [95]. Right, detail of a cartoon showing street sale of theriac in Paris, 1764.

Bibliothèque Nationale de France, Inv.-No. G 160302, with permission.

founded in 1600, practically ruled India from 1757, and became the largest player in the British global market. It exploited the Chinese desire for drugs: most Bengal opium was smuggled by the company to China, where the yearly import exceeded 1000 tons by 1830 [79]. The Qing government attempted to limit such imports in 1834, provoking the first opium war: British naval forces blocked Chinese ports, in 1842 the Peace of Nanking ceded five ports (and Hong Kong) to Britain. Most of the company's opium trade remained in Asia, but some ships made their way from Bengal and Burma around the Cape of Good Hope: in the port of London, 18 tons of opium were officially imported in 1831, rising to 88 in 1839 [80]. Much of this opium went into preparations for children. The French East Indies Company exported opium from India and Cambodia via Réunion to its Bretonian port Lorient (*l'orient*). The customs records show that 114 tons of opium were received in France from 1827 to 1836 [3]. The Dutch East India Company transported opium from Batavia (Indonesia) via South Africa to Amsterdam. Opiates were freely available all over Europe. Patent drugs, preservatives, or nostrums were sold over shop counters, by quacks, or by street vendors (Fig 6.11.4, right), with the contents, strength, and risk remaining a mystery to the customer. In Thuringia, Stemler found in 1820 'sleeping powders or Nicolai's Rest very common especially among manual workers, who can devote little time to their infants' [81]. From France, Arnould Frémy reported in 1841 [82]: 'In Lille, the female factory workers buy a certain amount of theriac for their infants.' Americans received opium mainly from Turkey; from 1850 to 1877, 2403 tons of opium were imported to the USA, not including morphine salts and proprietary drugs [83].

In England, the fathers of communism were shocked by widespread infant doping. Friedrich Engels, who had lived in Manchester for 2 years, decried the misery of the working class in 1845 [84]: 'One of the most injurious of these patent medicines is a drink prepared with opiates, chiefly laudanum, under the name Godfrey's Cordial. Women who work at home, and have their own and other people's children to take care of, give them this drink to keep them quiet, and, as many believe, to strengthen them. They often begin to give this medicine to newly-born children, and continue, without knowing the effects of this "heart's-ease", until the children die.' Karl Marx wrote his *Capital* in London in 1867 [85]: 'Every phenomenon of the factory districts is here reproduced, including, but to a greater extent, ill-disguised infanticide, and dosing children with opiates.'

Regulating prescriptions

In Britain, the 1868 Pharmacy Act regulated some advertising texts and put an end to the street and grocery-store sale of opiates, but pharmacies sold the specifics as freely as before. Throughout the 19th century, governments paid lip service to the abuse, hesitating to kill the goose that laid the golden eggs. As late as 1912, the International Opium Convention signed at The Hague established 'an international obligation to control domestic as well as foreign trade of opium'. Reluctantly, governments implemented the Convention in national legislations, as did the US via the Harrison Act 1914 [86], France and the Netherlands in 1915, Britain by the Dangerous Drugs Act in 1920, and Germany by the *Opiumgesetz* in 1929.

Opiate use today

Opium and its derivatives are no longer considered an appropriate treatment for teething or excessively crying babies. Presently, they are used in two conditions: the first is acute pain, as in surgery and other painful procedures. For this indication (and in addition to acetaminophen), morphine or fentanyl are recommended by American and European guidelines [87, 88]. The second indication is neonatal abstinence syndrome [89]. The prevalence of opiate use during pregnancy has been estimated to be 1–2%, with regional peaks up to 20%. Addicted pregnant women usually are substituted with methadone, buprenorphine, or slow-release morphine [90]. Neonatal consequences of maternal substance use include an increased rate of preterm delivery and low birthweight, withdrawal symptoms, persisting neurobehavioral problems, and an increased risk for sudden infant death. Neonatal abstinence syndrome is usually treated with phenobarbitone or opiates [91]. Exposure to opiates *in utero* or in early infancy is known to be detrimental to the developing nervous system. There is increasing concern that methadone maintenance during pregnancy and postnatal use of morphine may adversely affect infants' neurodevelopment [89]

Conclusion

Throughout history and in many cultures, opium was used extensively for infants even though its severe and fatal side effects were well known. In many cases, baby drugging may have been disguised infanticide, accepted more or less by society. Physicians were ambivalent to opium in infants, but on the whole promoted its use. Countries holding monopolies on trade and import tolerated its abuse for centuries. Even when it became obvious that opium intoxication was an important cause of infant mortality, governments were reluctant to pass laws to effectively curtail the use of this drug during early infancy.

REFERENCES

1. Brownstein MJ: A brief history of opiates, opioid peptides, and opioid receptors. PNAS 1993;**90**:5391–3.
2. Krikorian AD: Were the opium poppy and opium known in the Ancient Near East? J Hist Biol 1975;**8**:95–114.
3. Chevallier A: Notice historique sur l'opium Indigène. Paris: Remquet, 1852: p. 5.
4. Macht DI: The history of opium and some of its preparations and alkaloids. JAMA 1915;**64**:477–81.
5. Kritikos PG, Papadaki SP: The history of the poppy and of opium and their expansion in antiquity in the eastern Mediterranean area. Bull Narcot 1967;**19**:5–10, 17–38.
6. Berridge V, Edwards G: Opium and the people. London: Allen Lane, 1981: p. 97–109.
7. Lomax E: The uses and abuses of opiates in nineteenth century England. Bull Hist Med 1973;**47**:167–76.
8. Kramer JC: Opium rampant: medical use, misuse and abuse in Britain and the West in the 17th and 18th centuries. Br J Addict Alcohol Other Drugs 1979;**74**:377–89.
9. Newman JD: The infant cry of primates. In: Lester BM, Boukydis CFZ: Infant crying. New York: Plenum, 1985: p. 307–23.

10. Darwin C: The expression of emotions in man and animals. In: Francis Darwin: Works of Charles Darwin. 2. ed. London: Murray, 1890: Vol. **23**, p. 371.
11. Bowlby J: The nature of the child's tie to his mother. Int J Psychoanal 1958;**39**:350–73.
12. Barr RG, Konner M, Bakeman R, Adamson L: Crying in !Kung San infants. Dev Med Child Neurol 1991;**33**:601–10.
13. Maestripieri D, Jovanovic T, Gouzoules H: Crying and infant abuse in rhesus monkeys. Child Dev 2000;**71**:301–9.
14. Frodi A: When empathy fails. In: Lester BM, Boukydis CFZ: Infant crying. New York: Plenum, 1985: p. 263–77.
15. Joachim H: Papyros Ebers. Berlin: Reimer, 1890: p. 169.
16. Hippocrates: Works, Volume IV. Aphorisms, III, 24–25. Loeb's Classical Library. London: Heinemann, 1931: p. 130.
17. Green RM: A translation of Galen's Hygiene (de sanitate tuenda). Springfield, IL: Thomas, 1951: p. 28.
18. Radbill SX: The first treatise on pediatrics: booklet on the ailments of children and their care. Arch Pediatr 1971;**122**:369–76.
19. Gruner OC: A treatise on the canon of medicine of Avicenna, incorporating a translation of the first book. London: Luzac & Co., 1930: p. §711–9.
20. Bagellardo P: Opusculum recens natum de morbis puerorum (1st ed. 1472). Lyon: Barbou, 1538: p. 4, 31, 43.
21. Metlinger B: Regiment der jungen Kinder. Augsburg: Zainer, 1473: Vol. cap. 3, p. Fol. 31.
22. Roelans von Mecheln C: Das Buch der Kinderkrankheiten (1485). Edited by: Hermann Brüning. Wissenschaftliche Zeitschrift der Universität Rostock. Rostock: Universität Rostock, 1953: Vol. **3**, p. 38, 63.
23. Rößlin E: Der Swangern Frauwen und hebammen Rosegarten (Engl. transl. Thomas Reynald 1540). Facsimile Antiqua Verlag Wutöschingen 1993. Straßburg: Flach, 1513: p. 94.
24. Austrius S: De infantium morborum. Basiliae: Westheimer, 1540: p. 46, 170.
25. Phaire T: The boke of children, 1553. Edinburgh: Livingstone, 1955: p. 28–38.
26. Vallambert Sd: Cinq livres de la manière de nourrir et gouverner les enfants dès leur naissance. Reprint Droz, Genève 2005. Poitiers: Manefz et Bouchetz, 1565: p. 142, 267, 351.
27. Mercuriale G: De puerorum morbis tractatus locupletissimi. Frankfurt: Wechelius, 1584: p. 200–22, 324.
28. Guillemeau J: De la grossesse et accouchement des femmes. Paris: Jost, 1643: p. 593, 645, 658.
29. Sylvius de le Boe F: Praxeos medicae liber quartus. De morbis infantum. Amstelodami: Wolfgang, 1674: p. 3–152.
30. Harris W: A treatise of the acute diseases of infants (1st ed. 1689). London: Astley, 1742: p. 74, 91–106.
31. Ettmüller M: Etmullerus abridg'd (1st ed. 1688). 2. ed. London: Bell & Wellington, 1703: p. 620–32.
32. Kräutermann V: Aufrichtig getreuer, sorgfältiger und geschwinder Kinder-Artzt. Franckfurth: Beumelburg, 1740: p. 204, 240.
33. Armstrong G: An account of the diseases most incident to children (1st ed. 1767). 2. ed. London: Cadell, 1783: p. 171.
34. Girtanner C: Abhandlung über die Krankheiten der Kinder. Berlin: Rottmann, 1794: p. 113–7.
35. Underwood M: A treatise on the diseases of children. London: Mathews, 1784: p. 272.
36. Temkin O: Soranus' Gynecology. Baltimore, MD: The Johns Hopkins Press, 1956: Vol. Book II, p. 107, 113–22.
37. Paré A: The generation of man (1st ed. Paris 1573). London: Cotes & Du-gard, 1649: Vol. **67**, p. 603, 614, 647.
38. Eminent Physician: The nurse's guide. London: Brotherton & Gilliver, 1729: p. 28–39, 58.
39. Hamilton A: A treatise of midwifery. Edinburgh: Dickson & Co, 1781: p. 384–5.
40. Reese DM: Report in infant mortality in large cities, the sources of its increase, and means for its diminution. Philadelphia, PA: Collins, 1857: p. 11.
41. Routh CHF: Infant feeding and its influence on life. 3. ed. New York: Wood, 1879: p. 31–3, 104, 117.
42. Pliny the Elder: Natural history. Oxford: Oxford University Press, 2004: Vol. **32**, p. 26.
43. Smith H: Letters to married women on nursing. 6. ed. London: Kearsley, 1792: p. 147.
44. Rosen von Rosenstein N: Anweisung zur Kenntnis und Chur der Kinderkrankheiten (1st Swedish ed. 1764). 4. ed. Göttingen: Dieterich, 1781: p. 47–55, 64.
45. Clarke J: Commentaries on some of the most important diseases of children. London: Longman & Co, 1815: p. 31–3, 70–3.
46. Guthrie L: Discussion of teething and its alleged troubles. BMJ 1908;**2**:468–71.
47. West C: Lectures on the diseases of infancy and childhood. 5. ed. London: Longman & Co, 1865: p. 20, 555.
48. Buchan W: Domestic medicine. 10. ed. London: Strahan, Cadell, 1788: p. 38.
49. Hügel FS: Die Findelhäuser und das Findelwesen Europas. Wien: Sommer, Leopold, 1863.
50. Nichols RH, Wray FA: The history of the foundling hospital. London: Oxford University Press, 1935.
51. Dupoux A: Sur les pas de monsieur Vincent. Trois cents ans d'histoire parisienne de l'enfance abandonnée. Paris: Revue de l'assistance publique, 1958.
52. Ruland L: Das Findelhaus, seine geschichtliche Entwicklung und sittliche Bewertung. Berlin: Heymann, 1913: p. 26.
53. Jordan TE: The keys of paradise: Godfrey's Cordial and children in Victorian Britain. J R Soc Health 1987;**107**:19–22.
54. The slaughter of the innocents. The New York Times, 17 February 1859:4.
55. Bellow F: New York as a nursing mother to her foundlings. Harper's Weekly, 26 February 1859;**3**:144.
56. Struve CA: Ueber die Erziehung und Behandlung der Kinder in den ersten Lebensjahren. 2. ed. Hannover: Hahn, 1803: p. 158–62.
57. Dubé LF: Les sirops calmants—La cause du mal. Bull Med Quebec 1915;**17**:92–6.
58. The Analytical Sanitary Commission: Opium. Laudanum-poison. Lancet 1853;**61**:116–7.
59. Bause GS: McMunn's elixir of opium. Anesthesiology 2010;**113**:272.
60. Paris JA: Pharmacologia, in two volumes. 6. ed. London: Phillips, 1825: Vol. **2**.
61. Taylor AS: On poisons, in relation to medical jurisprudence and medicine. Philadelphia, PA: Lea & Blanchard, 1848: p. 465–517.
62. The Analytical Sanitary Commission: Opium and its adulterations. Lancet 1854;**63**:165–8.
63. Claudii Galeni Pergameni: De theriaca, ad Pisonem commentariolius. Basileae: Cratandrus, 1531: p. Fol. 81r.
64. Cook J: A plain account of the diseases incident to children with an easy method of curing them. London: Dilly, 1769: p. 9, 56.
65. Hall M: The effects of the habit of giving opiates on the infantine constitution. Edinb Med Surg J 1816;**12**:423–8.

66. Kelso JJ: Case of poisoning in a child from four drops of Laudanum. Lancet 1837;**29**:304–7.
67. Editorial: Death of a child from the administration of syrup of poppies. Lancet 1838;**30**:239–40.
68. Jeffreys J: Observations on the improper use of opium in England. Lancet 1840;**35**:382–3.
69. Palmer R, Coroner: Poisoning by laudanum synonymous with accidental death. Lancet 1840;**34**:384.
70. Everest G: Poisoning with a minim and a half of laudanum. Lancet 1842;**37**:758.
71. Smith E: Poisoning of an infant by one-twentieth of a grain of opium. Lancet 1854;**63**:419.
72. Lodge RT: On a case of poisoning of an infant by syrup of poppies. Lancet 1858;**72**:7.
73. Bull T: The maternal management of children in health and disease. 2. ed. Philadelphia, PA: Lindsay and Blakiston, 1853: p. 171–2.
74. Rose L: Massacre of the innocents: infanticide in Great Britain, 1800–1939. London: Routledge and Kegan Paul, 1986: p. 12.
75. Hufeland CW: Über den Missbrauch des Opiums bey Kindern, nebst der Geschichte einer Opiatvergiftung am ersten Tage des Lebens. Journal der practischen Arzneykunde und Wundarzneykunst 1800;**11**:143–54.
76. Herapath WB: Case of poisoning by laudanum in infancy, successfully treated by keeping up artificial respiration by means of the galvanic battery. Lancet 1852;**59**:303–5.
77. Kirk G: Poisoning by laudanum in an infant; effects of galvanism. Lancet 1853;**61**:80.
78. Down JLH: Observations on an ethnic classification of idiots. Lond Hosp Rep 1866;**3**:259–62.
79. Hartwich C: Das Opium als Genussmittel. Neujahrsblatt der Naturforschenden Gesellschaft (Zürich) 1898;**100**:12–54.
80. Paris JA: Pharmacologia. 9. ed. London: Highley, 1843: p. 175.
81. Stemler JG: Entwurf einer physisch-medizinischen Topographie von Zeulenroda. 2. ed. Neustadt: Wagner, 1820: p. 37.
82. Frémy A: L'enfant de fabrique. In: Encyclopédie morale du dix-neuvieme siecle. Paris: Curmer, 1841: Vol. **1**, p. 257–80.
83. Haller JS: Opium usage in the nineteenth century therapeutics. Bull New York Acad Med 1989;**65**:591–607.
84. Engels F: The condition of the working class in England. London: Penguin, 2009: p. 134.
85. Marx K: Capital: a critical analysis of capitalist production. London 1887. In: Marx K, Engels F: Gesamtausgabe (MEGA). New York: International, 1967: Vol. **9**, p. 344–8, 652.
86. Simrell EV: History of legal and medical roles in narcotic abuse in the U.S. Public Health Rep 1968;**83**:587–93.
87. Batton DG, Barrington KJ, Wallman C: Prevention and management of pain in the neonate: an update. Pediatrics 2006;**118**: 2231–41.
88. Lago P, Garetti E, Merazzi D, et al.: Guidelines for procedural pain in the newborn. Acta Paediatr 2009;**98**:932–9.
89. Mactier H: Neonatal and longer term management following substance misuse in pregnancy. Early Hum Dev 2013;**89**: 887–92.
90. Minozzi S, Amato L, Bellisario C, et al.: Maintenance agonist treatments for opiate-dependent pregnant women. Cochrane Database Syst Rev 2013;**12**:CD006318.
91. Osborn DA, Jeffery HE, Cole MJ: Opiate treatment for opiate withdrawal in newborn infants. Cochrane Database Syst Rev 2010;**10**:CD002059.
92. Opium, the poor child's nurse. Harper's Weekly 29 January 1859;**3**:80.
93. Ottmann J, lithographer. Advertising trade card for Mrs. Winslow's soothing syrup. New York: Curtis & Perkins, Anglo-American Drug Company, 1885.
94. Winter F: Römische Skulptur. In: Kunstgeschichte in Bildern. Prometheussarkophag. Leipzig: Kröner, 1925: Vol. **1**, p. 419.
95. Brunschweig H: Liber de arte distillandi de compositis. Strassburg: Grüningen, 1512: p. Fol. 317r.

PART 7
Disease

7.1 **Innocent blood: haemorrhagic disease of the newborn** *291*

7.2 **Yellow brains and blue light: neonatal jaundice** *297*

7.3 **Weak giants: infants of diabetic mothers** *305*

7.4 **Filth, impurity, and threat: meconium** *311*

7.5 **Necrotizing enterocolitis: 150 years of fruitless search for the cause** *317*

7.6 **Better baby bones: attacking rickets and scurvy** *325*

7.7 **Curse on two generations: congenital syphilis** *333*

7.8 **Thrush: nightmare of the foundling hospitals** *339*

7.9 **Systemic infection: sepsis** *345*

INTRODUCTION

Neonatal diseases are frequent and were often lethal. With their great vulnerability, newborns illustrate the impact of social conditions on morbidity and mortality. The main diseases were incomplete postnatal adaptation, infections due to poor hygiene, gastroenteritis caused by artificial nutrition, prematurity and its disorders, and birth asphyxia and brain damage. Industrialization and maternal factory work impeded breastfeeding, while poor housing and scanty sunlight promoted rickets. Necrotizing enterocolitis became a major problem when low birthweight infants overcame their pulmonary immaturity and survived the first days of life. Congenital syphilis was believed to be transmitted during conception or from breast milk. Thrush ravaged the institutions where infants were hospitalized. Until refrigeration and hospital hygiene were introduced, gastrointestinal infections were severe and frequently lethal in foundling hospitals. With the discovery of pathogenic microorganisms and development of antibiotics, systemic sepsis lost its near-total mortality in the 20th century.

7.1

Innocent blood
Haemorrhagic disease of the newborn

Introduction

Helplessly watching a newborn infant bleed to death was a worrisome although common experience: before prophylaxis, the incidence of severe bleeding was 0.25–1.7% [1]. The Jewish prophet Ezekiel (571 B.C.E.) attributed haemorrhage to God's wrath [Ezekiel 35:6]: 'Therefore, as I live, saith the Lord God, I will prepare thee unto blood, and blood shall pursue thee: since thou hast not hated blood.' And the law of Moses admonished [Deuteronomy 19:10] 'that innocent blood be not shed in thy land, which the Lord thy God giveth thee'. The Babylonic Talmud (2nd century C.E.) decreed: 'If she circumcised her first child and he died, and a second one also died, she must not circumcise her third child' [2], which has been related to haemophilia. As a genetic disorder that afflicted the royal houses of Europe [3], the history of haemophilia has been extensively described [4, 5]. The chronicle of neonatal haemorrhagic disease is less known. The following chapter attempts to close this gap.

Early reports, different diseases

Obstetricians observed bleeding neonates, as did François Mauriceau [6]: 'On April 10, 1682, I delivered a woman of a strong healthy girl without any violence at birth … during the first day she vomited some phlegm mixed with blood, after which she threw up, during two days, a totally blackish matter which I believed could only originate from bile of this color, or from pure intestinal meconium, or even of blood, discharged by the efforts of vomiting, which had stayed for some time in the fundus of the stomach, acquiring this blackish color. But whatever the cause, the infant remained stable.' Veit Riedlin, surgeon in Ulm, wrote in 1709 [7]: 'The midwife visited a merchant's wife, who had delivered a healthy term girl 7 days before. With the first meconium the newborn excreted some blood, its amount increased greatly, and at the age of 24 hours the diapers were blood stained nearly every hour … the girl was so weak that [the midwife] did not believe she would survive another day.' Eisenach physician Johann Storch described in 1726 [8]: 'A farmer's child, initially healthy. On the 9th day bloody stools and vomitings occurred; the parents collected the vomited blood in a diaper, that the father presented with several clots weighing 1–2 loth [15–30 g].' Unexpectedly, the infant survived, but 'its color remained cachectic and pale as death'. Haemorrhages from mouth, nose, skin, anus, navel, and internal organs were regarded as different diseases, and usually attributed to birth trauma.

A specific disorder of newborns

Hospitalization allowed larger series to be observed, and by the end of the 18th century it was known that neonates could bleed without any trauma. In London, obstetrician Michael Underwood described 'an oozing of blood [from the navel], which has sometimes continued for months, and in some instances, in such quantity as to prove alarming to the friends of the child … The little vein from whence the blood issues, lies always so deep that it cannot be conveniently cauterized … the haemorrhage has always returned' [9]. In 1825, Carl Gustav Hesse, surgeon in Altenburg, grouped together two cases of haematemesis, six of melaena, and seven of their combination, and distinguished by origin [10]: 'I regard vomiting of blood and *melaena* as one disease … The main issue is if the blood originated from the infant's stomach or gut (*Haematemesis et Melaena vera*) or if [maternal blood] was swallowed before being vomited or excreted in the stools (*Haematemesis et Melaena spuria*).' Among Charles Billard's Parisian cases were several forms of haemorrhage [11]: 'Baby girl Delarue was deposited in front of the Foundling Hospital on March 27, 1826. A leaflet attached to her arm indicated that she was three days old. She was large and strong, her skin yellowish, respiration weak, her cry barely audible. Face, trunk, legs and arms were covered with purplish blood spots, whose size varied from a pinpoint to a lentil. Their unequal distribution and the yellow color between them gave her a tigered aspect. She remained exhausted for two days, drank some drops of milk, cried and breathed weakly, and died on the evening of the 29th.' The autopsy revealed a stomach and gut filled with blood. Billard found this disease (possibly immune thrombocytopenia) 'analogue to that observed by Werlhof in adults' and clearly distinguished it from 'passive intestinal hemorrhage', of which 'I have collected 15 cases, 6 male and 9 female, 8 aged 1–6 days, 4 aged 6–8 days, and 3 aged 10–18 days'.

Fréderic Rilliet observed gastrointestinal haemorrhage in twins in Geneva [12]: 'On January 30, 1846, I was called to see a newborn said to be in greatest danger ... The little boy [a twin born at term 9 hours before] had released meconium after half a teaspoon of castor oil had been given ... two hours later released a stool abundant with pure blood, liquid and mixed with clots ... at 1 pm a third stool rich in blood ... I placed a cold vinegar compress on the abdomen and prescribed rathany [a root extract] enemas, which were immediately returned together with a large quantity of blood ... on February 8, he had completely recovered .... —The firstborn infant still in an alarming state, I was called to the second infant at 6 pm who vomited blood and had passed several stools with liquid blood ... I ordered rhatany enemas but he yielded, like his brother, abundant sanguinolent stools ... same symptoms as in the first case: paleness, getting cold, small pulses, shivering limbs ... improved on February 2 and recovered completely, but remained pale and weak as his brother ... None of the mother's or father's family ever suffered hemorrhages ... the infants, with greatest analogy, had a marked hemorrhagic predisposition.'

In the Vienna Foundling Hospital, Alois Bednar observed 17 cases of gastrointestinal bleeding in 1851 [13] and in Boston Francis Minot gathered 52 cases of navel bleeding from the literature in 1852 [14], confirming an 'association of jaundice with hemorrhagic diathesis'. In 1855, Stephen Smith of New York [15] compiled 75 cases of umbilical haemorrhage from the literature: 'The most common cause is a vitiated state of the blood due to jaundice, or a transmitted hemorrhagic or syphilitic dyscrasia.' In 1871, Ludwig Grandidier of Kassel tabulated 220 cases of 'voluntary' umbilical haemorrhage in a book [16]: 'Its main cause is most probably diminished fibrin leading to impaired clotting ... only rarely caused by hereditary hemophilia ... rather connected with the transition from fetal to respiratory life.' In 1894, Charles Townsend grouped 50 cases observed at the Boston Lying-in Hospital—haemorrhages from gut, stomach, mouth, nose, navel, skin and 7 more locations—under the term 'hemorrhagic disease of the newborn' [17].

Cholestasis and coagulation

John Cheyne, physician in Edinburgh, described haemorrhage with cholestasis in 1802 [18]: 'G.H.'s daughter, five days old, was remarkably stout and healthy, when born; but on the third day after birth, her skin became jaundiced ... [day 13], the child is becoming soft and emaciated, her stools are white, her urine stains the linen very deeply ... [day 16], no change in the jaundice; her stools and urine are much like they were. Last night she had a slight bleeding from the umbilicus ... [day 17], a great hemorrhage from the umbilicus, and the child died this morning in consequence of it.' Dissection of the infant (Fig. 7.1.1A) revealed the liver 'full and firm, and of dark green earthen colour. The gall bladder was empty and contracted ... the ducts also contracted, firm, white, and like an artery, and contained no bile ... The bleeding proceeded from the unhealthy change produced in the blood by the reception of the bile.'

The association between bleeding and cholestasis was firmly established in 1850, when Charles West, founder of the London Hospital for Sick Children, wrote [19]: 'One remarkable phenomenon attending these cases [congenital absence of the biliary ducts] is the tendency to hemorrhage by which they are characterized.' Also in 1850, Henry Bowditch of the Massachusetts General Hospital saw combined haemorrhage from umbilicus, in skin, and in stool of two infants [20]: 'No coagula, or tendency to coagulate, was shown.' Heinrich Finkelstein of Berlin held melaena and umbilical haemorrhage for different diseases, both due to impaired coagulability [21]. The understanding of neonatal haemorrhages was greatly enhanced when Paul Morawitz discovered the coagulation cascade in 1904 [22]. In 1910, Schwarz and Ottenberg reported prolonged coagulation in two newborn infants with haemorrhage due to infection and concluded [23]: 'Impaired blood coagulation is the immediate cause of uncontrollable hemorrhages in the newborn. It is probably due to destruction of, or interference with the production of thrombokinase.' In 1911 in New York, Schloss and Commiskey measured coagulation time in seven bleeding infants and suggested [24] 'incomplete, instead of delayed, coagulation is the underlying cause'. In 1912, Whipple postulated melaena to be due to a lack of prothrombin [25]. However, it was not until 1937 that Brinkhous and co-workers [26] proved hypoprothrombinaemia in a bleeding infant. In a prospective study performed in Minneapolis in 1920 [27], Frederick Rodda detected prolonged coagulation during the first 10 days in infants who developed cerebral haemorrhages.

Early treatment

The disease's lethality amounting to 70% encouraged heroic therapy. In 1894, Paul Carnot described the haemostyptic ability of gelatine [28], and soon bleeding infants were treated with subcutaneous gelatine injections [29, 30], which, as Elis Lövegren in Helsinki found, shortened the coagulation time [31]. In 1905, Emile Weil demonstrated that small injections of fresh animal serum controlled bleeding in haemophiliacs [32], and soon bleeding neonates were treated with subcutaneous injections of rabbit [33] or horse [34] serum. On 8 March 1908, Samuel Lambert saved a moribund infant by direct blood transfusion in New York [35]: 'On the [5th day] the case seemed hopeless. The baby's skin was waxen white and the mucus membranes without color; the nasal bleeding was continuous; the vomited matter contained food curls, dark blood, and at times bright clots; the stools were frequent and contained bright red blood ... her pulse weak, counting 150 ... It was decided to attempt a direct transfusion of blood from the father by end-to-end anastomosis of his left radial artery and the girl's popliteal vein.' Fresh blood instantly normalized coagulation, shock, and anaemia, and transfusion was repeated by others [36, 37]. It required surgical skill and became easier with Bernheim's cannula [38]: 'January 1, 1912, I was called ... the baby had two more stools of this same bright red, practically unclotted blood. He looked colorless, his breathing was laboured, while the pulse at the wrist was almost imperceptible. Transfusion was unusually difficult because of the minuteness and delicacy of the child's vessels ... Because of its size, the femoral vein of the infant was selected ... For emergency I believe that a cannula in

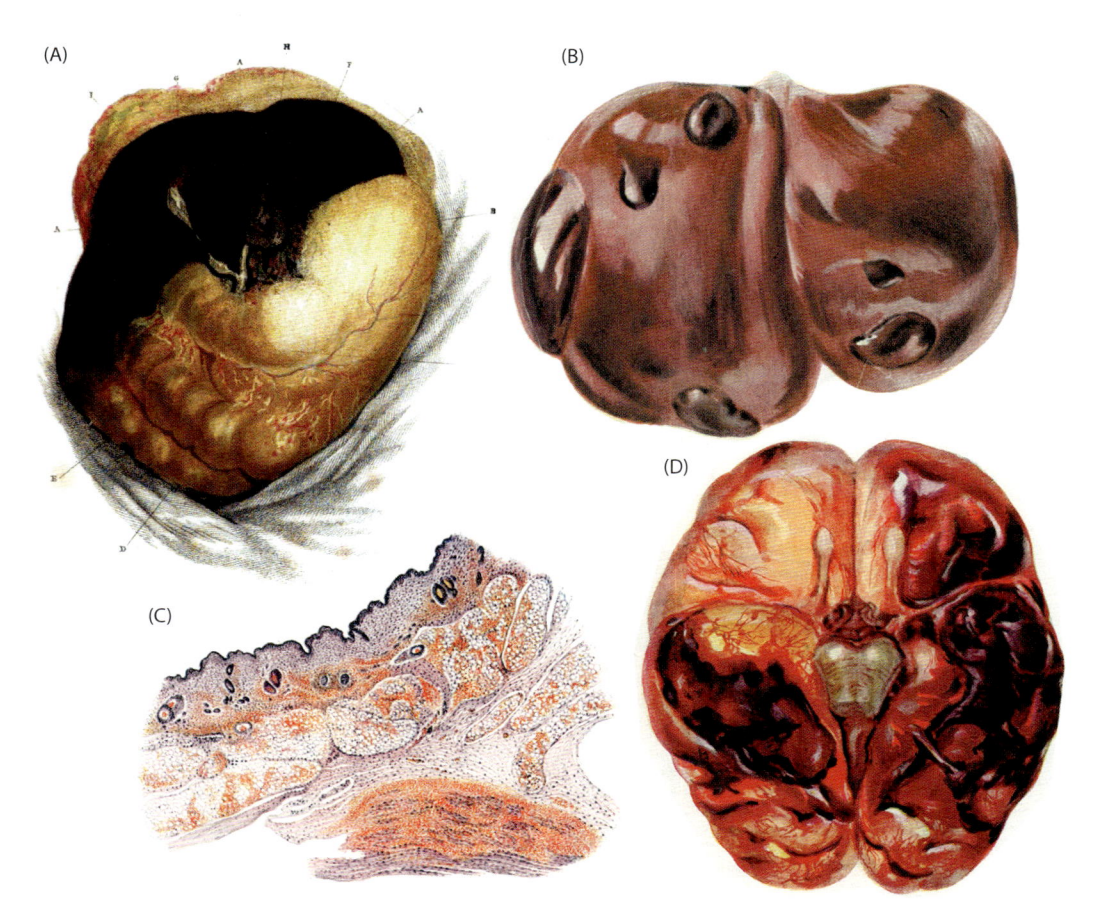

Fig. 7.1.1 Case reports of neonatal haemorrhages: A, Cheyne 1802 [18], abdominal situs of a girl who died on day 17 from severe umbilical haemorrhage. Liver is hard, gall-bladder and bile ducts hypoplastic; B–D, various haemorrhages described by Ylppö 1919 [55]; B, subcapsular liver haemorrhages in a preterm infant who died at 3 hours of age; C, microscopic view of a subcutaneous haemorrhage in a preterm girl who died at 25 hours of age; D, subarachnoidal haemorrhage in a 3-week-old infant with haematemesis.

two pieces [Fig. 7.1.2] one of which can be rapidly inserted into the artery of the donor, and the other into the vein of the recipient is best.'

Vitamin K

Vitamin K was discovered by biochemist Henrik Dam in 1935 at the University of Copenhagen. He observed haemorrhages in skin and organs of chicks on a fat-free diet [39]. This condition was cured by administering an ether extract of hempseed later shown to contain phylloquinone, and the active ingredient was named vitamin K_1 ('K-oagulation'). In 1939, the biochemist Edward Doisy in St. Louis elucidated its structure and succeeded in synthesizing various forms [40]. The same year, William Waddell reduced the mean coagulation time of ten newborns treated with vitamin K to 2.4 min as compared to 5.1 min in untreated control infants [41]. Moreover, he stopped the haemorrhages in three bleeding neonates with oral vitamin K [42]. In 1941, Beck and co-workers found that when vitamin K was given to the mother during labour, the fall in prothrombin was eliminated in 99% of the infants and the incidence of the disease reduced by 75% [43]. In 1943, Dam and Doisy were awarded the Nobel Price for discovering and characterizing vitamin K.

The Synkavit disaster

Water-soluble vitamin K analogues were better absorbed, and dose-finding studies with menadione (vitamin K_3) showed 1–2 μg per day sufficient to maintain adequate prothrombin levels in the newborn infant [44]. But the popular fallacy 'If a little is good, a lot should be better' once more proved disastrous: on 26 March 1955, Anthony Allison reported from Oxford [45]: 'I have recently investigated a small series of cases of kernicterus and haemolytic anaemia in premature infants whose only treatment had been relatively high doses of a water-soluble vitamin-K analogue [Synkavit] … 5 mg per day by injection are quite adequate for treating haemorrhagic disease of the newborn. There is, however, a widespread tendency to use much higher doses in the belief that this vitamin is innocuous under all circumstances.' Three weeks later, Bernard Laurance confirmed from Derby [46]: 'The routine care in this unit was modified recently and the dose of water-soluble vitamin K [Synkavit] was increased from 10 mg once on admission to 10 mg three times a day for three days. To my dismay, shortly after the introduction of this routine, six babies developed clinical signs of kernicterus and subsequently died between the ages of 6 and 13 days.' Another nine weeks later, Mary Crosse, who directed the Birmingham premature special care unit

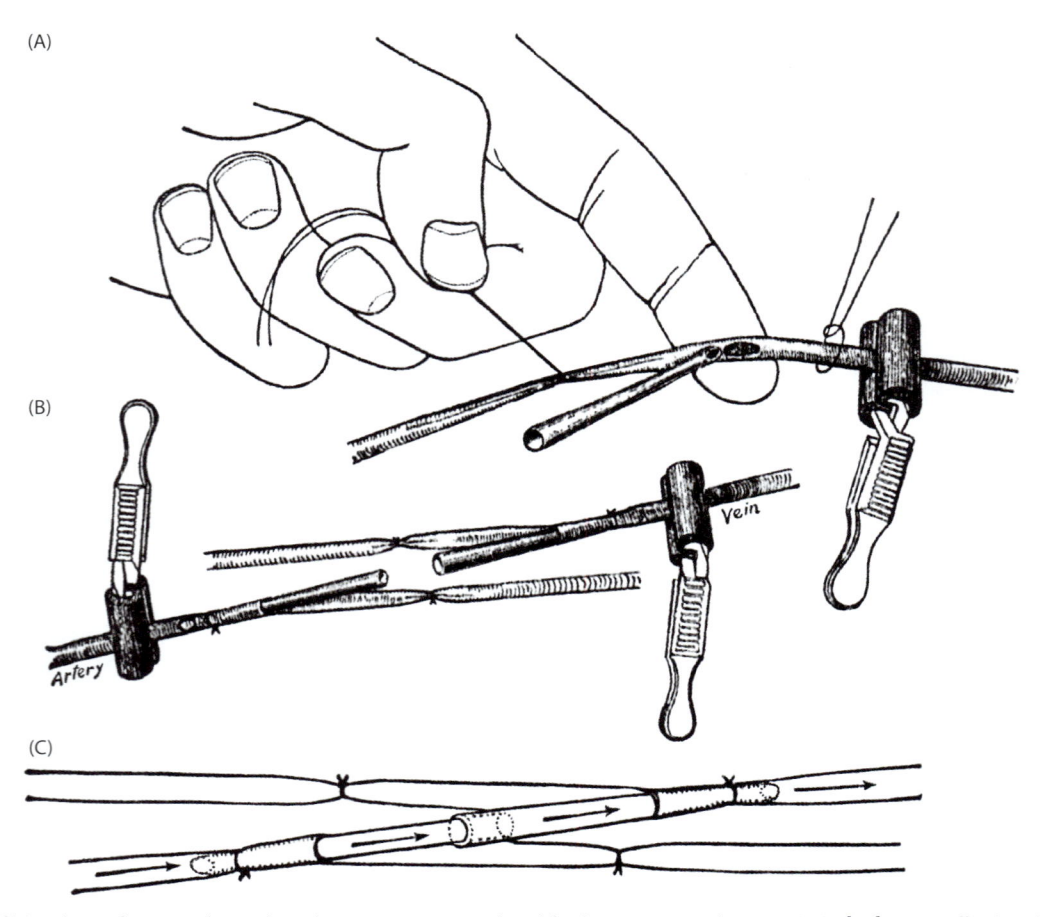

Fig. 7.1.2 Steps of blood transfusion with Bernheim's emergency cannula in life-threatening melaena in 1912 [38]: A, paraffin-lined recipient piece being inserted into infant's femoral vein; B, donor piece fixed in father's radial artery (left), recipient piece fixed in infant's vein (right); C, blood flow after connection of the two cannula pieces.

since 1931 reported a series of 60 premature infants with kernicterus observed within ten years [47]: 'In 1947, at a total Synkavit dose of 1–2 mg, kernicterus occurred in 0.8% of preterm infants. In 1949, at a dose of 10 mg, the incidence was 1.6%, and in 1953 the incidence [of kernicterus] rose fourfold [to 4.1%] when the dose of vitamin K was increased [to >30 mg].' Synkavit was withdrawn and in 1961, the American Academy of Pediatrics recommended [48]: 'The margin of safety is almost certainly greatest with vitamin K_1 (phytonadione) which is therefore considered the drug of choice. A single parenteral dose of 0.5 to 1.0 mg or oral dose of 1.0 to 2.0 mg is probably adequate for prophylaxis.'

Modern prophylaxis

Most, but not all neonatal haemorrhages result from diminished prothrombin, factor VII, and factor IX. This group was renamed 'vitamin K deficiency bleeding' and it became obvious that vitamin K would not help alleviate other disorders like septic consumption coagulopathy, immune thrombocytopenia, haemophilia, or traumatic haemorrhage. Infants of less than 27 weeks' gestation who received 1.0 mg intramuscular vitamin K at birth, have markedly longer prothrombin time and activated partial thromboplastin time than term infants [49]. As with other prophylactic measures in infants (immunization, vitamin D, etc.) and disregarding the evidence, opposition to vitamin K persisted and the need for its universal use at birth continued to be questioned. In 1992, Bristol epidemiologist Jean Golding reported an association between intramuscular but not oral vitamin K administration and cancer in childhood and concluded 'It may be prudent to use oral rather than intramuscular vitamin K' [50]. Several countries changed their policies accordingly, experiencing various incidences of late vitamin K deficiency bleeding in conjunction with various protocols of repeated oral application [51]. Goldings findings were not confirmed by other studies [52–54], but the sensationalistic debate in the media undermined the public confidence in vitamin K altogether, and haemorrhagic disease of the newborn has returned.

Conclusion

Haemorrhagic disease, for centuries a major threat for the newborn, was largely eliminated by vitamin K. Several lessons can be learned from its history: discovery of the coagulation cascade unified previously distinct disorders based on organ manifestation, and enabled other diseases unrelated to vitamin K to be distinguished. The enthusiasm for Synkavit shows how 'new' treatments tend to be overused, omitting properly controlled trials and dose-finding studies.

Long-standing debate about vitamin K prophylaxis revealed deep scepticism towards preventive measures in infants, and indeed it remains difficult to understand why evolution endowed the human infant with faulty coagulation.

REFERENCES

1. American Academy of Pediatrics Vitamin K Taskforce: Controversies concerning vitamin K and the newborn. Pediatrics 1993;**91**:1001–2.
2. Epstein I: Tractate Yebamoth. Hebrew-English Edition of the Babylonian Talmud. London: Soncino, 1994: p. Fol. 64b, 25–6.
3. Rogaev EI, Grigorenko AP, Faskhutdinova G, et al.: Genotype analysis identifies the cause of the "royal disease". Science 2009;**326**:817.
4. Ingram GIC: The history of haemophilia. J Clin Path 1976;**29**:469–79.
5. Schramm W: The history of haemophilia—a short review. Thromb Res 2014;1–6.
6. Mauriceau F: Observations sur la grossesse et l'accouchement des femmes. Paris: Libraires Associés, 1738: Vol. **2**, p. 8, 42, 249.
7. Riedlin V: Curarum medicarum, millenarius. Ulm: Kuhn, 1709: p. 314.
8. Storch JHP: Dritter Medicinischer Jahrgang oder observationes clinicae. Leipzig: Eysseln, 1726: p. 734.
9. Underwood M: A treatise on the diseases of children. London: Mathews, 1784: p. 171.
10. Hesse CG: Von dem Bluterbrechen und der Melaena der Neugeborenen. Allgemeine Medizin. Annalen des 19 Jahrhundert 1825:721–44.
11. Billard CM: Traité des maladies des enfants nouveau-nés et à la mamelle. Paris: Baillière, 1828: p. 93.
12. Rilliet F: Mémoire sur les hémorrhagies intestinales chez les nouveau-nés. Gaz Med Paris 1848;**18**:1029–33.
13. Bednar A: Die Krankheiten der Neugeborenen und Säuglinge. Wien: Gerold, 1850: Vol. **1**, p. 38.
14. Minot F: On hemorrhage from the umbilicus in new-born infants. Am J Med Sci 1852;**24**:310–20.
15. Smith S: Remarks on hemorrhage from the umbilicus of infants. NY J Med 1855;**15**:73–94.
16. Grandidier L: Die freiwilligen Nabelblutungen der Neugeborenen. Cassel: Kay, 1871: p. 77–83.
17. Townsend CW: The haemorrhagic disease of the new-born. Arch Pediatr 1894;**11**:559–65.
18. Cheyne J: On the bowel complaints more immediately connected with the biliary section. Edinburgh: Mundell, 1802: p. 8–10, plate V.
19. West C: Lectures on the diseases of infancy and childhood. Philadelphia, PA: Lea and Blanchard, 1850: p. 354.
20. Bowditch HJ: On hemorrhage from the umbilicus, in new-born children; with cases. Am J Med Sci 1850;**37**:63–70.
21. Finkelstein H: Lehrbuch der Säuglingskrankheiten. 2. ed. Berlin: Springer, 1921: p. 379.
22. Morawitz P: Beiträge zur Kenntnis der Blutgerinnung. Dt Arch Klinische Medizin 1904;**79**:1–28, 215–33, 432–42.
23. Schwarz H, Ottenberg R: The hemorrhagic disease of the newborn. Am J Med Sci 1910;**140**:17–29.
24. Schloss OM, Commiskey LJ: Spontaneous hemorrhage in the new-born. Am J Dis Child 1911;**1**:276–98.
25. Whipple GH: Hemorrhagic disease—septicemia, melena neonatorum and hepatic cirrhosis. Arch Int Med 1912;**9**:365.
26. Brinkhous KM, Smith HP, Warner ED: Plasma prothrombin level in normal infancy and in hemorrhagic disease of the newborn. Am J Med Sci 1937;**193**:475–80.
27. Rodda FC: The coagulation time of blood in the new-born with especial reference to cerebral hemorrhage. JAMA 1920;**75**:452–7.
28. Carnot P: Sur les propriétés hémostatiques de la gelatine. Bull Soc Biol 1896;**48**:758–9.
29. Fuhrmann E: Beiträge zur Gelatinebehandlung bei Melaena. Münchner Med Wochenschr 1902;**48**:1459–61.
30. Reuss A: Die verschiedenen Melaenaformen im Säuglingsalter. Erg Inn Med Kinderheilk 1914;**13**:574–615.
31. Lövegren E: Erfahrungen und Studien über Melaena neonatorum. Jahrb Kinderheilk 1913–1914;**78/79**:249–77, 708–14.
32. Weil PE: L'hémophilie: pathogénie et sérothérapie. Presse Méd 1905;**13**:673–6.
33. Bigelow EB: Serum treatment of hemorrhagic disease of the newborn. JAMA 1910;**55**:400–2.
34. Reichard VM: Spontaneous hemorrhage of the newborn with recovery. JAMA 1912;**59**:1539.
35. Lambert SW: Melaena neonatorum with report of a case cured by transfusion. Med Rec (New York) 1908;**73**:885–7.
36. Swain HF, Jackson JM, Murphy FT: A case of hemorrhagic disease in the newborn with direct transfusion from the father. Boston Med Surg J 1909;**161**:407–9.
37. Mosenthal HO: Transfusion as a cure for melaena neonatorum. JAMA 1910;**54**:1613.
38. Bernheim BM: An emergency cannula. Transfusion in a thirty-six-hour old baby suffering from melaena neonatorum. JAMA 1912;**58**:1007–8.
39. Dam H: Hemorrhages in chicks reared on artificial diets: a new deficiency disease. Nature 1935;**133**:909–10.
40. MacCorquodale DW, Cheney LC, Binkley SB, et al.: The constitution and synthesis of vitamin K1. J Biol Chem 1939;**131**:357–70.
41. Waddell WW, Guerry D: Effect of vitamin K on the clotting time of the prothrombin and the blood. Part 1. JAMA 1939;**112**:2259–63.
42. Waddell WW, Guerry D: The role of vitamin K in the etiology, prevention, and treatment of hemorrhage in the newborn infant. Part 2. J Pediatr 1939;**15**:802–11.
43. Beck AC, Taylor ES, Colburn RF: Vitamin K administration to the mother during labor as a prophylaxis against hemorrhage in the newborn infant. Am J Obstet Gynecol 1941;**41**:765–75.
44. Sells RL, Walker SA, Owen CA: Vitamin K requirement of the newborn infant. Proc Soc Exper Biol Med 1941;**47**:441–5.
45. Allison AC: Danger of vitamin K to newborn. Lancet 1955;**265**:669.
46. Laurance B: Danger of vitamin-K analogues to newborn. Lancet 1955;**265**:819.
47. Crosse VM, Meyer TC, Gerrard JW: Kernicterus and prematurity. Arch Dis Child 1955;**30**:501–8.
48. American Academy of Pediatrics Committee on Nutrition: Vitamin K compounds and the water-soluble analogues. Pediatrics 1961;**28**:501–7.
49. Neary E, Okafor I, Al-Awaysheh F, et al.: Laboratory coagulation parameters in extremely premature infants born earlier than 27

gestational weeks upon admission to a neonatal intensive care unit. Neonatology 2013;**104**:222–7.
50. Golding J, Greenwood R, Birmingham K, Mott M: Childhood cancer, intramuscular vitamin K, and pethidine given during labour. BMJ 1992;**305**:341–6.
51. Cornelissen M, von Kries R, Loughnan P, Schubiger G: Prevention of vitamin K deficiency bleeding: efficacy of different multiple oral dose schedules of vitamin K. Eur J Pediatr 1997;**156**:126–30.
52. Ansell P, Bull D, Roman E: Childhood leukaemia and intramuscular vitamin K. BMJ 1996;**313**:204–5.
53. McKinney PA, Juszczak E, Findlay E, Smith K: Case-control study of childhood leukaemia and cancer in Scotland: findings for neonatal intramuscular vitamin K. BMJ 1998;**316**: 173–7.
54. Passmore SJ, Draper G, Brownbill P, Kroll M: Case-control studies of relation between childhood cancer and neonatal vitamin K administration. BMJ 1998;**316**:178–84.
55. Ylppö A: Pathologisch-anatomische Studien bei Frühgeborenen. Zeitschr Kinderheilk 1919;**20**:212–431.

7.2

Yellow brains and blue light
Neonatal jaundice

Introduction

Jaundice of the newborn was described in the *Sakikku* tablet 40, a book on medical diagnoses from the Hammurabi epoch (ca. 1750 B.C.E.) [1]. Aspects of early 19th-century history of neonatal jaundice were reported by Roberts [2] and Hansen [3]. What this chapter adds are descriptions of fetal dropsy in the 17th century and of kernicterus in the work of Antoine Dugès [4]. The chapter focuses on the stepwise conquering of rhesus erythroblastosis, and on the introduction of phototherapy. Jaundice due to liver or metabolic diseases, and blood group incompatibilities other than rhesus have been omitted.

Jaundice of the newborn: a disease?

'Physiologic' jaundice occurs in virtually every newborn. Franciscus Sylvius, professor of anatomy in Leiden, wrote in 1671 [5]: 'Many infants are born with jaundice, or it erupts shortly after birth.' Johannes Juncker, physician at the Foundling Hospital of Halle, confirmed in 1718 [6]: 'In infants, the yellow color (*icteroides corporis*) is common and not at all dangerous.' Giovanni Battista Morgagni, anatomist in Padova, discerned physiologic and pathologic jaundice of the newborn in 1769 [7]: 'The cause is uncertain, when infants newly born are affected with a very considerable jaundice: for with a kind of slight jaundice, almost all of them are attack'd a little after birth.'

In December 1785, with the monarchy already shaken by Queen Marie-Antoinette's necklace affair, the Paris Royal Society of Medicine announced a competition 'to describe the jaundice in newborns, and to distinguish circumstances in which medical help is required from those in whom the natural course can be awaited'. Jean Baptiste Baumes from Nîmes won the competition with his 56-page treatise 'On the jaundice in newborns', published in 1788 a few months before the storming of the Bastille [8]. He described ten cases, beginning with his own daughter and ending with a boy who died at 4 weeks of age after prolonged jaundice and in whom the autopsy revealed enlarged liver and obstructed bile canals. Baumes concluded: 'The icterus in newborns can be caused by meconium retention, thickened stool in the duodenum, a spasm of the bile canals ... All these causes act differently but trigger the same effect.' Meconium retention was also believed to be the main cause of jaundice by other early 19th century investigators [9, 10]. Doctors in foundling hospitals associated neonatal jaundice with birth and transport to the hospital: skin contusion and haematoma resorption, postnatal hypothermia, and sclerema [11–13]. In 1633, Daniel Sennert described obstructive jaundice of the newborn [14]: 'If the bile, which stimulates the bowel's excretion, does not flow into the gut, the stool is not colored, but white or ash-like, and the infant's body becomes yellow.' However, later investigators did not discern jaundice with and without liver disease, and Eugène Bouchut wrote in 1867 [15]: 'Jaundice in the newborn always results from a moderate or severe liver inflammation'. Immature liver function was proposed by Arvo Ylppö in 1913 [16] and identified as a deficiency in glucuronyl transferase [17]. A hematogenous theory of neonatal jaundice was proposed by Anselmino and Hoffmann 1930 [18]: with increasing oxygenation at birth, fetal erythrocytes are in excess and are dissolved by haemolysis, which explains the increased formation of bilirubin during the first weeks of life.

Jaundice in the preterm infant

At the Stuttgart Katharina Hospital, the obstetrician Johann Adam Elsässer wrote in 1835 [19]: 'Preterm infants are jaundiced more intensely and longer than term infants.' In the 1950s it became clear that kernicterus may occur in preterm infants without haemolysis [20]. The maximum serum bilirubin concentration correlated inversely with the baby's birthweight. Today, kernicterus is predominantly a disorder of preterm infants. Sadly, it must be reported that iatrogenic damage contributed to several epidemics of kernicterus when, in uncontrolled hyperactivity, drugs interfering with bilirubin metabolism were administered to preterm infants, that is, high-dose synthetic vitamin K [21], sulfisoxazole [22], and benzyl alcohol [23]. Long debated was the question whether a jaundiced term infant without haemolysis will ever develop kernicterus. The evidence is weak [24].

Hydrops fetalis/habitual jaundice/haemolytic disease

In 1643, Naples surgeon Marco Aurelio Severino described and depicted [25] a stillborn infant of 8 months, born with 'dilated

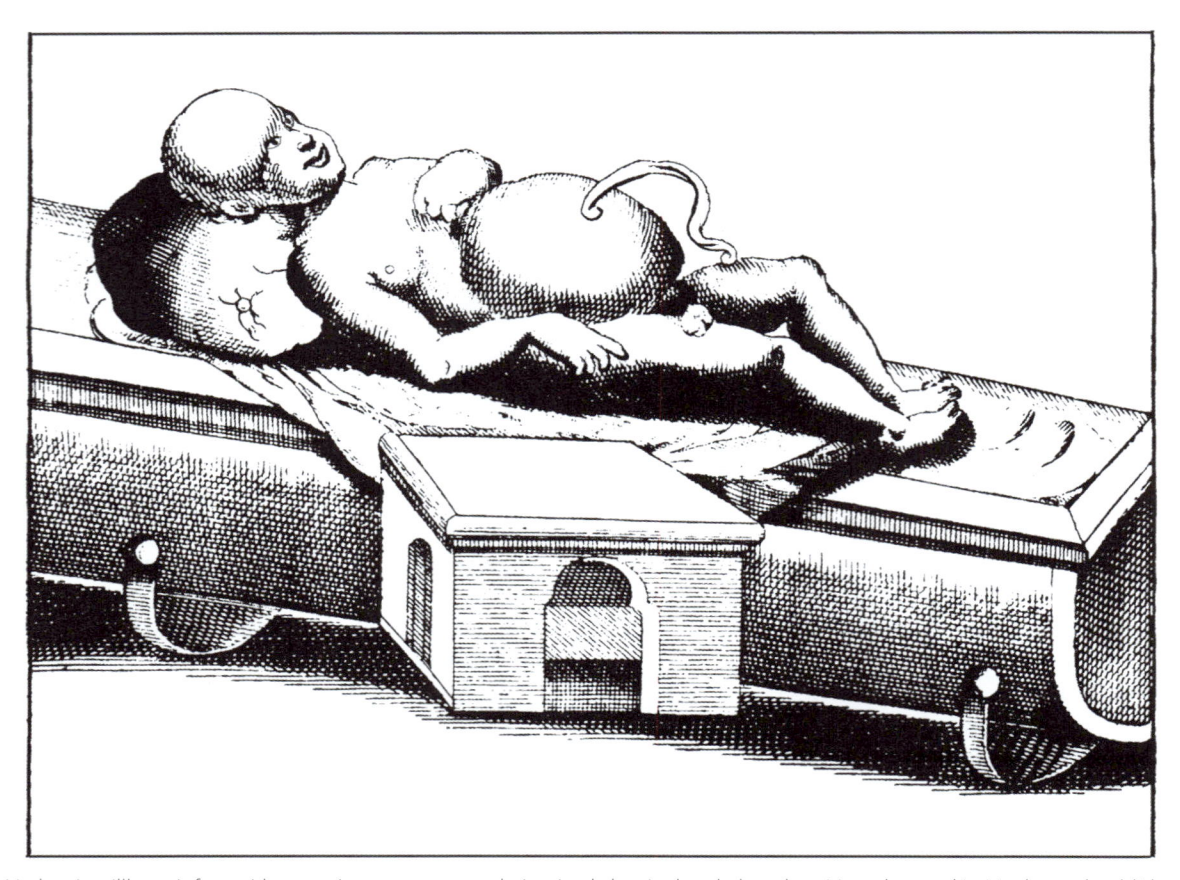

Fig. 7.2.1 Hydropic stillborn infant with excessive water accumulation in abdominal and pleural cavities, observed in Naples and published by Severino in 1643 [25].

abdomen that exceeded the baby's size'. At autopsy 'a large quantity of silverish water gushed out … also the thoracic cavity was entirely filled with this liquid' (Fig. 7.2.1). Other cases of hydropic neonates, reported during the 17th century, were believed to result from maternal jaundice [26], maternal imagination [27], or toxic mixture of the maternal blood [28]. In 1673, Johann Horst reported a hydropic and jaundiced newborn whose mother had already lost two infants with the same symptoms [29].

John Clay of Birmingham studied two cases of fetal hydrops and assumed in 1859 [30] 'a kind of toxin acting upon the fetus' and believed the dropsy 'not due to the state of the placenta, but produced by the condition of the mother's blood'. In *The Diseases and Deformities of the Foetus*, John Ballantyne of Edinburgh devoted 80 pages to general dropsy in 1892 [31]: '[Mrs A's] two first pregnancies resulted in the birth of full-time healthy infants … Her 3rd to 8th pregnancies terminated prematurely, the infants were stillborn … During the 9th gestation … between the 8th and 9th month premature labour set in and a male infant with general dropsy was born [Fig. 7.2.2, left]. There had been hydramnios in a very marked degree … The infant's heart beat for a few minutes after birth, but there was no attempt at respiration. This fetus was examined by the frozen sectional method [Fig. 7.2.2, right] … The most remarkable condition was the presence in the abdomen of a large quantity of transparent fluid of a light yellow colour, containing no flakes of lymph.'

Up to 1891, Mrs A had three more pregnancies, all of which resulted in stillborn dropsical infants. Ballantyne meticulously analysed the literature consisting of 65 cases and concluded 'only one was primiparous, all the others multiparous, and usually had a large number of gestation': 'The disease is due to a chain of factors and a blood disease of the fetus.' It was clear at the start of the 20th century that a dangerous or fatal jaundice could kill several or all infants in the same family, and series of 'familial' or 'habitual' icterus were published [32–36]. As measuring bilirubin, let alone conjugated bilirubin, was not yet possible, some of these series [29, 37] may have been hepatic or metabolic disease, but the majority must have been rhesus incompatibility: infants died early with seizures, or survived the first days with anaemia. With the chemical reaction discovered by Hymans van den Bergh, bilirubin measurement became possible [38], and in 1913, Ylppö classified four degrees of neonatal jaundice [16], according to the skin's appearance and the measured biliary pigments in stool, urine, and blood (Fig. 7.2.3).

For centuries, haemolytic disease of the newborn was perceived as three different syndromes: hydrops, jaundice, and anaemia. The unity of the three syndromes as 'erythroblastosis fetalis' was fully understood in 1932 [39]. In 1940, Landsteiner and Wiener discovered the rhesus factor [40], and in 1941 Levine demonstrated that rhesus antibodies caused the disease [41]: 'Presumably, the immunizing property in the fetal blood must be inherited by the

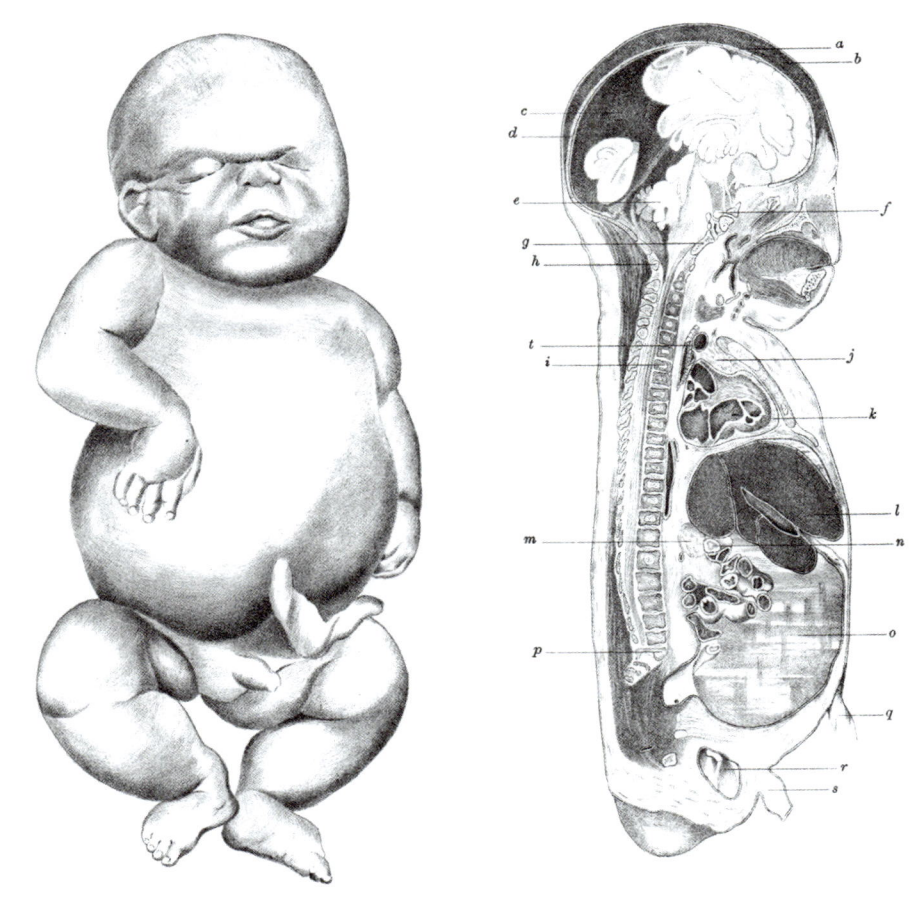

Fig. 7.2.2 Generalized dropsy of an infant published by Ballantyne in 1892 [31]. Left: swollen abdomen and generalized oedema. Right: vertical frozen section of the same infant showing scalp oedema (a), fluid in pericardium (k), and abdomen (o).

father.' About 16% of European and North American inhabitants are rhesus negative, which put 11% of all couples at risk for rhesus-sensitization.

Kernicterus

Roman physician Domenico Panaroli associated jaundice with neurologic symptoms in 1652 [42]: 'We saw the jaundiced newborn son of a barber, with great stiffness, who soon thereafter passed away according to God's will.' Royal accoucheur André Levret came close to understanding haemolysis and kernicterus in 1766 [43]: 'It has become proverbial that the jaundice predicts future paleness... the infant becomes drowsy, has burning skin, closes its fists with the thumbs inside and it is difficult to open the contracted fists. This symptom precedes the generalized seizures which soon terminate the infant's life.' Yellow staining of the basal ganglions associated with neurologic symptoms was reported by Antoine Dugès at the Paris Maternité in 1821 [4]: 'On January 13, 1821, Madame Lachapelle delivered a large baby by forceps... [small haematoma]... 20th, considerable jaundice... 22nd, seizures increasing, weight loss, death on the 23rd... [autopsy] skin and subcutaneous fat of saffron color... the brain yellow-gray, the corpus nigrum (Soemmerring), the rhomboid corps of the olives, and the cerebellum of brilliant yellow... This jaundice of several essential parts of the brain, could it have caused the convulsions?' At the Paris Foundling Hospital, Charles Billard observed in 1828 [44]: 'I have remarked the yellow coloring which constitutes jaundice, in four instances, in the brain and spinal marrow. The brain, which was of moderate firmness, presented a uniform and bright yellow in two of these subjects, while the color was in isolated patches in the other two.'

In 1847, bilirubin crystals were identified in haematomas [45], and in 1875 Johannes Orth described pigment crystals in the brain, which he microchemically identified as bilirubin [46]: 'The yellow staining of the brain varied. In the cerebellum especially the granular layer was yellow... in Ammon's horn individual large cells were impregnated with yellow color... the nerve cells were stained in the basal ganglions exclusively.' Christian Schmorl described and depicted the location of the bilirubin pigment in Luys' bodies (subthalamic ganglion), nucleus dentatus, and olive (**Fig. 7.2.4**), coined the term *kernicterus* in 1904 [47], and observed: 'The pigment decomposes easily and the coloration disappears when the preparation is exposed to light for some time.'

In 1950, Zuelzer and Mudgett studied serology and pathoanatomy in 55 consecutive cases of kernicterus in Detroit, 21 of them with, and 34 without haemolysis, and concluded [48]: 'Kernicterus does not represent a specific entity. Prematurity, severe infections, diarrheal

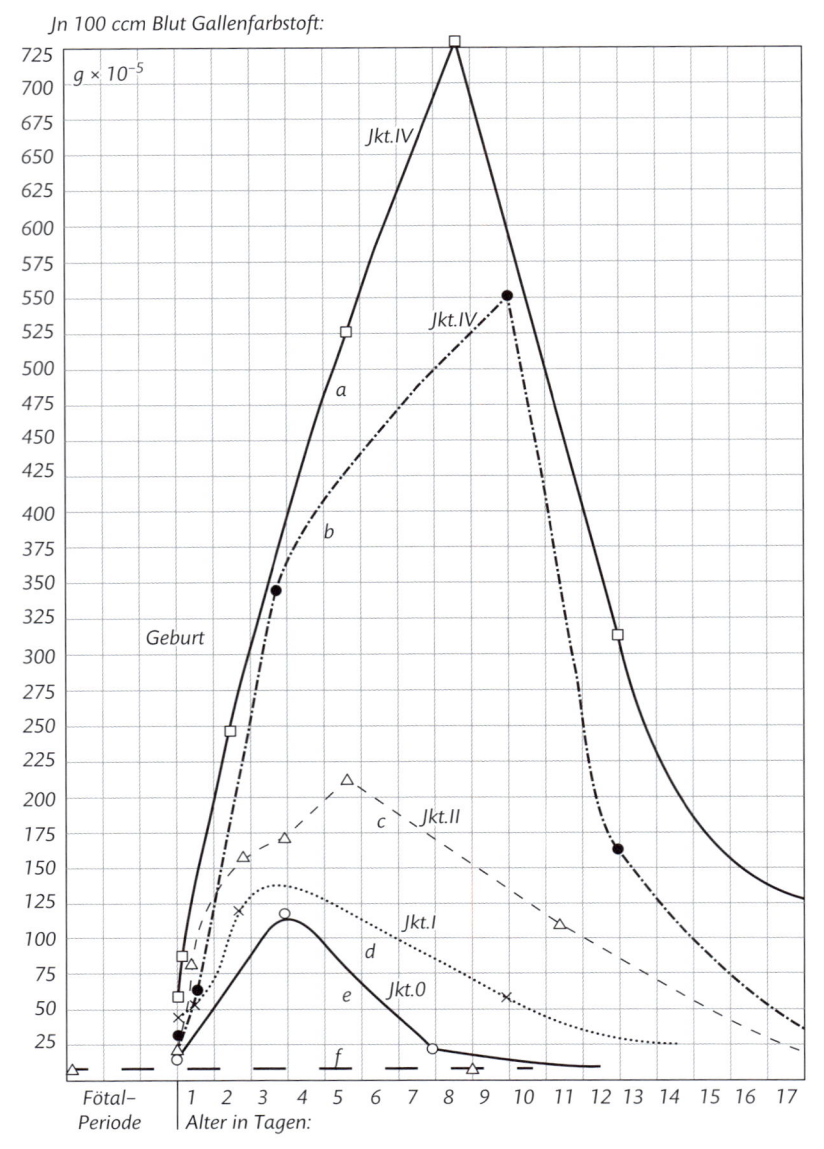

Fig. 7.2.3 Bile pigment (bilirubin plus biliverdin) concentration during the first 2 weeks of life in four infants with different degrees of jaundice (a–d), one non-icteric newborn (e), and the mothers of these infants (f, averaged), as published by Ylppö in 1913 [16].

disease, pulmonary and cerebral hemorrhage, and maternal diabetes were the chief conditions encountered in those cases of kernicterus in which erythroblastosis fetalis was excluded.'

Specific neurologic symptoms occur in most infants with bilirubin encephalopathy: head retraction, expressionless face, upward rolling of the eyes, refusal to suck, cyanotic attacks, and convulsions. Survivors suffered from athetosis and perceptive deafness [21]. In infants with haemolytic disease, Mollison and Cutbush [49] prognosticated the disease's severity by haemoglobin concentration in cord blood in 1951: 'As a subsidiary investigation … of 30 infants whose peak bilirubin concentration did not exceed 18 mg/100 mL, none developed kernicterus, whereas of 11 infants with peak bilirubin concentrations exceeding 18 mg/100 mL, five died of kernicterus and two others survived with signs of motor damage.' This smallprint subordinate clause was to become the indication for exchange transfusion even in term infants with non-haemolytic jaundice [50], when Hsia and co-workers published a retrospective analysis of 229 infants with erythroblastosis [51]: kernicterus developed in 18% of infants with serum bilirubin of 16–30 mg/dL and in 50% of infants with bilirubin concentration greater than 30 mg/dL. The Boston authors concluded: 'Kernicterus is unlikely to occur when the serum bilirubin remains below 20 mg/dL.' In the 1990s, having nearly fallen into oblivion, kernicterus returned because of lessened awareness when neonates were discharged ever earlier from the maternity wards with no means of monitoring their bilirubin at home [52].

Exchange transfusion

From 1919 to 1923, Bruce Robertson at the Toronto Hospital for Sick Children developed the technique of 'exsanguino-transfusion'

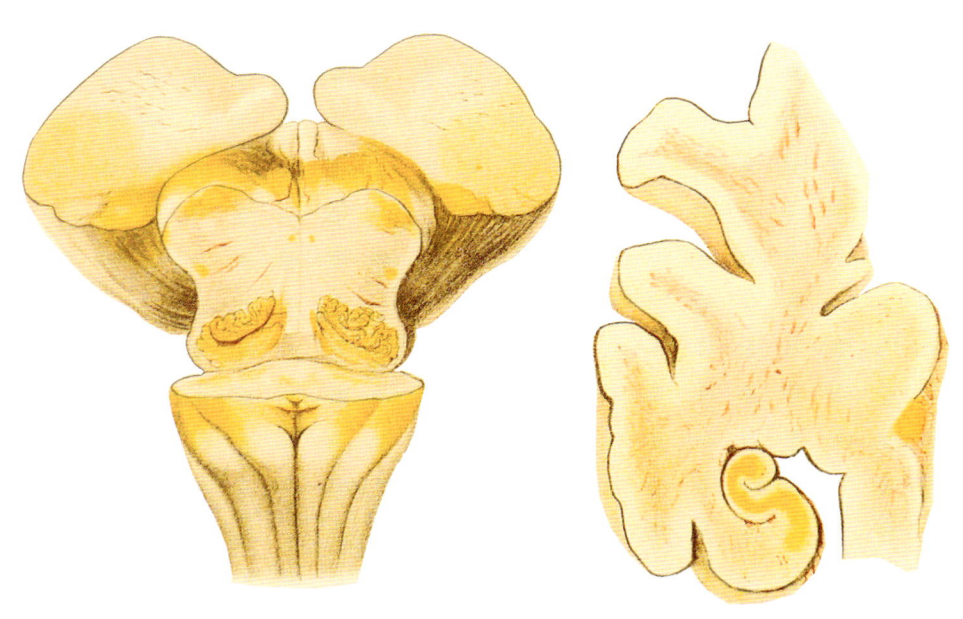

Fig. 7.2.4 Schmorl's kernicterus depiction of 1904 [47]. Left: dorsal view of brainstem, showing dark-yellow staining of the olive nucleus. Right: slice through the temporal lobe and hippocampus, showing dark-yellow staining of Ammon's horn.

via the sinus sagittalis with the aim to remove 'toxins' in poisoning, burns, and septicaemia [53]. In 1925, Alfred Hart, also in Toronto, successfully used the same technique in a severely jaundiced newborn of a family whose six infants had died [54]. In 1946, Harry Wallerstein reported on successful exchange transfusion—also via the sagittal sinus—in three infants with severe rhesus erythroblastosis [55], and in 1948 Arnold and Alford described replacement transfusion by access to the vena cava via the vena saphena in the groin flexure [56]. By using an elastic umbilical vein catheter, Louis Diamond and co-workers developed the technique that became the international standard for exchange transfusion in 1951 [57]. In the earliest era of neonatal intensive care, each perinatal centre had an 'erythroblastosis service' that performed hundreds of exchange transfusions per year [58]. In 1965, Wishingrad and co-workers published a randomized trial in infants with non-haemolytic jaundice and a bilirubin concentration above 18 mg/dL [59]: of 50 infants without exchange, one developed kernicterus; and of the 50 infants with exchange transfusion, one needed resuscitation during the procedure. In the clinical reality of preterm infants suffering from haemolytic disease, the mortality associated with exchange transfusion ranged from 2% to 7% [60, 61].

Phototherapy

As Schmorl's 1904 observation of bilirubin's destruction by light was ignored, phototherapy had to be reinvented half a century later. During the sunny summer of 1956, Sister Jean Ward, nurse-in-charge of the Premature Unit at Rochford General Hospital, Essex, wheeled some of the preterm infants into the courtyard [62], 'convinced that the combination of fresh air and warm sunshine would benefit them more than the stuffy overheated atmosphere of an incubator'. The nurse correctly observed that the skin jaundice faded away at sun-exposed areas. After the systematic sun exposure of 13 jaundiced infants, Richard Cremer and co-workers constructed the 'light cradle' for indoor use and demonstrated its effectivity in lowering serum bilirubin [63]. Controlled trials published from Uruguay in 1967 [64] and from Vermont in 1968 [65] proved the efficacy and safety of phototherapy, and phototherapy was introduced in most European and South American countries. But the available evidence failed to convince the American Academy of Sciences, who as late as 1974 ruled [66]: 'Exchange transfusion should still be considered mandatory when the usual criteria for it are met'. The opposition was led by Gerard Odell who as late as 1980 cautioned that free radicals could theoretically harm the infant receiving phototherapy [67], at a time when exchange transfusion in the preterm infant had a mortality of at least 2%.

Rhesus prophylaxis

Once the role of rhesus factor and isoimmunization was understood, progress was rapid. In 1945, Robin Coombs and co-workers developed the antiglobulin consumption test to diagnose erythroblastosis [68]. In 1961, Ronald Finn and Cyril Clarke in Liverpool demonstrated that the rhesus immunization of mothers can be prevented if fetal cells in their circulation are rapidly destroyed by anti-D immunoglobulin [69]. In New York, the group of Freda and Gorman had the same result in a study of male Sing-Sing prisoners [70]. The head-to-head race between Liverpool and New York continued until 1965, when both groups had developed effective preventions. An antepartum rhesus prophylaxis trial was initiated in 1968 in Manitoba, Canada by Bowman [71], anti-D immunoglobulin, and severe haemolytic disease was virtually eliminated within a few years (Fig. 7.2.5).

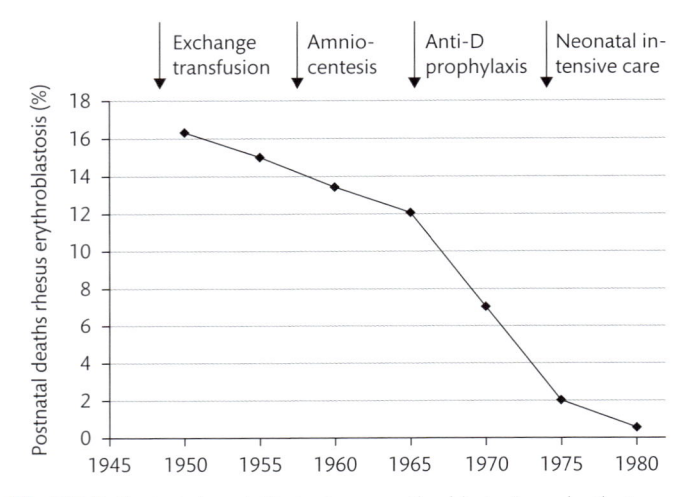

Fig. 7.2.5 Postnatal mortality in rhesus erythroblastosis, and milestones in eradicating this disease; drawn from data of Bowman 1977 [71] and Tovey 1986 [72].

Conclusion

Kernicterus had been known since 1821, but became widely acknowledged when in the 1950s greater numbers of preterm infants survived the first days of life. Once isoimmunization was understood, it took only 25 years to develop the prophylaxis of rhesus haemolytic disease by anti-D immunoglobulin. Excessive concern and theorizing delayed the introduction of highly effective and harmless phototherapy for 20 years. The debaters' different mentalities played as large a role as did scientific facts, and it was equally difficult to understand why the opposition dissipated. Diminished concern led to the re-occurrence of kernicterus in the 1990s, when neonates were discharged ever earlier from the maternity wards without monitoring their bilirubin values at home.

REFERENCES

1. Volk K: Kinderkrankheiten nach der Darstellung babylonisch-assyrischer Keilschrifttexte. Orientalia 1999;**68**:1–30.
2. Roberts GF: Comparative aspects of haemolytic disease of the newborn. London: Heinemann, 1957.
3. Hansen TWR: Pioneers in the scientific study of neonatal jaundice and kernicterus. Pediatrics 2000;**106**:e15.
4. Dugès A: Recherches sur les maladies les plus importantes et les moins connues des enfans nouveau-nés. Paris: Baillière, 1821: p. 32–4, 66, fig. 1.
5. Sylvius de le Boe F: Praxeos medicae liber primus. Lugduni Batavorum: Carpentier, 1671: p. 794.
6. Juncker J: Conspectus medicinae theoretico-practicae, tabulis 116. Halae: Impensis Orphanotrophi, 1718: p. 738.
7. Morgagni GB: The seats and causes of diseases investigated by anatomy (1st Latin ed. Venice 1761). London: Millar, 1769: Vol. **2**, p. 758, 766.
8. Baumes JBT: Traité de l'ictère ou jaunisse des enfans de naissance. 2. ed. Nismes: Castor Belle, 1788: p. 4–32.
9. Auvity J-P: Considérations générales sur les maladies propres aux enfans dans les premiers momens de leur vie. Paris: Didot Jeune, 1808: p. 15.
10. Gardien: Die Gelbsucht der Neugeborenen (Icterus neonatorum). Analekten über Kinderkrankheiten 1837;**4**:430–40.
11. Jörg JCG: Handbuch zum Erkennen und Heilen der Kinderkrankheiten. Leipzig: Cnobloch, 1826: Vol. **2**, p. 507–11.
12. Pieper PA: Die Kinderpraxis am Findelhause und in dem Hospital für kranke Kinder zu Paris. Göttingen: Dieterich, 1831: p. 187, 358.
13. Heyfelder JF: Beobachtungen über die Krankheiten der Neugeborenen. Leipzig: Hartmann, 1825: p. 60–3.
14. Sennert D: Tractatus de morbis infantium. In: Practicae medicinae liber quartus. Paris: Societas, 1633: p. 71–2.
15. Bouchut E: Traité pratique des maladies des nouveau-nés et des enfants a la mamelle et de la seconde enfance. 5. ed. Paris: Baillière, 1867: p. 638.
16. Ylppö A: Icterus neonatorum und Gallenfarbstoffsekretion beim Fötus und Neugeborenen. Zeitschr Kinderheilk 1913;**9**:208–318.
17. Brown AK, Zuelzer WW, Burnett HH: Studies on the neonatal development of the glucuronide conjugating system. J Clin Invest 1958;**37**:332–40.
18. Anselmino KJ, Hoffmann F: Die Ursachen des Icterus neonatorum. Arch Gynäkol 1930;**143**:477–99.
19. Elsässer JA: Erster Bericht über die Ereignisse in der Gebäranstalt und in der Hebammeneschule des Catharinenhospitals in Stuttgart. Schmidt's Jahrbücher 1835;**7**:314–22.
20. Aidin R, Corner B, Tovey G: Kernicterus and prematurity. Lancet 1950;**255**:1153–4.
21. Crosse VM, Meyer TC, Gerrard JW: Kernicterus and prematurity. Arch Dis Child 1955;**30**:501–8.
22. Silverman WA, Andersen DH, Blanc WA, Crozier DN: A difference in mortality rate and incidence of kernicterus among premature infants allotted to two prophylactic antibacterial regimens. Pediatrics 1956;**18**:614–25.
23. Jardine DS, Rogers K: Relationship of benzyl alcohol to kernicterus, intraventricular hemorrhage, and mortality in preterm infants. Pediatrics 1989;**83**:153–60.
24. Watchko JF: Vigintiphobia revisited. Pediatrics 2005;**115**:1747–53.
25. Severino MA: De recondita abscessuum natura libri 8. Francofurti: Beyer, 1643: p. 267.
26. Kerckring T: Spicilegium anatomicum. Amstelodami: Frisius, 1670: p. 118.
27. Seger G: Embryo hydropicus. Miscellanea curiosa medico-physica. Lipsiae: Trescher, 1670: Vol. **1**, p. 132–3.
28. Dorstenius JD: Foetu abortivo hydropico. In: Miscellanea curiosa. Norimbergae: Endter, 1684: Vol. **5**, p. 298–9.
29. Horst JO: Disputatio inauguralis medica, exhibens casum foetu abortivo icterico. (Gießen): Karger, 1673: p. 2–4.
30. Clay J: Über Anasarca des Foetus. Zeitschr der Kaiserl. Königl. Gesellschaft der Aerzte zu Wien 1859:200–3.
31. Ballantyne JW: The diseases and deformities of the foetus. Edinburgh: Olver and Boyd, 1892: Vol. **1**, p. 102–81, plates 1 and 2.
32. Blomfield JE: Congenital hepatic cirrhosis. BMJ 1901;**1**:1142.
33. Arkwright JA: A family series of fatal and dangerous cases of icterus neonatorum. Edinb Med J 1902;**12**:156–8.
34. Auden GA: A series of fatal cases of jaundice in the newborn. St Bart's Hosp Rep 1905;**41**:139–42.
35. Busfield J: A series of cases of icterus neonatorum in a family. BMJ 1906;**1**:20.
36. Pfannenstiel J: Über den habituellen Ikterus gravis der Neugeborenen. Münch Med Wochenschr 1908;**55**:2169–74.

37. Duguid WR: A series of cases of icterus neonatorum. BMJ 1906;**I**:319.
38. Hymans van den Bergh AA, Snapper J: Die Farbstoffe des Blutserums. Dt Archiv Klin Med 1913;**110**:540–61.
39. Diamond LK, Blackfan KD, Baty JM: Erythroblastosis fetalis and its association with universal edema of the fetus, Icterus gravis neonatorum and anemia of the newborn. J Pediat 1932;**1**:269–76.
40. Landsteiner K, Wiener AS: An agglutinable factor in human blood recognised by immune sera for rhesus blood. Proc Soc Exp Biol Med 1940;**43**:223.
41. Levine P, Katzin EM, Burnham L: Isoimmunization in pregnancy. Its possible bearing on the etiology of erythroblastosis foetalis. JAMA 1941;**116**:825–7.
42. Panaroli D: Natus ictericus. Observatio 44. In: Iatrologismorum seu medicinalium observationum pentecostae quinque. Romae: Franciscus Moneta, 1652: p. 273.
43. Levret A: L'art des accouchemens (1st ed. 1753). 3. ed. Paris: Didot Jeune, 1766: p. 76, 261, 445.
44. Billard CM: A treatise on the diseases of infants (1st French ed. 1828). 2. ed. New York: Langley, 1840: p. 506.
45. Virchow R: Die pathologischen Pigmente. Virchows Arch 1847;**1**:379–486.
46. Orth J: Über das Vorkommen von Bilirubinkrystallen bei neugeborenen Kindern. Virchows Arch 175;**63**:447–62.
47. Schmorl C: Zur Kenntnis des ikterus neonatorum, insbesondere der dabei auftretenden Gehirnveränderungen. Verh Dtsch Pathol Ges 1904;**6**:109–15.
48. Zuelzer WW, Mudgett RT: Kernicterus. Etiologic study based on an analysis of 55 cases. Pediatrics 1950;**6**:452–74.
49. Mollison P, Cutbush M: A method of measuring the severity of a series of cases of hemolytic disease of the newborn. Blood 1951;**6**:777–88.
50. Watchko JF: Bilirubin 20 mg/dL = vigintiphobia. Pediatrics 1983;**74**:660–3.
51. Hsia DY, Allen FH, Gellis SS, Diamond LK: Erythroblastosis fetalis. VIII. Studies of serum bilirubin in relation to kernicterus. N Engl J Med 1952;**247**:668–71.
52. Ebbesen F: Recurrence of kernicterus in term and near-term infants in Denmark. Acta Paediatr 2000;**89**:1213–7.
53. Robertson LB: Exsanguination-transfusion. Arch Surg 1924;**9**:1–15.
54. Hart AP: Familial icterus gravis of the newborn and its treatment. Can Med Assoc J 1925;**15**:1008–11.
55. Wallerstein H: Treatment of severe erythroblastosis by simultaneous removal and replacement of the blood of the newborn infant. Science 1946;**103**:583–4.
56. Arnold DP, Alford KM: A new technique for replacement transfusion in the treatment of hemolytic disease of the newborn infant. J Pediatr 1948;**32**:113–8.
57. Diamond LK, Allen FH, Thomas WO: Erythroblastosis fetalis. VII. Treatment with exchange transfusion. N Engl J Med 1951;**244**:39–49.
58. Crosse VM, Wallis PG, Walsh AM: Replacement transfusion as a means of preventing kernikterus of prematurity. Arch Dis Child 1958;**33**:403–8.
59. Wishingrad L, Cornblath M, Takakuwa T, Rozenfeld I, et al.: Prospective randomized selection for exchange transfusion with observations on the levels of serum bilirubin with and without exchange transfusion. Pediatrics 1965;**36**:162–72.
60. Boggs TR, Westphal MC: Mortality of exchange transfusions. Pediatrics 1960;**26**:745–55.
61. Jablonski WJ: Risks associated with exchange transfusion. N Engl J Med 1962;**266**:155–60.
62. Dobbs RH, Cremer RJ: Phototherapy. Arch Dis Child 1975;**50**:833–6.
63. Cremer RJ, Perryman PW, Richards DH: Influence of light on the hyperbilirubinemia of infants. Lancet 1958;**271**:1094.
64. Obes-Polleri J: La fototerapia en las hiperbilirubinemiae neonatales. Arch Pediatr Uruguay 1967;**38**:77–100.
65. Lucey JF, Ferreiro M, Hewitt J: Prevention of hyperbilirubinemia of prematurity by phototherapy. Pediatrics 1968;**41**:1047–54.
66. Behrman RE, Brown AK, Currie MR, et al.: Preliminary report of the committee on phototherapy in the newborn infant. J Pediatr 1974;**84**:135–43.
67. Odell GB: Neonatal hyperbilirubinemia. New York: Grune & Stratton, 1980: p. 115–34.
68. Coombs RRA, Mourant AE, Race RR: In-vivo isosensitization of red cells in babies with haemolytic disease. Lancet 1946;**247**:264–6.
69. Finn R, Clarke CA, Donohue WTA, et al.: Experimental studies on the prevention of Rh haemolytic disease. BMJ 1961;**1**:1486–90.
70. Freda VJ, Gorman JG, Pollack W: Successful prevention of experimental Rh sensitization in man with an anti-Rh gamma-2-globulin antibody preparation. Transfusion 1964;**4**:26–32.
71. Bowman JM, Chown B, Lewin M, Pollock J: Rh isoimmunization, Manitoba 1963–75. Can Med Assoc J 1977;**116**:282–4.
72. Tovey D: Haemolytic disease of the newborn—the changing scene. Br J Obstet Gynaecol 1986;**93**:960–6.

7.3

Weak giants
Infants of diabetic mothers

Introduction

Diabetes mellitus is an ancient disease, described since antiquity and regarded as a kidney disorder in the papyrus *Ebers* 1500 B.C.E. [1]. Fetal macrosomia, dreaded by midwives and obstetricians, has also been described for thousands of years. However, not until the 20th century began were the two problems interlinked. At the start of the 21st century, 0.6% of all births in Norway were complicated by maternal pregestational diabetes, and 1% by gestational diabetes [2]. In northern England, the prevalence of pregestational diabetes rose from 0.31% in 1996–1998 to 0.47% in 2002–2004 [3]. In Northern California the age- and ethnicity-adjusted incidence of gestational diabetes mellitus increased from 5.1% in 1991 to 7.4% in 1997 [4]. The recent increase in frequency was largely due to type 2 diabetes. Problems of infants of diabetic mothers were excellently reviewed by James Farquhar in 1959 [5], and the history of diabetes in pregnancy has been delineated by Jorge Mestman [6] and Harold Kalter [7]. The aim of the present chapter is to describe the process of understanding the problems of infants associated with maternal diabetes, and to explain why this process took so long.

Macrosomia

Before Caesarean section became an option, macrosomia was associated with difficult delivery and often forced the obstetricians to perform embryotomy or other mutilating surgery to save the mother's life. The condition was poorly defined, usually as birthweight above 4500 g (or 4000 g) at term. Fenton's growth chart reported a 97th centile of 4.5 kg at 40 weeks' gestation [8]. Soranus (200 C.E.) had grim experiences [9]: 'Causes of difficult labor, as far as the child is concerned, are the following: when it is extremely large, either in whole or in part, as it happens in those suffering from hydrocephalus ... If the fetus does not respond to manual traction, because of its size, or death, or impaction in any manner whatsoever, one must proceed to the more forceful methods, those of extraction by hooks and embryotomy.'

Physicians explained macrosomia by maternal imagination, as did Frederic Clauder in 1687 when describing the exceptionally large infant (**Fig. 7.3.1**) of a farmer's wife [10], who 'several months pregnant, fell in admiration when gazing at the nude torso of a handsome soldier'. In an appendix to his 'Art of midwifery', Hendrik Deventer of Den Haag explained in 1701 [11] several 'extraordinary means to save the mother [by embryotomy and hook] ... If you asked for and obtained consent to treat the child as dead ... this is the only way I have yet found'. At the start of the 20th century, several extensive series of 'giant babies' were described without even mentioning maternal diabetes, as did Henri Dubois in Paris 1897 [12], Jacobi in Mannheim in 1903 [13], and John William Ballantyne of Edinburgh in 1904 [14]. These authors related fetal macrosomia to postmaturity

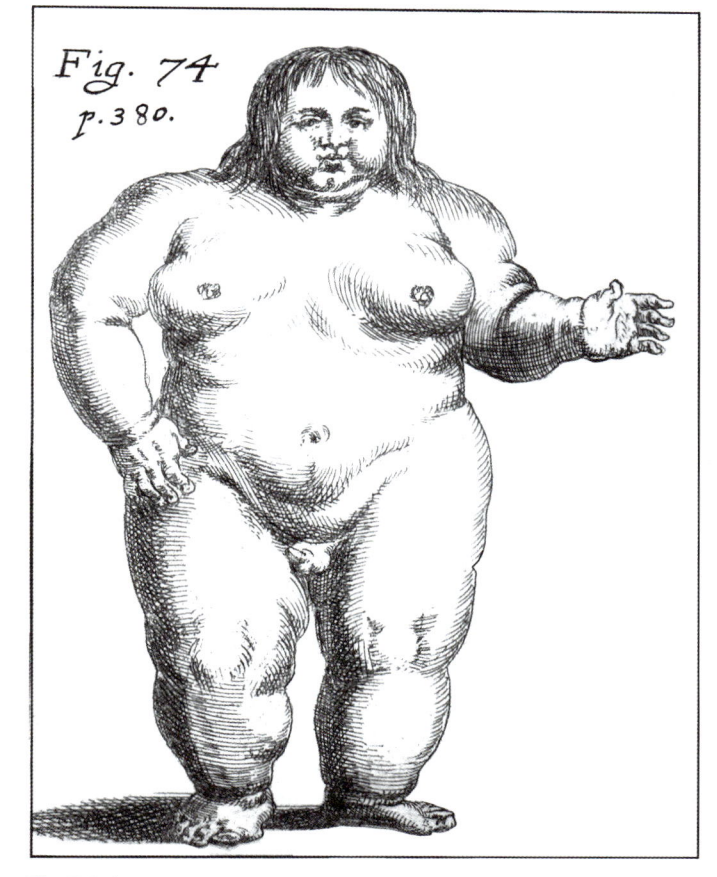

Fig. 7.3.1 Macrosomia in an infant born in 1687, believed by Clauder to be the result of maternal imagination (see text for details) [10].

or precocious puberty and discussed heredity and the risk of recurrence. The association with maternal diabetes was understood in 1909 by J. Whitridge Williams in Baltimore, who wrote [15]: 'It seems that the condition [diabetes] frequently predisposes to excessive development on the part of the child, which may give rise to serious dystocia and lead to its death during delivery'. In 1935, L. Fischer tabulated the birth weight of 49 infants born to diabetic mothers at a gestational age of 37–40 weeks: only 11 weighed below 4.0 kg, 18 weighed 4.0–4.9 kg, and 20 even 5.0 kg and more [16].

Maternal diabetes mellitus before insulin

In 1679, Oxford professor Thomas Willis observed that 'in the Diabetes, or Pissing Evil ... the urine is wonderfully sweet as it were imbued with Honey or Sugar' [17]. In 1776 in Liverpool, Matthew Dobson evaporated the urine of a diabetic man to a dry sweet cake, and concluded [18] 'the saccharine matter was not formed in the secretary organ, but previously existed in the serum of the blood'. Before the insulin era, few diabetic women conceived [19], and both maternal mortality and fetal loss were high. In 1823, the Berlin student Heinrich Bennewitz understood the essentials of diabetic fetopathy. His dissertation in Latin [20], abstracted in the *Edinburgh Medical and Surgical Journal* [21], contains a remarkable case description: 'At the age of 22, Friederica Pape became pregnant for the fifth time; hardly had the pregnancy begun when her thirst and diuresis reappeared ... The urine considerably exceeded in quantity the liquid drank, reaching a volume of 16 pounds per day ... It was sent to [the chemist Sigismund Friedrich] Hermbstaedt, who measured a sugar concentration of 2 ounces per civil pound [12.5 g/L] ... On December 29, 1823, the labour commenced prematurely ... the large female infant was difficult to extract because the arms were stuck besides the head and the umbilical cord compressed ... She moaned with a clear voice, but died thereafter and seemed a real Hercules, robust and sane, weighing 12 civil pounds [5600 g] ... After birth, the mother recovered rapidly and Hermbstaedt could no longer detect any more trace of sugar in her urine'. These measurements were pioneer work: Hermann Fehling did not publish his quantification of urine sugar with copper sulphate until 1849 [22]. Six years later, Paris obstetrician Hippolyte Blot found via this test that most pregnant and all delivered women have a certain 'physiological' amount of sugar in their urine [23].

Before insulin, however, diabetes in pregnancy remained rare. Apollinaire Buchardat of Paris wrote in his extensive monograph on diabetes in 1875 [24]: 'Among the great number of diabetic women in my consultation, I cannot remember a single one pregnant'. In 1882, Matthews Duncan published two cases of puerperal diabetes and tabulated another 13 from the literature [25]: 'They cannot be read without giving a strong impression of the great gravity of the complication'. Only five of the 15 women and six of the 22 infants had survived. In 1902, Ernest Herman attended a birth at the London Hospital where both a diabetic mother and her infant died [26] and concluded: 'The chances are two to one that the child will die in utero. Its life is therefore not of much account ... The early termination of pregnancy is the course which offers the greatest probability of benefit to the mother'. In 1908, Heinrich Offergeld of Frankfurt published a gruesome table of 57 pregnancies in diabetic women—at that time nearly the entire world literature [27]. Of the mothers, 17 had died during or shortly after delivery, and another 14 during the following months. Of the infants, 29 died before and nine after birth: only a third of the babies survived till the age of 1 year. In 1909, J. Whitridge Williams of Baltimore compiled a similar table of 66 cases from the literature: maternal mortality was 32%, fetal mortality 51% [15]. At that time, the Harvard Medical School founded the Department of Theory and Practice and appointed Elliott Joslin, who in 1915 deplored 'the gloomy outlook for pregnant women showing large quantities of sugar [in the urine]' [28]. He became a pioneer of diabetology and energetically promoted the introduction of insulin from 1922.

Birth trauma and asphyxia

François Mauriceau's observation no. 48 is one of many that illustrate the obstetrician's despair when delivering a giant baby [29]: 'On December 11, 1671, I delivered a woman of one of the largest infants ever seen, who presented by the buttocks and had voided much meconium the day before ... When I tried to free the leg, the mother suddenly moved and I broke the infant's thigh. After reducing the thigh I fixed the fracture with an appropriate bandage, and it healed perfectly within 25 days.' Yet not incarceration of the giant, but asphyxia and hyaline membranes were the main causes of death, as described by James Farquhar [5]: 'During their first 24 or more extra-uterine hours they lie on their backs, bloated and flushed, their legs flexed and abduced, their lightly closed hands on each side of the head, the abdomen prominent and their respiration sighing.'

Surfactant deficiency

Fetal lung maturation was noticeably retarded in diabetic pregnancy, as Farquhar reported [5]: 'Difficult respiration was observed in 21 [of 96 liveborn] babies ... Cyanosis of varying degree accompanied the forcible respirations, the sternal and costal indrawing and the strange tremulous expiratory whine which is known to the midwives as "murmuring".' Pulmonary hyaline membranes occurred in 80% or more of neonatal deaths in the large diabetic series of Priscilla White [30]. In 1973, Louis Gluck proved, by analysing the phospholipid pattern of amniotic fluid, that surfactant synthesis is seriously retarded in maternal diabetes [31], explaining respiratory distress syndrome in infants born at term.

Hypoglycaemia

Glucose tolerance diminishes during pregnancy, as proved by Marcel Brocard in 1898 [32]: 2 hours after ingesting 50 g of glucose, glucosuria occurred in 50% of pregnant and 11% of non-pregnant women. In 1920, Dubreuil and Anderodias found in a 5 kg newborn of a diabetic mother the islets of Langerhans double their normal size [33] (Fig. 7.3.2 left). In 1926, Gray and Feemster measured a blood sugar value of 67 mg/dL on the third day of life in a diabetic mother's infant [34]. In 1929, Holzbach suspected that [35] the fetal pancreas's augmented function persists for some time after birth, causing a low sugar concentration in the newborn's blood. In 1930, Pack and Barber confirmed islet hyperplasia and documented that

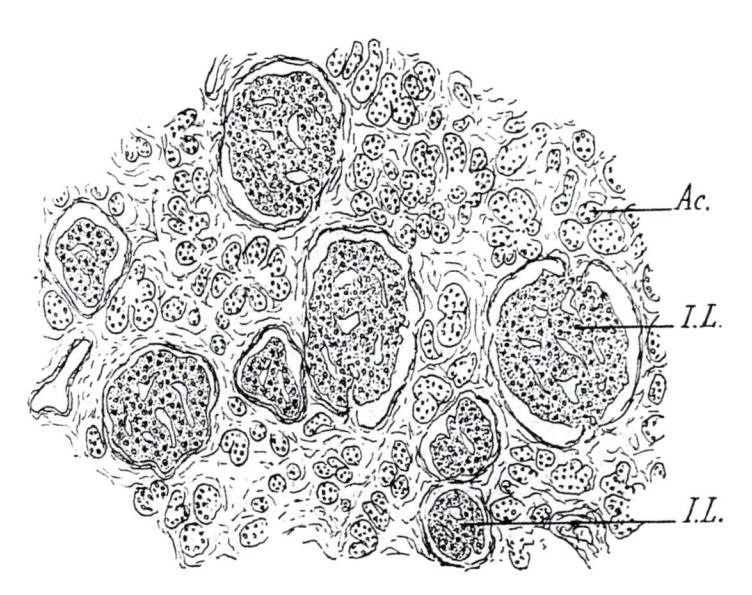

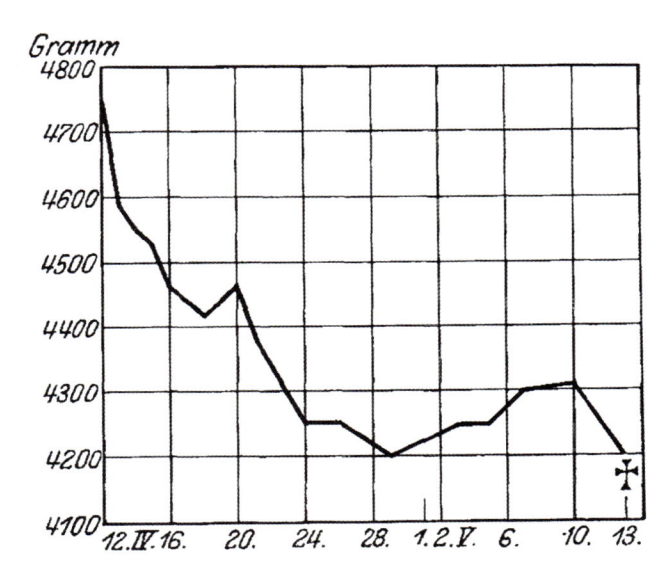

Fig. 7.3.2 Diabetic embryopathy and fetopathy. Left: giant islets of Langerhans (I.L.) in the pancreas of a 5050 g girl who died several minutes after birth and was born in 1920 by a diabetic mother who excreted 50–52 g/L urine. Ac, pancreatic glands. Case published by Dubreuil and Anderodias in 1920 [33]. Right: postnatal weight curve of a 4750 g girl born on 12 April 1929 to a diabetic mother, urine sugar excretion 50 g, blood sugar 120–300 mg/dL. The infant failed to thrive and died on the 32nd day of life. Postmortem examination revealed ventricular septum defect, abnormal pulmonary outflow tract, and severe muscular hypertrophy of the heart. Case published by Nevinny and Schretter in 1930 [46].

insulin may pass transplacentally from the fetus to the mother [36]. The oral glucose tolerance test during pregnancy was standardized by O'Sullivan in 1961 [37].

During the first hours after birth, the newborn infant's plasma glucose drops. As the islet size takes time to normalize, the blood sugar falls more consistently, more rapidly, and further in infants born to diabetic mothers than in normal babies of non-diabetic mothers [5]. In 1935, Reginald Higgons found in a diabetic mother's infant a sugar concentration of 47 mg/dL in blood drawn from the sinus longitudinalis by puncturing the fontanelle [38]. Micromethods were not available until 1950.

However, neonatal hypoglycaemia's definition remained controversial and guidelines for hypoglycaemia screening were not evidence based [39]. The study of Alan Lucas published in 1988 [40] revealed a 3.5-fold incidence of neurodevelopmental impairment in preterm infants when plasma glucose levels below 47 mg/dL (2.6 mmol/L) were recorded on 5 days. This value, although obtained from infants of less than 1850 g birthweight, has also been applied as the 'operational threshold' for infants of diabetic mothers [41].

Malformations

The risk of major non-chromosomal congenital malformations in infants exposed to pregestational diabetes is more than twice that in non-diabetic pregnancies [42–44]. Among 78 fetal deaths investigated in Boston in 1952, Priscilla White identified nine congenital anomalies [30]. A year later, London anatomist B.S. Cardell showed that the beta cells are chiefly involved, and a positive correlation between the volume of islet tissue and the size of the baby [45], and reported malformation rates of 25% and 20% at autopsy in babies of diabetic and non-diabetic women, respectively. In the population-based EUROCAT study, malformations in infants of diabetic mothers usually did not follow a specific pattern, the most frequent being congenital heart defects, the most specific caudal regression syndromes [44].

In 1930, Nevinny and Schretter published two cases from Innsbruck of diabetes in pregnancy [46]: a girl born measuring 61 cm and with a birthweight of 5730 g, who died on the 28th day of life; and another girl born measuring 58 cm and with a birthweight of 4750 g. Both infants failed to thrive, and postmortem examinations revealed cardiac malformations (Fig. 7.3.2, right).

Sacral agenesis was published by Otto in 1811 [47], Behn in 1827 [48], and Hohl in 1852 [49], usually under the terms *sirenomelia* or *monopodia*. In 1959, Blumel and co-workers published 50 cases of partial or total agenesis of the os sacrum bone [50]; in seven of them, the mother had had diabetes during pregnancy. In 1965, Rusnak and Driscoll reported three [51] and in 1966, Passarge and Lenz 43 infants of diabetic mothers presenting agenesis of the sacrum and coccyx [52].

The insulin era

In 1922, Frederick Banting and Charles Best isolated insulin in Toronto [53], the hormone became generally available from 1923, and since then the number of diabetic women becoming pregnant has increased. In 1924, George Graham, consultant at London's St Bartholomew's Hospital, reported a woman who had been treated with insulin before conception, received daily dosages increasing from 10 to 28 units during pregnancy, and gave birth to a healthy infant [54]. In 1925, Lindsay Peters reported from Alameda, California, the live birth of an infant at 35 weeks' gestation born to a woman with funnel pelvis and severe diabetes, who had been treated with 3 × 10 IU of insulin from week 24 [55]. Insulin immediately improved the mother's chances, but the infant's prognosis remained gloomy.

From 1923 to 1933, Eric Skipper observed 37 pregnancies of diabetic women at the London Hospital [19], and observed fetal mortalities of 45% and 25% in pregestational and gestational diabetes, respectively. In 1949 Priscilla White reported a series of 439 pregnant diabetics admitted to the Boston Lying-In Hospital since 1924 [56]. She defined six classes of diabetes in pregnancy: A, subclinical glucosuria; B, adult onset, duration less than 10 years; C, adolescent onset or duration 10–19 years; D, duration more than 20 years; E, vascular damage to pelvic vessels; and F, diabetic nephropathy [30]. She resumed: 'The perinatal, intrapartum, and neonatal death rate is 45%.' In Canada in 2010, infants of women with pregestational diabetes continued to carry more than twice the risk of perinatal death than those of women without diabetes [57].

Fetal programming

Fetuses exposed to maternal diabetes have a risk of developing diabetes later in life that exceeds that attributable to genetics. The explanation may be a mechanism called perinatal programming and described by Barker in infants with low birthweight [58]. It probably acts via epigenetic modification of the fetal genome and predisposes the children to develop metabolic syndrome: obesity, type 2 diabetes, hypertension, and cardiovascular disease [59]. In Denmark, the vicious circle 'diabetes begets diabetes' was described by Damm [60].

Conclusion

The history of diabetes in pregnancy appeared to be a success story initially: diabetic women were no longer excluded from reproduction, mothers and infants no longer threatened by early death. But a price has been paid: one century after insulin enabled successful pregnancy in diabetic mothers, gestational diabetes has become the most common medical complication of pregnancy, and its incidence continues to rise. All forms of maternal diabetes have serious and long-lasting health consequences for the infant. Fetal exposure to maternal diabetes is likely to remain a major public health problem for decades.

REFERENCES

1. Garrison FH: Historical aspects of diabetes and insulin. Bull NY Acad Med 1925;**1**:127–33.
2. Leirgul E, Brodwall K, Greve Geal: Maternal diabetes, birth weight, and neonatal risk of congenital heart defects in Norway, 1994–2009. Obstet Gynecol 2016;**128**:1116–25.
3. Bell R, Cresswell T, Hawthorne G, et al.: Trends in prevalence and outcomes of pregnancy in women with pre-existing type I and type II diabetes. BJOG 2008;**115**:445–52.
4. Ferrara A, Kahn HS, Quesenberry CP, et al.: An increase in the incidence of gestational diabetes mellitus. Obstet Gynecol 2004;**103**:526–33.
5. Farquhar JW: The child of the diabetic woman. Arch Dis Child 1959;**34**:76–96.
6. Mestman JH: Historical notes on diabetes and pregnancy. Endocrinologist 2002;**12**:224–42.
7. Kalter H: A history of diabetes in pregnancy. Dordrecht: Springer, 2012.
8. Fenton TR: A new growth chart for preterm babies: Babson and Benda's chart updated with recent data and a new format. BMC Pediatr 2003;**3**:13.
9. Temkin O: Soranus' Gynecology. Baltimore, MD: The Johns Hopkins Press, 1956: p. 37, 176, 189.
10. Clauder FW: Stupenda pueri recens nati obesitas ex matris gravidae impressione. Miscell Cur sive Ephemeridum Decur II 1687;**6**:380–1.
11. Deventer Hv: Neues Hebammen-Licht (1st Latin ed. 1701). 5. ed. Jena: Cröker, 1761: p. 261, 325, fig. 27.
12. Dubois H: Les gros enfants au point de vue obstetrical. Paris: Thèse de médicine, 1897.
13. Jacoby: Ueber den Riesenwuchs von Neugeborenen. Arch Gynäkol 1905;**74**:536–66.
14. Ballantyne JW: Manual of antenatal pathology and hygiene. The embryo. Edinburgh: Green, 1904: p. 105–28, 252–7.
15. Williams JW: The clinical significance of glycosuria in pregnant women. Am J Med Sci 1909;**137**:1–26.
16. Fischer L: Riesenkinder bei mütterlichem Diabetes. Zentralbl Gynäk 1935;**59**:249–60.
17. Willis T: Pharmaceutice rationalis. London: Dring, 1679: p. 79–85.
18. Dobson M: Experiments and observations on the urine in a diabetes. London: Cadell, 1776: p. 298–316.
19. Skipper E: Diabetes mellitus and pregnancy. A clinical and analytical study. Q J Med 1933;**2**:353–80.
20. Bennewitz HG: De diabete mellito, graviditatis symptomate. Berlin: Starck, 1824.
21. Bennewitz H: Symptomatic diabetes mellitus. (Osann's 12. Jahresbericht, p. 23). Edinb Med Surg J 1828;**13**:217–8.
22. Fehling H: Die quantitative Bestimmung von Zucker und Stärkemehl mittelst Kupfervitriol. Ann Chem Pharm 1849;**72**:106–13.
23. Blot H: De la glycosurie physiologique des femmes en couches, des nourrices, et d'un certain nombre de femmes enceintes. Paris: Masson, 1856.
24. Bouchardat A: De la glucosurie ou diabete sucré, son traitement hygiénique. Paris: Baillière, 1875: p. 176.
25. Duncan JM: On puerperal diabetes. Obstet Trans Lond 1882;**24**:256–85.
26. Herman GE: Diabetes and pregnancy. Edinb Med J 1902;**11**:119–23.
27. Offergeld H: Zuckerkrankheit und Schwangerschaft in ihren Wechselbeziehungen. Arch Gynäkol 1908;**86**:1160–209.
28. Joslin EV: Pregnancy and diabetes mellitus. Boston Med Surg J 1915;**173**:841–9.
29. Mauriceau F: Observations sur la grossesse et l'accouchement des femmes. Paris: Libraires Associés, 1738: Vol. **2**, p. 8, 42, 249.
30. White P: Pregnancy complicating diabetes. In: Joslin EP, Root HF, White P, and Marble A: The treatment of diabetes mellitus. 9. ed. London: Kimpton, 1952: p. 690–716.
31. Gluck L, Kulovich MV: Lecithin/sphingomyelin ratios in amniotic fluid in normal and abnormal pregnancy. Am J Obstet Gynecol 1973;**115**:539–46.
32. Brocard M: La glycosurie de la grossesse. Thèse de Paris, Paris. Compt Rend Soc Biol 1898;**7**(118).
33. Dubreuil G, Andérodias J: Ilots de Langerhans géant chez un nouveau-né issu de mère glycosurique. Compt Rend Soc Biol 1920;**83**:1490–3.

34. Gray SH, Feemster LC: Compensatory hypertrophy and hyperplasia of the islands of Langerhans in the pancreas of a child born of a diabetic mother. Arch Path Lab Med 1926;**1**:348–55.
35. Holzbach E: Diabetes und Schwangerschaft, hier besonders die hormonalen Beziehungen zwischen Mutter und Kind. Zentralbl Gynäk 1929;**53**:641–65.
36. Pack GT, Barber D: The placental transmission of insulin from fetus to mother. Am J Physiol 1930;**37**:271–4.
37. O'Sullivan JB: Gestational diabetes. N Engl J Med 1961;**264**:1082–5.
38. Higgons RA: Hypoglycemia in the new-born. Am J Dis Child 1935;**50**:162–5.
39. Harris DL, Weston PJ, Harding JE: Incidence of neonatal hypoglycemia in babies identified as at risk. J Pediat 2012;**161**:787–91.
40. Lucas A, Morley R, Cole TJ: Adverse neurodevelopmental outcome of moderate neonatal hypoglycaemia. BMJ 1988;**297**:1304–8.
41. Cornblath M, Hawdon JM, Williams AF, et al.: Controversies regarding definition of neonatal hypoglycemia. Pediatrics 2000;**105**:1141–5.
42. Jensen DM, Damm P, Moelsted-Pedersen L, et al.: Outcome in type 1 diabetic pregnancies: a nationwide, population-based study. Diabetes Care 2004;**27**:2819–23.
43. Evers IM, de Valk HW, Visser GH, et al.: Male predominance of congenital malformations in infants of women with type 1 diabetes. Diabetes Care 2009;**32**:1194–5.
44. Garne E, Loane M, Dolk H, et al.: Spectrum of congenital anomalies in pregnancies with pregestational diabetes. Birth Defects Res A Clin Mol Teratol 2012;**94**:134–40.
45. Cardell BS: The infants of diabetic mothers. A morphological study. J Obstet Gynecol Br Emp 1953;**60**:834–53.
46. Nevinny H, Schretter G: Zuckerkrankheit und Schwangerschaft. Arch Gynäkol 1930;**140**:397–427.
47. Otto AW: Monstrorum sex humanorum anatomica et physiologica disquisitio. Francofurti ad Viadrum: Apitz, 1811.
48. Behn HJ: De monopodibus. Dissertation inauguralis anatomico pathologica. Berolini: Augusti Petschii, 1827.
49. Hohl AF: Zur Pathologie des Beckens. Zwei Abhandlunge n. Leipzig: Engelmann, 1852.
50. Blumel J, Burke EE, Eggers GWN: Partial and complete agenesis or malformation of the sacrum with associated anomalies. J Bone Joint Surg 1959;**41A**:497–518.
51. Rusnak SL, Driscoll SG: Congenital spinal anomalies in infants of diabetic mothers. Pediatrics 1965;**35**:989–95.
52. Passarge E, Lenz W: Syndrome of caudal regression in infants of diabetic mothers: observations and further cases. Pediatrics 1966;**37**:672–5.
53. Banting FG, Best CH, Collip JB, Campbell WR, Fletcher AA: Pancreatic extracts in the treatment of diabetes mellitus. Preliminary report. Can Med Assoc J 1922;**12**:141–6.
54. Graham G: A case of diabetes mellitus complicated by pregnancy. Proc R Soc Med 1924;**17**:102–4.
55. Peters L: Report of results of insulin treatment in a case of pregnancy complicated by diabetes and funnel pelvis. Cal West Med 1925;**23**:1300–1.
56. White P: Pregnancy complicating diabetes. Am J Med 1949;**7**:609–16.
57. Feig DS, Gwee J, Shah BR, et al.: Trends in incidence of diabetes and serious perinatal outcomes. Diabetes Care 2014;**37**:1590–6.
58. Barker DJP, Winter PD, Osmond C, et al.: Weight in infancy and death from ischaemic heart disease. Lancet 1989;**II**:577–80.
59. Crume TL, Ogden L, Daniels S, et al.: The impact of in utero exposure to diabetes on childhood body mass index growth trajectories. J Pediatr 2011;**158**:941–6.
60. Damm P, Houshmand-Oeregaard A, Kelstrup L, et al.: Gestational diabetes mellitus and long-term consequences for mother and offspring. Diabetologia 2016;**59**:1396–9.

7.4

Filth, impurity, and threat
Meconium

Introduction: whence the impurity?

The term *meconium* for the thick, black-green matter that fills the fetal gut stems from the Greek word *mekon* (poppy juice, opium). In 350 B.C.E., Aristotle knew [1]: 'As soon as they are born they begin to cry and bring their hands to their mouth. They emit excrements, some immediately, others very soon, but all in the course of a day. This excrementitious matter is very abundant, considering the size of the child. Women call it the meconium. Its colour is like that of blood, and it is black and pitch-like. Afterwards it becomes milky, for the child immediately draws the breast.'

Romans called the newborn *sanguinolentus* (the blood-stained), and the *dies lustricus* (naming day) included rituals of purification (see Chapter 2.9). A century before oxygen was discovered, Michael Ettmüller believed that meconium is excreted immediately after birth [2], 'occasioned by the fresh air which rarifies and quickens the Blood and Spirits, and by consequence provokes the Stomach, Guts, and Bladder to expulsive Contractions'. Albrecht Haller explained the origin of meconium in 1779 [3]: 'All the excremental feces, which are collected in the fetus during the whole time of its residence in the womb, amount to no great quantity, as they are the remains of such thin nutritious juices, percolated through the smallest vessels of the uterus … But in the cavity of the intestines, there is collected together a large quantity of a dark green pulp, which may possibly be the remains of the exhaling juices.'

The following chapter addresses the real and imagined dangers associated with discharging meconium, and aims to explain the causes of hyperactivity in the context of these conditions.

Postnatal purgation

Not to be confused with cleanliness, purity is a religious term not defined by objective criteria, a spiritual status negotiated within societies. Impurity was a widespread status within the realm of sexuality, to which the newborn belonged. Rural Indian and other cultures dreaded the 'impurity and polluting effects of childbirth', and secluded mother and child [4]. In many religions, body secretions were regarded as impure or even dangerous, and meconium was the essence of impurity. Mother and child were secluded from society until meconium and lochial flows ceased. The Judeo-Christian concept of original sin reinforced the belief in the newborn's impurity.

Like many postnatal rituals, the custom to drive out the meconium was advantageous for the newborn by breaking the taboo on consuming the colostrum (see Chapter 6.1). Eighteenth-century authors asserted the meconium's dangerous potential, as did Michael Ettmüller in 1703 [2]: 'It is the Duty of Art to promote these Evacuations by exhibiting small quantities of a Mixture of solutive Syrup of Roses, Syrup of Cichory with Rhubarb and Sala's Emetic Syrup; and feeding it with the Beestings projected by Nature for that purpose.' *The Nurse's Guide* of 1729 had a different opinion of colostrum [5]: 'At this time (before this Refuse and Dregs of the blood are discharged), 'tis by no means proper to give them milk, for fear it should corrupt and curdle … A Decoction of Senna will gently carry off all the impurities that lie lurking in the most minute and remote Passages of the Body.'

Also lurking was an all-too-ready hyperactivity to remove the 'feculence' from the newborn's body. Laurence Heister, surgeon in Helmstedt, wrote in 1744 [6]: 'The newborn infants bring forth from their mother's womb an impurity called meconium, which is black and viscous filth, with which slime and other refuse stick on stomach and bowels. If not removed in time, it causes great aching and pain in the lower abdomen, (whereof they continuously whimper and cry), hiccups, jaundice, insomnia, unrest, nightmares, nay even seizures and nastiness, of which many infants die.' Friedrich Hoffmann, professor in Halle, reported in his textbook on newborn care in 1744 [7]: 'The Swedish women use purified cane sugar dissolved in sweet almond oil. French and Netherlands women give red wine with much sugar, and the Jews use honey mixed with butter.' This may have been derived from the prediction in Isaiah 7:14–15: 'Behold, a virgin shall conceive, and bear a son, and shall call his name Immanuel. Butter and honey shall he eat, that he may know to refuse the evil, and choose the good.'

William Buchan, physician at the Foundling Hospital at Ackworth, emphasized in 1769 [8]: 'The most proper medicine for expelling the meconium is the mother's milk, which is always, at first, of a purgative quality.' William Heberden Jr, physician at London's St George's Hospital, wrote in 1804 [9]: 'This should not be retained in the body, wherefore the first milk of all animals seems to have purgative ability. When two hours after birth nothing has been discharged, a dram of ricinus oil or three or four grains of rhubarb should be given ... often it is useful to apply an enema.' Anton Pieper, a visiting physician at the Paris Foundling Hospital for 6 months in 1829, criticized [10]: 'The custom of applying a laxative to each baby directly at admission to expel the meconium should not be neglected as a cause of thrush: each purgative irritates the very walls which it contacts.' The hunt is not over, in some Asian regions driving out the meconium remains routine care, and the glycerine clyster frequently used; various justifications were suggested or tested in clinical trials, including diminished jaundice [11] and improved feeding tolerance [12].

Fetal meconium passage, a bad omen

Obstetricians suspected the passage of meconium *before* birth to be threatening, as did Percival Willughby in 1672 [13]: 'I have observed that much moisture lying about the passage of the womb, doth much enfeeble the mother's expulsive faculty. It maketh the child sluggish, and the mother weake, and both their spirits drowned with humidity.' Cosme Viardel, surgeon in Paris, regarded prenatal meconium excretion a sign of fetal death in 1671 [14]: 'On the 10th August 1669 I delivered Mme Boulot ... My fingers stained with a blackish and saffron-like color, as is the usual aspect of *meconium*, the unclean humidity within the gut; therefore I recognized that the infant had voided the bowels and therefore must be dead.' This statement ignited vivid and persisting debates, not entirely academic, because declaring a fetus dead meant dismembering and extracting its parts with the hook. Mauriceau's response to Viardel reflects the competition among surgeons and midwives [15]: 'In this book, – which should rightly be called a cruel, horrible, malformed monster, a blind ogre that darkens the truth – he [Viardel] promotes a crude falsehood and error, which he then offers to the reader as irrefutable truth: namely that he claims it is a certain and undoubted sign of the unborn infant's death which nobody had observed before him, if it excretes meconium from its gut.' Hugh Chamberlen discreetly omitted this passage when translating Mauriceau's book into English in 1673 [16]. Guillaume Mauquest de la Motte, obstetrician in Valognes, tried to settle the controversy in 1722 [17]: 'In June 1686 I delivered ... The mother had voided much black matter ... The infant presented with the breech ... It is a near general rule that an infant is forced to evacuate when delivered from this position.' But the incorrect theory was in the world, often repeated, as by Michael Ettmüller 1703 [2]: 'Hence the voiding of 'em before Delivery is look'd upon as a Sign of a dead child: And their undue stay after the Birth taints the nourishment with a preternatural Acidity an is in good measure the Cause of all the tragical Symptoms that pursue our Infancy.'

Stuttgart obstetrician Christoph Völter wrote in 1722 [18]: 'The most certain sign [of the unborn child's death] is when from the anus a pitch-like matter escapes, though many infants die in whom this matter does not appear.' Paris Royal obstetrician André Levret ended the debate with a compromise in 1766 [19]: 'The child never excretes meconium while in its mother's womb except in extreme need, or when the body is compressed due to a bad position. When after the rupture of membranes the amniotic fluid is tainted by meconium, one can predict the infant will be born dead, but not in the second case [breech], in which it can be found living and well.'

Meconium aspiration

Meconium contains many substances derived from the digestive tract, such as desquamated cells, mucin, cholesterol, bile and bile acids, phospholipase, trypsin, lipase, and others [20, 21]. The highly active enzymes are not beneficial at all for the neonate's immature lung where meconium activates inflammatory mediators [22]. The vicious circle of meconium aspiration syndrome results, with the components mechanical obstruction, surfactant inactivation, atelectasis, and inflammation, which ultimately lead to hypoxia and pulmonary hypertension [23].

In 1798, Poul Scheel described seven stillborn or asphyxiated infants [24], whose trachea contained amniotic fluid, 'mixed with the content of the small intestine –chyme and mucus – and those of the large intestine, copious meconium'. Scheel already recommended intratracheal suctioning (see Chapter 2.4). In 1858 in Kiel, obstetrician Hermann Schwartz published observations on 59 cases of severe birth asphyxia [25]. He found discharged meconium before birth in two-thirds, and observed cases of severe meconium aspiration: 'Case 40: At 11 p.m. the membranes ruptured, and the amniotic fluid was discharged, very much mixed with meconium ... the female infant was apparently dead, began soon to breathe, but the respiration remained weak and rattling. She died one and a half hours after birth ... The post-mortem examination revealed well developed lungs, some parts containing air, some airless, trachea and bronchi were injected and filled with thick greenish mucus that could also be expressed out of the airless parts.'

Correctly associated with birth asphyxia, thick meconium in amniotic fluid was a threat for the newborn, although the frequency of meconium aspiration syndrome decreased during the 1990s, mainly due to fewer post-term deliveries [26]. But still in 2008, Avroy Fanaroff considered it a major problem [21]: 'An estimated 25,000 to 30,000 cases and 1,000 deaths related to meconium aspiration syndrome occur annually in the United States with many more cases in developing countries.' Much of the modern and persisting abhorrence of meconium may be due to this devastating disease. Some authors confused the harmless greenish staining of amniotic fluid that occurs in 10% of all deliveries, with the devastating 'pea-soup' aspiration of thick meconium. Despite lack of firm evidence, aggressive treatments relying on underpowered trials or anecdotal data were applied, such as corticosteroids, hyperventilation, tolazoline, suctioning of mouth and pharynx at birth, early laryngoscopy, lung lavage, inhaled nitric oxide, high-frequency oscillation, extracorporeal membrane oxygenation, and others. 'Expelling' the meconium, time-honoured since the 17th century, remained a form of hyperactivity to which Alex Robertson alluded ironically with the term 'the heroic years of neonatology' [27]. Only recently, meta-analyses of randomized trials yielded evidence on treating of meconium aspiration syndrome effectively [28, 29].

Meconium ileus and cystic fibrosis

The long-standing custom to withhold colostrum postponed meconium discharge for many infants, but for a special group of them, retained meconium proved disastrous. Hermann Boerhaave began his 1728 book on the diseases of children with the statement [30]: 'To new born Children happen Diseases peculiar to them, From the glutinous, caseous, and tough Filth, wherewith their Mouth, Gullet, Stomach, and Intestines are fill'd and obsessed.' Barthelemy Lafage wrote in 1812 [31]: 'This material, so useful for the fetus to maintain open the caliber of the gut, becomes very harmful in the baby who is born, if it is not expulsed within 24 hours after birth; it then acts like a foreign body and violent irritation.' In 1821, Antoine Dugès reported from the Paris Maternité an infant who died on the fifth day of life following meconium retention and distended belly [32]. The postmortem examination revealed 'a meconium-filled membraneous sac which had spirally convoluted around the ileum, strangling the gut' (Fig. 7.4.1, top right).

In 1859, George Barnes of Cheshire published the case of an infant who died at 48 hours of age, after 'no stool ... vomiting continually'. The postmortem examination revealed 'three to four inches upwards from the ileo-caecal valve, the contents of the bowel solid, and with difficulty protruded from the canal a mass large as a walnut ... death took place from the impaction of solid contents in the small bowel, immediately in front of the ileo-caecal orifice' [33] Later, Nobel Prize winner Karl Landsteiner described meconium ileus and correctly associated it with cystic fibrosis in 1905 [34] (Fig. 7.4.1): 'A flow of pancreas secretion is essential for the formation of normal meconium.' When tests were developed to quantify trypsin in duodenal fluid [20] and stool [35], it became obvious that most cases of meconium ileus and volvulus were caused by cystic fibrosis. The ΔF508 mutation on chromosome 7 that causes this disease occurred in Asia more than 52,000 years ago [36].

Meconium peritonitis

This disorder resulted when the dilated gut perforated during fetal life. In the abdominal cavity of a stillborn baby, Padovan anatomist Giovanni Battista Morgagni found in 1751 [37] 'a very great quantity of blood extravasated into the cavity of the belly ... all the intestines, and mesentery, which seem'd to be deficient, cover'd over with a pretty thick membrane'. Charles Billard, at the Paris Foundling Hospital, reported in 1828 [38] 'two infants who died during the first 24 hours of life ... with old and very firm adhesions between the gut's loops, and in one of them the anterior liver surface connected to the gut by four strong bands'. In Edinburgh, James Simpson encountered nine cases of fetal peritonitis in 1836–1838, compared their postmortem findings with 15 cases from the literature, and predicted cystic fibrosis with remarkable clairvoyance [39]: 'Peritonitis in the foetus ... may be excited by the derangements in some of the natural secretory and excretory actions of the foetal economy.' In 1850, Henrich described a case [40]: 'The child died on the fifth day. The postmortem examination showed the peritoneum transformed into a blackish paste ... stenosis 3 inches before the ileum ended.' From 1857, the St. Petersburg Foundling Hospital admitted 150,000

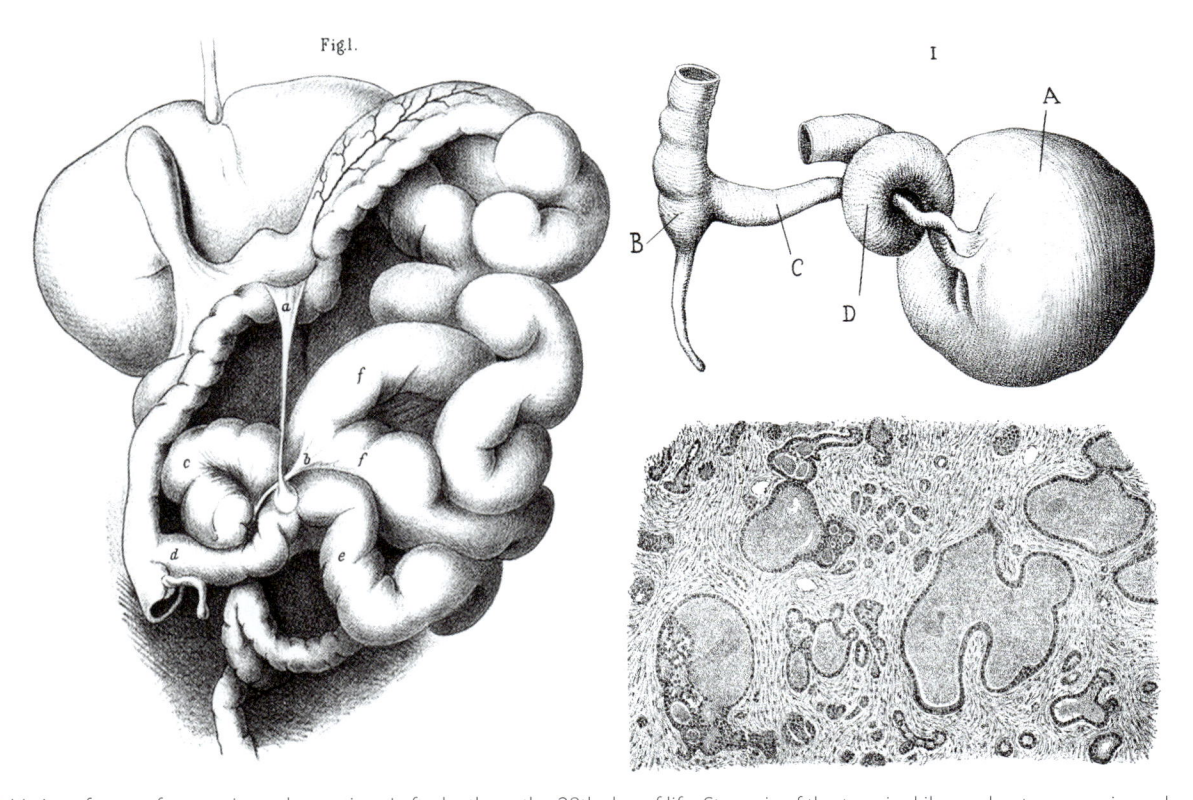

Fig. 7.4.1 Various forms of meconium obstruction. Left: death on the 28th day of life. Stenosis of the terminal ileum due to meconium plug, described by Theremin in 1877 [41]. Top right: death after 3 h of life. Malformation and peritonitis, published by Dugès 1821 [32]: A, sac filled with meconium; B, coecum and appendix; C, strangled ileum, lower end; D, spiral convolution of ileum (volvulus), upper part. Bottom right: death on fifth day of life. Meconium plug, the microscopic view of the pancreas shows dilated pancreatic ducts and cysts, published by Landsteiner 1905 [34].

newborn infants within 15 years. Among them, the physicians Karl Rauchfuß and Emil Theremin observed 12 cases of intestinal occlusion. Theremin believed the disorder to result from fetal peritonitis, not from malformation, and described strangulation by a peritoneal band (Fig. 7.4.1, left) [41].

Conclusion

Through the belief in birth-associated impurity, and analogous to menstrual blood and colostrum, meconium was loathed for being ugly, pathogenic, and dangerous. Like secluding mother and child, 'driving out' meconium was a millennium-old part of purification rites following birth, resulting in some protection for mother and baby. For centuries, 'expelling' the meconium was a postnatal routine with similarities to exorcism, or freeing the child from evil. The German term *Erbkoth* [42] was associated with *Erbsünde* (original sin). During the 'heroic' years of neonatology, invasive techniques were applied to remove meconium from the airways, a genuinely life-threatening condition, often without sound evidence or after underpowered, methodically flawed studies. Like cutting tongue-tie, shaping the head, and tight swaddling, the crusade against meconium was driven by the idea that something needs to be improved in the newborn.

REFERENCES

1. Aristotle: History of animals. In ten books. London: Bell, 1883: p. 191.
2. Ettmüller M: A compleat system of the theory and practice of physic (1st Latin ed. 1685). 2. ed. London: Bell & Wellington, 1703: p. 620–1.
3. Haller A: First lines of physiology. Edinburgh: Charles Elliot, 1779: p. 129, 461–6.
4. Bandyopadhyay M: Impact of ritual pollution on lactation and breastfeeding practices in rural West Bengal, India. Int Breastfeed J 2009;**4**:2.
5. Eminent Physician: The nurse's guide. London: Brotherton and Gilliver, 1729: p. 14.
6. Heister L: Practisches medicinisches Handbuch. Leipzig: Blochberger, 1744: p. 498.
7. Hoffmann F: Vernünfftiger Unterricht von heilsamer Vorsorge eines zur Welt gebohrenen und saugenden Kindes. Wittenberg und Zerbst: Zimmermann, 1744: p. 12–3.
8. Buchan W: Domestic medicine. Edinburgh: Balfour & Co, 1769: p. 578–9.
9. Heberden W: Morborum puerilium epitome. London: T. Payne, 1804.
10. Pieper PA: Die Kinderpraxis am Findelhause und in dem Hospital für kranke Kinder zu Paris. Göttingen: Dieterich, 1831: p. 187, 358.
11. Chen J, Ling U, Chen J: Early meconium evacuation: effect on neonatal hyperbilirubinemia. Am J Perinat 1995;**12**:232–4.
12. Shim S-Y, Kim H-S, Kim D-H, et al.: Induction of early meconium evacuation promotes feeding tolerance in very low birth weight infants. Neonatology 2007;**92**:67–72.
13. Willughby P: Observations on midwifery (1672). Edited from the original manuscript by: Henry Blenkinsop: Wakefield, Yorkshire: S.R. Publishers, 1972: p. 102, 120.
14. Viardel C: Anmerckungen von der weiblichen Geburt (1st French ed. 1671). Franckfurt: Zubrodt, 1676: p. 62.
15. Mauriceau F: Tractat von Kranckheiten schwangerer und gebärender Weibspersonen (1st French ed. 1668). Basel: Bertsche, 1680: p. 194, 226.
16. Mauriceau F: The accomplisht midwife, treating of the diseases of women with child. Translated by: Hugh Chamberlen: London: Darby, 1673.
17. Mauquest de la Motte G: Traité complet des accouchemens naturels, non naturels, et contre nature. Paris: Houry, 1722: p. 392–3, 636.
18. Völter C: Neueröffnete Hebammen-Schul. Stuttgart: Metzler, 1722: p. 153.
19. Levret A: L'art des accouchemens (1st ed. 1753). 3. ed. Paris: Didot Jeune, 1766: p. 76, 261, 445.
20. Hess AF: The pancreatic ferments in infants. Am J Dis Child 1912;**4**:205–18.
21. Fanaroff AA: Meconium aspiration syndrome: historical aspects. J Perinatol 2008;**28**:S3–7.
22. Lindenskov PHH, Castellheim A, Saugstad OD, Mollnes TE: Meconium aspiration syndrome. Neonatology 2015;**107**: 225–30.
23. Fox WW, Gewitz MH, Dinwiddie R, et al.: Pulmonary hypertension in the perinatal aspiration syndromes. Pediatrics 1977;**59**: 205–11.
24. Scheel P: Dissertation inauguralis de liquore amnii asperae arteriae foetuum humanorum. Hafniae: Christensen, 1798: p. 18–24, 48.
25. Schwartz H: Die vorzeitigen Athembewegungen. Ein Beitrag zur Lehre von den Einwirkungen des Geburtsactes auf die Frucht. Leipzig: Breitkopf und Härtel, 1858: p. 177.
26. Yoder BA, Kirsch EA, Barth WH, Gordon MC: Changing obstetric practices associated with decreasing incidence of meconium aspiration syndrome. Obstet Gynecol 2002;**99**:731–8.
27. Robertson AF: Reflections on errors in neonatology: II. The "heroic" years, 1950–1970. J Perinatol 2003;**23**:154–61.
28. Halliday HL, Sweer DG: Endotracheal intubation at birth for preventing morbidity and mortality in vigorous, meconium-stained infants born at term. Cochrane Database Syst Rev 2009;**1**:CD000500.
29. El Shahed AI, Dargaville PA, Ohlsson A, Soll R: Surfactant for meconium aspiration syndrome in term and late preterm infants. Cochrane Database Syst Rev 2014;**12**:CD002054.
30. Boerhaave H: Aphorisms (1st Latin ed. 1728). London: Bettesworth and Hitch, 1735: p. 396.
31. Lafage B: Essai sur les maladies des nouveau-nés. Paris: Didot Jeune, 1812: p. 14–5.
32. Dugès A: Recherches sur les maladies les plus importantes et les moins connues des enfans nouveau-nés. Paris: Baillière, 1821: p. 32–4, 66, fig. 1.
33. Barnes GR: Fatal obstruction of the bowel by meconium. Lancet 1859;**74**:663–4.
34. Landsteiner K: Darmverschluss durch eingedicktes Meconium: pankreatitis. Zentralbl Allg Pathol 1905;**16**:903–7.
35. Shwachman H, Patterson PR, Laguna J: Studies in pancreatic fibrosis. Pediatrics 1949;**4**:222–30.
36. Morral N, Bertranpetit J, Estivill X, et al.: The origin of the major cystic fibrosis mutation (DF508) in European populations. Nat Genet 1994;**7**:169–75.
37. Morgagni GB: The seats and causes of diseases investigated by anatomy (1st Latin ed. Venice 1761). London: Millar & Co, 1769: Vol. **3**, p. 567–8.

38. Billard CM: Traité des maladies des enfants nouveau-nés et a la mamelle (1st ed. 1828). 3. ed. Paris: Baillière, 1837: p. 478–84.
39. Simpson JY: Notices of cases of peritonitis in the fetus in utero. Edinb Med Surg J 1838;**15**:390–416.
40. Henrich: Innere Verwachsung des gewundenen Darms bei einem neugeborenen Kinde. Casper's Wochenschrift für die gesamte Heilkunde/Schmidt's Jahrbücher der gesammten Medizin 1850–1851:343.
41. Theremin E: Ueber congenitale Occlusionen des Dünndarms. Dt Zeitsch Chirurgie 1877;**8**:34–71.
42. Zückert JF: Unterricht für rechtschaffene Eltern, zur diätetischen Pflege ihrer Säuglinge. 2. ed. Berlin: Mylius, 1764.

7.5

Necrotizing enterocolitis
150 years of fruitless search for the cause

Introduction and epidemiology

Neonatal necrotizing enterocolitis (NEC) is an inflammatory disease of the gut with symptoms of abdominal distension, bilious vomiting, and bloody stools. It may proceed to septic shock, disseminated intravascular coagulation, peritonitis, and intestinal perforation. All parts of the gastrointestinal tracts may be involved, manifesting in multifocal haemorrhages, ulceration, and necroses. Almost exclusively a disorder of preterm infants, NEC was not acknowledged until special care units facilitated their survival. Presently, NEC has become the most common gastrointestinal emergency in neonates. This chapter focuses on the aetiology and diagnosis of NEC in preterm infants and omits discussion of animal models as well as prevention and therapy.

Early reports based on postmortem anatomy

In 1823, the Paris Athénée de Médecine offered a scientific prize to 'describe, following precise observations, the anatomic characteristics specific for inflammation of the gastrointestinal mucous membrane' [1]. The prize was won by the 24-year-old intern Charles Billard for his book entitled 'De la membrane muqueuse gastro-intestinale dans l'état sain et dans l'état inflammatoire'. At the Hôtel-Dieu of Angers he had not seen premature infants; the 81 observations in his 565-page book did not include neonatal NEC. But the prize, connected with membership to an academic society, allowed Billard to continue his medical training in Paris. He chose the Hôpital des Enfants Trouvés, which in 1826 admitted 5392 foundlings [2], giving him ample opportunity for clinical and postmortem observations in neonates. His next book [3] described a neonatal disease which he termed 'gangrenous enterocolitis': '50th observation. Caroline Jossey, nine days old, small and weak, is admitted to the ward for sick neonates on the 7th of November [1826]. She shows generalized redness of the integuments and oedematous extremities. The temperature of her skin is normal, her cry unaltered; her pulse irregular at a rate of 92 per minute. The infant has copious green-stained diarrhea. An intense perianal redness is noticed; the abdomen is swollen. On the 12th the green stool is mixed with streaks of blood ... On the 14th the infant yields a large amount of blood with the stool; her face is thin, livid and entirely distorted; she vomits the administered liquids; her extremities are cold and livid, her belly is tense; the heartbeat extremely slow; finally she dies in the evening yielding a large quantity of black liquid blood through the anus.—When opening the body on the next morning ... The duodenum is in healthy state, the terminal ileum is intensely red and swollen, its mucosa friable and the surface covered with blood. When these fluids are removed, the membrane looks rough and bloody; its surface furrowed by numerous wrinkles between which there are deep and black lines with the aspect of being burned by nitric acid. In addition to these blackish furrows, there are a large number of spots or ecchymoses with the same appearance in different regions of the colon. On these spots the mucosa is so soft that it turns to mash when scraped with the fingernail.'

Adam Elias von Siebold, directing the Obstetric Hospital of Berlin University since 1817, observed a preterm infant [4], which had some, but not all features of NEC: 'A stomach gangrenous at its small curvature with a perforation the size of a silver penny, containing a green liquid which, as the large curvature was unharmed, had not leaked into the peritoneal cavity. Also the duodenum's origin participated in the gangrenous metamorphosis ... It deserves mention that both from the mother's calculation and from the infant's aspect the birth had occurred about six weeks too early.'

Among 597 neonates admitted to the Vienna foundling hospital from 1846 to 1847, its director Alois Bednar [5] observed 25 infants with 'entero-colitis', of whom '8 were well nourished, 7 were premature and 10 were emaciated; 15 of them were between 3 to 10 days in age, four between 12 to 20 days, five between 22 to 30 days and one of 1 month and 22 days'. In 20 lethal cases, necropsy showed: 'The mucosa of small and large intestines swollen, injected, in the colon often a large number of millet-sized dirty-dark red spots ... In addition, the mucosa including the submucous tissue frequently corroded ... in many areas of the small intestine yellow-grey infiltrates with a tendency towards gangrene.' The critical scientist Bednar

---

Reproduced with permission from Obladen, M. Necrotizing enterocolitis—150 years of fruitless search for the cause. *Neonatology*, 96(4):203–210. Copyright © 2009 S. Karger AG, Basel

admitted: 'If we refrain from pure speculation, we are without any knowledge of a specific cause.'

Systematic observation in the first neonatal intensive care units

Arvo Ylppö, later director of the Helsinki University Children's Hospital, organized Germany's first special care unit for preterm infants at the Berlin Kaiserin Auguste Victoria Haus from 1912 to 1920, and described NEC in 1931 [6]: 'The mucosal hemorrhages and ulcers in some cases lead to bean-shaped swellings in certain sections of the small intestine. These swellings originate from extensive necrosis of the intestinal wall which gives way to increased gas pressure within the gut. From these necrotic parts of the gut easily arises peritonitis, and therefore it is not at all rare that we find peritonitis with hemorrhagic or purulent exsudation at postmortem examination of preterm infants. This is rarely diagnosed in vivo: It is so rapidly lethal, that the clinical symptoms are unspecific (vomiting, distended abdomen without clear tension of the abdominal wall).'

In 1907, Switzerland's first neonatal special care unit was founded—the Zurich Cantonal Infant Hospice Rosenberg. Heinrich Willi, its director since 1937, described 62 cases of 'malignant' enteritis occurring between 1941 and 1943 [7]: 'The following case is characteristic: Sch., Anna Lilli (J.-Nr. 159/40), born 10.6.1940, birthweight 1,110 g, vital. On the 2nd day of life severe oedema, spasmophilia, increasing icterus. On the 5th day asphyctic spell, recurring during the next day (heart malformation). At the beginning of July progressive pallor; stools become frequent, but did not raise concern as the infant nearly exclusively received wet nurses' milk. On the 8.7. vomiting; on the 11.7. ballooned, tense abdomen, bilious vomiting, decay, finally fecal vomiting. Death on the 12.7. Autopsy: Ulcerous and phlegmonous enteritis. Small intestine and coecum show numerous irregular round-oval defects with jagged and somewhat prominent margins, up to 8 mm in diameter. Enlarged mesenteric lymph glands. Fibrinous peritonitis. The heart shows hypoplasia of the tricuspid valve.' Among Willi's cases, 37 had a birthweight below 2500g; 12 were below 1500g. The disease occurred in clusters, as shown in Fig. 7.5.1, and he assumed: 'An indirect contact infection is most probable ... Our prophylactic measures had failed, due to the frequent overcrowding of our institution, which normally can provide for 44 infants.'

From 1948 to 1950, Kurt Schmidt and Karl Quaiser observed 85 mostly preterm infants in Graz, who died from a disease which they termed 'enterocolitis ulcerosa necroticans'. All had been breastfed [8, 9]: 'Pathoanatomically it is an exceptionally characteristic enterocolitis predominantly in the ileocoecum and the physiologic colon curvatures. It is frequently complicated by peritonitis due to transmigration or perforation. A specific pathogen could not be proven.' The distribution of necrotic lesions is shown in Fig. 7.5.2.

Before the advent of modern neonatal intensive care, NEC remained rare, as did the survival of very immature infants. Schaffer's 1965 issue of 'Diseases of the Newborn' did not mention it, and Beryl Corner, who in 1946 set up the preterm infants unit at Southmead Hospital in Bristol, emphasized [10]: 'We never saw a case of NEC prior to 1967, and we know it didn't exist, because of our very high postmortem rate and our very careful care of all babies. So we know it didn't exist, and seemed to occur when we started fairly extensive

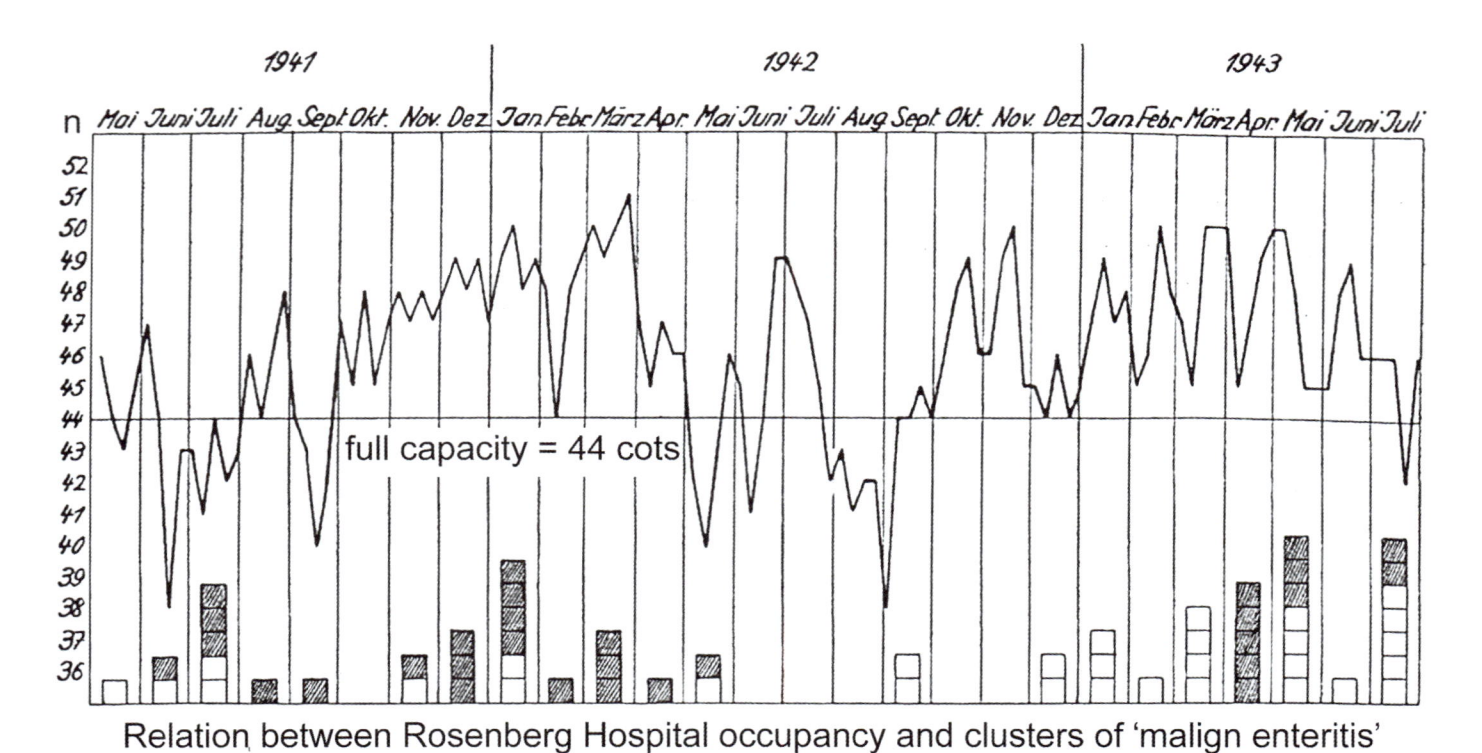

Fig. 7.5.1 Relation of occupancy in Willi's ward and occurrence of 'malignant' enteritis [7]. White squares, cases referred because of infection; hatched squares, in-house infection.
Adapted from Willi H: Über eine bösartige Enteritis bei Säuglingen des ersten Trimenons. *Ann Pediatr* 1944;162:87–112.

radiographic data to define three stages [19], which were further subdivided by Walsh and Kliegman [20], whose classification gained widespread acceptance. Paracentesis and lavage were proposed by Kosloske [21] to detect gangrene, peritonitis, and perforation.

Putative causes and pathogenesis

A frustrating aspect of NEC is the continuing lack of understanding of its aetiology, despite thoughtful and well-designed basic and clinical research for over a century. Clustering suggested nosocomial infection, with remarkable variation in incidence between hospitals [22]. An impressive list of aetiological proposals was published, some of which are shown chronologically in Table 7.5.1.

The disease became widely known when it attacked the New York Babies Hospital. A total of 64 neonates with NEC were observed from 1954 to 1974, prompting ten clinical papers from this institution. In addition to animal studies, they generated the hypothesis of mesenteric hypoperfusion as a major pathogenetic factor [28]: 'The noncontagious nature of the disease is evidenced by the lack of epidemics… All premature infants at Babies Hospital are fed cow's milk formula.' Santulli and co-workers specified [30]: 'Indirect injury to the mucosa may result from selective circulatory ischemia. This is the most acceptable theory of pathogenesis. It is supported by our clinical and pathological data.'

Most of the supposed pathogenetic factors featured in Table 7.5.1 act during the first days of life; NEC however, usually develops at two weeks of age and often catches by surprise infants who were postnatally stable and have left the intensive care unit when everyone believed the battle to be won. Monocausal explanations did not provide an accurate explanation of NEC's pathogenesis, and most researchers took refuge in more or less complex multifactorial models, as shown in Fig. 7.5.3 [47]. Immaturity, formula feeding, bowel ischaemia, diminished immune function, and infection with enterotoxin-producing bacteria all played a role, but their interaction and sequence remained elusive. It is remarkable that despite NEC's clinical similarity to clostridial infection, endemic occurrence, and different frequency among hospitals, only a few studies employed anaerobic culture techniques.

Related disorders and differential diagnosis

1. *NEC in term infants* accounts for less than 10% of cases. The onset is earlier and more rapid than in preterm infants, and predisposing disorders affecting the circulation are usually present. NEC in term infants has been linked to congenital heart disease and/or heart operation [48], perinatal asphyxia, polycythemia [49], exchange transfusion [50, 51], protracted diarrhoea with dehydration, maternal cocaine abuse, and exposure to HIV or antiretroviral medication.

2. *Appendicitis* has long been feared as a rare severe disorder of preterm infants: Isaac Abt, paediatrician at Chicago Northwestern University, found 20 cases under 3 months of age published before 1917 [52]. Additional cases were reported by Wilson [53], Engstrom [54], Meyer [55], Walker [56], and Hardman [57]. It is likely that this disease today is perceived as NEC.

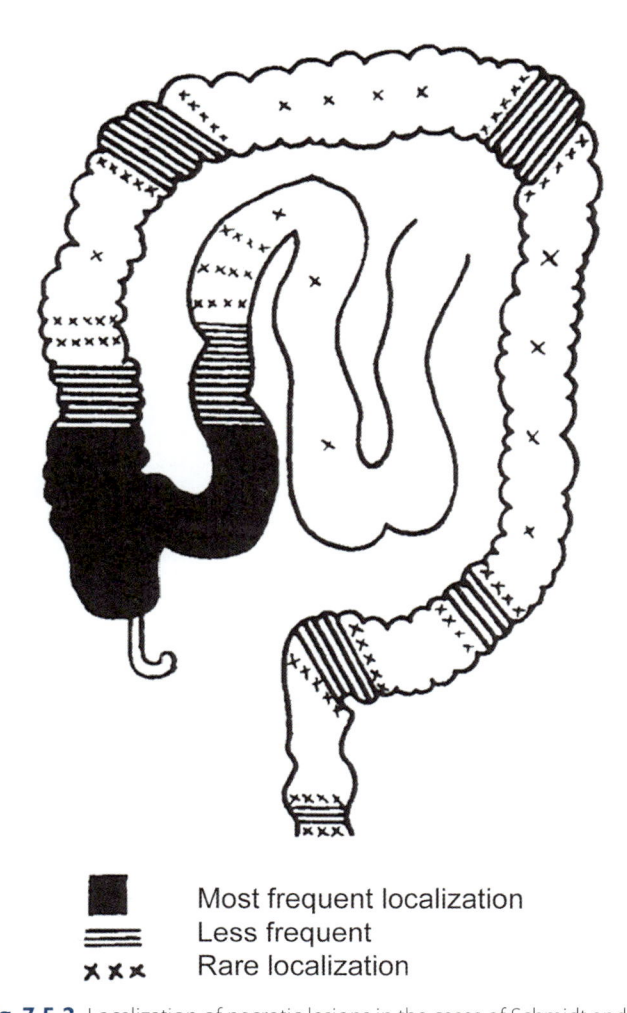

Fig. 7.5.2 Localization of necrotic lesions in the cases of Schmidt and Quaiser; black, frequent; hatched, less frequent; x, rare.
Adapted from Schmidt K: Über eine besonders schwer verlaufende Form von Enteritis beim Säugling, 'Enterocolitis ulcerosa necroticans.' I. Pathologisch-anatomische Studien. *Oesterr Z Kinderheilkd* 1952;8:114–136.

catheterization, venous catheterization, for all sorts of different purposes.' By the turn of the century, NEC had become the most important gastrointestinal emergency in infants worldwide, affecting 7% of very low birthweight infants in the US [11] and Canada [12] and killing approximately 500 infants per year in the US [13].

Diagnostic criteria

In 1899, Eugen Hahn observed pneumatosis intestinalis during a laparotomy [14]. In 1938, Botsford anatomically described it in six infants, among them a 4-week-old preterm infant [15]. Ann Arbor radiologist Arthur Stiennon saw pneumatosis on X-ray in 1951 [16] and proposed: 'From the mesenteric root gas can dissect, extend to the mesenteric insertion of the intestine and from here either dissect along the subserosal layers or, following the blood vessels…, enter the submucosa.' Pneumatosis portalis was described by Wolfe [17]; the whole spectrum of X-ray signs in NEC was characterized by Berdon [18]. In 1978, Bell combined historical, clinical, and

Table 7.5.1 Clinical series on preterm infants since Willi, with major suggestions for the pathogenesis of necrotizing enterocolitis

Proposed pathogenesis	Year	First author	Site	Cases	AC	Reference
Nosocomial infection	1944	Willi	Zurich	62	No	[7]
Air dissection at mesenteric root	1951	Stiennon	Ann Arbor	2	No	[16]
Endemic infection, probably virus	1952	Schmidt Quaiser	Graz, infants born 1948–1950	(85) 73	No	[8] [9]
Cluster within 53 days	1953	Refinetti	Sao Paulo	9	No	[23]
House endemy, viral	1955	Köttgen	Mainz	?	No	[24]
Endemic, ischaemia, Shwartzman reaction	1959	Rossier	Paris Hérold	15	No	[25]
Non-infectious aetiology, systemic hypoxaemia	1961	Singleton	Houston	10	Tns	[26]
Pseudomonas infection	1963	Waldhausen	Indianapolis	6	No	[27]
Reaction to endotoxin and deficient lysozyme; intestinal ischaemia; injury + bacteria + feeds	1964 1965 1967 1975	Berdon Mizrahi Touloukian Santulli	New York Babies', four reports, infants born since 1955	(21) (18) (25) 64	No Tns No Tns	[18] [28] [29] [30]
Mesenteric ischaemia, DIC	1969	Wilson SE	Los Angeles Children's	16	Tns	[31]
Circulation like reflex in diving mammals	1969	Lloyd	Detroit	87	No	[32]
Decreased mesenteric flow, umbilical/aortic catheters create spasm	1969 1970 1971 1971	Stevenson Hopkins Stevenson RS Bell	Seattle, four reports, infants born since 1962	(21) (13) (38) 43	No Tns No No	[33] [34] [35] [36]
Salmonella cluster	1972	Stein	Johannesburg	11	No	[37]
Endemic in summer, no agent found	1974	Virnig	St. Paul	21	Tns	[38]
Formula feeding, DIC, umbilical artery catheter	1975	Frantz	Minneapolis	54	No	[39]
Hyperosmolar feeding	1975	Book	Salt Lake City	16	No	[40]
Patent ductus arteriosus	1976	Siassi	Los Angeles USC	1	No	[41]
Gas-gangrene due to *Clostridium perfringens*	1976	Volsted Pedersen	Copenhagen	13	Yes	[42]
Clustering: enteric transmissible agent	1977	Book	Salt Lake City	74	No	[43]
Aetiology, pathophysiology unclear. Staging	1978	MJ Bell	St. Louis Children's Hospital	48	Yes	[19]
Clostridial infection in most severe cases	1978	Kosloske	Albuquerque	17	Yes	[44]
Indomethacin	1981	Nagaraj	Louisville	21	No	[45]
Intestinal flora changed by antibiotics	1982	Lawrence	Brisbane	2	No	[46]

AC, anaerobic culture from blood or peritoneal fluid; DIC, disseminated intravascular coagulation; no, no cultures reported; Tns, technique not stated.

3. *Focal intestinal perforation* was proposed to be different from NEC by Aschner and Deluga [58]. Also a disease of immature infants, it does not present with pneumatosis and the localized perforation is surrounded by normal tissue. Its pathogenesis is unknown as is that of NEC [59].

4. *Meconium plug/fetal peritonitis:* several commentators on this disease, which is not specific for preterm infants, were falsely credited for the 'first' NEC description. Simpson [60] published 23 instances of fatal peritonitis which began *in utero*; four other cases were reported by Zillner 1884 [61] and five more by the Prague pathologist Arnold Paltauf in 1888 [62]. Also, in Anton Genersich's much cited case of 1891, the perforation of the terminal ileum had occurred long before birth, the intraperitoneal masses were calcified, organized, and vascularized [63]. In 1905, ileus due to thickened meconium was correctly related to exocrine pancreatic insufficiency by former blood group discoverer and later Nobel Prize winner Karl Landsteiner in Vienna [64].

5. *Sepsis with ileus*: that neonatal sepsis can originate from the intestine was shown by Bonn obstetrician H. Cramer [65]. A pioneer in neonatology at Yale, Ethel Dunham showed that staphylococcal sepsis may trigger gastric perforation [66].

6. *Neonatal pseudomembranous colitis* is a complication of antibiotic treatment resulting from disrupted bacterial flora, overgrowth of *Clostridium difficile* in the colon, and release of toxins leading to mucosal damage and inflammation [67]. The pathogen's name alludes to painstaking culture techniques.

7. *Darmbrand (fire bowel)*: in 1918, Rudolf Jaffé described seven cases of lethal necrotizing and ulcerizing inflammation of the small intestine he had seen in severely undernourished Russian prisoners of war [68]. Expulsed from his Berlin chair of pathology in 1933, the Jewish scientist Jaffé escaped the Holocaust by emigrating to Venezuela, where he observed exactly the same necrotizing enteritis in cachectic natives in 1947 [69]. An epidemic of the same disease, termed 'darmbrand' was observed in northern Germany from 1946 to 1948, with 364 cases in Lübeck (among them 13 infants) and a high mortality [70–72]. It occurred in starving persons who had eaten a large meal. In 1948, Zeissler and co-workers found that darmbrand was due to *Clostridium perfringens* infection [73].

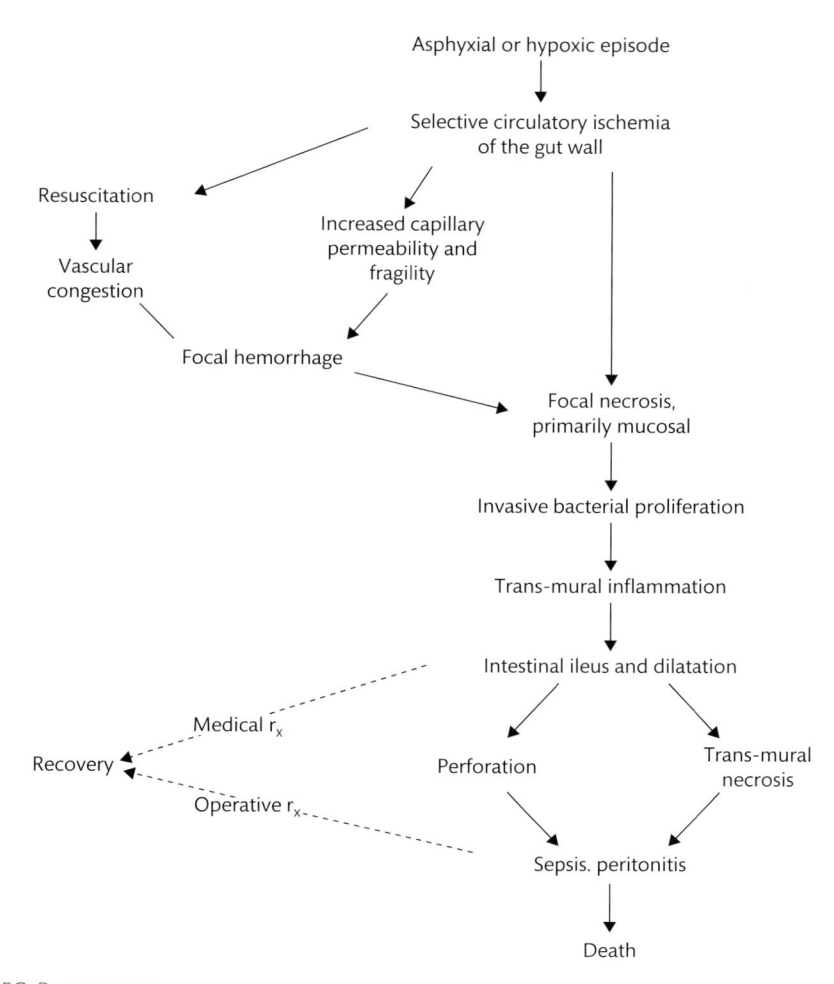

```
                    Asphyxial or hypoxic episode
                              │
                              ▼
                    Selective circulatory ischemia
                         of the gut wall
                    ↙         ↓         ↘
         Resuscitation   Increased capillary
              │          permeability and
              ▼             fragility
         Vascular              │
         congestion            ▼
              │         Focal hemorrhage
              └──────────────┐ │
                             ▼ ▼
                       Focal necrosis,
                       primarily mucosal
                              │
                              ▼
                   Invasive bacterial proliferation
                              │
                              ▼
                     Trans-mural inflammation
                              │
                              ▼
                    Intestinal ileus and dilatation
                    ↙         ↓         ↘
       Medical rₓ                      Trans-mural
  Recovery ◀─ ─ ─    Perforation        necrosis
           ◀─ ─ ─         ↘              ↙
       Operative rₓ      Sepsis. peritonitis
                              │
                              ▼
                            Death
```

Fig. 7.5.3 Pathogenesis of NEC. R$_x$, treatment.
Reproduced with permission from Touloukian, R., Posch, J., Spencer, R. The pathogenesis of ischemic gastroenterocolitis of the neonate. *J Pediatr Surg*, 7:194–205. Copyright © 1972 Elsevier.

8. *Pigbel* (*Enteritis necroticans*) is probably identical to darmbrand. It was published by Murrell and co-workers [74] to be the most frequent cause of death in children in the highlands of Papua New Guinea. Patchy enteral necrosis occurred after ritual pork feasts in protein-deprived persons who consumed sweet potatoes containing heat-stable trypsin inhibitors [75]. Given that the major source of defence against this toxin is adequate proteolysis in the gut, these children were specifically vulnerable to the beta toxins of *C. perfringens* contaminating the pork. The disease disappeared from New Guinea with beta toxoid vaccination. Pigbel has been observed in many underdeveloped regions and rarely in developed countries among diabetics [76, 77] and vegetarians [78]. Volsted Pedersen [42] first called attention to the striking clinical, radiological, and morphological similarities between pigbel and NEC.

Perspectives and conclusions

By 1978, most features of NEC had been described; however, despite extensive research no substantial progress has been made since then in understanding its pathogenesis. Surprisingly little effort has been made to distinguish NEC from other diseases and to elaborate its definition. Several related diseases are linked to enterotoxic clostridial infections, which were sometimes reported in NEC, but require anaerobic detection. NEC may be a pool of different disorders instead of a single entity. Although these disorders may lead to the same outcome, the underlying mechanisms vary greatly. It is unlikely that effective prevention will be established unless the disease is better understood.

REFERENCES

1. Billard CM: De la membrane muqueuse gastro-intestinale dans l'état sain et dans l'état inflammatoire. Paris: Gabon, 1825: p. IX.
2. Dupoux A: Sur les pas de monsieur Vincent. Paris: Revue de l'Assistance Publique, 1958.
3. Billard CM: Traité des maladies des enfants nouveau-nés et a la mamelle. Paris: Baillière, 1828: p. obs. 50.
4. Siebold AEv: Brand in der kleinen Curvatur des Magens eines atrophischen Kindes. J Geburtsh Frauenzimmer Kinderkrankh 1825;**5**:3–4.
5. Bednar A: Die Krankheiten der Neugeborenen und Säuglinge. Wien: Gerold, 1850: p. 101–3.

6. Ylppö A: Pathologie der Frühgeborenen einschließlich der "debilen" und "lebensschwachen" Kinder. In: Pfaundler M, Schlossmann A: Handbuch der Kinderheilkunde. 4. ed. Berlin: Vogel, 1931: Vol. **1**, p. 598.
7. Willi H: Über eine bösartige Enteritis bei Säuglingen des ersten Trimenons. Ann Pediatr 1944;**162**:87–112.
8. Schmidt K: Über eine besonders schwer verlaufende Form von Enteritis beim Säugling, "Enterocolitis ulcerosa necroticans." I. Pathologisch-anatomische Studien. Oesterr Z Kinderheilkd 1952;**8**:114–36.
9. Quaiser K: Über eine besonders schwer verlaufende Form von Enteritis beim Säugling, "Enterocolitis ulcerosa necroticans." II. Klinische Studien. Oesterr Z Kinderheilkd 1952;**8**:136–52.
10. Christie DA, Tansey EM: Origins of neonatal intensive care in the UK. London: Wellcome Trust, 2001: Vol. **9**, p. 24.
11. Guillet R, Stoll BJ, Cotten CM, et al.: Association of H2-blocker therapy and higher incidence of necrotizing enterocolitis in very low birth weight infants. Pediatrics 2006;**117**:e137–42.
12. Sankaran K, Puckett B, Lee DS, et al.: Variations in incidence of necrotizing enterocolitis in Canadian neonatal intensive care units. J Pediatr Gastroenterol Nutr 2004;**39**:366–72.
13. Holman RC, Stoll BJ, Clarke MJ, Glass RI: The epidemiology of necrotizing enterocolitis infant mortality in the United States. Am J Public Health 1997;**87**:2026–31.
14. Hahn E: Über pneumatosis cystoides intestinorum hominis und einen durch Laparotomie behandelten Fall. Dtsch Med Wochenschr 1899;**25**:657–60.
15. Botsford TW, Krakower C: Pneumatosis of the intestine in infancy. J Pediatr 1938;**18**:185–94.
16. Stiennon OA: Pneumatosis intestinalis in the newborn. Am J Dis Child 1951;**81**:651–63.
17. Wolfe JN, Evans WA: Gas in the portal vein of the liver in infants. Am J Roentgenol 1955;**74**:486–9.
18. Berdon WE, Grossman H, Baker DH, et al.: Necrotizing enterocolitis in premature infants. Radiology 1964;**83**:879–87.
19. Bell MJ, Ternberg JL, Feigin RD, et al.: Neonatal necrotizing enterocolitis. Therapeutic decisions based upon clinical staging. Ann Surg 1978;**187**:1–7.
20. Walsh MC, Kliegman RM: Necrotizing enterocolitis: treatment based on staging criteria. Pediatr Clin North Am 1986;**33**:179–201.
21. Kosloske AM, Lilly JR: Paracentesis and lavage for diagnosis of intestinal gangrene in neonatal necrotizing enterocolitis. J Pediatr Surg 1978;**13**:315–20.
22. Brown EG, Sweet AY: Neonatal necrotizing enterocolitis. New York: Grune and Stratton, 1980: p. 14.
23. Refinetti P, De Carvalho Pinto VA, Morales R de V: Perfuracao intestinal em recém-nascidos prematuros. Pediat Pratica (Sao Paulo) 1953;**24**:219–30.
24. Köttgen U, Braun E, Wengler G: Endemische ulzeröse Enteritis bei Frühgeborenen. Mschr Kinderhk 1955;**103**:226–30.
25. Rossier A, Sarrut S, Delplanque J: L'enterocolite ulcéro-nécrotique du prématuré. Ann Pédiatr 1959;**35**:1428–36.
26. Singleton EB, Rosenberg HM, Samper L: Radiologic considerations of the perinatal distress syndrome. Radiology 1961;**76**:200–12.
27. Waldhausen JA, Herendeen T, King H: Necrotizing colitis of the newborn. Surgery 1963;**54**:365–72.
28. Mizrahi A, Barlow O, Berdon WE, et al.: Necrotizing enterocolitis in premature infants. J Pediatr 1965;**66**:697–705.
29. Touloukian RJ, Berdon WE, Amoury RA, Santulli TV: Surgical experience with necrotizing enterocolitis in the infant. J Pediatr Surg 1967;**2**:389–401.
30. Santulli TV, Schullinger JN, Heird WC, et al.: Acute necrotizing enterocolitis in infancy. Pediatrics 1975;**55**:376–87.
31. Wilson SE, Woolley MM: Primary necrotizing enterocolitis in infants. Arch Surg 1969;**99**:563–6.
32. Lloyd JR: The etiology of gastrointestinal perforations in the newborn. J Pediatr Surg 1969;**4**:77–84.
33. Stevenson JK, Graham CB, Oliver TK, Goldenberg VE: Neonatal necrotizing enterocolitis: a report of 21 cases with fourteen survivors. Am J Surg 1969;**118**:260–72.
34. Hopkins GB, Gould VE, Stevenson JK, Oliver TK: Necrotizing enterocolitis in premature infants. Amer J Dis Child 1970;**120**:229–32.
35. Stevenson JK, Oliver TK, Graham CB, et al.: Aggressive treatment of neonatal necrotizing enterocolitis. J Pediatr Surg 1971;**6**:28–35.
36. Bell RS, Graham CB, Stevenson JK: Roentgenologic and clinical manifestations of neonatal necrotizing enterocolitis. Am J Roentgenol 1971;**112**:123–34.
37. Stein H, Geck J, Solomon A, Schmaman A: Gastroenteritis with necrotizing enterocolitis in premature babies. BMJ 1972;**2**:616–9.
38. Virnig NL, Reynolds JW: Epidemiological aspects of neonatal necrotizing enterocolitis. Am J Dis Child 1974;**128**:186–90.
39. Frantz ID 3rd, L'Heureux P, Engel R, Hunt CE: Necrotizing enterocolitis. J Pediatr 1975;**86**:259–63.
40. Book LS, Herbst JJ, Jung AL: Necrotizing enterocolitis in infants fed an elemental formula. J Pediatr 1975;**87**:602–5.
41. Siassi B, Blanco C: Patent ductus arteriosus. Pediatrics 1976;**57**:347–51.
42. Volsted Pedersen P, Hart Hansen F, Halveg AB, et al.: Necrotizing enterocolitis of the newborn—is it gas-gangrene of the bowel? Lancet 1976;**398**:715–6.
43. Book LS, Overall JC, Herbst JJ, et al.: Clustering of necrotising enterocolitis. N Engl J Med 1977;**297**:984–6.
44. Kosloske AM, Ulrich JA, Hoffman H: Fulminant necrotising enterocolitis associated with clostridia. Lancet 1978;**312**:1014–6.
45. Nagaraj HS, Sandhu AS, Cook LN, et al.: Gastrointestinal perforation following indomethacin therapy in very low birth weight infants. J Pediatr Surg 1981;**16**:1003–7.
46. Lawrence G, Bates J, Gaul A: Pathogenesis of neonatal necrotising enterocolitis. Lancet 1982;**1**:137–9.
47. Touloukian R, Posch J, Spencer R: The pathogenesis of ischemic gastroenterocolitis of the neonate. J Pediatr Surg 1972;7:194–205.
48. Polin RA, Pollack PF, Barlow B, et al.: Necrotizing enterocolitis in term infants. J Pediatr 1976;**89**:460–2.
49. Gunn T, Outerbridge E: Polycythemia as a cause of necrotizing enterocolitis. Can Med Assoc J 1977;**117**:438.
50. Corkery JJ, Dubowitz V, Lister J, Moosa A: Colonic perforation after exchange transfusion. BMJ 1968;**4**:345–9.
51. Friedman AB, Abellera RM, Lidsky I, Lubert M: Perforation of the colon after exchange transfusion in the newborn. N Engl J Med 1970;**282**:796–7.
52. Abt IA: Acute appendicitis in infancy. Arch Pediatr 1917;**34**:641.
53. Wilson WE: Appendicitis in the newborn. Proc R Soc Med 1945;**38**:186–7.
54. Engstrom CQ: Acute appendicitis in a premature infant aged 3 weeks. Acta Paediatr 1949;**37**:355–8.
55. Meyer JF: Acute gangrenous appendicitis in a preterm infant. J Pediatr 1952;**41**:343–5.
56. Walker RH: Appendicitis in the newborn infant. J Pediatr 1957;**51**:429–34.
57. Hardman RP, Bowerman D: Appendicitis in the newborn. Am J Dis Child 1963;**105**:99–101.

58. Aschner JL, Deluga KS, Metlay LA, et al.: Spontaneous focal gastrointestinal perforation in very low birth weight infants. J Pediatr 1988;113:364–7.
59. Mintz AC, Applebaum H: Focal gastrointestinal perforations not associated with necrotizing enterocolitis in very low birth weight neonates. J Pediatr Surg 1993;28:857–60.
60. Simpson J: Notices of cases of peritonitis in the foetus in utero. Edinb Med Surg J 1838;15:390–414.
61. Zillner E: Ruptura flexurae sigmoidis neonati inter partum. Virchows Arch Path Anat 1884;96:307–18.
62. Paltauf A: Die spontane Dickdarmruptur der Neugeborenen. Virchows Arch Path Anat 1888;111:461–74.
63. Genersich A: Bauchfellentzündung bei Neugeborenen in Folge von Perforation des Ileums. Virchows Arch Path Anat 1891;126:485–93.
64. Landsteiner K: Darmverschluss durch eingedicktes Meconium: pankreatitis. Zentralbl Allg Pathol 1905;16:903–7.
65. Cramer H: Gibt es vom Darm ausgehende septische Infektionen bei Neugeborenen? Arch Kinderheilk 1905;42:321–7.
66. Dunham EC, Shelton MT: Multiple ulcers of the stomach in a newborn infant with staphylococcus septicemia. J Pediatr 1934;4:39–43.
67. Donta ST, Stuppy MS, Myers MG: Neonatal antibiotic-associated colitis. Am J Dis Child 1981;135:181–2.
68. Jaffé R: Über nekrotisierende und ulceröse Entzündungen im Dünndarm. Med Klin 1918;14:904–12.
69. Jaffé R: Über nekrotisierende und ulceröse Entzündungen im Dünndarm (sog. Darmbrand). Virchows Arch Path Anat 1950;318: 23–31.
70. Jeckeln E: Über Darmbrand. Dtsch Med Wochenschr 1947;72: 105–8.
71. Hansen K, Jeckeln E, Jochims J, et al.: Darmbrand (enteritis necroticans). Stuttgart: Thieme, 1949: p. 65; figs. 22, 46.
72. Fick KA, Wolken AP: Necrotic jejunitis. Lancet 1949;253: 519–21.
73. Zeissler J: Zur Ätiologie der nekrotisierenden Enterocolitis. Med Klin 1948;43:341–3.
74. Murrell TGC, Roth L, Egerton J, et al.: Pig-bel: Enteritis necroticans. Lancet 1966;287:217–22.
75. Murrell TGC, Walker PD: The pigbel story of Papua New Guinea. Trans R Soc Trop Med Hyg 1991;85:119–22.
76. Severin WP, de la Fuente AA, Stringer MF: Clostridium perfringens type C causing necrotising enteritis. J Clin Pathol 1984;37: 942–4.
77. Petrillo TM, Beck-Sague CM, Songer JG, et al.: Enteritis necroticans (pigbel) in a diabetic child. N Engl J Med 2000;342:1250–3.
78. Farrant JM, Traill Z, Conlon C, et al.: Pigbel-like syndrome in a vegetarian in Oxford. Gut 1996;39:336–7.

7.6

Better baby bones
Attacking rickets and scurvy

Introduction

Evolution deprived us of our hairy coat when we migrated northwards after the Ice Age 20,000 years ago. We also lost our skin pigmentation while leaving Africa: white skin synthesizes vitamin D much faster than dark skin [1]. Enabling rapid growth during infancy, the newborn's skeleton, especially the long bones, are not yet fully mineralized, and the metabolically active epiphyseal growth zone is vulnerable to disease. During the 17th century, urbanization and female work in factories promoted malnutrition and a decline in breastfeeding. Its combination with smog-polluting use of brown coal and the crowding of poor people in the narrow streets of northern cities set the stage for an epidemic of infantile bone disease. The English literature of rickets was reviewed by Alfred Hess [2] and Mary Weick [3], and that of scurvy by Hess [4] and Elizabeth Lomax [5]. Focusing on the early literature, this chapter delineates causes of frequent bone diseases of infants and explains the coming and going of these diseases during the last four centuries.

Understanding rickets

Rickets is a lingering and usually painless disease of infancy caused by vitamin D deficiency and leading to bone deformities. It has been known since antiquity, but was rare. Soran's observation in the 2nd century C.E initiated the long-standing habit of tight swaddling [6]: 'If the child is too prone to stand up and desirious of walking, the legs may become distorted in the region of the thighs. This is observed to happen particularly in Rome; as some people assume, because cold waters flow beneath of the city and the bodies are easily chilled all over … When the child first begins to sit, one should support it by clothes or prop it up by holding it at its sides.' Seventeenth-century authors did not discern rickets, scurvy, and connatal syphilis, but related bone deformities to wrong swathing, and Jacques Guillemeau [7] admonished the nurses in 1620 'not to make him worse and deformed or misshapen … for in swathing they often bind and crush him so hard that they make him grow crooked … and make his ribs and breast stand out … and crooked legs, growing either inward or outward with their knees'.

Daniel Whistler, a British student, graduated in Leiden in 1645 under Joh. Polyander Kerchoven with a 14-page dissertation on 'The Rickets' [8]. He claimed the disease originated in England during 1619 and listed the following symptoms: (1) tension of the abdomen; (2) swelling of the ankles; (3) knots on the cartilaginous parts of the ribs; (4) all bones being soft as wax, bending under the body's weight; (5) enlarged head and sometimes hydrocephaly; (6) weakness and softness of skin and muscles; (7) delayed dentition; and (8) deformed chest wall. Whistler mentioned postmortem findings, believed the disease to result from slow moving circulation, and described its differences from scurvy and syphilis. His treatment proposals included king fern, raven's and frog's liver, and snail extract. In 1649, Arnold Boate, a Dutchman who lived in Dublin, described deformities of the chest and sternum under the term *tabes pectorea* [9], associated with bowed legs, deformed hips, and contracted pelvis, and believed the disease originated in the liver. In his 416-page monograph, Cambridge professor Francis Glisson described both rickets and scurvy in 1650 [10], listing many treatments and causes, including exposure to cold and deprivation of mother's milk. In 1669, John Mayow studied rickets in Oxford [11], concluding that the traction by muscles combined with the softness of bones caused the latter's deformities (Fig. 7.6.1). An oblique pelvis caused difficult birth, as described by Percival Willughby in Derby in 1672 [12] in a woman 'not well framed in the position of her [pelvic] bones. It was her sorrowful mishap always to have her children drawn away from her body by a chirurgion, that used to lay women … She had been afflicted, in her infancy, with the rickets. Shee had very great, swel'd ancle-bones, she went wadling, and her left leg was shorter than the other, and the middle of her back was much inverted.' A century later, Johann Böttcher stated in Königsberg in 1792 [13]: 'An evil complication [of the English disease] is a deformed pelvis in girls, which later hinders births.' In 1878, oblique pelvis remained the most frequent cause of difficult delivery when Karl Schröder classified 'rickety pelvises' from a Bonn collection of mothers who had died in childbirth [14] (Fig. 7.6.2).

An air-pollution disease rather than a vitamin deficiency, the rickets epidemic began with industrialization and urbanization during the 17th century. Breast milk contains five times more vitamin D than cow's milk, but the amount is still so low that sunlight irradiation is required to form the active

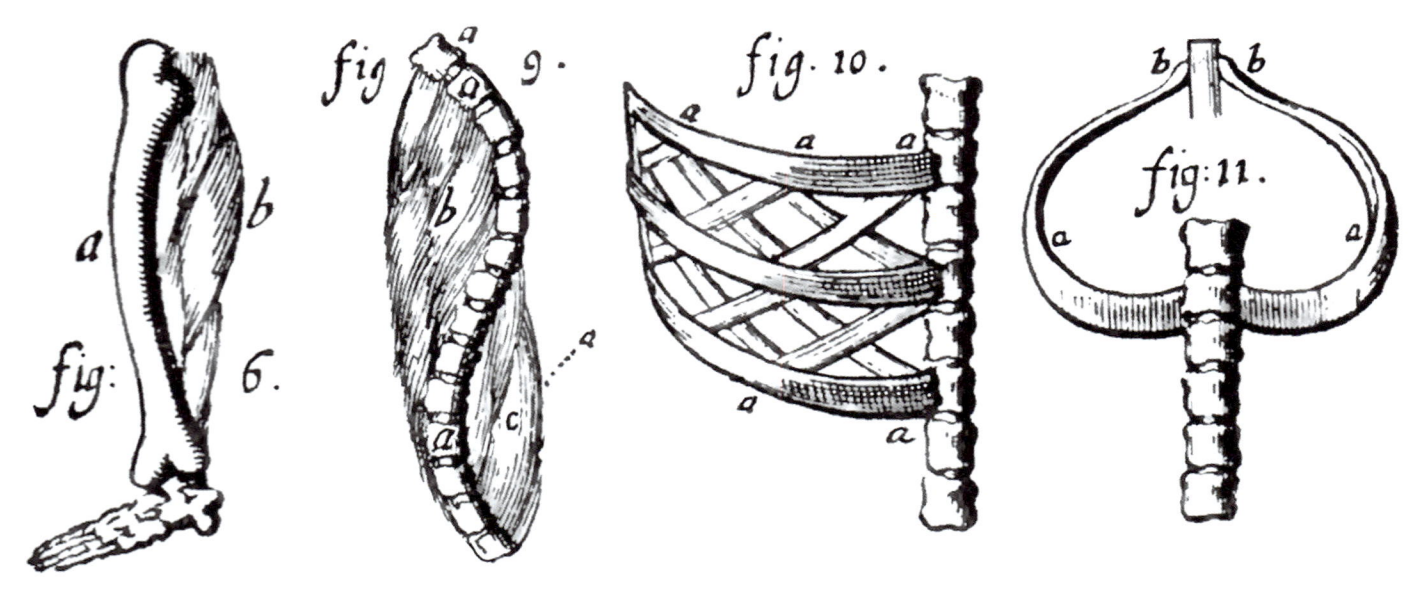

Fig. 7.6.1 Skeletal bending and mode of action depicted by John Mayow in 1674 as pathogenesis of rickets [11].

compound 1,25-dihydroxy-cholecaliciferol. City physician Georg Wendelstadt reported from his home town Wetzlar in 1801 [15]: 'Wetzlar has become famous by rickets: there are entire streets wherein house after house the wretched crippled by rickets are found... Rickets is a disease that affects children only between the ages of one and two years... According to our custom they are fed with pap and starch even in earliest infancy; as much is put in as can be forced down... the children must sit indoors, their digestion suffers severely... which ends in death, or if they continue to live, they develop thick joints, cease to be able to walk or have deformed legs. The head becomes large and the vertebral column bends.'

In 1843, Carl Ludwig Elsässer recognized seizures and craniotabes (softness of the occipital bones) as symptoms of rickets [16], uncertain, however, before age 4 months and in prematures [17]. In 1921, seizures were so frequent that Finkelstein described rickets

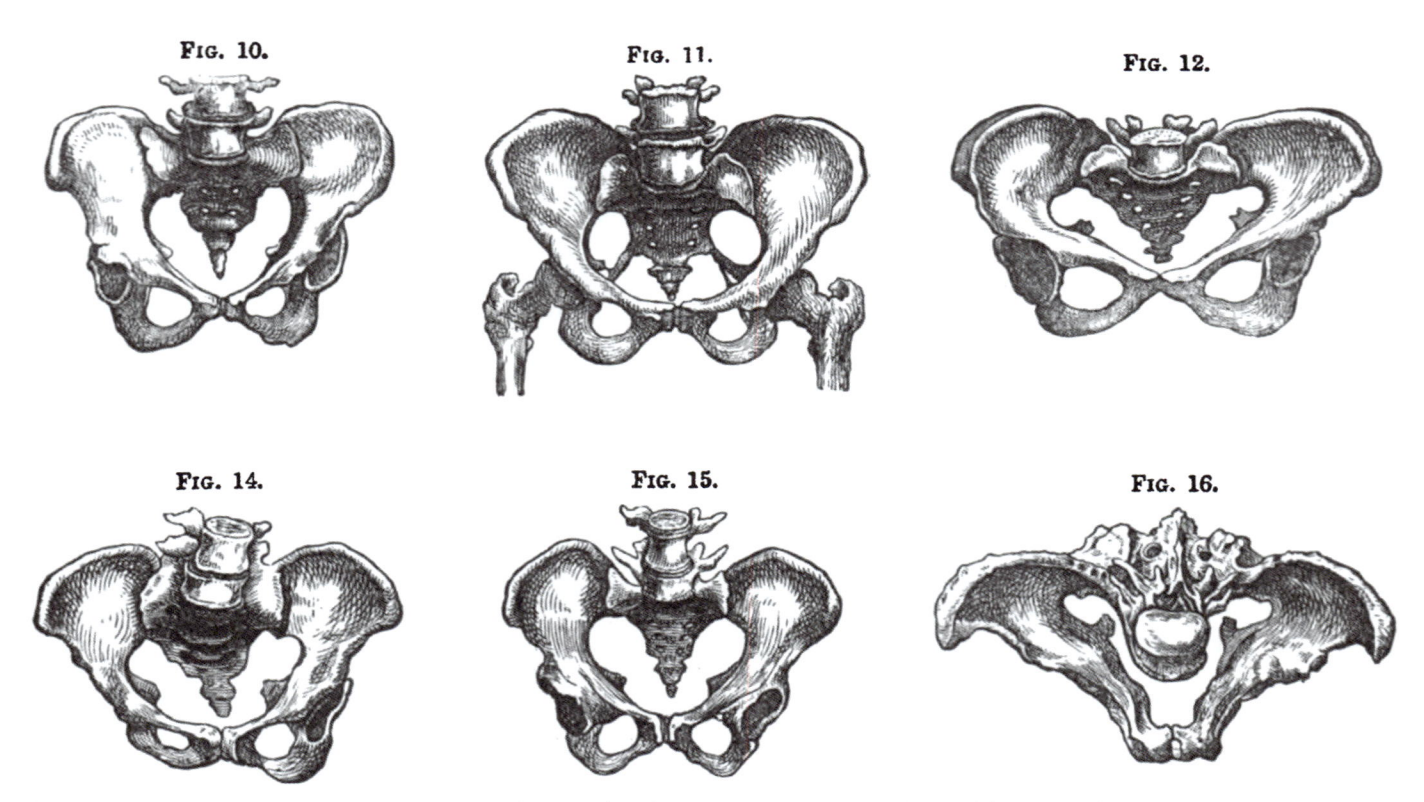

Fig. 7.6.2 Contracted rickety pelvises with obstetric diameters less than 9.5 cm. From women deceased during childbirth at the Bonn hospital, collected by Karl Schröder in 1873 [14].

under the heading *spasmophilia* [18]. Whereas most 19th-century authors equated fresh air and sunlight as beneficial for rickets, Theobald Palm, a medical missionary of Wigton, Cumbria, published a careful study in 1890 [19]: 'During my residence of over 9 years in Japan, in the course of which several thousands of patients came under observation ... I am unable to recall a well-marked case of rickets.' He made an inquiry among missionaries in China, Mongolia, India, Morocco, Sri Lanka (then Ceylon), and so on, and found that tropical 'countries which are grossly negligent of ordinary hygienic precautions, though they pay the penalty in other ways, are not scourged by rickets'. Palm proposed 'systematic use of sun-baths as a preventive and therapeutic measure in rickets' and foresaw that 'physiological chemistry may one day be able to inform us exactly what products of animal organisms are promoted by the action of sunlight'.

Ernst Buchholz from Hamburg reported successful treatment of 16 rickety children with electric light irradiation ('*Glühlicht*') in 1904 [20]. In 1921, 'fully three quarters of the infants in the great cities, such as New York, exhibit rachitic signs in some degree' [21]. From experiments with dogs, Edward Mellanby concluded in 1919 [22]: 'Rickets is a condition primarily due to the lack of an accessory factor in the diet.' In 1922, Elmer McCollum and co-workers in Baltimore demonstrated that the antirachitic activity of cod liver oil could survive both aeration and heating to 100°C and was not identical to vitamin A [23]. Vitamin D turned out to be a steroid hormone when analysed by Adolf Windhaus in 1930 [24].

Treating and preventing rickets

Cod liver oil was a popular nutrient among fishermen in many countries, and used as a remedy before the 18th century [25]. Thomas Percival of Manchester recommended it in 1771 to treat 'rheumatism' [26]. D. Schütte from Ründeroth near Cologne (then a vassal state of France) used it from 1814 for childhood rickets [27]. In France, cod liver oil was introduced to treat rickets in 1827 by Pierre Bretonneau [28]. With X-rays, a tool evolved enabling reliable diagnosis of rickets. On 25 January 1896, 2 days after Conrad Roentgen had presented his invention to the public, Gustav Gärtner, Vienna, used X-rays to diagnose rickets in a 4-year-old boy [29]. An X-ray apparatus, a 'generous gift from an unnamed lady,' was used in 1897 by Theodor Escherich at the Graz Foundling Hospital to monitor treatment with cod liver oil and phosphorus [30] (**Fig. 7.6.3**, left). World War I brought hunger and misery to children all over Europe and ample opportunity to study both rickets and scurvy of infancy [31, 32]. In autumn 1919, the London Lister Institute sent a group

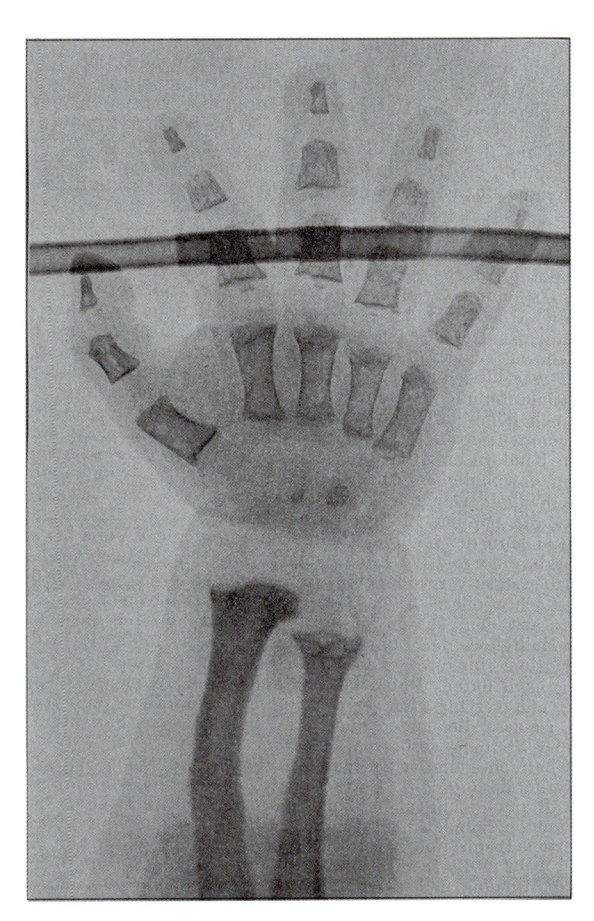

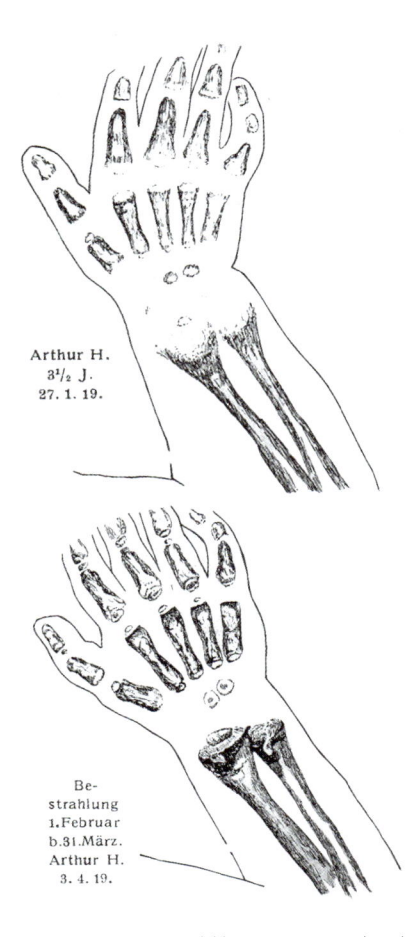

Fig. 7.6.3 Left: X-ray photograph taken on 3 April 1897 showing Franz Mauerhofer's left hand. The 2-year-old boy was treated with phosphorus and cod liver oil at the Anna Childrens' Hospital in Graz by Theodor Escherich [30]: 15 months after Röntgen's first publication and a few months after commercially produced X-ray apparatuses became available, this image shows osteolysis and cupping, fingers are fixed by a rubber band. Right: X-ray drawings of 1919 by Kurt Huldschinski of Arthur H's right hand before (top) and after (bottom) treatment with ultraviolet light [35].

of female researchers directed by Harriette Chick to Vienna to study and alleviate the rickets epidemic [33]. The ladies soon confirmed the therapeutic success of vegetables, fruit juice, and cod liver oil [34]. In post-war Berlin, Kurt Huldschinsky irradiated rickety infants with a mercury vapour lamp in 1919. Even without cod liver oil 'which is presently expensive and difficult to obtain … after two months of irradiation, the miserable, flaccid and delicate infants had become fresh and vigorous, they could all sit free and lift their head in the prone position' [35] (Fig. 7.6.3, right). Two days before signing the Versailles treaty, a German paper was appreciated reluctantly, a typical example of an untimely publication. In 1934, Huldschinsky, declared to be a Jew in 1933, emigrated to Egypt, where he died in 1940 [36]. Ultraviolet light therapy was reinvented by Alfred Hess in New York, who fed guinea-pigs irradiated phytosterol and wrote in 1925 [37]: 'It would seem quite possible that the cholesterol in the skin is normally activated by ultra-violet irradiation and rendered antirachitic … This point of view regards the superficial skin as an organ which reacts to particular light waves rather than as a mere protective covering.' With vitamin D fortification of baby formula, rickets disappeared, but a great part of the population remained vitamin D deficient [38].

Understanding infantile scurvy

Unlike rickets, scurvy is an acute and painful disease caused by vitamin C deficiency, with high mortality due to haemorrhages. Since antiquity, it was dreaded as a near-epidemic scourge among sailors, prisoners, armies, and besieged cities. In Germany, the disease was called Scharbock, in the Netherlands Scheurbuik. Infantile scurvy was rare before the 17th century, when most infants who were not breastfed died from gastroenteritis. A few cases from the Early Bronze Age have been unearthed in Britain [39], and a considerable proportion of children's skeletons of the 9th century C.E from Castel Tirolio, Italy, revealed bone lesions highly consistent with scurvy [40]. Greater numbers of infantile scurvy were observed and described in foundling hospitals and asylums, in wartime, and in regions where infants were breastfed for a short time only. Swelling, bleeding, and gum ulcers, associated with seizures and high mortality, were related to teething (see Chapter 6.11), and scurvy was misdiagnosed as *scrophula* or 'king's evil.' In Britain, scurvy seems to have masqueraded as 'difficult teething' or 'gangrene of the mouth,' as Still remarked [41], 'when the purple swelling over a tooth just coming was really due to the haemorrhage of infantile scurvy'. In 1702, Bartholomaeus Saviard, for 17 years surgeon at the Paris Hôtel-Dieu, wrote a chapter 'On scurvy … epidemic in the hospitals of the large cities', and distinguished infantile ('which attacks the gums and then proceeds to the muscles') and adult forms ('with black or livid spots on the legs and lower abdomen') [42]. William Cadogan reported from the London Foundling Hospital in 1750 [43]. 'Breeding teeth has been thought to be, and is, fatal to many children.' At the Hôtel-Dieu Hospital. M. Berthe observed 'scorbutic gangrene of the gums in infants' in 1754 [44], associated with 'extensive skin bleeding along the legs … could not be touched without causing pain'. Charles de Mertans reported from St. Petersburg in 1778 [45]: 'In the Foundling Hospital of which I was a physician, there were every winter many scorbutic infants … The usual symptoms were swelling of the gums, the nauseous breath, a great weariness and exhaustion; they used to become cachectic, and of a leaden colour … the gums and all the inside of the mouth became gangrenous … the legs were covered with scorbutic spots … most of them had their legs swelled … Even in this stage, dreadful as it was, they still took nourishment sufficient, but death soon put an end to their torments.' In the Paris Foundling Hospital in 1826, Charles Billard [46] 'saw an inflammation of the gums in an 18-month-old child in whom all milk-teeth had erupted. This inflammation was characterized by a red line along all teeths' neck.' In 1859, Königsberg physician Julius Möller described 'acute rickets' [47] whereas in 1871, Johan Ingerslev in Copenhagen clearly distinguished infant scurvy from rickets [48]. In 1983, Thomas Barlow at Great Ormond Street Hospital proved in a pathoanatomical study that scurvy differed from rickets [49] (Fig. 7.6.4) and warned 'that so-called "infant foods" cannot be trusted as sole aliment for any lengthened period'. In 1902, H. Neumann in Berlin demonstrated that the antiscobutic activity of milk is destroyed by excessive cooking [50]. With proprietary formula scurvy became epidemic, and in 1907, Jacob Bernheim observed a series of scurvy in infants nourished with *Berner Alpenmilch* in the Zürich Haus Rosenberg [51].

The 'antiscorbutic principle' was detected in Oslo by Axel Holst and Theodor Frölich in guinea pigs fed cereals [52]. Ascorbic acid plays a fundamental role in bone collagen synthesis and in the formation of blood vessel walls. Fresh cow's milk contains 1.5–2.0 mg of ascorbic acid per 100 mL, whereas human milk contains 8 mg per 100 mL [53]. In 1928, Albert Szent-Györgi isolated vitamin C [54], and received the Nobel Prize in Physiology or Medicine in 1937.

Treating and preventing scurvy

Charles De Mertans reported from the St. Petersburg Foundling Hospital in 1778 [45]: 'In autumn 1770, the foundling children, who remained in town to the number of a thousand [the greater part of the suckling children were at nurse in the country] … seeing that the remedies I had tried formerly were unsuccessful, I determined to give my patients those vegetables raw, while they had before used to eat boiled [sauerkraut, radishes, sweet turnips, carrots, and young onions] … In a few days after they had begun to eat the raw greens, all the bad symptoms decreased.' As Ruehl's incubator of 1835 [55], Doepp's report of 1835 [56], and Miller's recommendations for the care of premature infants [57], discoveries published from Russian foundling hospitals were not readily appreciated in western Europe. During the Napoleonic Wars, antiscorbutics became effective weapons. British navy sailors, supplied with lemon juice, were nicknamed 'limeys'; German soldiers were nicknamed 'krauts' [58]. In the Hebrew asylum in New York, Alfred Hess studied scurvy in infants fed pasteurized milk in 1914 [59] which could be cured by providing raw milk or orange juice. Harriette Chick proved in post-war Vienna that cow's milk has only minimal antiscorbutic activity [34], and lime only a tenth of the activity of fresh lemon

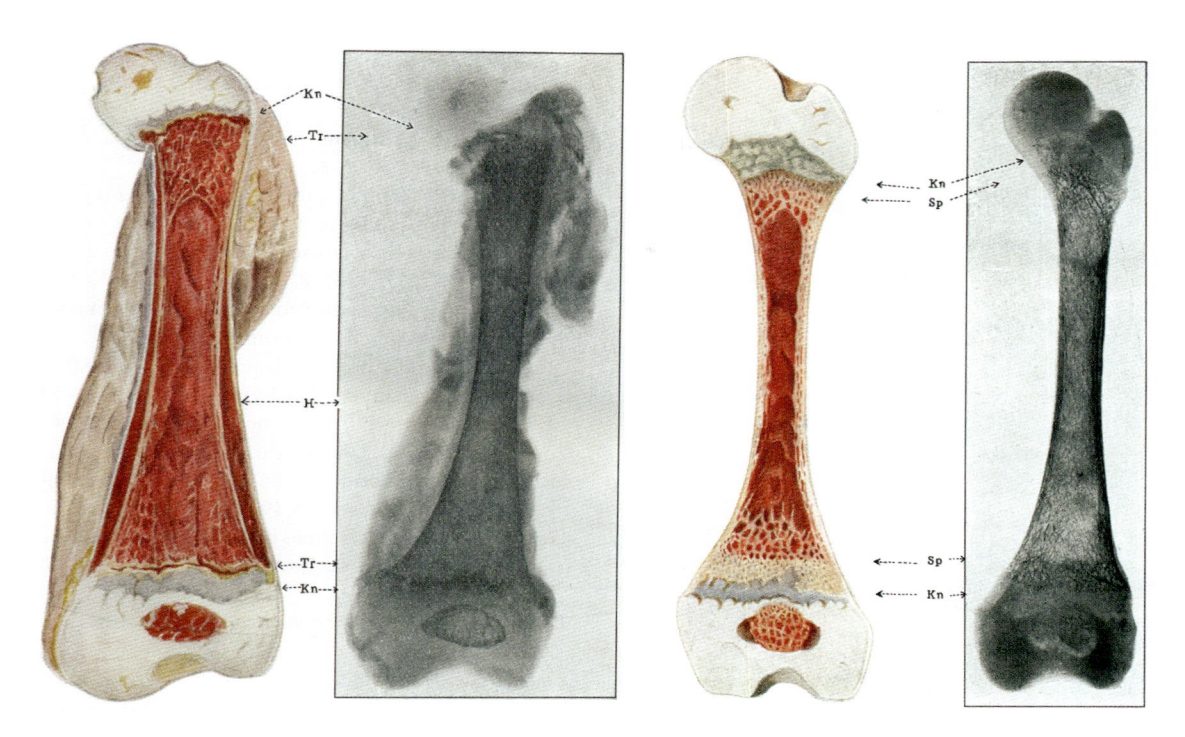

Fig. 7.6.4 Longitudinal cuts through and X-rays of the femur from an 8-month-old infant with scurvy (left) and of a 9-month-old boy with florid rickets (right). From Heinrich Finkelstein 1921 [18]. H, subperiosteal haematoma; Kn, epiphyseal growth zone; Sp, bone spongiosa; Tr, necrotic zone.

juice. Once baby formulas were enriched with vitamin C, the fight against scurvy seemed to have been won.

Osteogenesis imperfecta

Families with hereditary bone fragility were reported as early as 1788 [60]. In 1813, François Chaussier, Paris Maternité director, reported on a girl born with 113 fractures who died at 24 hours of age [61]. Eugène Bouchut depicted her and believed the fractures to result from 'fetal rickets' [62] (Fig. 7.6.5). Osteogenesis imperfecta ('brittle bone disease') is the most frequent heritable bone disorder. It is not a single disease, but a group of disorders caused by defective collagen formation. X-rays reveal single or multiple fractures, periosteal reaction, and callus formation. Fractures may occur with little or no trauma and parents have been unjustifiably accused of non-accidental injury [63].

Metabolic bone disease of prematurity

When in the 1970s premature infants under 28 weeks' gestation began to survive, many of them developed rib fractures, chest deformities, or the 'typical' flat preemie-head. Initially interpreted as 'rickets of prematurity', they were treated with high doses of vitamin D [64]. However, their vitamin D level was normal; it turned out they were lacking substrate: their usual protein, calcium, and trace element supply could not ensure these infants' rapid skeletal growth. By 1989, the incidence of 'osteopenia' was 55% in infants weighing less than 1000 g [65]. The disorder is far from conquered, the severity of metabolic bone disease is inversely proportional to the gestational age, and deteriorates through long-term parenteral nutrition, diuretics, caffeine, and steroid treatment [66]. Today, most immature infants receive 'breast milk fortifiers' to approximate the metabolic demands of their bones (see Chapter 6.9).

Extinct bone disease returns

Nutritional rickets never disappeared completely, but it had become rare thanks to widespread vitamin D prophylaxis during infancy. However, the disease recently returned in African and Arab children when families migrated north, and were unaware of the need for vitamin D supplementation in sun-deprived or air-polluted regions [67]. The disease was exacerbated by the excessive use of sunscreens and of clothing permitting minimal skin exposure to the sun, as well as the vegan nutrition of infants.

Conclusion

Although different in symptoms, rickets and scurvy were often confused. Both are results of malnutrition, both are secondary to or associated with the failure to breastfeed, and both worsen in wartime and in winter. Rickets became epidemic in the 17th century with industrialization and air pollution. A baby born in the autumn was almost certain to have rickets when 6 months old. Scurvy was

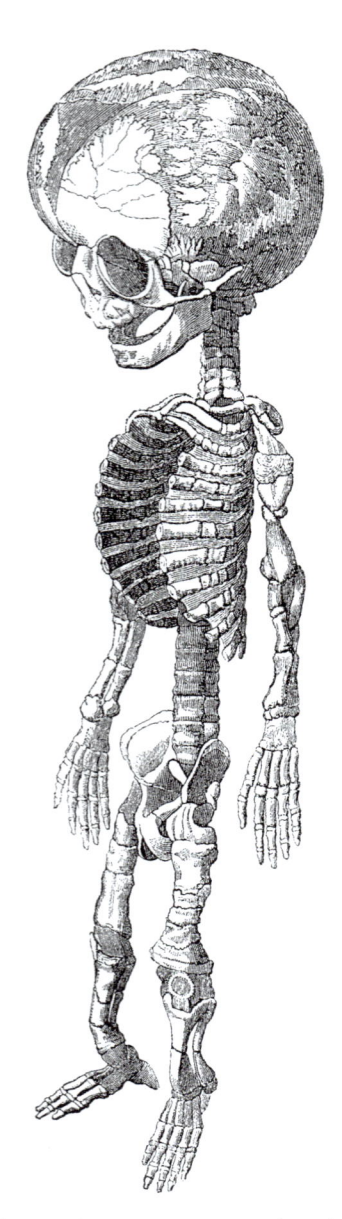

Fig. 7.6.5 A newborn with osteogenesis imperfecta, interpreted as 'fetal rickets', published by François Chaussier in 1813 [61] and depicted by Eugène Bouchut [62].

a long-known scourge in foundling hospitals and became epidemic at the start of the 20th century with the success of commercial formula. Both diseases became rare with adequate vitamin supplementation. The return of well-understood and easily preventable rickets in wealthy societies is scandalous and reveals organizational shortcomings within modern health systems.

REFERENCES

1. Harris SS, Dawson-Hughes B: Seasonal changes in plasma 25-hydroxyvitamin D concentrations of young American black and white women. Am J Clin Nutr 1998;**67**:1232–6.
2. Hess AF: Rickets including osteomalacia and tetany. Philadelphia, PA: Lea & Febiger, 1929.
3. Weick MT: A history of rickets in the US. Am J Clin Nutr 1967;**20**:1234–41.
4. Hess AF: Scurvy. Past and present. Philadelphia, PA: Lippincott, 1920.
5. Lomax E: Difficulties in diagnosing infantile scurvy before 1878. Med Hist 1986;**30**:70–80.
6. Temkin O: Soranus' Gynecology. Baltimore, MD: The Johns Hopkins Press, 1956: p. 79–117.
7. Guillemeau J: De la grossesse et accouchement des femmes. Paris: Jost, 1643: p. 551–87.
8. Whistler D: Disputatio medica inauguralis de morbo puerili Anglorum. Lugduni Batavorum: Box, 1645.
9. Boate A: De tabe pectorea. In: Observationes medicae de affectibus omissis. London: Newcomb, 1649: p. 44–53.
10. Glisson F: De rachitide sive morbo puerili, qui vulgo The Rickets dicitus, tractatus. London: Du-Gard, 1650.
11. Mayow J: On rickets (1st ed. 1668). In: Medico-physical works. Edinburgh: Alembic Club, 1957: p. 304–69.
12. Willughby P: Observations on midwifery (1672). Henry Blenkinsop: Wakefield, Yorkshire: S.R. Publishers, 1972: p. 109, 114, 120.
13. Böttcher JF: Von der Englischen Krankheit. Königsberg: Hartung, 1792.
14. Schröder K: A manual of midwifery including the pathology of pregnancy and the puerperal state. New York: Appleton, 1878: p. 227–45.
15. Wendelstadt GFC: Die endemischen Krankheiten Wezlars. Neues J Prakt Arzneikunde 1801;**12**:90–127.
16. Elsässer CL: Der weiche Hinterkopf. Stuttgart: Cotta, 1843.
17. Barenberg LH, Bloomberg MW: The significance of craniotabes and bowing of the legs. Am J Dis Child 1924;**28**:716–26.
18. Finkelstein H: Lehrbuch der Säuglingskrankheiten. 2. ed. Berlin: Springer, 1921: p. 149, 355, 542.
19. Palm T: The geographical distribution and etiology of rickets. Practitioner 1890;**45**:270–9, 321–42.
20. Buchholz E: Über Lichtbehandlung der Rachitis und anderer Kinderkrankheiten. Verh Dtsch Ges Kinderheilk 1904; **21**:116.
21. Hess AF: Newer aspects of some nutritional disorders. JAMA 1921;**76**:693–700.
22. Mellanby E, Cantag MD: Experimental investigation on rickets. Lancet 1919;**196**:407–12.
23. McCollum EV, Simmonds N, Becker JE, Shipley PG: An experimental demonstration of the existence of a vitamin which promotes calcium deposition. J Biol Chem 1922;**53**:293–312.
24. Windaus A, Linsert O, Lüttringhaus A, Weidlich G: Über das krystallisierte Vitamin D2. Justus Liebigs Ann Chem 1932;**492**:226–31.
25. Guy RA: The history of cod liver oil as a remedy. Am J Dis Child 1923;**26**:112–6.
26. Percival T: Observations on the medicinal uses of the oleum jecoris aselli, or cod liver oil. 4. ed. Warrington: Eyres, 1789: Vol. **2**, p. 354–62.
27. Schütte D: Beobachtungen über den Nutzen des Berger Leberthrans (Oleum jecoris aselli). Arch Med Erfahrung 1824;**45**:79–92.
28. Trousseau A: Rickets. In: Lectures on clinical medicine. Philadelphia, PA: Lindsay & Blakiston, 1873: Vol. **2**, p. 708–36.
29. Gaertner G: Über die Röntgen'sche Photographie als Hilfsmittel zum Studium normaler und pathologischer Ossificationsvorgänge. Wien Klin Rundsch 1896;**10**:165–7.

30. Escherich T: Die diagnostische Verwertung des Röntgen-Verfahrens bei Untersuchung der Kinder. Mitteilungen des Vereins der Ärzte in Steiermark 1898;**2**:1–7.
31. Tobler W: Der Skorbut im Kindesalter. Zeitschr Kinderheilk 1918;**18**:63–158.
32. Davidsohn H: Die Wirkung der Aushungerung Deutschlands auf die Berliner Kinder. Zeitschr Kinderheilk 1919;**21**:349–407.
33. Chick H: Study of rickets in Vienna 1919–1922. Med Hist 1976;**20**:41–51.
34. Chick H, Dalyell EJ, Hume M, et al.: The aetiology of rickets in infants: prophylactic and curative observations at the Vienna University Kinderklinik. Lancet 1922;**200**:7–11.
35. Huldschinski K: Heilung von Rachitis durch künstliche Höhensonne. Dtsch Med Wschr 1919;**26**:712–13.
36. Seidler E: Kinderärzte 1933–1945: Entrechtet—geflohen—ermordet. Bonn: Bouvier Verlag, 2000: p. 152.
37. Hess AH, Weinstock M, Helman FD: The antirachitic value of irradiated phytosterol and cholesterol. I. J Biol Chem 1925;**63**:305–9.
38. Holick MF: Vitamin D deficiency. N Engl J Med 2007;**357**:266–81.
39. Mays S: A likely case of scurvy from early Bronze Age Britain. Int J Osteoarchaeol 2008;**18**:178–87.
40. Paladin A, Wahl J, Zink A: Evidence of probable subadult scurvy in the Early Medieval cemetery of Castel Tirolo, South Tyrol, Italy. Int J Osteoarchaeol 2018;**28**:714–26.
41. Still GF: The history of paediatrics. London: Oxford University Press, 1931: p. 362.
42. Saviard B: Observation 128: Sur le scorbut. Nouveau recueil d'observations chirurgicales. Paris: Collombat, 1702.
43. Cadogan W: An essay upon nursing and the management of children. London: Roberts, 1750: p. 15, 18–27, 34.
44. Berthe M: Sur la gangrène scorbutique des gencives dans les enfans. Mém Acad Roy Chir 1774;**5**:381–96.
45. De Mertans C: Observations on the scurvy. Phil Trans R Soc Lond 1778;**68**:661–80.
46. Billard CM: Die Krankheiten der Neugeborenen und Säuglinge (1st French ed. 1828). Weimar: Industrie-Comptoir, 1829: p. 65, 228.
47. Möller JOL: Akute Rachitis. Königsberger Med Jahrb 1859;**1**:377–9.
48. Ingerslev JVC: Et tilfaelde af skorbug hos et barn. Hospitals-Tidende 1871;**14**:121–2.
49. Barlow T: On cases described as 'Acute Rickets' which are probably a combination of scurvy and rickets. Med Chir Trans 1883;**66**:159–220.
50. Neumann H: Bemerkungen zur Barlow'schen Krankheit. Dtsch Med Wochenschr 1902;**28**:628–30; 647–9; 213–15 V.
51. Bernheim-Karrer J: Säuglings-Scorbut bei Ernährung mit homogenisierter Berner Alpenmilch. Correspondenz-Blatt für Schweizer Ärzte 1907;**37**:593–8.
52. Holst A, Frölich T: Über experimentellen Skorbut. Zschr Hyg Infektionskr 1912;**72**:1–123.
53. Grewar D: Infantile scurvy. Clin Pediatr 1965;**4**:82–9.
54. Szent-Györgyi A: Observations of the function of peroxidase systems and the chemistry of the adrenal cortex. Biochem J 1928;**22**:1387–409.
55. Doepp P: Bemerkungen über einige Krankheiten der Säuglinge. Analekten über Kinderkrankheiten 1835;**1**:150–68.
56. Doepp P: Notizen über das kaiserliche Erziehungshaus (Findlingshaus) zu St. Petersburg. Hamburg: Hoffmann & Campe, 1835: Vol. **5**, p. 306–50.
57. Miller N. Th.: Die Frühgebornen und die Eigenthümlichkeiten ihrer Krankheiten. Jahrb Kinderheilk 1886;**25**:179–94.
58. Baron JH: Sailor's scurvy before and after James Lind—a reassessment. Nutr Rev 2009;**67**:315–32.
59. Hess AF, Fish M: Infantile scurvy. Am J Dis Child 1914;**8**:385–405.
60. Ekman OJ: Descriptio et casus aliquot osteomalaciae. Upsaliae: Inaug. Diss., 1788.
61. Chaussier F: Sur les fractures et les luxations observées chez des foetus encore contenus dans la matrice. Bull Ecole Med 1813;**II**:301–11.
62. Bouchut Eu: Traité pratique des maladies des nouveau-nés et des enfants a la mamelle et de la seconde enfance. 5. ed. Paris: Baillière, 1867.
63. Paterson CR: Osteogenesis imperfecta and other bone disorders in the differential diagnosis of unexplained fractures. J R Soc Med 1990;**83**:72–4.
64. McIntosh N, Livesey A, Brooke OG: Plasma 25-hydroxyvitamin D and rickets in infants of extremely low birthweight. Arch Dis Child 1982;**57**:848–50.
65. Koo WWK, Sherman R, Succop P, et al.: Fractures and rickets in very low birth weight infants. J Pediat Orthop 1989;**9**:326–30.
66. Ukarapong S, Venkatarayappa SKB, Navarrete C: Risk factors of metabolic bone disease of prematurity. Early Hum Dev 2017;**112**:29–34.
67. Kreiter SR, Schwartz RP, Kirkman HN, et al.: Nutritional rickets in African American breast-fed infants. J Pediat 2000;**137**:153–7.

7.7

Curse on two generations
Congenital syphilis

Introduction

Before penicillin removed its sting, congenital syphilis was frequent, dreaded, and lethal. Today, it affects a million pregnancies each year worldwide [1] and plays a role in every fifth perinatal death in sub-Saharan Africa [2]. In 2006, the World Health Organization launched a global effort to eliminate congenital syphilis [3]. Syphilis has been studied by historians more than other diseases [4–6], but few reports focused on the congenital form [7]. Much ink has been spilled speculating on the disease's origin. It was named the French, Spanish, Italian, American disease, and so on, and the epidemics of 1493 and 1496 were extensively reviewed. The 'new scourge' coincided with Columbus' return and perhaps more importantly, with the dissemination of the printing press: many diseases were first described in print in the early 16th century. In Gallo-Roman graves at Brény, Moreau found the skull of a 12-year-old child dated to the 7th century C.E. [8] displaying abnormalities which Parrot interpreted as syphilitic [9] (Fig. 7.7.1B). Pre-Wassermann reports on congenital syphilis must be interpreted with caution, as they often included gonorrhoea and soft chancre [10].

Classic publications

The neonatal form of the 'new' plague was recognized by Gaspard Torella in 1497 [11]: 'In suckling infants the first infection appears in the mouth or face; this results from infected breasts or from the nurse's face or mouth. The nurses often kiss the infants and I have frequently observed an infected infant transmit this disease to several nurses.' Jacopo Cattaneo [12] suggested in 1532 that maternal syphilis was transmitted in the birth canal, or from infected milk or breasts. Paracelsus [13] discerned three modes of transmission of the *French matter* to the neonate in 1536: '(1) during conception ... (2) after conception in a second infective coition ... (3) outside the mother's womb by poisoned milk.' Musa Brassavole [14] distinguished infection by (1) contact at birth, (2) suckling by an infected nurse, and (3) being itself infected, transmitting to another nurse. The most frequent maternofetal transmission was not thought of because the primary infection remained undiagnosed. Augier Ferrier [15] believed in 1564: 'The disease may be acquired in utero inherited from the father's seed; when the mother is infected at conception, formation of the fetal organs is severely disturbed.' In 1586, Guilleaume Rondelet [16] described 'a boy who at birth was totally covered by the pustules of *morbus gallicus*'. In 1776, royal physician Nils Rosén in Uppsala [17] referred to 'an instance of a chaste woman, who brought the disease on several lying-in women by sucking out their breasts, she not knowing herself to be infected'.

Glasgow obstetrician John Burns [18] noted in 1811: 'It often happens, that the child, though it have received the venereal disease in utero, is born alive, and has even no apparent disease on the skin, or in the mouth ... sometimes it has at the time of birth, or soon afterwards acquires, a wrinkled countenance, having the appearance of old age in miniature, so very remarkably, that no one who has ever seen such a child can possibly forget the look of the *petit vieillard* ... Copper coloured blotches, ending in ulceration, appear on the surface; or numerous, livid, flat, suppurating pustules, cover the surface; or many clusters of livid papulae appear, which presently have the top depressed, and then end in ulceration ... the disease generally appears within a fortnight after delivery, sometimes so early as the fourth day.'

Michael Underwood from London [19] and Henry Maunsell from Dublin [20] named the coryza (Fig. 7.7.1A) 'snuffles'. Infants were tormented by painful bone diseases, correctly interpreted by Bertin in 1810 as 'laminated periostosis'. From the Enfants Trouvés, François Valleix reported in 1835 [21]: 'Alexandrine Foulon was admitted to the infirmary on day ten of life because of some small pustules ... The next day, she could not move her left arm, and cried when one tried to move this limb. Assuming a cerebral lesion, leeches were applied behind each ear ... [died day 14, autopsy:] The upper part of the left humerus shows a kind of false joint entirely bathed in pus.' In 1870, Georg Wegner characterized syphilitic bone disease as osteochondritis, Jules Parrot named it *pseudo-paralysie* in 1872 [22]. Tardive congenital syphilis with interstitial keratitis, deafness, and upper incisors which 'are short, convergent, narrow from side to side at their edges, and show a

Reproduced with permission from Obladen, M. Curse on two generations: a history of congenital syphilis. *Neonatology*, 103(4):274–280. Copyright © 2013 S. Karger AG, Basel.

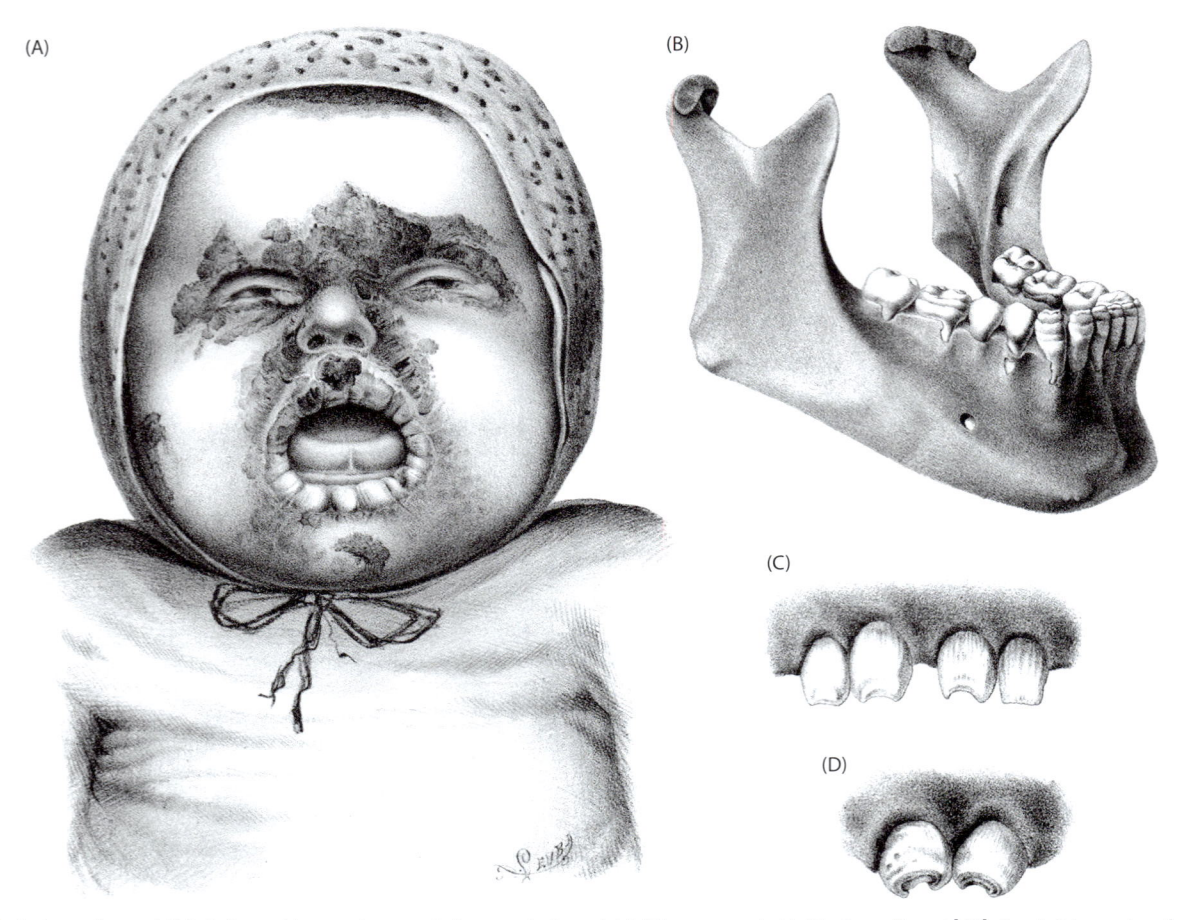

Fig. 7.7.1 A, face of a syphilitic infant with papulous and ulcerous lesions, labial fissures, and rhinitis, from Parrot [63]; B, adult lower jaw from the Merovingian period (7th century c.e.) unearthed near Brény/Aisne [8] and interpreted by Parrot as showing dental signs of connatal syphilis [9]; C and D, notched upper incisors of children 17 and 15 years old with *inherited* syphilis, published by Hutchinson 1863 [23].

vertical notch in each' (Fig. 7.7.1C, D) was described by Jonathan Hutchinson in 1863 [23].

The Infant Hospital in Vaugirard 1780–1793

In July 1780, Jean Lenoir, *Lieutenant Général de Police* in Paris, opened a hospice dedicated to the 'poor infants affected with venereal disease, who should be transferred there from Bicêtre, the Foundling Hospital, and the Hôtel-Dieu ... [It was] *enclosed*, with a large orchard allowing the sick mothers to walk, and providing the vegetables for their meals and the fodder for the animals required in the hospice' [24]. The *gastés* had beds for up to 71 syphilitic women and 64 syphilitic infants, stables for donkeys, goats, and cows, 'a large and clean dairy, and a horsedrawn carriage to pick up the infants from the said hospitals' [25, 26]. François Doublet became director in January 1781 and described the treatment installed by LeNoir and Colombier [27]: syphilitic women were treated with mercury orally and by friction. Their own infant, and a second syphilitic infant from the foundling hospital were believed to be cured by their milk. 'They consume more mercury than those not acting as wet nurses.' Within 10 years, 1463 'veneric' infants were referred to Vaugirard and 411 were born there by women regarded as syphilitic. Most infants were breastfed by nurses who received mercury: 1473 infants died (79%),

and 349 were discharged as 'healed' [26]. Syphilitic but breastfed infants survived longer than infants without syphilis but denied the breast: in 1800, the infant mortality at the Paris foundling hospital (then in the Port-Royal, former prison and even former monastery) was 92% [28].

The French Revolution advanced promiscuity, prostitution, and the abandonment of foundlings (now called *enfants de la patrie*). In 1790, the (former) Royal Society of Medicine advertised a price 'for whomever determined any reliable signs indicating infants born with the venereal disease; the circumstances in which it is communicated ... and how the infantile form of the disease should be treated'. Two authors applied: Pierre Mahon (published posthumously in 1804) [29] and René Bertin in 1810 [30], who reported: 'Marie Four ... had always been perfectly healthy until she nursed an infant from Paris, in whom gnawing chancres on the lips and pustules on the buttocks appeared fifteen days after birth ... Three weeks after starting to nurse this infant, she was attacked by fissures of both nipples and pustules on the left breast, which rapidly ulcerated ... She took fifty doses of VanSwieten's liqueur, and her infant took twenty doses: After two months all symptoms had completely disappeared in the nurse and her infant.' Too expensive in times of revolution and war, the Vaugirard hospice was closed in 1793 and the syphilitic infants and women transferred to the new *Hôpital des Vénériens* in the *Couvent des Capucins*.

Infected infants: the nursing dilemma

Feeding syphilitic infants, especially when abandoned, was difficult. Artificial feeding was often lethal, wet nursing transmitted the infection to the nurse and other infants. Already in 1664, Louis Guyon postulated [31]: 'To let a pocky infant spoil or infect a wet nurse is a matter worthy of punishment … I witnessed many lawsuits in Paris before the Civil Lieutenant of women suing parents for damages. They were sentenced right away to forfeit a certain sum of money … I gave goat's milk to a little girl of noble birth who had brought it from her mother's womb.' Still in 1874, laws in Denmark and other European countries forbade the transmission of the disease by and to wet nurses [32]. Jules Parrot opened the *nourricerie* in June 1881—wards designed to treat veneric foundlings [33] that were connected to stables where the infants were nourished with donkey milk (**Figs. 7.7.2** and **7.7.3**). At Parrot's institute, Anicet Wins studied the milk of various species in 1885. Low in casein and high in sugar, he found donkey milk resembled human milk more than cow's milk [34].

Infection versus heredity

John Hunter, surgeon in London [35], started the discussion in 1786: 'It is Also supposed, that a foetus, in the womb of a pocky mother may be infected by her. This I should doubt very much, both from what may be observed from the secretions, and from finding that even the matter from such constitutional inflammation is not capable of communicating the disease.' Around 1800, Lamarck reactivated Hippocratian ideas of the inheritance of acquired characteristics (epigenesis), and during most of the 19th century this theory was accepted. A vivid debate continued for a century: contagionists propagated exclusively maternal infection, hereditists believed in germinal transmission via paternal sperm, bypassing the mother. Fournier even regarded the transmission to a third generation as possible. Abraham Colles [36] stated in 1837 that 'a child born of a mother who is without any obvious venereal symptoms, and which, without being exposed to any infection subsequent to its birth, shows this disease when a few weeks old, this child will infect the most healthy nurse, whether she suckle it, or merely handle and dress it; and yet this child is never known to infect its own mother, even though she suckle it while it has venereal ulcers of the lips and tongue'.

Syphilis was believed to be a major cause of prematurity, and Arvo Ylppö, having found 29 cases among 668 preterm infants, complained in 1919 [37]: 'The widespread prejudice suspecting every preterm infant to be syphilitic is not supported by our data.'

Finally, the diagnosis

Breslau dermatologist Albert Neisser identified the gonococcus in 1879, and Berlin zoologist Fritz Schaudinn and dermatologist Erich Hoffmann *Spirochaeta pallida* in 1905, renaming it *Treponema pallidum* in the same year [38]. It was twice as large as the head of a human spermatozoon, which ended the theory of germinative transmission. Like many authors, Otto Heubner taciturnly changed the term *hereditary* into *congenital* syphilis in the 1911 edition of his textbook [39]. **Fig. 7.7.4** illustrates various manifestations of this devastating disease. In 1906, Wassermann, Neisser, and Bruck adapted Bordet and Gengou's (1901) complement fixation reaction to prove spirochete infections [40]. Despite an avalanche of publications and modifications, the test remained difficult to detect neonatal infection and treatment success. Fildes stated in 1915 [41]: 'The Wassermann reaction performed with umbilical cord blood is not diagnostic of syphilis in the infant, but of syphilis in the mother.' But

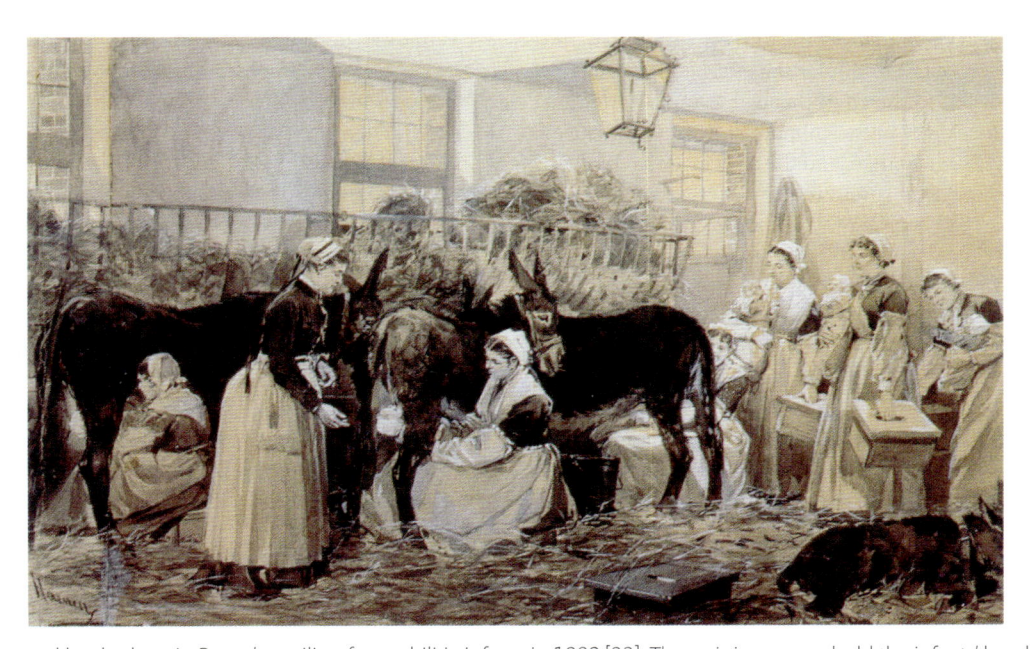

Fig. 7.7.2 Infants nursed by donkeys in Parrot's pavilion for syphilitic infants in 1882 [33]. Three sitting nurses hold the infants' heads with their right hand. Three more nurses with infants are waiting at the stable's entry.
Painting by Frédéric de Haenen, 1887. Paris, Musée de l'Assistance Publique, AP-HP/F.Marin, with permission.

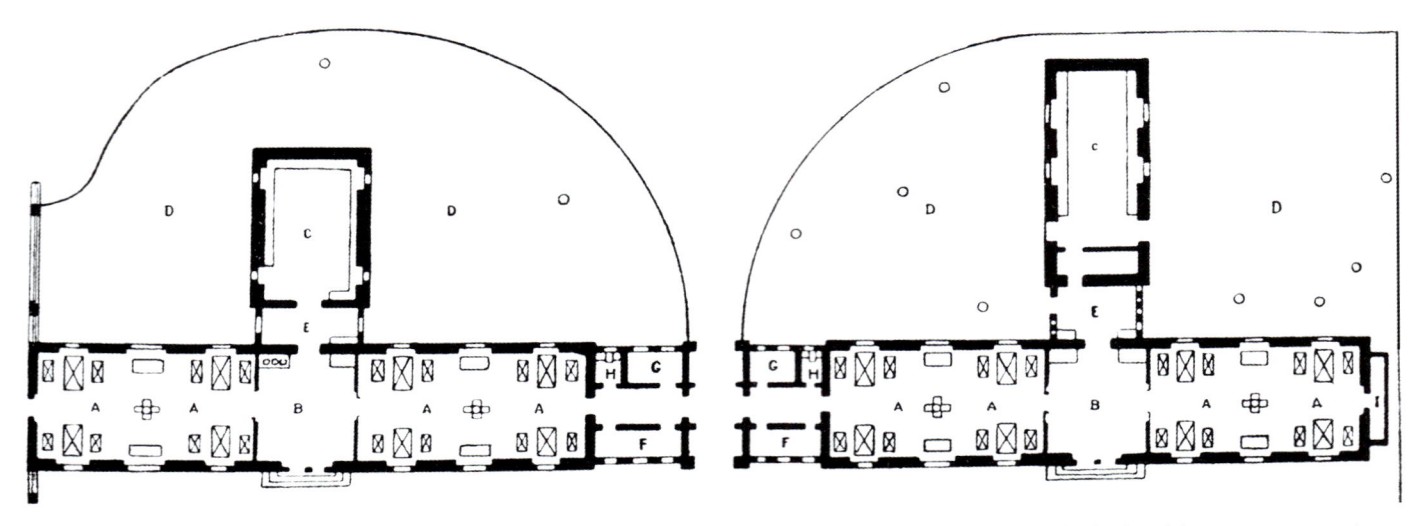

Fig. 7.7.3 Floor plan of Parrot's pavilion for syphilitic infants, opened in 1881 at the Paris Foundling Hospital. C, donkey's stables. Four nurses and eight infants were housed in each of the four rooms. Depicted by Nicolle 1891 [64].

the magnitude of the problem became visible: Churchill, studying 'at random' hospitalized children in Chicago [42] found a positive Wassermann reaction in 38%. De Buys and Loeber found a positive Noguchi reaction in 75% of inmates at the New Orleans Foundling Institution [43]. Three months after Conrad Röntgen published on X-rays, Schjerning and Kranzfelder described radiologic epiphyseal anomalies in congenital syphilis [44].

Mercury treatment

Following the Hippocratic rule 'heal suckling infants by treating the nurse' [45], mercury was given by indirect routes, as described by François Swediaur (first ed. 1798) [46]: 'The greatest part of children who we are consulted for, as infected with syphilis, have no visible sign of it when born … If the nipples of the nurse are ulcerated, or if there be any other impediment to hinder the effects of the mercury from being communicated to the child through the nurse, we must employ a she-goat or ass, a part of the animal's body must be shaved, and mercury ribbed in as with a man, and the milk given to the child.'

For direct treatment, Bertin 'preferred the myriate of mercury, combined with rhubarb, in a dose of a half grain, in a spoonful of soup … which is most successful in infants and which they tolerate best'. Zeissl described oral mercury treatment and sublimate-baths for neonates in 1858 [47] but the infants were not at all cured: 'May the reader be happier than I in the treatment of these decomposing fruits, poisoned in their seed.' Mercury unction of neonates was described by Wertheimber 1863 [48]. Proving, in retrospect, some efficacy of mercury, Jarisch [49] observed in 1895 'a reaction whereby in the first days of mercurial inunctions for syphilitic roseola there is an exaggeration of the clinical manifestations'.

Arsphenamine treatment

At the Wiesbaden congress on 19 April 1910, Frankfurt biochemist Paul Ehrlich (after having received the 1908 Nobel Prize in Physiology or Medicine for detecting the immune system) announced a new drug specifically synthesized against syphilis with his student and colleague Sahachiro Hata [50]. 'Compound 606', later called salvarsan, gave hope as a *therapia magna sterilisans*. Eighteen days later, Carl Noeggerath in Berlin started salvarsan in two infants born before Ehrlich's lecture: Hans M, 10 weeks old, received two injections of '606 Hata' and improved, but died at 10 months from bronchopneumonia; Otto W, 7 weeks old, received three injections … and improved markedly, but scarring at the gluteal injection site hampered mobility of his left leg. 'With this application, no infant escaped the serious and painful side effects at the injection site … therefore, from January 1911, I proceeded to intravenous injection … As injecting an arm vein is very difficult without phlebotomy, I exclusively injected the *scalp veins*. This performance requires some dexterity which can easily be learned on the rabbit's ear veins.' Of Noeggerath's 28 infants, nine died, and in most survivors the Wassermann reaction did not turn negative [51].

Within 15 months after its discovery, 101 publications on salvarsan in congenital syphilis appeared [52]. But it was not the magic bullet Ehrlich had hoped for. At New York Bellevue Hospital, Linnaeus La Fetra treated infants with salvarsan injections from June 1911 [53], whereas treatment at the New Orleans Foundling Institution in 1919 was still mercury given orally and as an ointment with a linen bellyband [43]. Prenatal therapy was more successful, and trials in Paris [54], Baltimore [55], and Copenhagen [56] reported more than 90% healthy infants when syphilitic mothers received a full course of arsphenamine during pregnancy. In Britain, salvarsan was received reluctantly [57], but in 1921 Findlay appealed to the British Ministry of Health to pass a law instituting the Wassermann test and prenatal treatment [58]. Up to the advent of penicillin, salvarsan was often combined with mercury or bismuth [59].

Penicillin treatment

When penicillin became available in 1943, Lentz and Ingraham in Philadelphia began to treat pregnant women and infected neonates

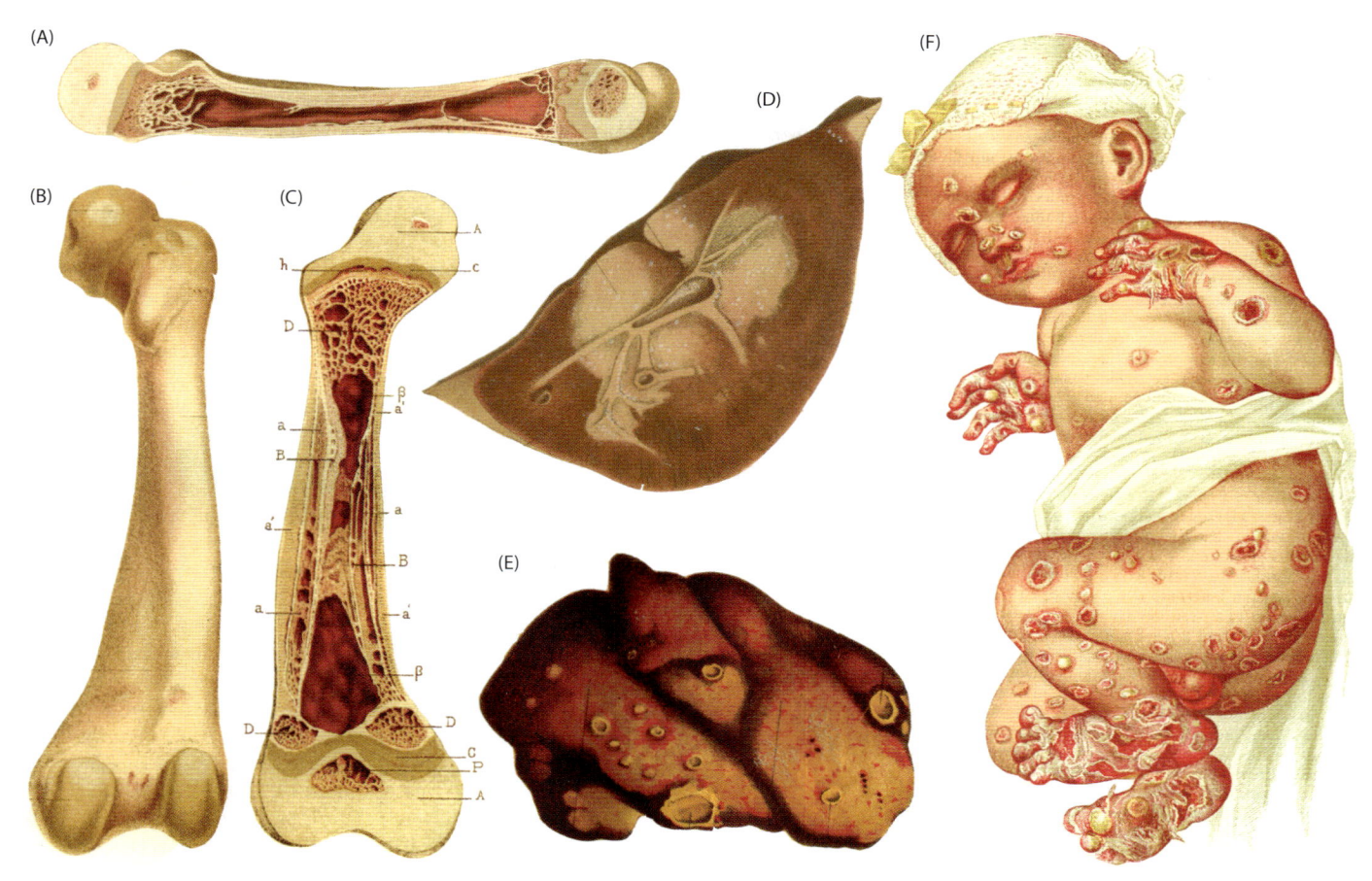

CHAPTER 7.7 Curse on two generations: congenital syphilis 337

Fig. 7.7.4 Pathologic changes due to congenital syphilis, A–E from Parrot 1886 [63]. A, humerus cut with diaphyseal lamellated periostitis; B, bowed femur thickened due to osteophyte; C, cut through the same femur showing lamellated periostitis and necrotic epiphyses; D, liver cut showing diffuse induration and gumma formation; E, lung surface with multiple gumma ulcers; F, papulo-pustulous syphilid as depicted by Friedinger and Mayr 1859 [65].

with the new drug. Whereas maternal treatment was highly effective, three of nine infants died, 'possibly not due to penicillin' [60]. A year later, the same group reported 34 'reactions' among 69 infants treated with penicillin [61]: the more powerful the drug, the more severe was the 'Jarisch Herxheimer reaction'. In Manchester, Holzel [62] observed 14 deaths among 32 infants treated during the first 3 months of life, 'in seven of them, the Jarisch Herxheimer reaction was a contributory cause of death'.

REFERENCES

1. Zhou Q, Wang L, Chen C, et al.: A case series of 130 neonates with congenital syphilis. Neonatology 2012;**102**:152–6.
2. Hossain M, Broutet N, Hawkes S: The elimination of congenital syphilis. Sex Transm Dis 2007;**34**:S22–30.
3. World Health Organization: Prevention of mother-to-child transmission of syphilis. Geneva: WHO Publications, 2006.
4. Sudhoff K: The earliest printed literature on syphilis: being ten tractates from the years 1495–1498. Florence: Lier, 1925.
5. Dennie CC: A history of syphilis. Springfield, IL: Thomas, 1962.
6. Quetel C: History of Syphilis. Baltimore: Johns Hopkins University Press, 1992: p. 1–342.
7. Kassowitz M: Die Vererbung der Syphilis. Wien: Braumüller, 1876: p. 1–140.
8. Moreau F: Fouilles du cimetière de Breny. Bull Soc Anthropol Paris 1880;**3**:630–3.
9. Parrot J: Une maladie préhistorique. Revue Scientifique de la France 1882;**30**:110–3.
10. Hudson EH: Historical approach to the terminology of syphilis. Arch Dermatol 1961;**84**:545–62.
11. Torella G: Tractatus cum consiliis contra pudendagram seu morbum gallicum. Romae: la Turre, 1497.
12. Cattaneo Lagomarsini J: Opus de morbo gallico. Taurini: Silva, 1532.
13. Paracelsus T: Vom Ursprung und Herkommen der Franzosen, 1536. In: Paracelsus, works in 5 volumes. Basel: Schwabe & Co., 1965: Vol. **2**, p. 367.
14. Brassavolus AM: De morbo Gallico liber. Venetiis: Zilettus, 1566: Vol. **1**, p. 564–610.
15. Ferrier A: De pudendagra, lue hispanica. Antverpiae: Nutius, 1564.
16. Rondelet G: De morbo Italico. Lugduni: Apud Guliel. Rouillium, 1586: p. 762–3.
17. Rosen von Rosenstein N: The diseases of children (1st Swedish ed. 1764). London: Cadell, 1776: p. 322.
18. Burns J: The principles of midwifery. 2. ed. London: Longman, & Co, 1811: p. 485–9.
19. Underwood M: A treatise on the disorders of childhood. 2. ed. London: Matthews, 1801: Vol. **1**, p. 53–8.

20. Evanson RT, Maunsell H: A practical treatise on the management and diseases of children. 4. ed. Philadelphia, PA: Barrington & Haswell, 1843: p. 352.
21. Valleix FLI: Observation et réflexions sur un décollement de plusieurs épiphyses des os longs. Arch Gen Med 1835;**37**:88–96.
22. Parrot J: Sur une pseudo-paralysie causée par une altération du système osseux chez les noueau-nés atteints de syphilis héréditaire. Arch Physiol Normale Pathol 1871–1872;**4**:319–333; 470–90; 612–23.
23. Hutchinson J: A clinical memoir on certain diseases of the eye and ear, consequent on inherited syphilis. London: Churchill, 1863: p. 205.
24. Colombier J: Hospice des pauvres enfans nouveaux-nés atteints du mal vénérien, situé a Vaugirard. Paris: Pierres, 1781: p. 1–30.
25. Delavierre Ph: L'hopital de Vaugirard: Dès origines a nos jours. Hist Sci Med 1978;**12**:153–61.
26. Piernas G: L'hospice de Vaugirard pour les 'enfans gastés et les femmes grosses'. Hist Écon Soc 2007;**26**:67–84.
27. Doublet F: Mémoire sur les symptomes et le traitement de la maladie vénérienne dans les enfans nouveaux-nés. Paris: Méquignon, 1781: p. 1–79.
28. Dupoux A: Sur les pas de monsieur Vincent. Paris: Revue de l'assistance publique, 1958: p. 179.
29. Mahon PAO, Lamauve L: Recherches importantes sur l'existence, la nature, et la communication des maladies Syphilitiques dans les Femmes enceintes, dans les Enfans nouveau-nés et dans les Nourrices. Paris: Buisson/Robert, 1804: p. 347–518.
30. Bertin RJ: Traité de la maladie vénérienne chez les enfans nouveau-nés, les femmes enceintes et les nourrices. Paris: Gabon, 1810: p. 186–7.
31. Guyon Dolois L: Le cours de médecine en françois. Lyon: Barbier, 1678: Vol. **2**, p. 27–8.
32. Meyer GS: Criminal punishment for the transmission of sexually transmitted diseases. Bull Hist Med 1991;**65**:549–64.
33. Parrot J: La nourricerie de l'hospice des enfants-assistés. Bull Acad Natl Med 1882;839–53.
34. Wins A-B: L'allaitement a la nourricerie de l'hospice des enfants-assistés. Paris: Inaug. Diss., 1885: p. 1–56.
35. Hunter J: A treatise on the venereal disease. London: Castle-Street, 1786: p. 398–9.
36. Colles A: Practical observations on the venereal disease, and on the use of mercury. Dublin: Waldie, 1837: p. 185.
37. Ylppö A: Zur Physiologie, Klinik und zum Schicksal der Frühgeborenen. Zeitschr Kinderheilk 1919;**24**:1–110.
38. Schaudinn FR, Hoffmann E: Vorläufiger Bericht über das Vorkommen von Spirochaeten in syphilitischen Krankheitsprodukten und bei Papillomen. Arbeiten aus dem Kaiserlichen Gesundheitsamte 1905;**22**:527–34.
39. Heubner O: Lehrbuch der Kinderheilkunde. 3. ed. Leipzig: Barth, 1911: Vol. **1**, p. 655–89.
40. Wassermann A, Neisser A, Bruck C: Eine serodiagnostische Reaktion bei Syphilis. Dtsche Med Wochenschr 1906;**32**:745–6.
41. Fildes P: The prevalence of congenital syphilis amongst the newly born of the East End of London. Br J Obstet Gynecol 1915;**27**:124–37.
42. Churchill FS: The Wassermann reaction in infants and children: a clinical study. Arch Pediatr Adolesc Med 1912;**3**:363–97.
43. DeBuys LR, Loeber M: Study in a foundling institution to determine the incidence of congenital syphilis. JAMA 1919;**73**:1028–31.
44. Schjerning Ov, Kranzfelder F: Verwerthbarkeit Röntgen'scher Strahlen für medicinisch-chirurgische Zwecke. Dtsch Med Wochenschr 1896;**14**:211–3.
45. Hippocrates: Opera omnia: des epidemies, part VI (Reprint ed. 1861, E. von Littré). Amsterdam: Hakkert, 1962: Vol. **5**, p. 323.
46. Swediaur FX: A comprehensive treatise upon the symptoms, consequences, nature, and treatment of venereal, or syphilitic, diseases. London: Longman & Co, 1819: Vol. **2**, p. 109–15.
47. Zeissl H: Ueber Syphilis congenita der Neugeborenen und der Säuglinge. Jahrb Kinderheilk 1858;**1**:55–63, 119–32.
48. Wertheimer A: Ueber die Behandlung der Syphilis congenita. Jahrb Kinderheilk 1863;**6**:11–17.
49. Jarisch A: Therapeutische Versuche bei Syphilis. Wiener Med Wschr 1895;**45**:721–4, 771–4, 826–9, 875–7, 927–9, 975–7, 1033–6.
50. Ehrlich P, Hata S: Die experimentelle Chemotherapie der Sprillosen. Berlin: Springer, 1910: p. 1–164.
51. Noeggerath CT: Klinische Beobachtungen bei der Salvarsanbehandlung syphilitischer Säuglinge. Jahrbuch Kinderheilk 1912;**75**:131–65.
52. Welde E: Die Behandlung der Lues congenita mit Salvarsan. Jahrb Kinderheilk 1911;**74**:322–40.
53. La Fetra LE: The employment of salvarsan in infants and young children. Arch Pediatr 1912;**29**:654–64.
54. Sauvage C: De l'emploi du Salvarsan chez les femmes enceintes syphilitiques. Ann Gynecol 2e Série 1913;**10**:49–56, 90–110.
55. Williams JW: Significance of syphilis in prenatal care and in the causation of fetal death. Bull Johns Hopkins Hosp 1920;**31**:141.
56. Boas H, Gammeltoft SA: Treatment of syphilis during pregnancy, with particular attention to the infants. Acta Gynecol Scand 1922;**1**:309–63.
57. Ross JE, Tomkins SM: The British reception of Salvarsan. J Hist Med All Sci 1997;**52**:398–423.
58. Findlay L: The ante-natal treatment of congenital syphilis with salvarsan and mercury. BMJ 1921;**2**:887–9.
59. Müller E: Die Behandlung der angeborenen Syphilis. In: Jadasson J: Handbuch der Haut- und Geschlechtskrankheiten 1926–1927:**19**:298–326.
60. Lentz JW, Ingraham NR, Beerman H, Stokes JH: Penicillin in the prevention and treatment of congenital syphilis. JAMA 1944;**126**:408–13.
61. Platou RV, Hill A, Ingraham NR, et al.: Penicillin in the treatment of infantile congenital syphilis. JAMA 1945;**127**:582.
62. Holzel A: Jarisch-Herxheimer reaction following penicillin treatment of early congenital syphilis. Br J Vener Dis 1956;**32**:175–80.
63. Parrot J: Maladies des Enfants: La Syphilis héréditaire et le rachitis. Paris: G. Masson, 1886: plates 1, 8, 9, 13, 22.
64. Nicolle EA: La nourricerie de l'hospice des Enfants Assistés (enfants syphilitiques et suspects). Paris: Inaug. Diss/Steinheil, 1891: p. 31.
65. Friedinger C, Mayr F, Zeissl H: Die Syphiliden im Kindesalter. Jahrb. Kinderheilk 1859;**2**:1–12.

7.8 Thrush
Nightmare of the foundling hospitals

Introduction

Neonatal mucocutaneous *Candida* infections are frequent and harmless, and modern physicians rarely recall that they were dreaded and lethal in the 19th century, hindering the foundation of hospital wards for sick infants.

Pre-foundling descriptions

In the history of any disorder, we are reminded that medical knowledge and the nature of disease change over time. Leven pointed out that retrospective diagnosis is a delicate matter which rapidly leads to misunderstandings [1]. The ancient Greek writers used the term *aphthai* in a different sense than we do, and did not strictly differentiate thrush, diphtheria, and stomatitis aphthosa [2]. Cornelius Celsus in Rome in the 1st century C.E. wrote [3]: 'Truly most dangerous are those ulcers which the Greeks call *aphthai*, to which infants frequently succumb, while they are less dangerous to adults. They begin at the gums, proceed towards the palate, occupy the entire mouth and finally descend to uvula and pharynx. It is difficult to cure the child and even more miserable the nursling, in whom the use of remedies is limited.'

Avicenna (11th century C.E.) believed [4]: 'Stomatitis is common among infants because the mucous membranes of their mouth and tongue are too delicate to bear touching, even by the wateryness of the milk, for it is this that is injurious to it, and gives rise to the aphthae.' Dubious terminology persisted throughout the Middle Ages. Eucharius Roesslin, a physician in Frankfurt, wrote in 1513 [5]: 'It occurs to the infant that multiple leaflets grow on the tongue and in the mouth. They result from acidity in the mother's milk.' Even though a disease of the poor, thrush was observed by Simon de Vallambert, physician to the duchess of Savoy and Berry, in 1565 [6], and believed to be caused 'by bad milk, either from the wet-nurse, or if the infant could not digest it, and it has been corrupted in the stomach, ascending and digesting the tender and vulnerable parts of the mouth'. Also, the royal midwife Louise Bourgeois blamed milk in 1609 [7]: 'I saw an infant of noble birth, breast-fed by a wet-nurse whose milk was old, thick and scarce, whose mouth, a few days after its birth, had been overheated by sucking to such a degree, that a white and thick chancre arose on its tongue and palate which spread to all gums, the entire mouth and throat, so that it was gripped by fever and could no longer suck.'

Endemic disease in foundling hospitals

Foundling hospitals proliferated in the 18th century, admitting thousands of neonates each year. Overcrowded and understaffed, without clean water or refrigeration, they were breeding grounds for nosocomial infections. Less than a third of foundlings survived their first year. Joseph Raulin, physician of Louis XV, wrote in 1769 [8]: 'Foundlings often die from contagious diseases, primarily from venereal diseases, without arising suspicion of such. Even when hidden, they infect the wet-nurse who then infects other infants whom she gives the breast … In Paris, there is a disease called *muguet* endemic in the Foundling Hospital and in the Hotel-Dieu, where the poor women deliver … Initially, there is slight redness of the palate and tongue, where small leaflets originate, which rapidly spread inside the entire mouth and palate, infecting the tongue and throat, and hindering swallowing; these leaflets then proceed into the stomach. The infants become weak and die rapidly.' The mortality of *muguet* in Paris was as high as 90%.

Michael Underwood, male-midwife in London, recognized involvement of the entire gastrointestinal tract in 1801 [9]: 'It has long been a received opinion that thrush must appear at the bottom, and many old nurses will not allow it to be cured if it does not … But the truth is that its appearance there is only a mark of the degree of the disease, or of the acidity that occasions it, and not in the least of its cure; and is not, therefore, generally to be wished for. The redness about this part is occasioned by the sharpness of the secretions in the bowels, and consequently of the stools, which slightly inflame and sometimes excoriate the bottom.'

PART 7 Disease

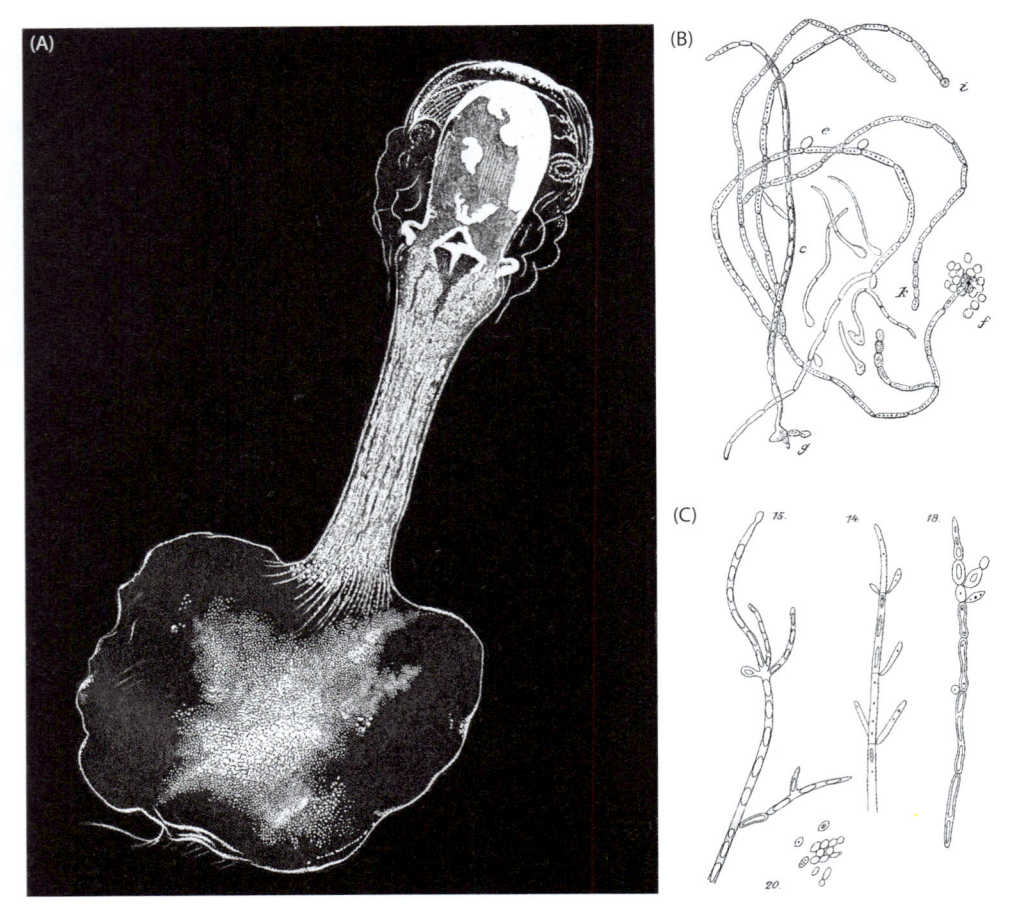

Fig. 7.8.1 A, postmortem view showing extensive thrush of tongue, oesophagus, and stomach; ink drawing from Billard's Atlas 1829 [44]; B, tubulous fibres (Gruby: Racines; Berg: Fibrilles) of thrush according to Robin 1853 [26] (c, ovoid cells; e, ramification erupting as a single cell; f, spores grouped at a tube extremity (chlamydospore); g, spore of origin; i, terminal spheric cell; k, articulating ovoid cells); C, segmented and unsegmented *Oidium albicans* hyphens (14–18) and spores (20) from the vagina, enlargement 400×, according to Haussmann 1872 [27].

Charles Billard, intern at the Hôpital des Enfants Trouvés, described clinical and postmortem findings in several infants with thrush, among them a girl with gastric *muguet* [10] (Fig. 7.8.1A): 'Louise Labry, 13 days old and of weak constitution, came into our care on July 8 [1826]. Her face had been pale for two days and she refused the breast of her wet-nurse … At arrival to the infirmary she showed severe redness of the oral mucosa and a thick layer of thrush spread on the internal surface of the cheeks and base of the tongue … On the 14th, yellowish substances were vomited, and the muguet formed a thicker layer … The skin was cold, the extremities livid, the pulse small. The child died in the evening.'

In St. Petersburg, thrush was also frequent, but not as lethal as in Paris [11]. The London physician William Heberden, Jr noted [12]: 'Among the French, and especially in their public hospitals, the thrush seems to be a more frequent, and a much severer disease, than in England.' In the Marseille Hospice de la Charité, *muguet* was also endemic, but its mortality was low, and the directing physician Vincent Seux explained in 1855 [13]: 'Of 401 cases which I observed within one year, I lost only 20 sick infants … During a visit at that hospital [Paris], Doctor Baron told me that whenever a newborn is affected by thrush, it is deprived of its wet-nurse, fearing that her breast be contaminated by the infant's mouth. It is understandable that this infant, being artificially nourished, will soon be affected by a severe *muguet* with enteritis, and will die.' Even during the 20th century, thrush remained a serious problem. Not a foundling hospital, but a modern special care nursery for preterm infants, the Simpson Memorial Maternity pavilion in Edinburgh was not spared the burden of thrush endemics and fatalities as reported by Ludlam and Henderson in 1942 [14]. Among 708 infants studied at the New York foundling hospital in 1958, diaper rashes were observed in 361 and skin cultures were positive for *C. albicans* in 205 infants [15].

Doubts about contagiosity

Theories of contagiosity have occupied physicians' minds since antiquity and have led to isolation. The Padovan professor and medical officer to the Council of Trent, Girolamo Fracastoro, described contagiosity per *contactum*, per *fomitem*, and per *distans* in 1546 [16] and even suggested that the infective material may augment by itself. He initiated the long-standing debate between *miasmaticians* and *contagionists*. Nobody, however, imagined infection by living organisms, and in the foundling hospitals, foul 'mephitic' air was held responsible for the endemic disease.

Before detecting the fungus, non-contagiosity of *muguet* was a kind of dogma at the Paris Hôpital des Enfants Trouvés, repeated by Véron 1825 [17]: 'The perfect health of many infants breast-fed by the same nurses or with the same vessels and spoons proves that this disease is not at all contagious'; and by Billard in 1829 [10]: 'Occurs mostly in those crowded in great numbers in one place, who are born weak and miserable, and who receive nourishment inappropriate for their age … I do not believe that oral thrush is contagious, and Baron rejects this opinion entirely, because he often saw healthy infants eating from the same spoon previously used to feed infants with *muguet*, and without acquiring the disease.' In 1838, François Valleix, faithful disciple of Broussais' doctrine, believed thrush was a form of enteritis, and devoted 292 pages to this disease [18], denying its contagiosity; he did not provide information beyond that published by Véron and Billard.

Detecting the fungus

In Bologna, Marcello Malpighi microscopically studied embryonic tissues and body fluids, discovering moulds in 1675 [19]. It is difficult for us to fathom that despite ample use in the *salons* of the 18th century, the microscope was little used in medical research. The Leipzig obstetrician Johann Christian Jörg was almost correct in 1826 [20]: 'The sponges [*Schwämme*] consist of whitish fibres similar to the mould on rotten bread, grow out point-by-point, and sometimes coat the entire surface.' Philipp Anton Pieper, working in the Enfants Trouvés in 1829, also approached the truth with his speculation [21]: 'The cheese-like covering, a formation of parasites, which in more than one respect is similar to some protophytes.'

However, the credit goes to David Gruby and Frederik Berg for having detected and correctly associated the first organism causing human disease. Having just immigrated to Paris and not yet authorized to practise medicine, Gruby conducted laboratory research in the Enfants Trouvés using a microscope and potassium hydroxide [22]: 'When a particle of this substance is placed under the microscope, one can see that it consists entirely of a mass of cryptogamic plants. To study the characteristics of these vegetations and their connection with the tissue on which they arise, one must observe the isolated cones which appear at the start of the disease. Each cone consists of a multitude of individuals equipped with roots, branches, and spores.' From October 1839 to July 1841, the Swedish physician Frederik Berg, designated director of the Stockholm orphanage, travelled through seven European countries studying infants' diseases and institutions for the care of foundlings [23]: 'My stay in Paris coincided with a remarkable period of advance in scientific research. Magendie had based new physiological views on vivisections and Longet further cultivated this field, Donné gave microscopical courses, the Hungarian Jew Gruby, a pupil of Berres in Vienna, had recently arrived in Paris, with far better training in the use of the microscope than Donné. With Gruby I entered into an agreement for the joint collection from the hospitals of objects for examination.' Returned to Sweden in autumn 1841, Berg gave his report [24] and published a monograph *Om torsk hos barn* in 1846 [25]. Christoph Robin named the fungus *Oidium albicans* [26]

and demonstrated different forms and spores (Fig. 7.8.1B). The Berlin obstetrician David Haussmann in 1870 [27] reported fungus spores in the mouth of infants whose mothers were suffering from mycotic vaginitis (Fig. 7.8.1C). The genus *Candida* was described by Utrecht botanist Christine Berkhout in her doctoral thesis in 1923 [28].

Towards effective topical treatment

Soran's warning against mouthwashing was reiterated by Felix Würz in 1563 [29, 30]: 'Some indiscreet people take wool, or rough linen, or the bath cloth out of the bath, feel with it to the throat, and so wash it saying how furr' d is this Child in the throat, I must wash off that white stuff, and rub it so hard that they pull off their subtle skin, even as a soft rind is peeled off the tree, which if once done, then the next day his mouth groweth more white …, and the more they continue their washing, the worse they make it. This great fault about the mouth washing, hath moved me to write this treatise, and I entreat all good people not to make use of such washing, and to warn others from it also: for the tongue doth cleanse itself, being a member which is still in motion, and groweth not wary.' However, mouthwashing remained in use, as shown in Van Puteren's 1889 recommendation in St. Petersburg [31]: 'The best means is said to consist in mechanically removing the thrush fungi by means of a brush. Any fears about inducing consecutive ulceration by brushing are altogether groundless.'

Astringents had been used since antiquity, and boric acid gained widespread acceptance, as explained by Underwood 1801 [9]: 'Borax is certainly one of the best; it may be mixed up with sugar, in the proportion of one part of the former to seven of the latter; a pinch of this put upon the child's tongue will be licked to all parts of the mouth.' Joseph Jakob von Plenk, professor at the Vienna Academy, recommended in 1807 [32]: 'Tortured by thirst the infant demands the breast frequently, but soon loses the nipple by crying, because the pains hinder sucking … Having applied mild laxatives and a lukewarm bath, one should paint the mouth twice daily with a solution of borax, white vitriol, or alum.' Joseph Parrot. director of the Paris Foundling Hospital from 1867, reported the wet nurses felt 'a veritable disgust to let their breast be sucked by an infant affected with thrush' [33], and mortality was high (Fig. 7.8.2). Treatment consisted of 'rubbing the buccal mucosa with a fine, dry cloth wrapped around the forefinger and of painting with rose honey and sodium borate'. Theodor Escherich, who directed the St. Anna Hospital in Graz from 1890, inserted crystalline boric acid with saccharin into a dummy, from which it continuously leaked into the infant's mouth [34]. However, McNeil reported side effects in 1912 [35], 'fits in addition to bowel trouble' in a 3-month-old infant after excessive exposure to borax and honey applied to the soothing teats: 'It would seem as if the commercial preparations are dangerously strong. Nurses and midwives should avoid using on their own responsibility preparations which may have such serious consequences.'

Stilling added gentian violet to the substances used to treat thrush in 1891 [36], while Peck and Rosenfeld added undecylenic acid in 1938 [37]. With the use of broad-spectrum antibiotics after World

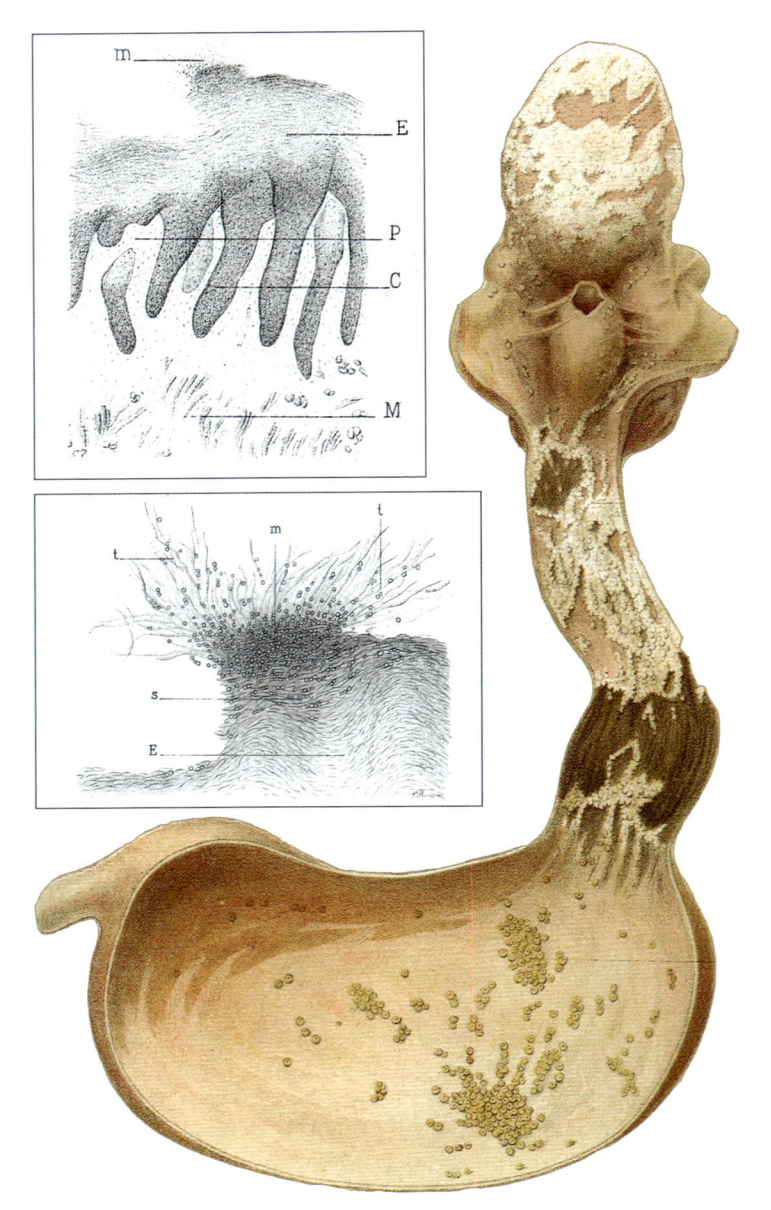

Fig. 7.8.2 Postmortem preparation showing thrush in the digestive tube, from Parrot 1877 [33]. Upper insert: microscopic detail, 35×; E, pavement epithelium; P, papillas; C, columns of mucous bodies; M, muscle. Lower insert: detail m from upper insert, enlargement 160×; t, arborescent mycelial vegetation; m, mass of spores; E, normal epithelium; s, epithelium separated by spores.

War II, fungus infections increased in frequency and severity and regained significance as a cause of mortality, necessitating research for antifungal substances. At the New York State Department of Health, a unique cooperation emerged between microbiologist Elizabeth Hazen in New York City and biochemist Rachel Brown in Albany. The two great old ladies examined thousands of soil samples for antibacterial and mycostatic properties. Fraction AN 48240 [38] was 'obtained from a soil actinomycete … extractable with alcohols from the surface growth on liquid medium and differs from other antibiotics within our knowledge. The latter agent, tentatively designated *fungicidin*, is effective in vitro against a large number of nonpathogenic and pathogenic fungi, including *Candida albicans*.' Effective *in vitro* (Fig. 7.8.3) and in infected mice [39], the substance was marketed by Squibb as *mycostatin*, later in honour of the two investigators' workplaces, *nystatin*. It was clinically tested in Cuba [40] and France, where Robert Debré and colleagues reported 'favorable results from mycostatin treatment' in 11 infants with severe or generalized candidiasis [41]. In a controlled trial, Harris and coworkers completely eradicated thrush from the Toronto nursery by preventive nystatin in 1958 [42]: 'Of the 714 infants treated, not one developed thrush during its hospital stay, and only three developed it within one week after discharge. Of the 728 control infants not treated, 18 developed thrush in the hospital and 13 in their first week at home.'

Elizabeth Hazen and Rachel Brown donated the royalties from their patent, more than US$13 million, to a foundation for the training of young microbiologists [43]. Their discovery ended the nightmare of thrush in the infant wards.

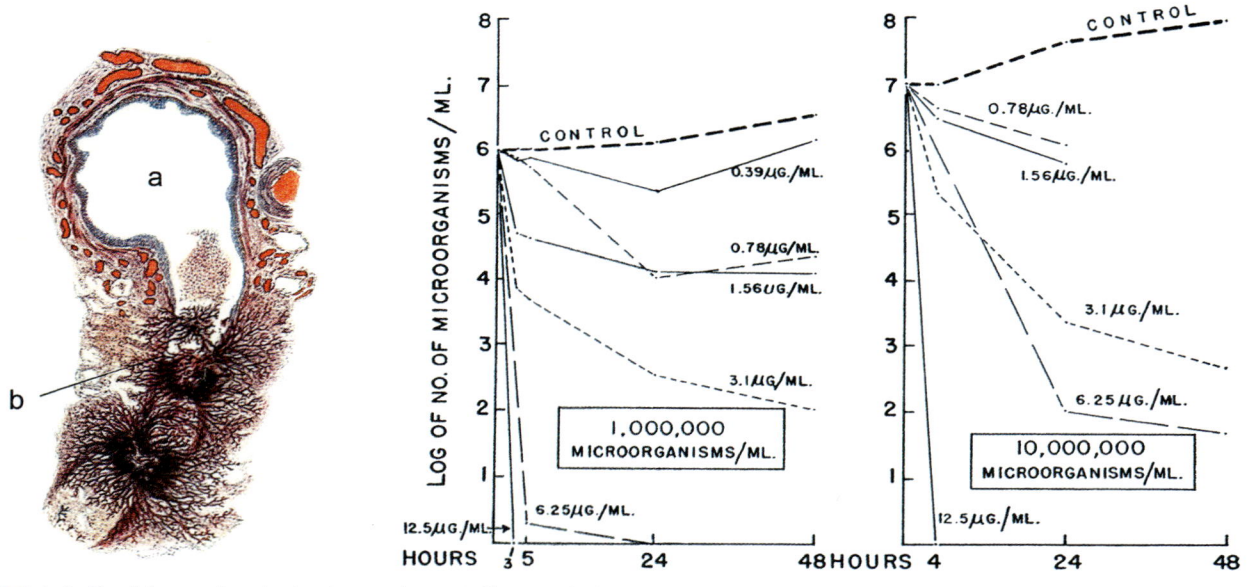

Fig. 7.8.3 Left: *Candida* mycelium in the deeper airways infiltrating the lung parenchyma, a, bronchiolus; b, ductus alveolaris. Microscopic preparation from Schlossmann 1906 [45]. Right: *in vitro* effect of *fungicidin* on the multiplication of *Candida neoformans*. A concentration of 12.5 µg/mL sterilized a solution with 10,000,000 micro-organisms/mL within 4 h.
Reproduced with permission from Hazen, E.L., Brown, R. Fungicidin, an antibiotic produced by a soil actinomycete. *Proc Soc Exp Biol Med*, 76:93–97. Copyright © 1951, © SAGE Publications.

REFERENCES

1. Leven K-H: Krankheiten: Historische Deutung versus retrospektive Diagnose. Medizingeschichte. Frankfurt: Campus, 1998: p. 153–85.
2. Hippocrates: Aphorisms. Loeb Classical Library 95. Cambridge, MA: Harvard University Press, 1979: Vol. **IV**, p. 131.
3. Celsus AC: De re medica libri octo. Lugduni Batavorum: Raphelengius, 1592: Lib. VI, p. 594.
4. Gruner OC: A treatise on the canon of medicine of Avicenna, incorporating a translation of the first book. London: Luzac, 1930: Book I, part 3, p. 374.
5. Rösslin E: Der Swangern Frauwen und hebammen Rosegarten. Straßburg: Flach, 1513: p. 84.
6. Vallambert Sd: Cinq livres de la manière de nourrir et gouverner les enfants dès leur naissance. Poitiers: Manefz et Bouchetz, 1565: p. 379.
7. Bourgeois L: Observations Diverses sur la Sterilite, Perte de Fruits, Foecondité, Accouchments, et Maladies de Femmes. Paris: Dehoury, 1609: p. 102.
8. Raulin J: Von Erhaltung der Kinder. Leipzig: Crusius, 1769: Vol. **2**, p. 165–7.
9. Underwood M: A treatise on the disorders of childhood. 2. ed. London: Matthews, 1801: Vol. **1**, p. 53–8.
10. Billard CM: Die Krankheiten der Neugeborenen und Säuglinge (1st French ed. 1828). Weimar: Industrie-Comptoir, 1829: p. 281.
11. Doepp P: Notizen über das kaiserliche Erziehungshaus (Findlingshaus) zu St. Petersburg. Hamburg: Hoffmann & Campe, 1835: Vol. **5**. p. 306–50.
12. Heberden W: An epitome of the diseases incident to children. London: Payne, 1807: p. cap. 10.
13. Seux V: Recherches sur les maladies des enfants nouveau-nés. Paris: Baillière, 1855: p. 197, 220.
14. Ludlam GB, Henderson JL: Neonatal thrush in a maternity hospital. Lancet 1942;**1**:64–70.
15. Vignec AJ: The role of candida albicans in the common skin disorders of infancy and early childhood. J Pediatr 1958;**53**:692–703.
16. Fracastoro H: De contagione et contagiosis morbis et eorum curatione. Venetiis: Giunta, 1546.
17. Veron L-D: Observations sur les maladies des enfans. Paris: Baillière, 1825: p. 25–44.
18. Valleix FLI: Clinique des maladies des enfants nouveau-nés. Paris: Baillière, 1838: p. 202–462.
19. Malpighi M: Anatome plantarum. Cui subjungitur De ovo incubato observationes. Londini: Martyn, 1675: tab. 95, fig. 1.
20. Jörg JCG: Handbuch zum Erkennen und Heilen der Kinderkrankheiten. Leipzig: Knobloch, 1826: Vol. **2**, p. 500.
21. Pieper PA: Die Kinder-Praxis im Findelhause und in dem Hospitale für kranke Kinder zu Paris. Göttingen: Dieterich, 1831: p. 169.
22. Gruby D: Recherches anatomiques sur une plante cryptogame qui constitue le vrai muguet des enfants. Compt Rend Acad Sci (Paris) 1842;**14**:634–6.
23. Berg F: Some extracts from Fredrik Theodor Berg's autobiographical memoranda. Acta Paediatr 1944;**32**:218–31.
24. Berg FT: Torsk i mikroskopiskt anatomiskt hänseende. (Thrush from the microscopical anatomical point of view). Hygiea 1841;**3**:541–50.
25. Berg FT: Om torsk hos barn. (On thrush in children). Stockholm: Hjerta, 1846.
26. Robin C: Histoire naturelle des végétaux parasites qui croissent sur l'homme et les animaux vivants. Paris: Baillière, 1853: p. 488.
27. Haussmann D: Die Parasiten der weiblichen Geschlechtsorgane des Menschen und einiger Thiere. Berlin: Hirschwald, 1870: p. 71–5, fig. 15–20.

28. Berkhout CM: De schimmelgeslachten Monilia, Oidium, Oospora, en Torula. Utrecht: Rijksuniversiteit, 1923.
29. Würtz F: Practica der Wundartzney.Annex: Ein schönes und nützliches Kinder-Büchlein. Basel: Henricpetri, 1563.
30. Ruhräh J: Pediatrics of the past. New York: Hoeber, 1925: p. 206.
31. Van Puteren MD: [On the treatment of thrush by brushings]. Vratch 1889;**41**:917.
32. Plenk JJv: Lehre von der Erkenntniß und Heilung der Kinderkrankheiten. Wien: Binz, 1807: p. 151.
33. Parrot J: Clinique des Nouveau-Nés: l'Athrepsie. Paris: Masson, 1877: p. 80, 444, tab. 1 and 6.
34. Escherich T: Der Borsäureschnuller, eine neue Behandlungsmethode des Soor. Therapie der Gegenwart, Neue Folge 1899;**1**:298–300.
35. McNeil AS: Borax and honey for bottle teats. Br J Nurs Suppl. 1912;78–9.
36. Stilling J.: Ueber Anilinfarbstoffe als Antiseptica. Naunyn-Schmiedeberg's Arch Pharmacol 1891;**28**:351–4.
37. Peck SM, Rosenfeld H.: The effects of hydrogen ion concentration, fatty acids and vitamin C on the growth of fungi. J Invest Dermatol 1938;**1**:237–65.
38. Hazen EL, Brown R: Two antifungal agents produced by a soil actinomycete. Science 1950;**112**:423.
39. Hazen EL, Brown R: Fungicidin, an antibiotic produced by a soil actinomycete. Proc Soc Exp Biol Med 1951;**76**:93–7.
40. Cardelle G: Moniliasis in childhood; diagnosis and treatment with mycostatin (nystatin). Rev Med Cubana 1955;**66**:653–71.
41. Debré R, Mozziconacci P, Drouhet E, et al.: Les infections a Candida chez le nourisson. Ann Paediat (Basel) 1955;**184**:129–64.
42. Harris LJ, Pritzker HG, Eisen A, et al.: The effect of nystatin (mycostatin) on neonatal candidiasis (thrush). Can Med Assoc J 1958;**79**:891–6.
43. Baldwin RS: The fungus fighters. Two women scientists and their discovery. New York: Cornell University Press, 1981.
44. Billard CM: Pathologisch-anatomischer Atlas. Weimar: Industrie-Comptoir, 1829: p. plate 1.
45. Moro E: Erkrankungen der Mundhöhle. In: Pfaundler M, Schlossmann A: Handbuch der Kinderheilkunde. Leipzig: Vogel, 1906: Vol. **II**, 1, p. 1–40.

7.9

Systemic infection
Sepsis

Introduction

Explaining sepsis in the era before microbiology resembles the metaphysical task of searching in a dark room for a black cat that isn't there. The task is even harder in newborns whose symptoms vary and the cardinal symptom, fever, is lacking. Sepsis definitions, never unanimously accepted [1], usually embraced both systemic inflammatory reaction and bacteraemia, but the interaction between these compounds remained obscure. Early-onset sepsis during the first 3 days is usually perceived to result from the mother, and late-onset sepsis to be hospital acquired. The history of sepsis in adults and in childbed has been described [2, 3]. The following chapter focuses on early-onset bacterial sepsis and on the newborn's particular disposition for atypical germs.

Antique theories of contagiosity

Egyptians purged their gut with enemas and passed laws against contaminating the rivers with human excrement. In the papyrus *Smith*, sepsis is mentioned as a complication of wound infection. The word *sepsis* is of Greek origin and means 'to rot'. Aristotle coined the term 'pepsis' (= fermentation), associated with concoction in the upper part of the body, and with good smell. 'Sepsis' (= putrefaction) was associated with rotting in the lower part of the body, and with a bad smell. He believed that small *animalculi* may originate spontaneously in rotting material [4].

Of course, the transmission of disease from one person to the other was known in antiquity, and was explained either by the *miasma* or by the *contagion* theory. Miasma was an external factor such as heat, cold, odour, or watching something ugly, which all had the ability to change or damage the body humours. The miasma was always transmitted by air. Contagion, somewhat different from the miasma, consisted of particles that reached the body by touch, ingestion, or via air, and were associated with dirt, but not with living microorganisms. A Hippocratic writer explained [5]: 'The influence of water on health is very great. Such as are marshy, standing and stagnant, must in summer be hot, thick and stinking, because there is no outflow; and as the sun heats them, they must be of bad color, unhealthy and bilious.' The disease most probably associated with these swamps was malaria: 'Those who drink it have large, stiff spleens ... their shoulders and faces are emaciated ... digestive organs very hot ... dysentery, diarrhea and long four-day fever ... the babies are big and swollen and become emaciated and miserable.'

Romans were familiar with contagiosity and contagion. Temples were established to venerate Juno, goddess of polluted air, under the name Mephitis. Pliny reported specific goddesses for infectious disease [6]: 'The exhalation of deadly vapours, emitted from caverns or from certain unhealthy districts ... are generally called vents, and, by some persons, Charon's sewers, from their exhaling a deadly vapour. Also at Amsanctum, in the country of the Hirpini, at the temple of Mephitis, there is a place which kills those who enter it'.

Roman architect Vitruvius Pollio defined suitable locations for cities in the 1st century C.E. [7]. His view of poisonous vapour originating from swamps and putrefying organic matter marks the change from the miasma to the contagion theory: 'When the morning breeze comes to the city with the rising sun, it transports the mist and the poisonous breath of the animals in the swamps, infects the inhabitants, and befouls the site.'

Personal hygiene

Since the 11th century, humans lived in ever-greater proximity to domestic animals, whose capacity for work was exploited and whose meat was consumed: camels, cows, goats, donkeys, or horses [8]. Thus, the streets were covered with manure, and millions of flies ensured that bacteria found their way into homes and baby food. Up to the Middle Ages and following Roman traditions, public bathrooms enabled people to clean the body, at least in the cities, where barbers and soap-boilers were licensed. When suspected of promoting promiscuity, plague and syphilis, the public baths fell from grace during the 16th century, and disappeared entirely during the 17th century, when shipbuilding caused a shortage of wood. Clothes and bodies were washed in the river, water was obtained from wells, often contaminated with faecal material, as no sewers existed (see Chapter 6.6). Although available since the Roman Empire, soap was seldom used throughout the Middle Ages, a parsimony that augmented the exposition to bacteria and exacerbated infant mortality [8]. Even when washing returned in the late 18th century, the connection between uncleanliness and infant death remained ignored.

Before microbiology: childbed fever

In 1794, Friedrich Benjamin Osiander described five newborns with generalized purulent vesicles 'and signs of putrid maceration, but born alive' (Fig. 7.9.1) [9]; only one survived. Puerperal fever was known as a killer of mothers and infants for thousands of years. It became a mass threat when lying-in hospitals were established in the 17th century, and soon epidemics of puerperal sepsis were reported from Paris, Stockholm, Vienna, and other cities. In 1795, Alexander Gordon suspected contagion when describing 77 women with puerperal fever observed in Aberdeen within 34 months, of whom 28 died [10]: 'Its cause has been referred to a noxious constitution of the atmosphere ... But it seized such women only, as were visited or delivered by a practitioner, or taken care of by a nurse, who had previously attended patients affected with the disease.' Gordon even traced the infection chain from patient to patient. 'It is a disagreeable declaration for me to mention, that I myself was the means of carrying the infection to a great number of women.'

In Boston, Oliver Wendell Holmes studied published series of endemic puerperal sepsis and recommended in 1843 [11]: 'A physician who attends cases of midwifery, should never take any active part in the post-mortem examination of cases of puerperal fever ... On the occurrence of a single case of puerperal practice, the physician is bound to consider the next female he attends as in danger of being infected by him.' Holmes was praised for his discovery and was promoted to professor and chair of anatomy and physiology at Harvard in 1847 [12]. In 1855 at the Paris Maternité, Paul Lorain studied the influence of maternal puerperal fever on the infant [13]: 'Of 193 infants born alive, 50 died of the very same affections which proved fatal to the lying-in women. The most frequent causes of death were peritonitis, numerous abscesses, purulent infection, phlegmonous swellings, erysipelas, and other septic conditions.'

In 1846, Ignaz Semmelweis was appointed assistant lecturer in the first obstetrics division at Vienna's General Hospital [14]. He recognized that in the first division (where medical students were trained) the prevalence of death from childbed fever was 16%, whereas in the second division (where midwives were trained) the prevalence was only 2% [15]. He assumed 'cadaverous particles, not cosmic or telluric' transferred by the physicians' and students' hands from the autopsies to the mothers during delivery. In May 1847, Semmelweis ordered the students to scrub their hands with chlorine, whereupon the mortality from puerperal sepsis fell immediately to 2% [16]. His colleague at the Vienna Foundling Hospital was Alois Bednar. Before describing the autopsy results of 87 newborns who had died from sepsis, Bednar noted in his monumental 'Diseases of the Newborn' [17]: 'The neonates owe their *dyscrasia* [imbalanced body humours] to the sepsis or inflammation of the uterus of their mothers, which these contract from hands contaminated with putrid cadaverous matter or other manure ... Neonatal sepsis has become rare which we owe to the beneficial discovery of Dr. Semmelweis in preventing puerperal sepsis.' But Bednar was but one of a handful of physicians who applauded Semmelweis: few episodes in the history of medicine are as shameful and tragic as the witch-hunt Semmelweis faced for telling an unpleasant truth. His suggestions for effective prevention were rejected by most of the medical community, and opposed by the German authorities Virchow and Scanzoni. He was fired from his hospital position, declared insane, and hospitalized in a psychiatric ward, where he died in 1865, 14 years before Louis Pasteur proved that living organisms, streptococci, cause childbed fever [18] and 1 year before Joseph Lister effected antisepsis by carbolic acid [19]. Today, puerperal sepsis no longer has epidemic dimensions, but it remained a threat, as shown by Jewett's 1968 report of a Boston endemic [20], where 20 mothers and five newborns suffered sepsis within 10 days.

Erysipelas

In the lying-in hospitals and foundling asylums, a severe disease was observed and named *Rose*, *Rotlauf*, *phlogosis*, and other names: redness of the skin, first located around the navel or genitalia, then migrating over large parts of the body (Fig. 7.9.2). The disease proved fatal within days. Michael Underwood termed it 'Erysipelas or St. Anthony's Fire' in 1801 [21], the latter term was also used for herpes zoster and ergot intoxication during the 18th century [22]. Underwood described erysipelas as 'a very dangerous species of inflammation, often met with in lying-in hospitals ... the ordinary time of its attack is a few days after birth, the progress is rapid, the skin turns of a purplish blue'. In 1821, Antoine Dugès reported that at the Paris Foundling Hospital erysipelas, under the name *enflure*, was 'sometimes epidemic,' and reported the case of a mother with

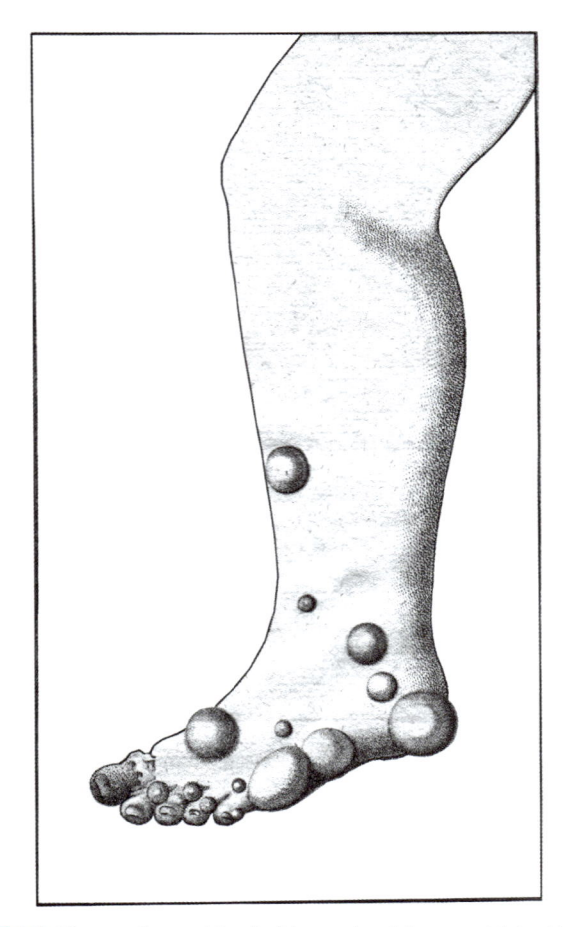

Fig. 7.9.1 'Connatal pemphigus' with purulent blisters published by Osiander in 1794 [9].

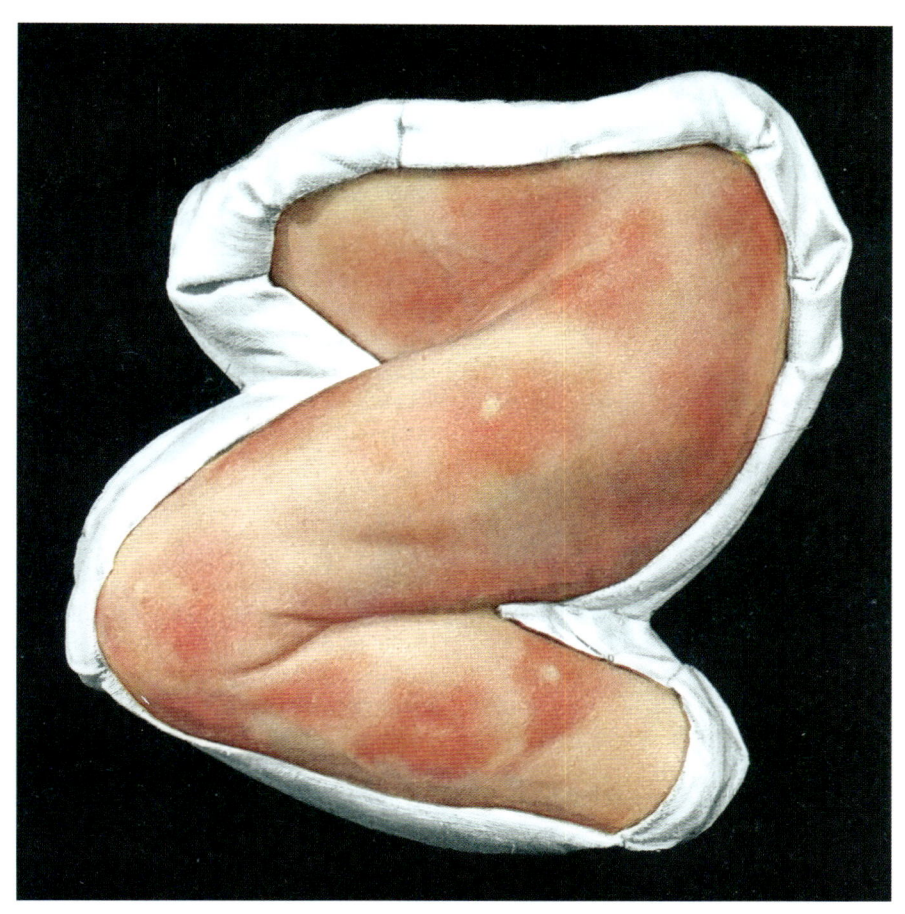

Fig. 7.9.2 Septic exanthema due to streptococci, with diffuse redness and oedematous spots, depicted by Finkelstein and co-workers in 1921 [63].

facial erysipelas who transmitted this disease to her infant [23]. After streptococci were identified, Friedrich Fehleisen proved in 1882 that in erysipelas the bacteria invaded the lymphatic vessels [24].

Buhl's disease, Winckel's disease

In 1861, the pathologist Ludwig Buhl described 'neonates … with cyanosis, jaundice, skin hemorrhages … the postmortem examination revealed acute fatty degeneration of liver, kidney and heart' [25]. Acute fatty degeneration in the newborn was also reported from New York [26] and Vienna [27]—'unclear etiology'. Retrospectively, we would classify the disorder as early-onset haemorrhagic sepsis without proof of the germ, but textbooks referred to Buhl's disease as late as 1962 [28]. In 1879, obstetrician Franz Winckel described an epidemic at the Dresden Lying in Hospital involving 23 infants suffering from cyanosis, haemolysis, jaundice, drowsiness, and skin haemorrhages; with two exceptions the infants died with seizures, mostly on day 4 [29] (Fig. 7.9.3). He named the disease 'afebrile icteric cyanosis'. In 1929, Hector Cameron classified 'types of septic infection in the newly born' and stated [30]: 'Buhl's disease and Winckel's disease still figure in textbook descriptions of neonatal disorders, but are in reality no more than particular manifestations of sepsis neonatorum.' As late as 1940, cases of Winckel's disease continued to be described in New York [31, 32].

Era of microbiology

In 1863, Louis Pasteur published his first paper on putrefaction [33], demonstrating that microbes are generated by microbes, not spontaneously as Aristotle had taught. Pasteur proposed his germ theory of disease caused by microorganisms and in 1879 proved that puerperal fever is caused by streptococci [18]. With microbiology advancing, Theodor Escherich (then at the Hauner Childrens' Hospital in Munich) characterized the normal bacterial flora of infants in 1886 [34], and proved their rapid colonization after birth. In 1919, Arvo Ylppö [35] and in 1948, Ethel Dunham [36] demonstrated that premature infants are peculiarly susceptible to septic infections. The main germs were streptococci, staphylococci, *Escherichia coli*, *Pseudomonas*, and *Klebsiella*. Changes in the bacterial spectrum from 1933 to 1957 were reported from New Haven [37].

Listeriosis

Listeria monocytogenes was identified in rabbits in 1926 [38], and in 1934, the bacterium was cultivated from the blood of three newborns with lethal sepsis [39]. An epidemic involving 15 newborns with septic symptoms and death during the first days of life occurred in Halle in 1951. It was associated with *L. monocytogenes* [40], and all infants had similar lesions: fine focal granulomas. In Canada's

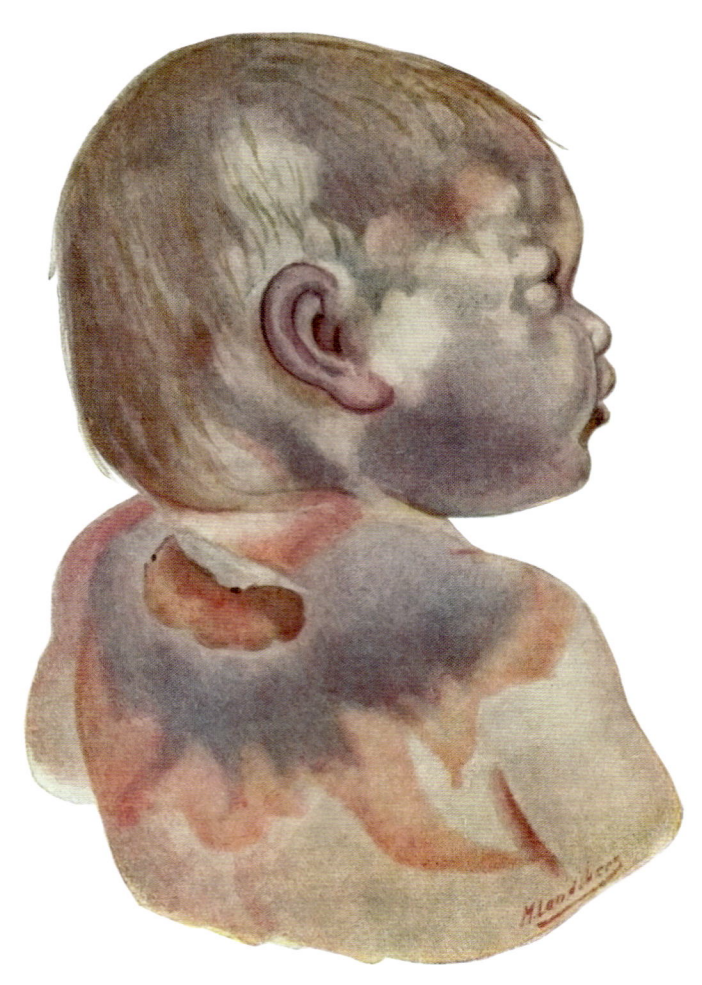

Fig. 7.9.3 Sepsis with haemoglobinuria, skin haemorrhage, and necrosis in a 7-day-old girl with streptococcal sepsis, interpreted as Winckel's disease by Finkelstein in 1921 [64].

maritime provinces, a listeriosis outbreak with 34 perinatal cases was transmitted by food (coleslaw) to the pregnant mothers [41]. The incidence of listeriosis has dropped dramatically since 1992 [42].

Group B streptococcal sepsis

Streptococci were identified in Switzerland as the cause of *Gälti* (purulent mastitis) in cattle and goats in 1887, and accordingly were named *Streptococcus agalactiae* [43, 44]. In 1933, Rebecca Lancefield classified streptococci serologically [45], and in 1935 she described that puerperal infections of the uterus were caused by group A streptococci, whereas group B strains usually were isolated from mothers with afebrile puerperium [46]. The belief in a 'harmless saprophyte' waned when in 1938 Rowdon Fry published the fate of three mothers who had died from puerperal sepsis caused by group B streptococci [47]. In the 1940s, group B streptococci emerged as a pathogen of newborns in New Haven [37], and by 1962, they had become the most common cause of neonatal sepsis in Boston, accounting for 25% of such infections [48]. The disease presented in 2 of 1000 live births, either within hours of birth and respiratory distress, or as meningitis in the late neonatal period [49]. By 1972,

one in four Texan women, pregnant, non-pregnant, and nurses in neonatal intensive care units, were colonized with group B streptococci [50]. Maternal colonization, however, did not predict neonatal infection [51].

From community-based studies, Barbara Stoll calculated the impact of neonatal infections in less developed countries such as sub-Saharan Africa, India, Southeast Asia [52]: 9–54% of neonatal deaths were due to infections, and the incidence of neonatal sepsis was 2.4–21 per 1000 live births, whereas in the US, the rate of early-onset sepsis was 0.98 per 1000 live births [53]; group B streptococci remained the most frequent pathogen in term, and *E. coli* the most significant pathogen in preterm infants. Group B streptococcal sepsis has become rare with routine screening of all mothers before birth, and antibiotic application at least 4 h before delivery [54].

Antibiotics: blessing and curse

The discovery of penicillin in 1928 [55] and of sulphonamides in 1932 [56] turned the usually deadly sepsis in the neonate into a treatable disease, and modern antibiotics further improved babies' chances of survival. In the 1950s, preterm infants were treated prophylactically with antibiotics, when born after prolonged rupture of membranes. In 1949, a new antibiotic came on the market: chloramphenicol, highly effective against *Haemophilus*, passing easily into the cerebrospinal fluid, but not studied in neonates. The result was, once more, an iatrogenic catastrophe: the 'grey baby syndrome'. The recommended daily dose was 100 mg/kg, but more than 220 mg/kg had been administered before a fatal collapse in three infants was noticed in Cincinnati which resembled septic shock [57]: abdominal distension, vomiting, progressive pallid cyanosis, circulatory collapse, irregular respiration, and death within a few hours of symptom onset [58]. After case reports from several countries, a controlled trial was finally conducted in 1959 in preterm infants born after prolonged rupture of the fetal membranes [59]: the mortality was 18% in two groups without, and 66% in two groups with chloramphenicol. The chloramphenicol toxicity in neonates turned out to be due to diminished glucuronidation during the first days of life [60].

In the 1970s, resistant bacterial strains emerged and late-onset nosocomial sepsis became frequent in newborns undergoing intensive care: hospital bacteria had allied dangerously with indwelling devices, particularly central venous catheters. Between hospitals, the frequency varied from 5 to 15 bloodstream infections per 1000 central-line days [61]. Surveillance programmes helped to reduce both the use of central lines and the device-associated rate of nosocomial sepsis. Group B streptococci isolated from neonates still were susceptible to penicillin in the 1990s, but 20% and 7% had become resistant to erythromycin and clindamycin, respectively [62].

Conclusion

Neonatal sepsis was understood at the same time as puerperal sepsis, from which it often resulted. Why was, in the same decade, the important but unpleasant discovery that puerperal sepsis was transmitted from patient to patient by the physician, accepted in Boston but rejected in Vienna? Different handling of the shocking news illustrates how sociocultural attitudes promote or hinder scientific progress: 28-year-old resident physician Semmelweis, of Hungarian origin, was abandoned and derided by his colleagues, his findings and conclusions ignored in the conservative and backward Austrian Empire that trusted in authorities. The 34-year-old junior professor Holmes, integrated in the academic and literary elite of Boston, was—after some debate—applauded and promoted. Group B streptococci rarely attacked adults or older children; but under the immunological characteristics of pregnancy and birth, they became the predominant infectious agents. The catastrophic dimension of 'grey baby syndrome' was due to three reasons: (1) administering a new drug to newborns without a controlled trial; (2) preventive use in a large number of infants; and (3) a 'much-helps-more' mentality that led to toxic overdoses. Much of the present-day fear of air pollution may have its roots in the deeply ingrained age-old idea of miasma.

REFERENCES

1. Wynn JL, Wong HR, Shanley TP, et al.: Time for a neonatal-specific consensus definition for sepsis. Pediatr Crit Care Med 2014;**15**:523–8.
2. Charles D, Larsen B: Streptococcal puerperal sepsis and obstetric infections. Rev Infect Dis 1986;**8**:411–22.
3. Majno G: The ancient riddle of sepsis. J Infect Dis 1991;**163**:937–45.
4. Aristotle: Generation of animals. Loeb Classical Library 366. Cambridge, MA: Harvard University Press, 2007: Vol. **3**, p. 762a.
5. Hippocrates: Airs, waters, places. Loeb Classical Library. London: Heinemann, 1957: Vol. **1**, cap. 7, p. 83–5.
6. Plinius GS: Naturgeschichte. Stuttgart: Metzler, 1840: Vol. **2**, cap. 95, p. 227.
7. Pollio MV: De architectura. Lugduni: Tornaesius, 1552: Vol. **1**, cap. 4, p. 17.
8. Braudel F: Die Geschichte der Zivilisation. 15. bis 18. Jahrhundert. München: Kindler, 1971: p. 355, 371.
9. Osiander FB: Denkwürdigkeiten für die Heilkunde und Geburtshülfe. Göttingen: Vandenhoek-Ruprecht, 1794: Vol. **1**, p. 383–423.
10. Gordon A: A treatise on the epidemic puerperal fever of Aberdeen. London: Robinson, 1795: p. 36.
11. Holmes OW: The contagiousness of puerperal fever. N Engl Q J Med Surg 1843;**1**:503–30.
12. Tubbs RS, Shoja MM, Loukas M, Carmichael SW: Oliver Wendell Holmes (1809–1894). Clin Anat 2012;**25**:992–7.
13. Lorain P: La fièvre puerpérale chez la femme, le foetus, et le nouveau-né. Paris: Baillière, 1855: p. 8–17.
14. Adriaanse AH: Semmelweis: the combat against puerperal fever. Eur J Obstet Gynecol 2000;**90**:153–8.
15. Semmelweis IP: Die Aetiologie, der Begriff und die Prophylaxe des Kindbettfiebers. Leipzig: Hartleben, 1861.
16. Semmelweis IP, [Anonymous]: Höchst wichtige Erfahrung über die Aetiologie der in Gebäranstalten epidemischen Puerperalfieber. Zeitschr der KK Ges Aerzte Wien 1847;**4**:242–4.
17. Bednar A: Die Krankheiten der Neugeborenen und Säuglinge. Wien: Gerold, 1853: p. 1–98, 4–240.
18. Pasteur L: Septicémie puerpérale. Bull Acad Méd, 2e série 1879;**8**:505–8.
19. Lister J: On the antiseptic principle in the practice of surgery. Lancet 1867;**II**:353–6.
20. Jewett JF, Reid DE, Safon LE, Easterday CL: Childbed fever—a continuing entity. JAMA 1968;**206**:344–50.
21. Underwood M: A treatise on the disorders of childhood. 2. ed. London: Matthews, 1801: Vol. **1**, p. 53–8.
22. Burserius von Kanilfeld JB: Anleitung zur Kenntnis und Heilung der fieberischen Ausschlagskrankheiten. Frankfurt: Krieger, 1789: Vol. **1**, p. 19, 52.
23. Dugès A: Recherches sur les maladies les plus importantes et les moins connues des enfans nouveau-nés. Paris: Baillière, 1821: p. 19–23.
24. Fehleisen F: Die Aetiologie des Erysipels. Berlin: Fischer, 1883.
25. Buhl L: Die acute Fettdegeneration der Neugeborenen. In: Hecker C, Buhl L: Klinik für Geburtskunde. Leipzig: Engelmann, 1861: p. 296–300.
26. Jacobi MP: Acute fatty degeneration of new-born. Am J Obstet Dis Women Child 1878;**11**:3–16.
27. Reuss ARv: Die Krankheiten des Neugeborenen. Berlin: Springer, 1914: p. 418.
28. Ewerbeck H: Der Säugling. Berlin: Springer, 1962: p. 246.
29. Winckel F: Über eine bisher nicht beschriebene endemisch auftretende Erkrankung Neugeborener. Dtsch Med Wochenschr 1879;**5**:303–307, 415–8, 447–50.
30. Cameron HC: Some types of septic infection in the newly-born. Lancet 1929;**213**:1127–30.
31. Polayes SH, Kramer B: Winckel's disease. J Pediatr 1933;**2**:482–6.
32. Glaser J, Epstein J: Winckel's disease. Am J Dis Child 1940;**60**:1375–80.
33. Pasteur L: Recherches sur la putréfaction. Compt Rend Acad Sci 1863;**56**:1189–94.
34. Escherich T: Die Darmbakterien des Neugeborenen und Säuglings. Fortschr Med 1886;**3**:515–22; 547–54.
35. Ylppö A: Zur Physiologie, Klinik und zum Schicksal der Frühgeborenen. Zeitschr Kinderheilk 1919;**24**:1–110.
36. Dunham EC: Premature infants. Children's Bureau Publication Nr. 325. Washington, DC: Federal Security Agency, 1948: p. 241.
37. Nyhan WL, Fousek MD: Septicemia of the newborn. Pediatrics 1958;**22**:268–78.
38. Murray EGD, Webb RA, Swann MBR: A disease of rabbits characterised by a large mononuclear leucocytosis. J Path Bact 1926;**29**:407–39.
39. Burn CG: Unidentified grampositive bacillus associated with meningo-encephalitis. Proc Soc Exp Biol Med 1934;**31**:1095–7.
40. Reiss HJ, Potel J, Krebs A: Granulomatosis infantiseptica, eine durch einen spezifischen Erreger hervorgerufene fetale Sepsis. Klin Wochenschr 1951;**29**:29.
41. Schlech WF, Lavigne PM, Bortolussi PM, et al.: Epidemic listeriosis—evidence for transmission by food. N Engl J Med 1983;**308**:203–6.
42. Lee B, Newland JG, Jhaveri R: Reductions in neonatal listeriosis. J Infect 2016;**72**:317–23.
43. Nocard M, Mollereau R: Sur une mammite contagieuse des vaches laitières. Ann Inst Pasteur 1887;**1**:109–26.
44. Hess E, Borgeaud A: Eine kontagiöse Euterentzündung, gelber Galt genannt (mastitis catarrhalis infectiosa). Schweiz Arch Tierheilk 1888;**30**:157–79.
45. Lancefield RC: A serological differentiation of human and other groups of hemolytic streptococci. J Exp Med 1933;**57**:571–95.
46. Lancefield RC: The serological differentiation of pathogenic and non-pathogenic strains of hemolytic streptococci from parturient women. J Exp Med 1935;**61**:335–49.
47. Fry RM: Fatal infections by haemolytic streptococcus group B. Lancet 1938;**231**:199–201.

48. Eickhoff TC, Klein JO, Daly A.K., et al.: Neonatal sepsis and other infections due to group B beta-hemolytic streptococci. N Engl J Med 1964;271:1221–8.
49. Franciosi RA, Knostman JD, Zimmerman RA: Group B streptococcal neonatal and infant infections. J Pediatr 1973;82:707–18.
50. Baker CJ, Barrett FF: Transmission of group B streptococci among parturient women and their neonates. J Pediatr 1973;83: 919–25.
51. Regan JA, Klebanoff MA, Nugent RP, et al.: Colonization with group B streptococci in pregnancy and adverse outcome. Am J Obstet Gynecol 1996;174:1354–60.
52. Stoll BJ: The global impact of neonatal infection. Clin Perinatol 1997;24:1–21.
53. Stoll BJ, Hansen NI, Sanchez PJ, et al.: Early onset neonatal sepsis. Pediatrics 2011;127:817–26.
54. Schrag SJ, Zell ER, Lynfeld R, et al.: A population-based comparison of strategies to prevent early-onset group B streptococcal disease in neonates. N Engl J Med 2002;347:233–9.
55. Fleming A: On the antibacterial action of cultures of a Penicillum. Br J Exp Path 1929;10:226–36.
56. Domagk G: Ein Beitrag zur Chemotherapie der bakteriellen Infektionen. Dtsch Med Wochenschr 1935;61:250–3.
57. Sutherland JM: Fatal cardiovascular collapse of infants receiving large amounts of chloramphenicol. AMA J Dis Child 1959;97:761–7.
58. Krieger E: Chloramphenicol therapy: a warning. Canad Med Assoc J 1961;84:550–1.
59. Burns LE, Hodgman JE, Cass AB: Fatal circulatory collapse in premature infants receiving chloramphenicol. N Engl J Med 1959;261:1318–21.
60. Nahata MC, Powell DA: Bioavailability and clearance of chloramphenicol after intravenous chloramphenicol succinate. Clin Pharmacol Ther 1981;30:368–72.
61. Gaynes RP, Martone WJ, Culver DH, et al.: Comparison of rates of nosocomial infections in neonatal intensive care units in the United States. Am J Med 1991;91:192S–6S.
62. Lin FYC, Azimi PH, Weisman LE, et al.: Antibiotic susceptibility profiles for group B streptococci isolated from neonates, 1995–1998. Clin Infect Dis 2000;31:76–9.
63. Finkelstein H, Galewski EE, Halberstaedter L: Hautkrankheiten und Syphilis im Säuglings- und Kindesalter. 2. ed. Berlin: Springer, 1921: p. 8.
64. Finkelstein H: Lehrbuch der Säuglingskrankheiten. 2. ed. Berlin: Springer, 1921: p. 379–80.

PART 8
Early death

8.1 **From right to sin: laws on infanticide in antiquity** 353

8.2 **From sin to crime: laws on infanticide in the Middle Ages** 359

8.3 **From crime to disease: laws on infanticide in the modern era** 365

8.4 **Despising the weak: long shadows of infant murder in Nazi Germany** 371

8.5 **Cot death: history of an iatrogenic disaster** 377

8.6 **Theirs is the kingdom of heaven: infant mortality statistics** 383

8.7 **For whom no bell tolled: infant burials** 391

8.8 **Revived for paradise: respite sanctuaries** 397

INTRODUCTION

Part 8 of this book deals with death in infancy. In antiquity, the killing of infants was frequent and more or less tolerated by societies, but natural infantile mortality also exceeded 40%, leading to incredible indifference of families and health professionals. With Christianization, infanticide became forbidden in most European states. Believing that an infant deprived of baptism is denied access to paradise, draconic punishment of women who killed their infants was introduced in the Middle Ages. In many cultures, stillborn and deceased neonates were not buried in normal cemeteries but in infant necropolises or the parental house. All over Europe, sanctuaries were established where stillborn or deceased neonates were 'revived' to be baptized, buried in sacred ground, and promised a life in paradise. In the second half of the 20th century, a cot death epidemic followed the recommendation of prone sleeping.

8.1 From right to sin
Laws on infanticide in antiquity

Introduction

Infanticide is common among primates, extinguishing firstborns, especially infants born by females with whom the (new) heard leader did not have intercourse [1]. It was a behaviour common to all human cultures, but for various reasons and in various forms. Infanticide is influenced by fertility control, sex preference, socio-economic situation, societal and religious attitude towards illegitimate pregnancy, and the state's interest reflected by the law. To get rid of superfluous offspring, various methods evolved: (1) adoption, usually to a wealthy childless family; (2) abandonment at a church door or foundling institution; (3) oblation ('offering') to a monastery [2]; (4) exposure in a hostile environment; and (5) direct killing (infanticide). Undesired infants included the legitimate of the poor, the illegitimate of the rich, the malformed of all, girls in cultures where dowry was mandatory, twins, and prematures.

Aims and focus

This is the first of three chapters investigating how infanticide legislation reflected the attitude of states towards the newborn and how societies valued the health and safety of infants. Chapters 8.1–8.3 focus on written laws concerning postnatal infanticide by the child's own mother. Other forms of child killing, although important but without specific laws, have been omitted, such as ritual or religious sacrifice [3, 4], immurement of live infants in buildings [5], suicide by proxy [6], postneonatal homicide of older children, and state-organized murder of handicapped infants [7]. Abortion has also been excluded and twin infanticide has been treated separately (see Chapter 4.1). Sources include court records, historic reports, demographic statistics, and analyses of inscriptions and gravestones. In the legislative context, antiquity is defined herein up to the Justinian enactments in 534 C.E.

Frequency and sex ratio

Estimating the frequency of infanticide is notoriously unreliable, as the neonate's corpse decays rapidly and court records represent but the tip of the iceberg. Dickemann estimated that 5–50% of infants born in recent agrarian cultures fell victim to infanticide [8]. Tarn found 118 sons and 28 daughters in 79 families living in Miletos in 228–220 B.C.E. [9]. Normally, slightly more males are born than females (106:100), but due to elevated male mortality, the natural sex ratio in adults is expected to be below 100. Table 8.1.1 shows sex ratios from different cultures and epochs, high ratios suggesting the possibility of selective female infanticide. As Hirschfeld and colleagues pointed out [10], unbalanced sex ratios must be interpreted with caution, as they may be influenced by cultural and economic factors, especially in data collected for tax purposes.

The Orient

In East Asian societies, selective female infanticide was the rule, despite formal interdiction by the law [21]. In the Zhou dynasty, the statesman Guan Zhong (died 645 B.C.E.) appointed guardians to ensure that orphans were provided for, and remitted taxes contributing to their support [22]. Confucianism, Chinese belief since the 5th century B.C.E., attributed little value to women. In the 3rd century B.C.E., philosopher Fung You-Lan reported [23]: 'A father and mother when they produce a boy congratulate one another, but when they produce a girl they put her to death ... This is because the parents think of their later convenience, and calculate about what is profitable in the long run.' In 235 B.C.E., the Han law decreed [24]: 'Unauthorizedly to kill a child (is punished by) tattooing and [hard work]. When the child is newly born and has strange things on its body, as well when it is deformed, to kill it is not to be considered a crime.' In Japan, infanticide was called *mabiki* (thinning rice seedlings) since antiquity, and was more or less legal until replaced by liberalized abortion in 1948. In India, female infanticide resulted from the low esteem of girls in Hinduism, and by the need to pay a dowry by the bride's to the groom's family. It could amount to several annual family incomes, and easily ruined a wealthy family of a girl, let alone of several [25]. Mesopotamian societies worshipped the mother goddess Ishtar. The birth of malformed infants prognosticated bad omens, but neither the Summa Izbu nor the Hammurabi Code suggest that Babylonians killed malformed infants. Adoption

Table 8.1.1 Sex ratios in *adult* populations (unless specified otherwise by *italics*), obtained from various epochs and study methods

Time	Material studied	N	Males/100 females	Reference
2,000,000–30,000 B.C.E.	Fossils of Pithecanthropus, Neanderthal, Palaeolithic *Homo*	122	148	[11]
4500–3300 B.C.E.	Skeletons from Paloma, Peru: adults >15 years	49	227	[12]
228–220 B.C.E.	Anatolian-Greek tombstone inscriptions in Miletos	146	421	[9]
3rd century B.C.E.	Burned bones of (sacrificed?) *neonates* in urns of Carthago cemetery	67	68	[4]
50 B.C.E.–200 C.E	City of Rome, tombstone inscriptions	8065	131	[13]
757–855 C.E.	Carolingean tax registry, 20 German villages	1061	119	[14]
801–829 C.E.	St. Germain/Paris polyptich, estate and population register	8304	110–253	[15]
1066–1509	*Children* of the 18 first Kings of England	94	109	[16]
1377	Poll tax during the great plague, 12 English locations	12,515	99	[16]
1733–1734	Parochial registry of the Serbian sector of Belgrade	1172	106	[17]
1792–1840	*Birth* registry of rural Liaoning, China	1871	214	[18]
1812	Government report on Jádejá villages in Kathiawar, India	458	527 (!)	[19]
1902	Demographic data of *children*, 3 Netsilik Inuit locations	287	202 (!)	[20]

and sale of infants 'raised from the dog's mouth' (foundlings) were common and regulated by clay tablet contracts [26]. Egyptian society was, to some degree, matriarchal. The goddesses Isis, Hathor, Nekhebet, Meskhenet, and Taweret were believed to protect childbirth and the neonate. Diodorus Siculus reported the punishment of parents in Egypt before Roman rule [27]: 'Parents that killed their children were not to die, but were forced for three subsequent days and nights to hug them continually in their arms, and had a guard all the while over them.' Also Claudius Aelianus described infant protection in Egypt in the 5th century B.C.E. [28]: 'It was a law, that a Theban could not expose his child on waste land. But if the father of the infant was very poor, whether the child was male or female, he had to take it immediately after birth in its clothing to the magistrates, who turned it over to the person who accepted the lowest payment. A contract was made ... whereby [the adopter] pledged to foster the child, and retain it as a slave when it grew up, receiving its services as the reward for having reared it.' Hebrews strictly condemned any practice of infanticide: 'But the midwives feared God, and did not do as the king of Egypt had commanded them, but let the boys live' [Exodus 1:17]. Describing Jews, Tacitus emphasized [29]: 'Population growth is one of their concerns; in fact it is a sacrilege to kill any infant which is born in excess; and they believe in the immortality of the soul.' By *excess* Romans meant any infant born to a *paterfamilias* who already had an heir by birth or adoption. The Jewish attitude was adopted in Christianity: 'And who so shall receive one such little child in my name receiveth me.' [Matthew 18:5].

Greek and Macedonian era

The third 'Homeric' *Hymn to Apollo*, written in the 6th century B.C.E., described Hera's attempt to kill her clubfooted infant, shown in **Fig. 8.1.1** [30]: 'But my son Hephaestus whom I bare was weakly among all the blessed gods and shrivelled of foot, a shame and disgrace to me in heaven, whom I myself took in my hands and cast out so that he fell in the great sea.' Stone-carved in the 5th century B.C.E., the Cretan Law of Gortyna [31] (**Fig. 8.1.2**, left) obliged the (divorced) woman to 'carry [the newborn] to the husband, in the presence of 3 witnesses; and if he do not receive the child, it shall be in the power of the mother either to bring up or expose.' Aristotle proposed in his *Politics* in the 4th century B.C.E. [32]: 'Let there be a law that no deformed child shall be reared; but on the ground of number of children ... there must be a limit fixed to the procreation of offspring, and if any people have a child in excess of these regulations, abortion must be practised on it before it has developed sensation and life.' Greeks usually did not rear more than one daughter [9], and during the Alexandrian Empire, Polybius associated infanticide with population decline [33]: 'In our own time the whole of Greece has been subject to a low birth-rate and a general decrease of the population, owing to which cities have become deserted and the land has ceased to yield fruit, although there have neither been continuous wars nor epidemics ... If [men] married, [they did not wish] to rear the children born to them, or at most one or two of them, so as to leave these in affluence.'

Roman Empire: *patria potestas*

In 451 B.C.E., the Law of 12 Tables commanded: 'A dreadfully malformed child shall be quickly killed' [34]. *Patria potestas* originated at the same time, which mainly regulated inheritance, but included the father's right to kill his children, *jus vitae ac necis*: 'The children whom we have begotten in lawful wedlock are under our power ... The power which we have over our children is peculiar to the citizens of Rome' [35]. The mother had no influence on this decision. Paternal rejection usually resulted from an abundance of (female) children; the infant's malformation; suspected maternal adultery; and birth on *dies ater* (fateful day) [36]. *Patria potestas* could be enacted from afar: In June of 1 B.C.E., the Roman soldier Hilarion sent a papyrus letter from Alexandria to his wife Alis in Oxyrhynchus, 300 km upstream of the Nile [37]: 'I urge you, care for the [elder] child, and if I soon get pay, I will send it to you. If perhaps you give birth, then if it is male, let it be; if it is female, throw it out' (**Fig. 8.1.2**, centre). *Patria potestas* was considered obsolete in late antiquity [38], but it prevented effective legislative protection of the newborn for centuries. Next to exposure, a typical Roman method

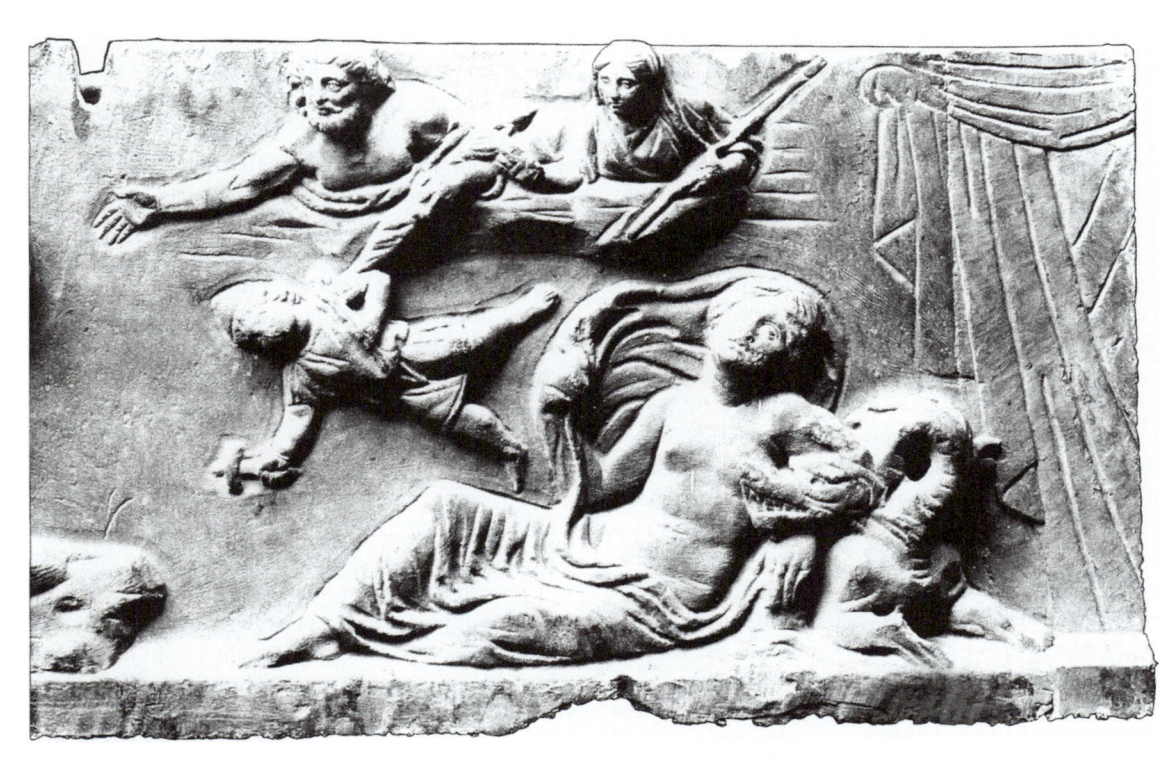

CHAPTER 8.1 From right to sin: laws on infanticide in antiquity 355

Fig. 8.1.1 Hera and Zeus throw their clubfooted son Hephaistos into the sea. Marble temple frieze from Ostia, 2nd century B.C.E. Rome, Museo Ostiense, inv. 148 & 18853, with permission.

of infanticide was drowning in a bucket, as reported by Seneca in the 1st century C.E. [39]: 'Unnatural progeny we destroy; we drown even children who at birth are weakly and abnormal. Yet it is not anger, but reason that separates the harmful from the sound.' Soranus of Ephesus taught in Rome in the 2nd century C.E. [40]: 'The infant which is worth rearing will be distinguished by the fact that its mother spent the period of pregnancy in good health, for conditions which require medical care, also harm the fetus. Second, by the fact

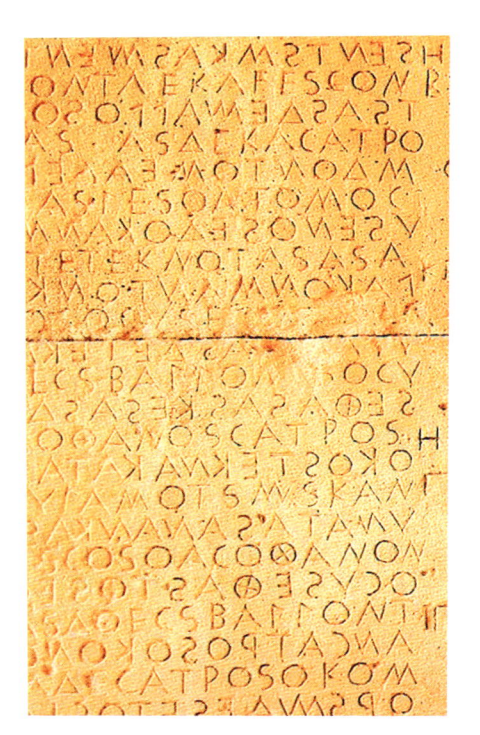

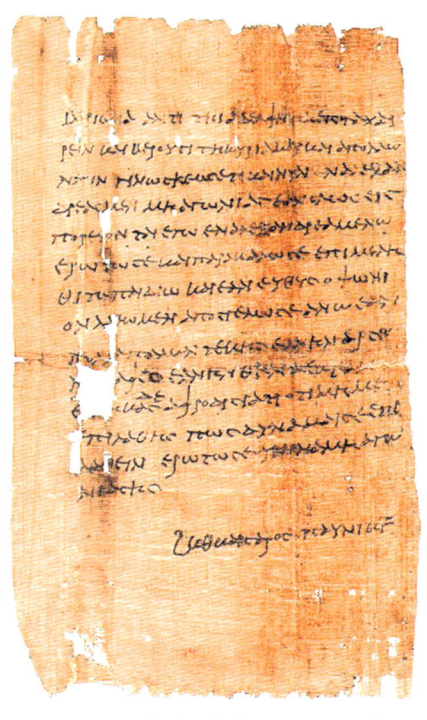

Fig. 8.1.2 Early documents of infant exposure and protection. Left: detail of stone-carved Law of Gortyna/Crete in Greek Bustrophedon text (5th century B.C.E.), regulating the exposure of infants [31]. Centre: Hilarion's papyrus letter (1 B.C.E.) from Alexandria/Roman Egypt, ordering his wife to kill the expected newborn if female (Papyrus Oxyrhynchus 744, Thomas Fisher Rare Book Library, University of Toronto). Right: detail of bronze tablet from Veleia/Emilia-Romagna of 103 C.E. The Latin inscription regulated the support of poor or exposed infants by Trajan's alimentation law [43].

that it was born at the due time, best at the end of nine months, and if it so happens, later; but also after only seven months … Also by the fact that it is perfect in all its parts, members and senses … And by conditions contrary to those mentioned, the infant not worth rearing is recognized.' Obviously, many newborns did not meet all these criteria, as Tertullian complained in 197 c.e. [41]: 'How many of you [Guardians of the Roman Empire] might I deservedly charge with Infant-murther? And not only so, but among the different Kinds of Death, for choosing some of the cruellest for their own Children, such as drowning, or starving with Cold or Hunger, or exposing them to the Mercy of Dogs.'

Change began when Trajan extended the *alimentaria* instituted by Emperor Nerva: governmental loans were given to landowners in small inland towns of Italy, the interest of 5% per year was used to maintain children of poor families [42]. The goal was to raise the birth rate and reduce infanticide. A large bronze tablet from Veleia (Fig. 8.1.2, right) explains that Trajan loaned the sum of 1.044 million sesterces (HS), equalling the price of 500 slaves, to this small community in 103 c.e. From the annual interest of 52,200 HS, '245 legitimate boys are to receive 192 HS each, 34 legitimate girls 144 HS each, 1 illegitimate boy 144 HS and 1 illegitimate girl 120 HS' [43] (Fig. 8.1.2, right). On the tablet follow 52 lists of proprietors and their mortgaged estates. In 104 c.e., Trajan wrote to Pliny the Younger [44]: 'Children born free, then exposed by their parents, and afterwards taken up by others and educated in slavery … you must not deny their freedom; nor ought they to pay for their maintenance, in order to enjoy their liberty.' But in no way did the law protect sick or malformed infants. Julius Paulus decreed in 230 c.e. [45]: 'Not among children rank those born untoward the human frame, e.g. if a woman brings forth a malformed or monstrous infant.' Another law, the *Lex Pompeia de parricidiis* passed in the consulship of Pompeius, 52 b.c.e., inflicted a singular punishment on the most horrible of crimes [35]: 'Who hastened the death of a parent or child, or of any other relation whose murder is legally termed parricide, whether he acts openly or secretely … He will be punished, not by the sword, nor by fire, nor by any ordinary mode of punishment, but he is to be sown up in a sack with a dog, a rooster, a viper, and an ape, and inclosed in this horrible prison thrown into the sea, or into a river.' Most probably parricide law was not applied to neonates until the Milan edict, when Emperor Constantine adopted the Christian faith and issued a series of laws to stop infanticide: in 313 c.e. he authorized the sale of infants [46]. His law of 315 c.e. 'intended to keep the parents' hands away from infanticide' [47]: 'Immediate and sufficient aid be given by magistrates to parents who produced children that they were too poor to bring up.' In 319, the *Lex Pompeia* was extended to include newborns. In 374 c.e., co-emperors Valentinian, Valens, and Gratian formally outlawed infanticide: 'Who committed the crime of killing a newborn shall know that he will be punished by death' [48]. In 410 c.e. the Visigoths sacked Rome. The collapsing Roman Empire could not reinforce Constantine's laws and handed infanticide over to the church, like other *carnal delicts*. The Justinian plague of 541 c.e. marked the end of antiquity.

Celtic and Germanic peoples

In his *Germania*, Tacitus, somewhat astonished, reported in the 4th century c.e. [49]: 'To limit the number of children or to kill an offspring born after the first is considered a sacrilege, and good morals there [in Germania] are stronger than good laws are elsewhere.' Despite Tacitus' benevolent judgement, several Germanic tribes practised infanticide, as Friesians and Visigoths. Infanticide was so common among the latter that King Chindasvinth (in 643 c.e.) announced severe penalties on perpetrators [50]. The *Lex Visigothorum* ordered that killing of a newborn by the mother be punished by death or blinding, regardless of the baby's legitimacy [51, 52]. The Salian-Frankish code of 507 c.e. decreed [53]: 'He who kills an infant in its mother's womb *or before it has a name* shall be liable to pay one hundred solidi.' The penalty for killing a free Frank was 200, a Roman aristocrat 300 solidi.

Social birth, the permit to live

In the absence of laws, rites evolved to protect the newborn during the dangerous days after birth. Romans and Inuit linked the right to live with *naming* an infant (*dies lustricus*), an act deeply rooted in most cultures (see Chapter 2.7) [54]. The Salic Law 511 c.e. also offered less protection to a newborn until a name was given [55], whereas for some Germanic tribes the right to life was associated with the start of oral feedings.

Conclusion

The literature of antiquity, without feelings of guilt about abandoning or killing infants, seems callous today. *Patria potestas* was a privilege of Roman males, whereas abortion or postnatal infanticide by females was regarded as immoral and was forbidden. Raising foundlings to become slaves, gladiators, or prostitutes was motivated by profit rather than mercy. The frequency of infanticide and its influence on demography is difficult to evaluate because the infant mortality rate was very high anyway. Laws intended to protect the life of infants were issued by the Roman emperors after Christianization. As unmarried women continued to be defamed and punished, such legislation was ineffective.

REFERENCES

1. Hrdy SB: Infanticide as a primate reproductive strategy. Am Sci 1977;**65**:40–9.
2. Boswell JE: Expositio and Oblatio: the abandonment of children and the ancient and medieval family. Am Hist Rev 1984;**89**:10–33.
3. Brown S: Late Carthaginian child sacrifice and sacrificial monuments in their Mediterranean context. Sheffield: Academic Press, 1991.
4. Schwartz JH, Houghton F, Macchiarelli R, Bondioli L: Skeletal remains from Punic Carthage do not support systematic sacrifice of infants. PLoS One 2010;**5**:e9177.
5. Beilke-Voigt I: Das 'Opfer' im archäologischen Befund. In: Berliner Archäologische Forschungen. Rahden/Westfalen: Leidorf, 2007: Vol. **4**.
6. Stuart K: Suicide by proxy. Cent Eur Hist 2008;**41**:413–45.
7. Benzenhöfer U: Genese und Struktur der 'NS-Kinder- und Jugendlicheneuthanasie'. Mschr Kinderheilk 2003;**151**:1012–9.

8. Dickeman M: Demographic consequences of infanticide in man. Ann Rev Ecol Syst 1975;6:107–37.
9. Tarn WW: Hellenistic civilization. 3. ed. London: Arnold, 1952: p. 100–2.
10. Hirschfeld LA, Howe J, Levin B: Warfare, infanticide, and statistical inference. Am Anthropol 1978;80:110–5.
11. Vallois HV: The social life of early man: the evidence of skeletons. Chicago, IL: Aldine, 1961: p. 214–35.
12. Benfer RA: The preceramic period site of Paloma, Peru. Latin Am Antiq 1990;1:284–318.
13. MacDonell WR: On the expectation of life in ancient Rome and in the provinces of Hispania and Lusitania, and Africa. Biom Trust 1913;9:366–80.
14. Inama-Sternegg K-T: Deutsche Wirtschaftsgeschichte. Vol. 1. Leipzig: Duncker & Humblot, 1879: Vol. 1, p. 514.
15. Coleman E: Infanticide in the Early Middle Ages. In: Stuard SM: Women in medieval society. Philadelphia, PA: University of Pennsylvania Press, 1976: p. 47–70.
16. Russell JC: British medieval population. Albuquerque: University of New Mexico Press, 1948: p. 148–65.
17. Laslett P, Clarke M: Houseful and household in an eighteenth-century Balkan city. In: Household and family in past time. Cambridge: Cambridge University Press, 1972: p. 375–400.
18. Lee J, Campbell C: Fate and fortune in rural China. Cambridge: Cambridge University Press, 1997: p. 96.
19. Wilson J: History of the suppression of infanticide in Western India. Bombay: Smith & Co., 1855: p. 28–46, 198.
20. Weyer EM: The Eskimos: their environment and folkways. New Haven, CT: Yale University Press, 1932: p. 293.
21. Lee JZ, Wang F: One quarter of humanity: Malthusian mythology and Chinese realities. Cambridge, MA: Harvard University Press, 1999: p. 177.
22. Mungello DE: Drowning girls in China. Lanham, MD: Rowman & Littlefield, 2008.
23. Fung Y-L: A history of Chinese philosophy. Princeton, NJ: Princeton University Press, 1952: Vol. 1, p. 327.
24. Hulsewe AFP: Remnants of Ch'in law. Leiden: Brill, 1985: p. 125–39.
25. Anderson S: The economics of dowry and brideprice. J Econ Perspect 2007;21:151–74.
26. Wunsch C: Findelkinder und Adoption nach neubabylonischen Quellen. Arch Orientforsch 2001;50:174–244.
27. Diodorus Siculus: The bibliotheca historica. London: Oxford University Press, 1957.
28. Aelianus C: Historical miscellany. Loeb Classical Library 486. Cambridge, MA: Harvard University Press, 1997: Vol. 2, p. 71.
29. Tacitus C: Historiae/les histoires. Liber 5, cap. 5.3. 4. ed. Paris: Les Belles Lettres, 1956.
30. Hesiod: To Pythian Apollo. Loeb Classical Library 57. Cambridge, MA: Harvard University Press, 1959: p. 316–7.
31. Merriam AC: Law code of the Kretan Gortyna. Part 1. Am J Archaeol 1885;1:324–50.
32. Aristotle: Politics. Loeb Classical Library 21. London: Heinemann, 1950: Vol. 7, chapter 14, p. 1335b (lines 19–21).
33. Polybius: The histories. Loeb Classical Library 161, Vol. 6. London: Heinemann, 1927: Vol. 36, cap. 17, p. 383.
34. Scott SP: The civil law. Cincinnati, OH: Central Trust, 1932: Vol. 1, p. Art. 1.
35. Justinian: The institutions. 2. ed. London: Parker, 1859: Vol. 1, title 9, p. 103; 597.
36. Peters R: Der Schutz des neugeborenen, insbesondere des mißgebildeten Kindes. Stuttgart: Enke, 1988: Vol. 18, p. 8.
37. McKechnie P: An errant husband and a rare idiom (P.Oxy. 744). Zeitschr Papyrol Epigr 1999;127:157–61.
38. Arjava A: Paternal power in late antiquity. J Roman Stud 1998;88:147–65.
39. Seneca LA: Moral essays. Loeb Classical Library 310. London: Heinemann, 1928: p. 145.
40. Temkin O: Soranus' Gynecology. Baltimore, MD: The Johns Hopkins Press, 1956: p. 79, 93, 110.
41. Tertullianus QSF: The apologies. In two volumes. Translated by: William Reeves. London: Churchill, 1716: p. 189–90.
42. Duncan-Jones R: The purpose and organisation of the alimentaria. Pap Br Sch Rome 1964;32:123–46.
43. Bormann E: Inscriptiones Aemiliae Etruriae Umbriae Latinae. In: Corpus Inscriptorum Latinarum. Berlin: Reimer, 1888: Vol. 11, part 1, p. 208–25.
44. Trajan to Pliny: Epistle LXI from Rome. The letters of Pliny the Younger. London: Vaillant, 1751: Vol. 2, p. 391.
45. Paulus J: Sententiae, 4,9: 3–4. Corpus Juris Civilis. Heidelberg: Müller, 1995: Vol. 2, p. 120.
46. Harris WV: Child-exposure in the Roman Empire. J Roman Stud 1994;84:1–22.
47. Theodosiani: Libri XVI cum constitutionibus Sirmondianis. Dublin: Weidmann, 1971: Vol. XI, title 27, p. 616.
48. Justinian: Codex (Reprint Frankfurt/Main 2011). Vico-Verlag. Nurimbergae: Petreius, 1530: Vol. IX, Titel 17, p. 455.
49. Tacitus: Germany. Cap. 23. Warminster: Aris & Phillips Ltd, 1999: p. 37.
50. Beck TR, Dunlop W: Elements of medical jurisprudence. 2. ed. London: John Anderson, 1825: p. 132–55.
51. Zeumer K: Leges Visigothorum. In: Leges Nationum Germanicarum. Hannover: Hahn, 1902: Vol. VI,3,7, p. 262.
52. Closmann K: Die Kindstötung historisch-dogmatisch dargestellt. Erlangen: Diss. Jur., 1889: p. 9–10.
53. Drew KF: The laws of the Salian Franks. Philadelphia, PA: University of Pennsylvania Press, 1991: p. 106.
54. Balikci A: Female infanticide on the arctic coast. Man NS 1967;2:615–25.
55. Eckhardt KA: Pactus Legis Salicae. In: Leges Nationum Germanicarum. Hannover: Hahn, 1962: Vol. 4,1, p. 90.

8.2

From sin to crime

Laws on infanticide in the Middle Ages

Introduction: background and aims

As in Chapter 8.1, this chapter investigates the history of the legislation concerning postnatal infanticide with the aim to shed light on the changing attitudes of societies towards the (illegitimate) newborn infant. From a legislative perspective, the Middle Ages are defined herein from the Justinian Code 534 C.E. to the Constitutio Carolina 1532 C.E.

Byzantine Empire

Between Constantine's and Charlemagne's empires, the great migrations shifted peoples from Asia and Germany into the Roman Empire, Huns and Franks to Germany and France, Anglo-Saxons to Britain, and Visigoths to Spain and Italy. The cultural and legislative achievements of the Roman Empire eroded. The Justinian enactments provided some protection for the neonate but were only partly enforced. Responsibility for *carnal* delicts—including fornication, abortion, and infanticide—was handed over from the states to the church. Ecclesiastical thinking focused on the infant's soul rather than its life. From the 7th to the 9th century, the spread of Islam heralded the decline of the Byzantine Empire. From the 11th to the 13th centuries the crusades struck the Mediterranean area. But more than these man-made apocalypses, the great plague of 1348, which killed 40% of the population between the Atlantic and the Urals [1], led governors to rethink the protection of newborn infants: manpower shortage became a political issue. It is tempting to speculate that child protection followed major wars and epidemics [2].

Church councils and canon law

Canon law spared life and limb, but absolution required public penance. Women guilty of infanticide were excluded from the sacraments and community life, and had to stand in front of the parish church on Sundays with a candle in hand, showing a crib as an emblem of their sin [3]. For infanticide, the Council of Elvira (300 C.E.) demanded lifelong penance, but in 314 C.E. the Council of Ancyra reduced the penance to 10 years [4]. The council of Vaison-1 enacted in 442 C.E. [5]: 'Whoever takes up an abandoned child shall bring it to the church where the fact will be certified. Next Sunday the priest will announce ... and the parents will be given ten days to claim their infant.'

St. Augustine's doctrine (412 C.E.) that infants who die unbaptized are excluded from resurrection triggered long-standing debates. In 1265, Thomas Aquinas—himself *oblated* at 5 years of age—described the *limbus puerorum*, a location where these infants live untormented in a state of perpetual bliss: 'The souls of children dying with original sin know happiness in general, but not in particular [since they are deprived of the vision of God]. As they have no knowledge of the loss of glory, they do not grieve over it.' [6]. However, the Council of Florence decreed in 1439 [7]: 'The souls of those who depart this life in original sin alone, go down straightway to hell to be punished.' This hindered burial in sacred ground and turned infanticide—which deprived the neonate of baptism—from a sin to the most heinous of all crimes. In 1546, the Council of Trent confirmed the decree and added [8]: 'The prevarication of Adam ... has transfused into the whole human race sin, which is the death of the soul.' This influenced legislation throughout Europe.

Italy: infanticide prompted foundling hospitals

Small foundling houses had long existed: in Milan from 787, Bergamo from 982, Siena from 1000, and Padua from 1049 C.E. The more illegitimate birth and infanticide were criminalized, the more the church felt the need to offer alternatives to unmarried mothers. In 1198, a few months after ascending the papal throne, Innocent III donated the Hospital of the Holy Spirit in the Saxon District of Rome to Guy de Montpellier with the specific mandate to transform it into a foundling hospital, including a baby *torno*. The Pope had allegedly been astounded by the number of drowned newborns

---

Reproduced with permission from Obladen, M. From sin to crime: laws on infanticide in the middle ages. *Neonatology*, 109(2):85–90. Copyright © 2016 S. Karger AG, Basel.

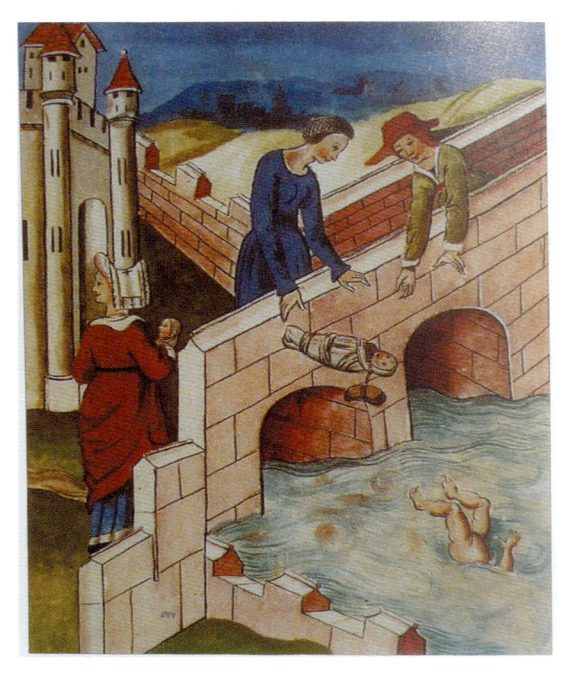

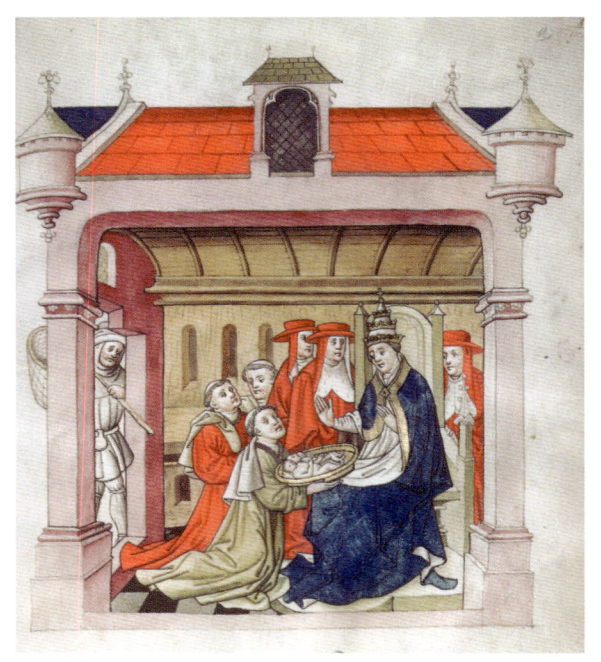

Fig. 8.2.1 Miniatures from the Manuscript A4 of the Archives Hôpitalières de Dijon, painted around 1460, showing the foundation of the Roman Ospedale Santo Spirito in 1198. Left: folio 7: 'How the sinners after delivery make disappear the proof of their dishonesty.' Right: folio 11. 'How the fishermen bring the infants pulled out of the Tiber to Pope Innocent [III], who thereby is much scared' [9].
Archives Hospitalières de Dijon, with permission.

that fishermen had been pulling out of the Tiber and bringing unto him (Fig. 8.2.1). Later popes enlarged the institution, which became an important site of neonatal research up to modern days [9]. In Florence, Bologna, Paris, London, St. Petersburg, and many other cities, widespread infanticide motivated the church to establish large foundling hospitals.

Holy Roman-German Empire

Similar to the Roman rite of name-giving (*dies lustricus*), Germanic tribes attributed a right to live to the beginning of oral nutrition. It is detailed in Bishop Liudger's biography, whose mother escaped infanticide thanks to a mouthful of honey in the 8th century, 'as it was the pagans' custom that boys or girls whom they wanted to kill had to be put to death before earthly food had been given' [10]. During the 13th century, secular jurisdiction took over the responsibility of punishing infanticide. One example is the *Schwabenspiegel*, issued in 1287 [11]: 'To kill a child, however young it may be, is manslaughter and shall be punished by beheading.' And: 'If a man is in genuine need, he is allowed to sell his child, but neither to the whorehouse nor to be killed.' Legislators, however, regarded infanticide the individual crime of a heartless woman, and ignored the social and cultural framework, and the need to limit offspring in agrarian societies. In the century between the Florence decree of 1439 and the Carolina of 1532, infanticide laws proliferated [12–14]. Believing in deterrence, European legislators competed for the most dreadful death penalties: drowning, sacking, impaling, and burying alive, penalties almost exclusively applied to unmarried women who had killed their infant. Infanticide as a female crime to be punished by drowning was specified in the Basel Law in 1426: 'She shall be thrown into the Rhine' [15]. Flowing water was believed to purify and carry away the blood-stained aura of the delinquent. Sacking, the exacerbated form of drowning, was adapted in Leipzig in 1548 from the Roman *poena culei*: '[The child murderess] was united in a sack with a dog, a rooster, a snake, and a cat instead of an ape, and drowned in water' [16]. The child's interests were irrelevant and preventive factors were neglected. Reasons given to intensify the death penalty included: (1) fornication, leading to pregnancy; (2) parricide, the murder of a close relative; (3) cruelty, based on the infant's helplessness; (4) intent or premeditation, based on concealing pregnancy; and (5) and foremost: depriving the infant of baptism and salvation.

Burying alive was the punishment in several countries. Tyrolean law ordained in 1499 [17]: 'A woman who destroys [*verthut*] her infant shall be buried alive in the earth and a stake impaled through her body.' In 1507, the Bamberg Law (*Constitutio Bambergensis*) ruled [18]: 'A woman who secretly and maliciously kills her infant who has received life and limb: these usually are buried alive. But to avoid despair, the evildoers may be drowned, if there is water in the juridicial district. However, where this crime is frequent, we allow the traditional punishment by burying alive and impaling.'

In 1532, Habsburg Emperor Karl V unified various regional legal systems within the Holy Roman Empire, which included today's Germany, Austria, Switzerland, Hungary, Czechia, Slovakia, Burgundy, Northern Italy, Western Poland, Netherlands, Belgium, and Luxemburg. With book printing, this system of law, called Constitutio Carolina, disseminated rapidly. Its section 131, identical to the Bambergensis (as previously mentioned), decreed that a woman who has concealed pregnancy and birth and claims the infant to have been stillborn, 'shall be forced by torture to confess the truth' [19].

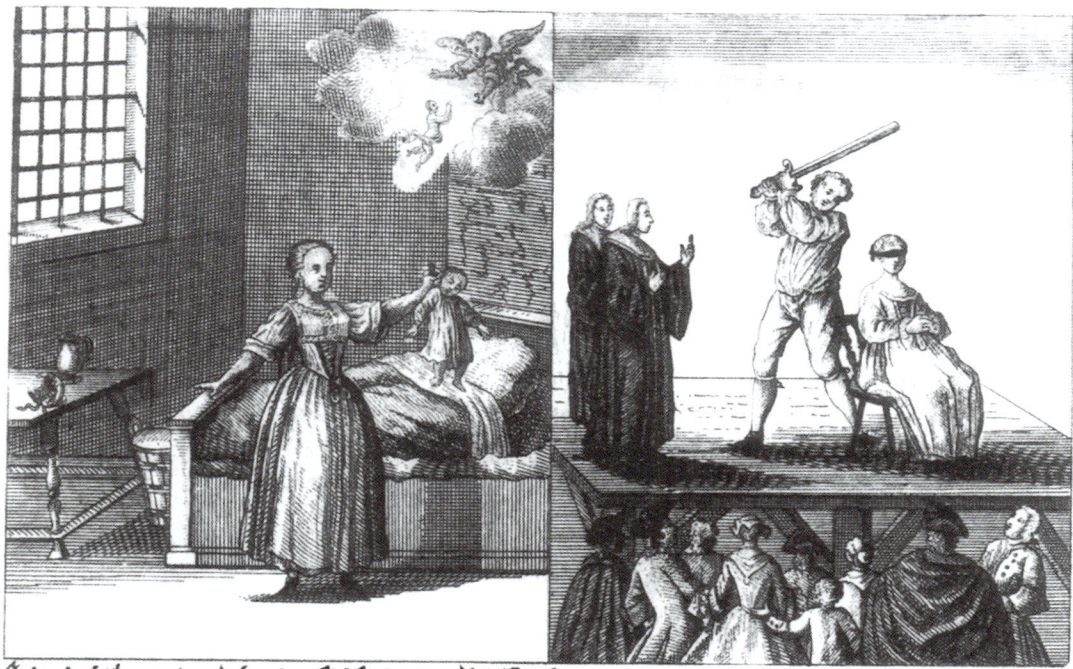

Fig. 8.2.2 Detail of an Augsburg leaflet describing child murder and execution of Maria Elisabeth Beckensteiner in 1742. Already several months old and baptized, the infant's soul rises to heaven.
Staats- und Stadtbibliothek Augsburg, graph. 29/123, with permission.

The reversed burden of proof, torture, and cruel executions failed to deter: in 1598, the city council of Nuremberg learned 'in very sad mood … that recently within and outside of the city dead newborn infants were found in streams and lakes' and asked the population to report the child murderesses for a reward of 50 guilders [20]. The number of Nuremberg women executed for infanticide remained unchanged at around two per year throughout the 17th century [21]. Well into the 18th century, verdicts usually condemned the mothers. The crime alone, not circumstances or motives, counted to determine guilt. Confession was forced by the threat of torture, and young women were often helpless. No questions were posed about the fathers, nor about the difficulties of unambiguous proof. Court hearings and research increasingly focused on the mother's claim that her infant had already been dead at birth. During the 17th century, drowning was gradually replaced by sword execution. A Christian funeral was possible only after sword execution, albeit not in consecrated earth [22]. Executions remained a carefully staged public spectacle, as shown in the broadside leaflet on child murderess Maria Elisabeth Beckensteiner in 1742 (**Fig. 8.2.2**).

France

The Frankish-Salian Law decreed in 511 C.E.: 'He who kills an infant in its mother's womb or before it has a name shall be liable to pay one hundred solidi.' To kill a free Frank cost 200 and a Roman aristocrat 300 solidi [23]. In 830 C.E., the penitential of Halitgar, written in Cambrai, repeated the decrees of Ancyra and Elvira [24]: 'If anyone of the women who have committed fornication slays those who are born or attempts to commit abortion, the original regulation forbids communion to the end of life … We determine that they shall do penance for a period of ten years, according to rank, as the regulations state.' In 1556, Henri II issued an edict that reversed the presumption of innocence, somewhat resembling the Carolina: [25]: 'Each woman convicted of having concealed and not declared her pregnancy and childbirth … and when thereafter the [dead] infant is found deprived of baptism and burial, this woman shall be regarded as having committed homicide of her infant, and shall receive the death penalty, and with such rigor as the particular features of the case deserve.' Renewed in 1685, this decree was read from the pulpit every 3 months and prevailed until 1791 [26]. The particular rigour of the penalty is illustrated by an Ensisheim verdict of 1570 ordering the executioner to lay 'the sentenced Agatha R. alive into her grave, and to place two thorny bushes, one beneath and one upon her; but before shield her face with a bowl through which a tube reaches into her mouth, to prolong suffering; then he should jump onto her thrice and cover her with earth' [27]. In Switzerland, infanticidal mothers were buried alive in exactly the same manner [28].

Britain

The Celtic-Irish penitential, written before 591 C.E., decreed [29]: 'To kill an infant before baptism is a major crime, as it destroys the soul... A cleric who does not support the infant of a poor woman shall do penance at water and bread for a whole year.' Anglo-Saxons were Christianized around 600 C.E., but already in pagan times despised unmarried mothers [30]: 'If either wife or maid were found in dishonesty, her clothes were cut off round about her, beneath the girdle-stead, and she was whipped, and turned out to be derided of the people.' After Christianization, infanticide was regarded a sin rather than a crime, threatened with church penalties similar to those for fornication. Theodore of Canterbury's penitential of 673 C.E. ordained [24]: 'An adulterous woman shall do penance for seven years... If a mother slays her child, she shall do penance for fifteen years, and never change except on Sunday... If a poor woman slays her child, she shall do penance for seven years.' When *overlaying* became a frequent excuse for infanticide of legitimate infants, the Statutes of Winchester I ruled [1224 C.E.]: 'Under threat of excommunication women should be restrained from keeping their children close in bed lest they smother them while in sleep' [31]. After the split from the Roman Church, England had to pass state laws, and the 'Act to prevent the destroying and murdering of bastard children' was passed by Parliament in 1623 (Public Act, 21 James I, c. 27). It was even harsher than the Carolina, and also reversed the burden of proof [32]: 'Whereas many lewd Women that have been delivered of Bastard Children, to avoyd their shame and to escape punishment, doe secretlie bury, or conceale the Death of their Children ... doe alleadge that the said childe was borne dead ... in every such Case the Mother soe offending shall suffer Death as in the case of Murther except such Mother can make proffe by one Witnesse at the least, that the Child was borne dead.' As in German and French laws, this offence related to illegitimate infants only. In the 17th century, Greater London's high courts had a rate of 1.35 indictments for infanticide per 100,000 inhabitants per year [13].

Asia

The Great Qing Legal Code (624 C.E.) prescribed beating or putting to death offending parents. However, Chinese laws did not protect neonates effectively and infanticide remained frequent. In 1659, Emperor Choen Tche decreed [33]: 'If a mother and father destroy the child to which they have given life, how can they help but see in that act a blot in the celestial harmony? ... The mandarins have prohibited this custom and measures must be taken to bring this prohibition to the knowledge of all.' Jesuits came to China in the 16th century and reported from Kiang-son how neonates were being traditionally killed via a procedure called *iam modom* (to feed the bucket) [34] (**Fig. 8.2.3**). In India, (female) infanticide has been embedded for millennia in the social structure of the upper castes, for whom dowries were expensive. It seems that no law interdicted infanticide. Europeans sent their daughters into nunneries for similar reasons.

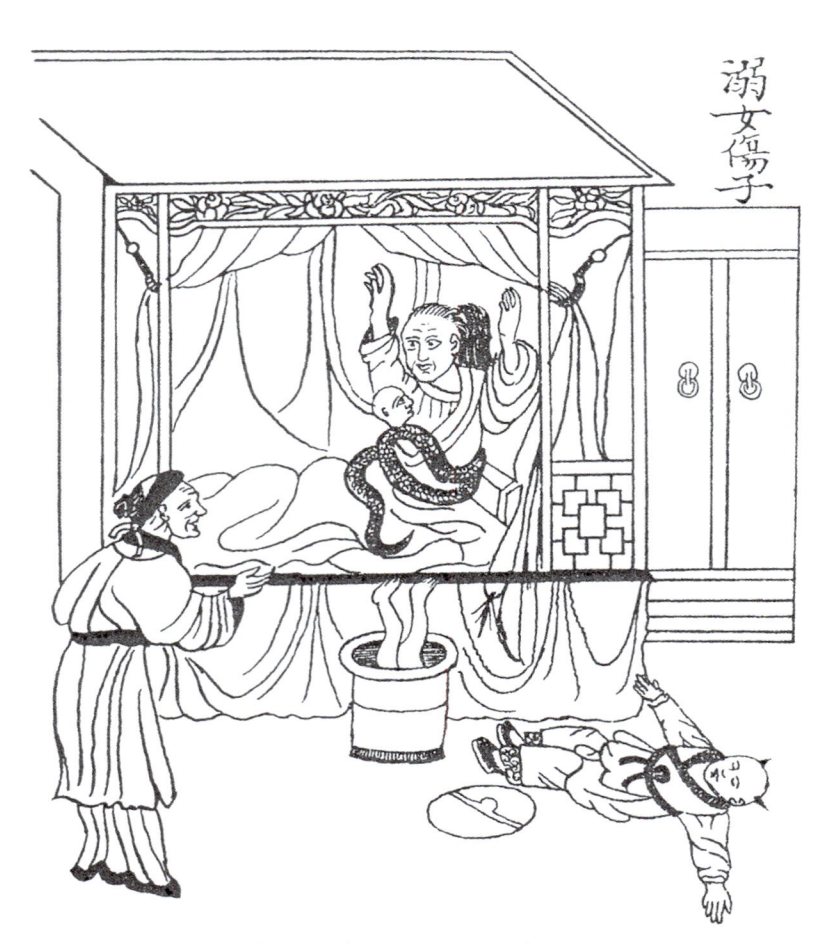

Fig. 8.2.3 Missionary Gabriel Palatre's view of traditional female infanticide in China. The mother-in-law had forced the mother to drown two girls in a bucket. The family is punished by the birth of a monstrous snake-tailed infant. The mother, grandmother, and 7-year-old son die from shock [34].

Arabia

Dowry was also a problem in Arabian culture, making daughters' marriage prohibitively expensive. Pre-Islamic Arabians buried their daughters alive. During Umar's Caliphate (634–644 C.E.), a Bedouin won the title *Muhy'l Maw'udát* (he who brings the buried girls to life) [35]. Koran sura 16:60 described the habit: 'For when the birth of a daughter is announced to any one of them, dark shadows settle on his face, and he is sad: He hideth him from the people because of the ill tidings: shall he keep it with disgrace or bury it in the dust?' And sura 17:31 outlawed infanticide: 'Kill not your children for fear of want: for them and for you we will provide. Verily, killing them is a great wickedness.'

Conclusion

The analysis of medieval history uncovers ambivalence in the legal protection of the newborn infant's life, which under canon law was incomplete. What mattered was to save its soul—only a living infant could be baptized. Christian churches defamed illegitimate birth, which probably augmented the crime. From the 10th century C.E., widespread infanticide led to the establishment of foundling hospitals. The driving force of legislation changed from purification and averting God's wrath in the 15th century to deterrence in the 16th, and retaliation in the 17th century. Not until the 18th century was the motive to effectively prevent infanticide addressed by legislators. The frequency of infanticide decreased when foundling hospitals—not necessarily successfully—were allowed to deal with unwanted infants in a way acceptable to church and society.

REFERENCES

1. Bulst N: Der schwarze Tod. Saeculum 1979;**30**:45–67.
2. Dwork D: War is good for babies and other young children. London: Tavistock, 1987.
3. Trexler RC: Infanticide in Florence. Hist Child Q 1973;**1**:98–116.
4. Schannat JF, Hartzheim J: Conciliae Germaniae. Cologne: Krakamp, 1759: Vol. **1**, p. 148.
5. Munier C: Concilia Galliae: A. 314–A. 506. In: Corpus Christianorum, Series Latina 148. Turnholti: Brepols, 1963: p. 100–1.
6. Thomas Aquinas: On evil. Question 5, article 3. Notre Dame, IN: University of Notre Dame Press, 1995: p. 220.
7. Tanner NP: Decrees of the Ecumenical Councils. Washington, DC: Georgetown University Press, 1990: p. 528, 666.
8. Buckley TA: Canons and decrees of the Council of Trent. London: Routledge, 1851: p. 21–4.
9. De Angelis P: L'Ospedale Apostolico di Santo Spirito in Saxia nella Mente e nel Cuore dei Papi. Rome: Editrice Italia, 1956: p. 19.
10. Altfridi: Die Vitae Sancti Liudgeri (ca. 840 C.E.), lib. I, cap. 6. Münster: Theissing'sche Buchhandlung, 1881: Vol. **4**, p. 10–1.
11. Lassberg FLAv: Der Schwabenspiegel: oder Schwäbisches Land- und Lehen-Rechtbuch (Manuscript of 1287). Tübingen: Fues, 1840: p. 149, 152.
12. Coleman E: Infanticide in the Early Middle Ages. In: Stuard SM: Women in medieval society. Philadelphia, PA: University of Pennsylvania Press, 1976: p. 47–70.
13. Hoffer PC, Hull NEH: Murdering mothers: infanticide in England and New England, 1558–1803. New York: New York University Press, 1981: p. 13–21.
14. Peters R: Der Schutz des neugeborenen, insbesondere des mißgebildeten Kindes. Stuttgart: Enke, 1988: Vol. **18**,
15. Urban P: Die Kindesaussetzung, Rechtsgeschichtliche Entwicklung, Dogmatik und Bekämpfung. Bonn: Nolte, 1936.
16. Wächtershäuser W: Das Verbrechen des Kindsmordes im Zeitalter der Aufklärung. Berlin: Schmidt, 1973: p. 67.
17. Feucht D: Grube und Pfahl. Ein Beitrag zur Geschichte der deutschen Hinrichtungsbräuche. Tübingen: Mohr, 1967.
18. Schwarzenberg J, Bauer H: Bambergische Peinliche Halsgerichtsordnung, 1507. Dettelbach: Röll, 2009.
19. Karl V: Des allerdurchleuchtigsten großmechtigste vnüberwindtlichsten Keyser Karls des fünfften: vnnd des heyligen Römischen Reichs peinlich gerichts ordnung. Mainz: Schöffer, 1533.
20. Dülmen Rv: Frauen vor Gericht: Kindsmord in der frühen Neuzeit. Frankfurt: Fischer, 1991: p. 30, 49–51.
21. Bode G: Die Kindstötung und ihre Bestrafung im Nürnberg des Mittelalters. Arch Strafrecht Strafprozess 1914;**61**:430–81.
22. Dülmen Rv: Theater des Schreckens. 3. ed. München: Beck, 1988: p. 174.
23. Drew KF: The laws of the Salian Franks. Philadelphia, PA: University of Pennsylvania Press, 1991: p. 106.
24. McNeill JR, Gamer HM: Medieval handbooks of penance. New York: Columbia University Press, 1938: p. 304.
25. Seresia A: De l'acte de naissance de l'enfant naturel. Bruxelles: Lesigne, 1869: p. 10.
26. Beck TR, Dunlop W: Elements of medical jurisprudence. 2. ed. London: Anderson, 1825: p. 132–55.
27. Stöber A: Merkwürdige Strafarten welche in ältern Zeiten im Elsass angewandt wurden. In: Alsatia. Jahrbuch für elsässische Geschichte. Mülhausen: Rißler, 1851: p. 36–45.
28. Osenbrüggen E: Das Alamannische Strafrecht im deutschen Mittelalter. Schaffhausen: Hurter, 1860: p. 229–30.
29. Bieler L: Penitentialis Vinniani, Canon XLVII. In: The Irish penitentials. Dublin: Institute for Advanced Studies, 1963: p. 92–3.
30. Verstegan R: A restitution of decayed intelligence, in antiquities, concerning the most noble, and renowned English Nation (1st ed. 1606). 3. ed. London: Newcomb, 1653: p. 45.
31. Moseley KL: The history of infanticide in western society. Issues Law Med 1986;**1**:345–61.
32. Damme C: Infanticide: the worth of an infant under law. Med Hist 1978;**22**:1–24.
33. Payne GH: The child in human progress. New York: Putnam, 1916: p. 56–8.
34. Palatre G: L'Infanticide et L'Oeuvre de la Sainte-Enfance en Chine (first published Shanghai 1878). Ann Oeuvre Sainte-Enfance 1913;**65**:214–6.
35. Nicholson RA: A literary history of the Arabs. Cambridge: Cambridge University Press, 1930: p. 243.

8.3

From crime to disease
Laws on infanticide in the modern era

Introduction

After describing the laws of Antiquity and of the Middle Ages (see Chapters 8.1 and 8.2), this chapter delineates the legislative efforts by modern states to protect the life of (illegitimate) infants. It covers the time from the Constitutio Carolina in 1532. Again, it excludes abortion and child murder beyond the neonatal period. Gutenberg, Columbus, and Luther had marked the beginning of a new age, but the spirit of the Middle Ages still hovered over European legislators during the 16th century. Church penance revealed some mildness, but the laws of the secular state punished the 'child murderess' in the most sadistic ways. Views changed gradually when the social causes of infanticide emerged.

Defaming the unmarried mother and her child

Many cultures excluded unmarried mothers from society and their children from honest professions. Jewish legislation ordered [Judges 11:1]: 'Thou shalt not inherit in our father's house; for thou art the son of a strange woman.' British Saxons whipped and derided illegitimate mothers [1]. But the Christian church made fornication a crime, punishable by canon law. Throughout Europe, 'fallen' women with extramarital relations were pilloried and whipped (Fig. 8.3.1, left) and had to do public penance. Domestic servants lost their position, and daughters of farmers and tradesmen were expelled. A life in poverty or prostitution was the consequence. The church propagated to expose 'bastard children' at church doors or in *tornos* (turntables) of the foundling hospitals. The few survivors had next to no chance to escape the lower class. Regarded as 'infamous', they were excluded from workers' guilds, higher schools, and heritage. Today, we can barely imagine how much shame burdened extramarital pregnancy.

From the age of Enlightenment, philosophers, poets, and social scientists began to influence public opinion and court judgement. A mentality named *Sturm und Drang* advanced legislation reform, especially Heinrich Wagner's tragedy *The Child Murderess* in 1776 [2] (Fig. 8.3.1, right). In his poem *Infanticide*, Friedrich Schiller blamed the never prosecuted fathers [3]:

> 'Alas! poor babe, thou seekest him in vain
> And other children may enjoy his smiles
> And thou shalt curse the passing hour, whose stain
> Thy memory with the Bastard's name defiles.'

Swiss educator Johann Heinrich Pestalozzi's book on infanticide [4] stated: 'Put away the sword of your executioners, Europe! In vain it slaughters the murderesses! ... Prejudiced against girls and lenient against young men, the jurisdiction violates its duties, destroys the confidence in justice and drives the unfortunate to infanticide.' In 1808, Johann Wolfgang Goethe made the Frankfurt child murderess Margareta Brandt a central character in his drama *Faust*, the most frequently cited work of German literature.

Sexual exploitation of the lower class

Thoughtful analyses of preserved court records have been published by Adriano Prosperi [5], who studied the case of Lucia Cremonini, hanged in Bologna in 1710, and by Rebekka Habermas [6], who studied the case of Anna Margareta Brandt, decapitated in Frankfurt in 1772. Domestic servants and slaves, the classic victims of seduction and abuse, formed the largest group of infanticidal mothers [7]. Often the employer or his son had impregnated the poor girl, without fatherly affection towards the child. The housemaid was fired when her pregnancy became known.

Understanding disguised infanticide

Killing an illegitimate infant was usually the response to enormous social, religious, and economic pressure. Despite dreadful public punishments, the crime remained frequent: within 150 years, from 1570 to 1720, the number of women executed for infanticide was 60 in Gdánsk and 51 in Nuremberg [8], yielding an average of one execution per 100,000 inhabitants per year. As the crime was easily

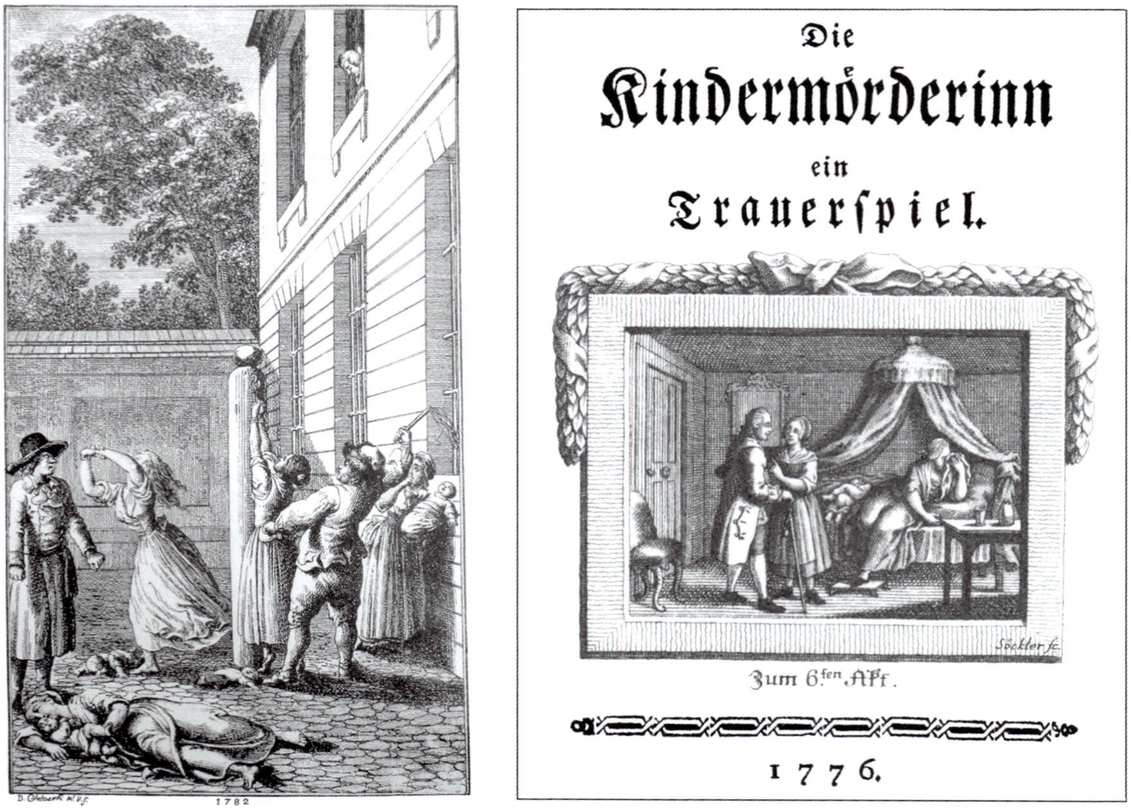

Fig. 8.3.1 Frontispieces of *Sturm und Drang* literature on infanticide. Left: 'Public whipping of unmarried mothers', copper etching by Daniel Chodowiecki, Berlin, 1782 [51]. Right: tragedy *The Child Murderess* by Heinrich Wagner, 1776 [2].

hidden and somewhat tolerated societally, the actual number of infanticides cannot be derived from this figure. Foundling homes and commercial wet nursing were associated with elevated infant mortality, and people realized there was no substantial difference between immediate and disguised infanticide in these institutions, which society and the church had tolerated for centuries. Direct infanticide, however, invariably led to capital punishment. When its motives—poverty, shame, despair, and saving honour—became understood in the late 18th century, the image of the child murderess changed from *lewd harlot* to *seduced victim*.

Viability and stillbirth: loopholes in the law

Section 131 of the Carolina referred to infants having received *Leben und Gliedmaß* (life and limb). This and similar clauses in other legislation alluded to stillbirth, malformation, and immaturity, and allowed foregoing prosecution. It is safe to assume that many malformed infants were killed by their parents or the midwife, as admitting the birth of a *monstrum* was especially dangerous: Zedler's Lexikon of 1739 repeated the belief that malformations resulted from sodomy [9]: 'Such monsters should be put away as they result from bestial indecency ... Having delivered a monster unlike the human frame, the mother can hardly escape the suspicion of having intercoursed with an animal.' As late as 1759, a commentary to the Carolina admonished 'to diligently investigate the causes of such [monstrous] birth, which may lead to prosecution for brutish sodomy' [10]. Sodomy was subject to the death penalty, and killing malformed infants was tacitly accepted by most cultures. The author was unable to find any reports of court trials for killing malformed infants.

The lung flotation test

A liveborn infant was a precondition for indictment, and most perpetrators claimed her infant had been stillborn. Since Galen, to live meant breathing [11]: 'As the [newborn] animal breathes ... the nature of the lung's flesh changes from being red, heavy, and dense to become white, light, and loose-textured.' For his dissertation on respiration, Jan Swammerdam of Amsterdam constructed a machine in 1667 to measure inspiratory pressure in isolated neonatal lungs (Fig. 8.3.2A): 'They never sink in water once the animal has breathed' [12]. In 1675, Carl Rayger concluded from autopsy of stillborn twins [13]: 'If the lung has breathed once after birth, the retained air prevents sinking in water.' On 11 October 1681, the body of a dead newborn was found near Leipzig. In the trial against the 15-year-old mother, Anna Voigt, the city physician Johann Schreyer interpreted the fact that the baby's lung sank in water as 'solid proof that the infant never lived outside the mother's body' [14]. Expert reports were requested from the universities of Leipzig and Frankfurt which confirmed, and of Wittenberg, which contradicted Schreyer's view. Debates persisted up to 1687 when, without torture, Anna Voigt was sentenced to 8 weeks imprisonment, not for infanticide,

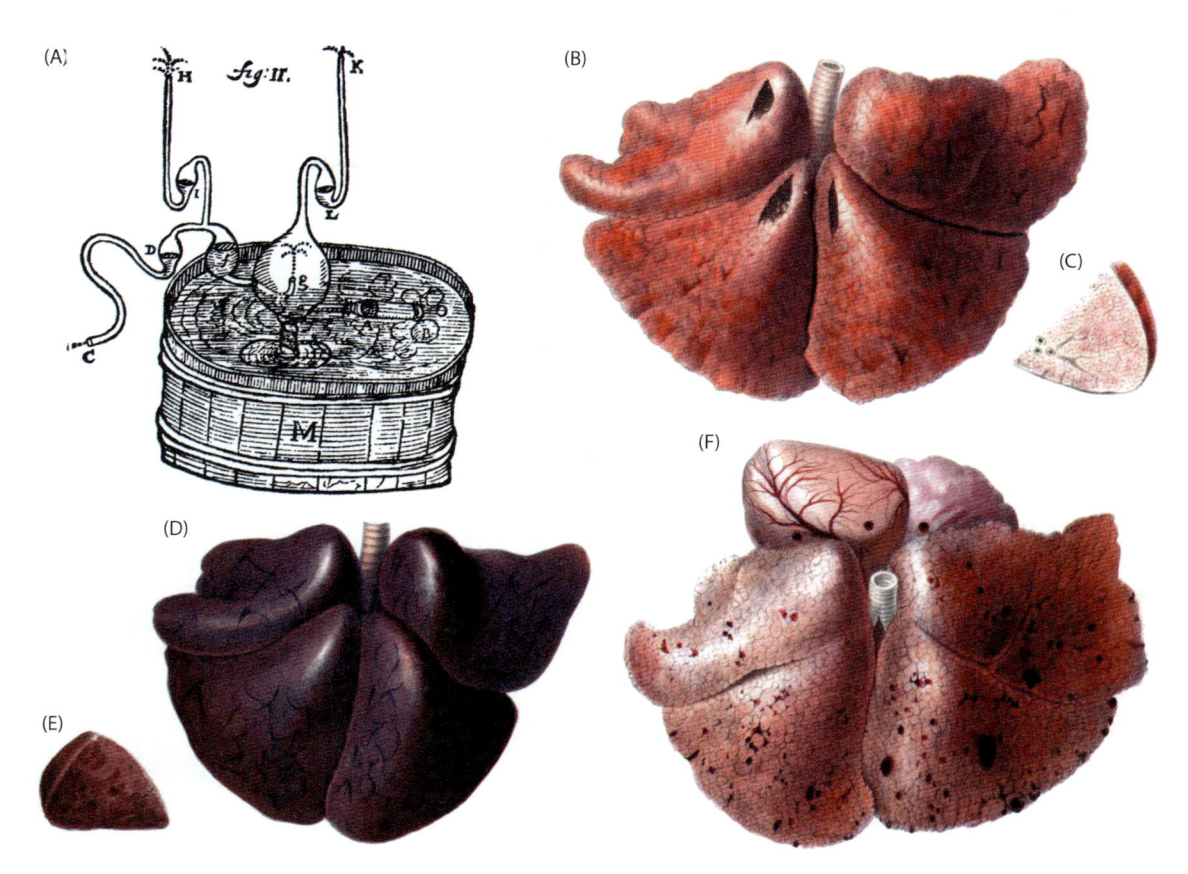

Fig. 8.3.2 A, machine for underwater measurements in isolated lungs, by Jan Swammerdam, 1667 [12]; B–F, lungs and segments of neonatal lungs, by Ambroise Tardieu, 1868 [52]: B, lung of term infant born alive and having breathed, filled with air; C, segment of B; D, lung of stillborn term infant without respiration; E, segment of D; F, thoracic organs of infant born alive and breathing and who died as infanticide victim by suffocation. Disseminated small haemorrhages under pleura and pericardium.

but for concealing her pregnancy [15]. In 1704, Leipzig professor Johannes Bohn doubted the reliability of the test [16]: 'Lungs submerged in water do neither acquit the *infanticida* nor spare her the torture.' Aware of its ambiguity, Groningen professor Peter Camper pinpointed the floating test's purpose in 1770 [17]: 'To spare the prisoner torture, as long as the physicians consider the infant stillborn.' The debate on the *docimasia pulmonum* (**Fig. 8.3.2 B–F**) continued for two centuries, as described by Krammer [18].

Law reforms: maternities and 'housemaid acts'

One of the first legislative acts of Prussian King Frederick II was to replace drowning by decapitation as the punishment for infanticide in 1740. Even when in 1765 infanticide had become frequent, Frederick did not return to an aggravated death penalty, but decreed 'persons impregnated outside marriage remain free of punishment and reproach … By threat of punishment, parents and employers must refrain from all hardness, which might incline fallen women to despair and commit an even greater evil' [19] (**Fig. 8.3.3**). The General State Law for Prussia of 1794 dedicated no fewer than 96 paragraphs to preventing and punishing infanticide [20]: section 894 ordered that institutions for unmarried pregnant women be established and midwives had to accept women and their infants 'without argument'. The Berlin *Gebärhaus* opened in 1751. In Hesse-Cassel, a law of 1761 ordered that 'to prevent child-murder, a delivery- and foundling hospital be attached to the present orphanage … to raise its funds, a lottery is set up … the unmarried mothers exempted from public church penance … not charged for baptism or burial'. Lying-in hospitals, simultaneously schools of midwifery, were founded in London in 1767, Vienna in 1784, Göttingen in 1791, and Paris in 1795. In 1871, section 217 was incorporated in German law, ordering 'a woman who intentionally kills her illegitimate infant in or shortly after birth, is to be punished with incarceration for three years' [7]. After a century of debate on the diminished protection of the neonate, this so-called *housemaid act* was repealed in 1997.

Britain

King James' law of 1623 was even harsher than the Carolina: when a birth was concealed, the child was presumed born alive. Despite the law and public executions, infanticide and exposure remained so frequent that Captain Thomas Coram, commuting from Rotherhithe to London in 1720, often saw exposed or dead infants, which motivated him to establish the London Foundling Hospital [21]. The Ellenborough's Act of 1803 repealed the cruel law [22]: 'The murderesses of bastard children are to be tried by the same rules of evidence as in other trials of murder.' Formally, the death penalty persisted,

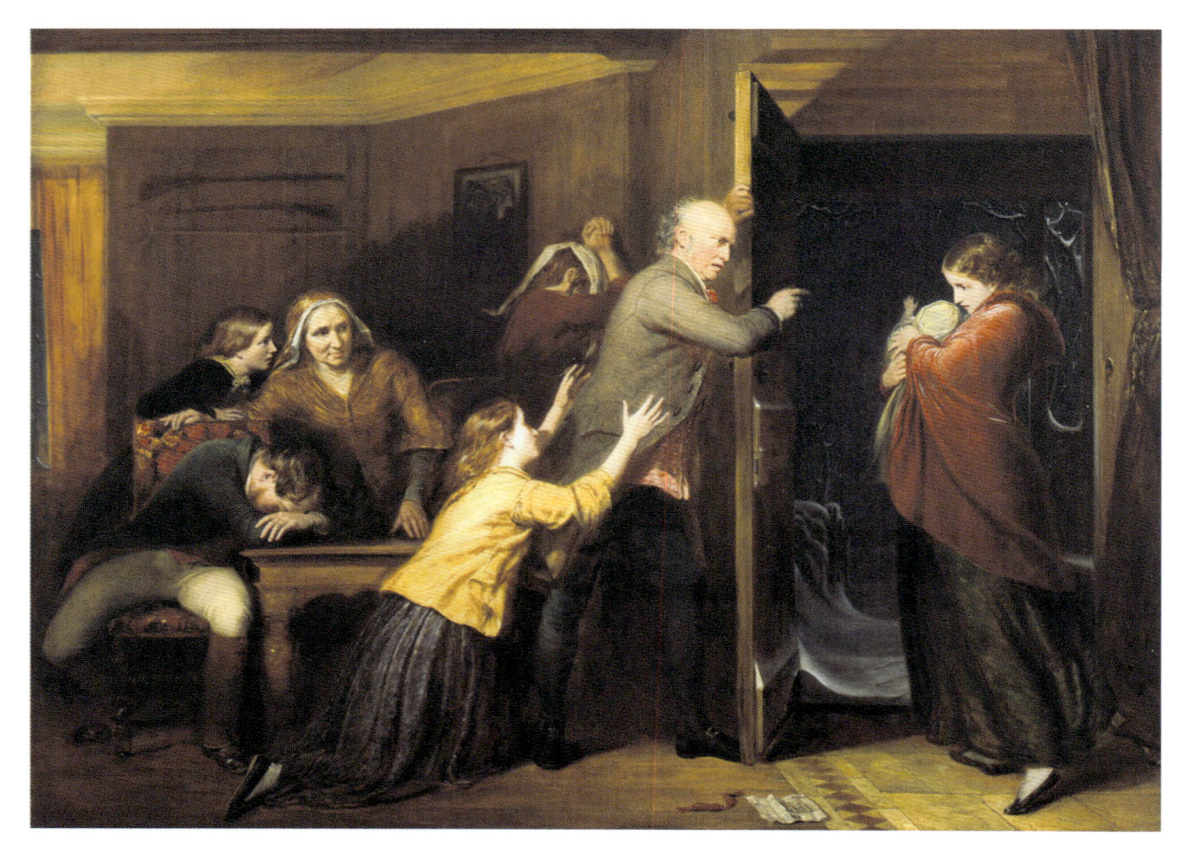

Fig. 8.3.3 *The Outcast*. Painting by Richard Redgrave, 1851.
© Royal Academy of Arts, London; photographer: John Hammond, with permission.

but no woman has been executed for infanticide since 1849 [23]. In June 1863, the *Morning Star* asserted that infanticide was a 'national institution' [24]. In debates on the Infant Life Protection Bill of 1872, it was acknowledged that the 'Bastardy Laws' themselves were causing infanticide [25]. In 1922, an infanticide bill allowed the judge any verdict from life imprisonment to conditional discharge when the mother 'had not fully recovered from giving birth' [26]. The law still called for the death penalty, but courts no longer passed such verdicts, termed 'divorce between law and public opinion' by Davies [23]. Its actual version of 1938 still distinguished infanticide from murder, assuming a 'disturbed balance of mind' shortly after birth.

Unlike Britain, the US passed no federal laws against infanticide, and most child murder cases were—and are—treated as homicide. In 1851, an infant mortality rate of 50% was considered normal among American slaves [27]. In 1868, the Working Women's Association successfully acted to save Hester Vaughan, a domestic servant in Philadelphia who had been impregnated by her employer, dismissed from her position, and sentenced to be hanged when found with her dead infant. The campaign shed light on the unfair treatment of women by the law, led to Vaughan's acquittal, and strengthened the American feminist movement [28].

France

The edict of 1556 had ordered unmarried women to report their pregnancy, 'condemning to death every woman convicted of having concealed her pregnancy and put to death a bastard-child' [29]. Article 302 of the penal code of 1810 stated 'every person guilty of assassination, parricide, infanticide, or poisoning shall suffer death' [30]. Fodéré specified in 1813: 'The murder of a newborn infant is called infanticide... will be punished... irrespective of the conditions.' In 1811 Napoléon decreed that a turntable had to be installed in each foundling hospital, and from 1826 to 1835, 1.2 million of *enfants trouvés et abandonnés*, a third of all births, were admitted to the foundling hospitals of France [31]. During the same time, the French courts sentenced 1084 accusations of infanticide: 521 acquitted, 19 death penalty, 76 lifelong forced work, 108 temporary forced work, 15 imprisonment, and 345 short custody. In 1876–1885, the number of infanticide trials in France had risen to 1956 [32]. In 1901, the French Parliament substituted the death penalty for infanticide with 5 years' imprisonment [33]. From 1994, France no longer distinguished infanticide from homicide [34].

In Asia, fighting infanticide meant fighting the dowry system. Traveller John Barrow reported from China in 1804 [35]: 'It is part of the duty of the police of Pekin to employ certain persons to go their rounds, at an early hour in the morning, with carts, in order to pick up such bodies of infants as may have been thrown out into the streets in the course of the night. No inquiries are made, but the bodies are carried to a common pit without the city walls... Twenty-four infants were, on the average, in Pekin, daily carried to the pit of death... The Chinese, in like manner, have no positive law against infanticide.' In the absence of laws, the British Bengal governor Jonathan Duncan concluded obscure 'agreements' with the

Rajkumars in 1789: alluding to the Holy Scripture Brahma Vaivartta Puràna, it sentenced infanticidal parents 'to suffer in the Hell called Kal Sooter for as many years as there are hairs on that [killed] female's body … and at rebirth become a leper' [36]. The Female Infanticide Act of 1870 was not more successful [37].

Privileged delict or curtailed protection?

Jurisdiction became more and more indulgent, in line with the public mind. Today, most nations' laws treat infanticide as a less severe crime than other forms of homicide. Many reasons have been offered for this discrepancy, including: (1) social circumstances—poverty, education, young age, and dependency; (2) defaming extramarital pregnancy and fear of the parents; (3) psychotic instability due to pregnancy, pain, or lone delivery; (4) doubtful proof, especially concerning premeditation and intent; (5) curtailed protection of the newborn due to helplessness and diminished awareness; and (6) diminished protection of the illegitimate child, who is, in Immanuel Kant's words, 'born outside the law, which means marriage, therefore also outside the law's protection' [38].

Some modern philosophers debated the question as to whether it is morally permissible to kill severely defected infants and attributed a diminished moral status to the newborn. Especially for malformed, premature, or disabled infants, the right to live has been reduced: Melbourne utilitarian Peter Singer regarded self-awareness more important for personhood than belonging to the human species, and denied personhood to severely impaired infants [39]. Houston ethicist Tristram Engelhardt justified the concept of 'wrongful life' when the infant's 'existence itself is a tort or injury to the person' [40]. Boulder philosopher Michael Tooley suggested that 'the capacity for thought emerges only after birth' [41]. He conceded that only if an immaterial soul is assumed, humans have an unconditional right to live, which follows Aristotle's dilemma of when this soul enters the body or if the zygote has a soul. Most philosophers agree that the infant's moral status changes at birth [42] and physicians admit that predicting the infant's quality of life is unreliable [43].

Out of her mind

Jean-Etienne Esquirol, Parisian pioneer of psychiatry, wrote in 1819 [44]: 'False shame, embarrassment, fear, poverty, and crime are not the only causes of infanticide; delirious confusion of the mind may guide the mother's sacrilegious hands.' In his book *Madness of Pregnancy*, Esquirol's student Louis-Victor Marcé described the case of Rosalie Prunot, who was acquitted in 1847 in Reims [45]. After World War II, infanticide was further 'psychiatrized' as denial and/or concealment of pregnancy, a heterogeneous condition occurring in 0.26% of all deliveries [46]. Various mental disorders have been identified in half of the women [47, 48]. Understanding the psychosocial framework has largely extinguished infanticide as a special delict in criminal law. Today, infanticide is rare in most countries—not so undesired children: even in the US and Europe, where modern contraception is available, 49% of pregnancies were unintended in 2006 [49, 50].

Conclusion

Realizing that infanticide was frequent in most cultures does not mean that it was ethically acceptable. Whereas infant abandonment was tolerated more or less, no culture explicitly allowed newborn infants to be killed. But it seems likely that the newborn infant enjoyed little protection by law and society. Adoption and paternal obligation to pay maintenance have done more for children than draconic criminal laws. Within the last three centuries, the legal interpretation of infanticide changed from serious crime to privileged offence. Frequent law reforms reveal the ambivalence of societies towards extramarital sexuality, illegitimate motherhood, immaturity, sex, malformation, and religion, all of which played specific roles in the history of the infant's legal protection. The debate as to whether infanticide essentially differs from murder never came to an end. Ethical dilemmas resulting from this ambivalence extend into our time and undermine consensus on abortion and end-of-life decisions in neonates.

REFERENCES

1. Verstegan R: A restitution of decayed intelligence, in antiquities, concerning the most noble, and renowned English Nation (1st ed. 1606). 3. ed. London: Newcomb, 1653: p. 45.
2. Wagner HL: Die Kindermörderin: Ein Trauerspiel. Leipzig: Schwickert, 1776.
3. Schiller F: The infanticide (1782). In: Poems. London: Heinemann, 1901: p. 20–3.
4. Pestalozzi JH: Ueber Gesetzgebung und Kindermord. Frankfurt: Buchhandlung der Gelehrten, 1783: p. 4, 150.
5. Prosperi A: Die Gabe der Seele. Geschichte eines Kindsmordes. Frankfurt: Suhrkamp, 2007.
6. Habermas R: Das Frankfurter Gretchen. Der Prozess gegen die Kindsmörderin Susanna Margaretha Brandt. München: Beck, 1999.
7. Michalik K: Kindsmord. Sozialverhalten und Rechtsgeschichte der Kindstötung. Pfaffenweiler: Centaurus, 1997: p. 448–60.
8. Dülmen Rv: Frauen vor Gericht: Kindsmord in der frühen Neuzeit. Frankfurt: Fischer, 1991: p. 30, 49–51.
9. Zedler JH: Grosses vollständiges Universallexikon. Reprint Graz 1982: Leipzig: Zedler, 1739: Vol. **21**, columns 486–91.
10. Frölich von Frölichsburg JC: Commentarius in Kaysers Carl des Fünfften und des h. Röm. Reichs Peinliche Halsgerichts-Ordnung. Ulm: Wohler, 1759: Vol. **2**. Titul 11, Art. 14, p. 174.
11. Galen: On the usefulness of the parts of the body. Ithaca, NY: Cornell University Press, 1968: Vol. **2**, book 15, cap. 6, p. 670.
12. Swammerdam J: Tractatus physico-anatomico-medicus de respiratione usuque pulmonum (1st ed. 1667). Lugduni Batavorum: van der Linden, 1679: p. 41.
13. Rayger C: Observatio CCII quibusdam in dissectione recens natorum observatis. In: Miscellanea curiosa medico-physica. Frankfurt: Gleditsch, 1688: Vol. **6 and 7**, p. 295–7.
14. Schreyer J: Erörterung und Erläuterung der Frage, ob es ein gewiss Zeichen, wenn eines todten Kindes Lunge im Wasser untersincket, dass solches in Mutter-Leibe gestorben sey? Zeitz: Ammersbacher, 1690.
15. Blumenstok L: Zum 200jährigen Jubiläum der Lungenprobe. Vjschr Gerichtl Med NF 1883;**38**:252–69; **39**:1–11.

16. Bohn J: De officio medici duplici, clinici nimirum ac forensis. Lipsiae: Gleditsch, 1704: p. 662–70.
17. Camper P: Abhandlung von den Kennzeichen des Lebens und des Todes bey neugebornen Kindern. Frankfurt: Brönner, 1777: p. 80–8.
18. Krammer L: Streit und Widerstreit um die Beweiskraft der Lungenschwimmprobe in geschichtlicher Darstellung. Sudhoffs Arch Gesch Med 1933;**26**:253–76.
19. Walcher K: Das Neugeborene in forensischer Hinsicht. Berlin: Springer, 1941: p. 3–7.
20. Hattenhauer H: Allgemeines Landrecht für die preußischen Staaten von 1794. 2. ed. Neuwied: Luchterhand, 1994: p. 707–11.
21. Brownlow J: The history and design of the foundling hospital. London: Warr, 1858.
22. Jackson M: Infanticide. Historical perspectives on child murder and concealment, 1550–2000. Aldershot: Ashgate, 2002.
23. Davies DS: Child-killing in English law. Mod Law Rev 1937;**1**:203–17.
24. Behlmer GK: Deadly motherhood: infanticide and medical opinion in Mid-Victorian England. Hist Med Allied Sci 1979;**34**:403–27.
25. Pinchbeck I, Hewitt M: Children in English society. London: Routledge & Kegan Paul, 1973: Vol. **2**, p. 598.
26. Damme C: Infanticide: the worth of an infant under law. Med Hist 1978;**22**:1–24.
27. Steckel RH: A dreadful childhood: the excess mortality of American slaves. Soc Sci Hist 1986;**10**:427–65.
28. Beisel N, Kay T: Abortion, race, and gender in nineteenth-century America. Am Sociol 2004;**69**:498–518.
29. Seresia A: De l'acte de naissance de l'enfant naturel. Bruxelles: Lesigne, 1869: p. 10.
30. Vallaud D: Le crime d'infanticide et l'indulgence des cours d'assises en France au XIXème siecle. Soc Sci Inf (Paris) 1982;**21**:475–99.
31. Remacle B-B: Des hospices d'enfans trouvés en Europe. Paris: Treuttel et Würtz, 1838: p. 221.
32. Lalou R: L'infanticide devant les tribunaux français (1825–1910). Communications 1986;**44**:175–200.
33. Donovan JM: Infanticide and the juries in France, 1825–1913. J Fam Hist 1991;**16**:157–76.
34. Tursz A, Cook JM: A population-based survey of neonaticides using judicial data. Arch Dis Child Fetal Neonatal Ed 2011;**96**:F259–63.
35. Barrow J: Travels in China. London: Cadell, 1804: p. 167–73.
36. Wilson J: History of the suppression of infanticide in Western India. Bombay: Smith & Co., 1855: p. 28–46, 198.
37. Vishwanath LS: Female infanticide. The colonial experience. Econ Political Wkly 2004;2313–8.
38. Kant I: Metaphysik der Sitten. In: Weischedel W: Immanuel Kant. Werke in 6 Bänden. Hamburg: Hoffmann & Campe, 1799: Vol. **4**, p. 458.
39. Singer P: Practical ethics. Cambridge: Cambridge University Press, 1979.
40. Engelhardt HT Jr: Euthanasia and children: the injury of continued existence. J Pediatr 1973;**83**:170–1.
41. Tooley M: Infanticide. In: La Follette H: The international encyclopedia of ethics. Malden, MA: Wiley-Blackwell, 2013: Vol. **5**, p. 2604–7.
42. Levy N: The moral significance of being born. J Med Ethics 2013;**39**:326–9.
43. Shinwell ES: Ethics of birth at the limits of viability: the risky business of prediction. Neonatology 2015;**107**:317–20.
44. Esquirol E: De l'aliénation mentale des nouvelles accouchées et des nourrices (1819). In: Des maladies mentales considérées sous le rapport médical, hygiénique et médico-légal. Paris: Baillière, 1838: p. 230–73.
45. Marcé LV: Traité de la folie des femmes enceintes, des nouvelles accouchées et des nourrices. Paris: Baillière, 1858: p. 141–4.
46. Wessel J, Büscher U: Denial of pregnancy: population based study. BMJ 2002;**324**:458.
47. Brezinka C, Huter O, Biebl W, Kinzl J: Denial of pregnancy. J Psychosom Obstet Gynecol 1994;**15**:1–8.
48. Vellut N, Cook JM, Tursz A: Analysis of the relationship between neonaticide and denial of pregnancy using data from judicial files. Child Abuse Negl 2012;**36**:553–63.
49. Finer LB, Zolna MR: Unintended pregnancy in the United States. Contraception 2011;**84**:478–85.
50. Singh S, Sedgh G, Hussain R: Unintended pregnancy: worldwide levels, trends, and outcomes. Stud Fam Plann 2010;**41**:241–50.
51. Chodowiecki D. Whipping of illegitimate mothers (Copper etching, frontispiece). In: Salzmann CG: Carl von Carlsberg. Über das menschliche Elend. Leipzig: Crusius, 1783: Vol. **1**.
52. Tardieu A: Etude médico-légale sur l'infanticide. Paris: Baillière, 1868: p. 50–3, plates 1–3.

8.4

Despising the weak
Long shadows of infant murder in Nazi Germany

Introduction

Whereas the killing of mentally ill adults in Nazi Germany has been thoroughly described [1], the systematic killing of handicapped children became clarified later: it was performed more secretly, and most documents were destroyed at the regime's collapse. German courts prosecuted child killing half-heartedly, and the testimony of the accused, the main source of historic research, played down the crime. After the war, paediatricians, nurses, and midwives involved in reporting or killing infants united in an alliance of silence. Finally, in 1999, the German Society of Paediatrics appointed a historical commission to elucidate its inglorious role during the Nazi time. Recent historical research, including the work of E. Seidler, T. Beddies, L. Pelz, G. Aly, U. Benzenhöfer, and S. Topp, saved the memory of this crime from oblivion.

The present chapter aims to trace the long-term influence of Nazi ideology on the development of neonatal medicine in post-war Germany, omitting actions T4 and 14f13 as well as the killing of foreign slave labourers' babies through wilful neglect [2] and outlining the child murder programme only briefly. The term 'euthanasia' is avoided, as it was misused by the Nazis to disguise the murder of the handicapped. The Greek term means 'good death' and describes the help given to a dying person on her or his request. Planned and done clandestinely, without legal justification, without parental consent, and for economic reasons, the Nazi killing programme was not 'mercy death', but plain murder.

Forerunners and public debate

In 1859, Charles Darwin published his epochal book on the origin of species, and soon others applied his findings to human societies. In 1865, Darwin's cousin Francis Galton developed the idea that human abilities are inherited, and that by combining them the human race can be improved, a process for which he coined the term 'eugenics'. In Germany, this idea was taken up by zoologist Ernst Haeckel in 1868; he justified the idea of killing as an act of mercy with the utilitarian argument of saving public and private money. In 1895, the Austrian psychologist Adolf Jost postulated a (voluntary) right to die when the 'worth' of a human life becomes negative for the individual or community. The German biologist Alfred Ploetz amalgamated racial biology, genetics, and nationalism in 1895. He speculated that war, revolution, and welfare support of the weak would lead to racial degeneration. He founded the term 'racial hygiene' and a society with the same name, believing in the 'superiority of the Nordic race'. Ploetz proposed that weak or malformed infants be killed 'gently' following evaluation by a committee of physicians.

Adalbert Czerny, Berlin chair of paediatrics from 1913, fixed social Darwinist principles within German paediatrics, believing 'infant mortality is a selection, it befalls inferior constitutions' [3], based education on obedience rather than empathy, and rejected premature infants' special care ('much money keeps few infants alive') [4].

Exerting greatest influence on the public debate was a small tract in 1920 by the renowned expert in constitutional law Karl Binding and the psychiatrist Alfred Hoche [5]. Binding proposed legalizing suicide and suggested the existence of 'a human life, that has so much lost the law's protection that its prolongation is worthless, both for its bearer and for society'. Hoche specified that this would include the incurably mentally ill, qualifying them as 'mentally dead', and severely malformed infants. He coined the term 'ballast existence' and bemoaned the expense for their 'unproductive' care. Fuelled by poverty, unemployment, and the belief that in World War I 'the best' had been lost and the gene pool would deteriorate, the ensuing debate seized much of the population. In 1925, Ewald Meltzer, director of the Saxonian asylum Katharinenhof, rejected the arguments of Binding and Hoche, insisting that the mentally handicapped are self-aware and do have the capacity to enjoy life [6]. He queried the parents of his mentally handicapped patients, and was shocked to learn that 73% would agree to the painless termination of their child's life.

These examples illustrate the atmosphere in which German paediatrics fought for independence from internal medicine. The new specialty evolved in surroundings that despised the weak.

Reproduced with permission from Obladen M. Despising the weak: Long shadows of infant mortality in Nazi Germany. Copyright 2019, Arch Dis Child Fetal Neonat Ed. 101(3): F190–194. Copyright © 2019 BMJ, London, UK.

Nationalism was common in 19th-century Europe and was particularly pronounced in Germany, which had not been united until 1871. But even the Social Darwinists Haeckel, Binding, and Hoche maintained the individual's desire to end his or her life as the main prerequisite for legal permits.

Expelling Jews: the protectors disappear

On 7 April 1933, 2 months after seizing power, the Nazi government passed the 'Law for the Restitution of Professional Civil Service', which expelled Jews from scientific positions. For most, dismissal meant humiliation and persecution, flight or emigration, poverty or death. For neonatal medicine in Germany, it meant decapitation: half of German paediatricians, but nearly all neonatal specialists were Jews. Eduard Seidler published detailed information on the fate of over 700 Jewish paediatricians [7], some of whom are listed in Table 8.4.1. Together with the Jewish scientists, their topic of interest disappeared from academic medicine, and special care units for 'weaklings' were closed. In Leipzig, Siegfried Rosenbaum was replaced by the Nazi Werner Catel, who worried about the 'threatening extinction of the German Volk' [8].

On 14 July 1933, the 'Law for the Prevention of Hereditarily Diseased Offspring' was passed, which mandated the sterilization of those regarded as having 'hereditary diseases' or being 'racially inferior'. German physicians had to sign the receipt of the law commentary. Most conditions listed were congenital, but not hereditary. Stigmatizing children with malformation, epilepsy, or mental retardation, this law influenced professional and public opinion, weakened the right to live for these individuals, and paved the way towards their elimination.

A planned crime

No law was ever passed to justify the killings. In a letter backdated to 1 September 1939 (the onset of World War II), Hitler ordered that 'certain physicians be personally authorized so that incurable patients can, after thorough evaluation of their condition, be granted a mercy death'. Killing handicapped children was organized in Hitler's Chancellery by Hans Hefelmann. On 8 August 1939, the secret edict IVb 3088/39-1079Mi was circulated to governmental health authorities: 'To clarify scientific questions concerning congenital malformation and retarded mental development', midwives, obstetricians, and paediatricians should report 'neonates and infants with severe congenital disease' to the regional health offices. The report form specified who was meant: (1) idiocy and mongolism; (2) microcephaly; (3) progredient hydrocephaly; (4) malformation of any kind, specifically limbs, head, or spine; and (5) palsies, including Little's disease. For each report, the midwife received 2 Reichsmark. Under the cover name 'Reich Committee for Scientific Registration of Congenital Severe Disorders' ('Reichsausschuss') an office was founded in Berlin tasked with deciding on the incoming reports. Reviewers were Werner Catel, director of the Leipzig University Children's Hospital; Ernst Wentzler, director of a private Berlin children's hospital; and Hans Heinze, director of the Department of Child Psychiatry at Görden, Brandenburg. When each of them had marked a '+' on the report form, the death sentence was spoken.

The mode of operation of the 'Reichsausschuss' and the network of more than 30 'Children's Special Departments' ('Kinderfachabteilungen') established throughout Germany and the occupied countries has been described by Klee [10] and Topp [11]. The 'treatment' consisted of administration of sedatives, usually phenobarbital at a dose depressing respiration. Not recorded in the chart, it led to a slow death disguised as natural (pneumonia). Food was withheld in some institutions. The median time interval between admission to the 'Special Department' and death was 1.4 months [12]. Parents were informed after their child's burial; no consent was acquired before using the body (brain) for research purposes. Thomas Beddies recently illustrated some victims' fate in an exhibition 'Remembering the Children' [13]; Ernst Klee reported a typical course [10]: 'Ilse Z. was born on April 21, 1940, with Down's syndrome and clubfeet. The day after her birth, the midwife reported her to the local health authority and received two Reichsmark. The public health officer sent the report to the Reichsausschuss on May 8, which ordered observation of the child's development. In October, the public health officer reported to Wentzler: "physical appearance of Mongoloid Idiocy". On February 21, 1941, a health nurse brought Ilse to the "Special Department" in Eglfing-Haar. On April 5,1941, she was dead.'

Sascha Topp [11] identified 93 physicians personally involved in killing in the 'Special Departments'. Many more paediatricians were involved in reporting handicapped infants to the 'Reichsausschuss'. Table 8.4.2 shows that they were not second-class physicians, but qualified paediatricians, among them eminent scientists, presidents, and honorary members of the German Society of Paediatrics. Heinze's first 'Special Department' in Görden served as the central training institution to teach doctors how to kill [12]. The age of the admitted children was gradually raised until 1944 and the justification shifted from diminished suffering ('mercy death') to economic arguments ('useless eaters'). The role of nurses and midwives in the child murder programmes has recently been described by Susan Benedict and Linda Shields [14]. About 10,000 children were killed in the 'Reichsausschuss' programme [11, 15]. Until now, no evidence has been found of protest or opposition by individuals or scientific societies.

Failed criminal prosecution

When the Allies returned jurisdiction to Germany in 1949, silence fell on the subject of child murder. Criminal proceedings were opened, but few verdicts were passed, most court trials against physicians were discontinued. The accused, defending themselves with Binding's and Hoche's arguments, were usually accorded 'an error about illegality without fault of their own'. Obviously, post-war judges equated a backdated letter of Hitler with the law. In 1968, the 'Law on Regulatory Offences' turned murderers into accomplices, whose crimes could no longer be prosecuted. The witness records, however, became the main source of rediscovery. It was neither historians nor physicians but two journalists who first tackled the crime and named perpetrators and victims: Ernst Klee [16] and Götz Aly [17].

Table 8.4.1 Some Jewish university teachers whose research focused on newborns or infant nutrition, and who lost their supervisory or teaching positions in 1933

Name, birth–death	Position	Achievements/research in neonatal medicine before 1933	Fate from 1933
Albert Eckstein 1891–1950	Düsseldorf	1923 H Freiburg; 1932 Dir UCH Düsseldorf; biology of the neonate; encephalopathies; hospital infection	1935 Turkey
Stefan Engel 1878–1968	Dortmund	1910 H Düsseldorf; 1912 *Textbook of Infant Care* (12 eds); 1917 *Textbook of Infant Nutrition*; 1918 Dir CH Dortmund	1936 UK
Berthold Epstein 1890–1962	Prague	1924 H Prague; candidiasis, hospital infections; 1920 Foundling Hospital Prague; 1922 Prague University; fled to Norway	1942 Concentration camp
Heinrich Finkelstein 1865–1942	Berlin	1899 H Berlin; infantile otitis media; 1905 *Textbook of Infant Diseases*, 4 eds; 1918 Dir Friedrich Hospital. Editor of *Zeitschrift für Kinderheilkunde*	1936 US, Chile
Ernst Freudenberg 1884–1967	Marburg	1917 H Heidelberg; rickets, tetany; 1922 Dir UCH Marburg; 1929 Physiology and pathology of digestion in infancy; 1937 Dismissed; 1938 Dir UCH Basel	1938 Switzerland
Werner Gottstein 1894–1959	Berlin	1927 H Freiburg; infections; 1930 Standards for establishing infant wards; 1931 Dir Kinderheim Charlottenburg	1938 US
Paul György 1893–1976	Heidelberg	1923 H Heidelberg; 1922 *Textbook of Paediatrics*; 1929 Treatment and prevention of rickets; 1931 Biotin; 1933 Vitamin B_2; 1934 Vitamin B_6	1933 UK, US
Richard Hamburger 1884–1940	Berlin	1923 H Berlin; 1928, Prof. at Charité; infant nutrition, rickets. Dismissed already in 1932 on Bessau's initiative	1933 UK
Rudolf Hess 1886–1962	Bremen	1916 H Strassburg; 1921 Dir CH Frankfurt; 1928 Dir CH Bremen; 1933 dismissed; 1945 returned as Dir CH Bremen	1944 Concentration camp
Walter Heymann 1901–1985	Freiburg	1931 H Freiburg: infant nephrology, rickets, vitamin D metabolism	1933 US
Kurt Huldschinski 1883–1940	Berlin	No H; osteogenesis imperfecta; 1919 Detected action of ultraviolet light on rickets; 1926 Heubner Prize	1934 Egypt
Paul Karger 1892–1976	Berlin	1924 H Berlin; 1930 Prof. at Charité; focused on sleep, neuropathies, X-ray diagnostics, infantile surgery	1937 Canada
Leopold Langstein 1876–1933	Berlin	1908 H Berlin; 1911 Dir KAVH; ward for preterm infants; 1914 *Textbook of Infant Nutrition and Metabolism; Atlas of Hygiene*	1933 Suicide
Bruno Leichtentritt 1888–1966	Breslau	1922 H Breslau; vitamin deficiency syndromes; public health; 1926 Prof; 1928 Dir Health Insurance Agency of Silesia	1938 US
Franz Lust 1880–1939	Karlsruhe	1913 H Heidelberg; tetany; social paediatrics; 1918 *Textbook of Paediatrics* (>20 eds, translations until 1939); 1919 Prof; 1920 Dir CH Karlsruhe	1938 Concentration camp
Ludwig Ferdinand Meyer 1879–1954	Berlin	1913 H Berlin; physiology and pathology of infants, infant nutrition, immunity, infection; 1918 Dir Waisenhaus Berlin; 1933 Dir Kaiserin Friedrich Hospital Berlin	1935 Palestine
Ernst Moro 1874–1951	Heidelberg	1906 H München; 1911 Prof Heidelberg; tuberculosis test; neonatal reflexes; Editor, *Yearbook of Paediatrics*	1936 Retired
Arnold Orgler 1874–1957	Berlin	1917 H Berlin; rickets; nutrition; twins; 1923 Dir CH Berlin-Neukölln	
Siegfried Rosenbaum 1890–1969	Leipzig	1925 H Leipzig; biochemistry of gastroenteritis; 1919 Breslau: 1922 KK Leipzig; 1925 Physiology and pathology of the infant stomach; 1932 Dir UCH Leipzig	1933 Palestine
Erwin Schiff 1891–1971	Berlin	1921 H Berlin; 1925 Prof at Charité; biochemistry of metabolism in infants; connatal muscular weakness; dehydration; dismissed by Bessau already in 1932	1938 US
Arthur Schlossmann 1867–1932	Düsseldorf	1894 Founded first German Infant Hospital in Dresden; 1898 H Dresden; 1906 (with Pfaundler) *Handbook of Paediatrics* (2nd ed. 1931); 1906 Dir UCH Düsseldorf	1932 Retired
Gustav Tugendreich 1876–1948	Berlin	No H; 1906 Dir Infant Hospital Prenzlauer Berg; social hygiene, infant protection; Textbook: *Illness and Social Situation*	1937 UK, US

Dir, director, CH, children's hospital; H, habilitation, academic qualification for university teaching, similar to PhD; Prof, professor; UCH, university children's hospital.
Source: Data from Seidler [7] and Fischer [9].

Post-war teaching and research

It is a sad fact that paediatricians involved in child murder, without feelings of guilt, continued to teach and train students, nurses, and physicians and to organize research after the Nazi regime. Textbooks, purged of antisemitic and racist passages, reappeared and continued to convey little compassion for the weak, the malformed, and handicapped: as late as 1966, the Keller–Wiskott textbook rejected operating for spina bifida 'when palsies are present', or hydrocephalus, 10 years after the development of the Spitz–Holter drainage [18]. The 1971 edition of the *Handbook of Paediatrics* classified treating infants

Table 8.4.2 Some physicians and university teachers involved in Nazi child-murder before, and in academic research or teaching after 1945

Person	Before 1945	After 1945	Reference
Wilhelm Bayer 1900–1972	1934 Dir CH Hamburg-Rothenburgsort; 1940 Established and directed KFA	1945 Suspended; 1949 Trial: discontinued; worked as editor, from 1952, private paediatric practice in Hamburg; 1960 Textbook: *The Infant's First Year*	[11]
Georg Bessau 1884–1944	1915 H; 1922 Dir UCH Leipzig; 1932 Dir UCH Charité Berlin; tuberculosis-experiments with RA infants. Cooperation with KFA Berlin-Wittenau	Died in 1944 Pupils: Catel, Schönfeld	[11]
Werner Catel 1894–1981	1926 H Leipzig; 1932 Prof Charité Berlin; 1933 Dir UCH Leipzig. Installed a KFA in this hospital. 1939 RA reviewer. 1939 *Textbook of Child Care*	1947 Acquitted. Dir Tbc-Hospital Mammolshöhe; 1954–1960 Dir UCH Kiel. *Textbook of Child Care*, 11th ed 1977. 1944 Textbook: *Differential Diagnostic Symptomatology of Diseases of Childhood*, 3rd ed. 1964	[15] [21]
Johann Duken 1889–1954	1924 H Jena; 1933 UCH Giessen; 1937 Dir UCH Heidelberg; cooperation with KFA Eichberg and Wiesloch	1945 Suspended by Allies; 2 years prison because of SS membership. 1948 Trial: discontinued	[17]
Heinrich Gross 1915–2005	1940 Assistant, 1941, Dir. KFA Vienna-Spiegelgrund	1948 2 years; prison; 1968 Dir Ludwig Boltzmann Institute for Brain Malformations; published 34 papers on brains of killed infants up to 1989	[11]
Julius Hallervorden 1882–1965	1929 Prosecutor in Brandenburg; 1933 SS member; 1938 Prof and Dir Kaiser Wilhelm Institute Berlin; studied brains and was involved in the killing of infants	1949–1956 Dir department of brain research, Max-Planck Institute Giessen. Brains of murdered infants were studied in Frankfurt up to 1990	[17]
Hans Heinze 1895–1983	1938 Dir KFA Görden—training centre for 'euthanasia' doctors; 1939 RA reviewer. Cooperation with Hallervorden; 1941 President, German Society for Child Psychiatry; 1943 Prof	1946 7 years' prison; 1954 Dir Child Psychiatry Wunstorf; 1960 Retired	[11] [22]
Jussuf Ibrahim 1877–1953	1904 H Heidelberg; 1915 Dir UCH Würzburg; 1917 Dir UCH Jena; neurology chapter in Feer's textbook. Cooperation with KFA Stadtroda	Remained Dir UCH Jena up to his death. This hospital was named after Ibrahim until 2000	[23]
Walter Keller 1894–1967	1927 H Heidelberg; 1938 Prof UCH Giessen; 1942 Polio transmission experiments	1945 2 years' prison because of SS membership, 1949 Dir UCH Freiburg; 1961 *Textbook of Paediatrics* (with Wiskott), 6th ed. 1991	[24]
Albert Viethen 1897–1978	1932 H Freiburg; 1934 UCH Heidelberg; 1939 Dir UCH Erlangen. Cooperation with KFA Ansbach	1945 2 years' prison because of SS membership; 1948 Trial: discontinued; 1949 Dir CH Berchtesgaden; 1951 Teaching licence renewed; 1962 Retired	[25]
Ernst Wentzler 1891–1973	Dir CH Berlin-Frohnau; 1939 RA reviewer	Paediatric practice in Hannoversch-Münden	[26]
Hans-Rudolf Wiedemann 1915–2006	1944 H Jena, cooperation with KFA Stadtroda	1950 Prof Bonn; 1952 Dir CH Krefeld; 1961 Dir UCH Kiel; 1976 *Atlas of Clinical Syndromes*; 6th ed. 2010; 1960 *Textbook of Skeleton Malformations*	[21] [27]
Alfred Wiskott 1898–1978	Dir UCH München. Cooperation with killing-institution München Eglfing-Haar	1961 *Textbook of Paediatrics*, 6 eds. up to 1991	[11] [17]

CH, children's hospital; Dir, director; H, habilitation, academic qualification for university teaching, similar to PhD; KFA, 'children's special department'; Prof, professor; RA, 'Reichsausschuss'; UCH, university children's hospital.

with Down's syndrome 'a wasted effort' [19]. Another generation of students, paediatricians, and nurses was exposed to the inhumane and degrading terminology that lingered in textbooks and hospitals. It related to preterm infants: 'Lebensschwäche' (debility), 'Aufzucht' (breeding), 'Defektheilung' (defective recovery), 'Risikokind' (at-risk child), 'Krüppel' (cripple), 'Krampfkind' (seizured), and so on. And it related to malformed infants: 'Abartigkeit' (deviance), 'Wolfsrachen' (cleft palate), 'Froschkopf' (frog-head, anencephalus), 'Gargoylismus' (Hurler face), 'Monstrum' (monster), and so on. Catel still advocated the killing of handicapped infants in 1964 [20]: 'They have no soul, are inhuman, and will never become human.' His textbook of child care remained the standard for children's nurses well into the 1980s.

Julius Hallervorden continued research on the brains of murdered children when his institute moved to Giessen in 1949, renamed Max Planck Institute for Brain Research. Heinrich Gross, who studied the victims' brains in Vienna up to 1989, had the Ludwig Boltzmann Institute for Abnormalities of the Nervous System established. While in the US the National Institute of Child Health and Human Development and in the UK the Medical Research Council substantially sponsored research of major neonatal problems, German Research Foundation —itself involved in Nazi research programmes—continued to promote genetic projects.

Absent neonatology in the 1960s

There was reluctance or sheer unwillingness to keep infants less than 1500 g alive throughout the 1960s. Although it needs considerable insensitivity to watch an infant die from respiratory distress, opposition against artificial ventilation of neonates persisted for many years—because it required intensive care units. From the 1960s, long-term ventilation was applied to neonates in many countries, especially in preterm infants with respiratory distress

Table 8.4.3 Health statistics related to infant welfare in 22 OECD states in the year 1970

Country	IMR	PNMR	GDP	THE	Country	IMR	PNMR	GDP	THE
Australia	17.9		4653	5.7	Italy	29.6	31.7	3574	5.2
Austria	27.0	20.5	3846	5.3	Japan	13.1	21.7	3203	4.6
Belgium	20.5		3959	4.1	Luxemburg	24.9	24.9	5874	3.7
Canada	18.8	22.0	4532	7.0	Netherlands	12.7	18.8	4328	5.9
Denmark	14.2	18.0	4354	5.9	Norway	12.7	19.3	3322	4.5
Finland	13.2	17.2	3354	5.7	Portugal	58.0	38.9	1980	2.8
France	18.2	23.7	3693	5.8	Spain	28.0		2801	3.7
Germany (West)	23.4	26.8	3969	6.3	Sweden	11.0	16.5	4838	7.1
Greece	29.6	27.8	3085	5.7	Switzerland	15.1	18.3	6940	4.9
Iceland	11.7	18.6	3851	5.0	UK	20.2	25.1	3772	4.5
Ireland	19.5	24.6	2397	5.3	US	19.8		5245	7.3

IMR, infant mortality rate: deaths of children under 1 year of age per 1000 liveborn infants; PNMR, perinatal mortality rate: number of stillborns from 22 completed weeks of gestation plus deaths in the first week of life per 1000 live births; World Health Organization data [30]; GDP, gross domestic product per capita (US$, current exchange rate, current purchasing power parity); THE, total health expenditure in percent of GDP; OECD data [31].

syndrome. Pioneers of this treatment included C.A. Smith, M.E. Avery, L. Gluck, and M. Stahlman in the US; P. Swyer, L. Stern, and R. Usher in Canada; B. Corner, L. Strang, and E.O. Reynolds in the UK; A. Minkowski, J.P. Relier, and M. Dehan in France; L.S. Prod'Hom and P. Dangel in Switzerland; A. Okken in the Netherlands; P. Karlberg in Sweden; and N. Räihä in Finland. On 18–20 April 1969, Alexandre Minkowski organized the Paris symposium on artificial ventilation in the newborn with about 40 contributions from all over the world [28]. But none came from Germany, as there were few neonatologists, and newborn infants were seldom ventilated. In Mainz, Germany's first intensive care unit—for newborns and older children—opened in 1965. Dominik K, the first Heidelberg neonate to survive artificial ventilation, was born in August 1971. In the same year, the *Handbook of Paediatrics* claimed [19]: 'The discussion on indication, benefit and complications of prolonged ventilation [in respiratory distress] is not finished.' Most textbooks devoted more space to describing poor long-term results than to describing therapies. In 1975, the German Society of Paediatrics recommended establishing neonatal intensive care units, albeit combined with paediatric intensive care units [29]. As late as 1980, fewer than ten neonatal intensive care units existed, located near the delivery room. Not surprisingly, (West) Germany's infant mortality rate was 23.4 in 1970—rank 17 among 22 member states of the Organisation for Economic Co-operation and Development (OECD) (Table 8.4.3). At that time Germany was wealthy, ranking 9/22 in gross domestic product and 4/22 in health expenditures.

Malformed infants were treated reluctantly. De Rudder observed a 'remarkable' sevenfold 'increase' of severe malformations in West Germany after 1945 [32]. Parts of this 'increase' may be due to improved diagnostics, poor nutrition, and post-war folate deficiency, but a greater part was probably infants previously classified as stillborn. In East Germany, the infant mortality rate was falsified by defining life birth as heartbeat *and* respiration, and by drowning immature infants at birth [33]. In the Magdeburg region, the prevalence of severe malformations rose threefold after the reunification in 1990 [34]. A part of this 'rise' may be attributable to improved diagnostics and higher maternal age, but many will have previously been declared stillborn.

Delayed effect: a blocked ethical debate

Ethical principles quite naturally diverge, and free societies debate them prior to practicable legislation. In Germany, such discussions are burdened with the unatoned murder of the handicapped during the Nazi regime and often reveal a strange ambivalence: bashful or timid debates continue for years, frequently becoming emotional or even hysterical, and rarely leading to durable consensus. Most Germans approve aborting severely malformed fetuses following elaborated prenatal diagnosis—but legislation justifies abortion when the mother's life is threatened. Most Germans want the right to end their own life voluntarily—but legislation forbids physicians to assist. Most Germans agree that severely sick infants should not die on a ventilator—but legislation leaves parents and doctors alone in that situation.

Conclusion

State-organized murder of handicapped infants was not the crime of a few mad Nazi henchmen, but rooted in the feelings of an indoctrinated population and in the paediatric profession's value system. Both evolved in close neighbourhood to eugenics in a society that exchanged respect for the individual's dignity for the alleged state's interests. Despising the weak was an enduring legacy of Nazism that, among other problems, may have delayed the introduction of neonatology in Germany and other countries. This is a hypothesis: to prove or disprove it will take historians a generation of effort. A century of utilitarian thinking reveals striking parallels between Binding and Hoche in 1920; Catel in 1961; Engelhardt in 1973 and Singer in 1979: they all denied intrinsic human dignity and equated personhood with self-awareness, which led them to justify the extinction of the severely mentally impaired.

REFERENCES

1. Burleigh M: Death and deliverance: 'Euthanasia' in Germany c. 1900–1945. Cambridge: Cambridge University Press, 1994.
2. Brand G: The Velpke baby home trial. In: War crimes trials, Vol. **7**. London: Hodge, 1950: p. 1–356.
3. Czerny A: Was ist bei Kindern angeboren, was erworben? In: Adam C, Kirchner M: Der Wiederaufbau der Volkskraft nach dem Kriege. Jena: Fischer, 1918: p. 157–63.
4. Czerny A: Die Pädiatrie meiner Zeit. Berlin: Springer, 1939: p. 65.
5. Binding K, Hoche A: Die Vernichtung lebensunwerten Lebens. Ihr Maß und ihre Form. Leipzig: Meiner, 1920.
6. Meltzer E: Das Problem der Abkürzung 'Lebensunwerten' Lebens. Halle: Marhold, 1925: p. **VIII**, 128.
7. Seidler E: Kinderärzte 1933–1945: Entrechtet—geflohen—ermordet. Bonn: Bouvier, 2000.
8. Catel W: Die Pflege des gesunden und kranken Kindes. 2. ed. Leipzig: Thieme, 1942: p. 381.
9. Fischer I: Biographisches Lexikon der hervorragenden Ärzte der letzten fünfzig Jahre. Berlin: Urban & Schwarzenberg, 1932.
10. Klee E: 'Euthanasie' im NS-Staat: Die 'Vernichtung lebensunwerten Lebens'. 9. ed. Frankfurt: Fischer, 1999: p. 298.
11. Topp S: Der 'Reichsausschuss zur wissenschaftlichen Erfassung erb- und anlagebedingter schwerer Leiden'. In: Beddies T, Hübener K: Kinder in der NS-Psychiatrie. Berlin-Brandenburg: be.bra Wissenschaft Verlag, 2004: p. 17–54.
12. Pelz L: Kinderärzte im Netz der 'NS-Kindereuthanasie' am Beispiel der 'Kinderfachabteilung' Görden. Monatsschr Kinderheilk 2003;**151**:1027–32.
13. Beddies T: 'Was habt ihr mit meinem Kind gemacht, das ist ja mein Kind gar nicht mehr!...'—Zeitzeugnisse. Monatsschr Kinderheilk 2011;**159**:6–8.
14. Benedict S, Shields L: Nurses and midwives in Nazi Germany: The 'euthanasia programs'. New York: Routledge, 2014.
15. Benzenhöfer U: Genese und Struktur der 'NS-Kinder- und Jugendlicheneuthanasie'. Mschr Kinderheilk 2003;**151**:1012–9.
16. Klee E: Dokumente zur 'Euthanasie'. Frankfurt: Fischer, 1985.
17. Aly G: Der saubere und der schmutzige Fortschritt. In: Reform und Gewissen. 'Euthanasie' im Dienst des Fortschritts. Berlin: Rotbuch, 1985: p. 9–78.
18. Keller W, Wiskott A: Lehrbuch der Kinderheilkunde. 2. ed. 1966: Thieme, 1966: p. 137.
19. Opitz H, Schmid F: Handbuch der Kinderheilkunde. Berlin: Springer, 1971: p. Vol. **1**, pt. 1, p.722; Vol. 1, pt. 2, p.377.
20. Renner H: Aus Menschlichkeit töten? Spiegel-Gespräch mit Professor Dr Werner Catel über Kinder-Euthanasie. Der Spiegel 1964; 41–7.
21. Petersen H-C, Zankel S: Werner Catel—ein Protagonist der NS-'Kindereuthanasie' und seine Nachkriegskarriere. Med Hist J 2003;**38**:139–73.
22. Nedoschill J, Castell R: Der Vorsitzende der Deutschen Gesellschaft für Kinderpsychiatrie und Heilpädagogik im Zweiten Weltkrieg. Prax Kinderpsychol Kinderpsychiatrie 2001;**50**:228–37.
23. Zimmermann S: Die medizinische Fakultät der Universität Jena während der Zeit des Nationalsozialismus. Habilitationsschrift: Berlin: Verlag Wissenschaft und Bildung, 2000: p. 160–7.
24. Topp S: Geschichte als Argument in der Nachkriegsmedizin. Göttingen: V&R Unipress, 2013: p. 131.
25. Bussiek D, Castell R, Rascher W: Albert Viethen (1897–1978), Direktor der Universitätskinderklinik in Erlangen 1939–1945. Monatsschr Kinderheilk 2004;**152**:992–1003.
26. Beddies T: Der Kinderarzt und 'Euthanasie'-Gutachter Ernst Wentzler. Monatsschr Kinderheilk 2003;**151**:1020–6.
27. Bericht der Kommission zur Untersuchung der Beteiligung von Prof. Dr Jussuf Ibrahim an der Vernichtung 'lebensunwerten Lebens' während der NS-Zeit. Jena: Friedrich Schiller Universität, 2000: p. 33. http://www.verwaltung.uni-jena.de/unimediajena/ibrahim/ (accessed 5 November 2015).
28. Minkowski A, Swyer P: Symposium on artificial ventilation, Paris, April 18–20, 1969. Biol Neonat 1970;**16**:1–375.
29. Schäfer KH: Von der Deutschen Gesellschaft für Kinderheilkunde beschlossene Richtlinien für die Betreuung von Risikoneugeborenen. Monatsschr Kinderheilk 1975;**123**:41–4.
30. World Health Organization: World health statistics annual. Geneva: World Health Organization, 1970: Vol. **1**, p. 10–4.
31. Huber M: Health expenditure trends in OECD countries, 1970–1997. Health Care Financ Rev 1999;**21**:99–117.
32. de Rudder B: Zur Frage einer Zunahme schwerer Mißbildungen. Dtsch Med Wschr 1959;**84**:1809.
33. Bezirksgericht Erfurt: AZ 1U 38/92. 'Stellen Sie 'nen Eimer hin'. Der Spiegel 1992;**46**:63–5.
34. Rösch C, Steinbicker V: Fehlbildungserfassung in der Region Magdeburg. Demogr Mitteil Johann Peter Süssmilch Gesell Demogr 1997;**17**:5–9.

8.5

Cot death
History of an iatrogenic disaster

Introduction

Finding one's own baby dead in the crib is a ghastly experience that parents of all times had to endure. As other causes of infant mortality waned, cot death began to attract medical interest in the 19th century. When its frequency actually rose during the 1970s, it became one of the most researched paediatric topics. Its recent history has been described by Russell-Jones [1], Norvenius [2], Poets [3], Dally [4], Högberg and Bergström [5], and Gilbert and co-workers [6], and is therefore abbreviated here. This chapter adds an earlier perspective and a focus on the reasons for recommending prone sleep. The old term 'cot death' is preferred to the modern term 'sudden infant death syndrome', as the latter's definition changed and as a syndrome is a set of several concurrent symptoms.

Antique bed sharing and blame

Mesopotamian cultures feared that the lion-headed goddess Lamashtu lurked at night for a chance to destroy infants (see Chapter 2.7). Jews assumed a more natural explanation, as expressed in 1 Kings 3:17–19: 'And the one woman said [to Solomon], O my lord, I and this woman dwell in one house; and I was delivered of a child with her in the house. And it came to pass the third day ... this woman's child died in the night; because she overlaid it.' Infanticide and accidental death were barely distinguishable, and families were blamed when their baby died. Diodorus Siculus reported from Egypt [7]: 'In the case of parents who had slain their children, the offenders had to hold the dead body in their arms for three successive days and nights, under the surveillance of a state guard ... which brought with it pain and repentance to turn them from such deeds.' Soranus (teaching in Rome 200 C.E.) accused drunkenness [8]: 'Seized by a sleep from which she is hard to awaken, she leaves the newborn untended or even falls down upon it in a dangerous way.' Soranus also opposed bed sharing: 'Besides, the newborn should not sleep with her, especially in the beginning, lest unaware she roll over and cause it to be bruised or suffocated. For this reason the cradle should stand either alongside the bed, or if she wants to have the newborn still nearer, the crib should be placed upon the bed.'

Smothering, overlaying, and punishment

In many societies, only the rich could afford cradles, and sleeping in the mother's straw bed was a sheer need during winter. The Catholic Church did not believe in the accidental character of smothering and for a millennium issued threats, as did the Council of Mainz in 852 [9]: 'Who carelessly oppresses his infant or lets it suffocate by the weight of the bed cover, must suffer penance on bread and water ... for 40 days and abstain from the spouse. Thereafter he must do penance on holidays for three years. If the child was oppressed before baptism, the penance is 60 days and five years, respectively.' This decree was reinforced by the Councils of Worms in 868, Tours in 1163, and York in 1236; but overlaying remained so frequent, that the 4th Provincial Council of Milan decreed in 1576 [10]: 'Any woman who kept an infant less than one year old in her bed, without the *caution* the bishop has ordered, is ipso facto excommunicated, and will not be absolved unless she submits to severe and visible penance.' The *caution* was a device invented in Florence, which Zückert described [11]: 'No mother or wet-nurse shall put a baby to her breast, unless it is safely enclosed in a case called *arcuccio* [little arch].' Outside Italy, the device was more discussed than used, and no specimen seems to have survived. In 1731, Oliver St. John sent a drawing of the box from Florence to the London Royal Society (Fig. 8.5.1A) [12]. Uppsala professor Nils Rosenstein wrote in 1764 [13]: 'In Sweden near 700 infants are suffocated each year. In Florence a cradle named arcuccio has been ordered for prevention, in which bended rods keep the bedcovers distant. The Lapponic cradle [Fig. 8.5.1B] evolved for the same purpose.' In his last work *On Education*, Königsberg philosopher Immanuel Kant wrote in 1803 [14]: 'The most suitable arrangement would be a kind of box covered with leather straps [Fig. 8.5.1C], such as the Italians use and call *arcuccio*. The child is never taken out of this box, even when nursed by its mother. This protects the child from

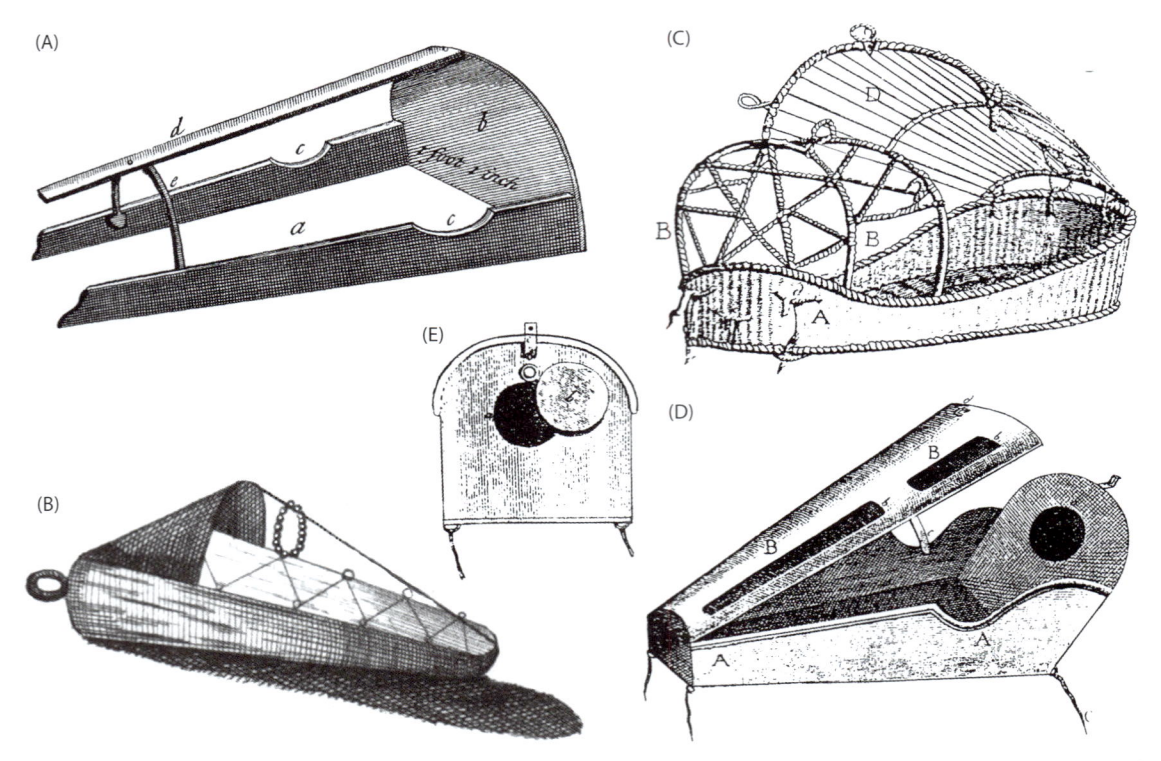

Fig. 8.5.1 Devices constructed to protect the sleeping infant. A, arcuccio, manufactured in Florence, described by Oliver St. John 1731 [12]: 'When I consider how many are charged overlaid in the Bills of Mortality, I wonder that the Arcutios, universally used here, are not used in *England*.' B, Lapponian cradle published by Knut Leem in 1767 [80]; C and D, two Danish models of 1770 [2]; E, head board of device D.

the chance of being smothered when sleeping with its mother at night, while here many children lose their lives in this way.' The General State Law for the Prussian States of 1794 [15] prohibited 'mothers and wet-nurses from taking children less than two years into their beds at night. Those doing such, forfeit jail or corporal punishment, depending on the circumstances'.

Accidental mechanical suffocation

Unexpected death without suffocation was rarely described. On 29 November 1459, 4-month-old Joachim de France was found dead in his cot. He was the elder son of Charlotte de Savoye and the Dauphin, future King Louis XI. The cause of death remained obscure, and Simon de Vallambert, personal physician of the Duchess of Savoye, suggested that the prince 'lacked fresh air and was kept too warm' [16]. 'Near-miss' cot death was also long known; Jean Janin of Paris published an example in 1772 [17]: 'A nurse had the misfortune to stifle in his bed her nurse-child … I found the little victim without any sign of life, pulseless arteries, no respiration, the face livid, the eyes open and dull … [the baby] was rubbed with fine linen, some puffs of tobacco smoke were blown up his nostrils. To this succeeded blowing into the mouth … recovered within half an hour.' In 1892, police surgeon Charles Templeman of Dundee linked cot death to social problems [18]: 32% of his 258 cases were 'born illegitimate' and 46% occurred on Sunday morning to parents 'receiving their week's wages on Saturday and going to bed more or less intoxicated'. Alluding to frequent infanticide throughout history (see Chapter 8.3), Asch hypothesized in 1968 [19]: 'A large percentage of "crib deaths" are actually infanticides.'

The thymus hypothesis

Accidental 'overlaying', 'smothering', or 'suffocation' were considered natural causes of death, and entered as such in the mortality statistics. In the 19th century, these terms became unacceptable for physicians and lawmakers, and 'natural' explanations were sought.

The term 'sudden and unexplained death' was coined by Samuel Fearn in 1834 [20]: 'It seemed impossible that the child could have been suffocated … I became at a loss on how to account for the death.' But instead of confessing doubts, a fatal disease was invented. Forensic doctor Joseph Schallgruber reported in 1823 [21]: 'I rescued the honor and freedom of two women', stating that 'enlarged thymus is the internal cause of suffocation in early age'. Johann Kopp termed the disorder 'asthma thymicum' in 1830 [22] and despite Friedleben's extensive analysis of 1858 [23], 'there is no asthma thymicum', influential teachers associated enlarged thymus with cot death, as did Virchow [24], Grawitz [25], Jacobi [26], Osler [27], and Holt [28]. In 1889, the Austrian pathologist Arnold Paltauf defined thymic enlargement as part of an abnormal constitution later called 'status thymo-lymphaticus' [29, 30]. In Cincinnati, the 'enlarged' thymus of a 2-month-old boy with stridor was 'successfully' irradiated in 1905 [31], 9 years after the discovery of X-rays. This treatment was enthusiastically adopted by many hospitals, and persisted even after World War II [32]. In

1950, Duffy and Fitzgerald reported on 28 children under 18 years, treated for thyroid cancer in New York from 1932 to 1948 [33]: ten had been irradiated for 'enlargement of the thymus' at age 4–16 months, as was 'a large number of children'. In 1961, Theodore Winship compiled a list of 277 children with thyroid carcinoma, of whom 80% had received 'X-ray therapy for a so-called enlarged thymus' [34]. Already in 1931, the British Status Lymphaticus Investigation Committee had concluded [35]: 'There is no evidence that so-called "status thymo-lymphaticus" has any existence as a pathological entity.'

Prone sleeping: propaganda and protagonists

Infant sleep position was debated before cots became available. Skulls were shaped by sleep positioning throughout millennia (see Chapter 5.2). The Hippocratian work *Airs, Waters and Places* described 'longish' head shape as 'noble' in the 4th century B.C.E. [36]. In his main work published in 1543, Belgian anatomist Andreas Vesalius noted [37]: 'Germans are often seen with compressed occiput and a wide head because as infants they always lie on their backs and are tied to the sides of their cradles … The Belgians as a rule retain longer heads … because their mothers … let them sleep on their side.' During the 16th and 17th century back versus lateral, but never prone sleep position was debated. In Orleans, Vallambert taught in 1565 [16]: 'He must be protected from bending his neck during sleep. It is good to lay him down on his back … or to turn him a little bit to the side.' Venetian author Scipione Mercurio insisted in 1595 [38]: 'The face should be directed towards heaven; because when forced to lie on its side, the ribs, still tender and soft, may easily be deformed.' *The Nurses Guide*, London, recommended in 1729 [39]: 'So long as a child takes no other Nourishment but milk,' tis better he should be laid to sleep on his Back, than either of his sides … a nurse should not take a child to Bed with her, before he has his Hands and Feet at Liberty, for fear she should happen in a deep sleep to lye upon him.' In the 'Child's Pavilion' of the 1873 Vienna World Exposition, the recommended supine sleep position was demonstrated by plaster models [40].

The prone position became custom in the US between world wars. In 1931, New York paediatricians Hess [41] and Greene [42] rediscovered Vesalius' finding of 1543 that sleep position influences skull shape, and declared positional flattening of the skull 'a new syndrome' that required 'correction and prevention'. Soon prone sleeping predominated in the US whereas in Europe the habit shifted slowly from supine to prone after 1960. Alleged benefits heralding this shift are compiled in **Table 8.5.1**.

Sheffield paediatrician Kenneth Holt, using the Gesell test during a fellowship in Iowa City, where 80% of babies slept in the prone position, wrote in 1960 [46]: 'In their early motor behavior the American babies were more advanced in the prone position but less well developed in the supine position than would be expected of English babies.' In 1961, an editorial in the *British Medical Journal* stated [54]: 'There is virtually no risk of suffocation when babies are placed in the prone position—provided, of course, there is no pillow.'

Alarms unheard: early whistle-blowers

With 849 cases in 1930, accidental mechanical suffocation was a leading cause of infant death in the US [55]. In 1944, Harold Abramson reported an increase in this accident from 692 infants in 1933 to 1333 in 1942 in the registration states of the US [56]. He found 68% in the 'face-down posture', blamed 'loose pillows, improperly applied blankets and mattress coverings', and recommended 'the routine nursing practice of placing infants in the prone position be avoided except during such times as the babies are constantly attended'. A year later, William Davison, coroner of Birmingham, published that among 210 infants who died in 1938–1944 while asleep [57], he observed 'mechanical suffocation' in only six, but 'quite a number were found prone with the face turned into the pillow'. In 1965, Carpenter and Shaddick compared 110 cases of cot death that occurred in 1958–1961 in London and Cambridge with 196 controls

Table 8.5.1 Protagonists of prone sleeping for healthy term infants, with their claimed advantages. None of these recommendations was based on a controlled trial, some of them even provided no data at all

Authors	Year	Location	Claim/reasoning	Reference
R.S. Illingworth	1954	Sheffield, UK	Soothes '3-month colic'	[43]
P. Erlacher	1959	Vienna, Austria	Less aspiration, less hip dislocation	[44]
H.G. Keitel et al.	1960	Philadelphia, PA, US	Less diaper rash, less crying, fewer scratch marks	[45]
K.S. Holt	1960	Sheffield, UK	Advanced motor development	[46]
H. Mau	1969	Tübingen, Germany	Less scoliosis	[47]
J. Gleiss	1969	Oberhausen, Germany	Less aspiration, less hip dislocation	[48]
E. Reisetbauer and H. Czermak	1972	Vienna, Austria	Orthopaedic and developmental advantages, prevents scoliosis	[49]
Y. Brackbill et al.	1973	Washington, DC, US	Sleep more, cry less, move less	[50]
V.M. Hewitt	1976	Victoria, Australia	Less aspiration of milk	[51]
J. Blumenthal and G.T. Lealman	1982	Bradford, UK	Less gastro-oesophageal reflux in low birthweight infants	[52]
K. Palmén	1984	Göteborg, Sweden	Less hip dislocation	[53]

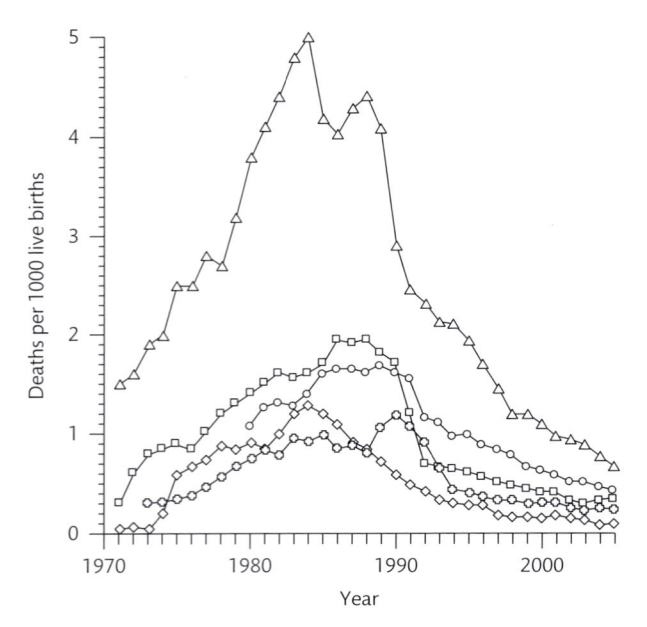

Fig. 8.5.2 Epidemic of cot death 1971–2005 in five countries with risk reduction campaigns, death rate per 1000 live births. Symbols and (start of regional campaign): triangles, New Zealand (1990); squares, England and Wales (1990); circles, Germany (1991); diamonds, Netherlands (1989); crosses, Sweden (1992). Data are from the registrar general/national statistic offices [5, 67, 68, 75, 81]. 'Sudden infant death syndrome' became a registrable cause of death in 1971. Data must be interpreted with caution, as definitions changed repeatedly and were not applied uniformly.

[58]: 'Cases were found face downwards rather more frequently than would be expected … from controls, the difference being statistically significant.'

Tragically, these warnings were ignored or forgotten. Prone sleeping was recommended to improve comfort, psychomotor development, or head shape, while a worldwide deadly epidemic surged: tens of thousands of infant deaths were associated—if not caused—by the unwarranted recommendation of prone sleeping. Fig. 8.5.2 shows the epidemic's coming and going in five countries.

Defining a 'new' syndrome

In 1969, during the second international conference, Bruce Beckwith defined a 'syndrome' [59]: 'Sudden death of an infant, unexpected by history, in which a thorough postmortem examination fails to demonstrate an adequate cause.' The definition was modified repeatedly, the San Diego revision of 2004 [60] added 'review of the circumstances of death', but did not define 'thorough' postmortem examination.

To explain a disease that by definition is unexplained, is intrinsically and logically demanding. However, many researchers took the plunge. When cot death became more and more frequent, theories proliferated. In 1973, Beckwith assembled 73 single-cause theories proposed up to that date—prone sleeping not being among them [61]. Hundreds more were to follow, derived from incomplete observations or underpowered series and derided by Bergman [62] as 'crib death theory-of-the-month-club'. The most bizarre and influential was Steinschneider's theory of 'prolonged central apnoea' [63], believed for 20 years and quoted 404 times between 1974 and 1996 [64]. This paper heralded the institution of baby sleep laboratories and the prescription of home monitors. When the mother Waneta Hoyt was sentenced for fivefold murder of her infants in April 1995, the editor of *Pediatrics* published a 'very important erratum': 'This is an incredible story. The whole apnea home monitoring … began with Steinschneider's original paper.'

Risk reduction campaigns

The cot death epidemic was broken thanks to epidemiologic research. As Ruth Gilbert demonstrated [6], the association between prone sleeping and cot death was significant by 1970, after the case–control studies of Carpenter [58] and Froggatt [65] had been published. But it took another 18 years, ten more case–control studies, and tens of thousands of dead babies before interventions were initiated (Fig. 8.5.2). In 1988, Susan Beal observed [66] that in Australia the prevalence of prone sleeping and incidence of cot death were decreasing. The Netherlands campaign headed by Adèle Engelberts and Guus de Jonge in 1989 reduced the prone sleeping rate from 60% to 10% [67]. Edwin Mitchell led the New Zealand intervention [68], focusing on reaching the vulnerable Maori subpopulation. The UK campaign was headed by Peter Fleming [69]: within 4 years the cot death rate in England and Wales fell by 75% [70]. In Germany, a regional campaign was initiated by Gerhard Jorch [71], the Swedish campaign was led by Göran Wennergren [72]. These campaigns did not just propagate supine sleeping, but included a smoke-free environment, breastfeeding, and avoiding overheating. Wherever prone infant sleep disappeared, cot deaths ceased. The US, where the epidemic began, reacted reluctantly. In 1992, the American Academy of Pediatrics recommended [73]: 'The weight of evidence implicated the prone position as a significant risk for SIDS [sudden infant death syndrome]', but 'there are still good reasons for placing certain infants prone'. In the US, 54% of all infants and 75% of those second- and thirdborn were put to sleep prone in 1995 [74], and the rate of sudden infant death syndrome was 0.87 per 1000 live births [75]. As late as 2016, the American Academy of Pediatrics recommended among 18 other measures [76]: 'Back to sleep for every sleep.'

Perhaps part of the rise in the 1970s and part of the decrease in the 1990s resulted from reclassification due to changes in the 'sudden infant death syndrome' definition. However, the changes largely paralleled postneonatal infant mortality [77]. Smoke-free homes accounted for up to 20% of the reduction [78]. A causal relation between prone sleeping and cot death has not been proven, and it remains unclear how prone sleeping harms babies: airway obstruction, rebreathing hypercapnia, overheating, myocardial hypoxia, or other factors? But the near-total disappearance of the disease following the back-to-sleep campaigns strongly supports a cause-and-effect relation.

Conclusion

How could the epidemic of cot death rage for three decades in the modern world of science-oriented medicine? The recipe had at least five ingredients: (1) the paediatricians' old sin of introducing interventions without controlled trials and follow-up; (2) euphemistically motivated replacement of the blunt 'accidental suffocation' by 'sudden infant death syndrome'; (3) support of Steinschneider's unproven hypothesis of central apnoea by companies interested in selling monitors; (4) the historical amnesia of modern science that ignored valuable studies from the past and fostered the belief that cot death is a 'novel' disease; and (5) overestimating laboratory and underrating epidemiologic research prolonged the epidemic. The fact that nearly the entire world followed wrong advice is disquieting, and deserves deeper study beyond the scope of this chapter. Even if painful, causes and mechanisms of the 18-year delay between Carpenter's [61] and Froggatt's [68] findings, and Beal's [69] and Engelbert's [70] consequences must be understood: this will not revive the infants who died between 1970 and 1988. But it may help to avoid future disasters in a field of medicine exposed to an ever-increasing amount of information.

'Sudden infant death syndrome' does not exist in the form discussed since Beckwith's definition in 1969. The majority of cases during the 1970-2000 epidemic seem to have been accidental suffocation due to prone sleeping. In infant history, medical treatments frequently went in wrong directions. But in cot death, error, prejudice, emotion, and wishful thinking accumulated irrationally. For decades, the motive to console the parents with a 'natural' explanation for their child's death superseded medicine's primary duty to prevent the accident. In his pioneering *Treatise on Acute Diseases of Infants*, Cambridge lecturer Walter Harris stated in 1689 [79]: 'A physician ought not to glory in the Invention of *Hypotheses*, but in the success of his *Practice*.'

REFERENCES

1. Russell-Jones DL: Sudden infant death in history and literature. Arch Dis Child 1985;**60**:278–81.
2. Norvenius SG: Some medico-historic remarks on SIDS. Acta Paediatr Suppl 1993;**389**:3–9.
3. Poets CF: Status thymo-lymphaticus, apnoea, and sudden infant death—lessons learned from the past? Eur J Pediatr 1996;**155**:165–7.
4. Dally A: Status lymphaticus: sudden death in children from 'Visitation of God' to cot death. Med Hist 1997;**41**:70–85.
5. Högberg U, Bergström E: Suffocated prone: the iatrogenic tragedy of SIDS. Am J Public Health 2000;**90**:527–31.
6. Gilbert R, Salanti G, Harden M, See S: Infant sleeping position and the sudden infant death syndrome. Int J Epidemiol 2005;**34**:874–87.
7. Diodorus Siculus: Bibliotheca historica. Loeb Classical Library Vol. **279**. London: Heinemann, 1933: Vol. **I**, p. 77.7.
8. Temkin O: Soranus' Gynecology. Baltimore, MD: Johns Hopkins Press, 1956: p. 79, 93, 110.
9. Concilium Moguntinum (852, 3 Oct). In: Boretius A, Krause V: Capitularia Regum Francorum. Hannover: Hahn, 1897: Vol. **2**, p. 184–9.
10. Acts of the 4th Provincial Council of Milan 1576 Pars 2. Lugduni: Anisson and Posuel, 1683: Vol. **1**, p. 110.
11. Zückert JF: Unterricht für rechtschaffene Eltern, zur diätetischen Pflege ihrer Säuglinge. 2. ed. Berlin: Mylius, 1771: p. 149.
12. St. John O, Graham R: An extract of a letter from Oliver St. John, Esq. dated from Florence, November the 30th, 1731. Phil Trans 1731;37:256.
13. Rosen de Rosenstein N: Traité des maladies des enfans (1st Swedish ed. 1764). Paris: Cavelier, 1778: p. 16.
14. Kant I: On education (1st ed. Köningsberg 1803). Boston, MA: Heath, 1900: p. 38–9.
15. Königreich Preußen: Allgemeines Landrecht für die Preussischen Staaten (1st ed. 1794). Berlin: Pauli, 1796: Vol. **4**, p. 1282.
16. Vallambert S: Cinq livres de la manière de nourrir et gouverner les enfants dès leur naissance. (Reprint Droz, Genève 2005). Poitiers: Manefz et Bouchetz, 1565: p. 141.
17. Janin J: Réflexions sur le triste sort des personnes, qui sous une apparence de mort, ont été enterrées vivantes. Paris: Didot Le Jeune, 1772: p. 62–6.
18. Templeman C: Two hundred and fifty-eight cases of suffocation of infants. Edinb Med J 1892;**38**:322–9.
19. Asch SW: Crib deaths. Their possible relation to postpartum depression and infanticide. Mt Sinai J Med 1968;**35**:214–20.
20. Fearn SW: Sudden and unexplained death of children. Lancet 1834;**23**:246.
21. Schallgruber J: Abhandlungen im Fache der Gerichtsarzneykunde. Grätz: Christoph Penz, 1823: p. 76, 91.
22. Kopp JH: Asthma thymicum. In: Denkwürdigkeiten in der ärztlichen Praxis. Frankfurt: Kettembeil, 1830: Vol. **1**, p. 1–46.
23. Friedleben A: Die Physiologie der Thymusdrüse in Gesundheit und Krankheit. Frankfurt: Rütten, 1858.
24. Virchow R: Die krankhaften Geschwülste. 30 Vorlesungen. Berlin: Hirschwald, 1864–1965: Vol. **2**, p. 613.
25. Grawitz P: Cases of sudden death in nursing infants. JAMA 1888;**11**:853–6.
26. Jacobi A: Contributions to the anatomy and pathology of the thymus gland. Trans Assoc Am Phys 1888;**3**:297.
27. Osler W: The principles and practice of medicine. New York: Appleton, 1892: p. 580.
28. Holt LE: The diseases of infancy and childhood. New York: Appleton, 1898: p. 43.
29. Paltauf A: Über die Beziehungen der Thymus zum plötzlichen Tod. 1. Teil. Wien Klin Wochenschr 1889;**2**:877–81.
30. Paltauf A: Über die Beziehungen der Thymus zum plötzlichen Tod. 2. Teil. Wien Klin Wochenschr 1890;**3**:172–5.
31. Friedlander A: Status lymphaticus and enlargement of the thymus; with report of a case successfully treated by the X-ray. Arch Pediatr 1907;**24**:490–501.
32. Clark DE: Association of irradiation with cancer of the thyroid in children and adolescents. JAMA 1955;**159**:1007–9.
33. Duffy BJ, Fitzgerald PJ: Thyroid cancer in childhood and adolescence. Cancer 1950;**3**:1018–32.
34. Winship T, Rosvoll RV: Childhood thyroid carcinoma. Cancer 1961;**14**:734–43.
35. Young M, Turnbull HM: An analysis of the data collected by the status lymphaticus investigation committee. J Pathol Bacteriol 1931;**34**:213–58.
36. Hippocrates: Airs, waters and places. Loeb Classical Library. London: Heinemann, 1957: Vol. **1**, p. 111.
37. Vesalius A: De humani corporis fabrica (1st ed. Basel 1543). Basel: Oporinus, 1555: p. 23.
38. Mercurio S: Kinder-Mutter oder Hebammen-Buch (1st Latin ed. Venice 1595). Wittenberg: Mevius, 1671: p. 293.
39. Eminent Physician: The nurse's guide. London: Brotherton and Gilliver, 1729: p. 46.
40. Ploss H: Das kleine Kind vom Tragbett bis zum ersten Schritt. Leipzig: Grieben, 1881: p. 12.
41. Hess AF: Nonrachitic soft chest and flat head. A new syndrome. Arch Pediatr Adolesc Med 1931;**41**:1309–16.

42. Greene D: Asymmetry of the head and face in infants and in children. Arch Pediatr Adolesc Med 1931;41:1317-26.
43. Illingworth RS: Three months' colic. Arch Dis Child 1954;29:165-74.
44. Erlacher P: Muss das Menschenkind auf dem Rücken liegen? Wien Klin Wochenschr 1959;71:937-8.
45. Keitel HG, Cohn R, Harnish D: Diaper rash, self-inflicted excoriations, and crying in full-term newborn infants kept in the prone or supine position. J Pediatr 1960;57:884-6.
46. Holt KS: Early motor development. Posturally induced variations. J Pediatr 1960;57:571-5.
47. Mau H: Säuglinge sollten in Bauchlage großgezogen werden. Münch Med Wochenschr 1969;111:471-6.
48. Gleiss J: Die Vor- und Nachteile der Bauchlage bei Neugeborenen und jungen Säuglingen. Dtsch Med Wschr 1969;94:2449-52.
49. Reisetbauer E, Czermak H: Die Körperlage des Säuglings. Pädiat Prax 1972;11:5-14.
50. Brackbill Y, Douthitt TC, West H: Psychophysiologic effects in the neonate of prone versus supine placement. J Pediatr 1973;82:82-4.
51. Hewitt VM: Effect of posture on the presence of fat in tracheal aspirate in neonates. Aust Pediatr J 1976;12:267-71.
52. Blumenthal I, Lealman GT: Effect of posture on gastro-oesophageal reflux in the newborn. Arch Dis Child 1982;57:555-6.
53. Palmén K: Prevention of congenital dislocation of the hip. Acta Orthop Scand Suppl 208 1984;55:1-65.
54. Editorial: Prone or supine? BMJ 1961;1:1304.
55. Gafafer WM: Time changes in the mortality from accidental mechanical suffocation among infants under 1 year old in different geographic regions of the United States, 1925-32. Public Health Rep 1936;51:1641-6.
56. Abramson H: Accidental mechanical suffocation in infants. J Pediatr 1944;25:404-13.
57. Davison WH: Accidental infant suffocation. BMJ 1945;251-2.
58. Carpenter RG, Shaddick CW: Role of infection, suffocation, and bottle-feeding in cot death. Br J Prev Soc Med 1965;19:1-7.
59. Beckwith JB: Discussion of terminology and definition of the sudden infant death syndrome. Seattle, WA: University of Washington Press, 1970: p. 14-22.
60. Krous HF, Beckwith JB, Byard RW, et al.: Sudden infant death syndrome and unclassified sudden infant deaths. Pediatrics 2004;114:234-8.
61. Beckwith JB: The sudden infant death syndrome. Curr Probl Pediatr 1973;3:3-36.
62. Bergman AB, Beckwith JB, Ray CG: The apnea monitor business. Pediatrics 1975;56:1-3.
63. Steinschneider A: Prolonged apnea and the sudden infant death syndrome. (Editor: Very important erratum: Pediatrics 1994, 944). Pediatrics 1972;50:646-54.
64. Bergman AB: Wrong turns in sudden infant death syndrome research. Pediatrics 1997;99:119-21.
65. Froggatt P: Epidemiological aspects of the Northern Ireland study. Seattle, WA: University of Washington Press, 1970: p. 32-43.
66. Beal S: Sleeping position and sudden infant death syndrome. Med J Aust 1988;149:562.
67. Engelberts AC, de Jonge GA: Choice of sleeping position for infants: possible association with cot death. Arch Dis Child 1990;65:462-7.
68. Mitchell EA: International trends in postneonatal mortality. Arch Dis Child 1990;65:607-9.
69. Fleming PJ, Gilbert R, Azaz Y, et al.: Interaction between bedding and sleeping position in the sudden infant death syndrome. BMJ 1990;301:85-9.
70. Blair PS, Sidebotham P, Berry PJ, et al.: Major epidemiological changes in sudden infant death syndrome. Lancet 2006;367:314-9.
71. Jorch G, Findeisen M, Brinkmann B, et al.: Bauchlage und Plötzlicher Säuglingstod. Dtsch Ärztebl 1991;88:A4266-72.
72. Wennergren G, Alm B, Öyen N, et al.: The decline in the incidence of SIDS in Scandinavia and its relation to risk-reducing campaigns. Acta Paediatr 1995;37:117-35.
73. AAP Task Force on Infant Positioning and SIDS: Positioning and SIDS. Pediatrics 1992;89:1120-6.
74. Chessare JB, Hunt CE, Bourguignon C: A community based survey of infant sleep position. Pediatric Research in Office Practices Network. Pediatrics 1995;96:893-6.
75. Hauck FR, Tanabe KO: International trends in sudden infant death syndrome: stabilization of rates requires further action. Pediatrics 2008;122:660-6.
76. AAP Task Force on Sudden Infant Death Syndrome: SIDS and other sleep-related infant deaths: updated 2016 recommendations for a safe infant sleeping environment. Pediatrics 2016;138:e20162938.
77. Mitchell EA: SIDS: past, present and future. Acta Paediatr 2009;98:1712-9.
78. Behm I, Kabir Z, Connolly GN, Alpert HR: Increasing prevalence of smoke-free homes and decreasing rates of sudden infant death syndrome in the United States. Tob Control 2012;21:6-11.
79. Harris W: A treatise of the acute diseases of infants (1st Latin ed. London 1689). Translated into English by: John Martyn. London: Astley, 1742: p. XVII.
80. Leem K: Beskrivelse over Finmarkens Lapper, deres Tungemaal, Levemaade og forrige Afgudsdyrkelse. Koebenhavn: Kongel Wäysenhuses Bogtrykkerie, 1767: p. 133.
81. Gilbert R.: The changing epidemiology of SIDS. Arch Dis Child 1994;70:445-9.

8.6 Theirs is the kingdom of heaven
Infant mortality statistics

Introduction

One in three newborns failed to survive up to their first birthday for thousands of years. Today, we find it difficult to understand how societies coped with such mortality levels, and how families could helplessly watch the loss of their offspring. Since 1850, a sharp and sustained decline in infant mortality caused a demographic revolution and the need for birth control. The history of infant mortality was described in Britain by Hugh Ashby in 1915 [1], in the US by Robert Woodbury in 1926 [2], and in several other countries by Henri Seibert in 1940 [3] and Alain Bideau in 1997 [4]. The present chapter aims to delineate the origins of birth registration and demography, and to show how the publication of mortality rates improved infants' fate and became the benchmark of a state's social well-being. It also seeks to shed light on some major causes of infant loss.

The chapter is restricted to infant mortality because this parameter has been consistently defined for 150 years. Where not indicated otherwise, data are reported as infant mortality rates (IMRs), defined as death before 1 year of age, per 1000 live births (‰). Neonatal and perinatal mortality have been omitted because stillbirth as well as the start and end of the perinatal period were poorly defined and many states did not follow the World Health Organization definitions.

Before birth registration: pioneers of statistics

Historic sources of infant mortality were methodically flawed which led to systematic undercounting. Parish records counted baptisms, not births. Bishop Basileus of Caesarea wrote in 370 C.E. [5]: 'Be inscribed in our book, that you may be transcribed to heaven's register.' Church records did not target historical demography, but rather religious discipline and civil control. In 1563, the Council of Trent regulated their contents [6]. Most statistics classified prematures as 'miscarriages', for which no registration was required. Infanticide was frequent, especially among unmarried mothers (see Chapters 8.2 and 8.3), and malformed infants [7]. Housefather-books were kept by privileged families only, and the meticulous reports of the foundling hospitals aimed to justify the costs of these charitable institutions [8–10]. Analysis of skeletons and teeth allows us to estimate infant mortality, but many infants were not buried in regular cemeteries (see Chapter 8.7). Regional migration from countryside to cities and international migration from poor to rich countries led to rural under- and urban over-registration: sometimes the number of buried infants exceeded the number of infants born. Altogether, at least every fourth deceased infant was not registered.

Infant mortality was bemoaned in Britain by Captain John Graunt in 1676 [11] and in Ireland by Surveyor General William Petty in 1683, possibly in mutual cooperation [12]. Graunt was not happy with the data quality: 'The weekly bills of mortality extant at the parish clerks begin the 29th of December 1603, being the first year of King James his reign, since when a weekly account has been kept there of burials and christenings ... In the matters of infants I would desire but to know clearly, what the searchers mean by infants, as whether children, that cannot speak, as the word infant seems to signify, or children under two or three years old; although I should not be satisfied, whether the infant died of wind, or of teeth [confused with scurvy], or of the convulsion, &c.' William Farr compiled abstracts for the General Register from 1837 for 40 years, describing increased mortality in infants born outside of marriage and in males as compared to females, and reported, among many other details, 'drainage of the refuse previously retained in the houses has been an advance on the previous state of things' [13].

In Prussia, Johann Peter Süßmilch, Berlin pastor, evaluated church records in 1741 [14]. In his 1400-page work he described many relationships in dozens of tables. Knowing that the church did not record all deliveries, he related infant deaths to all deaths, finding a first-year liveborn death incidence of 243‰ in 1746. Süßmilch constructed lifetables for Augsburg from 1501, Breslau from 1556, Rome from 1601, and for many other regions, with first-year mortality higher in the cities than on the countryside, and little change between 1540 and 1740.

Population-based statistics were kept in Sweden since 1749. Frederic Berg, chair of paediatrics at the Karolinska Institute, became director of the central bureau of statistics in 1853 [15]: 'I ought to abandon the pursuit of a profession in which I had been so bitterly disappointed.' Belgian astronomer Adolphe Quetelet compared lifetables in 1864 and found 'considerable differences' in infant mortality, highest in Bavaria and lowest in Sweden, with England, Belgium, France, and the Netherlands in between [16].

PART 8 Early death

Luigi Bodio directed the Italian Royal Statistical Office from 1872, and made it a European reference centre. 'Bodio's tables' are the basis of Table 8.6.1 and Fig. 8.6.1 [17]. In the US, infant mortality was poorly documented: in 1900, the Census Bureau only includes ten states; coverage remained incomplete until 1933, when Texas joined the 'registration states'.

Table 8.6.1 Infant mortality rates per 1000 liveborn infants, both sexes, trend in 50-year steps during the last 150 years

Country/state	1860	1908	1960	2010
Europe				
Austria	258	204	38	4
Belgium	174	147	31	4
Bulgaria		170	45	11
Denmark	138	123	22	4
Finland	(172)	(128)	21	2
France	166	(132)	27	3
Germany			East 39 West 34	3
Prussia	218	173		
Württemberg	324	184		
Bavaria	316	217		
Baden	272	168		
Saxonia	276	201		
Thuringia	221			
Greece	(138)		40	3
Hungary	(212)	199	48	5
Iceland	(240)	(106)	13	2
Ireland	99	97	29	3
Italy	214	153	44	3
Netherlands	(182)	125	17	4
Norway	107	76	18	3
Poland			57	5
Portugal	(150)		78	3
Romania	(250)		76	11
Russia (West)	265	260	35	9
Slavonia/Serbia	247	s.u.	87	
Spain	(193)	173	44	4
Sweden	137	85	17	2
Switzerland	198	108	21	4
Turkey				12
UK				5
Scotland	125	121	26	
England & Wales	153	120	22	
Yugoslavia/Serbia		s.o.	87	
Africa				
Algeria			118	31
DR Congo			144	112
Egypt			121	19
Libya				13

Table 8.6.1 Continued

Country/state	1860	1908	1960	2010
Morocco			(149)	30
South Africa				41
Tunisia			109	14
Americas				
Argentina			59	12
Brazil				17
Canada			27	5
Chile			128	8
Cuba				5
Mexico			75	14
United States			26	7
Uruguay			49	9
Venezuela			45	16
Asia and Australia				
Australia	(135)	(126)	20	4
China			31	16
India		(246)	146	48
Iraq			39	31
Israel			31	4
Japan	(236)	(162)	31	2
New Zealand	(95)	(75)	23	5
Philippines			73	23
Singapore			35	2
Vietnam			36	19

1860, Bodio, reflecting the pre-statistics situation [17]; 1910, data from Falkenberg [45], situation before World War I, sewage and clean water generally available; 1960, United Nations data, neonatology becoming a specialty [46]; 2010, World Health Organization, data at the end of the 'heroic' years of neonatology [47]. Data in brackets: Phelps 1908 [48] or Bideau 1997 [4].

Definitions and international comparison

Although the death of infants has attracted scientists since antiquity, governments became interested during the 18th century, their motive being a population census for tax purposes, military recruitment, school organization, and food supply. William Buchan, former physician at the Foundling Hospital in Ackworth, wrote in 1769 [18]: 'The annual registers of the dead shew, that at least one half of the children born in Great Britain die under twelve years of age. This may appear a natural evil; but whoever accurately examines the matter, will find that it is an evil of our own making.'

Population-based civil registration of births and deaths was introduced in the middle of the 19th century, enabling international comparison (Fig. 8.6.1): The current definition of IMR was used as early as 1741 [14] but was not commonly accepted until 1880 [19]. The oldest data were limited to geographical areas such as Geneva, Bologna, Paris, and London [4]. International comparison of IMRs became possible after World War II when the World Health Organization defined livebirth (any sign of life), preterm (<37 weeks), and low birthweight (<2500 g) [20]. East European countries

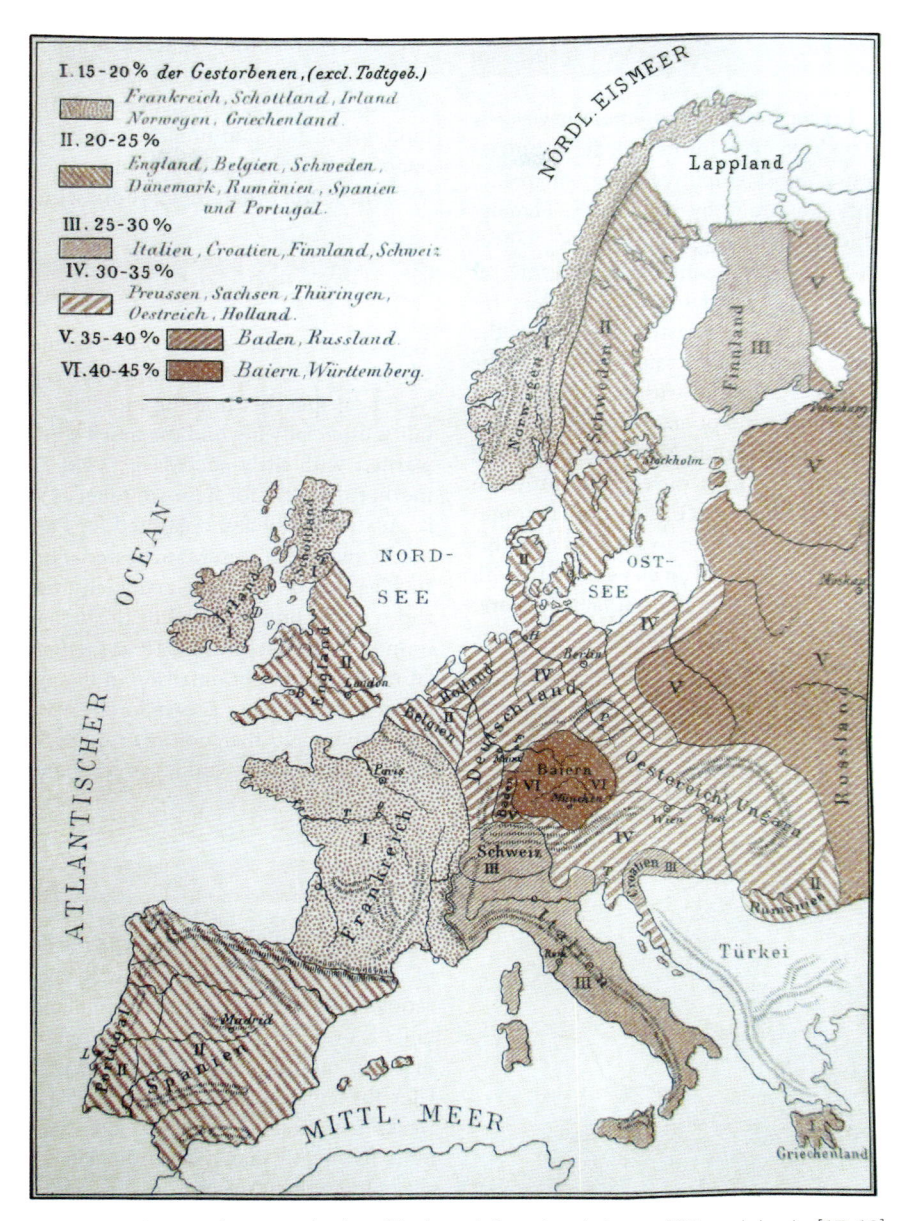

Fig. 8.6.1 Bodio's map of Europe 1878 showing first-year deaths of liveborn infants in relation to 100 total deaths [17, 19].

doctored their results with their definitions of live birth. In the Soviet Union, survival for an entire week was required for live birth before 28 weeks, or birthweight below 1000g, and the World Health Organization definitions were adopted as late as 2010 [21]. In East Germany, two signs of life (heartbeat and respiration) were required to register a liveborn infant [22]. Neonatal and perinatal mortality rates reflected the impact of fetal death and prematurity, but were plagued by underreporting and ambiguous definitions: when the State of Georgia linked infant birth and death certificates, it became evident that 21‰ of neonatal deaths in 1974–1977 had not been reported, mainly in rural areas, unmarried mothers, and African American infants [23]. Many states continued to apply highly different definitions of fetal death and stillbirth [24]. After an analysis in the Netherlands and Belgium, Marc Keirse complained in 1984 [25]: 'It is in the comparison between countries that the use and interpretation of crude perinatal mortality data reach summits of simplicity … a high percentage of obstetricians did not comply with their own country's regulations for registration of birth and perinatal death … systematic underreporting of very immature infants … Perinatal mortality rates do not contain what they purport to contain.'

Table 8.6.1 shows that the IMR fell dramatically everywhere, and even in the least developed populations, today's infant and child mortality is low by historical standards. Ranking lists revealed that the states' efforts to reduce IMR had varying success: the Nordic states were always ahead with the lowest IMRs. During the first half of the 20th century, Japan, Australia, and Russia significantly improved their ranking, as did Portugal and Singapore during the second, whereas the US fell from 6th to 27th place in international IMR ranking [26, 27].

Social class and marital status

Social inequality was best studied in countries where it was the lowest. It played an important role even in the Nordic countries [28]. In the mid-19th century, most employees worked in factories, and most of the work was done by machinery. Females took part in industrial production, reducing their infants' chances to survive. For the years 1817 to 1824, Louis-René Villermé reported that within the city of Paris, mortality under 1 year (as part of total mortality) depended on the quarter: whereas in the well-to-do 1st arrondissement the mortality rate was 168‰, the poor 12th arrondissement's was 252‰, and within the latter, the Rue Mouffetard 'one of those where the poorest live' even had a rate of 326‰ [29]. A century later, Arthur Newsholme showed that within the city of Manchester the IMR varied from 110‰ in Rusholme to 242‰ in Crumpsall (Fig. 8.6.2) [1]: 'There is something wrong in these places, and we must set to work to find this out and correct it.' In 1922, Ashby associated an elevated IMR with poverty, alcoholism, crowded conditions, maternal factory work, and illiteracy: 'In those counties [of England and Wales] where the marriage document is signed with a X, instead of a signature, there is the highest infant mortality.'

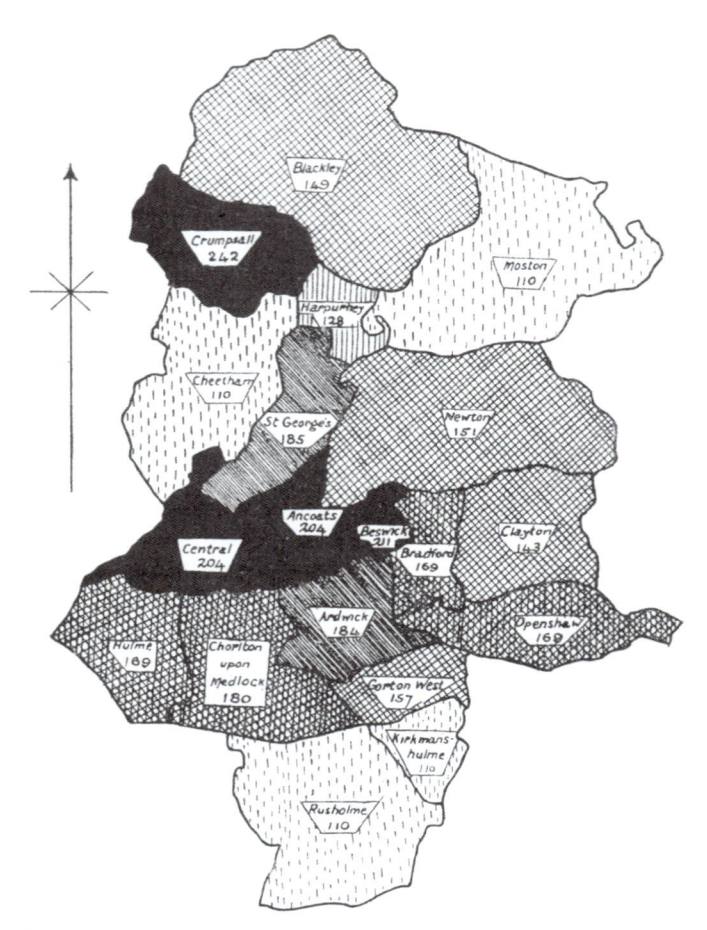

Fig. 8.6.2 Infant mortality rates in 1911 in different areas of Manchester. Data from Newsholme [42], depicted by Ashby in 1915 [1]. The darker the shading, the higher the mortality.

Unmarried mothers suffered a higher infant mortality than married women. In line with medieval church penalty, 'illegitimacy' was stigmatized, and societies did little to alleviate the unmarried mother's social condition. In Sweden and Denmark, infants born out of wedlock had a 70–80% higher IMR during the second part of the 19th century than infants born within wedlock [30].

Season and nutrition

When breastfeeding went out of fashion in the 17th century (see Chapters 6.2 and 6.4), 'summer diarrhea' or 'cholera infantium' or 'watery gripes' became the most important cause of infant mortality, especially beyond the first 4 weeks of age. William Cadogan warned with little success in 1748 [31]: 'I would advise every mother that can, for her own sake, as well as her Child's, to suckle it.' As drastically demonstrated for Paris during 1899 (Fig. 8.6.3), Ashby reported from Manchester [1]: 'During a hot, dry summer such as that of 1911, the artificially-fed babies got epidemic diarrhoea by the hundreds, while the breast-fed ones remained almost immune.' The decline in IMR in England and Wales is shown in relation to changes in nutrition in Fig. 6.8.2 in Chapter 6.8. Crucial improvements were access to clean water, separate sewage, pasteurization, and the cooling of milk. Street railways and automobiles reduced horse traffic, street manure, and thus the urban fly population.

The weaker sex

In 1752–1755, Süßmilch recorded a male-to-female ratio at birth of 105:100 and male mortality exceeding the female by 20%. These ratios were the same in 1915 in England [1]: 'The male infant mortality is over 20% greater than the female: it is, however, during the first two months of life that the males die so often.' One century later, the female advantage remained visible in infants born at 22–25 weeks' gestation who received intensive care [32]: females survived more frequently than males, equivalent to a difference in gestational age of more than 1 week.

Birth rate and prematurity

In 1893, Philip Biedert described 'a certain parallel between the infant mortality rate and birth rate' [33] depicted for some European states in Fig. 8.6.4. Ashby confirmed in 1915 [1]: 'The fact came to light from vital statistics in Ireland and in the different counties of England, that a high birth rate is generally associated with a high rate of infant mortality. This, however, is not improbably due to the fact that large families are most common among the very poor.' Considered stillborns or abortuses, preterm infants were rarely mentioned in early statistics. Moreover, prematurity, weakness, and birth asphyxia were barely distinguished. In 1902, Ballantyne stated [34]: 'The weight of the premature infant varies from 3 to 4 1/2 lb [1380–2419 g], and their length is about 16 in [41 cm].' The 2500 g cut-off was used by Miller in 1886 [35], Hahn in 1901 [36], and Ylppö in 1919 [37]. Once the IMR fell below 50‰ after World War II, preterm infants became the key factor in child loss.

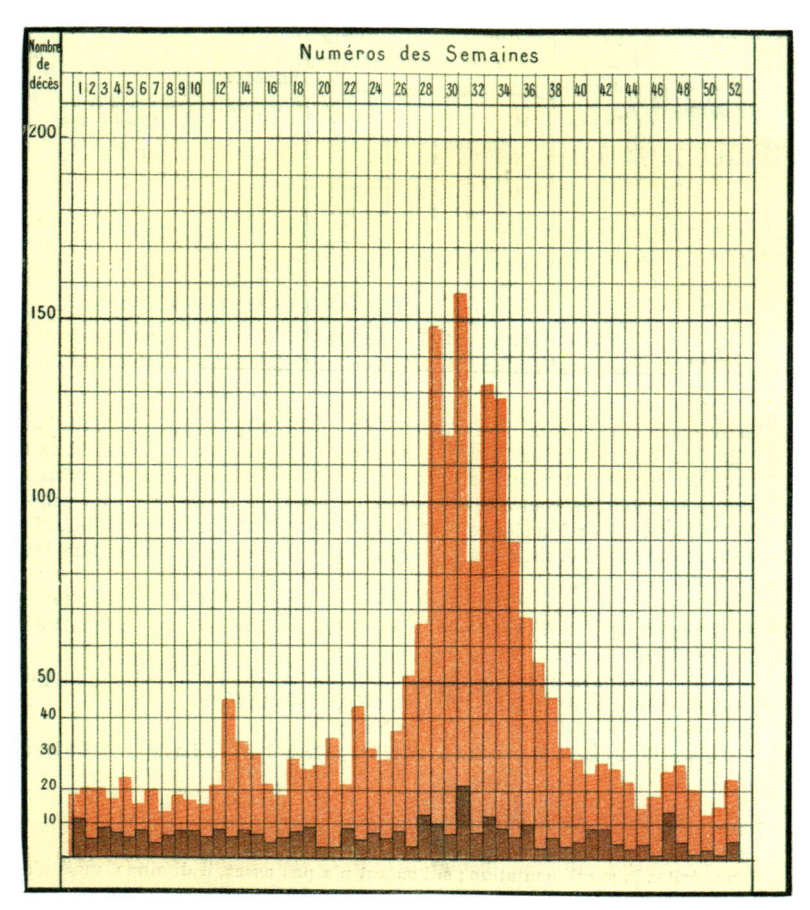

CHAPTER 8.6 Theirs is the kingdom of heaven: infant mortality statistics 387

Fig. 8.6.3 First-year deaths due to gastroenteritis by week during 1899 in the city of Paris (absolute numbers), published by Planchon in 1900 [43] and depicted by Budin in 1900 [44]. Of 2840 infants who died during the first year of life, the cause of death was gastroenteritis in 1470. Red columns, bottlefed infants (n = 1331); brown columns, breastfed infants (n = 139).

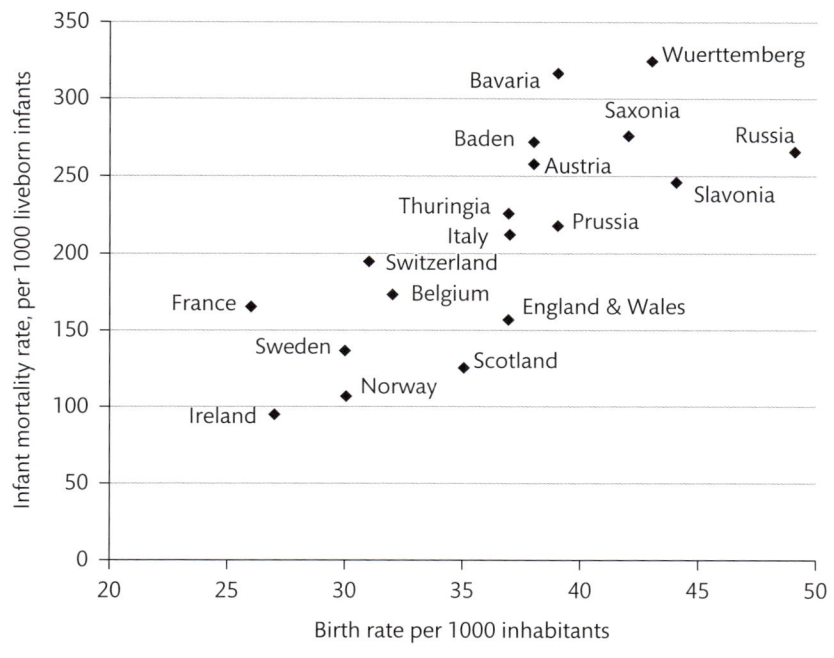

Fig. 8.6.4 Correlation of infant mortality rate (per 1000 live births) and birth rate (per 1000 inhabitants) in some European states from 1866 to 1878, published by Biedert in 1893 [33].

By 1941, 50% or more of first-year mortality was directly attributable to prematurity.

Ethnic group and racism

Attitudes towards race and ethnicity played a complex role in the history of US infant mortality [2]. Only the state of Massachusetts had reliable vital registration before 1890. In Boston, 1909 infant mortality was analysed 'by race', not yet by skin colour, but based on the parents' family name [38]: they reported an IMR of 263‰ for the Jewish, 240‰ Italian, 175‰ Irish, and 162‰ for the American 'race.' The IMR was 101‰ from 1915 to 1918, and Raymond Pearl found 'the mean rates of infant mortality are something like twice as high for the colored population than for the white population' [39]. This gap remained unchanged for 100 years. After a history of slavery, black skin was a proxy of poverty. Infants of African-born American black women had birthweights closer to infants born to white women than to infants born to US-born black women [40]. Instead of hunting the preterm birth gene, research should clarify whether the living conditions of African American women adversely affect pregnancy [27], or whether latent racism discourages them from obtaining prenatal care [41].

Legislation for child protection

After a series of 'baby-farming' scandals and an initiative of Lord Shaftsbury, the British parliament passed the Registration Bill in 1871, which however did not require the registration of stillbirths. In France, the Loi Roussel in 1874 regulated care by wet nurses, established infant counselling services, and provided clean milk (*gouttes de lait* movement). Bodio's Istituto Centrale di Statistica strongly promoted the lowering of infant mortality in Italy. In Germany, the maternity protection law of 1878 granted mandatory time off for 3 weeks after childbirth, later supplemented with dismissal protection before and breastfeeding breaks after birth. In an atmosphere of rising nationalism in Europe, efforts to reduce infant mortality were fuelled by widespread fear of 'depopulation', especially within the competition between Germany and France. The International Congresses for the Study and Prevention of Infant Mortality took place in Paris in 1905, Brussels in 1907, and Berlin in 1911, the latter already a political event in the pre-war atmosphere of ambivalence and distrust. In the US, private philanthropy, especially Nathan Straus' depots of pasteurized milk, reduced the threat of summer diarrhoea. In 1912, a federal law established the US Children's Bureau, which developed guidelines for the care of preterm infants and training programmes for midwives. In 1921, the Sheppard Towner Act established child and maternal health care services, but was soon vilified as a 'socialist threat' and repealed in 1929.

Conclusion

Despite methodical flaws, publishing national and regional vital statistics accelerated the change in infant death from a universal to an exceptional event. Mortality decreased dramatically in the late 19th century due to improved hygienic conditions, sewage removal, refrigeration, and pasteurization. In the early 20th century, mother–infant clinics, health visitors, the supply of clean milk, and public health measures contributed to the decline in infant mortality. It was not until after World War II that prematurity became the main cause of infant mortality, and that medicine could claim the lion's share for lowering the IMR. In the US, where most of the scientific progress in neonatology has been achieved, infant mortality remained relatively high, mainly among African Americans. In this regard, 'race' is a social construct rather than a biological fact. Infant mortality is a social system disease and health systems must adapt to the needs of the very population they serve.

REFERENCES

1. Ashby HT: Infant mortality. Cambridge: Cambridge University Press, 1915: p. 18–26, 44, 184, 217.
2. Woodbury RM: Infant mortality and its causes. Baltimore, MD: Williams & Wilkins, 1926.
3. Seibert H: The progress of ideas regarding the causation and control of infant mortality. Bull Hist Med 1940;**8**:546–98.
4. Bideau A, Desjardins B, Brignoli HP: Infant and child mortality in the past. Oxford: Clarendon, 1997.
5. Basilius: Des heiligen Kirchenlehrers Basilius des Großen ausgewählte Schriften. München: Kösel & Pustet, 1925: Vol. **2**, p. 313.
6. Börsting H: Geschichte der Matrikeln von der Frühkirche bis zur Gegenwart. Freiburg: Herder, 1959.
7. Rose L: Massacre of the innocents: infanticide in Great Britain, 1800–1939. London: Routledge and Kegan Paul, 1986.
8. Gaillard AH: Recherches administratives, statistiques et morales sur les enfants trouvés. Paris: Leclerc, 1837.
9. Hügel FS: Die Findelhäuser und das Findelwesen Europas. Wien: Sommer, Leopold, 1863.
10. Dupoux A: Sur les pas de monsieur Vincent. Paris: Revue de l'Assistance Publique, 1958.
11. Graunt J: Natural and political observations on the bills of mortality (Reprinted ed. 1662). In: A collection of the yearly bills of mortality, from 1657 to 1785 inclusive. London: Millar, 1759: p. 9–16.
12. Petty W: Another essay in political arithmetic concerning the growth of the city of London (Reprinted ed. 1683). In: A collection of the yearly bills of mortality from 1657 to 1758 inclusive. London: Millar, 1759: p. 63–76.
13. Susser M, Adelstein A: An introduction to the work of William Farr. Am J Epidemiol 1975;**101**:469–76.
14. Süssmilch JP: Die göttliche Ordnung in den Veränderungen des menschlichen Geschlechts (1st ed. 1741). 2. ed. Berlin: Buchladen der Realschule, 1762: Vol. **2**, p. 315–23, App. p. 35–51.
15. Berg F: Some extracts from Fredrik Theodor Berg's autobiographical memoranda. Acta Paediatr 1945;**32**:218–31.
16. Quetelet A: Sur la mortalité pendant la première enfance. Bull Acad R Belg 1864;**17**:9–16.
17. Bodio L: Il movimento della populazione in Italia e in altri Stati d'Europa. Archivio di Statistica, 1876: Vol. **1**, p. 119–205.
18. Buchan W: Domestic Medicine. Edinburgh: Balfour, 1769: p. 2.
19. Pfeiffer L: Die Kindersterblichkeit. In: Gerhard C: Handbuch der Kinderkrankheiten. 2. ed. Tübingen: Laupp, 1882: Vol. **1**, part 2, p. 206–70.

20. World Health Organization: Expert committee on health statistics, report of the second session. Expert group on prematurity. WHO Tech Rep Ser 1950;27:1–11.
21. Masuy-Stroobant G, Gourbin C: Infant health and mortality indicators. Their accuracy for monitoring the socio-economic development in the Europe of 1994. Eur J Popul 1995;11:63–84.
22. Mallik S: Lebendgeburt und Totgeburt in der DDR. Motive und Konsequenzen der Neudefinition von 1961. Der Gynäkologe 2013;46:858–64.
23. McCarthy BJ, Terry J, Rochat RW, et al. The underregistration of neonatal deaths: Georgia 1974–77. Am J Public Health 1980;70:977–82.
24. Joseph KS, Kinniburgh B, Hutcheon JA, et al.: Rationalizing definitions and procedures for optimizing clinical care and public health in fetal death and stillbirth. Obstet Gynecol 2015;125:784–8.
25. Keirse MJNC: Perinatal mortality rates do not contain what they purport to contain. Lancet 1984;323:1166–9.
26. David R, Collins J: Disparities in infant mortality: what's genetics got to do with it? Am J Public Health 2007;97:1191–7.
27. Matoba N, Collins J: Racial disparity in infant mortality. Semin Perinatol 2017;41:354–9.
28. Arntzen A, Andersen AMN: Social determinants for infant mortality in the Nordic countries, 1980–2001. Scand J Public Health 2004;32:381–9.
29. Villermé L-R: De la mortalité dans les divers quartiers de la ville de Paris. Annales d'Hygiène Publique et de Medicine Légale 1830;3:294–341.
30. Edvinsson S, Gardarsdottir O, Thorvaldsen G: Infant mortality in the Nordic countries, 1780–1930. Contin Chang 2008;23:457–85.
31. Cadogan W: An essay upon nursing and the management of children. London: Roberts, 1750.
32. Tyson JE, Parikh NA, Langer J, et al.: Intensive care for extreme prematurity-moving beyond gestational age. N Engl J Med 2008;358:1672–81.
33. Biedert Ph: Die Kinderernährung im Säuglingsalter und die Pflege von Mutter und Kind. 2. ed. Stuttgart: Enke, 1893: p. 16.
34. Ballantyne JW: The problem of the premature infant. Br Med J 1902;1:1196–200.
35. Miller NT: Die Frühgebornen und die Eigenthümlichkeiten ihrer Krankheiten. Jahrb Kinderheilk 1886;25:179–94.
36. Hahn C: Des prematurés: caractères, prognostic, traitement. Paris: Steinheil, 1901: p. 173.
37. Ylppö A: Über die Mortalität und Pathologie der Frühgeburten und Neugeborenen. Monatsschr Kinderheilk 1937; Bd. 69, Heft 5,6:407–15.
38. Cabot RC, Richie EK: The influence of race on the infant mortality of Boston in 1909. Boston Med Surg J 1910;162:199–202.
39. Pearl R: Biometric data on infant mortality in the United States birth registration area, 1915–1918. Am J Hyg 1921;1:419–39.
40. David RJ, Collins JW: Differing birth weight among infants of U.S.-born blacks, African-born blacks, and U.S.-born whites. N Engl J Med 1997;337:1209–14.
41. Salm Ward TC, Mazul M, Ngui EM, Bridgewater FD, Harley AE: 'You learn to go last': perceptions of prenatal care experiences among African-American women with limited incomes. Matern Child Health J 2013;17:1753–9.
42. Newsholme A: Second report on infant and child mortality. London: Parliamentary papers. 42th report of Local Government Board, 1912.
43. Planchon P: Resultats obtenus a la consultation des nourrissons de la Clinique Tarnier, pendant les mois de Juin, Juillet, Aout et Septembre 1899. L'Obstetrique 1900;5:35–50.
44. Budin P: Le Nourrisson. Paris: Octave Doin, 1900.
45. Falkenburg PH: Morbidität, Mortalität und Geburtenziffer in den verschiedenen Ländern. In: Keller A: Bericht über den III. Internationalen Kongress für Säuglingsschutz (Gouttes de lait). Berlin: Stilke, 1912: p. 1111–26.
46. United Nations: Demographic yearbook 1961. Special topic: mortality statistics. 13. ed. New York: United Nations, 1961: p. 222–35.
47. World Health Organization: World health statistics 2012. Life expectancy and mortality. Geneva: WHO Press, 2012: p. 51–60.
48. Phelps EB: A statistical study of infant mortality. Publ Am Stat Assoc 1908;83:233–72.

8.7

For whom no bell tolled
Infant burials

Introduction: disappeared and forgotten

Burial rites reveal great diversity across the world's societies. Two elements must be discerned: (1) interment, the corpse's disposal, either by cremation or burial, and (2) funeral, a rite of passage. Most families suffered the loss of one child or more before the 20th century, half of all pregnancies ended in perinatal death [1]. Theoretically, there should be many infant tombs: assuming a lifetime average of eight pregnancies per woman and an infant mortality rate of 50%, at least two-thirds of all gravesites should contain infants. However, this is not the case. Most archaeological studies mentioned no infant burials at all. Françoise Le Mort reported a Neolithic graveyard in Cyprus containing 45% newborns and infants [2]. Iowa anthropologist Kathryn Kamp realized that archaeology had grossly neglected infancy and asked [3]: 'Where have all the children gone?'

Early records of births and deaths must be read judiciously as the former were often limited to births among married couples and the latter to church records of baptized infants. Immature or malformed infants were often not baptized, not mentioned in records nor buried in sacred ground, and soon fell into oblivion. This absence of commemoration suggests an ambiguous perception of the newborn, similar to the unborn, stillborn, and preterm babies who had yet to be named, all of whom were attributed partial personhood prior to the life-granting, name-giving rite of passage (see Chapter 2.9). Considering mainly archaeological evidence, the present chapter examines infant burials and how they varied in different societies. It disregards the extensive literature on parental grief and seeks to explain how infant burials differed from those of older children or adults, and to understand why infant graves were either rare or remained ignored.

Archaeological evidence and prehistoric graves

To identify gestational age and to discern fetuses from liveborn infants, traditional archaeological tools are of limited value. Sparsely mineralized neonatal bones decay rapidly, and long bone size is a poor measurement for neonates: it enables us to determine gestational but not postnatal age, and therefore cannot distinguish fetal and postnatal death. As teeth develop within a fairly predictable timetable, archaeologists relied on dental enamel [4]. This requires looking for the tiny tooth buds by sieving, and permits us to date postmenstrual age at death. Microscopic analysis of deciduous teeth allows fetal death and demise in the postnatal period to be distinguished by identifying the neonatal line in sliced sections [5].

A well-preserved infant grave in Dederiyeh, Syria, revealed that late Neanderthals (100,000–50,000 before present) disposed of the corpse in a cave [6]. A palaeolithic grave of twin newborns, covered with a mammoth scapula, was dated to 26,580 before present by Einwögerer [7] (**Fig. 8.7.1**).

In the pre-pottery Neolithic cemetery of Khirokita, Cyprus (7th millennium B.C.E.), where one of the largest series of infant burials has been unearthed, infants were buried in the same way as adults: no gravesite area was reserved for neonates [2]. However, when cities originated in Mesopotamia in the fifth millennium B.C.E., funeral rites and burial places evolved differently for infants and older children or adults [8]. When pottery developed, jar burials became the prevailing mortuary practice. Containers for the corpse concealed the decay process, kept the deceased from being eaten by scavengers, prevented the soul's restless transmigration, and provided a place for commemoration. The practice of interring infants in ceramic pots within the settlement, whereas adults were placed in formal cemeteries outside the habitation area, began during the Mesolithic (8500–6500 B.C.E.) and spread from Mesopotamia to Greece and further west during the Neolithic period [9]. Georgiadis [10] suggested that the infant was perceived as a 'protective spirit' important for the family's well-being [11]. Frank Hole found most Mesopotamian adults were interred in clearly defined cemeteries outside the residential areas and infants were relegated to sub-floor disposal in their natal homes [12]. He suggested this resulted from 'their transitory role and relative insignificance'. Neolithic graves sometimes contained artefacts; for babies these were beads, small ceramic vessels, or feeding jars [8], suggesting ritual burial.

In the settlements of Neolithic pottery users in the Danube Gorges (7500–5000 B.C.E.), many newborn and infant burial sites have been found located beneath red limestone house floors. They did not go *ad patres* but remained within the house, perhaps to strengthen social relations within the family. From the late Neolithic period (4400–2300 B.C.E.), grave goods (glass beads, obsidian pearls) were added, which were believed to secure the household's future wealth

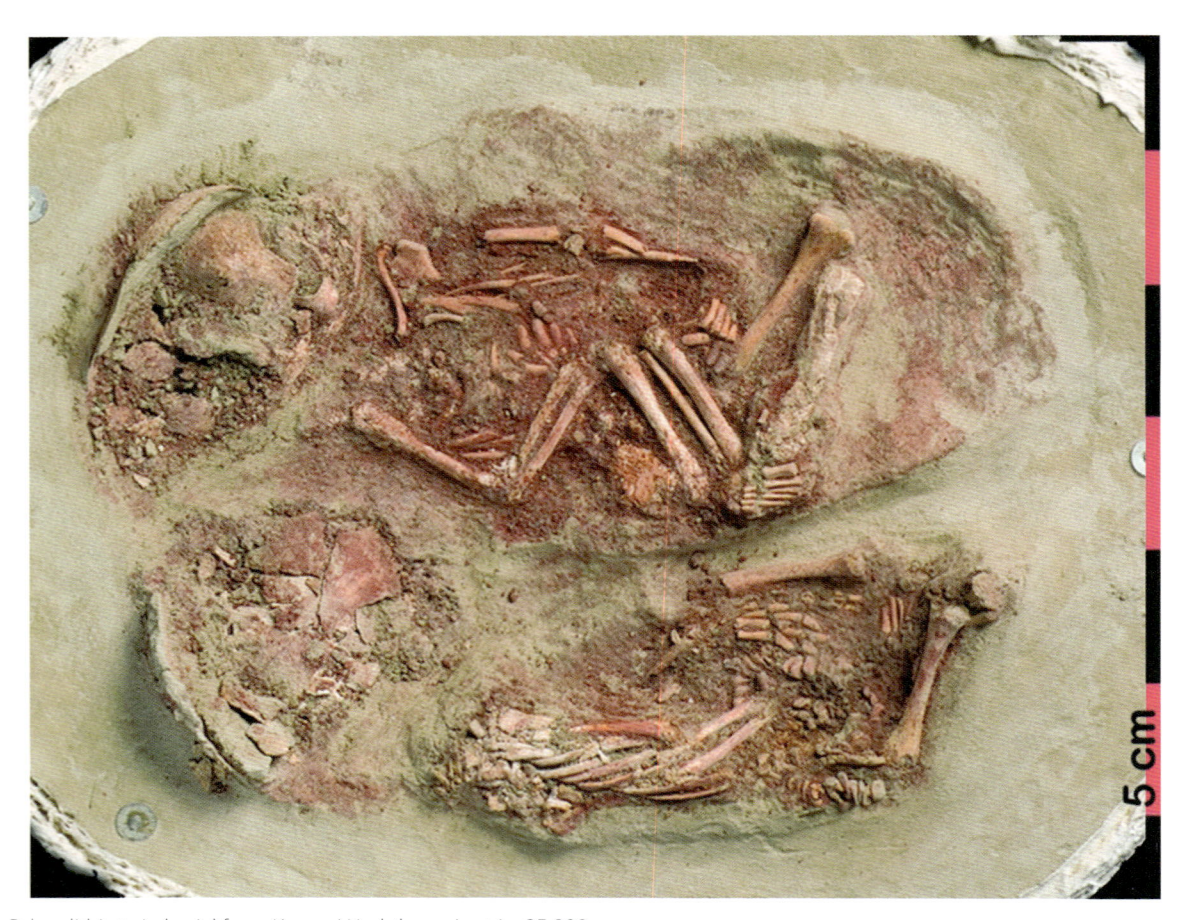

Fig. 8.7.1 Palaeolithic twin burial from Krems-Wachtberg, Austria, 25,000 B.C.E.
Reproduced with permission from Einwögerer, T., Friesinger H., Händel, M., et al. Upper Palaeolithic infant burials. *Nature*, 444:285. Copyright © 2006 Springer.

[13]. In central Thrace, Bulgaria, pot interment within the settlement persisted unchanged for millennia [14].

Various patterns of infant burial evolved in Asia. In the prehistoric gravesite of Khok Phanom Di, Thailand, 51 newborn skeletons from 4000–3500 B.C.E. have been examined: the infants were fullterm and buried not in jars, apart from the adults jars [15]. About 4000 years later in Kiangan, Northern Philippine Archipelago, children older than 2 years were buried outside the village, like the adults, whereas newborn infants were buried in jars or supine under house foundations [16].

Antique infant cemeteries

In Egypt, pot burials were introduced for infants from 3500 B.C.E. [17]. A switch from pot to coffin interment occurred 500 years later in the Naqada II culture [18]. Infanticide, common in ancient Greece, is not known to have been practised in dynastic Egypt, but infants and neonates were not deemed a social person deserving an adult-style burial [19]: 'Not yet complete, they were buried individually and provided with some basic grave goods, but no lasting monument. This level of provision was all that was practicable in view of the high infant mortality rate.' In Roman Egypt (100–450 C.E.), fetuses and newborns were wrapped in linen and buried among the adults, heads facing to the west [20]. Their gestational age distribution did not differ from the natural expected mortality distribution.

Inhumation was a Greek and Near East custom, whereas cremation was a Roman and Germanic custom. No infant graves have been found in Greece dating before 750 B.C.E. At that time, the societal role of the infant changed, and after 700 B.C.E., infants usually had their own cemetery. Athenians used a specific type of water-amphora (*lutrophoros*) for infant burial [21]. On the remote Dodecanese island of Astypalaia, Greece, two ancient graveyards were excavated, in use from 750 to 100 B.C.E. Clearly separated from the adjacent adult cemetery Katsalos, over 2700 infant graves have been identified in Kylindra, making it the largest ancient children's cemetery in the world [4]. The infants had been buried in large commercial pots or amphoras. Most of the infants ranged from 37 to 42 postfertilization weeks; indeed, many were preterm. Kylindra was reserved for newborns, and it is very unlikely that infant corpses were shipped there from other islands.

Throughout the Roman Empire, the Law of the Twelve Tables requiring burial or burning of dead persons outside of settlements [22] did not apply to infants: newborn burial sites have not yet been found in Roman Italy [1]. Mourning for deceased newborns was unusual, as Cicero related in 44 B.C.E. [23]: 'If a young child dies, the survivors ought to bear his loss with equanimity; that if an infant in the cradle dies, they ought not even to utter a complaint.' However, in the *Aeneid*, written ca. 25 B.C.E., Virgil bewailed the fate of those not ferried across the River Styx and condemned to a marginal existence [24]:

> 'Before the gates, the cries of babe's new born
> Whom fate had from their mothers torn
> Assault his ears: then those whom form of laws
> Condemn'd to die, when traitors judg'd their cause.'

Plinius described the Roman rite in 75 c.e. [25]: 'It is not the custom in any Country to burn in a Funeral Fire the dead Body of an Infant before the Teeth are come up.' Perceived as 'bad deaths', newborns were lumped together with persons who committed suicide, and those who died a violent death, such as soldiers killed in action: the Roman Empire expanded by warfare. In Roman France, an exceptional cluster of infant graves was found at Nuits St. Georges, Burgundy [1], containing 109 adult burials and 113 prematures or neonates, located near a sanctuary.

Mass graves and public pits

At the Athenian Agora, at least 449 fetal and neonatal skeletons were detected in a well in use from 165 to 150 b.c.e. [26]. From skeletal malformations and the presence of dog bones and household pottery, it has been suspected that the babies were victims of infanticide or sacrifice. But the rate of 15% preterms makes a natural cause of death more probable, a well being an easy cheap place for Athenian midwives to dispose of the bodies.

Romans had to buy the gravesites along the streets outside of the city and also in later times, *loculi* of the Christian catacombs were for the rich Romans. The poor left no memorial and were disposed of, together with dead animals, in public mass graves [27]. Over 10,000 epitaphs have survived in the western part of the Roman Empire: few of them commemorated children, and none newborn infants. Collective pits outside the city were called *puticuli* (putor = stench). Of many hundred *puticuli* in the Esquiline cemetery, Roman archaeologist Rodolfo Lanciani brought to light 75 in 1888 [28], each 12 feet square and 30 deep, containing the remnants of human corpses, animals, and household refuse. Between 130 and 300 c.e., the preference for inhumation migrated from Hellenistic to Roman areas [21], and with Christianization infants—when baptized—were also buried. From the number and size of the *loculi* (rectangular niches in the catacomb tuff stone), it has been calculated that 35% of Roman newborns died within their first year of life [29], but this number is underestimated: in addition to the *loculi*, they were often buried in groups in the larger family graves (*cubicula, arcosolia*).

In Roman Britain, graves of neonates were found from the 5th century c.e., obviously under the influence of Christianization [30]. Burial clubs arranged collective tombs (*columbaria, cubicula*) for those who wanted to escape the humiliation of a mass grave but who could not afford an individual gravesite. In Britain, the burial sites of 261 premature and term infants have been analysed from 71 settlements, usually located near hearths, doorways, and hypocausts [31]. Grave goods for babies consisted of a standard deposit of black mineral jewellery, a coin (for the ferryman), a small jet bear (for protection), and a pottery beaker (for nutrition) [32]. In Christianized Ireland, unbaptized infants were buried in *cillini*, separate grounds outside the church enclosure [33]. In Ashkelon, Israel, an infant cemetery from the 5th century c.e. holding over 100 newborns was detected, all less than a week old and possibly killed after birth [34].

Funeral customs for infants

Individual death threatens the continuity of human culture. As a protective strategy, ritual patterns emerged seeking to attest to the immortal soul of the deceased, and to facilitate its transition to the afterlife. These rites generally involved viewing of the deceased, prayer and religious service, procession to the gravesite, and burial. Additional features varied widely depending on the region, family wealth, and religion. This is not the place to describe cultural differences in funeral rites [11]. Suffice it to say that for deceased newborn infants, the adult rite was often applied in a shortened or simplified form. Roman customs included the funeral procession of the relatives, placing an image of the deceased in a wooden shrine at home, and the *lamento*, an open and dramatic expression of grief. Neither of these customs were practised for dead babies, 'they did not have a social personality which justified individual commemoration' [27]: Christians abandoned the death knell, restricted the procession to the inner family, and shortened the duration of wearing black (Fig. 8.7.2). Greek Orthodox Christians omitted the vigil and church service. The Muslim rite included washing, anointing and shrouding the corpse, and a prayer that asked the baby—believed to have died in a state of innocence—to intercede in heaven on their parents' behalf [35]. Hindu rites required washings, covering the corpse with a shroud, and extended purification, but deceased infants did not incapacitate their survivors to the same degree [36, 37]. Still, in the early 20th century in the Albanian mountains, children aged under 2 years were buried without any ceremony and without the usual weeping [38]: they were carried to the cemetery in their cradle, which was turned around and left on the grave for some days. Protecting the baby's corpse from animals was important in African societies: quite recently, the Samburu (Kenya) exposed dead adults and older children under a tree to scavengers, whereas infants were buried under the sleeping hides in the hut [39].

Insured to be buried

Well into the 19th century, many families lost one child a year and the mother's life was endangered with every further pregnancy. Besides causing emotional distress and being a social tragedy, a child's death was a financial catastrophe. The costs of funeral and mortuary rites were high, and greatly influenced by socioeconomic hierarchy [40, 41]. In 1843, the actual cost for a child's funeral varied from £1 (20 shillings) to 30 shillings in Britain, more than the average labourer's monthly income [42]. Modern economics did not shy away from exploiting infant and children's mortality. By setting off the costs of maintenance and future earnings in 1853, William Farr calculated a human infant to be worth £0.39, a 10-year-old £6.67, and a 20-year-old £14.10 [43]. 'Friendly' Societies were organized in the early 19th century [44] and 'burial clubs' provided funds for funeral expenses. However, a 'vicious perversion of their function developed' [45, 46]. To the Houses of Parliament, Edwin Chadwick

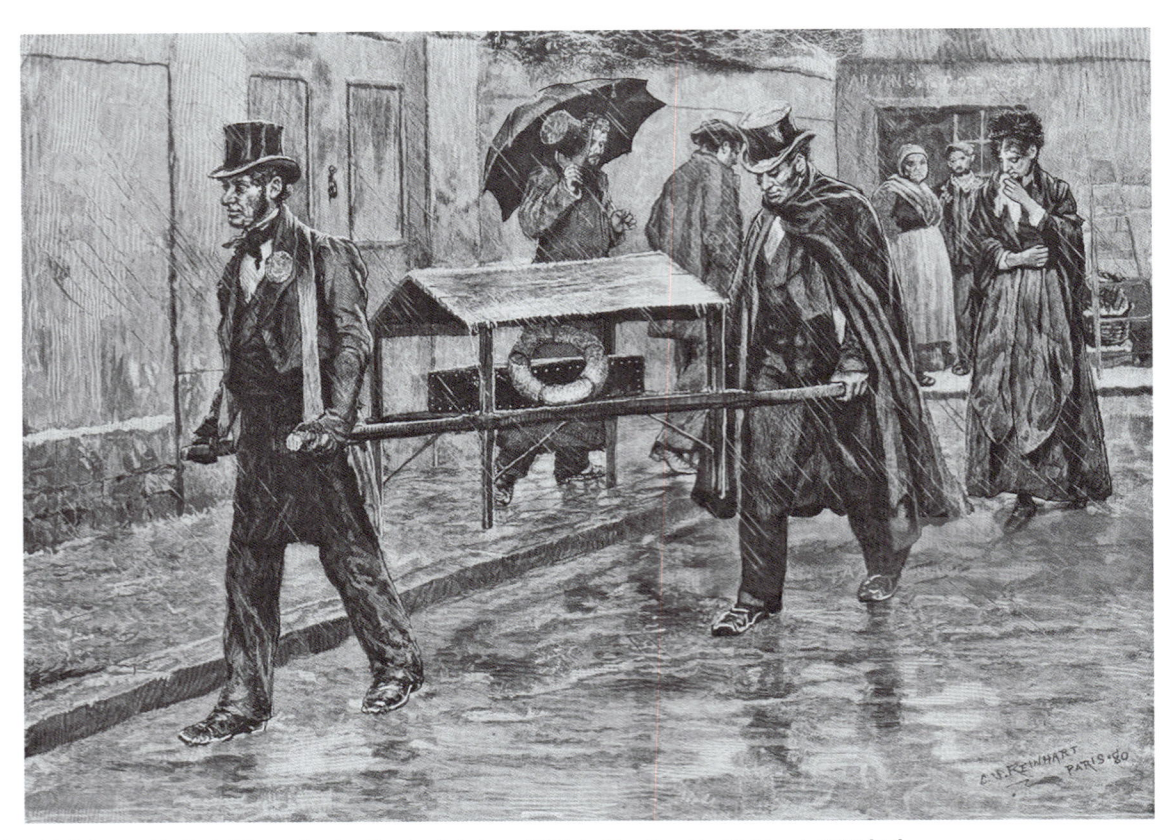

Fig. 8.7.2 'A Child's Funeral in Paris.' Engraving by Charles Reinhart, 1880, in *The Graphic*, 31 March 1883 [57].

reported a child from Manchester in 1843 [42]: 'Mr Gardiner, the clerk to the Manchester Union ... assigned the death to wilful starvation: ... The child had been entered in at least ten burial clubs; and its parents had six other children, who only lived from nine to eighteen months respectively. They had received 20£. from several burial clubs for one of these children ... post-mortem examination stated: Died through want of nourishment ... [Even though] the man enforced payments upon his insurances from ten burial clubs, and obtained a total sum of 34£. 3s. for the burial of this one child.'

Under the heading 'Premiums for Infanticide', a *Lancet* editorial on 28 September 1861 [47] reported that in the Preston district, 'while infants of labouring men outside the clubs die at a rate of 36% before reaching five years, children of the same age who are insured in the burial clubs die at the rate of 62 to 64% ... There is only one remedy for this large and perpetually active cause of infant mortality: it is the abolition of burial clubs'. In May 1866, the Harveyan Society formed a committee on infanticide, chaired by Tyler Smith, who in January 1876, among other suggestions, postulated 'that no infant or very young person be allowed to be entered as a member of burial clubs or to become the subjects of life assurance' [48]. Still in 1882–1891, 28% of 258 infants who died from 'overlaying' were insured [49]. The Children Act of 1908 finally ruled that 'no life insurance of any of these infants [nursed for rent] is allowed' [50].

In the US, infant life insurance remained common until today. Despite fervent debates since 1873 [51], 'we should shrink with horror from applying life insurance to infants, though the hopes that cluster around them may easily be conceived to have a money value', life insurance even was available in 1986 for infants with severe cardiovascular malformations [52]. The debate on children's life insurance reflects the transformation of the child from an object having pecuniary value to an individual with its own dignity, a process termed 'sacralization' by Zelizer [53].

From the Middle Ages until now there has been debate about whether stillborns or deceased preterm infants deserve the costs for funeral and gravesite. In 1527, German engraver Barthel Beham depicted 'The Miser and the Untimely Birth', a father who tries to keep his money [54] (Fig. 8.7.3). The toad sitting on his right shoulder was a popular medieval symbol representing gluttony and avarice [55]. The recent cost of infant death in the US exceeded $2000 for the funeral and $8000 for bereavement leave [56]. Economic arguments continue to play an important role in the debate on mortuary practices for stillborns, baby-fields, and commemoration sites for preterm infants.

Conclusion

Mortuary practices have been age dependent at all times. Prehistoric newborns were buried apart from adults, often within the house, and once they became available, in pots. Burying deceased newborns within the settlement was a worldwide and persistent phenomenon, preserved for six millennia. There are various reasons why infants were denied a normal burial: their death was frequent, gravesites were rare, and the funeral costs considerable. Newborns, especially when preterm or malformed, were regarded as unfinished,

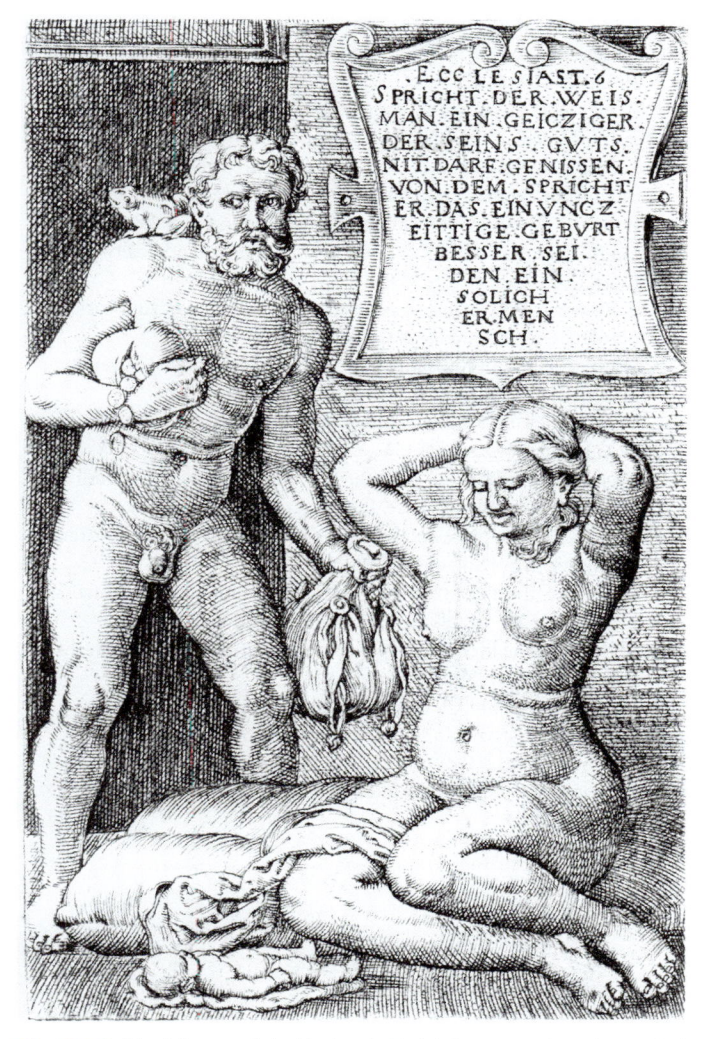

Fig. 8.7.3 'The Miser and the Untimely Birth.' Copper etching by Barthel Beham, 1527: the toad on the father's shoulder was a medieval symbol for avarice and demonic punishment [54].

endowed with partial or no personhood, and of limited societal importance. Dead infants were perceived as dangerous, as their soul may wander around and threaten other members of the community, or were considered protective for the family, and therefore kept close to the house.

REFERENCES

1. Carroll M: Infant death and burial in Roman Italy. J Roman Archaeol 2011;**24**:99–120.
2. Le Mort F: Infant burials in pre-pottery neolithic Cyprus: evidence from Khirokitia. In: Babies reborn. Infant/child burials in pre- and protohistory. Oxford: BAR Publishing, 2008: p. 23–32.
3. Kamp KA: Where have all the children gone? J Archaeol Method Theory 2001;**8**:1–34.
4. Hillson S: The world's largest infant cemetery and its potential for studying growth and development. Hesperia supplements. Princeton, NJ: American School of Classical Studies at Athens, 2009: Vol. **43**, p. 137–54.
5. Smith P, Avishai G: The use of dental criteria for estimating postnatal survival in skeletal remains of infants. J Archaeol Sci 2005;**32**:83–9.
6. Akazawa T, Muhesen S, Dodo Y, et al.: Neanderthal infant burial. Nature 1995;**377**:585–6.
7. Einwögerer T, Friesinger H, Händel M, et al.: Upper Palaeolithic infant burials. Nature 2006;**444**:285.
8. Brereton G: Cultures of infancy and capital accumulation in pre-urban Mesopotamia. World Archaeol 2013;**45**:232–51.
9. Bacvarov K: A long way to the west: earliest jar burials in southeast Europe and the Near East. Oxford: BAR Publishing, 2008: p. 61–70.
10. Georgiadis M: Child burials in Mesolithic and Neolithic Southern Greece. Child Past 2011;**4**:31–45.
11. Huntington R, Metcalf P: Celebrations of death: the anthropology of mortuary ritual. Cambridge: Cambridge University Press, 1979.
12. Hole F: Patterns of burial in the fifth millennium. In: Henrickson EF, Thuesen I: Upon this foundation. Copenhagen: Museum Tusculanum Press, 1989: p. 149–80.
13. Boric D, Stefanovic S: Birth and death: infant burials from Vlasac and Lepenski Vir. Antiquity 2004;**78**:526–46.
14. Mishina T: A social aspect of intramural infant burials' analysis. In: Babies reborn. Oxford: BAR Publishing, 2008: p. 137–46.
15. Halcrow SE, Tayles N, Livingstone V: Infant death in late prehistoric Southeast Asia. Asian Perspect 2008;**47**:371–404.
16. Lauer AJ, Acabado SB: Infant death and burial practices in late prehistoric Kiyyangan village. National Museum Journal of Cultural Heritage 2015;**1**:31–7.
17. Power RK, Tristant Y: From refuse to rebirth: repositioning the pot burial in the Egyptian archaeological record. Antiquity 2016;**90**:1474–88.
18. Midant-Reynes B: The prehistory of Egypt. Malden, MA: Blackwell, 2000.
19. Harrington N: Children and the dead in New Kingdom Egypt. In: Mairs R, Stevenson A: Current research in Egyptology. Oxford: Oxbow Books, 2005: p. 52–65.
20. Tocheri MW, Dupras TL, Sheldrick P, Molto JE: Roman period fetal skeletons from the east cemetery of Kellis, Egypt. Int J Osteoarchaeol 2005;**15**:326–41.
21. Morris I: Death-ritual and social structure in Classical Antiquity. Cambridge: Cambridge University Press, 1992: p. 27, 52, 89.
22. Scott SP: The civil law. Cincinnati, OH: Central Trust, 1932: Vol. **1**, Art. 1.
23. Cicero MT: Tusculan disputations. New York: Harper, 1877: Vol. Book 1, chapter 39, p. 50–1.
24. Publius Vergilius Maro: The aeneid. London: Whittingham, 1810: Vol. **6**, lines 426–9.
25. Plinius the Elder: Natural history. London: Wernerian Club, 1847: Vol. **2**, p. 192–9.
26. Liston MA, Rotroff SI: Babies in the well. In: Parkin T, Evans-Grubbe J: Oxford handbook of childhood and education in the classical world. Oxford: Oxford University Press, 2013: p. 62–81.
27. Letts M: Death in Rome. In: Hopkins K: Death and renewal. Cambridge: Cambridge University Press, 1983: p. 201–28.
28. Lanciani R: Ancient Rome in the light of recent discoveries. London: Macmillan, 1888: p. 65.
29. Timmermans M: Roma subterranea. The catacombs of late antique Rome. Inaug. Diss. Leiden: Faculty of Archaeology, 2012.
30. Watts D: Infant burials and Romano-British Christianity. Archaeol J 1989;**146**:372–83.

31. Wang H, Liddell CA, Coates MM, et al.: Global, regional, and national levels of neonatal, infant, and under-5 mortality during 1990–2013. Lancet 2014;**384**:957–79.
32. Crummy N: Bears and coins: the iconography of protection in Late Roman infant burials. Britannia 2010;**41**:37–93.
33. Finlay N: Outside of life: traditions of infant burial in Ireland from cillin to cist. World Archaeol 2000;**31**:407–22.
34. Smith P, Kahila G: Identification of infanticide in archaeological sites. J Archaeol Sci 1992;**19**:667–75.
35. Hedayat K: When the spirit leaves: childhood death, grieving, and bereavement in Islam. J Palliat Med 2006;**9**:1282–91.
36. Orenstein H: Death and kinship in Hinduism. Am Anthropol 1970;**72**:1357–77.
37. Mines DP: Hindu periods of death 'impurity'. Contrib Indian Sociol 1989;**23**:103–30.
38. Cozzi E: Malattie, morte, funerali nelle montagne d'Albania. Anthropos 1909;**4**:903–18.
39. Spencer P: Nomads in alliance. London: Oxford University Press, 1973: p. 107–8.
40. Ariès P: Geschichte der Kindheit. 6. ed. München: Deutscher Taschenbuch Verlag, 1984: p. 92–111.
41. Kamp KA: Social hierarchy and burial treatment. Cross Cult Res 1998;**32**:79–115.
42. Chadwick E: A supplementary report on the results of a special inquiry into the practice of interment in towns. London: Clowes, 1843: p. 64–5.
43. Farr W: On the equitable taxation of property. Quarterly Journal of the Statistical Society 1853;**XVI**:1–44.
44. Gorsky M: The growth and distribution of English friendly societies in the early nineteenth century. Econ Hist Rev 1998;**51**: 489–511.
45. Baines MA: Infant alimentation; or artificial feeding, considered in its physical and social aspects. Lancet 1869;**1**:33–4.
46. Forbes TR: Deadly parents: child homicide in eighteenth- and nineteenth-century England. J Hist Med Allied Sci 1986;**41**:175–99.
47. Editorial: Premiums for infanticide. Lancet 1861;**78**:299.
48. Smith T: Report of the Committee of the Harveian Society on infanticide. Lancet 1867;**89**:61–3.
49. Templeman C: Two hundred and fifty-eight cases of suffocation of infants. Edinb Med J 1892;**38**:322–9.
50. Ashby HT: Infant mortality. Cambridge: Cambridge University Press, 1915: p. 18–26, 44, 184, 217.
51. Wright E: Politics and mysteries of life insurance. Boston, MA: Lee and Shepard, 1873.
52. Truesdell SC, Skorton DJ, Lauer RM: Life insurance for children with cardiovascular disease. Pediatrics 1986;**77**:687–91.
53. Zelizer VA: The price and value of children: the case of children's insurance. Am J Sociol 1981;**86**:1036–56.
54. Pauli G: Barthel Beham: ein kritisches Verzeichnis seiner Kupferstiche. Der Geiz (1527). Strassburg: Heitz, 1911: p. 41/IV, item 38-II.
55. Tudor AP: The medieval toad: demonic punishment or heavenly warning? French Stud Bull 1996;**17**:7–11.
56. Fox M, Cacciatore J, Lacasse J: Child death in the United States: productivity and the economic burden of parental grief. Death Stud 2014;**38**:597–602.
57. Reinhart C: A child's funeral in Paris. The Graphic 1880;**27**:696.

8.8 Revived for paradise
Respite sanctuaries

Introduction: pilgrimage of dead babies

It seems incredible that at a time of high perinatal mortality, thousands of parents all over Europe carried the corpses of their dead newborns over long distances, summer or winter, usually on foot, in an attempt to save the infant's soul. Such pilgrimages led to sanctuaries where the infant was revived, baptized, and buried. The institutions and their activities were studied in France by Saintyves [1] and Gélis [2], in Switzerland by Vasella [3] and Ulrich-Bochsler [4], and in Germany and Austria by Kindermann [5] and Prosser [6]. Focusing on signs of life in the 'revived' infants, the present chapter describes the rite of revival baptism in some famous sanctuaries, its religious impact on the families, and the political consequences in the Reformation.

The soul in limbo: theological views

The idea that the soul continues to live after death evolved in antique cultures for individuals who were socially integrated. Egyptians longed to be reborn with the sun god; Buddhists believed the rebirth cycle ends by achieving *nirvana*; Greeks wished to be ferried over the *Styx* into the underworld; Romans to rejoin *ad patres* their families and ancestors; and Christians to rise *ad sanctos* to join the saints in paradise. These goals were pursued by complex burial rites denied to newborn infants who died before the integrating rite of passage (see Chapter 2.7). A sign of social stigma, they were not buried in regular cemeteries. Tertullian predicted for them an uncertain fate [7]: 'Detained in these infernal regions with the *Ahori*, or souls which were prematurely hurried away; or else a very bad thing to be there associated with the *Biaeothanati*, who suffered violent deaths.'

During the first centuries of Christianity, infants were not baptized. The custom originated when St Augustine proclaimed the dogma of original sin in 412 C.E. [8]: 'Infants who die unbaptized are damned, but receive the mildest punishment in hell.' Scholasticism perceived St Augustine's position as insufficient, and Thomas Aquinas alleviated the problem somewhat by dividing the underworld into four levels in 1254 [9]: '(1) Below is the hell of the condemned souls unable to see God nor ever hoping for salvation, and being bodily punished. (2) Above that is limbo [*limbus puerorum*] in which the [children's] souls cannot see God and are forever without salvation, but without bodily pain. (3) Further up is purgatory, where the souls cannot see God, and suffer pain, but can hope for salvation. (4) At the top is the hell of the Holy Fathers [*limbus patrum*] in which the souls cannot see God, but are not punished and can hope for salvation.'

The *limbus puerorum* was understood as lasting forever, the paradise remained inaccessible, as did a decent grave. Durandus' *Rationale* stated in 1294 [10]: 'Only a baptized Christian ought to be buried in a Christian cemetery … The stillborn child, not having been baptized, is buried outside of sacred ground'—the lonesome duty of the father or midwife. No name was given, and neither church record nor gravestone remembered the child. Parental anguish was augmented by the decision of the Council of Mainz in 813 to baptize only at Easter or Pentecost [11]. In 1439, the Council of Florence rejected the limbo doctrine [12]: 'The souls of those who depart this life in actual mortal sin, or in original sin alone, go down straightaway to hell to be punished, but with unequal pains.' In 1547, the Council of Trent allowed midwives to baptize infants in an emergency.

To escape such merciless dogma, the baptism of stillborn infants evolved in the 15th century as a service to console parents and enrich monasteries. The Church was not amused, the Synod of Langres decreed in 1452 [1]: 'We condemn and detest the abuse introduced since some time that infants who are suffocated at birth and those who are stillborn are carried to a church where they are exposed for a certain number of days and nights before the images of saints. Initially cold and stiff as a board, they receive the Holy Baptism and an Ecclesiastical funeral once they are softened by the coal-fire or by candles and lamps, they resume for some time a livid color, blood flows from their nose … the veins of their temples or neck show some movement; they open and close an eye, and reveal some breathing visible by a feather placed under their nose.' The decree was confirmed at the Synod of Sens in 1524. The reformers rejected the limbo doctrine. Cranach's picture of 1538 (Fig. 8.8.1) reflects a contemporary topic described in chapter 22 of the

---

Reproduced with permission from Obladen, M. Revived for paradise: a history of respite sanctuaries. *Neonatology*, 113(3):249–255. Copyright © 2018 S. Karger AG, Basel.

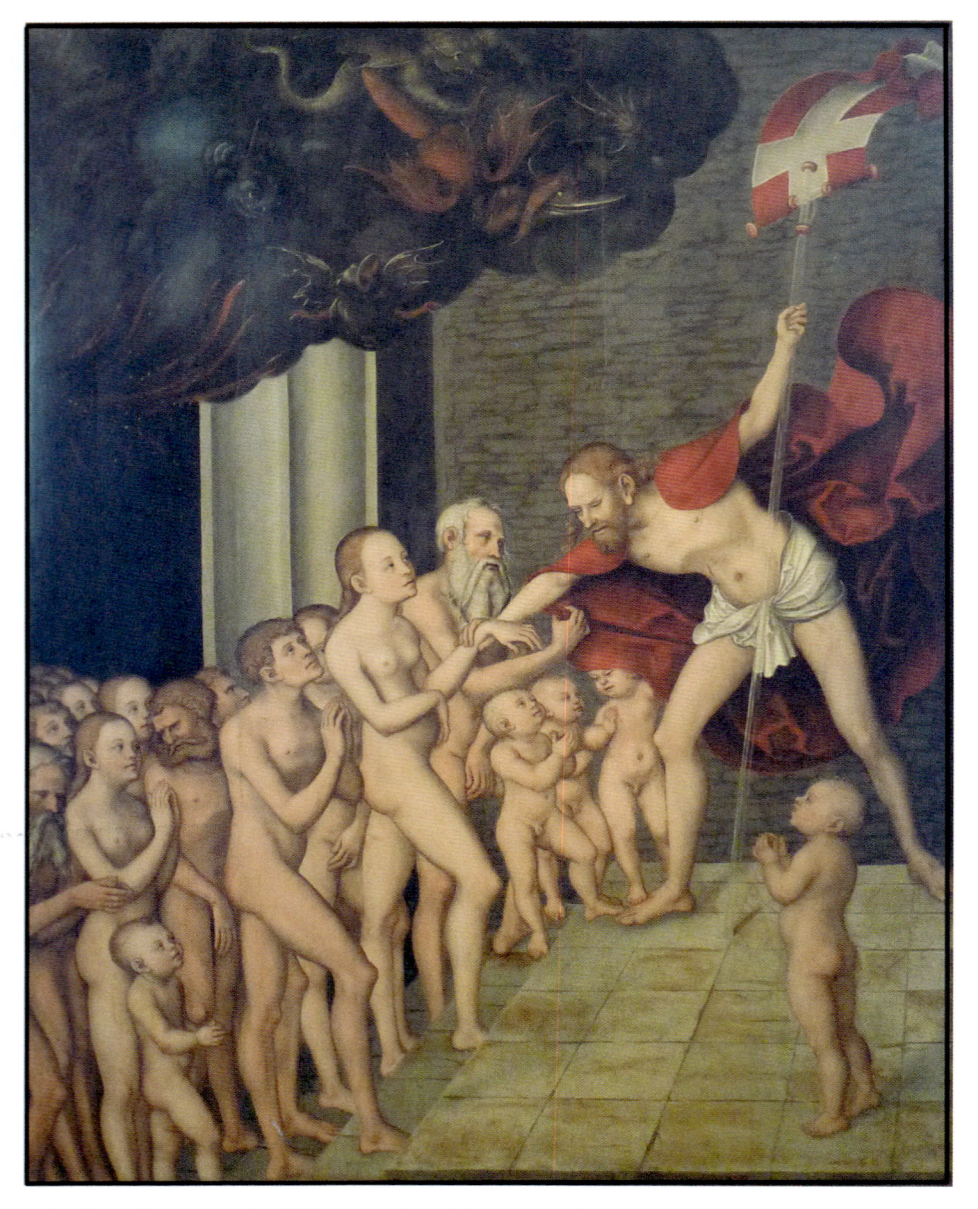

Fig. 8.8.1 Lucas Cranach the Elder: *Christ in Limbo*, 1538. Cranach's religious topics depicted issues of the Protestant Reformation. As described in the (apocryphal) gospel of Nicodemus, Christ descended into an edge of hell to resurrect the Holy Fathers from the *limbus patrorum* and the innocent infants from the *limbus puerorum*. Berlin, Jagdschloss Grunewald. Inv. Nr. GK I/2271.
© Prussian Palaces and Gardens Foundation, with permission. Photographer: Wolfgang Pfaundler.

(apocryphal) gospel of Nicodemus: Christ's descent into limbo to rescue the ancient Holy Fathers and innocent infants condemned for original sin only.

Nameless and unburied: popular beliefs

Whereas theologians debated the limbo doctrine for centuries, it remained unacceptable for the common people, even more so as deceased unbaptized infants were considered threatening. They were believed to find no rest and to ally with soldiers killed in action and persons who committed suicide, forming the 'Wild Hunt', a sinister procession erring about noisily during certain nights [13].

Of pre-Christian origin, this myth was widely adopted all over medieval Europe (*Chasse Sauvage, Mesnie Hellequin, Wildes Heer, Odins Jakt*). In 1021, bishop Burchard of Worms had reason to forbid the following custom [14]: 'When a child dies unbaptized, [some women] remove the little corpse to a secret place, pierce the body with a wooden stake and claim if they didn't this, the infant could arise and harm many.'

The Catholic world dreaded the sacramentally unprotected death. In despair, the anguished parents made incredible efforts, either the father alone, or the mother who just had given birth. The poor could not afford carriages and usually walked long distances, with the infant's decomposing corpse smelling worse from day to day. The route went uphill, as most sanctuaries were in remote mountain regions, the miraculous image often being associated with a chapel, monastery, or cemetery. The pilgrimage was dangerous, the Thirty Years War and subsequent conflicts devastated Europe. Moreover, the economic burden was high: in 1697, Gabriel d'Emiliane described the 'revivification' of stillborn twins, 'several days old, all livid and black, and largely decayed' in Notre Dame de St. Benigne in Dijon [15]: 'The parents, belonging to a wealthy Dijon family, had paid for over 200 masses at one ecu [about €12.50] each … The smell in the church became intolerable … the priest interrupted his prayer, pronouncing on the infants: I baptize you.' In all of Europe, the late Middle Ages saw pilgrimages to supposedly miraculous images. Of more than regional importance for infant revivification were the Alpine sanctuaries Schruns, Brixen, Imst, Riffian, Trens, Lausanne, Disentis, and Oberbüren. Dozens of sanctuaries in France were described by Gélis [2].

Oberbüren: profit, reformation, and iconoclasm

Located 25 km from Bern, the respite sanctuary Oberbüren became active in 1482. Thousands of stillborns and deceased neonates accumulated at St. Mary's: the chapel's yearly income rose from 534 pounds [about €70,000] in 1492 to 2344 pounds [about €300,000] in 1504 [3]. The small town of Büren also prospered from the pilgrimages, and had to regulate markets and lodging for the pilgrims. Abuse of the miraculous images triggered the iconoclastic fury that accompanied the Swiss and Flemish Reformation. For the reformed churches, baptism was no longer required for a baby to obtain salvation and burial in sacred ground. In 1528, the reformer Berchtold Haller wrote to Ulrich Zwingli [3] 'that due to the miracle-works 30,000 pounds [about €4 million] have been collected in Oberbüren'. Immediately after the Bern Disputation, the district council decided to remove the images from the churches 'within 8 days', and soon the Oberbüren image was removed [16]. This did not stop the pilgrims, and in 1532 the church was torn down to its fundaments. As late as 1997, modern archaeological excavation revealed the remnants of 250 infant corpses [4]. In December 1563, the last session of the Council of Trent restored 'due honor and veneration' of the images of saints, particularly in churches [17], 'because they set God's miracles before the eyes of the faithful'.

After the reformation

Miracle paintings, healing wells, and pilgrimages persisted, and even proliferated in Catholic regions after the Council of Trent. Jesuit William Gumppenberg's *Atlas Marianus* listed 1200 miraculous locations in 1672 [18]. In 1695, the Theatine Giovanni Bagatta systematically catalogued 10,000 approved miracles, including revivals of stillborns [19]. But the custom became increasingly clandestine when the Rituale Augustanum declared in 1704 [20]: 'The priest should not permit the transfer of obviously dead infants to pious places called *thaumaturgas* [miraculous]'. **Fig. 8.8.2** illustrates a typical revivification scene on a votive tablet. The stillborn infant has been placed on the altar before the miraculous image. A sufficient number of trustworthy witnesses, more men than women, has gathered in prayer, waiting for the infant 'to sign'. The midwife among them is equipped with a bottle of holy water to christen the child immediately.

A long journey to St Hippolyte

The distance and duration of the pilgrimage to a respite sanctuary is documented in a letter by Prince Anton Florian of Liechtenstein to his brother, the governing Prince Maximilian Jacob [21]: 'When my wife [Eleonora Barbara] gave birth to a stillborn daughter [in Vienna on 17 November 1687] during my absence in Pressburg, I was bereaved even more as she had been buried without holy baptism, therefore deprived of seeing God … [At my return] she had been underneath the ground for 13 days, I had her exhumed laboriously and ordered Mr Chassignet to bring her to Imst to St. Hippolyte's reliquary [ca. 550 km] … Once the third mass was held, her blackish-yellow death-color changed into a natural and vital one and the corpse ceased to smell.' The princess was then baptized by a Capucin and buried in the church's crypt. An inscription on the copper coffin confirms that she 'had been exposed at St. Mary's and St. Hippolyte's Altar, and was baptized on 06.12.1687, having shown signs of life.' Of course, travelling 550 km within 5 days was no option for the poor.

Ursberg: marketing heaven

The Premonstratensian monastery, Ursberg, in Swabia used a wooden crucifix to revive stillborn infants from 1686 and it soon became Europe's largest sanctuary for respite baptism: around 600 dead babies were brought there per year [6]. When in 1727 a baby was transferred from Worms, 300 km away, the bishop of Speyer complained in Rome, and the Holy Office ordered the bishop of Augsburg, responsible for Ursberg, to set an end to the abuse. But the lucrative custom persisted, as did the dispute among Premonstratensians, the Bishop of Augsburg, and the Holy Officium. The 50-year-conflict has been detailed by Kindermann [5]. When Pope Benedict XIV ascended the Holy Chair in 1740, support for miracles and sanctuaries waned, and he declared [22]: 'Doubtful signs of life that do not prove revivification are: skin color change from pale to red; change from rigidity to flexibility; blood flow from the nose; drops of sweat on forehead and stomach … These effects can be ascribed to the warmth of candles or the heating system of the sanctuary … We consider only crying and sounds of respiration as valid signs of revivification.' Other signs of life considered valid in Ursberg included loss of the cadaveric smell and altered transparency of the eyes [23]. To prove respiration, a feather was placed on the infant's mouth: if it moved thanks to the charcoal fire, this was interpreted as 'sign of life' [6]. When the Premonstratensians failed to stop reviving dead babies, the Pope sent an investigative committee in 1750, headed by the learned Dominican Eusebius Amort, who prohibited revivification baptism and recommended not accepting any more dead infants in Ursberg. Engaged by Benedict XIV, the Inquisitor Cangiamila referred to respite sanctuaries when he wrote in 1765 [24]: 'Those sin gravely who pretend a stillborn infant is alive, either by letting it move via tricks or drugs, or by inventing a miraculous resurrection

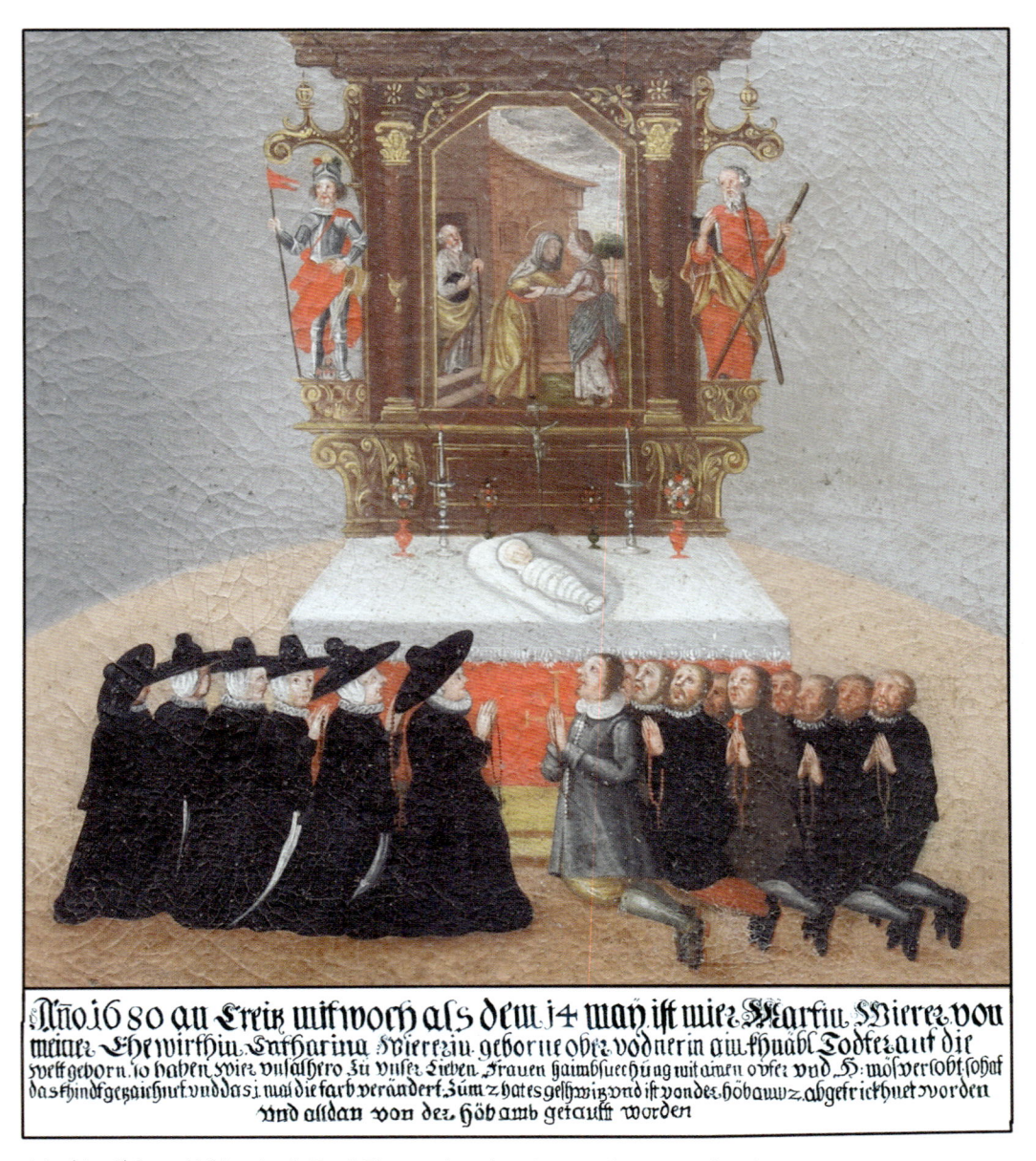

Fig. 8.8.2 Votive tablet (detail) from Abfaltersbach, Tyrol. The text describes the son of Martin and Catharina Wiehrer, stillborn on 14 May 1680. He was transferred to the sanctuary 'Mary's visitation', where an offering and Holy Mass were promised. The child 'signed' and changed colour. Thereafter he 'sweated' and was dried and baptized by the midwife.
© Museum Schloß Bruck, Lienz, Austria. Inv.-Nr. MSB-66, with permission.

by the saints, in order to baptize it to console the parents and bury it in a sacred place.' The Ursberg monastery was closed down in 1803.

Cheerless infants and eaves graves

With infant mortality between 300‰ and 400‰ and maternal mortality between 10% and 30% in the 18th century (Fig. 8.8.3, left), many families faced the alternative of losing a child to limbo or hell, or of gaining an angel in heaven as an advocate for sinful adults (Fig. 8.8.3, right). Up to the early 19th century, stillborn infants were called 'cheerless' (*unfrölich*), as defined in the German Dictionary begun by Jacob und Wilhelm Grimm in 1838 [25]. Baptized and unbaptized infants were still buried apart. The official 1795 birth record of Memmingen (Bavaria) revealed among 262 newborn infants 16 who were 'cheerless' (= stillborn and unbaptized) and one who was 'found dead' [26].

Similar to intrauterine- and revival-baptism, eaves-drip graves were another opportunity to open heaven's gate for a dead newborn. The custom in Switzerland, performed secretly, was described in 1838 by Jeremias Gotthelf, himself a priest in the Bern region [27]: 'The gravedigger had made the little grave in the eaves, not deep ... The closer to the church the child is buried, the more it is protected from earthly ghosts ... When the priest blesses the holy water, all water in and around the church is sanctified, and the rainwater running down the eaves reaches the buried child who

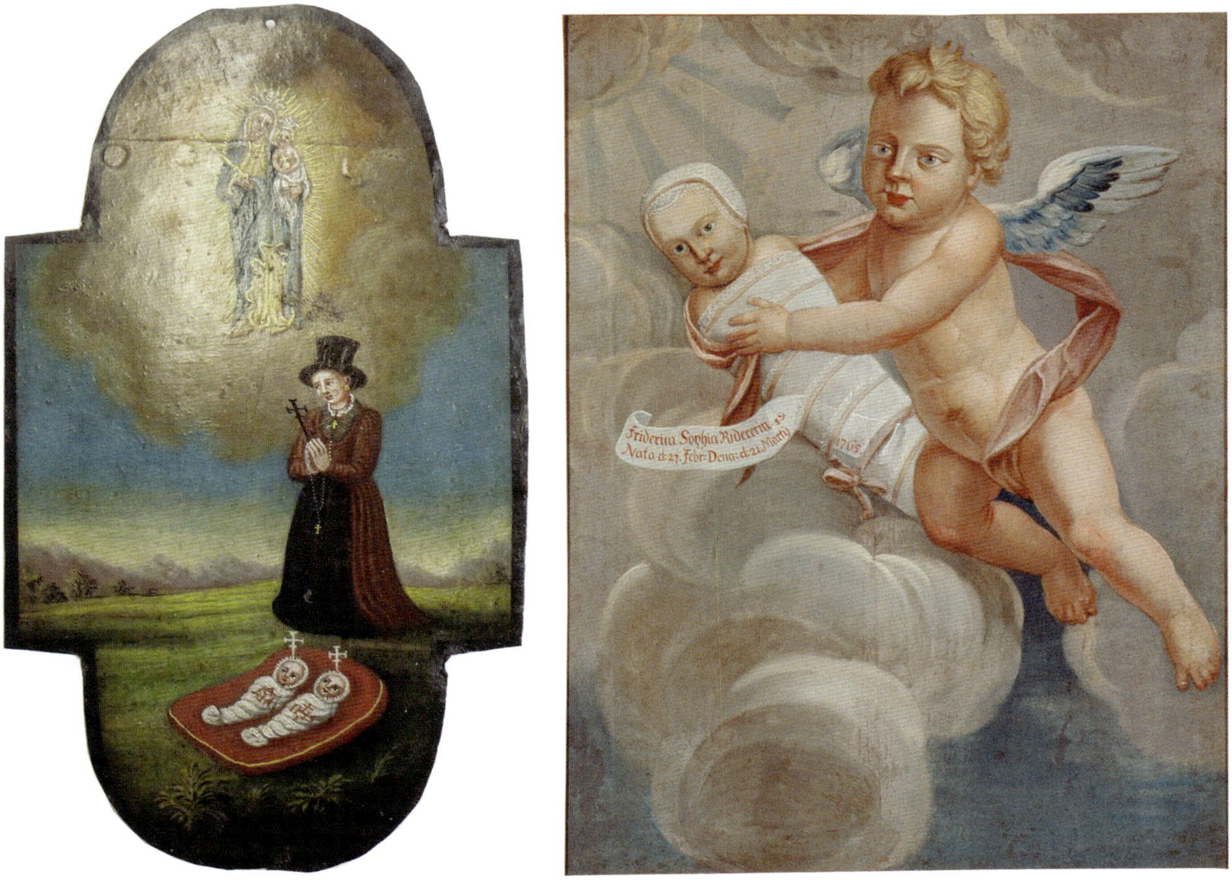

Fig. 8.8.3 Left: Votive tablet from Brixen depicting twins [ca. 1720]. The infants' white crosses indicate that they died baptized and their souls rose to heaven. The mother's black cross indicates that she also died, but must spend some time in purgatory. Museum Hofburg Brixen/Bressanone, Italy. Right: Epitaph for Friderica Sophia Riderer, born 27 February died 21 March 1765, transferred to heaven by an angel.
Left: Hofburg Brixen, with permission. Right: Kassel, Museum für Sepulkralkultur, Inv. Nr. M 1979/123, with permission.

is thereby baptized as valid as in the church.' Archaeologists have discovered neonates' graves in the eaves of several churches in the canton of Bern. Anglo-Saxon England was Christianized during the 7th century. From then up to the 11th century, archaeologists have identified eaves-drip burials: large clusters of fetuses, preterm, and term newborns were found within 1.5 m of many church walls [28].

Conclusion

Persisting all over Europe for 500 years, respite sanctuaries illustrate the failure of the doctrine of original sin, which was unbearable for the pious. The dogma of no mercy and the trivialization of piety then triggered the Reformation, and the commercialized abuse of miraculous images ignited the iconoclasm.

Centuries of debate on what constitutes 'valid' signs of life did not advance a scientific definition. Discerning stillborn and liveborn remained virtually impossible before the stethoscope was introduced in 1819. The debate resumed in the 19th century to determine who was eligible to legally inherit. In 1913, the American Public Health Organization decreed [29]: 'No child that shows any evidence of life after birth should be registered as stillbirth', defining life as 'action of heart, breathing, or movement of voluntary muscle'. In 1950, the World Health Organization defined signs of life in the newborn 'who after separation from its mother, breathes or shows any other evidence of life, such as beating of the heart, pulsation of the umbilical cord, or any definite movement of voluntary muscles' [30].

Although newborns were considered 'unfinished', the institution of respite sanctuaries endured for centuries. It was part of mankind's longing for a safe place in the afterlife, a strategy to cope with the hardships of an earthly and early death.

REFERENCES

1. SaintYves P: Les resurrections d'enfants morts-nés et les sanctuaires a 'répit'. Rev Ethnogr Sociol 1911;**9**:65–74.
2. Gélis J: De la mort a la vie. Les 'sanctuaires a répit'. Ethnologie Français 1981;**11**:211–24.
3. Vasella O: Über die Taufe totgeborener Kinder in der Schweiz. Zeitschr Schweiz Kirchengesch 1966;**60**:1–75.
4. Ulrich-Bochsler S, Gutscher D: Wiedererweckung von Totgeborenen. In: Schlumbohm J, Duden B, Gélis J, Veit P: Rituale der Geburt. München: Beck, 1998: p. 244–68.
5. Kindermann M: Die Ursberger Bedingungstaufe. Krumbacher Heimatblätter 1998;**12**:38–71.

6. Prosser M: Erweckungstaufe. Bayerisches Jahrbuch für Volkskunde. München: Bayerische Akademie der Wissenschaften, 2003: p. 101–38.
7. Tertullianus QSF: A treatise on the soul/De anima. Amsterdam: Meulenhoff, 1947, chap. 57.
8. Augustinus A: De peccatorum meritis et remissione, et de baptismo parvulorum (412 c.e.). Patrologia Latina. Paris: Migne, 1845: Vol. **44**, p. 120.
9. Thomas Aquinas: In quattuor libros sententiarum. In: Opera omnia. Stuttgart: Frommann, 1980: Vol. **1**, p. 336.
10. Thibodeau TM: The rationale divinorum officiorum of William Durand of Mende (1294). New York: Columbia University Press, 2007: p. 57.
11. Concilium Moguntiacum (813): De sacramento baptismi uniformiter celebrando. In: Acta conciliorum et epistolae decretales ac constitutiones. Paris: Typographia Regia, 1714: Vol. **4**, p. 1010.
12. Tanner NP: Decrees of the Ecumenical Councils. Washington, DC: Georgetown University Press, 1990: p. 528, 666.
13. Lecouteux C: Das Reich der Nachtdämonen. Angst und Aberglaube im Mittelalter. Düsseldorf: Artemis & Winkler, 2001: p. 163–72.
14. Burchardus Vormatiensis: Decretorum liber decimus nonus: de poenitentia (1021). Patrologia latina. Paris: Migne, 1853: Vol. **140**, p. 974.
15. D'Emiliane G: Histoire des tromperies des prestres et des moines (1st ed. Rotterdam 1693). Rotterdam: Acher, 1710: p. 17–21.
16. Gisi LM: 'Darumb vast hinus mit, doch mit gschickte!' Ikonoklastisches Handeln während der Reformation in Bern 1528. Zwingliana 2003;**30**:31–63.
17. Invocation, veneration and relics of saints and sacred images. In: Buckley TA: Canons and decrees of the Council of Trent. London: Rutledge, 1851: p. 214.
18. Gumppenberg W: Atlas Marianus. Monachii: Jaecklin, 1672.
19. Bagatta JB: Admiranda orbis Christiani. Augustae Vindelicorum: Bencard, 1695: p. 542.
20. Rituale Augustanum: $5: De Subjecto Baptismi. Anno 1752 Romae correctius editi: Augustae Vindelicorum: Labhart, 1764: p. 8–9.
21. Wilhelm G: Taufe totgeborener Kinder: ein Beispiel aus dem Fürstenhaus. Jahrb Hist Ver Furst Liechtenstein 1982;**82**:253–9.
22. Benedictus XIV Papa: De synodo diocesana libros priores novem. Bassano: Venetiis Remondini, 1767: Vol. **11**, p. 129.
23. Rückert G: Zur Taufe toter Kinder. Jahrbuch für Volkskunde 1937;**2**:343–6.
24. Cangiamila FE: Embryologia sacra sive de officio sacerdotum, medicorum, et aliorum circa aeternam parvulorum in utero existentium salutem. 3. ed. Augustae Vindelicorum: Mauracher, 1765: p. 776.
25. Grimm J, Grimm W: Deutsches Wörterbuch. Leipzig: Hirzel, 1936: Vol. **11**, chap. 3, p. 592.
26. Ehrhart G: Physisch-medizinische Topographie der königl. baier. Stadt Memmingen. Memmingen: Rehm, 1813: p. 27.
27. Gotthelf J: Wie die Leute den lieben Gott kennen (1838). In: Freuden und Leiden eines Schulmeisters. Bern: Schmidt & Francke, 1898: Vol. **2**, chap. 16.
28. Craig-Atkins E: Eavesdropping on short lives. In: Hadley DM, Hemer KA: Medieval childhood. Oxford: Oxbow Books, 2014: p. 95–113.
29. Hemenway HB, Davis WH, Chapin CV: Definition of stillbirth. Am J Public Health 1928;**18**:25–31.
32. World Health Organization Expert Committee on Health Statistics (1950): Report of the second session; expert group on prematurity. WHO Technical Report Series 25/27. Geneva: World Health Organization, 1950.

APPENDIX 1
Methodical limitations

Like every scientific endeavour, this historical research has limitations and is not free of bias:

1. *Bibliography*: many medical publications contain a historical introduction in which citations of the older medical literature are incorrect for various reasons—different book editions were confounded, book pages were omitted, journals were cited either by volume or by year but not both. Not seldom, the historian's first duty was violated, namely to go *ad fontes* to study the original reports. This is especially annoying as, despite progress in the field of scientific bibliography, many old sources are still difficult to find. With the ongoing digitization of ancient books, the access to early sources will become easier: a major aim of this book is to provide entrance keys to these valuable sources, and references were scrutinized. To avoid footnotes, two or three references to the same source may be indicated by their corresponding page numbers.

2. *Selection bias*: the material is voluminous, and I had to be selective. 'The secret of being boring is to say everything' (Voltaire). The author of a history of science assumes a heavy responsibility to be fair in selecting the material for inclusion. As much as possible, literal or translated citations were used in this book. Sometimes, quoting some more words than I did may have changed the citation's meaning. I tried to avoid making value judgements and forwarding personal opinions.

3. *Publication bias*: as medical history relies so heavily on printed sources, one gets the wrong impression that many discoveries were made in the 16th century. The truth is that at that time, it was the printing press that accelerated the spread of new and old knowledge. And in medicine of all periods, success was more likely to be published than failure.

4. Publication must not be confused with *reception*, which often lagged way behind. But the intense exchange of thought within the small international scientific community and the speed of expanding knowledge must not be underestimated. The reception of new knowledge by scientists does not mean that many patients benefited from progress made, as in centuries without health insurance usually only the wealthy received treatment. Despite active and international contact, some important discoveries were made nearly simultaneously in different parts of the world.

5. *Language bias*: considerable effort has been made to access English, French, Greek, Latin, Italian, and German sources. Neither word-by-word nor free translation of the assumed meaning were appropriate. I sought to capture the meaning of the statement at the time of publication. If necessary, non-English terms are kept in *italics*, whereas modern transcriptions are identified by [square brackets]. Chinese, Japanese, Indian, and Arabian sources are perforce under-represented.

6. Language bias must not be confused with *linguistic bias*: in living languages the meaning of a word root changes over time, and will not remain constant for centuries. A frequent example in this book is the Greek-Roman root γένεο generare. It appears in the English terms genus—gentle—general—generic—genetic—gendarme—gender—congenital—genitals—genocide—gentleman—generosity—generate—generalize—engender and others. Drug names may have been used for millennia (as *theriac*), which does not mean that their composition was constant. An example where the term for the same condition changed is *apparent death* versus *asphyxia*.

7. *Confirmation bias* is an inherent part of human reasoning: it describes the seeking of evidence that is part of already existing knowledge, belief, or prejudice. For the historian, it becomes especially virulent when reporting on current events. Time must prove which of the more recent developments are historic, therefore the work of living authors and research in which I have participated myself was usually omitted. This resulted in a cut-off around 1970, the time when I began working in neonatology.

8. The *illustrations* also deserve a word of caution. Infant descriptions in medical texts are scanty, and usually not illustrated. Therefore, attention was paid to the paintings of infants in contemporary works of art. The reader must understand, however, that the iconographic evidence is ambivalent because it was usually not the artist's intent to document the infant's state—which was often not understood—but rather to furnish a portrait or to fulfil a religious duty.

APPENDIX 2

Early special care baby units and their scientific achievements

Introduction

Hospital care for sick neonates is a recent accomplishment. Reasons for the delayed development were manifold; sanitary conditions were poor, and sewerage and plumbing were not installed in most European cities until between 1840 and 1870, finally allowing access to clean water. Microorganisms as pathogens were not known before 1841 [1]. Washing hands and diapers with disinfecting agents was gradually introduced after 1867 [2]. Other obstacles were the need for wet nursing by women residing in the hospital, ignorance about breast milk substitutes, and difficulties in obtaining and storing bottled milk. Last, but not least, hospital infant care was not covered by health insurance providers, as Oswald Vierordt, director of the Heidelberg Luisenanstalt, complained in 1904 [3]: 'Infants remain in the situation of the poor before the advent of health insurance: their treatment depends on municipal, parochial, or private charity.'

The history of neonatal intensive care after World War II has been documented [4–6]. Earlier reports on children's hospitals often disregarded the fact that these institutions did not admit sick neonates and bypassed wet nursing. 'Even after children's hospitals were established, infants under two years were seldom accepted' [7]. The aim of this chapter is to identify sites of neonatal care at the beginning of the 20th century. Another aim of this tabulation is to provide access to contemporary reports on the work going on in these units.

Methods

Hospital wards for preterm and sick neonates, from which more than one researcher had published on neonates before the Great Depression (1929), were tabulated (Table A2.1). Precursor units were omitted when no information was available on neonatal treatment. The first column lists the hospital's founding date and location, the second the date from which neonatal treatment was reported. References authored by the protagonists were preferred to historic reviews. Other sources include comparisons of institutions published by Hügel in 1848 and 1863 [8, 9], Rauchfuss in 1877 [10], Eröss in 1886 [11], and Deutsch in 1900 [12], reports by travelling scientists [13–15], and hospital news appearing in the *Archiv für Kinderheilkunde* from 1880 to 1918.

Infirmaries in foundling hospitals

Abandoning neonates was common in antiquity, and foundling asylums have existed since Bishop Datheus opened the Milan institution in 787 C.E. Not intended for the sick, they admitted neonates for a few days and organized their foster care in the countryside. Connected to maternity hospitals for unmarried women, they provided some social support in exchange for wet-nursing services. Initiated by private or clerical charity, some foundling hospitals were famous for their architecture, art collections (Rome, Florence, Moscow), or orchestras (Venice, London). In France, they became sites of research, when in 1811 Napoleon ordered infirmaries to be installed in each foundling hospital, including resident wet nurses and in-house physicians. Specialized units evolved for surgery on congenital malformations and treatment of ophthalmia and of suspected congenital syphilis. Mortality ranged from 50% to over 90%. Separate statistics for the in-house babies and those farmed out for foster care masked the fact that three out of four foundlings did not survive their first year.

Weakling wards in maternity hospitals

With the development of heated chambers and closed incubators, prematures were given a chance to survive. Wards for preterm

---

Reproduced with permission from Obladen, M. Early neonatal special care units and their achievements. *Neonatology*, 102(2):89–97. Copyright © 2012 S. Karger AG, Basel.

Appendix 2

Table A2.1 Early neonatal special care units, their research topics, and major achievements in the care of sick neonates

City, name of hospital, founding date, address	Neonates treated from	Pioneers	Affiliation period	Main achievements and research topics related to the care of neonates	Historic sources
Basel 1862 Kinderspital Rheinufer/1906 Säuglingsheim	1907	Emil Wieland Emil Feer Ernst Freudenberg	1894–1938 1894–1907 1938–1954	Ward for prematures, types of congenital rickets Gastroenteritis; League of Infant Protection Rickets, ultraviolet radiation	[16]
Berlin 1899 Kinderasyl Kürassierstr./ Waisenhaus Jacobstrasse	1901	Heinrich Finkelstein Iwan Rosenstern Ludwig F. Meyer	1901–1918 1907–1914 1905–1924	Protein-enriched milk, chronic malnutrition Metabolism in undernutrition Immunity; nutrition and metabolism	[17] [18]
Berlin 1909 Kaiserin Auguste Victoria Haus Heubnerweg	1909	Arthur Keller Leo Langstein Adalbert Reiche Arvo Ylppö Lotte Landé	1909–1911 1909–1933 1911–1918 1912–1920 1917–1920	High-risk maternity unit within infant hospital Bilirubin metabolism, preterms, intraventricular haemorrhage Fetal opiate action, preterm follow-up Preterm: diseases, pathology, growth and nutrition Anaemia of prematurity	[19] [20] [21] [22]
Birmingham 1911 Sorrento Maternity Hospital Wake Green Rd.	1929	Victoria M. Crosse W.F. Young Thomas C. Meyer	1929–1961 1938–1942 1955–1956	Premature infants' kernicterus, retinopathy cause Neonatal kidney function, urea clearance Kernicterus following high-dose vitamin K	[23] [24] [25]
Bordeaux 1689 Foundling Hospital/Clinique Chirurgicale	1841	E. Lebariller Jean-Loui Denucé	1856 1857	Thrush: clinical forms, contagiosity, and treatment Open Berceau-type incubator	[26] [27]
Boston 1869 Infants' Hospital, Blossom Street/Longwood Ave.	1881	Thomas M. Rotch Charles W. Townsend William E. Ladd Louis K. Diamond	1880–1914 1894–1905 1914–1945 1932–1968	Percentage feeding, mobile incubator, milk lab Haemorrhagic disease of the newborn Surgery for congenital malformations Erythroblastosis fetalis, exchange transfusion	[28, 29] [30]
Cassel 1761 Foundling Hospital/ Collegium Carolinum	1763	Georg W. Stein Friedrich B. Osiander Samuel Soemmerring	1761–1788 1780–1782 1779–1784	Instruments for body measurements; breast pump Resuscitation with tobacco clyster Systematic of congenital malformations	[31, 32] [33] [34]
Chicago 1913 Michael Reese/1922 Sarah Morris Hospital, Groveland/ Ellis Ave.	1913	Isaac Abt Julius Hess Iris M. Chamberlain	1912–1939 1921–1941 1927	Wet nursing of preterm infants; textbook Water jacket incubator, closed incubator bed Report on 266 preterm infants and 79 autopsies	[35] [36] [37]
Copenhagen 1759 Maternity/1879 Queen Louise Children's Hospital	1879	Poul Scheel Harald Hirschsprung Svend Gammeltoft	1802–1811 1870–1904 1919–1949	Endotracheal intubation of asphyctic neonates Megacolon, pyloric stenosis, oesophageal atresia Forms of congenital syphilis	[38] [39]
Dublin 1757 Foundling Hospital/ Rotunda Maternity O'Connell Street	1932	Brian D. Crichton W. Robert Collis	1925–1941 1932–1957	Causes of infant mortality Management and prognosis of the preterm infant, textbook of neonatal paediatrics	[40] [41]
Dresden 1897 Säuglingsheim Wormser Strasse	1898	Arthur Schlossmann Heinrich Peters Hans Rietschel	1897–1906 1902 1907–1917	Specific hospital for sick infants, infection control Incubator with electric heating, artificial nutrition Causes of hospital mortality Training programme for nurses; summer mortality	[42] [33] [43]
Edinburgh 1879 Royal Maternity and Simpson Memorial Hosp.	1910	John W. Ballantyne Francis J. Browne W.S. Craig	1890–1919 1919–1926 1927–1939	Fetopathies, hydrops fetalis, pre- and postmaturity Organization of 'no-man's land', antenatal care Classification of intracranial haemorrhages	[44] [45] [46]
Florence 1444 Spedale degli Innocenti Piazza dell' Annunziata	1895	Vittorio Bosi Giuseppe Mya Germano Guidi Carlo Comba	1879–1996 1890–1911 1895–1898 1911–1941	Air-conditioned heated room for preterms Bureau of Infant Welfare, megacolon congenitum Incubator room, systemic *Candida* infection Public health activities, infectious diseases	[47] [48]
Graz 1875 Landesfindelanstalt/ Annaspital, Mozartgasse	1899	Theodor Escherich Ernst Moro Meinhard Pfaundler	1890–1902 1898–1902 1902–1906	Bacterial enteritis, heated chamber for preterm infants, X-ray diagnosed rickets, borax thrush dummy Nutrition and development of preterm infants Chemical analysis of infants' blood, gastric capacity.	[49] [50, 51] [52]
Heidelberg 1885 Luisenheilanstalt Luisenstrasse/Vosstrasse	1904	Oswald Vierordt Ernst Moro Paul György	1890–1906 1911–1936 1920–1933	Couveuse unit, hygienic conditions of bottle-feeding Infant nutrition, gastroenteritis, body startle reflex Vitamin D prophylaxis of rickets	[3] [53] [54]
Helsinki 1917 Lastenlinna, Childrens' Castle, Stenbäckinkatu	1920	Arvo Ylppö Eero Löfqvist Erkki I. Sinkko	1920–1957 1931 1937	Infant protection, care for preterm infants Statistical studies on preterm infants Infant mortality and human milk vitamin C content	[55] [56]
Lyon 1858 Hospice de la Charité, Place Antonin Poncet	1830	Pierre E. Martin C. Richard (Nancy) Jean L. Brachet	1811–1835 1823–1839 1818–1837	Fetal disorders, inflammatory disposition of neonate Classification of malformations, incubator for prematures Hydrocephalus, infant convulsions	[57] [58] [59]

Table A2.1 Continued

City, name of hospital, founding date, address	Neonates treated from	Pioneers	Affiliation period	Main achievements and research topics related to the care of neonates	Historic sources
Moscow 1763 Imperial House of Education, Miassnitzkaja/ Nikolai Hospital	1891	Andreas H. Kronenberg H. Blumenthal Nikolaus Th. Miller Nil F. Filatow	1847 1861 1865–1886 1881–1902	Thrush pathogenesis Causes of infant mortality Report on diseases in 6036 preterm infants Infectious diseases, directed Chludow hospital	[60] [61] [62]
Munich 1846: v. Hauner'sches Kinderspital Goethestr./Lindwurmstr	1910	Heinrich v Ranke Meinhard Pfaundler Ernst Moro	1886–1905 1906–1939 1907–1911	Aetiology of spina bifida Maternal–fetal antibody transfer, body measurements Carrot soup in gastroenteritis	[63] [64]
New Haven 1913 Yale School of Medicine, Dept. Pediatrics Cedar St.	1921	Ethel C. Dunham Maude M. Eliot Arnold Gesell P.F. McAlenny	1920–1935 1921–1935 1915–1948 1935	Prematurity, septicaemia, Children's Bureau Vitamin D rickets prevention, Children's Bureau Behavioural patterns, mental development Study of 244 premature infants	[65]
New York City 1887 Babies' Hospital/Lexington Ave/55th Street	1902	Abraham Jacobi Luther E. Holt Linnaeus E. LaFetra	1870–1910 1889–1923 1904–1919	Diarrhoea, foundling mortality, Brain development Milk station, percentage feeding, diseases of infancy Infection, pyuria	[66] [67]
Paris 1638 Hôpital des Enfants Trouvés, Rue d'Enfer	1814	Gilbert Breschet J. François Baron Prosper S. Denis Charles M. Billard David Gruby Joseph Parrot Victor Hutinel	1812–1835 1822–1847 1825–1827 1826–1828 1839–1841 1867–1883 1890–1907	Congenital malformations, ward for ophthalmia Auscultation of the neonate, hydrocephalus Tentorium rupture, cerebral malacia, thrush, jaundice Systematics of respiratory disorders Thrush germ identified 'athrepsie', pavilion for congenital syphilis Circulation, antisepsis, isolation boxes	[68] [15] [69] [70] [71] [72] [73]
Paris Maternité, pavillon des débiles, Bd. Port-Royal	1893	Stéphane Tarnier Pierre Budin Adolphe Auvard	1867–1897 1875–1907 1883–1905	Gavage feeding, closed incubators League against infant mortality, Gouttes de lait Incubator with mobile heating elements	[74] [75, 76] [77]
Philadelphia 1855 Children's/1911 Babies', Lombard St.	1911	Charles A. Fife Emily P. Bacon Charles Chapple John F Sinclair	1911–1932 1925–1938 1929–1957 1914–1940	Nutrition of atrophic infants, social services Health education, visiting nurses. Climatized incubator, isolette Feeding the newborn	[81]
Prague 1781 Königlich-Boehmische Landesfindelanstalt	1864	Gottfried Ritter Alois Epstein R.W. Raudnitz Julius Eröss Rudolf Fischl	1864–1880 1875–1918 1883–1910 1886–1887 1887–1918	Staphylococcal scalded skin syndrome Septicaemia, hospitalism, hygiene, icterus Haemorrhagic disease, international comparison Surrounding temperature in premature infants Reasons for hospital infection, infant nutrition	[82] [83] [84] [85]
Stockholm 1785 Allmänna Barnhuset	1841	Fredrik T. Berg Hjalmar Abelin Adolf Kjellberg Isak Jundell	1841–1854 1855–1882 1861–1884 1895–1922	Characterization of thrush, sudden infant death Causes of infant mortality Diet in acute neonatal gastroenteritis Pathogenesis of gonoblenorrhoea	[1] [86]
St. Petersburg 1770 Imperial House of Education, Bobrinsky Palais	1835	Philipp Doepp W. Fröbelius Carl A. Rauchfuss Nicolai P. Gundobin	1829–1842 1863–1882 1858–1907 1888–1908	Incubator care, drainage of cephalhematoma Pneumonia, survival statistics, vaccination Congenital heart malformations, ductus arteriosus Organ measurements	[78, 79] [80]
Strasbourg 1837 Säuglingsheilstätte/Clinique infantile Hôpital Civil	1901	Ferdinand Siegert Paul Rohmer	1896–1904 1919–1947	Social support for the neonate; hypothyreosis Synthesis of vitamin C in infants	[87]
Toronto 1875 Hospital for sick Children, College Street	1914	Alan Brown W. Edward Gallie Frederick Tisdall Alfred P. Hart	1918–1951 1918–1947 1921–1949 1921–1951	Milk pasteurization, protein milk powder Surgery Nutrition research, vitamin-enriched baby cereal *Pablum* Exchange transfusion in haemolytic disease	[88] [89] [90]
Vienna 1784 Foundling Hospital, Alserstr.	1818	Alois Bednar Max Zarfl	1844–1861 1901–1926	Diseases of the newborn, clinical-pathological view Congenital tuberculosis	[91] [92]
Vienna 1850 Anna Hospital Alsergrund	1904	Theodor Escherich August v Reuss Jr	1902–1911 1911–1930	Incubator room, society for infant protection Continuous positive airway pressure, textbook on diseases of the neonate	[93] [94]
Zurich Haus Rosenberg	1908	Jacob Bernheim Heinrich Willi	1908–1937 1937–1970	Neonatal jaundice, vitamin deficiencies Pyloric stenosis, necrotizing enterocolitis, reflexes	[95] [96]

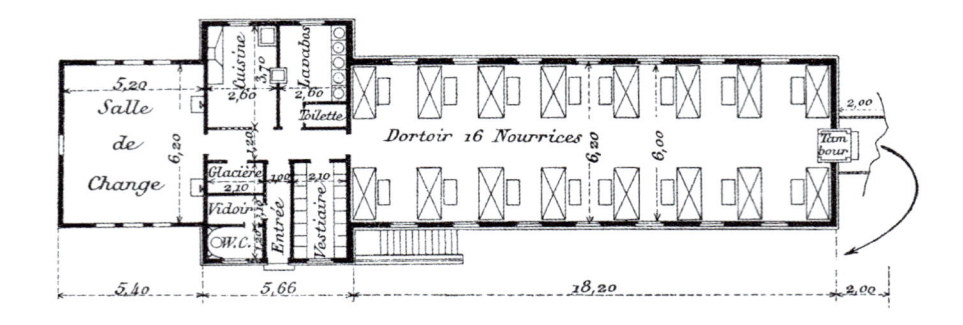

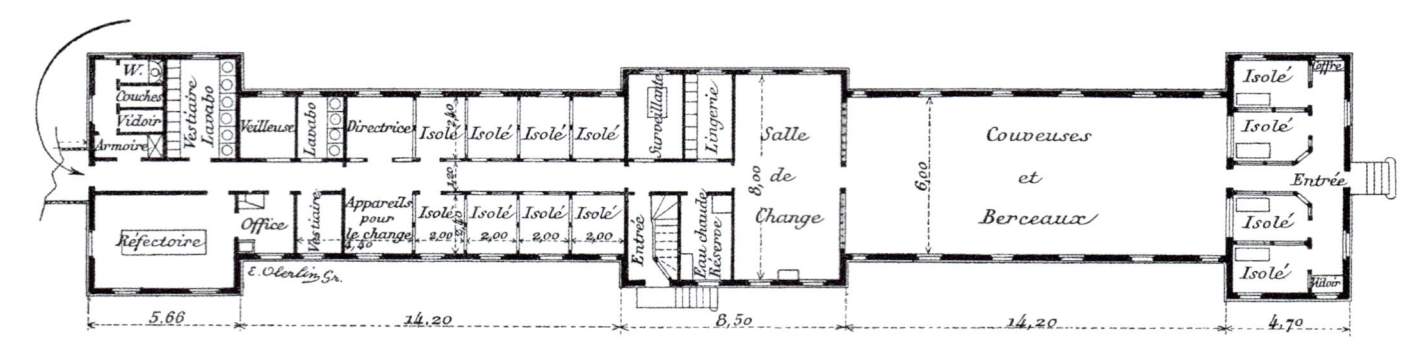

Fig. A2.1 Weaklings' pavilion (*pavillon des débiles*) at the Paris Maternité in service since 1893, with Budin's enlargement of 1897 [76]. Three sections were strictly separated. Top: sleeping room for up to 16 wet nurses with their infants, with dressing room, washbasins, kitchen, cool room and icebox for sterilized milk. Bottom right: large room for up to 16 healthy prematures in heated cots and closed incubators, room for washing and dressing the weaklings, plus four isolation chambers. Bottom left: eight isolation rooms for sick and suspect infants, supervising nurses' office, nurses' dining room, linen and cloak rooms, chambers for scales, bathtubs, breast pumps, glasses, and other equipment.

infants were established in maternity hospitals (Fig. A2.1), and early 'neonatologists' were obstetricians (Scheel, Stein, Martin, Runge, Reuss, Credé, Tarnier, Budin, Pinard, Crosse). They had no formal training in neonatal care and left most decisions to the nurses, albeit deploring 'midwifepower' [11]. As late as 1916, the Edinburgh obstetrician John Ballantyne called the field of neonatal medicine a 'no-man's land' [44]. The history of the incubator has been recounted by Baker [97]. From 1910, however, the incubator fell from grace: petrol heating and uncontrolled temperature had caused accidents and wooden devices could not be properly disinfected. Couney's incubator spectacles prompted the 'protest that human infirmities do not constitute a fit subject for the public showman to exploit' [98]. The importance of light in ricket prevention became known in 1919 [99], and in 1925, the Berlin paediatrician Adalbert Czerny, influential opponent of neonatal medicine, cheered: 'No need any more to write about incubators, because they are outdated' [100]. The advent of public health institutions shifted attention from treatment to prevention.

Wet nursing in children's hospitals

Hospitals for sick children were founded in developed countries during the 19th century, usually against resistance from internal medicine. The dispensary, earliest help for sick children of the poor, was unsuitable for neonates. Franz Hügel listed 28 children's hospitals in 1848, of which only the traditional foundling institutions in Paris and Stockholm admitted infants [8]. In 1877, Carl Rauchfuss compiled a list of more than 50 children's hospitals in Europe, none of which admitted neonates [10]. When Arthur Schlossmann, who had collected a large sum of donations, built a hospital for sick infants in Dresden in 1898, he had to name it *baby home* instead of *hospital* [101]. Based on wet nursing and heated rooms, Theodor Escherich installed wards for premature infants in the children's hospitals in Graz in 1899 [49] and Vienna in 1904 [93] (Fig. A2.2), which became a model for many other hospitals. As late as 1928, Zürich paediatrician Emil Feer demanded 'to establish specialized units for infants, with a milk kitchen and in-house wet-nurses' [102].

Political framework and funding

During the 19th century, most governments were more inclined to invest taxpayer money in armies than in children's hospitals. It was left to the persuasiveness of certain charismatic personalities to evoke feelings of charity in the wealthy and the public for the endangered infant. Social Darwinism unleashed prejudices towards the sick, malformed, or preterm infant, hindering the neonate from

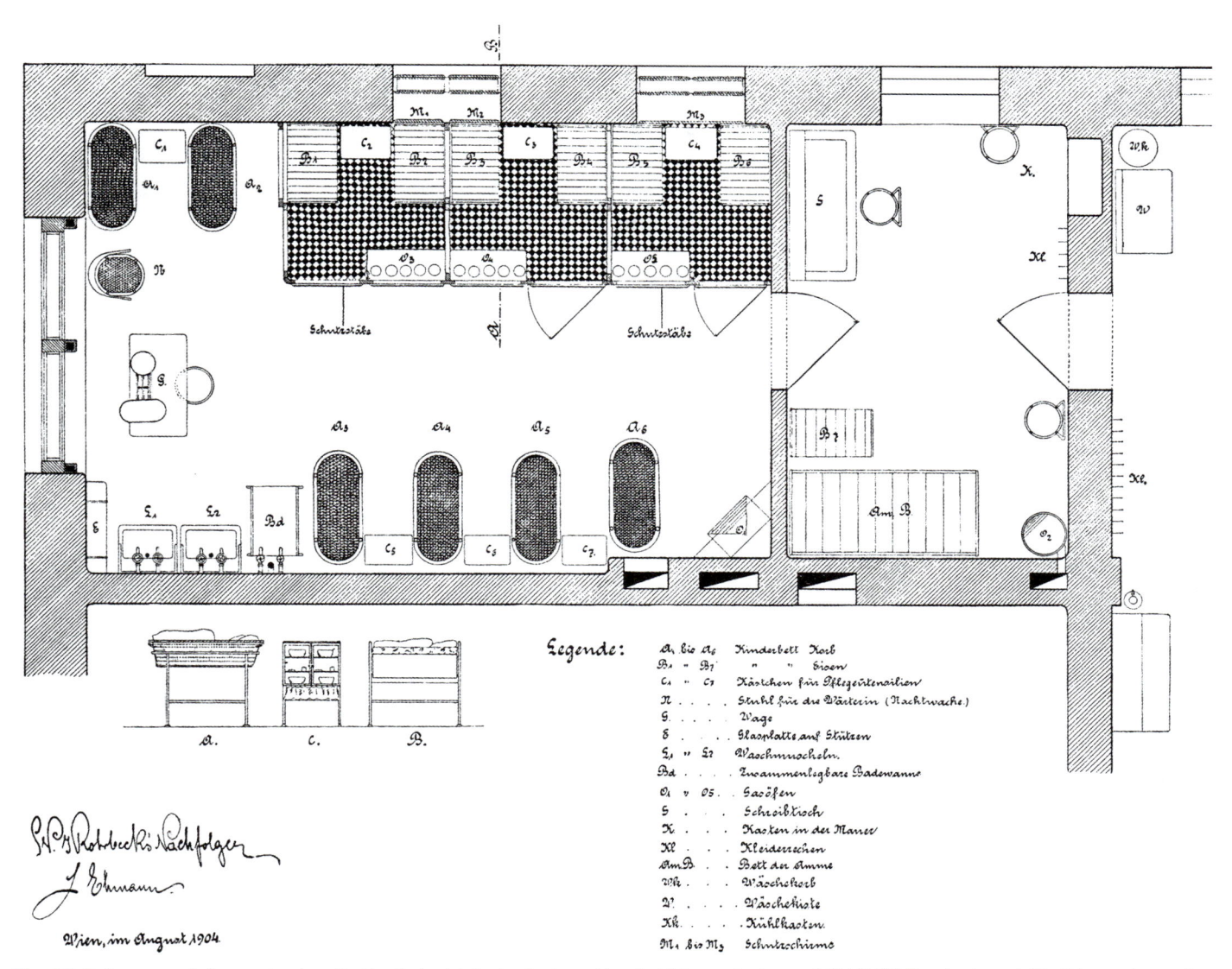

Fig. A2.2 Premature infant station installed by Escherich in the St. Anna Hospital, Vienna, in August 1904 [105]. Two beds each (B₁–B₆) were located in three heated rooms with shielded windows. Six other cots (A₁–A₆) were located in the larger room. O₁–O₅, gas heated ovens; C₁–C₇, separate utensils for each infant; Bd, folding bathtub; N, night nurse's chair. Outside the room were facilities for gowning (Kl), documentation (S), the wet nurse (AmB), and her infant (B₇)

becoming a 'normal' patient up to the present day. Wars aggravate shortness of resources, malnutrition, and poverty. However, following wars or declining birth rates, governments invested in measures to reduce infant mortality [103]. The commitment to preterm and malformed infants, however, varied considerably among nations, as discussed during the international *Gouttes de lait* congresses [104]. Many of the pioneers in neonatal medicine were Jewish scientists and physicians. Some examples from the table are Isaac Abt, Jacob Bernheim, Alois Epstein, Heinrich Finkelstein, Ernst Freudenberg, Paul György, Julius Hess, Abraham Jacobi, Leo Langstein, Ludwig F. Meyer, and Arthur Schlossmann. With the persecution of Jews and the discrimination against disabled infants, Nazi Germany halted the progress of neonatal medicine in large parts of Europe. Modern neonatal special care emerged in North America (Fig. A2.3).

Conclusion

Neonatal medicine evolved earlier in sites where foundling hospitals had established the infrastructure of wet nursing and sanitary installations. We cannot help but admire the courage, ingenuity, and frustration tolerance of the pioneers who overcame the problems resulting from: (1) ignorance of microorganisms, inadequate hygiene, and lack of clean water; (2) artificial feeding, especially in summertime; (3) prejudices against prematurity, congenital disorder, and

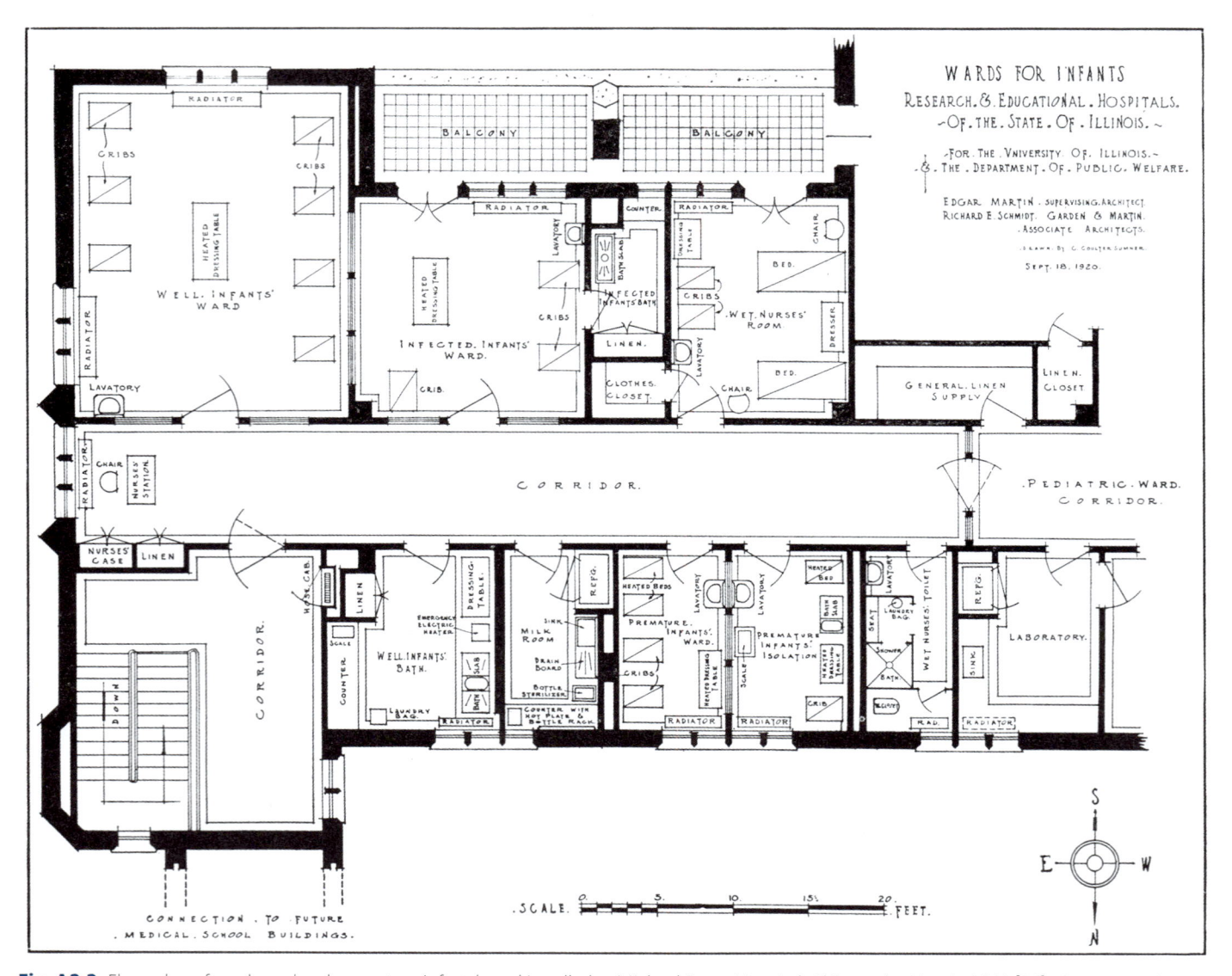

Fig. A2.3 Floor plan of newborns' and premature infants' ward installed at Michael Reese Hospital, Chicago, by Hess in 1920 [36]. This unit marks the transition from care in a superheated room (Escherich type, see Fig. A2.2) to individually heated cribs. Cross-infection was prevented by strictly separated departments for well babies, infected infants, premature infants, and infected prematures. Also separated was the living room for two wet nurses and their infants.

illegitimacy; and (4) competition for resources within notoriously underfinanced health systems.

REFERENCES

1. Berg FT: Torsk i mikroskopiskt anatomiskt hänseende. [Thrush from the microscopical anatomical point of view]. Hygiea 1841;**3**:541–50.
2. Lister J: On the antiseptic principle in the practice of surgery. BMJ 1867;**II**:246–8.
3. Vierordt O: Die Säuglingsabteilung, Säuglingsambulanz und Milchküche der Luisenheilanstalt zu Heidelberg. Stuttgart: Moritz, 1904.
4. Christie DA, Tansey EM: Origins of neonatal intensive care in the UK. In: Wellcome Witnesses to Twentieth Century Medicine. London: Wellcome Trust Centre for the History of Medicine, 2001: Vol. **9**.
5. Philip AG: The evolution of neonatology. Pediatr Res 2005;**58**:799–815.
6. Dunn PM: The birth of perinatal medicine in the United Kingdom. Semin Fetal Neonatal Med 2007;**12**:227–38.
7. Radbill SX: A history of children's hospitals. Am J Dis Child 1955;**90**:411–6.
8. Hügel FS: Beschreibung sämmtlicher Kinderheilanstalten in Europa. Wien: Kaulfuß, 1848.
9. Hügel FS: Die Findelhäuser und das Findelwesen Europas. Wien: Sommer, 1863.
10. Rauchfuss C: Die Kinderheilanstalten. In: Handbuch der Kinderkrankheiten. Tübingen: Laupp, 1877: Vol. **I**, p. 464–528.
11. Eröss J: Die Kinderspitäler Mittel-Europas nach Reisenotizen. Arch Kinderheilk 1886;**7**:44–65.

12. Deutsch E: Die Lage der Frühgeborenen in den Geburtsanstalten. Arch Kinderheilk 1900;**28**:245–63.
13. Otto K: Reise durch die Schweiz, Italien, Frankreich, Großbritannien und Holland, mit besonderer Rücksicht auf Spitäler. Hamburg: Campe, 1825.
14. Horn W: Reise durch Deutschland, Ungarn, Holland, Italien, Frankreich, Großbritannien und Irland. In: Rücksicht auf medizinische und naturwissenschaftliche Institute. Berlin: Enslin, 1831: Vol. **1**.
15. Pieper PA: Die Kinderpraxis am Findelhause und in dem Hospital für kranke Kinder zu Paris. Göttingen: Dieterich, 1831: p. 10–39.
16. Hottinger A: Über die Aufzucht frühgeborener Kinder im Basler Kinderspital. Basel: Karger, 1927.
17. Finkelstein H: Ärztlicher Bericht. In: Brugger P: Die Bekämpfung der Säuglingssterblichkeit. Leipzig: Duncker und Humblot, 1905: p. 49–89.
18. Waisenverwaltung des Magistrats: Die Säuglingsfürsorge der Haupt- und Residenzstadt Berlin. Berlin: III Internationaler Kongress für Säuglingsschutz, 1911.
19. Keller A: Aufgaben des Kaiserin Auguste Victoria Hauses. Festschrift. Berlin: Stilke, 1909.
20. Langstein L: Das Kaiserin Auguste Victoria Haus zur Bekämpfung der Säuglingssterblichkeit im Deutschen Reiche. Die Naturwissenschaften 1919;**7**:467–71.
21. Ylppö A: Zur Physiologie, Klinik und zum Schicksal der Frühgeborenen. Zeitschr Kinderheilk 1919;**24**:1–110.
22. Landé L: Beitrag zur Hämatologie, Ätiologie und Therapie der Frühgeburtenanämie. Zeitschr Kinderheilk 1919; **22**:295–336.
23. Crosse VM: The premature baby. 3. ed. London: Churchill, 1952: p. 114.
24. Young WF, Hallum JL, McCance RA: The secretion of urine by premature infants. Arch Dis Child 1941;**16**:243–52.
25. Meyer TC, Angus J: The effect of large doses of 'Synkavit' in the newborn. Arch Dis Child 1956;**31**:212–5.
26. Lebariller E: Sur le muguet des enfants nouveau-nés. J Med Bord 1856;2e série:672–86.
27. Denucé J-L-P: Berceau incubateur pour les enfants nés avant terme. J Med Bord 1857;**2**:723–4.
28. Rotch TM: Pediatrics. The hygienic and medical treatment of children. Edinburgh: Pentland, 1896: p. 288–317.
29. Rotch TM: The development of the hospital. Boston Med Surg J 1914;**170**:483–5.
30. Townsend CW: The hemorrhagic disease of the newborn. Arch Pediatr 1894;**11**:559–65.
31. Stein GW: Kurze Beschreibung einer Brust- oder Milchpumpe. Marburg: Academische Buchhandlung, 1774: p. 49, 64–8.
32. Stein GW: Kurze Beschreibung eines Baromacrometers und eines Cephalometers. Marburg: Academische Buchhandlung, 1789: p. 105–32.
33. Osiander FB: Beobachtungen, Abhandlungen und Nachrichten. Tübingen: Cotta, 1787: p. 273–84.
34. Soemmerring ST: Abbildungen und Beschreibungen einiger Misgeburten, die sich ehemals auf dem anatomischen Theater zu Cassel befanden. Mainz: Universitätsbuchhandlung, 1791.
35. Abt I: The technic of wetnurse management in institutions. JAMA 1917;**69**:418–20.
36. Hess JH: Premature and congenitally disabled infants. London: Churchill, 1923: p. 136.
37. Hess JH, Chamberlain IM: Premature infants. Am J Dis Child 1927;**34**:571–84.
38. Scheel P: Commentatio de liquoris amnii asperae arteriae. Hafniae: Brümmer, 1799.
39. Thamdrup E: Paediatri i Danmark. Copenhagen: Laegeforeningens forlag, 1994: p. 11–30.
40. Crichton B: Infant mortality in Dublin. Ir J Med Sci 1925;**4**:302–5.
41. Solomons B, Dowse RV, Seager PNL, et al.: Report of the Rotunda Hospital, 1932–1933. Ir J Med Sci 1934;**6**:331–86.
42. Schlossmann A: Zur Frage der natürlichen Säiglingsernährung. Arch Kinderheilk 1900;**30**:288–382.
43. Schlossmann A, Peters H: Über Häufigkeit und Ursachen des Todes bei der Anstaltsbehandlung kranker Säuglinge. Arch Kinderheilk 1902;**33**:246–84.
44. Ballantyne JW: Where obstetrics and paediatrics meet: infant welfare. Int Clin (Phila) 1916;**26**:93–106.
45. Johnstone RW: The Simpson memorial maternity pavilion, Edinburgh. Br J Obstet Gynecol 1939;**46**:1020–6.
46. Craig WS: Intracranial haemorrhage in the new-born. Arch Dis Child 1938;**13**:89–124.
47. Bosi V, Guidi G: Le sale incubatrici nella nuova science del brefotrofio. La Pediatria Napoli 1895;**3**:65.
48. Henderson CR: Infant welfare: methods of organization and administration in Italy. Am Sociol 1911;**17**:289–302.
49. Escherich T: A description of a new incubator employed in the children's hospital at Graz. Albany Med Ann 1900;Sept:1–4.
50. Escherich T: La valeur diagnostique de la radiographie chez les enfants. Revue mensuelle des maladies de l'enfance 1898;**16**:233–44.
51. Escherich T: Die Einrichtung der Säuglings-Abtheilung im Anna-Kinderspitale. Mittheilungen des Vereines der Ärzte in Steiermark 1902;**37**:45–7.
52. Pfaundler M: Physikalisch-chemische Untersuchungen an Kinderblut. Verh Dtsch Ges Kinderheilk 1904;**21**:24.
53. Moro E: Das erste Trimenon. Münch Med Wschr 1918;**42**:1147–50.
54. György P: Die Behandlung und Verhütung der Rachitis und Tetanie. Erg Inn Med Kinderheilk 1929;**36**:752–966.
55. Löfqvist E: Klinisch-statistische Untersuchungen über Frühgeborene. Acta Obstet Gynecol Scand 1931;**11**:5–165.
56. Sinkko EI: Über die Beziehung der Säuglingssterblichkeit und der Mortinatalität der Kinder zu den Schwankungen im C-Vitamingehalt der Muttermilch. Acta Paediatr 1937;**21**:407–27.
57. Martin PE: Mémoires de médecine et de chirurgie pratique sur plusieurs maladies at accidens graves, qui peuvent compliquer la grossesse, la parturation et la couche. Paris: Baillière, 1835.
58. Richard (de Nancy) CJF: Traité pratique des maladies des enfants. Paris: Baillière, 1839.
59. Montfalcon JB, Poliniere: Hygiène de la ville de Lyon. Lyon: Savy, 1845.
60. Kronenberg AH: Bemerkungen über den Soor. Journal für Kinderkrankheiten 1847;**8**:81–90.
61. Blumenthal H: Das kaiserlich Moskowische Erziehungshaus. Jahrb Kinderheilk 1861;**4**:79–89.
62. Miller NTh: Die Frühgebornen und die Eigenthümlichkeiten ihrer Krankheiten. Jahrb Kinderheilk 1886;**25**:179–94.
63. Pfaundler M: Die Antikörper-Übertragung von Mutter auf Kind. Arch Kinderheilk 1908;**47**:260.
64. Moro E: Karottensuppe bei Ernährungsstörungen der Säuglinge. Münch Med Wschr 1908;**31**:1637–40.
65. Dunham E: Mortality among prematurely born infants. J Pediatr 1936;**9**:17–22.
66. Jacobi A: History of pediatrics in New York. Arch Pediatr 1917;**34**:144–9.

67. Babies' Hospital of the City of New York: Annual reports 1903–1910. New York: Babies' Hospital, 1903.
68. Heyfelder JF: Beobachtungen über die Krankheiten der Neugeborenen. Leipzig: Hartmann, 1825: p. 63-5.
69. Denis P-S: Recherches d'anatomie et de physiologie pathologique sur plusieurs maladies des enfants nouveau-nés. Commercy: Denis, 1826.
70. Billard CM: Die Krankheiten der Neugeborenen und Säuglinge (1st French ed. 1828). Weimar: Industrie-Comptoir, 1829.
71. Obladen M: Thrush—nightmare of the foundling hospitals. Neonatology 2011;**101**:159–65.
72. Parrot J: Clinique des Nouveau-Nés: l'Athrepsie. Paris: Masson, 1877.
73. Dupoux A: Sur les pas de monsieur Vincent. Paris: Revue de l'assistance publique, 1958: p. 284–317.
74. Henry M: Fondation du pavillon des enfants débiles a la maternité de Paris. Revue mensuelle des maladies de l'Enfance 1898;**16**:142–54.
75. Budin P: Le Nourrisson. Paris: Doin, 1900: p. 111.
76. Budin P: Service des enfants débiles a la maternité. Année 1895. In: Femmes en couches et Nouveau-Nés. Paris: Doin, 1897: p. 389–405.
77. Auvard A: De la couveuse pour enfants. Arch Tocologie 1883;**14**:577–609.
78. Doepp P: Notizen über das kaiserliche Erziehungshaus (Findlingshaus) zu St. Petersburg, 1830–1833. Hamburg: Hoffmann & Campe, 1835: Vol. **5**, p. 306–50.
79. Doepp P: Notizen über das kaiserliche Erziehungshaus (Findelhaus) zu St. Petersburg, 1834–1840 umfassend. St. Petersburg, Leipzig: Hoffmann & Campe, 1842: Vol. **6**, p. 129–77.
80. Gundobin NP: Die Besonderheiten des Kindesalters. Berlin: Allgemeine Medizinische Verlagsanstalt, 1912.
81. Chapple CC: Controlling the external environment of premature infants in an incubator. Am J Dis Child 1938;**50**:459–60.
82. Epstein A: Studien zur Frage der Findelanstalten unter besonderer Berücksichtigung der Verhältnisse in Böhmen. Prague: Beyer, 1882: p. 13–36.
83. Epstein A: Statistische und hygienische Erfahrungen aus der k. böhm. Findelanstalt in Prag im Quinquennium 1880–1884. Arch Kinderheilk 1886;**7**:87–116.
84. Eröss J: Untersuchungen bezüglich der Temperaturverhältnisse und der Indicationen der künstlichen Erwärmung frühzeitig geborener Kindere. Arch Gynecol Obstet 1886;**27**:350–78.
85. Steinert E: Beiträge zur Frage des Hospitalismus und der Rolle der individuellen Pflege für das Gedeihen im Säuglingsalter. Zeitschr Kinderheilk 1921;**28**:255–94.
86. Abelin H: Ueber die Sterblichket unter jungen Kindern und über einige Ursachen derselben. Journal für Kinderkrankheiten 1864;**43**:159–200.
87. Rohmer P, Sanders U, Bezzsonoff N: Synthesis of vitamin C by the infant. Nature 1934;**134**:142–3.
88. Brown A, MacLachlan IF: Protein milk powder. Can Med Assoc J 1919;**9**:528–37.
89. Tisdall FF, Drake TGH, Brown A: A new cereal mixture containing vitamins and mineral elements. Am J Dis Child 1930;**40**: 791–9.
90. Hart AP: Familial icterus gravis of the newborn and its treatment. Can Med Assoc Journal 1925;**15**:1008–11.
91. Nebgen S, Kasper HU, Schafer D, et al.: Bednar's aphthae in neonates. Neonatology 2010;**98**:208–11.
92. Bednar A: Die Krankheiten der Neugeborenen und Säuglinge. Wien: Gerold, 1850–1853.
93. Escherich T: Die neue Säuglingsabteilung im St.-Anna-Kinderspital in Wien. Wiener Klin Wochenschr 1905;**18**:977–82.
94. Reuss ARv: Die Krankheiten des Neugeborenen. Berlin: Springer, 1914.
95. Bernheim J: Ueber Ikterus beim Neugeborenen. Schweiz Med Wochenschr 1928;**58**:1125–9.
96. Willi H: Über eine bösartige Enteritis bei Säuglingen des ersten Trimenons. Ann Pediatr 1944;**162**:87–112.
97. Baker JP: The machine in the nursery. Baltimore, MD: Johns Hopkins University Press, 1996.
98. Editorial: The danger of making a public show of incubators for babies. Lancet 1898;**151**:390–1.
99. Huldschinsky K: Heilung von Rachitis durch künstliche Höhensonne. Dtsch Med Wschr 1919;**26**:712–3.
100. Czerny A, Keller A: Des Kindes Ernährung, Ernährungsstörungen und Ernährungstherapie. 2. ed. Leipzig: Deuticke, 1925: Vol. **1**, part 2, p. 1017.
101. Schlossmann A: Die Entwicklung der Versorgung kranker Säuglinge in Anstalten. Erg Inn Med Kinderheilk 1923;**24**: 188–209.
102. Feer E: Bau und Einrichtung des Kinderkrankenhauses. Monatsschr Kinderheilk 1928;**41**:227–41.
103. Dwork D: War is good for babies and other young children. London: Tavistock, 1987.
104. Report on the 3rd International Congress on Infant Protection (Gouttes de lait), Berlin 1911. Berlin: Stilke, 1912.
105. Rommel O: Frühgeburt und Lebensschwäche. In: Pfaundler M, Schlossmann A: Handbuch der Kinderheilkunde. Leipzig: Vogel, 1906: Vol. **I**, p. 491–506.

APPENDIX 3

Synchronoptic timetable

Table A3.1 shows the neonate's progress within the cultural environment. It contains events that influenced the infant's position in society and its chance of surviving. Any selection of facts must be incomplete and imperfect owing to the inclusion or exclusion of events, people, works, and publications.

Table A3.1 The neonate's progress within the cultural environment

Sociocultural/political development; legislation concerning newborns	Scientific and technology milestones, institutions concerning newborns	Progress in fetal/neonatal medicine; publications concerning newborns
2500 B.C.E. Mesopotamian incantations and rituals to protect newborns	3400 B.C.E. Writing evolved in Sumeria and Egypt	45,000 B.C.E. Iraq: Neanderthals shaped infant's heads. Practice persisted in many cultures
2000 B.C.E. Egypt: malformed infants (anencephaly, achondroplasia) venerated and embalmed	1750 B.C.E. Wet nursing regulated in Hammurabi law 1550 B.C.E. Egypt: papyrus *Ebers*; opiates against excessive crying	1500 B.C.E. Shuma Izbu: Cuneiform catalogue of Babylonian and Assyrian omens for many congenital malformations
1600–200 B.C.E. Phoenician–Punic cult of (firstborn) infant sacrifice. Forbidden by laws of Moses 700 b.c.e. Rome: Law of Numa Pompilius: postmortem sectio in mother compulsory	650 B.C.E. Ninive, Assyrian Empire: more than 20,000 books in cuneiform tablets collected in Ashurbanipal's library 500 B.C.E. Athens, *Amphidromia*: ritual acceptance and name-giving on fifth day	500 B.C.E. Hippocratic Corpus, Kos: *The eight months' infant*. Calculation of gestational age. Fetal somersault. 360 B.C.E. Plato, Athens: *The laws*. Recommend tight swaddling for 2 years
450 B.C.E. Roman Law of Twelve Tables ordered the killing of malformed infants	400 B.C.E. Highly sophisticated metal tools in Latène culture	350 B.C.E. Aristotle, Athens: *History of animals. Generation of animals*. Tongue-tie
264–146 B.C.E. Punic wars, Carthago destroyed	50 B.C.E. Egypt: Cleopatra ordered the study of fetuses of executed pregnant women	
103 C.E. Trajan's alimentary law: financial support for children in poor regions		163 C.E. Galen of Pergamon, Rome: *Usefulness of the parts. On hygiene. On forming the fetus*
315 C.E. Emperor Constantine, Rome: Christianization of Roman empire. State law to maintain poor and exposed infants	272 C.E. Egypt: Alexandria library destroyed, scientific literature lost 324 C.E. Roman capital moved to Constantinople	98–138 C.E. Soranus of Ephesus, Rome: *Gynecology*: on midwifery and newborn care
410/455 C.E. Sack of Rome by Visigoths and Vandals	442 C.E. Council of Vaison offers protection to foundlings	412 C.E. Saint Augustine's dogma of original sin placed unbaptized deceased infants in hell
533 C.E. Emperor Justinian, Constantinople: set an end to the father's right to kill his offspring. Foundlings no longer enslaved	622 C.E. Mohammed's flight from Mecca to Medina. Begin of the spread of Islam	300/442 C.E. Councils of Elvira/Vaison forbade infanticide and ordered to protect foundlings
800 C.E. Charlemagne coronated as Holy Roman Emperor	787 C.E. Archbishop Datheus founded Milan asylum for abandoned infants	660 C.E. Paul of Aegina, Alexandria: *Surgical procedures for congenital malformations*
1096–1099 First Crusade 1163 Council of Tours:	910 Benedictine abbey Cluny 968 Cordoba: Arabian university with large library 970 Byzantine encyclopaedia *Souda* 1198 Rome Hospital Santo Spirito	900 Rhazes, Persia: *liber ad Almansorem* ca. 1000 Ibn-Sina (Avicenna), Hamadan: *Canon medicinae*
1292 Marco Polo's China travel	1158 Bologna University 1180 Montpellier University 1200 Salerno School of Medicine 1222 Padova University 1243 Salamanca University 1249 Oxford University	1250 Trotula: ensemble of three *Treatises on diseases of women* 1254 Thomas Aquinas: *Limbo doctrine*: painless edge of hell for unbaptized dead infants
1299 After defeating Genova, the Republic of Venice became leading power in the Mediterranean	1296 Bernard de Gordon: Caesarean section in deceased mother 1348 Plague killed 25 million Europeans	1310 Translation of Galen's *De usu partium* into Latin by Nicolas of Reggio

(continued)

Table A3.1 *Continued*

Sociocultural/political development; legislation concerning newborns	Scientific and technology milestones, institutions concerning newborns	Progress in fetal/neonatal medicine; publications concerning newborns
1337–1453 Hundred Years' War in France and England	1439 Strasbourg cathedral finished, highest building of mankind	
1424 Midwives' rule of Brussels 1437–1440 European famine 1451 Midwives' rule of Regensburg 1453 Osmans conquer Constantinople, end of Byzantine Empire	1445 Florence Foundling Hospital degli Innocenti 1450 Johann Gutenberg, Mainz: printing with moveable type 1457 Freiburg University	1473 Bartholomäus Metlinger, Augsburg: *Regimen of young infants*
1484 Pope Innozent VIII, *summis desiderantes*, established inquisition 1486 *Malleus maleficarum*: start of the European witch hunt	1437–40 European famine followed crop failures 1472 Copernicus' planetary system 1492 Columbus's first landing, begin of the *conquista*	1473 Paulus Bagellardus, Padova: *Little booklet of infants' diseases*
1517 Martin Luther, Wittenberg, publishes his theses triggering the Reformation	1510 Leonardo da Vinci, *Codex Windsor*: studies of pregnant uterus and fetus	1513 Eucharius Rösslin: *Der Swangern Frawen und Hebammen Rosegarten*
1520 Ferdinand Magellan travelled around the world	1536 Paris: Hospice de Enfants-Dieu, for orphans and foundlings	1544 Thomas Phaire, *The boke of children*
1534 Henry VIII founds Anglican church to obtain divorce 1545–1563 Council of Trent 1558–1603 Reign of Elizabeth I in England	1543 Andreas Vesalius, Padua: *De humani corporis fabrica* 1573 Ambroise Paré: *Generation of man/treaty of monsters*	1564 Cesare Aranzio, Bologna: *De humano foetu*. Ductus venosus and arteriosus described 1565 Simon Vallambert, Orleans: *De la manière*. Syphilitic infant may infect the nurse
1562 Mesoamerica: start of organized slave trade. Inca Empire extinguished by *conquista* and smallpox	1593 Galileo Galilei, Padua: water thermometer 1594 Padova Anatomical Theatre	1583 Girolamo Mercuriale, Padova: *De puerorum morbis tractatus*. Resuscitation
1608 Venice Senate: severe punishment for failed Caesarean delivery in a dead mother 1618–1648 Thirty Years' War in Europe	1610 Galileo observes Jupiter moons with telescope 1633 René Descartes: *On man and on the formation of the fetus*	1609 Louise Bourgeois, Paris: *Observations* 1612 Felix Würtz, Basel: *The children's book*
1620 Maximum of transatlantic slave-trade from Africa to America	1640 St. Vincent de Paul and Mme Legras open the Foundling Hospital of Paris	1628 William Harvey, London: *On the motion of the heart and blood in animals*. 1651 *De generatione*
1643–1715 Reign of Louis XIV in France	Before 1650 William Chamberlen: obstetric forceps (published by Edmund Chapman in 1733)	1645 Daniel Whistler, Leyden: *De morbo puerili Anglorum*; 1650 Francis Glisson, London: *De rachitide*
1666 Great Fire of London	1670 Isaac Newton, a former preterm infant, founded differential calculation and laws of gravity	1668 François Mauriceau: *Treatise on pregnant women and deliveries* 1672 Isbrand Diemerbroeck: *Anatomy*. Correct description of placental circulation
1683 Maximum of Turkish expansion in Europe	1674 Antonie van Leeuwenhoek, Delft: microscope detected bacteria and cells	1689 Walter Harris, London, *Treatise*: calcium salt for infantile convulsions 1690 Justine Siegemund: *The Brandenburg court midwive*
1716 Midwives' rule of New York	1717 Gabriel Fahrenheit, Den Haag: mercury thermometer	
1740 Pope Benedict XIV regulated conditions for emergency baptism	1741 Thomas Coram: London Foundling Hospital. 1742 Georg F. Händel: Messiah to benefit London Foundling Hospital	1733 James Calder, Edinburgh: duodenal atresia 1735 Carl Linné: *Systema naturae* 1740 Johann Peter Süßmilch, Berlin: population statistics
1751 Inquisitor Francesco Cangiamila, Palermo: *Embryologia sacra*: church rules for baptism and neonatal resuscitation	1752 Benjamin Franklin, Philadelphia: lightning conductor	1752 William Smellie, London: *Treatise on the theory and practise of midwifery* 1759 Herman Boerhaave/Gerard van Swieten: *Infants' diseases* 1759 Angélique Le Boursier Du Coudray: *Art of obstetrics*
1761 Jean Jacques Rousseau: emile, or education 1756–1763 Seven-Years' War	1763 Moscow Foundling Hospital 1769 James Watt, Glasgow: improved steam engine starts Industrial Revolution 1770 St. Petersburg Foundling Hospital	1764 Nils Rosen von Rosenstein, Upsala: *Treatise on children's diseases*; 1753 Georg Roederer, Göttingen; and 1775 Georg W. Stein, Cassel: *Neonatal body measurements*
1776 Philadelphia: Declaration of Independence signed 1782 Last European 'witch' executed in Switzerland	1772 Carl Scheele, Göteborg, and 1775 Joseph Priestley, Birmingham, independently discovered oxygen 1782 Harvard Medical School	1780 François Chaussier, Dijon/Paris: oxygen-supplied ventilator for neonates; 1806 Silver endotracheal tube for newborns 1784 Michael Underwood, London: *Treatise on diseases of children*
1789 French Revolution 1789 US Constitution ratified 1791 Human Rights Declaration 1796–1815 Napoleonic Wars. Holy Roman Empire dissolved.	1785 Antoine Lavoisier, Paris, named oxygen 1793 Paris: surgeons incorporated in medical faculty 1798 Paul Scheel, Copenhagen: elastic endotracheal tube for neonates	1788 Jean Baptiste Baumes, Montpellier: *Treatise on jaundice of newborn infants* 1788 Hezekiah Beardsley, New Haven: *Hypertrophic pyloric stenosis of infancy*

Table A3.1 Continued

Sociocultural/political development; legislation concerning newborns	Scientific and technology milestones, institutions concerning newborns	Progress in fetal/neonatal medicine; publications concerning newborns
1811 Napoleon's decree on organization and financing the foundling hospitals 1815 Waterloo battle ends Napoleon's expansion in Europe	1792 Dr Brand, Leiden: Caesarean delivery, mother and child survived 1800 London: Royal College of Surgeons; 1800 Alessandro Volta, Pavia: electric battery 1802 New England Journal of Medicine	1812 Marie Anne Boivin, Paris: *Mémorial de l'art des accouchemens* 1819 Elias v Siebold, Würzburg: preterm delivery in obstructed pelvis
1815 Congress of Vienna redistribution of European states 1818 Steamship Savannah crosses Atlantic 1829 Paris Academy verdict against artificial ventilation for resuscitation	1804 François Chaussier director of the Paris Maternité 1819 René TH Laennec, Paris: stethoscope. 1822 François Baron: neonatal version 1822 MJ Lejumeau de Kergaradec, Paris: obstetric stethoscope	1828 Charles Michel Billard, Paris: *Treatise on the diseases on neonates and infants* 1835 Eduard Jörg, Leipzig: *The fetal lung in the child who is born*
1845–1851 Irish famine 1849 Paris: Assistance Publique founded	1841 Fredrik Berg and David Gruby, Paris: identified thrush fungus, first pathogen microbe 1847 Ignaz Semmelweis, Budapest: antisepsis in the delivery room	1845 Ernest Bouchut, Paris: *Treatise on the diseases of newborns and infants* 1850 Alois Bednar, Vienna: *Treatise on the diseases of newborns and infants*
1848 British Public Health Act improved sewage and water supply	1854 New York Nursing and Child Hospital; Children's Hospital Philadelphia 1856 Gail Borden, Galveston: patent on milk condensation 1860 Abraham Jacobi: paediatric chair in New York	1857 Jean-Paul Denucé, Bordeaux: *Berceau incubator for preterm infants*
1861–1865 US Civil War	1859 Ferdinand Carré, Paris: absorption refrigerator 1863 Louis Pasteur, Paris: one-time heating reduces bacterial growth	1859 Charles Darwin, London: *The origin of species* 1886 Franz v. Soxhlet, Munich: apparatus to pasteurize milk
1870 Unification of Italy 1870–1871 German-French War 1871 Unification of Germany	1863 Casimir Davaine, Paris: bacteria can cause diseases 1867 Joseph Lister, Glasgow: antisepsis	
1873 France: Loi Roussel 1875 Paris metre convention harmonized mass and length units in Europe	1867 Henri Nestlé, Vevey: powdered infant food 1878 Joseph W Swan, Gateshead UK: long-lasting electric lightbulb 1882 Robert Koch, Berlin: tuberculosis bacilli (Nobel Prize 1905) 1885 Carl Benz, Mannheim: auto-mobile with combustion engine	1875 Johannes Orth, Berlin: *Bilirubin crystals in neonates with kernicterus* 1880 Philipp Biedert, Hagenau: *Treatise on infant nutrition* 1884 Stéphane Tarnier, Paris: closed incubator
1890 USA Milk Commission: *Clean Milk Crusade on the American Continent*	1893 Stéphane Tarnier, Paris: the weaklings' pavilion. Incubators 1895 Wilhelm C Roentgen, Würzburg: X-rays (Nobel Prize 1901) 1897 Emil Fischer, Berlin: caffeine synthesis (Nobel Prize 1902)	1891 John Ballantyne, Edinburgh: Royal Maternity Hospital. Several books on fetal/neonatal medicine 1894 C.W. Townsend, Boston: *Hemorrhagic disease of newborn*
1893 Pierre Budin, Paris, *Gouttes de lait* = Society for Social Hygiene for Infants	1898 Arthur Schlossmann, Dresden: hospital for sick infants 1898 Theodor Escherich, Graz: Annaspital with heated chamber for preterm infants	1898 L. Emmett Holt, New York: *Diseases of infancy and childhood* 1898 Max Rubner: energy quotient by calorimetry
1903 Kitty Hawk, NC: Wright brothers fly heavier-than-air plane	1900 Karl Landsteiner, Vienna: ABO blood groups (Nobel Prize 1930)	1900 Infant mortality rates: Finland 153, France 160, Germany 229, Italy 174, Netherlands 155, Russia 253, Sweden 99, Switzerland 150, UK 141, US 140
1905 Paris: 1st International Congress to prevent infant mortality (Gouttes de lait) 1907 Brussels: 2nd International Congress to prevent infant mortality (Gouttes de lait) 1911 Berlin: 3rd International Congress to prevent infant mortality	1907 Jacob Bernheim, Zürich: Infant Hospital Rosenberg 1909 Leo Langstein, Berlin: Kaiserin Auguste Victoria Haus, hospital for sick and preterm infants	1900 Pierre Budin, Paris: *The nursling* 1910 Paul Ehrlich; *Salvarsan against syphilis* (Nobel prize 1908). 1914 August Reuss, Vienna: *Diseases of the newborn* 1919 Arvo Ylppö, Berlin: *Three treatises on preterm infants*
1912 US Children's Bureau 1914–1918 World War I 1917 Russian revolution: Tsar's regime replaced by communists	1915 Julius Hess, Chicago: incubator unit at Michael Reese Hospital 1921 Oxygen administration became standard for preterm infants with apnoea	1922 Julius Hess, Chicago: *Premature and congenitally disabled infants*
1921 US: Sheppard-Towner Bill guaranteed healthcare for poor mothers and infants	1927 Philip Drinker, Boston: iron lung 1928 Alexander Fleming, Oxford: penicillin (Nobel Prize 1945)	1925 Alfred Hart, Toronto: exchange transfusion for familial jaundice (erythroblastosis) 1930 Nicholson Eastman, Baltimore: *Fetal blood studies*
1929 Great Depression, unemployment rates up to 33% in US	1929 Kurt v. Neergaard, Basel: surface tension of lung alveoli 1930 American Academy of Pediatrics	1932 Louis K Diamond, Kenneth Blackfan, and James M Batty, Boston: *Hydrops fetalis, icterus gravis, and anemia of the newborn are all 'erythroblastosis fetalis'*

(continued)

Table A3.1 *Continued*

Sociocultural/political development; legislation concerning newborns	Scientific and technology milestones, institutions concerning newborns	Progress in fetal/neonatal medicine; publications concerning newborns
1933 Nazi Regime in Germany. Jewish scientists prosecuted. From 1939, organized murder of handicapped infants	1936 Henrik Dam, Copenhagen, and Edward A. Doisy, St. Louis: coagulation Vitamin K (Nobel Prize 1943).	1939 Philip Levine, Rufus E. Stetson, Newark: rhesus factor
1939–1945 World War II	1941 Konrad Zuse, Berlin: software-controlled computer	1942 Theodore Terry, Boston: *Retrolental fibroplasia in preterm infants* 1944 Heinrich Willi, Zürich: *Necrotizing enterocolitis* 1944 Alfred E. Barclay, Kenneth J. Franklin, Oxford: *The foetal circulation*
1943 Ethel Dunham, Washington Childrens' Bureau: *Standards and recommendations for the hospital care of newborn infants*	1944 Alfred Blalock, Baltimore: subclavian-pulmonary shunt in tetralogy of Fallot 1940–1960 Retrolental fibroplasia blinded over 10,000 children worldwide due to unrestricted oxygen	1946 Clement A. Smith, Boston: *The physiology of the newborn infant* 1946 Joseph Barcroft, Cambridge: *Researches on pre-natal life* 1947 Helen B. Taussig, Baltimore: *Congenital heart malformations*
1945 Division of Europe, Cold War 1948 National Health Service, UK 1948 Geneva: World Health Organization	1946 Louis K. Diamond: exchange transfusion through the umbilical vein to treat erythroblastosis fetalis	1951 Victoria M. Crosse, Birmingham, and Kate Campbell, Melbourne: *Oxygen responsible for retrolental fibroplasia*
1949 Nuremberg and following trials acquitted German physicians who had killed handicapped babies	1952 James Watson and Francis Crick, Oxford: double-helix structure of DNA (Nobel Prize 1962) 1953 Leland C. Clark, Yellow Springs, OH: PO_2 electrode	1952 Virginia Apgar, New York: score for evaluating the condition of the newborn 1953 Poul Astrup, Copenhagen: developed blood gas analysis during polio epidemic
1956 Egypt took over Suez Canal	1956 John Clements, Edgewood, MD: surfactant function and action 1957 Alexandre Minkowski, Paris: editor, *Biology of the Neonate* 1958 John W. Severinghaus, Bethesda: PCO_2 electrode	1956 Eugen Spitz, John D Holter, Philadelphia: cerebral shunt 1957 Gösta Rooth, Lund: neonatal PO_2 measurement. 1958 Richard J Cremer, Rochford, Essex: *Light effect on hyperbilirubinemia*
1957 European Economic Community established	1958 Ian Donald, Glasgow: B-mode obstetric ultrasound 1959 Jerome Lejeune, Paris: trisomy 21 in Down syndrome 1960 Louis Gluck, New Haven CT: neonatal intensive care unit at Yale	1958 L. Stanley James: acid–base status of human infant 1958 Geoffrey Dawes, Oxford: *Pathophysiology of fetal asphyxia*
1961 Russia puts astronaut Juri Gagarin into orbit around earth	1963 Sune Bergstrom, Stockholm, and 1971 John Vane, London: prostaglandin metabolism (Nobel Prize 1982) 1966 Osmund Reynolds, London: neonatal intensive care unit at University College Hospital	1959 Mary Ellen Avery and Jere Mead, Boston: *Surfactant deficiency causes RDS* 1960 Alexander Schaffer, Baltimore, coined the terms *neonatology* and *neonatologist*
1961–1963 John F. Kennedy US president. Founded National Institute for Child Health and Development	1963 Robert Guthrie (Albany, NY): test for detecting phenylketonuria in the newborn period	1957–1962 Thalidomide catastrophe: around 10,000 infants with malformed limbs 1963 Lula Lubchenco, Denver: charts of fetal growth
1967 Christiaan Barnard performed human heart transplantation	1968 Claudine Amiel-Tison, Paris: neurological assessment of gestational age 1968 Louis Gluck, San Diego: LS-ratio to assess pulmonary maturity	1969 Dietrich Lübbers, Renate Huch, Albert Huch, Marburg: transcutaneous PO_2 1971 George Gregory et al., San Francisco: *Continuous positive airway pressure for RDS*
1981 Oxford database on perinatal trials; later Cochrane collaboration	1972 Bengt Robertson, Stockholm: porcine surfactant	1975 Michael Heyman, San Francisco: indomethacin for ductus closure
1989 Fall of the Berlin Wall, end of the Cold War	1980 Richard R. Ernst, Zurich: magnetic resonance spectroscopy (Nobel Prize 1991)	1980 Tetsuro Fujiwara, Tokyo *Surfactant substitution in preterm infants with RDS* 1984 Edward M Connor, *Maternal-infant HIV-transmission reduced by zidovudine* 1992 John P Kinsella et al., Denver: *Inhaled NO for persisting pulmonary hypertension*
1992 Maastricht treaty transforms European Economic Community in European Union	2000 Francis Collins and Craig Venter: mapping the human genome	2000 Infant mortality rates: Finland 3.8, France 4.5, Germany 4.4, Italy 4.5, Netherlands 5.1, Russia 20.5, Sweden 3.4, Switzerland 5.3, UK 5.6, US 6.9

Glossary of abbreviations and medical and foreign language terms

Abdomen, abdominal related to the belly
Abstinence syndrome symptoms in a baby whose mother is habituated to opiates
Acardius twin fetus without a heart
Accoucheur French: obstetrician, male midwife
Acidosis excessive acidity in blood or tissue
Acrid sharp or biting taste or smell
Adaptation adjusting to (postnatal) conditions
Adrenal concerning the hormone-producing adrenal glands
Aetiology origin and causes of diseases
Ailment disorder
Alimentary concerning food or digestion
Alkali basic ionic salt, yielding pH above 7.0 when dissolved in water
Alveolus, alveolar air exchange pockets in the lung
Amino acids protein compounds
Amnion internal membrane surrounding the unborn and forming the amniotic cavity
Amniotic fluid watery liquid in which the fetus is suspended
Amulet object believed to protect from danger or disease
Analeptic drug that stimulates the central nervous system
Anastomosis communication between vessels
Anencephaly congenital absence of the brain
Angioma benign tumor from blood vessels
Animatio Latin: ensoulment
Ankyloglossia tongue-tie
Anodyne quieting, relieving pain
Antigen protein which, introduced into the body, stimulates the production of antibodies
Aorta main trunk of the arterial system
Apgar score a point system to rapidly tally the newborn's health at birth
Aphthae white specks on mouth and tongue of infants with thrush
Apnoea, apnoic temporary cessation of breathing
Apocryphical Christian gospel not included in the New Testament
Apoptosis programmed cell death

Aqueous watery
Arcuccio Italian: structure to prevent overlaying the baby
Artery, arterial blood vessel carrying blood away from the heart
Artefact man-made object
Ascites excess fluid accumulated in the peritoneal cavity
Asphyxia lack of oxygen with increase of carbon dioxide
Asphyxia livida/pallida asphyxia with blue/pale skin color
Atelectasis incomplete expansion of the lungs
Atresia absence or narrowing of a body channel
Autopsy examination of a dead body (also postmortem)

Balia Italian: wet nurse
Baptism Christian rite using water for ritual purification
Basal concerning the lower part of a structure
Basal ganglia part of the brain
B.C.E. before current era; before birth of Jesus Christ
Beestings first milk secreted after birth (colostrum)
Biberon French: feeding bottle
Bilirubin reddish-yellow pigment in bile and blood
Birth asphyxia condition resulting from lack of oxygen
Blastocyst early stage of the embryo, formed 4 days after fertilization
Blemmyes legendary creatures lacking a head
Bovine concerning cows
Bradycardia slow heart rate
Breech lower part of the trunk
Breech birth delivery of a baby bottom-first
Bronchopulmonary dysplasia chronic lung disorder of preterm infants
Bronze Age prehistoric era of human history when metal began to be widely used (3300–1200 B.C.E.)
Bull, encyclica Papal letter concerning Catholic doctrines

Calorimeter apparatus for measuring heat generation
Candida albicans a yeast causing localized or systemic infection (thrush)
Canon law a body of laws made by ecclesiastical authority

Cardiac concerning the heart
Cardiotocography, CTG electronic recording of fetal heartbeat and uterine contractions before birth
Casein protein in milk
c.e. current era, after the birth of Jesus Christ
Cephalhematoma bleeding outside the skull, beginning at birth
Cerebral concerning the brain
Cerebral palsy movement disorder resulting from trauma to the immature brain
Chalcolithic prehistoric era of human history from 4500 to 2300 b.c.e. (also: Copper Age)
Changeling sick child believed to have been switched for a stolen baby
Chemoreceptor a sensory cell that converts a chemical substance into a biological signal
Cholera infantum diarrhea in infants
Cholestasis arrested bile flow
Chorion external membrane surrounding the unborn. In the placenta, its villi enable transfer of substances between mother and fetus
Chromosome threadlike body carrying the genes
Circumcision removal of the foreskin from the human penis
Coagulopathy disease affecting blood coagulation
Coagulum clot of milk or blood
Codex bound manuscript volume
Cognitive concerning mental abilities
Colostrum first milk secreted after birth, with immune function
Congenital condition present at birth, regardless of causation
Conjoined identical twins sharing parts of the body
Contagion infectious matter
Contagiosity state of being able to transfer an infection
Corpus collection of books concerning a specific era or topic
Cotyledon part of the placenta with circumscribed fetal circulation
Council an ecclesiastical assembly deciding doctrinal matters
Couveuse French: incubator, heated bed
Cuneiform tables Sumerean or Babylonic clay tablets with text

Debility weakness
Dehydration abnormal loss of water from the body
Dental, dentition concerning teeth, breeding of teeth
Dextrine polysaccharide obtained by heating of starch
Diacodium sirup made from poppy juice
Diaphragm membrane separating adjacent regions (e.g. midriff)
Diarrhea Abnormally loose stool
Diploid cell with two chromosome sets, e.g. 46 in humans
Dispensary outpatient department of hospital providing free treatment
Dissociation process of splitting molecules into smaller particles
Diuretic drug that promotes the secretion of urine
Dizygotic twins resulting from two different fertilized eggs; also called non-identical or fraternal

DNA deoxyribonucleic acid, material carrying the genetic information
Docimasia French: lung flotation test
Doctrine a principle or policy taught or advocated although not proven
Dorsal situated at the back
Down's syndrome disorder resulting from an extra chromosome (trisomy 21)
Dry nursing taking care of an infant but not suckling it (= hand feeding)
Ductus arteriosus connection between main lung artery and aorta
Dyspnea difficult breathing, shortness of breath

Electroencephalography, EEG record of the brain's electrical activity, usually with multiple electrodes placed on the scalp
Elizabethan era epoch from 1558 to 1603 in British history
Embryo the unborn from day 15 after fertilization up to the end of organ formation (day 56)
Encephalitis inflammation of the brain tissue
Encephalopathy generalized disorder of the brain
Endemic disease peculiar to a certain geographical region
Endogenous caused by factors inside the organism
Endothelium cell layer that lines the inner surface of blood vessels
Enfants trouvés French: foundlings
Enlightenment philosophical movement in the 18th century valuing the power of human reason and education
Ensoulment theological doctrine that ascertains a time at which the unborn is endowed with a soul
Enteral concerning the gut or digestion
Enterocolitis infection or inflammation of the bowel
Epidemic disease affecting many persons simultaneously
Epigenetic theory assumption, that environmental factors acting on an individual may become inheritable
Epilepsy brain diseases with recurrent seizures
Epistemology branch of philosophy concerned with the theory of knowledge
Epithelium cell layer that covers the outer surface of organs and skin
Ethnology branch of anthropology that analyses and compares human cultures
Evaporation drawing moisture from a substance, as by heat
Evidence based treatment or intervention based on well-designed research
Exorcism a magic formula or spell to expel demons or devils
Extremely low birthweight birthweight less than 1000 g

Farinaceous mealy, containing flour
Fertilization union of oocyte and sperm, usually occurring in fallopian tube
Fetopathy disorder of the unborn fetus
Fetus, foetus the unborn from day 56 after fertilization to birth

Folate vitamin B$_9$ required for red cell formation and neural tube closure
Foramen ovale opening between the left and right heart atrium
Forceps an instrument used to extract the infant during birth
Formula baby milk with defined combination of ingredients
Fortifier supplement added to human milk for the nutrition of preterm infants; contains protein, minerals, and trace elements
French Revolution historic epoch from 1789 to 1799
Frenotomy operation whereby the band of the tongue is cut
Fructose fruit sugar, monosaccharide of many fruits

Galactopoiesis secretion of milk
Gametes mature reproductive cells (oocyte, sperm)
Gastroenteritis inflammation of stomach and gut
Gavage French: tube feeding
Glucocorticoids a group of steroid hormones produced by the adrenal glands
Glucose blood sugar, main source of energy metabolism
Glycogen branched polysaccharide, the energy storage form of glucose
Gonadotropins hormones secreted by anterior pituitary regulating reproductive functions
Goutte de lait French: milk drop (dispensary for infants)
Gruel liquid food made by boiling oatmeal in water or milk
Gumma syphilitic excrescence
Guttus Latin: drop. A vessel to feed infants

Habilitation academic qualification corresponding to PhD
Haemangioma benign tumour composed of blood vessels and endothelia
Haematemesis vomiting blood
Haematoma localized collection of blood outside vessels
Haemoglobin oxygen-transporting metalloprotein in red blood cells
Haemolysis rupture of red blood cells releasing haemoglobin
Haemolytic disease disease that destroys red blood cells
Haemophilia genetic blood clotting disorder
Haemorrhage bleeding
Haemorrhagic disease disorder with excessive bleeding
Hand feeding dry nursing; artificial feeding with a bottle
Haploid cell with a single set of chromosomes, e.g. 23 in humans
Hellin's rule mathematical model to calculate the frequency of multiple birth
Hemiplegia paralysis of one side of the body
Hepar, hepatic concerning the liver
Hereditary trait or disease passed from parents to offspring by specific sequences in the DNA code within a chromosome
Hippocratic concerning a collection of Greek medical texts from the 5th to the 3rd century B.C.E.
Holoprosencephaly malformation in which the forebrain fails to develop into two hemispheres

Horus falcon-headed Egyptian deity
Hyaline membrane disease respiratory distress syndrome. Today: surfactant deficiency
Hydrocephaly excess fluid accumulation in the brain ventricles
Hypoplasia incomplete development of an organ
Hypoxia oxygen deprivation
Hypoxic-ischaemic brain damage brain injury resulting from lack of oxygen or perfusion

Iconoclasm 16th century movement destroying religious images and opposing their veneration
Icterus, jaundice yellow discoloration of the skin due to excess of bilirubin
Imagination doctrine the belief that maternal mental processes may cause malformations in the fetus
Implantation attachment of the blastocyst to the uterus mucosa
IMR infant mortality rate: number of infants deceased up to 1 year of age, per 1000 liveborn infants
Incidence probability of a condition's occurrence during a specified time period in a population
Infanticide killing of unweaned or otherwise maternally dependent offspring
Intestinal related to the gut
Intracranial situated within the head
Intubation introduction of tube into a hollow organ (windpipe)
Iron Age prehistoric era of human history from 1200 to 350 B.C.E.
Ischaemia locally deficient blood flow to tissue

Jurisdiction court's authority to decide a case

Kernicterus German: destruction of basal ganglia by bilirubin

Lactation breast milk production
Lactogenesis mammary gland transformation to produce milk
Lactose milk sugar, disaccharide composed of glucose and galactose
Lateral situated on a side
Laudanum tincture of opium
Legislation law enacted by a governing body
Lesion localized organ injury
Lethality death rate of a disease; also: fatality
Leukomalacia injury to the brain's white matter
Limbus puerorum, limbo edge of hell, abode of unbaptized infants
Litigation taking a conflict to court in order to obtain a judgement
L/S ratio (lecithin/sphingomyelin) test of amniotic fluid to assess fetal lung maturity

Malrotation failure of the embryo's internal organs to rotate normally
Maltose malt sugar, disaccharide composed of two glucose residues

Glossary of abbreviations and medical and foreign language terms

Mammalia animals that nourish their young with milk
Maternal concerning the mother
Meconium black tarry substance in the fetal gut, excreted within the first days after birth
Melaena passing tarry stools due to presence of blood
Meneur French: a man transporting foundlings to caregivers at the countryside
Meningocele spinal malformation with the membrane sac protruding between the vertebrae
Menstrua Latin: monthly discharge of blood from uterus
Mercury quicksilver
Mesolithic prehistoric era of human history from 10,000 to 5000 B.C.E.
Miasma, miasmatic foul air believed to cause disease
Microcephaly abnormally small head with diminished brain
Microvilli microscopic protrusions that increase the cell surface
Middle Ages, medieval historic period from 5th to 15th century
Miswatching the belief, that maternal visual impressions may cause malformations in the fetus
Mithridate drug mixture believed to act as poison antidote
Mongolism previous name for Down's syndrome
Monochorionic shared chorion sac in monozygotic twins
Monozygotic twins resulting from a single fertilized egg; also called identical
Morbidity prevalence of a disease in a specific population
Morphine opium's main active alkaloid
Mortality deaths in a defined population (e.g. infants up to 1 year of age)
Mucus, mucosal viscous matter discharged from nose, lungs, etc.
Muguet French: thrush. A fungal yeast infection
Myocardial concerning the heart muscle

Naevus Latin: birthmark: circumscribed chronic lesion on skin
Neanderthals species of archaic humans extinct 40,000 years ago
Necropolis ancient cemetery distant from a city
Necrotizing local process leading to tissue death
Neolithic prehistoric era of human history, from 6500 to 3500 B.C.E.
Neonatal period after birth up to day 28 of life
Neural tube embryonal structure that develops into brain and spinal cord
Nourrice French: wet nurse

Odds ratio statistic that quantifies the strength of an association
Oedema abnormal accumulation of water in the body
Oesophageal atresia congenital absence of an opening in the gullet
Oligohydramnios shortage of amniotic fluid
Omphalo- concerning the navel
Ontologic related to the philosophical study of being
Ophthalmia severe eye inflammation
Opium dried juice of unripe poppy capsules
Osmosis dissolved molecules moving through a semipermeable membrane
Ovulation release of an egg from the ovary

-pagus combining suffix specifying the site of attachment in conjoined twins
Palaeolithic prehistoric era of human history, from 2.5 million to 10,000 B.C.E.
Palsy paralysis, often accompanied by weakness and loss of feeling
Panada semi-liquid food made by boiling bread in broth or milk
Pap semi-liquid food made by boiling flour in water or milk
Papulous circumscribed, solid elevations of the skin
Parenteral outside the alimentary canal, usually by intravenous route
Pasteurization heating food (e.g. milk) to a specific temperature to reduce germs
Patent ductus arteriosus unclosed connection between aorta and pulmonary artery
Pathogen microorganism causing a specific disease
PDA patent ductus arteriosus
Pelvis ring of bones supporting the back and abdomen
Penance punishment for a sin, imposed by the church
Perfusion passage of blood through an organ's circulatory system
Perinatal concerning events that occur to the infant after 28 weeks of pregnancy and within the first week after birth
Peritoneum, peritoneal membrane lining the cavity of the belly and covering the intestines
Periventricular referring to the white matter around the brain ventricles
Pharyngeal referring to the throat
Phlegm liquid secreted by mucous glands. In ancient medicine one of the four humours that had to be balanced to stay healthy
Phototherapy applying light to the skin to break down bilirubin in jaundice
Pigbel infectious disease of the gut in a person who eats much meat following a period of starvation
Pineal gland endocrine gland of the brain that produces melatonin
Placenta tissue consisting of blood vessels across which nutrients and oxygen pass to the fetus
Pleistocene geological epoch from 2.5 million to 11,700 years ago (ice age)
Plethoric full of blood
Pneuma Greek: warm air, but also spirit
Pneumothorax abnormal air leak into pleura space between lung and chest wall
Polyhydramnios excess of amniotic fluid
Polyovulation release of several eggs at the same time
Postmenstrual number of weeks/days since first day of last menstruation
Postnatal concerning events that occur to the infant after birth

Postpartum concerning events that occur to the mother after birth

Post-term extension of pregnancy beyond 42 weeks of gestation

Pox, pocky concerning syphilis

Pre-embryo the unborn from fertilization until appearance of the primitive streak (day 15)

Preformationism theory that organisms originate from their miniature versions (homunculi) in the egg (ovists) or in the sperm (animalculists)

Premature, preterm born before 37 weeks of pregnancy are completed

Prenatal concerning events that occur before birth

Prevalence proportion of total disease cases in a population at a given time

Proboscis elongated trunk-like appendage from the front replacing the nose in certain malformations

Prognosis forecast of a disease's probable course

Prostaglandins group of hormones acting on smooth muscles and vessels

Prothrombin blood-clotting protein formed by the liver

Pulmo, pulmonary concerning the lungs

Pulmonary stenosis narrowed pulmonary outflow tract of the right heart

Purgation cleaning, also in a ritual sense

Pus whitish yellow substance consisting of white blood cells

Quadruplets four infants born by the same mother at the same time

Quickening time when fetal movements are first felt by the mother

Quintuplets five infants born by the same mother at the same time

Quran, Koran main religious text of Islam, arranged in 114 surae

Rachitic affected by rickets

RDS respiratory distress syndrome = surfactant deficiency

Reformation religious movement in the 16th century aiming to reform the Roman Catholic Church, established Protestant Churches

Renaissance era of revival in art and science, from 14th to 17th century

Respiratory distress syndrome respiratory failure in preterm infants due to surfactant deficiency; formerly hyaline membrane disease

Resuscitation emergency procedure restoring ventilation and circulation

Retinopathy non-inflammatory disease of the light-sensitive layer of the eye

Rhesus factor specific antigen on the surface of red cells

Rickets bone disease due to vitamin D deficiency and few sunlight

Rituale book defining specific rites of a religion

Sanguinolent tinged with blood

Scholasticism method of reasoning based on deduction, developed in the 12th century

Scurvy disease of gums, bones, and skin due to vitamin C deficiency

Sedation reduction of sensitivity via sleep-inducing drugs

Seizures nervous activity (convulsion, loss of conscience) due to abnormal electric discharges in the brain

Sepsis, septicaemia generalized blood-borne infection of the entire organism

Septuplets seven infants born by the same mother at the same time

Sextuplets six infants born by the same mother at the same time

Singleton newborn who is not a twin or other multiple birth

Sonography diagnostic imaging technique using ultrasound

Spectroscopy measuring the wavelength to identify materials

Spina bifida embryonic failure to close the neural tube

Sterilization elimination of all microorganisms

Stillbirth birth of a dead child

Substitute taking the place of another

Superfecundation fertilization of two ova by separate coital acts

Surfactant surface active agent covering the lung's air cells

Swill milk milk derived from sick cows fed residual distillery mash

Syngamy fusion of gamete nuclei with formation of the diploid zygote

Syphilis sexually transmitted disease caused by *Treponema pallidum*

Tachycardia excessively rapid heartbeat

Teratology science dealing with malformations

Teratoma tumour originating in embryonal period with tissues derived from more than one germ layer

Téterelle French: milk pump

Thaumaturga Greek: wonder-working image

Theriac mixture of 50 ingredients including opium and viper flesh

Thrombin enzyme catalysing the conversion of fibrinogen to fibrin

Thrombocytopenia abnormally low number of blood platelets

Thrombokinase coagulation factor 10

Thrombus blood clot in a vessel

Thrush fungal yeast infection of mucous membranes

Tiralatte Italian: breast pump

Tire-tête French: hook. A device to extract the dead infant at birth

Torah, Pentateuch Hebrew: the five books of the sacred scriptures (Genesis, Exodus, Leviticus, Numeri, Deuteronomium)

Torno Italian: rotating box for anonymous admission of a baby to a foundling hospital. Also tour, ruota

Toxoplasmosis infection of the fetus with the parasite *Toxoplasma gondii*

Transcription first step of gene expression with DNA copied into RNA

Triglycerides main constituents of body fat

Tube, endotracheal catheter introduced into the windpipe

Tudor era epoch from 1485 to 1603 in British history

Twin reversed perfusion condition developing when monozygotic twins share a placenta and an artery of one connects to a vein of the other

Twin–twin transfusion condition developing in twins sharing a placenta when blood from one twin (donor) is diverted into the other (recipient)

Ulcer, ulcerous relating to a discontinuity of skin or mucous membrane

Umbilicus, umbilical relating to the navel

Urethra canal conveying the urine from the bladder

Utilitarian referring to ethical doctrine that bases virtue on utility

Valois era epoch from 1328 to 1589 in French history

Veda canonical collection of prayers in Hindu sacred writings before 500 B.C.E.

Vein, venous blood vessel carrying blood towards the heart

Venereal, veneric related to sexually transmitted diseases

Ventilator machine designed to move air or oxygen into the lung

Ventricular septum muscular wall separating left and right heart chambers

Vernix caseosa creamy white substance covering the fetus towards term

Viability ability to maintain itself; in premature babies, lowest gestational age or birthweight at which survival is possible

Villi root-like extensions augmenting the surface

Vitalism doctrine starting in the 18th century that the organism lives due to a vital principle distinct from physicochemical forces

Vitium cordis organic heart defect

Vulcanization improving strength of rubber by heating with sulphur

Watery gripes diarrhoea

Wet nurse a woman employed to breastfeed another's baby

Withdrawal symptoms occurring when opiates are discontinued: irritability, tremor, seizures, sneezing, poor feeding, loose stools

Zygote a single diploid cell formed by the union of the haploid male and female gametes

Biographical notes on frequently cited authors

Abbott, Maude E. *St. Andrews, Quebec, Canada 1869, †Montreal 1940.
1925 Assistant professor at McGill University, Montreal. 1924 *The clinical classification of congenital cardiac disease. Int Clin 4;156–188*. 1936 *Atlas of congenital cardiac disease. New York: American Medical Association*.
Biography: Dobell ARC: Maude Abbott. Clin Cardiol 1988;11:658–9.

Aegineta, Paulus *Aegina 625, †Alexandria 690.
Practised in Alexandria. Surgical procedures for congenital malformations in the sixth book of *Seven books of medicine (Engl. ed. Francis Adams 1844, Sydenham Society)*.
Biography: Gurunluoglu R et al.: Paul of Aegina: landmark in surgical progress. World J Surg 2003;27:18–25.

Aitken, John *Date and place of birth unknown. †Edinburgh 1790.
1770 Fellow of Edinburgh Royal College of Surgeons. 1785 Lecturer on Anatomy, Surgery and Midwifery. 1784 Described neonatal asphyxia in *Principles of midwifery. Edinburgh, Lying-in Hospital*.
Biography: Kaufman MH: John Aitken (d. 1790)—grinder or scholar? J Med Biography 2003;11:199–205.

Apgar, Virginia *Westfield, NJ 1909, †New York City 1974.
1938 Director of the Division of Anesthesia at Columbia University. Developed a score to evaluate the newborn after birth: 1953 *A proposal for a new method of evaluation of the newborn infant. Curr Res Anest Analg 32:260-267*. 1955 *A study of the relation of oxygenation at birth to intellectual development. Pediatrics 15:653–62*.
Biography: James LS: Memories of Virginia Apgar. Teratology 1974;10:213–5.

Aranzio, Giulio Cesare *Bologna 1530, †Bologna 1589.
1556 Professor Of Surgery and Anatomy, University of Bologna. 1564 *De humano foetu, Bononiae: J. Rubrius*. Therein: description of ductus arteriosus, ductus venosus, foramen ovale, and separate maternal and fetal circulation in the placenta. Coined the term 'hepar uterinum' for the placenta and denied connections between maternal and fetal blood.
Biography: Gurunluoglu R et al.: Giulio Cesare Arantius (1530–1589): a surgeon and anatomist. Ann Plast Surg 2008;60:717–22.

Aristotle (Aristoteles) *Stageira, Greece 384 B.C.E., †Chalkis 322 B.C.E.
367 B.C.E. Philosopher and natural scientist in Platon's Academy in Athens. *History of animals*; *Parts of animals*; *Generation of animals*.
Biography: Gracia D: The structure of medical knowledge in Aristotle's philosophy. Sudhoff's Arch 1978;62:1–36.

Armstrong, George *Castleton 1719, †London 1789.
1745 Practised in London. 1767 *An account of the diseases most fatal to infants. London: Cadell*; described pyloric stenosis, postnatal hypothermia, handfeeding. 1769, opened the London 'Dispensary for the Infant Poor'.
Biography: Dunn PM: George Armstrong (1719–1789) and his Dispensary for the Infant Poor. Arch Dis Child Fet Neonat Ed 2002;87:F228–31.

Astrup, Poul Björndahl *Copenhagen 1915, †Copenhagen 2000.
Laboratory chief of Blegdamshospitalet; guided artificial ventilation by blood gas analysis during polio epidemic 1952–1953. 1954 *Laboratory investigations during treatment of patients with poliomyelitis and respiratory paralysis. Br Med J 1:780–6*.
Biography: Astrup P, Severinghaus J. The history of blood gases, acids and bases. Copenhagen: Munksgaard, 1985.

Auvard, Alfred Pierre Victor *Corrèze, France 1855, †Paris 1941.
1879 Intern at the Maternité in the Port Royal Hospital. Developed several incubator types with Stéphane Tarnier. 1883 *De la couveuse pour enfants. Arch Tocologie 14:577–609*. 1890 *Le Nouveau-Né: Physiologie—hygiène—allaitement. Paris: Doin*.
Biography: Vignes H: Necrologue pour Alfred Auvard. Presse Méd 1941;49:85.

Avery, Mary Ellen *Camden, NJ 1927, †West Orange, NJ 2011.
1959 Discovery of surfactant deficiency in respiratory distress syndrome (with Jere Mead) *Surface properties in relation to atelectasis and hyaline membrane disease. Am J Dis Child 97:517–23*. 1965 *The lung and its disorders in the newborn infant. Philadelphia, PA: Saunders*. 1974 Chair of pediatrics at Harvard Medical School.
Biography: Pincock S: Mary Ellen Avery. Lancet 2012; 379:610.

Biographical notes on frequently cited authors

Avicenna (Abu Ali al Husayn Ibn Sina) *Buchara/Persia 980, †Hamadan/Persia 1037.
997 Physician to King Mansur of Buchara. Moved to Hamadan, Physician to King al-Dawlah. *Al-Qanun fi al-Tibb (Canon of medicine)*, English ed. Gruner OC, London: Luzac, 1930.
Biography: Gohlman WE: The life of Ibn Sina: Albany, NY: State University of New York Press, 1974.

Bagellardo, Paulus *Flumine, Venice 1410, †Venice 1492.
Professor in Padova, Pisa, and Rome. 1472 *Libellus de egritudinibus infantium*, Padova: Valdezoccho.
Biography: Ruhräh J: Pediatrics of the past. New York: Hoeber, 1925: p. 28.

Baker, Sara Josephine *Poughkeepsie, NY 1873, †Princeton, NJ 1945.
1908 Developed and directed the New York City bureau of maternal and child hygiene. Developed home nurse and teaching programmes to improve sanitation, breast feeding, and nutrition. 1920 *Healthy babies: a volume devoted to the health of expectant mother and the care and welfare of the child*. Minneapolis, MN: Federal Publishing.
Biography: autobiography 1939: Fighting for life. New York: Macmillan. Parry MS: Sara Josephine Baker (1873–1945). Am J Public Health 2006;96:620–1.

Ballantyne, John William *Esbank, Midlothian 1861, †Edinburgh 1923.
1885 Obstetrician at the Royal Maternity Hospital Edinburgh. 1891 *An introduction to the diseases of infanca*. Edinburgh: Oliver & Boyd. 1892 *Diseases and deformities of the foetus*. Edinburgh: Oliver & Boyd; described general dropsy of the fetus. 1894 *Deformities of the embryo*. Edinburgh: Oliver & Boyd. Founded and edited the journal *Teratologia*. 1902 *The problem of the premature infant. BMJ 1196–200*.
Biography: Reiss HE: John William Ballantyne 1861–1923. Hum Reprod Update 1999;5:386–9.

Ballexserd, Jacques *Geneva 1726, †Paris 1774.
1762 *Dissertation sur l'éducation physique des enfans depuis leur naissance*. Paris: Vallat-la-Chapelle. 1772 *Dissertation sur les causes principales de la mort d'Enfans*. Marseille: Mossy. Propagated maternal breastfeeding instead of wet-nursing.
Biography: Morsier G: Jacques Ballexserd, the physician from Geneva (1726–1774) and the physical education of children. Clio Med 1974;9:311–5/

Barclay, Alfred E. *Manchester 1876, †Oxford 1948.
1912 *X-ray diagnosis and treatment*. London: Business IMP. 1936 Radiologist at Nuffield Institute, Oxford. 1944 (with KJ Franklin and MML Prichard) *The foetal circulation and cardiovascular system, and the changes that they undergo at birth*. Oxford: Blackwell.
Biography: Edling, L: Alfred Ernest Barclay: in memoriam. Acta Radiol 1949;32:1–10.

Barcroft, Joseph *Down County, Ireland 1872, †Cambridge 1947.
1900 King's College, Cambridge. High-altitude cardiopulmonary physiology. Placental and fetal oxygen transport. 1917 *Respiratory Functions of Blood*. Cambridge: Cambridge University Press. 1947 *Researches on Prenatal Life*. Springfield, IL: Thomas.
Biography: Boyd R et al.: Sir Joseph Barcroft, Cambridge and intergenerational science. Int J Dev Biol 2010;54:257–68.

Baron, Jacques Francois *Paris 1782, †Paris 1849.
1814 Physician-in-chief of Paris Foundling Hospital. 1815 *Observation sur une hydrocephale chronique … Bull Fac Med*, 5. 1811 Adapted Laennec's stethoscope to neonates. 1826 *Observation d'obliteration de l'intestin par vice de conformation. Bull Sci Med IX*.
Biography: Hirsch, A: Biographisches Lexikon. Wien. Urban & Schwarzenberg 1929, Vol. 1 p. 341.

Bartholin, Thomas *Copenhagen 1616, †Copenhagen 1680.
Extensive studies in Leyden, Basel, and Padova. 1646 Professor of anatomy in Copenhagen; 1661 Tobacco-smoke clyster for resuscitation. 1654–1661 *Historiarum anatomicarum Cent. I–VI*: multiple congenital malformations described.
Biography: Hill R: The contributions of the Bartholin family to the study and practice of clinical anatomy. Clin Anat 2007;20:113–5.

Bauhin, Caspar *Basel 1560, †Basel 1624.
1577 Studied in Padova. 1589 Professor of Anatomy in Basel. 1614 Classified congenital malformations: *On hermaphrodites and monsters*. Opppenheim: Galleri. 1619 Rector of Basel University.
Biography: Fuchs-Eckert, HP: Die Familie Bauhin in Basel. Bauhinia 1979;6/2:311–29; 1981;7/2:45–62.

Baumes, Jean Baptiste Timothée *Lunel, France 1756, †Montpellier 1828.
1782 Physician in Nîmes. 1785 *L'ictère des nouveaux-nés, et les circonstances ou cet ictère exige le secours de l'art*. Nismes: Castor Belle. 1790 Professor at Montpellier. 1805 *Traité des convulsions dans l'enfance*, Paris: Méquignon.
Biography: Kellaway S et al.: Jean Baptiste Timothée Baumes. In: Ashwal S ed.: Founders of child neurology. San Francisco, CA: Norman Publishing, 1990: p. 97–102.

Bednar, Fedor Alois *Potterstein, Bohemia 1816, †Vienna 1888.
1848 Director of the Vienna Foundling Hospital. 1856 Lactose. 1850–1853 *Die Krankheiten der Neugeborenen und Säuglinge. 4 vols.* Vienna: Gerold. Introduced hand disinfection in 1847 which drastically reduced the incidence of sepsis. 1851 He was not kept on as director.
Biography: Abt IA: The influence of pathology on the development of pediatrics. Am J Dis Child 1927;34:1–22.

Berg, Frederik Theodor *Göteborg, Sweden 1806, †Stockholm 1887.
1839–1841 Study journey to various European foundling hospitals. 1841 Discovery of the thrush fungus (together with D. Gruby at Paris). 1841 *Torsk i mikroskopiskt anatomiskt hänseende Hygiea 1841;3:541–50* (Thrush from the microscopical anatomical point of view). 1842 Appointed to direct the Stockholm Foundling Hospital. 1845 Professor of paediatrics at Royal Karolinska Medico-Surgical Institute Stockholm. 1853 Secretary-General of the Central Bureau of Statistics. Left paediatrics, but published infant mortality rates in European countries.
Biography: Berg F: Some extracts from Frederik Theodor Berg's autobiographical memoranda. Acta Paediatr 1945;32:218–31.

Bernheim-Karrer, Jakob *Zürich 1868, †Bern 1958.
1892 Zürich Children's Hospital. 1898 Office in Zürich. 1907 *Säuglings-Scorbut bei Ernährung mit homogenisierter Berner Alpenmilch. Correspondenz-Blatt Schweizer Ärzte 37:593–8.* 1908 director of the newly founded Cantonal Infant Hospital Rosenberg. 1928 *Über Ikterus bei Neugeborenen. Schweiz Med Wochenschr 58:1125–9.*
Biography: Didierjean B: Geschichte der Neonatologie in Zürich. Zürich: Juris Druck Verlag, 1979.

Biedert, Philipp *Niederflörsheim, Alsace 1847, †Haguenau, Alsace 1916.
1877 Hagenau District Hospital. 1903–1912 Director of Public Health Service in Alsace-Lorraine; 1874 Development of the fat-enriched formula *Ramogen*. 1880 *Die Kindernahrung im Säuglingsalter. Stuttgart: Enke.*
Biography: Selter P: Philipp Biedert. Dtsch Med Wochenschr 1916;42:1390.

Billard, Charles Michel *Pelouailles, France 1800, †Angers 1832.
1824 Intern at the Hôtel-Dieu in Angers; 1825 *De la membrane muqueuse gastro-intestinale. Paris: Gabon.* 1826 Intern at the Paris Foundling Hospital. 1828 *Traité des Maladies des Enfants Nouveau-Nés et a la Mamelle, Paris: Baillière.*
Biography: Beckwith JB: Charles-Michel Billard (1800–1832): Pioneer of infant pathology. Pediatr Dev Pathol 2002;5:248–56.

Bodio, Luigi *Milano 1840, †Rome 1920.
1867 Professor of Statistics in Venice. 1872 Director, Royal statistical office. 1876 *Del movimento della popolazione in Italia e in altri Stati d'Europa, Arch Statist 1:119–205.* 1878 Comparative statistics of infant mortality in Italy and in the European states. 1909 President of the International Statistical Institute.
Biography: Gilman FH: Luigi Bodio. Publ Am Stat Assoc 1910;12:283–5.

Boerhaave, Herman *Voorhout, Leiden 1668, †Leiden, Netherlands 1738.
1709 Combined chair of medicine and botany at Leiden University. Introduced physiology into clinical teaching. 1709 *Aphorisms*, translated and commented by Gerhard van Swieten in 1742. Set an end to the belief in a direct vascular connection of uterus and breast.
Biography: Sigerist HE: A Boerhaave pilgrimage in Holland. Bull Hist Med 1939;7:257–75.

Boivin, Marie-Anne Victoire *Montreuil, France 1773, †Paris 1864.
1801 Midwife in chief at the Paris Maternité; standard teaching book for midwifes. 1812 *Mémorial de l'art des accouchemens (4th ed. 1879).* 1828 Honorary MD degree of Marburg University.
Biography: Blanvalet-Boutouyrie S: Naître a l'hôpital au XIXe siècle. Paris: Belin, 1999.

Borden, Gail *Norwich, NY 1801, †Borden, TX 1874.
1839 Customs collector in Galveston, Texas. 1849 Production of meat biscuit. 1856 *Concentration of sweet milk and extracts. US-patent No. 15553.* 1858 Borden Condensed Milk Company moved to Litchfield, Connecticut, and 1860 to New York. 1865 *Improvement in condensing milk. US-patent No. 2103.* 1866 Anglo-Swiss Condensed Milk Company in Cham, Switzerland. Pioneered use of glass milk bottles in 1885.
Biography: Frantz JB: Gail Borden. Dairyman to a nation. Norman, OK: University of Oklahoma Press, 1951.

Bouchut, Eugène *Paris 1818, †Paris 1891.
1844 Paris Hotel-Dieu Hospital. 1845 *Traité pratique des maladies des nouveau-nés, des enfants a la mamelle et de la seconde enfance. Paris:Baillière (7th ed. 1879).* 1856 Hôpital Necker-Enfants Malades. 1858 New technique for orotracheal intubation with a metal tube. 1864 *Histoire de la médecine et des doctrines médicales. Paris: Baillière.* 1872 Physician of the Paris Hospital for Sick Children.
Biography: Sperati G et al.: Bouchut, O'Dwyer and laryngeal intubation in patients with croup. Acta Otorhinolaryngol Ital 2007;27:320–3.

Bourgeois, Louise dite Boursier *Faubourg St. Germain, Paris 1563, †Paris 1636.
1601 Royal midwife to Marie de Medici and other aristocrats. 1609 *Observations diverses sur la stérilité, perte de fruict, fécondité, accouchements et maladies des femmes et enfants nouveaux naiz, Paris: Saugrain.*
Biography: Perkins W: Midwifery and medicine in early modern France: Louise Bourgeois. Exeter: University of Exeter Press, 1996.

Brown, Rachel Fuller *Springfield, MA 1898, †Albany, NY 1980.
Biochemist at New York State Department of Health. Developed antifungal Nystatin treatment together with E. Hazen. 1950 *Two antifungal agents produced by a soil actinomycete. Science 112:423.* 1951 *Fungicidin, an antibiotic produced by a soil actinomycete. Proc Soc Exp Biol Med 76:93–7.*
Biography: Baldwin RS: The fungus fighters: Ithaca, NY: Cornell University Press, 1981.

Buchan, William *Ancrum, Scotland 1729, †London 1805.
1758 Practice in Yorkshire. 1759 Physician at the Foundling Hospital in Ackworth, Yorkshire. 1761 *On the preservation of infant life.* 1769 *Domestic medicine. Edinburgh: Balfour.* Described opium intoxication in neonates.
Biography: Dunn PM: William Buchan (1729–1805) and his Domestic Medicine. Arch Dis Child 2000;83:F71–3.

Budin, Pierre Constant *Enencourt, France 1846, †Marseille 1907.
1872 Obstetrician at the Paris Maternité. 1895 Director of the ward for premature infants. 1872 Infant Mortality Prevention Programme *Goutte de lait.* 1897 *Femmes en couches et Nouveau-Nés; Paris: Doin* (58 papers on perinatal medicine); 1900 *Le Nourrisson; Paris: Doin.* 1905 *Manuel pratique de l'allaitement.*
Biography: Toubas PL: Pierre Budin: promoter of breastfeeding in 19th century France. Breastfeed Med 2007;2:45–9.

Burns, John *Glasgow 1774, †Portpatrick 1850.
1809 Discerned neonatal jaundice with and without obstruction: *Principles of Midwifery.* 1815 Chair of Surgery, University of Glasgow. 1817 *The principles of midwifery; including the diseases of women and children.* London: Longman.
Biography: Dunn PM: John Burns (1774–1850) and neonatal jaundice. Arch Dis Child 1989;64:1416–7.

Biographical notes on frequently cited authors

Butterfield, L. Joseph   *Terre Haute, IN 1926, †Denver, CO 1999.
1965 Director of Newborn Center at Denver Children's Hospital. 1972 Regionalization program for perinatal centers. 1973 *Regionalization for respiratory care. Pediatr Clin North Am 20:499–505*.
Biography: Sunshine P: L. Joseph Butterfield: a man for all seasons. J Perinatol 1999;19:176–8.

Cadogan, William   *Cardiff 1711, †London 1797.
1747 Bristol infirmary. 1748 *An essay upon nursing, and the management of children from their Birth to three years of age. London: Roberts (10th ed. 1772)*. Promoted breastfeeding, opposed swaddling. 1749 Director of the London Foundling Hospital.
Biography: Rendle-Short J: William Cadogan—eighteenth-century physician. Med Hist 1960;4:288–309.

Campbell, Kate   *Hawthorn, Australia 1899, †Camberwell, Australia 1986.
1922 Residency at Melbourne Hospital. 1927 Victorian Bay Health Center. 1947 *A guide to the care of the young child. Melbourne: Department of Health*. 1951 Associated retrolental fibroplasia with oxygen therapy: *Intensive oxygen therapy as a possible cause of retrolental fibroplasia; Med J Austral 1951;2:48–50*. 1965 Consultant in paediatrics.
Biography: McCalman J: Campbell, Dame Kate Isabel (1899–1986). Austr Dict Biograph 2007;17.

Cangiamila, Francesco Emanuele   *Palermo 1702, †Palermo 1763.
Theologian, Inquisitor of Sicily. 1745 *Embriologia sacra, ovvero dell'uffizio de' sacerdoti, medici, e superiori circa l'eterna salute de' bambini racchiusi nell' utero. Palermo, Giuseppe Cairoli*. Translated into Latin 1751, French 1762.
Biography: Knapp L: Theologie und Geburtshilfe. F.E. Cangiamila's Sacra Embryologia. Prague: Bellmann, 1908.

Capuron, Joseph   *Larroque-Saint-Cernin, France 1767, †Paris 1850.
Surgeon and obstetrician at Montpellier and Paris. 1806 *Dictionary of medicine*; classification of brain hemorrhages of the newborn. 1813 *Traité des maladies des Enfans. Paris: Crullebois*.
Biography: Hirsch A: Biographisches Lexikon. Wien, Urban & Schwarzenberg 1929, Vol. 1, p. 826; Sarrut G: Biographies des hommes du jour. Paris: Pilout, 1838: Vol. 4. p. 50–1.

Chapple, Charles C.   *Billings, MT 1904, †Lincoln, NE 1979.
1928 Philadelphia children's hospital. Developed the closed, thermocontrolled Isolette Incubator. 1938 *Controlling the external environment of premature infants in an incubator. Am J Dis Child 50:16–17*.
Biography: Cone, TE: History of the care and feeding of the premature infant. Boston, MA: Little, Brown & Co., 1985: p. 70–3.

Chaussier, Francois   *Dijon, France 1746, †Paris 1828.
1780 Physiologist in Dijon, work with oxygen. 1781 *Reflexions sur les moyens propres a déterminer la respiration dans les enfants qui naissent sans donner aucune signe de vie; Vol. 4. Paris: Histoire et Mémoires de la Société Royale de Médecine, années 1780–1781:346–54*. 1794 Reorganization of the Paris Medical Faculty, together with Fourcroy; from 1804 director of the Paris Maternité. Multiple courses and papers addressed to midwifes; bag ventilation, oxygen, and endotracheal intubation in neonatal asphyxia.
Biography: Stofft H: La mort apparente du nouveau-né en 1781 et en 1806. L'oeuvre de Francois Chaussier. Hist Sci Med 1997;31:341–9.

Chick, Harriette   *London 1875, †Cambridge 1977.
1902 Royal commission on sewage disposal. 1905 Lister Institute London. 1915 Lister Institute Elstree. 1919 Went to Vienna to lead a team researching the relation of nutrition to infant rickets and scurvy. 1922 *The aetiology of rickets in infants: Lancet 200:7–11*. 1934 Secretary of the League of Nations Health Committee. 1949 Dame of the British Empire. 1976: *Study of rickets in Vienna. Med Hist 20:41–51*.
Biography: Carpenter KJ: Harriette Chick and the problem of rickets. J Nutr 2008;138:827–32.

Clarke, John   *Northamptonshire 1760, †London 1815.
1783 Licentiate in midwifery at the London College of physicians; obstetrician and teacher. 1803 *The London Practice of Midwifery*. 1815 *Commentaries on some of the most important diseases of children. London, Longman, Hurst & Co*.
Biography: Hunter KR: Dr John Clarke: licentiate in midwifery. Clin Med 2002;2:153–6.

Clements, John Allen   *Auburn, NY 1923.
1951 US Army Chemical Center in Edgewood; detected the physical properties of surfactant. 1956 *Dependence of pressure-volume characteristics of lungs on intrinsic surface active material. Am J Physiol 187:592*. 1957 *Proceedings of the Society of Experimental Biology and Medicine*. 1961 Cardiovascular Research Institute, San Francisco.
Biography: Rockafellar, NM: Interviews with John Clements MD. UCSF Oral History Program, Vol. 19, 1998.

Comroe, Julius H.   *York, PA 1911, †San Francisco 1984.
1946 Chairman Department of Physiology of University of Pennsylvania. 1958 Director, Cardiovascular Research Institute San Francisco; *The lung: clinical physiology and function tests*; 1965 *Physiology of respiration. Chicago, IL: Year Book Medical Publishers*. 1977 *Retrospectroscope. Insights into Medical Discovery. Menlo Park, CA: Von Gehr*.
Biography: Cardiovascular Research Institute: The first twenty-five years 1958–1983. San Francisco, CA: UCSF, 1983.

Corner, Beryl Dorothy   *Bristol 1910, †Bristol 2007.
1937 Bristol Children's Hospital. 1939 National survey into rickets. 1946 Opened and directed neonatal intensive care unit at Southmead Hospital, Bristol.
Biography: Watts G: Beryl Dorothy Corner. Pioneering paediatrician and one of the founders of UK neonatology. Lancet 2007;369:986.

Crosse, Victoria Mary   *Rye, Sussex 1900, †Birmingham 1972.
Trained in obstetrics. 1931 Founded the Premature Baby Unit at Sorrento Hospital Birmingham. 1945 *The premature baby. London: J & A Churchill*. Reported toxicity of vitamin K. 1955 *Kernikterus and prematurity. Arch Dis Child 30:501–8*.
Biography: Dunn P: Dr. Mary Crosse, OBE, MD (1900–1972) and the premature baby: Arch Dis Child Fetal Neonat Ed 2007;92:F151–3.

Davies, Pamela Anne   *Southsea, Hampshire 1924, †Oxford 2009.
1958 Radcliffe infirmary, Oxford; 1964 (with Victoria Smallpeice) *The immediate feeding of babies weighing 1,000–2,000 g with breast milk. Proc Roy Soc Med 43:1173–5*. 1966 Hammersmith Hospital London. 1972 *Medical care of newborn babies. Philadelphia, PA: Lippincott*. 1994 *Neonatal meningitis. London: Mac Keith*.
Biography: Wigglesworth J: Pamela Anne Davies. Br Med J 2009;339:4345.

Dawes, Geoffrey S. *Mackworth, Derbyshire, UK 1918, †Oxford 1996.
1948 Director of the Nuffield Institute of Medical Research, Oxford. 1958 Outlined cardiorespiratory changes during asphyxia. 1964 *The effect of alkali and glucose infusion on permanent brain damage in rhesus monkeys asphyxiated at birth. J Pediatr 65:801–23.* 1968 *Foetal and neonatal physiology; a comparative study of the changes at birth.* Chicago, IL: Year Book Medical Publishers.
Biography: Hansen MA: Tribute to Professor Geoffrey Dawes. Pediatr Res 1996;40:767–71.

Day, Richard L. *Manhattan, NY 1905, †Westbrook, CT 1989.
1933 Babies Hospital NY. 1935 Columbia University. 1943 *Regulation of body temperature of premature infants. Am J Dis Child 65:376–98.* 1953 Chairman of Pediatrics, Brooklyn, New York. 1965, Director, Planned Parenthood International; 1969 Chair of Pediatrics, Pittsburgh University. 1968 Mt. Sinai Hospital, Columbia University.
Biography: Silverman WA: Richard L. Day (1905–1989). J Pediat 1995; 127:503–5.

Denis, Prosper-Sylvain *Commercy, France 1799, †Toul 1863.
1823 Intern at the Paris Foundling Hospital, performed many autopsies of newborns. Description of tentorium laceration and pathogenesis of intracranial hemorrhage. 1826 *Recherches d'anatomie et de physiologie pathologiques sur plusieurs maladies des enfans nouveau-nés. Commercy: Denis.* 1843 Military Hospital of Toul; 1856 Biochemical analysis of body fluids.
Biography: Minel, in: Union Méd Nouv Sér XIX; 1863, p. 127.

Denucé, Jean-Louis-Paul *Ambares, Gironde 1824, †Bordeaux 1889.
1854, Professor of surgery, Ecole de Medecine de Bordeaux; double-walled open incubator. 1857 *Berceau incubateur pour les enfants nés avant terme. J Med Bordeaux 2:723–4.*
Biography: Feret E: Statistique Génerale de Gironde, t. 3: Biographie. Bordeaux: Masson, 1989: p. 184.

Diamond, Louis K. *Kishinev, Bessarabia 1902, †Los Angeles, CA 1999.
1929 Harvard University. 1942 Director of hematology at Boston Children's Hospital. 1932 *Erythroblastosis fetalis and its association with universal edema of the fetus, icterus gravis neonatorum and anemia of the newborn. J Pediatr 1:269–309.* Developed exchange transfusion via umbilical vein: 1948 *Replacement transfusion as a treatment for erythroblastosis fetalis. Pediatrics 2:520–4.*
Biography: Mentzer WC: Louis Diamond and his contribution to hematology. Br J Haematol 2003;123:389–95.

Diemerbroeck, Isbrand van *Montfoort 1609, †Utrecht 1674.
1636 Practitioner in Nimwegen. 1646 Monograph on the plague. 1649 Professor of anatomy in Utrecht. 1672 *Anatome corporis humani,* Utrecht: description of placental circulation and of congenital diaphragmatic hernia.
Biography: Hirsch A: Biographisches Lexikon. Wien, Urban & Schwarzenberg 1930, Vol. 2, p. 265.

Doepp, Philipp *Wesenberg, Estonia 1793, †Jamburg (today Kingissepp), Russia 1855.
1829 Head physician at the St. Petersburg Foundling Hospital; incubator care; drainage of cephalhematoma. 1835 *Notizen über das kaiserliche Erziehungshaus (Findlingshaus) zu St. Petersburg,* *die Jahre 1830–1833 umfassend.* Hamburg: Hoffmann & Campe, 1835: Vol. 5, p. 306–50.
Biography: Hirsch A: Biographisches Lexikon. Wien, Urban & Schwarzenberg 1990, Vol. 2, p. 282.

Doublet, Francois *Chartres 1751, †Paris 1795.
1776 Charité Paris; 1781 Director of the Hospice for Syphilitic Infants in Vaugirard. Treatment of congenital syphilis by applying mercury to a syphilitic wet nurse. 1781 *Mémoire sur les sympomes et le traitement de la maladie vénérienne dans les enfans nouveau-nés. Paris: Méquignon.* 1785 *Observations dans le Département des Hôpitaux Civils. Journal de Médecine January:102–47.*
Biography: Sherwood J: Infection of the innocents. Montreal: McGill University Press, 2010: p. 38–40.

Down, John Langdon *Torpoint, Cornwall 1828, †Teddington 1896.
Studied pharmacy, from 1853 medicine. 1858 Medical superintendent of the Royal Earlswood Asylum for Idiots. Described trisomy 21 in 1862. *Observations on an ethnic classification of idiots. Lond Hosp Rep 3:259–62.* 1876 *The education and training of the feeble in mind.* London: Lewis.
Biography: Ward OC: John Langdon Down: the man and the message. Down Sdr Res Pract 1999;6:19–24.

Drillien, Cecil Mary *Taunton, Somerset 1917, †Edinburgh 2006.
1944 Trials on the use of penicillin at Directorate of Biological Research. 1952 Department of Child life and health, Edinburgh University. 1964 *The growth and development of the prematurely born infant.* Edinburgh: Livingstone. 1971 Consultant in Dundee.
Biography: Drummond, M: Cecil Mary Drillien. BMJ 2006;333:1274.

Drinker, Philip *Haverford, PA 1894, †Fitzwilliam, NH 1972.
1921 Harvard School of Public Health. 1928 invention of iron lung. 1929 (with LA Shaw) *An apparatus for the prolonged administration of artificial respiration. I. A design for adults and children. J Clin Invest 7:229–47.* The device was used in neonates by Murphy DT et al. in 1931: *The Drinker Respirator Treatment of the immediate asphyxia of the newborn. Am J Obstet Gynecol 21:528–36.*
Biography: Sherwood RJ: Obituary: Philip Drinker 1894–1972. Ann Occup Hyg 1973;16:93–4.

Dubowitz, Lilly M. *Budapest, Hungary 1930, †London 2016.
1938 Emigration to Shanghai, later to Australia and London in 1956. 1973 Department of Child Health in Sheffield. 1970 Neurological score: *Clinical assessment of gestational age in the newborn infant; J Pediatr 77:1–10.* The Hammersmith neurological examination: 1981 (with her husband Victor Dubowitz) *The neurological assessment in the preterm and full-term infant.* London: MacKeith.

Dufour, Léon *St. Lo, France 1856, †Fécamp 1928.
1889 Hôpital de Fécamp. 1894 Comité des oeuvres de la Goutte de Lait. Infancy Museum in Fécamp.
Biography: Sautereau M: Aux origines de la pédiatrie moderne: Le Docteur Léon Dufour et l'oeuvre de la 'Goutte de lait' (1894–1928). Ann Normand 1991;41:217–33.

Dugès, Antoine Louis *Mézières, Ardennes 1797, †Montpellier 1838.
1817 Intern at Paris Maternity Hospital. Described meconium ileus and bilirubin-encephalopathy in 1821: *Recherches sur les maladies les plus importantes et les moins connues des enfans nouveau-nés.* Paris:

Bailliere. 1825 Professor of obstetrics at University of Montpellier. 1826 *Manuel d'obstétrique.*
Biography: Dechambre A: Dugès (Antoine-Louis). Dictionnaire encyclopédique des sciences médicales 1884;64:642.

Dunham, Ethel Collins *Hartford, CT 1883, †Cambridge, MA 1969. 1920 Instructor of Pediatrics at Yale Medical School; multiple papers on premature infants. 1935 Chief of child development at the Children's Bureau Washington; reports on infant mortality and morbidity. 1943 Guidelines: *Standards and recommendations for the hospital care of newborn infants.* 1948 *Premature Infants: A Manual for Physicians.* Washington, DC: Children's Bureau.
Biography: Gordon HH: Presentation of the John Howland Medal to Dr. Ethel C Dunham. JAMA Pediatr 1957;94:367–71.

Eastman, Nicholson Joseph *Crawfordsville, IN 1895, †Minnesota 1973. 1928 Johns Hopkins. 1930 *Foetal blood studies, I. The oxygen relationship of umbilical cord blood at birth. Bull Johns Hopkins Hosp 47(4):221–30.* 1933 Professor at Peking University. 1935 Obstetrician-in-chief, Johns Hopkins. 1954 *Mount Everest in utero. Am J Obstet Gynecol 67:701–11.* 1955 *The etiology of cerebral palsy. Am J Obstet Gynecol 69:950–61.* 1963 *Expectant motherhood.*
Biography: Bayes M: Tribute to Dr. Nicholson J. Eastman. J Nurse Midwifery 1973;18:5.

Eliot, Martha May *Dorchester, MA 1891, †Cambridge, MA 1978. 1921 Yale University. 1923 Study on the prevention of rickets with cod liver oil. 1951 National Children's Bureau. 1956 Chair of child and maternal health at Harvard. 1967 *The United States Children's Bureau. Am J Dis Child 114:565–73.*
Biography: Lesser A: Martha May Eliot. J Pediatr 1993;123:162–5.

Elsässer, Carl Ludwig *Neuenstadt/Linde 1808, †Untertürkheim 1874. Obstetrician at Katharinen Hospital Stuttgart. Studies on neonatal jaundice 1835: *Schmidt's Jahrbücher 7;314–322.* Study on craniotabes: 1843 *Der weiche Hinterkopf.* Stuttgart: Cotta. 1853 Court physician. Study on neonatal jaundice.
Biography: Ruhräh J: Carl Ludwig von Elsässer 1808–1874. Am J Dis Child 1935;49:1008–11.

Enhörning, Göran *Birkdale, England 1924, †Vero Beach, FL 2013. 1961 Karolinska Institutes Stockholm. 1971 Professor of Obstetrics, Toronto. Groundbreaking research on pulmonary surfactant. Studies with Bengt Robertson. 1973 *Pharyngeal deposition of surfactant in the premature rabbit fetus. Biol Neonat 22:126–32.* 1985 Randomized trial.
Biography: Curstedt T, Halliday HL, Speer CP: A unique story in neonatal research: the development of a porcine surfactant. Neonatology 2015;107:321–9.

Epstein, Alois *Kamenice, Czechia 1849, †Prague 1918. 1875 At the Prague Foundling Hospital, since 1881 as its director. Introduced antisepsis into infant care. 1900 *Die neugebaute deutsche Abteilung und Kinderklinik der kgl. böhm. Landesfindelanstalt. Prager med Wochenschr;* 1916 *Über die Notwendigkeit eines systematischen Unterrichtes in der Säuglingspflege an Hebammenlehranstalten.* Urban und Schwarzenberg. Work on sepsis.
Biography: Moll L: Alois Epstein. Zeitschr Kinderheilk 1919;23:1–4.

Escherich, Theodor *Ansbach, Bavaria 1857, †Vienna 1911. 1890 Director of the Annahospital and Foundling Hospital in Graz. 1902 Director of Anna Children's Hospital Vienna. 1886 *Die Darmbakterien des Neugeborenen und Säuglings. Fortschr Med 3:515–22, 547–54.* 1899 *Der Borsäureschnuller, eine neue Behandlungsmethode des Soor. Ther Gegenw NF 1:298–300.* 1900 *A description of a new incubator in the Children's Hospital at Graz. Albany Med Ann Sept:1–4.* 1905 *Die neue Säuglingsabteilung im St. Anna-Kinderspital in Wien. Wien Klin Wochenschr 18:977–82.*
Biography: Shulman ST et al.: Theodor Escherich: the first pediatric infectious diseases physician. Clin Infect Dis 2007;45:1025–9.

Ettmüller, Michael *Leipzig, Saxonia 1644, †Leipzig 1683. 1681 Chair of botany, surgery and anatomy at Leipzig University. Explained jaundice from meconium retention. 1688 *De morbis infantum (in Opera omnia, Vol. 4, 583),* Frankfurt: Zunneri.
Biography: Neue Deutsche Biographie, 1964. Vol. 6, Leipzig: Duncker & Humblot, p. 400f.

Fabricius ab Aquapendente, Hieronymus *Aquapendente, Orvieto 1533, †Padova, Venice 1619. Anatomist in Padova, focusing on embryology. 1600 *De formato foetu,* Venice, Franciscus Bolzettani. 1621 *De formatio ovi, et pulli.* Padova, Aloisi Buxii.
Biography: Adelmann HB: The embryological Treatises of Hieronymus Fabricius. Ithaca, NY: Cornell University Press, 1942.

Farr, William *Kenley, Shropshire 1807, †London 1883. 1837 Joined the General Register Office; established the *British Annals of Medicine, Pharmacy.* 1865 *On infant mortality, and on alleged inaccuracies of the census. J Statist Soc London 28:125–49.* Vital Statistics and General Science. Standardized and evaluated the national life tables, allowing mortality rates to be compared. 1866 *Mortality of children in the principal states of Europe. J Statist Soc Lond 29:1–12.*
Biography: Dupaqier M: William Farr. In: Hyde CC, Seneta E: Statisticians of the centuries. New York: Springer, 2001: p. 163–6.

Finkelstein, Heinrich *Leipzig, Saxonia 1865, †Santiago de Chile 1942. 1910 *Protein-enriched milk for preterm infants: Berlin Klin Wochenschr 25:1194.* 1910 *Ueber Eiweissmilch. Jahrb Kinderheilk 71;525 & 683.* 1911 Physiologic anaemia of newborns. 1905–1912 *Lehrbuch der Säuglingskrankheiten.* Berlin: Springer. 1918 Director of Emperor Frederick Hospital for Children in Berlin. 1938 Emigration to Chile after anti-Jewish pogrom.
Biography: Rosenstern I: Heinrich Finkelstein (1865–1942): J Pediatr 1956:49;499–503.

Flagg, Paluel Joseph *New York City 1886, †New York City 1970. 1916 Anaesthesiologist in charge at St. Vincent Hospital New York. 1922 *The art of anesthesia.* Philadelphia, PA: Lippincott. 1928 *Treatment of asphyxia in the newborn. JAMA 91:788–91.* 1931 *The treatment of postnatal asphyxia. Am J Obstet Gynecol 21:537–41.*

Fujiwara, Tetsuro *Morioka, Japan 1931. 1966 Research fellow in Forrest Adams' laboratory at Los Angeles, where bovine surfactant was developed. 1968 *'Alveolar' and whole lung phospholipids of the developing fetal lamb lung. Am J Physiol 215:375–82.* 1970 Associate professor at Akita University in Japan. 1980 First successful clinical trial: *Artificial surfactant therapy in hyaline-membrane disease. Lancet 315:55–9.* 1981 Chair of pediatrics at Iwate University, Marioka.

Biographical notes on frequently cited authors

Galen (Galenus) *Pergamon, Asia minor 129, †Rome 210.
Philosophy studies in Asia minor; 163 C.E. Court physician in Rome. Most influential physician of the antique world. *On the usefulness of the parts. On Hygiene. On properties of the foodstuffs. On forming of the fetus.* Described fetal circulatory shunts; animal milk feeding.
Biography: Leven KH: Antike Medizin. Ein Lexikon. München: Beck, 2005: p. 315–9.

Gennep, Arnold van *Ludwigsburg (then Württemberg) 1873, †Epernay 1957.
Ethnologist who developed the theory of important rites associated with steps in maturation and social acceptance. 1909 *Les rites de passage.* 1912 Chair of ethnology at Neuchatel, Switzerland.
Biography: Schomburg-Scherff, SM: Arnold van Gennep. München: Beck, 2004.

Girtanner, Christoph *St. Gallen, Switzerland 1760, †Göttingen 1800.
Private Scientist in Göttingen. 1794 *Abhandlung über die Krankheiten der Kinder.* Berlin, Rottmann. Studied fetal oxygenation in 1792: *Anfangsgründe der antiphlogistischen Chemie.* Several political writings.
Biography: Wegelin C: Christoph Girtanner. Neue Deutsche Biographie, Vol. 6. Leipzig: Duncker & Humblot, 1964: p. 411f.

Gluck, Louis *Newark, NJ 1924, †Laguna Hill, CA 1997.
1960 Designed the modern neonatal intensive care unit at Yale/New Haven. 1967 *The biochemical development of surface activity in mammalian lung. 1, The surface-active phospholipids. Pediatr Res 1:237–46.* 1969 University of California San Diego; lecithin/sphingomyelin ratio to diagnose surfactant deficiency.
Biography: Festschrift to Louis Gluck, MD. J Perinatol 1989;9:1–68.

Graunt, John *London 1620, †London 1674.
Statistician and founder of the science of demography. Longitudinal studies of the development of infant mortality. 1662 *Natural and political observations upon the bills of mortality.* London, John Martyn.
Biography: Heyde CC: John Graunt. In: Heyde CC et al.: Statisticians of the centuries. New York: Springer, 2001: p. 14–6.

Gruby, David *Kis-Ker, Hungary (now Dobro Polje, Serbia) 1810, †Paris 1898.
1839 Pathologist in Vienna with Rokitansky, expertise in microscopy. 1840 Emigration to Paris. 1841 Paris Foundling hospital. Detected (together with Frederic Berg) the thrush fungus in 1842: *Recherches anatomiques sur une plante cryptogame qui constitue le vrai muguet des enfants. Comptes Rendus Hebdomadaires Acad Sci (Paris)* 14:634–6.
Biography: Beeson BB: David Gruby, MD, 1810–1898. Arch Derm Syphil 1931;23:141–4.

Guillemeau, Jacques *Orléans 1549, †Paris 1613.
Student of Ambroise Paré. 1580 Surgeon and obstetrician at the Paris Hôtel-Dieu. 1609 *De la nourriture et gouvernement des enfants.* Surgeon of Charles IX and Henri III.
Biography: Siebold ECJ: Versuch einer Geschichte der Geburtshilfe, Tübingen: Pietzker, 1902: Vol. II, p. 84.

György, Paul *Nagyvarod, Hungary 1893, †Moristown, NJ 1976.
1920 Assistant, from 1927 professor of pediatrics at Heidelberg. 1933 *Über das Vitamin B2. Naturwiss* 21:560–70. 1933 Dismissed because of Jewish origin, escaped Nazi pogroms by emigrating to Cambridge. 1944 Professor of nutrition in pediatrics at Philadelphia School of Medicine.
Biography: Barness LA et al.: Paul György (1893–1976). A biographical sketch. J Nutr 1979;109:17–23.

Haller, Albrecht von *Bern 1708, †Bern 1777.
1725 Assistant of Boerhaave in Leiden. 1736 Chair of medicine, anatomy and botany in Göttingen. 1753 Return to Switzerland. 1766 *Elementa physiologiae corporis humani, vol 8: Fetus hominisque vita. Lugduni Batavorum, Haak.* 1774 *On generation.*
Biography: Buess, H: Albrecht von Haller and his Elementa Physiologiae as the beginning of pathological physiology. Med Hist 1959;14:175–82.

Hamilton, Alexander *Fordun, Scotland 1739, †Edinburgh 1802.
1780 Professor of Midwifery at Edinburgh University. 1781 *Treatise of midwifery … and treatment of children in early infancy.* Edinburgh: Dickson.
Biography: Former Fellows of the Royal Society of Edinburgh, 1783–2002. Biographical Index. Edinburgh: Royal Society of Edinburgh, 2006: p. 404.

Harris, Walter *Gloucester, England 1647, †Cambridge 1732.
Student of Sydenham. 1680 Lecturer at Cambridge College of Physicians. 1689 *De morbis acutis infantum.* London: Samuel Smith (English ed. London 1742). 1710 Lumleian Lecturer.
Biography: Ruhräh J: Walter Harris 1647–1732. Am J Dis Child 1929;38:1064–7.

Harvey, William *Folkestone, England 1578, †Roehampton, London 1657.
1599 Student of Fabricius in Padova; elucidated pulmonary circulation and fetal function of the ductus arteriosus. 1609 Physician at St. Bartholomew's Hospital London. 1628 *On the Motion of the Heart and Blood in Animals.* Frankfurt: William Fitzer. 1651 *On the Generation of Animals.* London: James Young. 1653 *Anatomical exercitations concerning the generation of living creatures.* London: James Young.
Biography: Wright T: William Harvey. A life in circulation. Oxford: Oxford University Press, 2013.

Hazen, Elizabeth Lee *Rich, MS 1885, †Seattle, WA 1975.
1944 Microbiologist at the New York office of the Division of Laboratories and Research, State Department of Public Health. With R. Brown in 1950: *Two antifungal agents produced by a soil actinomycete. Science* 112:423. 1951: *Fungicidin, an antibiotic produced by a soil actinomycete. Proc Soc Exp Biol Med* 76:93–7.
Biography: Baldwin RS: The fungus fighters. Ithaca, NY: Cornell University Press, 1981.

Herrgott, Alphonse *Belfort 1849, †Nancy 1927.
1887 Professor of obstetrics in Nancy. Fetal diseases. 1878 *Des maladies foetales qui peuvent faire obstacle a l'accouchement.* Paris. 1890 Founded infant consultation agency.
Biography: Couvelaire A: Alphonse Herrgott (1849–1927). Gynécologie et obstetrique 1927;16:445–7.

Hess, Alfred F. *New York City 1875, †New York City 1933.
Independent scientist doing research with his own funds. 1905 Practice in New York City; found that milk pasteurization increases

the risk of scurvy in 1914: *Infantile scurvy: the blood, the blood-vessels and the diet. Am J Dis Child 8:385–405.* 1929 Monograph on rickets: *Rickets, including osteomalacia and tetany. Philadelphia, PA: Lea & Febiger.*
Biography: Darby WJ, Woodruff CW: Alfred Fabian Hess—a biographical sketch. J Nutr 1960;71:3–9.

Hess, Julius H *Ottawa, IL 1876, †Los Angeles, CA 1955.
1911 *A study of the caloric needs of premature infants. Am J Dis Child 2:302–14.* 1922 Opened and directed the premature infants ward at Michael Reese Hospital, Chicago; developed closed incubator-bed with oxygen supply. 1922 *Premature and congenitally diseased infants. Philadelphia, PA: Lea & Febiger.* 1927 *Premature infants: a report of 266 consecutive cases. Am J Dis Child 34:571–84.*
Biography: Dunn PM: Julius Hess (1876–1955) and the premature infant. Arch Dis Child Fetal Neonat Ed 2001;85:F141–4.

Hippocratian Corpus *430 b.c.e., 350 b.c.e.
Collection of 60 Greek medical texts from three centuries. French edition in ten volumes, E. Littré 1961–1962. A part has been translated into English in the Loeb Classical Library. Especially relevant for neonates are the books: *Airs, waters and places*; *On dentition*; *On the nature of the child*; *On the eight-month infant*; *On superfetation.*
Biography: Jouanna J: Hippocrates. Baltimore, MD: Johns Hopkins University Press, 2001.

Holt, Luther Emmett *Webster, NY 1855, †Peking, China 1924.
1889 Director of Babies Hospital at Columbia University New York. 1894 *The Care and feeding of children. New York: Appleton.* 1896 *The diseases of infancy and childhood. New York: Appleton.* 1901 Chair of Diseases of Children.
Biography: Prudden TM: Luther Emmett Holt. Science 1924;59:452–3.

Huch, Albert *Duderstadt, Germany 1934, †Zürich, Switzerland 2009.
1967 Max Planck Institute for Respiratory Physiology, Göttingen. 1969 Department of obstetrics, Marburg. 1969 Developed transcutaneous PO_2 measurement together with his wife Renate Huch and with D.W. Lübbers: *Quantitative polarographische Sauerstoffdruckmessung auf der Kopfhaut des Neugeborenen. Arch Gyn 207:443–51.* From 1978 professor of obstetrics at Zurich University.
Biography: Dudenhausen JWD, Vetter K: Albert Huch: a life based on contradictions. Geburtsh Frauenheilk 2009;69(8):718–20.

Huldschinsky, Kurt *Gleiwitz, Silesia (then Germany) 1883, †Alexandria, Egypt 1940.
1911 Kaiserin Auguste Victoria Infant Hospital Berlin. 1919 Ultraviolet light for the treatment of rickets. *Heilung von Rachitis durch Ultraviolettbestrahlung. Dt Med Wschr 26;712–13.* 1934 Emigration to Egypt following anti-Jewish pressure in Nazi Germany.
Biography: Emed A: Kurt Huldschinsky (1883–1940). Harefuah 1999;137:80–1.

Hunter, John *East Kilbride, Scotland 1728, †London 1793.
1760 Army surgeon. 1768 Surgeon to St George's Hospital. 1776 *Double chambered bellows for artificial respiration. J Phil Trans 66:412.* 1790 Surgeon General. 1786 *On the structure of the placenta. In: Observations on certain parts of the animal oeconomy. London.* Together with his brother William: discovery of the intervillous space.
Biography: Moore W: The knife man. London: Bantam, 2005.

Hügel, Franz Seraph *Vienna 1808, †Vienna 1876.
1848–1863 director Children's Hospital Vienna-Wieden; 1848 *Beschreibung sämtlicher Kinderheilanstalten in Europa. Wien, Kaulfuss.* 1863 *Die Findelhäuser und das Findelwesen Europas. Wien: Sommer.*
Biography: Hirsch A: Biographisches Lexikon 1931, vol. 3, p. 324.

Jacobi, Abraham *Hartum, Westphalia 1830, †New York City 1919.
1850 Imprisoned for participation in the German Revolution. 1853 Emigration to New York City. 1870 Professor of Diseases of Children at Columbia University. 1888 Founded American Pediatric Society. Opposed percentage feeding. 1917 *History of pediatrics in New York. Arch Pediatr Jan–Feb:196–7.* 1898 *Therapeutics of infancy and childhood. Philadelphia, PA: Lippincott.*
Biography: Burke EC: Abraham Jacobi MD, Respectable Rebel. Pediatrics 1997;99:462–6.

James, L. Stanley *Te Awamuti, New Zealand 1925, †Center Harbor, NH 1994.
Emigrated to US. 1967 Professor of pediatrics assigned to anesthesiology at Columbia University, New York. 1972 Director of the Perinatal medicine division; 1958 *The acid-base status of human infants in relation to birth asphyxia and the onset of respiration. J Pediatr 52:379–394.*
Biography: James LS: Acidosis of the newborn and its relationship to birth asphyxia. In: Rooth G, Saugstad OD: The roots of perinatal medicine. Stuttgart: Thieme, 1985: p. 67–75.

Jörg, Eduard *Leipzig 1808, †Pennsylvania 1878.
Leipzig; research on atelectasis/respiratory distress syndrome in preterm infants. 1835 *Die Foetuslunge im geborenen Kinde. Grimma: Gebhardt.* 1848 Marine Hospital Cuba. Emigration to Pennsylvania. 1854 *Tropical diseases. Leipzig: Dürr.*
Biography: Jörg E: Briefe aus den Vereinigten Staaten. Leipzig: Weber, 1853.

Karlberg, Petter *Särna, Sweden 1919, †Göteborg 2006.
1954 Docent Pediatrics Karolinska Stockholm; 1953 *Determination of standard energy metabolism in normal infants. Acta Paediatr 42:576–80.* 1963 Professor of paediatrics Göteborg; research on respiratory control in premature infants. 1960 *The adaptive changes in the immediate postnatal period, with particular reference to respiration. J Pediatr 56:585–604.*
Biography: Kjellmer I, Wennergren G: Petter Karlberg (1919–2006), a curious scientist. Acta Paediatr 2016;105:1399–401.

Klaus, Marshall H. *Cleveland, OH 1927, †Palo Alto, CA 2017.
1966 *Oxygen therapy for the newborn. Ped Clin North Am 13:731–52.* Director, neonatal unit Stanford University. 1976 (with J. H. Kennell) *Maternal-infant bonding: St. Louis, MO: Mosby.* Professor and chair of pediatrics, Michigan University. 1973 (with A Fanaroff) *Care of the high-risk neonate. Philadelphia, PA: Saunders* (5 eds). 1985 *Your amazing newborn. Reading, MA: Addison-Wesley* (translated into seven languages). 1992 Founded Doulas of North America to support mothers in labour and postpartum.
Biography: Fanaroff AA: Marshal Klaus: the impact of a pioneer in neonatology. Pediatr Res 2017;83:6–8.

Lachapelle, Marie-Louise née Dugès *Paris 1769, †Paris 1821.
1795 Midwife-in chief at the Paris Maternité and School of Midwifery. Taught midwives to master forceps deliveries and endotracheal intubation of the neonate. 1819 *Observations sur differens cas d'accouchemens. Paris.* Textbook of midwifery which became standard throughout France. 1821, 1825 *Pratique des accouchemens* (posthumously edited by her nephew Antoine Dugès).
Biography: Chaussier F: Notice historique sur la vie et les écrits de Mme. Lachapelle. Paris: Huzard, 1823.

LaFetra, Linnaeus *Washington 1868, †New York City 1965.
1911–1920 Director, children's medical service, Bellevue Hospital New York City. Babies' Hospital New York; infections, congenital syphilis. 1912 *The employment of salvarsan in infants and young children.* Arch Pediatr 29:654–64. 1916 Room-sized incubator for premature infants: *The hospital care of premature infants.* Trans Am Pediatr Soc 28:90–101.

Landsteiner, Karl *Vienna 1868, †New York City 1943.
1898 Pathologist in Vienna. 1901 Description of three blood groups: *Wiener Klin Wochenschr 14:1132–4.* 1903 Habilitation. Described meconium ileus due to cystic fibrosis in 1905: *Zentralblatt Allg Pathol 16:903–7.* 1923 Rmigration to US, worked at New York Rockefeller Institute. 1930 Nobel Prize for Medicine or Physiology. 1940 (with A. Wiener) *Discovery of the Rhesus-factor: Proc Soc Exp Biol Med 43:223.*
Biography: Schwarz HP, Dorner F. Historical review: Karl Landsteiner and his major contributions to haematology. Br J Haematol 2003;121:556–65.

Langstein, Leopold *Vienna 1876, †Berlin 1933.
1909 Head physician. 1911 Director, Kaiserin Auguste Victoria Infant Hospital in Berlin. 1910 *Säuglingsernährung und Säuglingsstoffwechsel.* Wiesbaden: Bergmann. 1918 *Atlas der Hygiene des Säuglings und Kleinkindes.* Berlin: Springer. 1919 *Das Kaiserin Auguste Victoria Haus zur Bekämpfung der Säuglingssterblichkeit im Deutschen Reiche.* 1933 Anti-Jewish Nazi legislation forced him to quit his functions.
Biography: Stürzbecher M: Langstein, Leo. In: Neue Deutsche Biographie, Vol. 13. Berlin: Duncker & Humblot, 1982: p. 613 f.

Lathrop, Julia Clifford *Rockford, IL 1858, †Rockford, IL 1932.
1912–22 Director of the United States Children's Bureau. Training of social workers, improvement of birth registration. 1912 *The Children's Bureau.* Am J Sociol 18:318–30. 1919 *Income and infant mortality.* Am J Public Health 9:270–4. 1921 Sheppard-Towner Maternity and Infancy Act: federally funded social welfare measures for infants.
Biography: Addams J: My friend, Julia Lathrop. Urbana: University of Illinois Press, 2004.

Lavoisier, Antoine Laurent *Paris 1743, †Paris 1794.
1769 Tax office Ferme Générale. Private laboratory. 1772 Oxygen uptake in combustion (using ideas of Scheele and Priestley). 1777 Calorimetry to measure the heat production in cold surrounding. 1785 *Mémoire sur l'affinité du principe oxygine avec le différentes substances auxquelles il est susceptible de s'unir.* Hist Acad R Sci 530–40. 1789 *Traité élémentaire de Chimie. Paris.* 1794 Executed during the revolution.
Biography: EA Underwood: Lavoisier and the history of respiration. Proc R Soc Med 1943;37:247–62.

Le Boursier du Coudray, Angelique *Clermont-Ferrand, France 1712, †Bordeaux 1794.
1759 *Abrégé de l'art des accouchements.* Chalons-sur-Marne, Bouchard. Invented the obstetric mannequin 'The machine'. Royal brevet, travelled all over the country and trained midwives.
Biography: Gelbart NR: The king's midwife. Berkeley, CA: University of California Press, 1998.

Levret, André *Paris 1703, †Paris 1780.
1753 *L'art des accouchemens. Paris, Delaguette.* 1760 Royal accoucheur. 1781 *Observations sur l'allaitement des enfants. Paris, Méquignon l'aîné.*
Biography: Tshisuaka BI: André Levret. In: Gerabek WE et al.: Enzyklopädie Medizingeschichte. Berlin: de Gruyter, 2005: p. 847.

Liggins, Graham *Thames, New Zealand 1926, †Auckland 2010.
1968 Professor of Obstetrics, Auckland University; developed antenatal steroid treatment to accelerate lung maturation. 1968 *Premature parturition after infusion of corticotrophin or cortisol into foetal lambs.* J Endocrinol 42:323–9. 1972 (with R. Howie) *A controlled trial of antepartum glucocorticoid treatment for prevention of the respiratory distress syndrome in premature infants.* Pediatrics 50:515–25.
Biography: Gluckman P, Buklijas T: Sir Graham Collingwood (Mont) Liggins. Biogr Mems Fell R Soc 2013;59:193–214.

Lind, John *Stockholm 1909, †Stockholm 1983.
1957 Professor of paediatrics at Karolinska Institute Stockholm. 1949 (with Carl Wegelius) *Angiocardiographic studies on the human foetal circulation; a preliminary report.* Pediatrics. 1949;4:391–400.
Biography: Oh W: Professor John Lind. Neonatology pioneer. Neoreviews 2008;9:e279.

Little, William John *London 1810, †Malling, England 1894.
1838 Lecturer at the London Hospital Medical School. From 1843 series of 13 *Lectures on the Deformities of the Human Frame.* Lancet 44. 1845 Director of Royal Orthopaedic Hospital. Related cerebral palsy to perinatal events. 1861: *On the influence of abnormal parturition, difficult labours, premature birth and asphyxia neonatorum on the mental and physical condition of the child.* Trans Obstet Soc London 3:293–344.
Biography: Schifrin BS et al.: William John Little and cerebral palsy. Eur J Obstet Gynecol Reprod Biol 2000;90:139–44.

Lubchenco (Josephson), Lula O. *Turkistan, Russia 1915, †Denver, CO 2001.
Moved to US when 3 years old. 1943 Associate professor of pediatrics at Medical Center, Denver. 1969 Chair of pediatrics. 1963 *The high risk infant.* Philadelphia, PA: Saunders. Percentiles ('the Lulagram').
Biography: Nelson RA: Lula O. Lubchenco, MD. The oral history project. Elk Grove Village, IL: American Academy of Pediatrics, 2012.

Lucey, Jerold F. *Holyoke, MA 1926, †Sarasota, FL 2017.
1956 University of Vermont. 1972 Neonatal unit at University of Vermont. 1968 *Prevention of hyperbilirubinemia of prematurity by phototherapy.* Pediatrics 41:1047–54. 1974–2008, editor in chief of

Pediatrics. 1988 Founder and president, Vermont-Oxford Neonatal Network. 1995 Professor of neonatology.
Biography: First LR, Kemper AR: Carrying forward a legacy: a tribute to Jerold F. Lucey, MD, Pediatrics editor-in-chief (1974–2008). Pediatrics 2018;141: e20174216.

Lycosthenes (Wolffhart), Conrad *Rufach 1518, †Basel 1561.
1545 Diacon of St. Leonhard's church in Basel. Published a chronicle of congenital malformations in 1557: *Prodigiorum ac ostentorum chronicon = Wunderwerck oder Gottes unergründtliches vorbilden, Basel*.
Biography: Franck J: Konrad Lycosthenes. In: Allgemeine Deutsche Biographie, Vol. 19, Leipzig: Duncker & Humblot, 1884: p. 727f.

Macklin, Charles Clifford *Toronto 1883, †London, Ontario 1959.
Pioneer of surfactant research. 1921 Professor of histology and embryology at University of Western Ontario. 1946 *Residual epithelial cells on the pulmonary alveolar walls of mammals. Trans R Soc Can 40:93–111*. 1950 *The alveoli of the mammalian lung. Proc Inst Med 18:78–95*. 1954 *The pulmonary alveolar mucoid film and the pneumonocytes. Lancet 1:1099–104*.
Biography: Staub NC et al.: Charles Clifford Macklin, 1883–1959: an appreciation. Am Rev Resp Dis 1976;114:823–30.

Mahon, Paul Augustin-Olivier *Chartres, France 1752, †Paris 1800.
1795 Teacher of Legal Medicine; Physician-in-chief of the Paris Hospital for Venerics. 1804 *Maladies syphilitiques, et manière de les traiter, dans les femmes enceintes, dans les enfans nouveaux-nés et dans les nourrices. Paris: Buisson* (posthumously edited by L. Lamauve).
Biography: Coquillard I: [From sworn physicians at the Châtelet de Paris to forensic physicians. The birth of a professionalization (1692–1801)]. Hist Sci Med 2012;46:133–44.

Mauriceau, François *Paris 1637, †Paris 1709.
Obstetrician at Hotel Dieu, Paris. 1668 *Traité des maladies des femmes grosses, et accouchées. Paris: Henault* (English translation London 1672). 1670 Dispute with the Chamberlen family for not publishing their family secret, the obstetric forceps. 1694 Collected case reports: *Observations sur la grossesse et l'accouchement des femmes. Paris: Compagnie des Libraires*.
Biography: Karamanou M et al.: Practising obstetrics in the 17th century: François Mauriceau. J Obstet Gynec 2013;33:20–3.

Mayow, John *Cornwall 1641, †London 1679.
1669 Dissertation: *Respiration as a form of combustion: De sal-nitro et spiritu nitro-aëreo. Fetal gas exchange in the placenta. Oxford*. 1670 Practised in Bath; described mechanism of bone deformation in rickets in 1674 *De rhachitide. In: Tractatus quinque medico-physici. Oxford: Sheldon*.
Biography: Partington JR: The life and work of John Mayow. Isis 1956;47:217–30.

McNutt, Sarah J. *1839, †Albany NY 1930.
1887 Founder of New York Babies' Hospital; Neuropathology of birth injuries. 1885 *Double infantile spastic hemiplegia. Am J Med Sci 89:58*. 1885 *Seven cases of infantile spastic hemiplegia. Arch Pediat 2:20*.
Biography: Horn SS, Goetz CG: The election of Sarah McNutt as the first woman member of the American Neurological Association. Neurology 2002;59:113–7.

Meckel, Johann Friedrich Jr. *Halle 1781, †Halle 1833.
1802 *De cordis conditionibus abnormis*. 1805 Professor of anatomy in Halle. 1808 Combined chair of anatomy, surgery and obstetrics. Many papers on congenital malformations. 1812 *Handbuch der pathologischen Anatomie, Vol 1; Leipzig, Reclam*.
Biography: Wormer EJ: Johann Friedrich Meckel von Hemsbach. Neue Deutsche Biographie, Vol. 16. Berlin: Duncker & Humblot, 1990: p. 585.

Meigs, Arthur Vincent *Philadelphia, PA 1850, †Philadelphia 1912.
Pennsylvania Children's Hospital. 1885 *Milk analysis and infant feeding. Philadelphia, PA: Saunders*. Human milk only 1% protein: 1896 *Feeding in early infancy. Philadelphia, PA: Saunders*.
Biography: Cone TE: The doctors Meigs of Philadelphia and their contributions to infant feeding. In: History of American pediatrics, Boston, MA: Little, Brown & Cie, 1979: p. 135–6.

Meigs, John Forsyth *Philadelphia, PA 1818, †Philadelphia 1882.
1848 *A practical treatise on the diseases of children*. 1850 'Meigs' mixtures' (3.5% fat, 1.2% protein, 6.7% sugar, 0.25% ash).
Biography: Cone TE: The doctors Meigs of Philadelphia and their contributions to infant feeding. In: History of American Pediatrics, Boston, MA: Little, Brown & Cie, 1979: p. 135–6.

Mercuriale, Hieronymus *Forli, Papal States 1530, †Forli 1606.
1562 Physician at the Vatican. 1569 Professor in Padova and Pisa. 1583 *De morbis puerorum tractatus locupletissimus*. Skull percussion to diagnose hydrocephalus.
Biography: Boerner F: De vita, moribus, meritis et scriptis Hieronimi Mercuriali. Brunsvigiae: Keitelian, 1751.

Mercurio, Scipione Girolamo *Rome 1550, †Venice 1615.
Dominican monk in Milan. 1595 *La Commare o raccoglitrice, Venetia, Battista Cioti* (midwives' textbook); 1653 *Die Kinder-Mutter oder Hebammen-Buch*. From 1601 in Venice. 1604 *On popular errors in Italy*.
Biography: Siebold ECJ: Scipione Mercurio. In: Versuch einer Geschichte der Geburtshülfe. 2nd ed., Vol II. Tübingen: Pietzker, 1902: p. 136–40.

Minkowski, Alexandre *Paris 1915, †Paris 2004.
1947 Fellowship to study neonatology at Julius Hess' unit in Chicago. 1950 Returned to Paris. 1959 Founded journal *Biologia neonatorum*, since 1983 *Biology of the Neonate*, since 2007 *Neonatology*. 1966 Director of Neonatal Services at Port Royal Hospital; first ventilator unit for neonates in France.
Biography: Relier JP: Alexandre Minkowski, 1915–2004. Biol Neonat 2004;86:183. Autobiography: Le mandarin au pieds-nus. Paris: Editions Seuil, 1975.

Moro, Ernst *Laibach, Illyria (today Lubljana, Slovenia) 1874, †Heidelberg 1951.
1899 Assistant of Escherich in Graz; Munich; bacteriologic studies. 1907 Hauner Children's Hospital Munich. 1908 Percutaneous test for tuberculosis. 1911 Professor of paediatrics in Heidelberg; diagnostic test for tuberculosis; treatment of infantile diarrhoea with carrot soup; Moro reflex. 1919 Full professor in Heidelberg; married to a Jewish wife, he was forced out of office in 1936.

Biography: Weirich A et al.: Ernst Moro (1874–1951)—a great pediatric career started at the rise of university-based pediatric research but was curtailed in the shadows of Nazi laws. Eur J Pediatr 2005;164:699–706.

Nestlé, Henri *Frankfurt/Main 1814, †Glion, Switzerland 1890.
1867 Invention of *farine lactée*; 1875 Nestlé sold his factories, having become a millionaire. In 1905, Nestlé and Anglo-Swiss companies merged.
Biography: Pfiffner A: Henri Nestlé (1814–1890): Vom Frankfurter Apothekergehilfen zum Schweizer Pionierunternehmer. Zürich: Chronos, 1993.

Newsholme, Arthur *Haworth 1857, †Worthing 1943.
1875 St Thomas Hospital, London. 1889 *The elements of vital statistics*. Multiple papers on birth rate and infant mortality rate. 1908 President of the Society of Medical Officers of Health. 1919 *The historical development of public health work in England. Am J Publ Health 9:907–18*.
Biography: Eyler JM: Sir Arthur Newsholme and State Medicine, 1885–1935. Cambridge: Cambridge University Press, 1997.

Noeggerath, Carl T. *New York 1876, †Freiburg 1952.
1913 Professor of paediatrics at Freiburg University. 1912 Intravenous injection of Salvarsan in neonates: *Klinische Beobachtungen bei der Salvarsanbehandlung syphilitischer Säuglinge. Jahrb Kinderh 75:131–65*. 1913 Electrocardiogram in infants: *Electrokardiogramme schwächlicher Säuglinge. Zeitschrift Kinderheilk 6:369–42*.
Biography: Rominger E: Nachruf auf Carl T. Noeggerath. Zeitschrift Kinderheilk 1952;71:I–IV.

Parrot, Joseph Marie Jules *Excideuil, France 1829, †Paris 1883.
1867 Director of the Foundling Hospital Paris. 1872 Pseudoparalysis of the extremities in congenital syphilis; built a pavilion at the Foundling Hospital where syphilitic infants were nursed by donkeys. 1876 Chair of the History of Medicine. 1877 Chronic failure to thrive: *Athrepsia: Clinique des Nouveau-Nés: L'Athrepsie. Paris: Masson*. 1882 *La nourricerie de l'hospice des enfants-assistés. Bull Acad Méd 2e série:839–53*. 1886 *Maladies des Enfants. La Syphilis Héréditaire et la Rachitis. Paris: Masson*.
Biography: Gerabek WE et al.: Joseph Marie Jules Parrot. In: Enzyklopädie Medizingeschichte. Berlin: de Gruyter, 2005.

Paré, Ambroise *Laval, France 1510, †Paris 1590.
1552 Royal surgeon to Henry II; 1562 Royal surgeon to Charles IX. 1573 Two books on surgery: *1. De la génération de l'homme, et manière d'extraire les enfans hors du ventre de la mère, ensemble ce qu'il faut faire pour la faire mieux, et plus tost accoucher, avec la cure de plusieurs maladies qui luy peuvent survenir. 2. Des monstres tant terrestres que marins avec leurs portraits plus un petit traité des plaies faictes aux parties nerveuses. Paris: André Wechel*.
Biography: Paget S: Ambroise Paré and his times, 1510–1590. London: Putnam, 1903.

Pfaundler, Meinhard *Innsbruck, Austria 1872, †Ötztal, Austria 1947.
1904 *Physikalisch-chemische Untersuchungen an Kinderblut. Verh Dtsch Ges Kinderh 21:24*. 1906 Director of Munich University Hospital. 1906 (together with Schlossmann) Handbook of *Pediatrics*; nosocomial infections. 1907 *Über die Behandlung der angeborenen Lebensschwäche. Münch Med Wochenschr 54:1417–21*. 1936 Introduced the term perinatal: *Studien über Frühtod, Geschlechtsverhältnis und Selection. Zeitschrift Kinderheilk. 57:185–227*.
Biography: Wormer EJ: Meinhard Pfaundler von Hadermur. In: Neue Deutsche Biographie, Vol. 20. Berlin: Duncker & Humblot, 2001, p. 303f.

Phaire, Thomas *Norwich, Wales 1510, †Cardigan, Pembrokeshire 1560.
1545 *The Boke of Children. London?: Printer unknown*. 1547 Member of parliament.
Biography: Ruhräh J: Thomas Phair, the father of English Pediatrics. In: Pediatrics of the past, New York: Hoeber, 1925: p. 147ff.

Powers, Grover F. *Lafayette IN 1887, †New Haven CT 1968.
1921 Yale, from 1927 as chairman of pediatrics. 1926 Treatment shock in diarrhoea.
Biography: Gordon HH: Grover F. Powers—in memoriam. Yale J Biol Med 1969;42:39–44.

Prod'hom, Louis Samuel *Lausanne 1926, †Pully, Switzerland 2008.
Training in Boston; from 1960–1970 several papers on respiratory distress syndrome. 1970 'Pavillon des prématurés' Lausanne. 1980 Director of the division of neonatology at Lausanne University.
Biography: Micheli JL et al.: Samuel Prod'hom périnatologue. Paediatrica 2008;19:70–1.

Quetelet, Adolphe *Gent 1796, †Brussels 1874.
1827 *Recherches sur la population, les naissances, les deces, les prisons, etc. dans le Royaume des Pays-Bas*. 1828 Built an astronomical observatory in Brussels. 1835 *Sur l'homme et le developpement de ses facultés. Paris, Bachelier*. 1838 *De l'influence des saisons sur la mortalité des differens ages dans la Belqique*. 1841 Associate of the Royal Institute of the Netherlands. Compared lifetables and found considerable differences in infant mortality between European states. 1864 *Sur la mortalité pendant la première enfance. Bull Acad R Sci Belg 5:89–94*.
Biography: Sheynin OB: A. Quetelet as a statistician. Arch Hist Exact Sci 1986;36:281–325.

Raulin, Joseph *Ayguetinte France 1708, †Paris 1784.
1763 Accoucheur and professor in Paris. 1768–9 *De la Conservation des enfants, ou les Moyens de les fortifier, depuis l'instant de leur existence, jusqu'a l'âge de puberté. Paris: Merlin*.
Biography: Ruhräh J: Pediatric biographies. Chicago, IL, 1930, reprinted Am J Dis Child, pp 67–9.

Reuss, August Ritter von *Vienna 1879, †Vienna 1954.
Professor of pediatrics in Graz. Neonatal ward at the Obstetric Hospital, University of Vienna. 1914 *Die Krankheiten des Neugeborenen. Berlin, Springer*. Therein, continuous positive airway pressure described. 1924 Professor of paediatrics at Vienna University. 1929 *Säuglingsernährung, Berlin*; 1931 *Pathologie der Neugeburtsperiode, in: Handbuch Kinderh 4*.
Biography: Czeike F: August Reuss. In: Historisches Lexikon Wien, Vol. 4. Vienna: Kremayr & Scheriau, 1995.

Biographical notes on frequently cited authors

Reynolds, E. Osmund R. *Brighton 1933, †London 2017.
1962 Fellowship at Boston Children's Hospital. 1964 University College Hospital London; pioneer of artificial ventilation with lower pressure and prolonged inspiration (with S. Herman). 1973 *Methods for improving oxygenation in infants mechanically ventilated for severe hyaline membrane disease. Arch Dis Child 48:612–7.* 1976 Professor and director of neonatology; delayed brain destruction after asphyxia due to apoptosis.
Biography: Watts G: Osmund Reynolds, key figure in the foundation of UK neonatology. Lancet 2017;390:224.

Rhazes (Abu Bakr Muhammed ibn Zakariya al-Razi) *Ray, Teheran 864, †Teheran 925.
Structured and translated Galen's works; 1187 *Liber ad Almansorem, Pediatric Appendix*; translated into Latin by Gerhard von Cremona.
Biography: Ruhräh J: Rhazes (852–932 AD). In: Pediatrics of the past. New York: Hoeber, 1925: p. 19–21.

Ribemont, Alban-Alphonse *Vendôme 1847, †Paris 1940.
1878 Endotracheal tube for neonates: *Recherches sur l'insufflation des nouveau-nés et description d'un nouveau tube laryngien. Progrès Médical 16:293–5; 17:316–7; 19:355–7; 20:376–8; 21:395–6.* 1889 *De la maceration chez le foetus vivant. Paris.* 1898 Professor of obstetrics in Paris. 1914 *Traité d'obstetrique, Paris.*
Biography: Fischer I: Biographisches Lexikon. Wien, Urban & Schwarzenberg Vol. 2, p. 1291.

Riegel, Klaus Philipp *Schorndorf 1926, †München 2018.
1963 Lecturer, University Children's Hospital Tübingen. 1969 Associate professor at University of München. Founder of perinatal survey in Germany. Neonatalerhebung. 1972 *Perinatale Atmung: Physiologische Grundlagen und therapeutische Konsequenzen. Heidelberg: Springer.* 1985 *Perinatalrisiken und kindliche Mortalität und Morbidität. München: Ges. f. Strahlen- u Umweltforschung.*
Biography: Roehr CC, Versmold H: In memoriam Klaus P. Riegel—leading pediatrician, clinical scientist, and pioneer perinatal epidemiologist. Pediatr Res 2018;84:570–1.

Robertson, Bengt *Stockholm 1935, †Stockholm 2008.
From 1970 pathologist at St. Göran's Hospital Stockholm. From 1974 Professor of Perinatal Pathology at Karolinska Institute. Developed with Göran Enhörning a method to substitute natural surfactant in 1972: *Lung expansion in the premature rabbit fetus after tracheal deposition of surfactant. Pediatrics 50:709–82.* Randomized trial with Curosurf in 1988: *Pediatrics 82:683–91.*
Biography: Halliday HL, Speer CP: Bengt Robertson (1935–2008): a pioneer and leader in surfactant research. Neonatology 2009;95:VI–VIII.

Roederer, Johann Georg *Strasbourg 1726, †Paris 1763.
1746 Strasbourg School of Midwifery. 1751 Professor of obstetrics at Göttingen University. Systematic measurement of neonatal body weight: 1753 *Sermo de pondere et longitudine infantum recens natorum. Comment. Soc Reg Scient Gottingae 3:410–24.* 1753 *Elementa artis obstetricae in usum praelectionum academicarum.* 1758 Opposed the dogma of maternal imagination causing fetal disease.
Biography: Zimmermann V: Johann Georg Roederer. In: Neue Deutsche Biographie. Vol. 21. Berlin: Duncker & Humblot, 2003: p.709f.

Roelans von Mecheln, Cornelius *Mechelen, Brabant 1450, †Mechelen 1525.
1483 *Libellus egritudinum infantium.* 1498–1525 Hospital- and city-physician of Mechelen.
Biography: Ruhräh J. Cornelius Roelans (1450–1525). Pediatrics of the past. New York: Hoeber, 1925: p. 99–102.

Roesslin, Eucharius Rhodion *Waldkirch (then Austria) 1470, †Frankfurt/Main 1526.
Pharmacist in Freiburg. 1509 City physician in Frankfurt/Main. 1513 *Der Swangern Frauwen und hebammen Rosegarten.* Compilation from Corpus Hippocraticum, Soran, Aetius, and Avicenna.
Biography: Baas K: Eucharius Rösslins Lebensgang. Arch Gesch Med 1908;1:429–41.

Rosén von Rosenstein, Nils *Sexdrega, Sweden 1706, †Uppsala 1773.
1731 Teaching appointment at Uppsala University. 1764 *The diseases of children and their remedies. Stockholm, Salvius* (25 editions, ten translations, English ed. 1776).
Biography: Wallgren A: Nils Rosén von Rosenstein, a short biography. Acta Paed Suppl 1964;156:11–26.

Rotch, Thomas Morgan *Philadelphia, PA 1849, †Boston, MA 1914.
1881 Established the West End Nursery in Boston. 1888 Professor at Harvard Medical School, first pediatric chair with full faculty status in the US. Mobile incubator. The percentage method for infant feeding. 1896 *Pediatrics. The hygienic and medical treatment of children. Philadelphia, PA: Lippincott.* 1900 *Some important aspects connected with the scientific feeding of infants. New York: Knickerbocker.*
Biography: Talbot FB: Thomas Morgan Rotch. J Pediatr 1956;49:109–12.

Rubner, Max *München 1854, †Berlin 1932.
1877 Physiology Institute München. 1883 Habilitation. 1885 Chair of hygiene, Marburg University. 1891 Chair of hygiene, Berlin University. 1898 *Die natürliche Ernährung eines Säuglings. Zeitschr Biol 36:1–55.* 1902 Studies of nutrition in childhood.
Biography: Chambers WH: Max Rubner. J Nutr 1952;48:3–12.

Rudolph, Abraham M. *Johannesburg, South Africa 1924.
1951: Emigrated to US; trained in Boston Children's Hospital. 1960 Albert Einstein College New York. Developed many techniques for cardiac catheterization. 1966, Cardiovascular Research Institute at San Francisco; 1970 *The changes in the circulation after birth. Their importance in congenital heart disease. Circulation 41:343–59.* 1974 Textbook: *Congenital diseases of the heart: clinical-physiological considerations. Armonk, NY: Futura* (further eds. 2001, 2009).
Biography: Hoffman JI: Abraham Morris Rudolph: an appreciation. Pediatrics 2002;110:622–6.

Runge, Max *Stettin 1849, †Göttingen 1909.
1883 Professor of obstetrics in Dorpat; 1888 in Göttingen. Textbook of neonatology: 1885 *Die Krankheiten der ersten Lebenstage. Stuttgart, Enke* (other eds. 1893, 1906).
Biography: Zimmermann V: Heinrich Max Runge. In: Neue Deutsche Biographie, Vol. 22. Berlin: Duncker & Humblot, 2005: p. 264.

Ruysch, Frederik *The Hague 1638, †Amsterdam 1731.
1667 Prelector of the Amsterdam surgeon's guild. 1668 Chief instructor of the city's midwives; 1685 Professor of botany. One of the founders of teratology. 1701–1716 *Thesaurus anatomicus. Amsterdam: Johan Wolters*. 1720 *Adversariorum anatomico-medico-chirurgicorum, Amsterdam: Janssonio-Waesbergios*. Large collection of embalmed specimens of congenital malformations, sold to St. Petersburg in 1717.
Biography: Boer L et al.: Frederik Ruysch (1638–1731): historical perspective and contemporary analysis of his teratological legacy. Am J Med Gen A 2017;173:16–41.

Räihä, Niels C. R. *Helsinki 1930, †Lund 2013.
1970 *Artificial ventilation of the very small premature infant with respiratory insufficiency. Biol Neonate* 16:184–186. 1976 *Milk protein quantity and quality in low birthweight infants. I: Metabolic responses and effects on growth. Pediatrics* 57:659–74.

Schaffer, Alexander J. *Baltimore, MD 1902, †Baltimore 1981.
1924 Johns Hopkins Hospital/Harriet Lane Home; coined the term *neonatology*. 1960 *Diseases of the Newborn. New York: Saunders*.
Biography: Baker BM: Alexander J Schaffer. Trans Am Clin Climatol Assoc 1982;93:xl–xli.

Schatz, Friedrich *Plauen 1841, †Rostock 1920.
1868 Obstetric University Hospital Leipzig; 1872 University Rostock; 14 papers devoted to placental anastomoses and twin-twin transfusion syndrome: 1875–1910 *Die Gefäßverbindungen der Plazentakreisläufe eineiiger Zwillinge, ihre Entwicklung und ihre Folgen. Systematisches und alphabetisches Inhaltsverzeichnus. Arch Gynäk* 1900;60:559–84.
Biography: Ludwig H: Friedrich Schatz, Rostock (1841–1920): Über Zwillinge, Wehen und Schwangerschaftsdauer. Gynäkologe 2006;39:657–60.

Scheel, Poul *Itzehoe, Holstein 1783, †Copenhagen 1811.
Endotracheal intubation for resuscitation of the neonate in meconium aspiration: 1799 *On the properties and action of amniotic fluid in the trachea of human fetuses and in asphyxia of neonates. Copenhagen: Brummer (Latin)*. 1801 Court physician Copenhagen. 1802 Director of obstetric hospital. 1802 Blood transfusion, Copenhagen.
Biography: Gammeltoft SA et al.: The Gynecological and Obstetrical Society of Copenhagen. Acta Obstet Gyn Scand 1923;2:205–15.

Schlossmann, Arthur *Breslau, Silesia 1867, †Düsseldorf, Germany 1932.
Founded in 1898 the Infant Hospital of Dresden. Multiple papers on hospitals for infants, nutrition, and causes of infant mortality. 1900 *Zur Frage der natürlichen Ernährung des Säuglings. Arch Kinderh* 30:288. 1906 Director of the Children's Hospital at Düsseldorf University. Editor (with Pfaundler) *Handbook of Pediatrics. Leipzig: Vogel*.
Biography: Pfaundler M: Arthur Schlossmann [obituary]. Klin Wschr 1932;11:1246–7.

Schultze, Bernhard Sigmund *Freiburg, Baden 1827, †Jena, Germany 1919.
1854 Obstetric University Hospital Berlin. 1858 Professor of obstetrics in Jena. Worked on pathogenesis of hydrocephalus, spina bifida, and clubfoot. Introduced resuscitation by swinging the body: 1871 *Der Scheintod Neugeborener. Jena: Mauke*.
Biography: Henkel M: Bernhard Sigmund Schultze. Arch Gyn 1919;111:iii–xx.

Severinghaus, John Wendell *Madison, WI 1922.
1952: Research associate in physiology, University of Pennsylvania. 1956 Professor of anesthesiology, Cardiovascular Research Institute, San Francisco. 1956 *Accuracy of blood pH and PCO2 determinations. J Appl Physiol* 9:189–96. 1958 (with A.F. Bradley) *Electrodes for blood pO2 and pCO2 determination. J Appl Physiol* 13:515–20.
Biography: Astrup P, Severinghaus J. The history of blood gases, acids and bases. Copenhagen: Munksgaard, 1985.

Siegemund, Justine Dittrich *Rohnstock, Silesia 1636, †Berlin 1705.
1683 City midwife in Liegnitz; midwife to the court of Brandenburg. 1690 *Königlich Preussische und Chur-Brandenburgische Hof-Wehemutter. Cölln an der Spree, Liebpert*. (Translation 2005: *The court midwife. Chicago, IL: University of Chicago Press*.) Attacked Petermann, Frankfurt Faculty.
Biography: Siebold ECJ: Justina Siegemundin. In: Versuch einer Geschichte der Geburtshilfe. Tübingen: Pietzker, 1902: Vol. 2, p. 201–5.

Silverman, William A. *Cleveland, OH 1917, †Greenbrae, CA 2004.
1945 Joined pediatric team at Columbia University New York. 1955 Director of Neonatology division at Columbia. 1956 *A difference in mortality rate and incidence of kernicterus among premature infants allotted to two prophylactic antibacterial regimens. Pediatrics* 18:614–25. Propagated randomized studies to establish new forms of treatment: artificial ventilation. 1967 *A controlled trial of management of respiratory distress syndrome in a body-enclosing respirator. Pediatrics* 39:740–8; use of oxygen, temperature regulation. Emphasized the importance of iatrogenic disease in neonatology: 1980 *Retrolental fibroplasia: a modern parable. New York: Grune & Stratton*. 1985 *Human experimentation: a guided step into the unknown. Oxford: Oxford University Press*. Published multiple notes in *Pediatrics* under the pseudonym 'Submitted by Student'.
Biography: Watts G: William Silverman. BMJ 2005;330:257.

Sinclair, John C. *Regina 1933, †Toronto 2014.
1970 Professor of pediatrics at McMaster University, Hamilton, Ontario. Established evidence-based medicine in neonatology. 1992 (with M.B. Bracken) *Effective Care of the Newborn. Oxford: Oxford University Press*. 2003: *Cochrane neonatal systematic reviews: a survey of the evidence for neonatal therapies. Clin Perinat* 30:285–304.
Biography: The Cochrane Collaboration: In memoriam John Collison Sinclair MD: neonatologist. Cochrane Database, 2014.

Smallpeice, Victoria *London 1901, †Oxford 1991.
1947 Consultant to the Oxford Regional Hospital Board. 1964 Clinical director at Oxford Hospitals. Propagated early nutrition of preterm infants (with Pamela Davies): 1964 *Immediate feeding of premature infants with undiluted breast-milk. Lancet* 2:1349–52. 1965–1966 President of the paediatric section of the Royal Society of Medicine.
Biography: Davies PA: Gwladys Victoria Smallpeice. In: Life of the RCP fellows, London: Munks, 2009: Vol. IX, p. 479.

Smith, Clement A. *Ann Arbor, MI 1901, †Boston, MA 1988.
1931 Boston Children's Hospital. 1946 *The Physiology of the Newborn Infant. Springfield, IL: Charles Thomas.* 1961–1974 Editor of *Pediatrics.* 1960 Circulatory factors in relation to idiopathic respiratory distress in the newborn. *J Pediatr* 56:605–11. 1963 Professor of pediatrics at Boston Lying-In Hospital and Harvard University. 1965–1966, President of the American Pediatric Society.
Biography: Lucey J, Haggerty R: A tribute to Dr. Clement A. Smith. Pediatrics 1974;53:1.

Soemmerring, Samuel Thomas *Thorn, Poland 1755, †Frankfurt/Main 1830.
1779 Professor of Anatomy at Collegium Carolinum Kassel. 1784 Chair of Anatomy and Physiology University of Mainz. 1791 *Abbildungen und Beschreibungen einiger Misgeburten, die sich ehemals auf dem anatomischen Theater zu Cassel befanden. Mainz, Univ.-Buchhandlung.* 1804 Munich Academy of Sciences: invention of the telegraph.
Biography: Ruhräh J: Samuel Thomas Soemmerring (1755–1830). In: Pediatrics of the Past. New York: Hoeber, 1925: p. 437–9.

Soranus of Ephesus *Ephesus/Asia minor (today Turkey) 70, †Rome 130.
Studied in Alexandria. 98–117 Practised in Rome. *Gynecology* (English translation by O. Temkin, Baltimore 1956, Johns Hopkins University Press). This book exerted the greatest influence on neonatal care and nutrition for 1800 years.
Biography: Temkin O: Soranus' Gynecology. Baltimore, MD: Johns Hopkins University Press, 1956: p. xxiii–xlix.

Soxhlet, Franz *Brno (then Brünn), Czechia 1848, †München 1929.
1879 Professor of Chemistry at Munich Technical University. Research on sterilization of milk, inventor of the Soxhlet apparatus. 1886 *Über Kindermilch und Säuglingsernährung. Münch Med Wschr* 13:253–6; 276–8.
Biography: Gerabek WE: Franz Ritter von Soxhlet. In: Neue Deutsche Biographie, Vol. 24. Berlin: Duncker & Humblot, 2010: p. 606f.

Stern, Leo *Montreal 1931, †Providence RI 1989.
McGill University, Montreal; thermoregulation. 1965 *Environmental Temperature, Oxygen Consumption, and Catecholamine Excretion in Newborn Infants. Pediatrics* 36:367–73. 1987 (with Paul Vert) *Neonatal Medicine, Paris: Masson.* 1970 Description and utilization of the negative pressure apparatus. *Neonatology* 16:24–9. 1970 Results of artificial ventilation in the newborn. *Neonatology* 16:155–63.

Strang, Leonard B. *East Kilbridge, Scotland 1925, †Volx, France 1997.
1959 Hammersmith Hospital. 1961 Fellow at Harvard. 1967 Professor of paediatrics, University College Hospital London. Respiratory adaptation at birth.
Biography: Lloyd J: James Spence Medallist 1990: Professor Leonard B. Strang. Arch Dis Child 1990;65:1101–12.

Straus, Nathan *Otterberg (Palatinate) 1848, †New York City 1931.
Co-owner of New York department store Macy. From 1889, philanthropic activities, focusing on providing pasteurized milk for infants. Instituted milk depots. Statistics on infant mortality: 1911 Official delegate of the United States at the Berlin Congress of Infant Protection. 1913 *Disease in milk—the remedy: pasteurization.* New York: Dutton.
Biography: Miller J: Nathan Straus and the drive for pasteurized milk, 1893–1920. New York Hist 1993;74:159–84.

Swyer, Paul R. *London 1921, †Toronto 2019.
1954 Emigrated to Toronto, fellowship at the Hospital for Sick Children. Since 1960 artificial ventilation of intubated preterm infants. 1964 (with M. Delivoria-Papadopoulos) *Assisted ventilation in terminal hyaline membrane disease. Arch Dis Child* 1964;39:481–4. 1964 Director of the Division of Neonatology at HSC Toronto. 1975 *The intensive care of the newly born. Physiological principles and practice. Monogr Paediatr* 10:1–208. 1992 How small is too small? A personal opinion. *Acta Paed* 1992;81:443–5.
Biography: Reese CN, Reese J: Paul R. Swyer: the beginnings of Canadian neonatology at the Hospital for Sick Children in Toronto. J Perinatol 2018;38:297–305.

Sylvius (de le Boe), Franciscus *Hanau 1614, †Leiden 1672.
1639 Lecturer in Leiden; 1641 Medical practice in Amsterdam. 1658 Professor of medicine in Leiden. 1669 Established a chemical laboratory. 1671–1674 *Praxeos medicae idea nova, 4 vols Lugduni Batavorum, Carpentier.* 1682 *Of Children's diseases … as also a treatise of the rickets. London: George Downs.*
Biography: Van Gijn J: Franciscus Sylvius (1614–1672). J Neurol 2001;248:915–6.

Süßmilch, Johann Peter *Berlin 1707, †Berlin 1767.
1741 Army chaplain in Jena. 1742 Pastor in Berlin-Cölln. Analysis of church records, regional and international comparison of infant mortality, structure of life tables. 1742 *Die göttliche Ordnung in den Veränderungen des menschlichen Geschlechts [the divine order]. Berlin: Gohls.*
Biography: Birg H: Ursprünge der Demographie in Deutschland. Leben und Werk Johann Peter Süßmilchs. Frankfurt: Campus, 1986.

Tarnier, Etienne Stéphane *Aiseray, France 1828, †Paris 1897.
1858 *De la fievre puerpérale observé a la Maternité de Paris.* 1864 *Mémoire sur l'hygiene des hôpitaux de femmes en couches.* 1867 Surgeon-in-chief of the Paris Maternité. 1880 Applied closed wooden incubator (couveuse) for the care of preterm infants. 1877 Forceps. 1889 Professor of obstetrics at Paris University.
Biography: Dunn PM: Stéphane Tarnier (1828–1897), the architect of perinatology in France. Arch Dis Child Fet Neonat Ed 2002;86:F137–9.

Taussig, Helen Brooke *Cambridge, MA 1898, †Chester County, PA 1986.
1927 Johns Hopkins Hospital. 1930 Harriet Lane Home. 1944 With Alfred Blalock: palliative operation for tetralogy of Fallot; pioneered the use of X-ray for the diagnosis of congenital heart malformations. 1947 *Congenital malformations of the heart. New York: The Commonwealth Fund.* 1967 Initiated ban of thalidomide in the US and Europe.
Biography: McNamara DG et al.: Helen Brooke Taussig: 1898 to 1986. J Am Coll Cardiol 1987;10:662–71.

Underwood, Michael *Molesey, England 1737, †Knightsbridge, England 1820.
1779 Surgeon at the British Lying Hospital London. 1784 Licentiate in Midwifery. 1784 *A Treatise of the Diseases of Children With Directions For the Management of Infants from the Birth, especially such as are brought up by Hand. London: Mathews.* Eighteen editions, remained standard for over 60 years. 1796 Physician and accoucheur to the Princess of Wales; kept a daily record of his life extending to 122 volumes.
Biography: Still GF: Michael Underwood. In: The history of paediatrics. London: Dawson, 1965: p. 476–86.

Usher, Robert H. *Montreal 1929, †Montreal 2006.
1959 Director of the neonatal unit at McGill University Montreal. 1963 *Reduction of mortality from respiratory distress syndrome of prematurity with early administration of intravenous glucose and sodium bicarbonate. Pediatrics 32:966–75.* 1969 (with McLean): centiles for birthweight and body measures: *Intrauterine growth of liveborn Caucasian infants at sea level. J Pediatr 74:901–10.*
Biography: Dunn PM: Robert Usher. Br Med J 2006;332:1514.

Vallambert, Simon de *Avalon, France 1520?, †Poitiers 1570?
1558 Personal physician of the duchess of Savoye and Berry. 1565 *Cinq livres de la maniere de nourrir et gouverner les enfans des leur naissance. Poitiers: Marnefz et Bouchetz.*
Biography: Winn CH: Simon de Vallambert, Cinq livres … Edition critique. Genève: Librairie Droz, 2005.

Valleix, Francois Louis Isidore *Toulouse 1807, †Paris 1855.
Followed Billard and Berton as intern at the Paris Foundling Hospital. 1835 *De l'asphyxie lente chez les enfants nouveau-nés*; 1836 Physician to the Central Bureau. 1838 *Clinique des maladies des enfants nouveau-nés. Paris: Baillière*; described diagnostic nerve points. 1842 Hopital Ste. Marguérite, Hopital de la Pitié, Paris.
Biography: Bouillet MN, Chassang A: Isidore Valleix. In: Dictionnaire universel d'histoire et de géographie. Paris: Hachette, 1878.

Verheyen, Philip *Verrebroek (now Belgium) 1648, †Leuven 1710.
1683 Professor of anatomy in Leuve. 1689 Rector of Leuven University. 1693 Also Professor of surgery. 1693 *Corporis humani anatomiae. Leuven, Denique.* 1710 and 1726 *Supplementum anatomiae corporis humani … descriptio partium foetui et recenter nato propriarum. Bruxellis: t'Serstevens.* Therein description the fetal cardiovascular system, reference work until the middle of the 18th century.
Biography: Suy R: Philip Verheyen (1648–1710) and his Corporis Humani Anatomiae. Acta Chir Belg 2007;107:343–54.

Vesalius, Andreas *Brussels (now Belgium) 1514, †Zakynthos/Greece 1564.
1536 Padua. 1537 Professor and chair of anatomy and surgery at Padua University. 1538 *Tabulae Anatomicae Sex.* 1543 Went to Basel to edit his magnum opus *De humani corporis fabrica. Basel, Oporinus*; descriptions of endotracheal ventilation. 1544 Court physician to Emperor Charles V. 1555 Revised edition of the *Fabrica.* 1564 Pilgrimage to the Holy Land, died after shipwreck on the island of Zakynthos.
Biography: O'Malley CD: Andreas Vesalius of Brussels, 1514–1564. Berkeley, CA: University of California Press, 1964.

Villermé, Louis René *Paris 1782, †Paris 1863.
1814 Military surgeon. Studies in social epidemiology, factory and prison reform, and infant mortality. 1818 Secretary General of the Société Médicale d'Emulation. 1823 Academie Royale de Médecine. 1830 *De la mortalité dans les divers quartiers de la ville de Paris. Annales d'Hygiène publique et de Médecine Légale 3:294–341.*
Biography: Julia C: Louis-René Villermé (1782–1863), a pioneer in social epidemiology: J Epidemiol Community Health 2011;65:666–70.

Volpe, Joseph *Salem, MA 1938.
Washington University St. Louis. 1980 Classification system for periventricular leukomalacia; 1990 Pediatric neurologist in Boston. 1981 *Neurology of the newborn, Philadelphia, PA: Saunders* (six eds. up to 2018). 1984 Professor of pediatric neurology, Harvard Medical School. 2002 *Perinatal brain injury in the preterm and term newborn. Curr Opin Neurol 15:151–7.*

West, Charles *London 1816, †Paris 1898.
1842 Royal Dispensary for Women and Children in Lambeth. 1845 Lecturer in Obstetrics at Middlesex Hospital. 1848 *Lectures on Diseases of Infancy and Childhood. London: Longman.* 1852 Founded the Hospital for Sick Children in Great Ormond Street, remained its senior physician until 1875.
Biography: Besser FS: Notes on Dr. Charles West and his grave in Chislehearst (Kent). Hist Med 1975;6:47–50.

Wiedenmann, Barbara *Augsburg 1695, †Augsburg 1751.
1729 Midwife in Augsburg. 1738 Midwives' textbook: *Kurtze, jedoch hinlängliche und gründliche Anweisung Christlicher Hebammen. Augsburg, Lotter.* Propagated intrauterine baptism and designed a syringe for this purpose.
Biography: Winckel, F: Wiedenman(nin), Barbara. In: Allgemeine Deutsche Biographie. München: Duncker & Humblot, 1897: Vol. 42, p. 342–3.

Willi, Heinrich *Chur, Switzerland 1900, †Zürich 1971.
1937 Director of the Zurich Infant Hospital Rosenberg. Described Necrotizing enterocolitis: 1944 *Über eine bösartige Enteritis bei Säuglingen des ersten Trimenons. Ann Pediatr 162:87–112.*
Biography: Didierjean B: Geschichte der Neonatologie in Zürich. Zürich: Juris Druck & Verlag, 1979.

Willughby, Percival *Nottinghamshire 1596, †Derby 1685.
Oxford graduate, pupil of William Harvey. 1631 Settled in Derby in obstetric practice. His 1621 manuscript *Observations in midwifery* was published in the Netherlands in 1754 and in England in 1863.
Biography: Blenkinsop, H: Observations by Percival Willughby; edited from the original MS. Warwick: Shakespeare Printing Press, 1863.

Wolff, Caspar Friedrich *Berlin 1734, †St. Petersburg 1794.
Anatomist and embryologist. 1759 *Theoria Generationis. Halle: Hendelianis*; a classic in embryology, despite epigenetic argumentation. 1766 Academy of Sciences, St. Petersburg; 1768 *De formatione intestinorum, Petropolitanae, Acad. Sci.* Opposed preformationism and proposed the theory that organisms develop gradually. Long controversy with Haller.
Biography: Aulie RP: Caspar Friedrich Wolff and his 'Theoria Generationis' 1759. J Hist Med All Sci 1961;16:124–44.

Würtz, Felix *Basel, Switzerland 1518, †Basel 1576.
Barber surgeon in Basel. 1563 *Practica der Wundartzney (Treatise of Surgery)…* attached: *Kinderbüchlein.* (Engl. ed. 1656: The Children's book).
Biography: Ruhräh J: Pediatrics of the past. New York: Hoeber, 1925: p. 196.

Ylppö, Arvo *Akaa, Finland 1887, †Helsinki 1992.
1912 Fellowship at Kaiserin Auguste Victoria Haus Berlin. Fundamental monography on preterm infants: 1919 *Pathologisch-anatomische Studien bei Frühgeborenen. Zeitschrift Kinderheilk 20:213–431.* 1919 *Zur Physiologie, Klinik und zum Schicksal der Frühgeborenen. Zeitschrift Kinderheilk 24:1–178.* 1920 Mannerheim foundation for the protection of children. 1921 Docent. 1923 Professor at Helsinki University Hospital. Various chapters on neonates in *Pfaundlers Handbook of Pediatrics.*
Biography: Autobiography: Ylppö A: Mein Leben unter Kleinen und Großen. Lübeck: Hansisches Verlagskontor, 1987.

Index of Personal Names

Page locators given in italics are for figures; page locators in bold are for the biographies.

Abramson, H 37, 379
Abt, I 225, 230, 406, 409
Adams, F 93
Aetios of Amida 183, 189
Ahlfeld, F 80, 127, 139, 150, 184
Ainu, Japan 118
Aitken, J 19, 423
Akhenaton, Pharaoh 3, 155, *156*
Albertus Magnus 13, 213, 245
Alcmene *116*, 241
Aldrovando, U 58, *59*
Alemona, Goddess 11
Alexander of Tralles 178
Allison, A 293
Alunno, N *175*
Amalthea, Nymph 241, *242*
Amenhotep III, Pharaoh 115
Amort, E 399
Amphitryon 116
Anderson, B 260
Anglicus, B 213
Anselm of Canterbury 5
Anteverta, Goddess 57
Anthony, Saint 175
Anubis, God 3
Apgar, V 29, 30, *30*, 41, 168, 169, 416, **423**
Apollo, God 51, 117, 352
Apple, R 233, 262
Aranzio, GC 12, 17, 21, 96, **423**
Aristotle 65, 79, 137, 214, 221, 233, 311, 345, 347, **423**
    fetal life 4, 5, 8, 22, 16
    infant anatomy 96, 273
    lactation 213, 214, 221
    malformation 354
    meconium 311
    milk, animals 241
    procreation 115, 123
    resuscitation 25, 51
    twins 129
    viability 74
Armstrong, G 174, 176, 235, 253, 280, **423**
Ashby, HT 383, 386
Ashvins, Gods 117
Astrup, PB 416, **423**
Aspertini, A *179*
Assurbanipal, King 64, 197
Atkins, P 249, 250
Aton, Sun-God 3, *156*
Atwood, H 255
Augustine, Saint 5, 65, 95, 137, 241, 359, 397, 413
Aulus Gellius 57

Auvard, AP 73, 230, 231, 255, 266, **423**
Avery, ME 75, 86, 91, **423**
Avicenna 79, 173, 183, 213, 222, 280, 339, **424**
    breastfeeding 215, 217, 222, 280
    fetal nutrition 213
    imagination 183
    resuscitation 45
    seizures, teething 173
    tongue-tie 274
    umbilicus 52
    viability 79

Bagatta, G 399
Bagellardo, P 28, 33, 237, 280, **424**
Baines, MA 223
Baldini, F 247, 254, *255*
Baldung (Grien), H 145, *146*, 214
Ballantyne, JW 159, 406, 408, **424**
    fetal dropsy 298, *299*
    imagination 183
    macrosomia 305
    malformations 199
    prematurity 386
    viability 75, 83
Ballexserd, J 235, 236, **424**
Bancroft, H 65, 158
Banta, HD 30
Banting, F 307
Barclay, AE 416, **424**
Barcroft, J 20, *21*, 416, **424**
Barker, DJP 308
Barness, LA 261, 269
Baron, JF 340, 341, 407, **424**
Barrie, H 43
Barron, D 20
Barrow, J 368
Bartels, H 20
Barthe, A 147
Bartholin, C 12, *12*
Bartholin, T 39, 145, 184, **424**
Bartolomeo, M *167*
Baudelocque, JL 85, 116, 130, 235, 253, 255
Bauhin, C 197, *198*, 199, **424**
Baumes, JB 174, 176, 216, 297, **424**
Bazalgette, J 250
Beckensteiner, E 361, *361*
Beckwith, B 380, 381
Beddies, T 371, 372
Bednar, FA 53, 85, 107, 166, 292, 317, 346, 407, **424**
Beham, B 160, 394, *395*
Bell, AG 35, 87

Bell, B 29
Bell, MJ 319, 320
Beller, F 8, 169
Benda, G 269
Benedict XIV, Pope 33, 66, 399
Benirschke, K 120, 133, 140
Benjamin, H 269
Bennewitz, H 306
Berg, FT *340*, 341, 383, **424**
Berkhout, C 341
Bernard, C 14, 243
Bernheim, BM 292, *294*
Bernheim-Karrer, J 261, 328, 407, **425**
Bernstein, J 176
Bertin, R 333, 334, 336
Biedert, Ph 251, 261, 386, 387, **425**
Billard, CM 265, 291, 313, 317, 407, **425**
    cerebral bleeding 107
    ductus arteriosus 102, *103*
    jaundice, brain 299
    lung disorders 85
    scurvy 128
    thrush 330, *340*, 341
Binding, K 371, 372, 375
Blalock, A 416, 436
Bloch, I 147
Blondel, JA 187
Blumenbach, JF 188, 199
Blundell, J 46, 47
Bodin, J 147
Bodio, L 384, *385*, 388, **425**
Boe, Sylvius 12, 280, 297, **436**
Boerhaave, H 72, 214, 216, 313, **425**
Boivin, MAV 33, 46, 415, **425**
Boleyn, A 147
Borden, G 257, 259, *260*, 261, **425**
Borelli, G 18
Bosch, H 174, *175*.
Botallo, L 96, *97*
Bouchut, E 46, 73, 102, 107, 275, 297, 329, *330*, **425**
Bourgeois, L 26, 33, 129, 159, 215, 222, 274, 339, **425**
Bowditch, H 292
Bowlby, J 279
Bowman, JM 301, *302*
Boyssou, L 241, 242
Brachet, JL 131, 406
Brandt, AM 365
Brassavole, M 333
Breck, S 266
Breton, MV 253, *255*

Brissaud, E 167
Broussais, F 75
Brown, J 75
Brown, R 342, *343*, **425**
Brueghel, P 216
Buchan, W vii, 281, 311, 384, **425**
Buckley, W 251
Budin, PC 213, 251, 252, *387*, 407, 408, **425**
    artificial feeding 243, 266, *266*
    infant mortality 213
    pasteurization 250, *256*
    prematures' unit 71, 74, *81*, 408
Buhl, L 347
Bull, T 254, 284
Bunsen, R 19, 20
Burchard, Bishop 412
Burns, J 333, **425**
Burq, V 179, *179*

Cadogan, W 216, 217, 235, 328, 386, **426**
Caesar, GJ, Emperor 57, 241
Caldeyro-Barcia, R 30
Caldwell, F 230
Calvin, J 6, 66, 96, 174
Cameron, H 120
Cameron JR 59
Camper, P 236, 367
Cangiamila FE 6, 7, 33, 39, 45, 57, 137, 399, 414, **426**
Cantimpré, T 58, 137
Capper, A *81*, 168
Capuron, J 34, 74, 107, 168, 275, **426**
Carmentes, Goddesses 57
Carnot, P 292
Carpenter, W 13, 14, 103
Carré, F 254, 255, *256*
Casserio, G 17, *18*
Castara, M 205, *206*
Catel, W 166, 372, 374
Catozze, M 197, *200*
Cattaneo, J 333
Celsus, AC 273, 339
Chamberlen, H 26, *28*, 33, 312
Charles V, Emperor 95, 184, 360, 374
Chaussier, F 41, 74, 329, *330*, 414, **426**
    intubation 46, *46*, 87
    Maternité 39
    oxygen use 39
    ventilator 34, 39, 87, *88*
Cheselden, W 19, 97
Cheyne, J 292, *293*
Chick, H 328, **426**

Index of Personal Names

Clarke, C 177, 301
Clarke, J 54, 281, 284, **426**
Clauder, F *305*
Claudius, F 139, 140
Clément, J 26
Clements, JA 92, 93, 104, **426**
Coceani, F 99, 104
Coit, HL 250, 252
Colombo R 11, 96
Columbus, C 155, 333, 365, 414
Comroe, JH 85, 87, 93, 103, 104, **426**
Conduitt, J 79
Confucius 4, 353
Constantine, Emperor 25, 33, 221, 222, 356, 359, 413
Cook, J 284
Coombs, R 301
Cooper, A 139, 214, *215*
Cooper, W 147
Coram, T 367, 414
Cornblath, M 269
Corner, BD 318, 375, **426**
Coudray, A 414
Coutsoudis, A 262
Craig, WS 177, 406
Cranach, L 397, *398*
Credé, C *81*, 408
Cremer, R 301, 416
Crosse, VM 80, *81*, 293, 406, 408, **426**
Crow, H 119
Cruveilhier, J 107, *108*
Cullen, W 254
Cullough, M 281, *282*
Culpeper, N 235
Cunningham, HB *231*
Czerny, A 71, 217, 243, 371, 408

Dafoe, AR 125
Dalrymple, J 14
Dam, H 293
Dapper, O 118
Darwin, Ch 120, 157, 192, 279, 371, 415
Darwin, E 19
Das, K 140, *141*
Davenport, C 124
Davidson, M 269
Davies, PA 267, **426**
Davison, W 379
Dawes, GS 20, 30, 42, 101, **427**
Day, RL **427**
De Almagro, M 101, *102*
De Graeff, J 129, *131*
De Lee, J 47
Del-Rio, JM 174
Denis, PS 59, 168
Denman, T 72
Denucé, JP 406, 415, **427**
Denys, J *149*
Descartes, R 6, 186, *187*, 414
Deventer, H *60*, 305
Diamond, LK 301
Diemerbroeck, I 12, 18, 186, 414, **427**
Dimme, Demon 63
Dinouart, JA 40
Diodorus Siculus 354, 377
Dionne quintuplets 124, 125, 126
Dioscuri, 117
Dobbing, J 262
Dodd, L 248, 249, 257

Doepp, Ph 54, 260, 265, 328, 407, 427
Doisy, E 293, 416
Donald, I 87
Doublet, F. 334, **427**
Down, L 191, *192*, 193, 284, 372, 374, 416, **427**
Draeger, H 37
Drake, T 233, *234*, 237
Drillien, CM 267, **427**
Drinker, Ph 87, 415, **427**
Dubreuil, G 306, *307*
Dufour, L *234*, 250, 251, 254, **427**
Dugès, A 297, 299, *313*, 346, **427**
Duncan, A 207
Duncan, M 306
Dunham, EC 80, *81*, 320, 347, 407, **428**
Durand, P 257
Durand, W 397
Dwork, D 251

Eastman N. 29, **428**
Ebers Papyrus 33, 279, 305
Ehrlich, P 336, 415
Eldridge, DL 101, 102
Elsässer, JA 161, *161*, 287, **428**
Emiliane, G 399
Engelberts, A 380
Engelhardt, T 6, 8, 369, 389
Engelmann, F 41, *42*
Enhorning, G 93, **428**
Epstein, A *81*, 407, 409, 428
Eröss, G 405, 407
Escherich, Th 341, 406, 407, **428**
  bacteria, gut 238, 347
  Coli bacteria 255
  incubator room 408, *409*, *410*
  rickets therapy 327, *327*
Esquirol, JE 369
Ettmüller, M. 235, 280, 311, 312, **428**
Evans, E 192
Everaerts, A 13
Ezekiel, Prophet 51

Fabricius ab Aquapendente 96, 97, 147, 166, 274, *274*, **428**
Fabricius Hildanus 175; 186
Fallot, A 201, 416, 436
Fanaroff, A *81*, 312
Farr, W 383, 393, **428**
Fatio, J 34
Fauvel, H 248, 254
Fernel, J 12
Ferrarius, O 215, 228
Ferrier, A 333
Fildes, V 223, 235
Finkelstein, H 108, 222, 261, 326, 347, *347*, 373, 406, 409, **428**
  formula feeding 243, 250
  haemorrhages 292
  nasal feeding 266, *266*
  navel infection 53, *54*
  rickets 326, *329*
  scurvy *329*
  sepsis *348*
Finn, R 301
Flagg, P 29, 37, 48, *428*
Florian of Liechtenstein 399
Fomon, SJ 261
Ford, N 3, 6, 8

Foregger, R 48
Fores, S 27, *27*
Forsyth, D 244, 250
Fourcroy, JL 53
Fracastoro, G 340
Francesca, P *179*
François I, King 249
Frank, JP 159
Fraser, J 192, *193*
Frederick II, Prussian King 367
Freud, S 29, 168
Friedinger, C *337*
Friedman, W 104
Frölich, T 261, 328
Froggatt, P 380
Frugardi, R 228, *228*
Fujiwara, T 93, *93*, 416, **428**

Galen of Pergamon 25, 95, 96, 125, 166, 273, 277, 366, 413, **429**
  animal milk 233, 241
  imagination 183
  opiates 180, 279, 283
  physiology *5*, 17, 18
  pregnancy duration 71
  procreation 214
  soul 4, 5, 17
  umbilical vessels 11, 17, 96
  uterus-breast connection 13, 213, *214*
Gardanne, JJ 29, 54
Garnier, P 216
Garrod, A 193
Gedda, L 115
Gemzell, CA 126
Geoffroy, J *251*
Geoffroy St. Hilaire, E 138, 139, 145, 148, 187
Geoffroy St. Hilaire, I 147, 199
George III, King 26
Gersdorf, H 214
Gesner, C 241
Gibbs, F&E 177
Gibson, T 13
Girtanner, C 19, 28, 277, 280, **429**
Gleiss, J 267, 379
Glisson, F 325, 414
Gluck, L 92, 306, 375, **429**
Godfrey's cordial 280, 281, 283, 284, 285
Goethe, JW 29, 75, 194, 365
Golding, J 294
Gomez, PV, Bishop 59, 118
Goodhart, J 267
Goodlin, RC 30
Goodyear, C 207, 229, 254
Gorcy, PC 34
Gordon, A 346
Gordon, G 243, 250
Gordon, R 269
Gosse, LA 158, *158*
Gotthelf, J 400
Grandidier, L 292
Graunt, J 383, 429
Gregory GA 41, 87, 104, 416
Grien, HB 145, *146*, 214
Grimm, J&W 79, 400
Gross, R 103
Gruby, D *340*, 341, 407, 415, **429**
Gruenwald, P 91, 92
Guersant, P 208, 275

Guillemeau, J 26, 58, *60*, 217, 222, 234, 235, 280, **429**
Gumppenberg, W 399
Gundobin, NP 407
Guyon, L 335
György, P 406, 409, **429**

Habermas, J 7
Habermas, R 365
Haeckel, E 192, 371, 372
Hagen, JP 27, 274
Hahn, C 85, 108
Hahn, E 319
Hall, M 49, 284
Haller, A 18, 57, 147, 199, 311, **429**
  ductus arteriosus 97
  fetal nutrition 13
  irritability 29
  life, beginning 6
  uterus-breast connection 214
  viability 72
Haller, B 399
Hallman, M 92
Hamilton, A 223, 236, 280, **429**
Hammacher, K 30
Hammurabi, King 221, 297, 353, 413
Hannah, M 61
Hantzsch, JG *282*
Hardy, J 269
Harper's Weekly 281, *282*
Harris, JR 115, 117, 118
Harris, W 174, 175, 176, 223, 234, 237, 280, 281, 381, **429**
Hartley, R 247, *248*
Harvey, W 12, 17, 18, 79, 96, 166, 414, **429**
Hata, S 336
Hathor, Goddess 63, 241, 354
Hauner, A 237, 253
Haussmann, D 341
Hazen, E 342, *343*, **429**
Heberden, W 311, 340
Hefelmann, H 372
Heinze, H 372, 374
Heliodorus 185
Heister, L 311
Hellin, D 123
Helmont, JB 186, 235
Henke, A 174, 222, 235, 253
Hennig, C 247
Henry II, French King 361
Henry VIII, Engl. King 174, 414
Hephaistos, God 165, *355*
Hera, goddess 25, 241, 354, *355*
Heracles 116, *116*, 241
Herlin, F *64*
Hermbstaedt, S 306
Herodotus 137
Herrgott, A 251, 429
Hesiod 116
Hess, AF 250, 325, 328, **429**
Hess, JH 222, 269, 406, 410, **430**
  bed with oxygen *41*
  ductus arteriosus 103
  gestational age 72
  preterms, feeding 265, *266*, 267
  preterms, survival *81*
Hesse, CG 291
Hewitt, D 149
Heymann, MA 99, 104
Hildanus, F 175, 186
Hildegard von Bingen 5, 6, 95

Index of Personal Names

Hippocratian Corpus 72, 155, 165, 173, 174, 180, 214, 335, 345, 379, **430**
   cord ligation 25, 51
   dentition 175, 279
   fetal nutrition 11
   fetal respiration 17
   fetus, formed 8
   gestational age 71
   lactation 213
   quickening 8
   somersault 57, *58*
   superfetatio 116
   twins 115
Hoboken, N 12, *13*, 17
Hobrecht, J 250
Hoche, A 193, 371, 375
Hochheim, K 86
Hodgkin, T 139
Hofmann, JM 186
Holland, H 54
Holmes, OW 346, 349
Holst, A 261, 328
Holt, LE *73*, 174, 217, 222, 225, 238, 378, 407, **430**
Hon, E 30
Hoppe-Seyler, F 19
Horlick, J 260, 261
Horus, God 3, *4*, 115, 178, *178*
Huch, A 416, **430**
Hufeland, CW 28, 34, 75, 284
Huggett, A 14, 20
Huldschinski, K *327*, 373, **430**
Hunter, J 12, 34, 87, 335, 430
Hunter, W *12*, 13, 26
Hutchinson, J *334*

Icart, JF 25
Ingraham, NR 336
Innocent III, Pope 11, 359, *360*
Iphicles 116
Ishtar, Goddess 174, 353
Isis, Goddess 63, 241, 354

Jackson, JH 177
Jacobi, A 243, 250, 255, 261, 378, 407, 409, **430**
Jacquemet, E 230, *231*
James I, King 362, 367, 383
James, LS 30, *30*, 41, 416, **430**
Jeliffe, DB 262
Jörg, E 85, 86, *86*, 91, 101, 415, **430**
Jörg, JC 29, 167, 275, 341
John the Good, King 223
Jordaens, J *242*
Jordan, T 281
Joslin, E 306
Julius Caesar 71
Juno Lucina, Goddess 25, 57, 65
Jurine, L 238
Justinian, Emperor 67, 82, 353, 356, 359, 413

Kagan, BM 269
Kane, P 157, *157*
Kant, I 6, 369, 377
Kähler, D 138, *139*
Keirse, M 385
Kelsey, F 202
Kennedy, E 104
Kennedy, JF 103, 202, 416
Kergaradec, JA 30, 415

Ketham, J 214, *214*
King, R 92
Kirchhoff, G 19, *20*
Kite, C 45
Klaus, M 41, 92, **430**
Klee, E 372
Koch, R 35, 249, 255, 415
Koch-Hershenov, R 8
Koelliker, A *148*
Kolb, P 52, 119, *119*
Koplik, H 250, 252
Kopp, J 378
Kornmann, J 166, 174
Kräutermann, V 280
Kramer, H 174

Lachapelle, ML 33, 299, **431**
Laennec, RT 415, 424
La Fetra, L 336, 407, **431**
Lagercrantz, H 75
Lallemand, CF 130
Lamashtu, Goddess 63, *64*, 377
Lambert, S 292
Lancefield, R 249, 348
Lanciani, R 393
Landsteiner, K 298, 313, *313*, 320, 415, **431**
Langer, H 269
Langerhans, P 306, *307*
Langhans, T 14
Langstein, L 373, 406, 409, 415, **431**
Laplace, PS 91, 243, *244*
Larsson, KO *231*
Larsson, MN *231*
Lavoisier, AL 19, 39, 87, 243, *244*, 414, **431**
Lecornu, P 261
Leeuwenhoek, AL 185, 414
Lejeune, J 193, 416
Lentz, JW 336
Lenz, W 200, 201, 202, 307
Leonardo da Vinci 214, *214*, 414
Leroy d'Etiolles, JJ 34, 46, 85, 87, 91
Leslie, F 248, *249*
Leviton, A 169
Levret, A 33, 57, *75*, 130, 299, 312, **431**
Licetus, F 79, *80*, 184, *184*
Liebig, J 225, 243, 259, 260, 261, 267
Liggins, GM 92, 126
Linnaeus, C 214, 241, 414
Little, WJ 29, 31, 40, 168, *169*, **431**
Liudger, Bishop 360
Livius, T 183, *184*, 205
Lobstein, F 13, *14*
Longo, LD 11, 17
Lövegren, E 292
Louis XI, Fr. King 378
Louis XIV, Fr. King 26, 66, 224, 414
Lower, R 18
Lubchenco, LO 74, *75*, 416, **431**
Lucas, A 270, 307
Lucey, JF 301, **431**
Lucretius, T vii, 4
Lundeen, EC 269
Luther, M 6, 65, 137, 165, 166, 174, 186, 193, 197, 414
Lycosthenes/Wolffhart, C 124, 137, *138*, 145, *146*, 184, *184*, *185*, 197, **432**

Mackay, H 270

MacLennan, A 30
Magendie, F 34, 125, 341
Mahon, PA 334, **432**
Malpighi, M 13, 147, *148*, 341
Mangold, H 148
Mansel, J 5, *7*
Mantegna, A *166*, 191
Marcé, LV 369
Marchant 265
Marchini, G *177*
Marcot, E 147, 148
Marie-Antoinette, Queen 224, 297
Marlet, H *224*
Martin IV, Pope 184
Martiny, B 247, *248*
Maunsell, H 333
Mauriceau, F 28, 33, 58, 85, 165, 222, 235, 312, 414, **432**
   baptism, intrauterine 66, 67
   birth weight 73
   breast pump 229
   breech delivery *60*, 312
   haemorrhage 291
   macrosomia 306
   resuscitation 45
   tire-tête *26*
   tongue-tie 274, 275, *275*
   twins, placenta 129, *132*, 138
   viability 74, 107
Mauron, A 7
May, C 262
Maydl, K 208
Mayor, FI 30
Mayow, J 12, 17, 18, 28, 325, *326*, **432**
McBride, W 200, 202
McCollum, E 327
McCrackin, R 185
McLaren, D 223
McNutt, S 29, 168, **432**
McWhinnie, AM 207
Mead Johnson 261
Meckel, H 139, 140
Meckel, JF 138, 148, 149, **432**
Megenberg, K 185, 214
Meigs, AV 242, 260, 261, **432**
Meigs, JF 432
Meissner, FL 149, 159, 235, 253, 275
Mellin, G 260, 261
Mephitis, Goddess 345
Mercier, S 249
Mercuriale, H 173, 180, 274, 280, **432**
Mercurio, S 25, *58*, *60*, 186, 379, **432**
Mertans, C 328
Mery, J 138
Mesnard, J 229
Metlinger, B 180, 215, 216, 222, 228, 233, 235, 273, 280, 414
Miller, NT 80, 265, 328, 386, 407
Minkowski, A 375, 416, **432**
Minot, F 292
Mirandola, FP 124, *126*
Mitchell, A 192, *193*
Mitchell, E 380
Mitchell, J 247
Moeller, J 328
Mondino dei Luzzi 213
Monot, C 224
Morgagni, JB 97, 101, 149, 166, 187, 297, 313
Moro, E 277, 373, 406, **432**
Morse, A 14

Morse, JL 269
Morton, E 217
Morton, SG 157
Müller, J 188
Müller, M 262
Muralt, J *60*, 159, 215, 217

Naegele, FC 72, *75*
Naegele, H 29, *34*
Napoleon I, Emperor 39, 85, 192, 328, 368, 405, 415
Narmer, Pharaoh 3, *4*
Needham, W 11, 13, 18
Neergaard, K 91, *92*, 415
Nefertiti, Queen 156
Neisser, A 335
Nelson, J 235
Nelson, K 169
Nestlé, H 257, 259, 260, 261, 262, **433**
Nevinny, H 307, *307*
Newman, J 279
Newsholme, A 386, *386*, **433**
Newton, I 79, *80*
Newton, LH 262
Nicolle, EA 336
Nihell, E 27
Ninhursag, Goddess 63, 233
Nocart, M 249, 255
Noeggerath, CT 336, **433**
Noonan, J 3, 8

Oberwarth, E 80, 266
O'Dwyer, J 48
Ollivier d'Angers, CP 74, 149, 166
Oribasius 222
Orth, J 299, 415
Osiander, FB 39, *40*, 131, 346, *346*, 406
Osler, W 29, 108, 166, 168, 378
d'Outrepont, J 81

Palm, T 327
Paltauf, A 320, 378
Pape, K 109, *110*
Papile, LA 108
Paracelsus, T 147, 178, 279, 333
Paré, A *146*, 147, 185, 284, 414, **433**
   birth marks 186
   breech delivery 26
   dentition 281
   haemangioma 185, 186
   hooks, embryotomy 26
   malformations 146, 147, 183, 197, *200*
   multiple birth 124, *126*
   pap, panada 234, 235
   weaning 280
Parrot, JJ 107, *170*, 342, 407, **433**
   athrepsia (brain necrosis) 169, *170*
   cerebral haemorrhage 107, 108
   donkey pavilion 335, *335*, *336*
   pseudo-paralysis 333
   syphilis, organs 337
   syphilis, teeth 333, *334*
   thrush 341, *342*
Parsons, J 185
Passalacqua, J 145
Passini, F 265
Pasteur, L 250, 251, 255, 346, 347, 415
Pattle, RE 92

Index of Personal Names

Paul of Aegina 180, 273, 413, **423**
Persius 65
Pestalozzi, H 365
Petit, JL 275, *275*
Petty, W 383
Pfaundler, M 75, 81, *81*, 222, 406, 407, **433**
Phaire, T 166, 173, 176, 178, 180, 233, 280, **433**
Phanostrate 25
Pieper, PA 312, 341
Pignotti, M 82
Pildes, R 269
Pius IX, Pope 6
Plato 4, 8, 65, 165, 221, 413
Platter, F 191
Plempius, V 11
Plenk, JJ 40, 341
Pliny the Elder 11, 57, 67, 115, 123, 137, 183, 249, 281, 345, 356, 393
Ploetz, A 371
Ploss, HH 52, 242
Plutarch 65, 82, 221
Pollio, V 345
Postverta, Goddess 57
Powers, GF 242, 243, 260, **433**
Pratt, E 245, *255*
Priestley, J 19, 39, 86, 243, 414
Pugh, B 26, 45, *46*

Quaiser, K 318, *319*, 320
Quetelet, A 72, 383, **433**
Quing legal code 362
Quintero, RA 134, 141

Räihä, N 269, 375, **435**
Rang, BH 242
Rau, GM 34
Raulin, J 52, 74, 85, 235, 236, 339, **433**
Raynald, T 26
Redgrave, R *368*
Reese, D 248, 281
Regnault, HV 243, *244*
Reinhart, C *394*
Remus 117, *117*, 241
Reuss, A 40, 407, 408, 415, **433**
Reynolds, EOR 109, 375, **434**
Rhazes 173, 180, 279, 413, **434**
Ribemont, AA 46, 47, *47*, **434**
Richard de Nancy, C 80, 207, 230, 265, 406
Riderer, FS *401*
Riedel, JGF *157*
Riedlin, V 51, 291
Rilliet, F 292
Risiana, E 184
Robertson, A 312
Robertson, Bengt 93, 416, **434**
Robertson, Bruce 300
Robillard, E 93
Robin, C *340*, 341
Rodda, FC 292
Roederer, JG 73, 159, 187, 414, **434**
Roelans of Mecheln, C 173, 233, 280, **434**
Roentgen, WC *327*, 336, 415
Roesslin, E. 26, 33, *60*, *130*, 159, 215, 222, 233, 280, 339, 414, **434**
Romney, S 20
Romulus 117, *117*, 241
Rondelet, G 333

Roscoe, W 228
Rosenstein, NR 107, 176, 216, 222, 274, 281, 333, 377, 414, **434**
Rotch, TM 74, 174, 217, 243, 250, 260, 406, *434*
Rott, F 267
Roussel, T 224, 388, 415
Routh, CHF 176, 217, 224, 254, 262, 281
Rubens, PP *117*
Rubner, M 243, *244*, 415, **434**
Rudolph, AM 99, 103, 104, **434**
Rueff, J *26*, *130*,
Ruland, L 281
Ruysch, F 186
Ryff, W 159, 214, *214*

Sambon, L 227, *228*
Sanger, F 20
Santulli, TV 319, 320
Sass, HM 7, 8
Saugstad, O 41
Saviard, B 328
Savonarola, G 116
Scévole de St. Marthe 186
Schatz, F 132, 133, *133*, 140, *140*, **435**
Schaudinn, F 335
Schedel, H 137, *138*
Scheel, P 19, 45, 312, 406, 408, 414, **435**
Scheele, CW 19, 39, 243
Schenck, J 197, 205
Scherer, F 243, *244*
Schiller, F 365
Schlaginhaufen, O 124
Schleiden, M 14
Schlossmann, A *343*, 373, 406, 408, 415, **435**
Schmidt, K 318, *319*, 320
Schmorl, C 299, 301, *301*
Schmotzer, B 123, *125*
Schneider, K 173
Schultze, BS 35, *35*
Schurig, M 147
Schwartz, H 34, 312
Schwartz, P 108, 168
Scultetus, J *26*, 228, *229*, 274, *274*, *275*
Seguin, E 192, 194
Seidler, E 75, 371, 373
Semmelweis, I 346, 349, 415
Sendivogius, M 17, 39
Seneca 355
Sennert, D 297
Servetus, M 95, 96, 243
Seux, V 340
Severinghaus, JW 104, 416, **435**
Severino, MA 297, *298*
Sharp, J 216, 222
Sheppard Towner Act 225, 388, 415
Shiva, Hindu God 175, *176*, 183
Siebold, AE 72
Siebold, E 317, 415
Siegemundin, JD 27, 33, 274, 414, **435**
Silverman, WA ix, 93, **435**
Simon, F 242
Simon, J 208
Singer, C 5, *5*
Singer, J 14
Singer, P 7, 8, 369, 375
Smallpeice, V 267, **435**
Smellie, W 45, 85, 168, 235, 414

birth weight 72
breech head 161, *161*
forceps 27, *28*
imagination 147
seizures 177
twins, placenta 130
Smith, CA 86, 168, 281, 375, 416, **436**
Smith, H 236, 237, 241, 253, 281
Smith, P 126
Smith, S 292
Smith, T 394
Smithells, RW 151, 201
Snijder, G 227, *228*
Soemmerring, ST 131, 149, *149*, 299, 406, **436**
Soranus of Ephesus 65, 145, 215, 305, 325, 341, 413, **436**
  breastfeeding, doctrines 217, 233, 280
  breech delivery 58
  cord cutting 51, 52
  dentition 179, 180, 281
  head shaping 155
  imagination 183
  infant worth raising 25, 110, 355
  nose shaping 159
  overlaying 377
  swaddling 65, 165
  wet nursing 221, 222
Soxhlet, F 255, *256*, 261, 415, **436**
Spemann, H 148
Spieghel, A 12, 17, *18*, 51
Spielmann, JR 242
Spock, B 217
Sponsel, WE *231*
Sprenger, J 174
Stahl, GE 18, 29, 39
Stahlman, M 375
Stalpart, C 129, *132*, 149
Stalpart, P 13, 18
Stark, JC 206, *206*, 277
Stein, GW *72*, 73, 229, *230*, 406, 414, 422
Steinschneider, A. 380, 381
Stephanus, Saint *167*
Still, G 194, 328
Stoll, B 348
Storch, J 159, 175, 291
Strang, L 375, **436**
Straus, N 250, 251, 388, **436**
Struve, C 281
Süß von Kulmbach, H *160*
Süßmilch, JP 383, 386, 414, **436**
Sudhoff, K *228*
Suleman octuplets 126
Swammerdam, J 366, *367*
Swediaur, F 336
Sylvius de le Boe, F 12, 238, 297, **436**

Tacitus, C 241, 354, 356
Tarnier, St 407, 408, 415, **436**
Taussig, HB 202, 416, **436**
Taweret, Goddess 354
Templeman, C 378
Ten Rhyne, W *206*
Tertullian, QSF 5, 356, 397
Thannhauser, S 92
Theden, JCA 229, *230*
Theodore of Canterbury 362
Theremin, E *313*, 314

Thomas Aquinas 5, 8, 66, 359, 397, 413
Thore, AM 103
Tiedemann, F 139, 148, *148*
Todd, R 176
Tooley, M 6, 369
Tooley, W 104
Topp, S 371, 372
Torella, G 333
Touloukian, R 320, *321*
Townsend, C 292, 406, 415
Trajan, Emperor *355*, 356, 415
Trueheard 35, *36*, *46*, 47
Tutankhamun, Pharaoh *178*
Tyson, JE 83

Underwood, M 178, 235, 346, 414, **437**
  frenotomy 276
  milk composition 241
  navel bleeding 291
  opiates 280
  palsy, legs 29, 167
  resuscitation 42, 45, 48
  seizures 174, 176
  syphilis 333
  thrush 339, 341
Usher, RH 42, 269, 375, **437**

Valentine, Saint 175, **177**
Vallambert, S 215, 222, 378, 414, **437**
  artificial feeding 233, 234, 235
  balneum animale 34
  cerebral haemorrhage 107
  dentition 180
  opiates 280
  seizures 173
  thrush 339
Valleix, F 333, 341, **437**
Van der Weyden, R *64*
Vane, J 99, 416
Van Gennep, A 63, 429
Van Stipriaan Luiscio, A 241, 242
Variot, G 251
Vaughan, H 368
Veith, G 123
Verheyen, Ph 18, 28, *28*, 214, **437**
Vesalius, A. 45, 95, 96, 214, 379, 414, **437**
Vesling, J *97*
Viardel, C 119, 147, 312
Villermé, LR 386, **437**
Virchow, R 86, 97, 155, 162, 169, *170*, 250, 346, 378
Vishnu, Hindu God 3
Volpe, J 173, 174, 437
Von Euler, U 98
Vrolik, G 139, 187, 199
Vrolik, W 148, *150*, *184*, *200*, *207*

Waddell, W 293
Wallerstein, H 301
Ward, J 301
Wassermann, A 333, 335, 336
Waters, M 223
Wegner, G 333
Wells, G 112
Wendelstadt, G 326
Wendt, J 174, 275
West, C 222, 281, 292, **437**
West, WJ 177
Whipple, GH 292

Index of Personal Names

Whistler, D 325, 414
White, P 306, 307, 308
Whytt, R 107
Widdas, W 15
Wiedenmann, B 66, 67, 437
Wiehrer, M&C *400*
Wigglesworth, J 109, *110*
Willi, H 318, *318*, 320, 407, 416, **437**
Williams, C 262
Williams, JW 306
Williams, M 92
Willis, T 178, 306
Wills, L 151
Willughby, P 26, 58, 159, 312, 325, **437**

Wilson, GS 257
Wilson, PK 187
Wilson, SE 320
Winckel, F 347, *348*
Windship, C 254
Winslow, J 31
Winslow, JB 139, 187
Winslows Soothing 282, 283, *283*, 295
Winsor, C 223
Woillez, EJ 35, *36*
Wolff, CF 147, 148, *148*, 188, 198, **437**
Wolffhart / Lycosthenes, C 124, 165, 166, 174, *185*, 197, 414, **432**

amelia 197
anencephalus 145, *146*
blemmyes 137, *138*
malformations 184, *184*, *185*, 186
Woodbury, R 383
Wright, R 61
Wrisberg, HA 30
Würtz, F 159, 166, 414, *438*
Wydyz, H *282*

Ylppö, A 42, 80, 267, 318, 335, 347, 406, 415, **438**
acidosis 42
atelectasis 86, *87*

bilirubin, jaundice 297, 298, *300*
cerebral haemorrhage 109, *293*
oxygen therapy *41*
preterm infants 75, *81*, 108, 269
resuscitation 35, 40
rickets 269
Young, T 242

Zacchia, P 5, 8
Zeissler, J 320
Zeus, Greek God 116, *116*, 213, 241, *242*, 355
Zückert, JF 377
Zweifel, P 19, *20*, 21
Zwingli, U 399

Index of Locations

Page locators given in italics are for figures.

Abfaltersbach, sanctuary 399, *400*
Altdorf 186
Amarna 156
Amsterdam 136, 187, 199, *200*, 207, 227, *228*, 242, 285, 366
Ancyra, Council 359, 361
Angers, Hôtel-Dieu 317
Antilles 198
Apothetae 82
Arabia 363
Arslan Tash, Syria *64*
Ashkelon cemetery 393
Asia, infanticide 362
Astypalaia 392
Athens, Agora 393
Attica tombstones 166
Augsburg, executions 361
Aztecs 157

Babylonia 117, 123, 221
  clay Tablets *64*, 165, 197
  Talmud 3, 11, 291
Baltimore 269, 306, 327, 336, 416
Bamberg law 360
Basel 74, *81*, 91, 96, 159, 191, 360
Bavaria 74, 166, 178, 191, *276*, 384, *387*, 400
Belarus 262
Berlin 39, *72*, 74, 213, 225, 242, 244, 250, 251, 306, 328
  Charité 71, 97, 169, 188, 217, 317, 371
  Finkelstein 53, *54*, 250, 261, 266, 292, *329*, *347*, 348
  Ylppö 40, *41*, 75, *81*, 168, 267, *268*, 318
Bern, graves 399
  iconoclasm 413
Birmingham 87, 120, 191, 379, 406, 414, 416
  Sorrento Hospital 267, 293, 406
Bönnigheim 123; *125*
Bologna 12, 58, 147, 213, 228, 341, 360, 384
  death penalty 365
Bonn 320, 325, *326*
Bordeaux 224, 406, 415
Boston 61, 103, 133, 147, 177, 225, 255, 300, 307, 388
  Children's Hospital 169, 174, 217, 243, 249, *347*, 406
  Floating Hospital 225, 265, *266*
  Harvard University 74, 91, 168, 269, 306, 345, 346, 414,
  Lying-in Hospital 86, 249, 267, 269, 292, 308

Walker-Gordon Lab 243, 250, 260
Bovenau, Schleswig *66*
Breslau 137, *138*, 174, 243, 335, 373, 383
Bristol, Southmead Hospital 235, 294, 318
Britain 34, 35, 53, 244, 261, 267, 328, 336, 362, 368
  anencephaly 149, *150*
  industrialization 236, 325
  infant mortality 379, 383, 384, *385*, 393
  jurisdiction 82, 200, 223, 225, 285, 388
  milk politics 249, 250, 257
Brixen, pilgrimage 399, *401*
Brussels 72, *146*, 186, 225, 235, 251, 388, 414
Budapest 81, 415

Caesarea 383
Carthago, Council 65, 66, cemetery 354,
Castres 25, 124
Celtic Ireland 361
Cham, Switzerland 259, 261
Chicago 59, 98, 125, 161, 217, 225, 250, 269, 319
  Hess bed *41*
  Michael Reese hospital 265, 269, 406, *410*
  preterm infants 72, 81, *81*, 103
China 52, 285, 327, 354, 362, *362*, 368, 384
Cologne *81*, 175, 233, *234*, 327
Constantinople / Byzanz 359, 413
Cordova University 228,
Copenhagen 19, 45, 293, 320, 336, 406
Crete 241
Crimea 155
Cyprus 227, *234*, 391

Danube gorges 391
Dederiyeh, Syria 391
Derby 26, 58, 159, 237, 244, 293, 325
Dijon 39, *360*, 399
Dresden 251, 347, 373, 406, 408
Dublin 54, 281, 325, 333, 406

Earlswood, Surrey 192, *192*
Eaves graves 400
Edinburgh 29, 72, 107, 242, 267, 281, 284
  infant mortality 384, *385*, 387

Royal maternity 75, 159, 199, 298, 305, 408
Simpson memorial 59, 177, 313, 340
Egypt 79, 221, 328, *355*, 377, 392
  gods 63, 115, 178, 241
  mummies 145, 155
  papyri 33, 215, 279, 305, 345, 354
  pharaohs 3, *4*, 156, 221
  rites 3, 63, 178, *178*
England and Wales 27, 52, *150*, 248, 285, 305, 325, 354
  triplet rate 123
  mortality *81*, 262, *263*, 281, *380*, 384, 386, *387*
Ensisheim 361

Florence 222
  Arcuccio 377, *378*
  Council 5, 359, 360, 397
  Innocenti Hospital 405, 406
  legislation 360
France 52, 74, 85, *150*, 185, 191, 281, 285, 361
  artificial nutrition 233, 243, 247, 251, 255
  infanticide 361, 368
  mortality 375, 378, 383, 384, 387, 397
  resuscitation 33, *36*, 45, 46
  revolution 73, 223, 297
  wet nursing 221, *224*
Frankfurt/M 7, *167*, 168, 215, 306, 339, 365
  death penalty 365
Freiburg 81, 148, 197, *282*, 373, 414
  midwives order 25
Friedberg, Herrgottsruh 275, *276*

Gdánsk, death penalty 365
Geneva 96, 158, 233, 238, 292, 384
Georgia, mortality 385
Germany 35, 47, 52, 82, *234*, 247, 283, 318, 360, 375, *380*, 388
  doctrines 75, 193
  drug laws 200, 202, 272, 285
  infant mortality 375, 384, *385*, 389
  infanticide 360, 365, 367
  midwives 30, 33, 275
  Nazi era 7, 166, 193, 371
Giessen 374
Görden 372
Göttingen 73
Gortyna law 354, *355*
Graz 318
  Annaspital 327, 341

Foundling Hospital 327, 406, 408
Greece 74, 145, 191, 221, 354, 384, 391, 392

Haiti (St. Domingue) 53
Hamburg 200, 327, 374
Heidelberg 29, 47, *75*, 97, 277, 375, 405, 406
Helsinki 92, 267, 269, 292, 318, 406
Hermopolis 145
Hindu rituals 65, 175, *176*, 183

Imst, sanctuary 399
Inca, Peru 59, 101, 118, 155, 158, 172, 229
India 176, 353, 369
Ireland, mortality 384, 387

Japan 52, 80, 82, 115, 118; 327, 353, 375, 384

Kassel 72, 73, 149, 229, 292, *401*
Khoisan, South Africa 119
Königsberg 325, 328, 377
Krems-Wachtberg graves *392*
Kylindra 392

Lambach, Abbey 66
Langres, council 397
Lapponia, cradle *378*
Leiden 12, 18, 96, 214, 297, 325
Leipzig 27, 43, 66, *81*, 85, 123, 159, 166, 187, 244, 280, 360, 366, 372
Lesche, Greece 82
Lichtenstein castle 124
Lima Council 118, 157
Liverpool 29, 119, 151, 250, 301, 306
  milk quality 249, 250
London 13, 26, 29, 45, 73, 96, 109, 167, 235, 333
  Dispensary for the Poor 156, 176, 253, 280
  Foundling Hospital 216, 328, 367
  Great Ormond Street 292, 328, 437
  infant mortality 384
  milk quality 238, 249, 257, 281, New River 250
  St. Thomas Hospital 97
  survival, prematures *81*
Los Angeles 75
Lyon 131, 230, 265, 406
  Charité 406

Maeotian Lake 155
Mainz, Council 377

Index of Locations

Manchester 228, 237, 285, 327, 386, *386*, 394
Marburg 132
Marseille Charité 340
Massachusetts 229, 254, 292, 388
Maya, Mexico 65, 155, 229
Memmingen 400
Mesopotamia 63, 64, 233, 249, 353, 377, 391
Mexico 52, 65, 155, 191, 229, 233, 384
Milan
 Council 356, 377
 foundling hospital 359, 405, 413
Montpellier 148, 216, 359
Montreal 269, 437
Morocco 52, 65, 384
Moscow
 Foundling Hospital 80, 265, 279, 405, 407
 Nicolai Hospital 407
Munich 74, *81*, 200, 243, 255, 259
 Haunersches Spital 237, 347, 407

Nancy 251, 443
Naples, fish-monster *185*
Naqada 392
New Haven 30, 81, 347, 407
 Yale University 243, 260, 320
New York City 29, 41, 48, *81*, 161, 168, 230, 254, 281, 328, 342, 379, 407
 Babies Hospital 267, 319, 407
 Croton aqueduct 250
 infant mortality 81
 milk trade 248, *249*
New Zealand 52, 92, 380, 384
Nicaragua 158, 262
Nigeria, twins 117, 118, 123, 179
Nile valley 145, 155, 354
Nineveh library *64*, 165, 197
Nuremberg 29, 124, 137, *160*, *236*
 infanticide law 361, 365, 416

Oberbüren, image 399
Olmecs, Mexico 155
Orleans 173, 215, 235, 379
Oslo 41, *81*, 328

Oxford 18, 28, 30, 151, 228, 267, 293, 306, 325

Padova 28, 79, 159, 173, 340
 anatomy 17, 96, *97*, 148, 166, 187, 214, 274, 297, 313
 Scrovegni Chapel 159, *160*
Paris 26, 34, 39, 72, *75*, 87, 124, 145, 148
 Belleville dispensary *251*
 bureau des nourrices *224*
 donkey nourricerie 334, 335, *335*, *336*
 Enfants Trouvés 59, 103, 107, 166, 169, 265, 299, 312, 328, 334, *336*, 341, 346
 Maternité 46, 107, 266, *268*, 299, 313, 329, 346, 407, *408*,
 meter convention 73, 74
 mortality 213, 386
 prematures' unit 74, *266*, *387*, *408*
 Vaugirard Hospital 334
Passau, midwives rule 159
Peking, infanticide 368
Peking man 155
Philadelphia 157, 168, 242, 251, 260, 336, 368
Phoenicians 64
Prague *81*, 243, 292
Preston 394
Prussia 27, 28, 74, 229, 367, 378, 383, 384, *387*

Rapallo 79
Regensburg 52, 67, 166, 186
Reutlingen 186
Rochester 81
Rome 11, 25, 74, 117, 311, 339, 354, 355, 356, 359, 383
 catacomb graves 393
 cloaca maxima 249
 columna lactaria 223
 forum olitorium 223
 Galen teachings 4, *5*, 11, 13, 15, 71, 95, 183, 213, 284, *284*
 law of 12 tables 147, 354, 392
 Ospedale Santo Spirito 359, 360, *360*

Popes 11, 66, 67, 184, 359, 360, 399
 Soran teachings 51, 58, 65, 145, 155, 159, 165, 179, 183, 215, 377
 wet nursing 222
Roman Britain 393
Russia 74, 125, 265, 320, 328, 384, 385, *387*, 399, 415

Salerno Medical School 58, 183, 228
San Diego 104, 141, 380
San Francisco 75, *81*, 87, 92, 99, 103, 104
Saxon British law 73, 117, 191, 359, 362, 365
Saxony, Germany 82, 124
Schruns sanctuary 399
Sheffield 379
Shanidar, Iraq 155
Singapore 93, 262, 384, 385
Sinuessa 183, 205
South Africa 52, 118, 285, 384
Stockholm 75, 98, 341, 407
St. Petersburg 187, 360
 Foundling Hospital 54, 68, 97, 124, 261, 265, 313, 328, 341, 407
Strasbourg 13, 19, 139, 145, 242, 407
Stuttgart 198, 297, 312
Sulawesi 157, 158
Sumeria 63, 165, 233, 279, 413
Sweden 61, 74, 200, 375, 377, 379, 380, 383, 386, *386*, 387

Taygettos, Grece 25, 82
Tell al-'Ubaid 233
Thebes, Egypt 145
Thebes, Greece 116, 117,
The Hague 129
Toltecs, Mexico 191
Toronto 61, 99, 104, 109, 157, 233, 300, 307, 342, 407
Trens sanctuary 399
Trent, Council 5, 95, 340, 359, 383, 397, 399, 414
Tyrolia 124, 360, 400

United Kingdom *150*, 384
United States 30, 47, 53, 82, 115, 149, *157*, 193, 202, 230, 237, 312, 348, 369
 condensed milk 250, 260, 261
 infanticide law 368
 mass and length 74
 milk depots 224
 infant mortality 225, 375, 384, 388
 prone sleep 379, 380
 quadruplets 123, 124
 swill milk 248, *249*
Uppsala 126, 174, 176, 216, 274, 333, 377,
Ursberg, monastery 399, 400
Uttenheim altarpiece *236*

Vaison, Council 359, 413
Veleia tablet *355*, 356
Venice 405, 413
 Theriac market 280, *284*
Vevey, Switzerland 259, 261
Vienna 40, 53, *81*, 85, 132, 168, *267*, 320, 327, 328, 341,
 Anna Hospital 407, *409*
 Boltzmann Institute 374
 Foundling Hospital 53, 107, 166, 317
 General Hospital 159, 346
 incubator exhibition *267*
 mass and length 59, 73, 74
 survival preterms 81
Vienne, Council 5

Wallamet Indians 157
Washington 80, 379, 416
 Children's Bureau 80, 225, 388, 415
Wetzlar 326
Winchester statutes 362
Woolsthorpe 79

Yoruba, Nigeria 118, 119, *120*
Yucatan, Maya 65, 157, 158

Zurich 91, 147, 159, 166, 194, 215, 261, 320, 408, 415
 Rosenberg Hospital 318; 328, 407

Index of Subjects

Page locators given in italics are for figures.

abandoning 117, 165
Abendberg 192
abomination, twins 115–21
academy verdict 34, 46
acardius 137, *138*, *139*
accoucheur 26, *27*, 33, 46, 57, 66, 129, 130, 159, 229
acranius 137, *139*, 139
active transport 14, *15*
adoption 353, 354, 369
adultery, maternal 115, 120, 129, 185, 354
Agrippa 57
air-pipe 45, *46*
air pollution 325
albinism 185
alimentaria, law *355*, 356
alkali 42
amelia 197, *200*, 201
amulets 52, *64*, 65, 145, 165, 178, *178*, 179, *199*
anaemia 28, 133, 292, 293, 298, 406
analeptics 42
anencephaly 60, 139, *146*, *149*, *150*, 183, 413
ankyloglosson 273, 277
anodyne necklace 178
antibiotics 348
antibody transmission 297, 301
anticonvulsants 180
antiscorbutic principle 328
apparent death 25, 28, 29
appendicitis 319
arcuccio 377, *378*
artificial feeding 216, 225, 233, *234*, *237*, 243, 253, 261
 mortality 262, 335
 reasons 221, 234, 235, 263
 safety 225, 250
ascites, foetal 132, 297, 298, *298*
asphyxia 25, 28, *28*, 30, 33, 40, 306, 312
 brain damage 29, 107
 ductus 103, 168
 grades 29
 resuscitation 42, 47
 seizures 177
 treatment 30, 41, 42
asses' milk 242
assisted reproduction 126
asymmetry, head 161, *161*, 379
asylums 191, *192*, 225, 281, *282*, 328, 371
atelectasis 85, *86*, *87*, 91, 103, 312

baby farming 223, *282*, 388
bacteria 253, 254, 255, 270, *321*, 335
 milk 243, 248, 250, 255, 257, 270, 345
 sepsis 347, 348, 362
 umbilicus 51, 53, *54*
balia 222
balneum animale 34
baptism 5, 25, *64*, 65, 67, 361, 397
 conditional 66, 67, 137
 emergency 66, *66*, 67
 intrauterine 25, 67
 stillborns 138, 397, 400
barber surgeons 26, *27*, 33
bastards 185, 362, 365, 367, 368
bear child 129, 184, *185*
bed sharing 377
beggars' rules 186
bewitchment 59, 147, 165, 174, *175*, 197
biberon 254, *255*
bicarbonate therapy 30, 41, 42, 269
bile duct, obliteration 292, *293*, 297
bilirubin 297, 298, 299, *300*
biological facts 7
birth marks 183, 185, *195*
bladder, exstrophy 205–8, *206*
blastocyst 8
bleeding, see haemorrhage 291–5
blemmyes 137
blood coagulation 292
boanerges 115
Boke of Children 166
brachycephaly 161
brain, haemorrhage 107–10, *108*, *109*, *110*, 168, 177
breast, erotization 218, 230
breastfeeding 118, 158, 213, 215, 227, 243, 262, 280
breast pumps 227–32, *230*, *231*
breech delivery 29, 57–61, *60*, *144*, 312
 head shape 161, *161*
 infanticide 59
B streptococci 348
bubby pot *234*, 236
Buhl's diasease 347
burial 359, 391, *392*, 394, 399

calorimeters 243, *244*, 269, 415
Candida albicans 340, 341
cat head 145, *150*
cemeteries, infants' 155, 191, 391, *392*, 393

cerebellum, trauma 60, 108
cerebral haemorrhage 107–10, *108*, *109*, *110*, 168, 177
cerebral palsy 25, 30, 165–71, *169*
certified milk 247, 250
changeling 165, *167*, 193
childbed fever 346
Children's Bureau 80, 225, 388, 407, 415
chimpanzee 191
Chinook 157
cheerless infants 400
cholera infantum 237, 249, 260, 386, *387*
cholestasis 292
Christian rites *64*, 65, 137, 365, 397–401
chromosomes 193
chuchuru 59
circulation, fetal 95, 96, 132
circulation, placenta 25, *133*, *141*
circulation, pulmonary 5, 17, 101
circumcision 63, *64*, 67
cleft bladder 205
clostridium tetani 54
cod liver oil 81, 261, 327, *327*, 328
colostrum 176, 216, 227, 311
columna lactaria 25, 221, *223*
condensed milk 259, *260*
contagion theory 118, 335, 340, 345
contergan 200
continuous positive pressure 40, 41 *42*, 87, 104, *263*
conversion units 74
convulsions 168, 173, *176*, 177, *177*, 217, 300
 dentition 173
coral amulets 178, *179*
cord, umbilical 11, *12*, 51
 circulation 11, 17, 18, 51
 ligation 52
 stump care 52
 tetanus 53, 173
 vessels 12, 13, 138
corsets 228
cot death 377–81, *380*
cow's milk, chemistry 233, 235, 242, 248
cradleboards 157, 158
cravings, pregnancy 147, *187*, 188
cretinism 191, 192
crying 25, 39, 41, 82, 85, 157, 236, 265, 282, 379, 399
cyclopia 184, *184*

delayed feeding 216, 267
dentition, difficult 166, 173, 175, 280, *282*, 328
diabetes, maternal 300, 305, *307*, 308
diarrhoea 233, 237, 249, 260, 319, 386, *387*
diascordium 279, 280
dies lustricus 65, 311, 356
distaval 200
distress, respiratory 85, 87, 92, 102, 110, 306
dowry 353, 363, 368
donkey pavilion *335*, 336
dropsy, fetal 129, 132, 134, 297, *298*, *299*
drug approval 201
ductus arteriosus 95, 101
 anatomy 95, 103
 closure 21, 97, 101, 102
 intima cushions 98, *103*
 ligation 103
 persisting 101, 102
 prostaglandins 98, 104
dyspnoea 85, 86, 103, *110*

eaves graves 400
ectromelia 201
electroencephalogram 177
elephant head 183, *184*
embarrassment 230, *231*, 232
embryogenesis 3, 8, 147, 199
embryotomy *26*, 57, 61, 305
ensoulment 8
enterocolitis, necrotizing 317–21
epigenesis theory 148, 308, 335
erysipelas 346, *347*
erythroblastosis, fetal 297, 300, *302*, 415
ethical recommendations 82, 375
eugenics theory 120, 192, 371, 375
evaporizer 259, *260*
evil eye 65, 72, 165, 174, *175*, 178, *179*
excavations 191, 227, 233, 328, *334*, 391, 399
exchange transfusion 300, 301, *302*, 319
excommunication 65
exorcism 63, 66, 174, 314
exposed infants 25, *119*, 125, 193, *242*, *355*, 359, 367
extremities, malformed 197–202

farine lactée 259
feeding, artificial 216, 225, 233, 235, 237, *242*, 250, 253, 261, 262

Index of Subjects

feeding bottles 227, 234, 254, *266*
feeding horn 234, 253
fire-air 18, 19, 39
fish monster 184, *195*
flotation test 366, *367*
foetus
  asphyxia 168
  dropsy 129, 132, 297, *298*, *299*
  fractures 329
  growth charts 73, *75*, 268, 305
  monitoring 30
  nutrition 11–15
  respiration 17–21
  syphilis 333–7
folate deficiency 149, *151*
fontanelle, puncture *26*, 300, 307
foramen ovale, closure 95, 96, 97, 102
formula composition 243, 260, 261, 262, *263*, 270, 319
fortifyer, breastmilk 269
foundling hospitals 85, 102, 334, 339, 356, 359, 368
fractures, traumatic 60, 168, 269
French revolution 33, 73, 223, 297, 334
frenotomy 273, *274*, *275*
froggy 275, 277
frog head 146, *150*
funeral customs 393, *394*

galactophore 266, *266*
gastroenteritis 237, 249, 260, 386, *387*
gavage, feeding 81, 230, 265, *266*, 268
gene expression 20
gestational age 71
giant babies 305f, *305*
glass bottle 254, *255*
goitre 152, 186
goutte de lait 251, *251*
Gregorian calendar 79
growth, foetal 11, 73, *75*, 268, 305
growth, postnatal 59, *267*, 270, *329*
gruel 233, 235
gums, lancing 176, 177, 281
guttus 227, *228*

haemoglobin, fetal 19
haemolysis 297, 299, 347
haemophilia 291
haemorrhage 273, 291, *293*
  brain 107, 109
  frenotomy 275, *276*
  gastrointestinal 317
  prematures *108*
  scurvy 328
  sepsis 348
Hand of Ishtar 174
hare's brain 179, 280, 281
head shaping 155–62
heart terminology 96
hepar uterinum 11
heredity 124, 138, 147, 158, 176, *199*, 329, 335, 372
hermaphrodites 205
Hindu rites 57, 241, 353
hip dislocation 59, 379
holoprosencephaly *184*
homocysteine 151
hooks *26*

hyaline membranes 86, 92, 108, 306
hydramnios 60, 132, *133*
hydrops, foetal 29, 132, 134, 297, *298*
hygiene, personal 345
hypertrichosis 129, 184, *185*
hyperventilation 109, *110*
hypoglycaemia 306
hypothermia 35, *66*, 80, 267
hypothyreosis 191, 192, 407
hypsarrhythmia 178

ichthyosis 184, *185*
idiots, asylums 191, *192*, 281, 328
imagination, maternal 145, 183, *187*
impurity 311
incontinence apparatuses *296*, 207
incubator, prematures 40, 75, 79, 81, 85, 124, 265, *267*, 268, 405, 408
indomethacin 104
industrialization 236, 253, 259, 281, 325
infant cemeteries 392
infanticide, females 119, 353, *355*, 362, *362*, 369
infanticide, laws 353, 360, 362, 366, 369
infanticide, twins 118, *120*
infant mortality 59, 80, 213, 383
  birth rate 387
  England & Wales *263*
  gastroenteritis *387*
  OECD states 375
  social class 386
  statistics 383, *385*
  summer 213,
  150-year trend 384
inheritance 124, 138, 147, 158, 176, *199*, 329, 335, 372
injection studies *12*, 129, 131, *131*, 133, 137, 140
insulin 269, 306, 307, 308
intestinal perforation 320
intubation, larynx 35, 45, *46*, *47*
islets, pancreas *307*

jaundice 297, *300*
Jewish rites 63, 64
Jews, persecution 372, 373

Kalmuc idiocy 192, *193*
kernicterus 293, 297, 299, *301*

lactometers 247, *248*
lame children 25, 30, 165, *169*
laryngoscope 48
laser coagulation 134
laudanum 280, *282*, 283, 284
legislation, infanticide 353, 359, 365, 369
legislation, viability 82
liber scivias 6, 95
life insurance 393, 394
life, onset 3, 8
limbs, malformed 28, 168, 186, 197, 372
limbus puerorum 5, 66, 359, *397*, *398*
listeriosis 347
litigation 30
lockjaw 53, 54, 173
lung maturation 92, 106, 306, 416

macrosomia 305–8, *305*
malformations, congenital 29, 101, 145, 147, 151, 183, 184, 193, 197, 200
  causes *199*
  diabetes 307
  Down's syndrome 193
  extremities 197
  neural tube 8, 147, *148*
  skin 183, *185*
mammary gland *215*, 217
man-midwife 26, *27*, 33
mare's milk 117, 242
marketing formula 261
meconium 311
  aspiration 312
  fetal passage 312
  ileus 312
  obstruction 313
  peritonitis 313
melaena 291, *294*
meningocele 149
menstrual blood 11, 186, 213, *214*
mercury in syphilis 334, 336
merovingians 155, 334
mesolithic 391
metallotherapy 179
meter convention 73
miasma theory 238, 340, 345
midwifery 25, *27*, 60, 159, 168, 229, 234
milk
  adulterated 247, *248*
  animals 233, 241, 242
  certified 250
  depots 224
  fever 216
  myths 241
  pumps 227–32
  sterilized *256*
mithridate 279, 280, 281
mongolism 191
mortality, see infant 53, 83
mother's imagination 145, 183
moulding skull 159
mouth-to-mouth 33
multiple birth 115, 123
murder of disabled 371
muslim rites 4, 65, 185, 241, 393
myoclonic 174

nail milk test 221
nalorphine 43
name giving 63, 65, 115, 119, 356, 360, 391
nasal feeding *266*
nasogastric tube 81, 230, *267*
navel, see umbilicus
Nazi Germany 7, 120, 166, 193, 371, 375
Neanderthals 155, 354, 391
necrotizing enterocolitis 317–21
neolithic 155, *156*, 187, 191, 391
neural tube 8, 147, *148*
nose shaping 159, *160*
nursing 221
  office 224
  qualification 222
nutrition 213–18
  artificial 253–7

foetus 11
  milestones *263*
  parenteral 269
nystatin 342, *343*

octuplets 126
oligohydramnios 60
omphalitis 51, 53, *53*
omphalos ritual 51
ondine 266, *266*
opiates for infants 279
opium trade 284, *284*, 285
orangutan 191
original sin 5, 65, 311, 359, 397, 401
osteogenesis imperfecta 329, *330*
overlaying 362, 377, 378, 394
oxygen 19, *19*, 39, 101, 243
  discovery 15, *19*, 39, 87
  dissociation 14, 21, *21*
  foetus 17, 20, 168
  measurement 20, 29, 168, 416
  therapy 40, *41*, 87, 88, 102

palsy, cerebral 25, 30, 165, *169*
panada 233, 235
pancreas, fibrosis *313*
pancreas, islets *307*
pap 235, *236*, *237*
pasteurisation 250, 255, *256*
patria potestas 82, 354, 356
pelvis, rickety 326
pemphigus 346
penicillin 336, 348
percentage method 243
periostitis, syphilis 333, *337*
person, definitions 3, 8, 118
phlogiston theory 18, 39
phocomelia 197, *200*, 201
phototherapy 301
phrenology 157
pigbel 321
pituitary stalk 60
placenta 3, 11, 17
  anastomoses 129, 131, 133
  nutrition 11
  perfusion 137
  respiration 28
  twins 119, 129, *132*, *133*, 137, 183
pneuma doctrine 17
pneumothorax 34
podalic version 58
polyovulation 123
postverta 57
pot burials 392, 393
pregnancy 54, 57, 123, 200, 285
  concealed 361, 367, 369
  diabetic 305
  duration 71, 74, 82
  folate 151
  imagination 166, 183, 205
  interruption 194
prematurity 79, 107, 167, 265, *266*, 317, 329, 386
  bone disease 329
  brain injury 167
  ductus 102, *103*
  growth *267*, 268
  personhood 6, 25, 59
  viability 71, 74, 80, 366
prenatal diagnosis 194
priests *64*, 66, 67, 359, 399, 400

Index of Subjects

prisoners 250, 301, 320, 328
proboscis *184*
procreation, animals 147
prolactin 215
prone sleeping 379, *380*
prostitution 334, 356, 365
pulmonary circulation *5*, 17, 101
pulmo uterinus 17
purification 63, 65, 311

quadruplets 123
quickening 8
quintuplets 124, 126

racism 193, 372, 388
ranula 275, *275*
refrigeration 254, *256*
Reichsausschuss killings 372
reproduction, assisted 126
research funding 103
respiratory distress syndrome 85
   brain 110
   ductus 102
   grunting 33
   histology 8, 332
   surfactant 86, 91
   ventilation 41, 88
reversed perfusion 137
rhesus incompatibility 297, 299, 301, *302*
rickets 59, 161, 199, 269, 325, *326*, 327, *329*, 373
roentgen imaging 133, 327, *327*, *329*, 336, 378
rubber vulcanization 41, 47, 48, 207, 229, *230*, 254, *255*, 265, *266*

sal-nitro 18, 28
salvarsan 336
sanctuaries, revival 397
Saxon mirror lawbook *82*

scales, weighing 72, *72*, 73, *75*
Schwabenspiegel lawbook 360
scurvy, infantile 55, 257, 281, 325, 328, 329
sedation 279, 281, 372
seizures 168, 173, *175*, *176*, 177, *177*, 217, 300
sepsis 53, 249, 320, *321*, 345, *348*
septuplets 124
sewers 249, 260, 345, 384, 386
sex ratios 354
sextuplets 123
Shanidar man 155
Shumma Izbu 123, 353
skeleton, diseases 191, 325, 392, 393
sleeplessness 173, 202, 279, 280
social birth 63, 356
Social Darwinism 120, 192, 371, 408
somersault theory 57, *58*
soothers 281, *283*, 284, 294
spasm, infantile 174
spectroscope *20*
soul 3, 5, 8
sterilization *256*
sternocleidomastoid 59, 60
sudden infant death 377
suffocation 367, 378, 379, 381
summer diarrhoea 237, 249, 260, 386, *387*
superfecundation 116, 123
superstitions 11, 51, 52, 66, 72, 137, 145, 157, 165, 173, 185
supranatural disease 173
surfactant 85, 91
   composition 92
   deficiency 85, 86, 126, 306
   function 91, 92, *92*
   substitution 91, 92, *93*, 109, 110
survival, preterms 79
Susruta Samhita 57

swaddling 65, 165, *166*, 325
swill milk 247, 249
swingings 35, *35*
Synkavit 293, 294
syphilis 333, *334*, *337*, 405

tank ventilators 35
teats, feeding 207, 253–8, 260
teeth, connatal 59
teething 55, 166, 173, 175, 176, 280, 281, *282*, 328
teratology 148, 187, 198
teratoma 8, 186, *187*
tetanus 53, 54, 173, 178
téterelle 227, 230, *231*, 265
thalidomide 197
theriac 180, 279, 280, 283, *284*
thrombosis, purulent *54*
thrush 238, 339, *340*, *342*, 343
thymus 378
tiralatte 227, *228*, *229*
tire-tête *26*
tobacco smoke 39, *40*
tongue-tie 273, *274*, 277
torticollis 59, 60
transfusion 294
transport, active 14, *15*
treponema pallidum 335
triplets 123
trisomy 21 191
tube, tracheal *46*
twins 59, 115, 292
   abomination 115, 118
   frequency 123
   heavenly 117
   placenta 132, 138
   transfusion syndromes 129, 133, 137
   unequal 129
   zygosity 115
tyrosinase deficiency 185

udjat eye 178, *178*
ultrasound imaging 108, 133
ultraviolet light, rickets 328
umbilical cord, 12, 51, 132
   circulation 12, *13*, 17, 131, *139*
   cutting 51, 65
   ligation 52
   omphalitis *53*
   severing *53*
   stump care 52
   twins 119, 129, 130, 131, 138
urine drainage *296*, 207
uterine milk 13
uterus-breast connection 214

venereal disease 334, 339
ventilation, artificial 33, 37, 47, 87, 375
ventilators 34, *36*, 88
very low birthweight 71, 81, *81*, 101, 257, 267, 319
viability 71, 74, 366
vitalism theory 29, 34
vitamin B9, folate 149, *151*
vitamin C 261, 328
vitamin D 152, 261, 269, 326
vitamin K 293, 294
vulcanization, rubber 41, 47, 48, 207, 229, *230*, 254, 265, *266*
weaning 235, 236, 280
weighing 72, *72*, 73, *75*, 251, 267
wet nursing 215, 221–5, *224*, 225, 335
Winckel's disease 347
witchcraft 59, 147, 165, 174, *175*, 197
World Health Organization 54, 82
wry neck 59, 60

X-rays 133, 327, *327*, *329*, 336, 378